CECIL
ESSENTIALS
OF
MEDICINE

THOMAS E. ANDREOLI / CHARLES C. J. CARPENTER / FRED PLUM / LLOYD H. SMITH, JR.

SECOND EDITION

1990

W. B. SAUNDERS COMPANY

Harcourt Brace Jovanovich, Inc.

Philadelphia, London, Toronto, Montreal, Sydney, Tokyo

W. B. SAUNDERS COMPANY
Harcourt Brace Jovanovich, Inc.

The Curtis Center
Washington Square West
Philadelphia, PA 19106

Library of Congress Cataloging-in-Publication Data

Cecil essentials of medicine.

    Includes bibliographies and index.

    1. Internal medicine. I. Cecil, Russell L.
(Russell La Fayette), 1881–1965. II. Andreoli, Thomas E.,
1935–   III. Title: Essentials of medicine.
[DNLM: 1. Medicine. WB 100 C3882]
RC46.C42 1990 616
ISBN 0-7216-2614-9

88-30541

Listed here is the latest translated edition of this book together with the language of the translation
and the publisher:

Portugese — *first edition* — DISCOS CBS Industria e Comercio Ltda., Rio de Janeiro, Brazil

Editor: John Dyson

Designer: Lorraine B. Kilmer

Production Manager: Frank Polizzano

Manuscript Editor: Donna Walker

Illustration Coordinator: Joan Sinclair

Illustrator: Joan Sinclair

Indexer: Donna Walker

Cecil Essentials of Medicine   ISBN 0-7216-2614-9

Last digit is the print number: 9   8   7   6   5   4   3   2   1

CONTRIBUTORS

CARDIOVASCULAR DISEASES

WILLIAM M. MILES, M.D.

Assistant Professor of Medicine, Indiana University School of Medicine; Research Associate, Krannert Institute of Cardiology, Indianapolis. Staff Cardiologist, Indiana University Hospital and Roudebush Veterans Administration Medical Center, Indianapolis, Indiana.

DOUGLAS P. ZIPES, M.D.

Professor of Medicine, Indiana University School of Medicine; Senior Research Associate, Krannert Institute of Cardiology, Indianapolis. Attending Physician, Indiana University Hospital; Staff Cardiologist, Roudebush Veterans Hospital, Indianapolis, Indiana.

RESPIRATORY DISEASES

DAVID R. DANTZKER, M.D.

Professor of Internal Medicine and Director, Division of Pulmonary Medicine, University of Texas Health Science Center at Houston. Attending Physician, Hermann Hospital, Houston, Texas.

MARTIN J. TOBIN, M.D.

Associate Professor of Internal Medicine, University of Texas Health Science Center at Houston. Attending Physician, Hermann Hospital, Houston, Texas.

RENAL DISEASE

THOMAS E. ANDREOLI, M.D.

Professor and Chairman, Department of Internal Medicine, University of Arkansas College of Medicine. Chief of Medicine, University of Arkansas Hospital, Little Rock, Arkansas.

R. MICHAEL CULPEPPER, M.D.

Assistant Professor of Medicine, Medical College of Virginia, Richmond. Attending Physician, Department of Internal Medicine, Medical College of Virginia Hospitals; Consultant in Internal Medicine, McGuire Veterans Administration Hospital, Richmond, Virginia.

CATHERINE S. THOMPSON, M.D.

Assistant Professor of Internal Medicine, University of Texas Medical School at Houston. Attending Physician, Hermann Hospital, Houston, Texas.

EDWARD J. WEINMAN, M.D.

Professor of Internal Medicine and Director, Division of Nephrology, University of Texas Medical School at Houston. Attending Physician, Hermann Hospital, Houston, Texas.

GASTROINTESTINAL DISEASE

NATHAN M. BASS, M.D., Ph.D.

Assistant Professor of Medicine, University of California, San Francisco, School of Medicine. Attending Physician, University of California, San Francisco Hospitals and Clinics, San Francisco, California.

LLOYD H. SMITH, Jr., M.D.

Professor of Medicine and Associate Dean, University of California, San Francisco, School of Medicine. Attending Physician, University of California, San Francisco Hospitals and Clinics, San Francisco, California.

REBECCA W. VAN DYKE, M.D.

Assistant Professor of Medicine, University of California, San Francisco, School of Medicine. Attending Physician, University of California, San Francisco Hospitals and Clinics, San Francisco, California.

DISEASES OF LIVER AND BILIARY SYSTEM

NATHAN M. BASS, M.D., Ph.D.

Assistant Professor of Medicine, University of California, San Francisco, School of Medicine. Attending Physician, University of California, San Francisco Hospitals and Clinics, San Francisco, California.

REBECCA W. VAN DYKE, M.D.

Assistant Professor of Medicine and Attending Physician, University of California, San Francisco, School of Medicine. Attending Physician, University of California, San Francisco Hospitals and Clinics, San Francisco, California.

HEMATOLOGY

BABETTE B. WEKSLER, M.D.

Professor of Medicine, Cornell University Medical College, New York. Attending Physician, The New York Hospital—Cornell Medical Center, New York, New York.

ANNE MOORE, M.D.

Associate Professor of Clinical Medicine, Cornell University School of Medicine, New York. Attending Physician, New York Hospital—Cornell Medical Center, New York, New York.

ONCOLOGY

JEFFREY TEPLER, M.D.

Assistant Professor of Medicine, Cornell University Medical College, New York. Assistant Attending Physician and Director, Oncology Unit, The New York Hospital—Cornell Medical Center, New York, New York.

ANNE MOORE, M.D.

Associate Professor of Clinical Medicine, Cornell University School of Medicine, New York. Attending Physician, New York Hospital—Cornell Medical Center, New York, New York.

BABETTE B. WEKSLER, M.D.
Professor of Medicine, Cornell University Medical College, New York. Attending Physician, The New York Hospital—Cornell Medical Center, New York, New York.

METABOLIC DISEASES

PETER N. HERBERT, M.D.
Professor of Medicine, Brown University, Providence. Director, Division of Nutrition and Metabolism, The Miriam Hospital, Providence, Rhode Island.

DONALD HRICIK, M.D.
Assistant Professor of Medicine, Case Western Reserve University School of Medicine, Cleveland. Attending Physician, University Hospitals of Cleveland, Ohio.

ENDOCRINE DISEASES

KENNETH R. FEINGOLD, M.D.
Associate Professor of Medicine, University of California, San Francisco, School of Medicine. Chief, Endocrine-Metabolism Clinic, Veterans Administration Medical Center, San Francisco, California.

LAURENCE A. GAVIN, M.D.
Associate Professor of Medicine, University of California, San Francisco, School of Medicine. Associate Director, Diabetes Clinic, University of California, San Francisco Hospitals and Clinics. Attending Physician, Veterans Administration Medical Center, San Francisco, California.

MORRIS SCHAMBELAN, M.D.
Professor of Medicine, University of California, San Francisco, School of Medicine. Chief, Division of Endocrinology, San Francisco General Hospital, California.

ANTHONY SEBASTIAN, M.D.
Professor of Medicine, University of California, San Francisco, School of Medicine. Attending Physician, University of California, San Francisco Hospitals and Clinics, San Francisco, California.

DISEASES OF BONE AND BONE MINERAL METABOLISM

LLOYD H. SMITH, Jr., M.D.
Professor of Medicine and Associate Dean, University of California, San Francisco, School of Medicine. Attending Physician, University of California, San Francisco Hospitals and Clinics, San Francisco, California.

INFECTIOUS DISEASES

CHARLES C. J. CARPENTER, M.D.
Professor of Medicine, Brown University, Providence. Physician-in-Chief, The Miriam Hospital, Providence, Rhode Island.

JERROLD J. ELLNER, M.D.

Professor of Medicine, Case Western Reserve University School of Medicine, Cleveland. Attending Physician, University Hospitals of Cleveland, Ohio.

MICHAEL LEDERMAN, M.D.

Assistant Professor of Medicine, Case Western Reserve University School of Medicine, Cleveland. Attending Physician, University Hospitals of Cleveland, Ohio.

G. RICHARD OLDS, M.D.

Associate Professor of Medicine, Brown University, Providence. Director, International Health Institute, Brown University, Providence, Rhode Island.

KENNETH H. MAYER, M.D.

Associate Professor of Medicine, Brown University, Providence. Director, Infectious Diseases Division, Pawtucket Memorial Hospital, Pawtucket, Rhode Island.

MUSCULOSKELETAL AND CONNECTIVE TISSUE DISEASES

GEORGE HO, Jr., M.D.

Assistant Professor of Medicine, Brown University, Providence. Attending Physician, The Miriam Hospital, Providence, Rhode Island.

GARY M. KAMMER, M.D.

Associate Professor of Medicine, Case Western Reserve University, Cleveland. Attending Physician, University Hospitals of Cleveland, Ohio.

NEUROLOGIC DISEASES

FRED PLUM, M.D.

Anne Parrish Titzell Professor and Chairman, Department of Neurology, Cornell University Medical College, New York. Neurologist-in-Chief, The New York Hospital—Cornell Medical Center, New York, New York.

JEROME B. POSNER, M.D.

George C. Cotzias Professor of Neurology, Cornell University Medical College, New York. Attending Neurologist, Memorial Sloan-Kettering Cancer Center and The New York Hospital, New York, New York.

PREFACE

This Second Edition of CECIL ESSENTIALS OF MEDICINE renews and advances the goals of its predecessor. Specifically, we have attempted to provide, in this companion to the encyclopedic CECIL TEXTBOOK OF MEDICINE, a succinct and readable text that covers the indispensable elements of the principles and practice of the broad field of internal medicine. Thus this book especially addresses the needs of undergraduate students of the medical sciences, as well as other health care providers who wish to obtain a concise account of current knowledge and practices in internal medicine.

As with the First Edition of ESSENTIALS, this book contains 12 major sections focused either on different organ systems—for example, cardiac diseases and diseases of the nervous system—or on groups of diseases sharing a common theme—for example, infectious diseases and neoplastic disorders. Each section begins with a description of the pertinent signs and symptoms of disease followed by an account of relevant anatomic and physiologic considerations. A series of chapters follow that describe the relevant clinical and laboratory findings of disease states, as well as their therapy. Each of the sections has undergone critical scrutiny by external reviewers, and the editors have revised each section thoroughly to include the latest available information that pertains to the modern practice of internal medicine. Put another way, we intend that ESSENTIALS provide a "core" that students of medicine may digest and assimilate during the traditional undergraduate medical clerkship.

This Second Edition of ESSENTIALS, like its predecessor, includes original contributions by a small number of authors. Each chapter makes generous use of tabular and graphic illustrative material to facilitate the reader's learning. We are grateful to these authors, as well as to residents, fellows, and many colleagues at and outside of our own institutions for advising us on the content and for reviewing critically each of the chapters submitted for this edition.

We are especially grateful to Mr. John Dyson, Senior Medical Editor of the W.B. Saunders Company, for meticulous editorial assistance, and to Mrs. Lorraine Kilmer, Manager of Editorial/Design/Production of the W.B. Saunders Company, for her elegant contributions to the design and preparation of this Second Edition of ESSENTIALS. We also thank our able secretarial staffs, especially Ms. Clementine M. Whitman (Little Rock); Ms. Barbara S. Ryan (Providence); Mr. Lew Brockway (New York); and Ms. Judith A. Serrell (San Francisco).

THOMAS E. ANDREOLI
CHARLES C. J. CARPENTER
FRED PLUM
LLOYD H. SMITH, JR.

CONTENTS

III RENAL DISEASE

IV GASTROINTESTINAL DISEASE

V DISEASES OF THE LIVER AND BILIARY SYSTEM

VI   HEMATOLOGY

VII   ONCOLOGY

VIII   METABOLIC DISEASES

IX ENDOCRINE DISEASES

X DISEASES OF BONE AND BONE MINERAL METABOLISM

XI INFECTIOUS DISEASES

XII MUSCULOSKELETAL AND CONNECTIVE TISSUE DISEASES

XIII NEUROLOGIC DISEASES

SECTION
I
CARDIOVASCULAR DISEASES

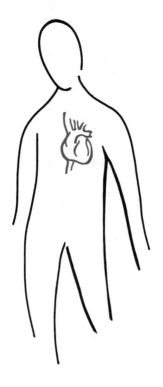

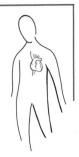

1

STRUCTURE AND FUNCTION OF THE NORMAL HEART AND BLOOD VESSELS

GROSS ANATOMY

About two thirds of the heart is left of the midline, resulting in an apical impulse normally palpated in the fourth to fifth left intercostal space at the midclavicular line. Two relatively thin-walled upper chambers, the right and left atria, and two thicker-walled lower chambers, the right and left ventricles, compose the heart (Fig. 1–1). The left ventricle has walls significantly thicker than those of the right ventricle because of the considerably higher systemic arterial pressure into which it pumps blood. The interventricular septum separates the two ventricles. The lower and much larger part of the interventricular system is termed the muscular interventricular septum and is composed of muscle the same thickness as that of the left ventricular free wall. The uppermost portion of the septum, termed the membranous interventricular septum, also forms a portion of the right atrial wall.

The tricuspid valve is a three-leaflet structure. The mitral valve has only two leaflets, a large anteromedial and a small posterolateral leaflet. A fibrous ring called the annulus supports each valve and forms a portion of the fibrous structural skeleton of the heart. Chords of fibrous tissue, the chordae tendineae, extend from the ventricular surfaces of both atrioventricular (AV) valves and attach to the papillary muscles. Papillary muscles are bundles of cardiac muscle (myocardium) arising from the interior of the ventricular walls. As the ventricles contract, the papillary muscles also contract, pulling taut the chordae tendineae and preventing the AV valves from prolapsing back into the atria and leaking. There are two papillary muscles in the left ventricle (anteromedial and posterolateral) and three in the right ventricle, connected via the chordae tendineae to each valve leaflet.

A somewhat different type of valve, the semilunar valve, separates the ventricles from their respective outflow tracts. The pulmonic valve is composed of three fibrous leaflets or cusps that are forced open against the walls of the pulmonary artery during ventricular ejection of blood but fall back into the pulmonary outflow tract during diastole, their free edges coapting to prevent blood from returning into the right ventricle. The aortic valve is a thicker but similar three-valved structure. The aortic wall behind each aortic valve cusp bulges outward, forming three structures known as sinuses of Valsalva. The left and right coronary arteries emerge from the aortic wall of two of these sinuses of Valsalva. The two most anterior aortic cusps are known as the left and right coronary cusps because of the respective origins of the left and

right coronary arteries, while the remaining posterior cusp is known as the noncoronary cusp.

The pericardium, a double-layered fibrous structure, encloses the heart. The visceral layer is immediately adjacent to the heart and forms part of the epicardium (outer layer) of the heart. The parietal layer is exterior to the heart and is separated from the visceral layer by a thin film of lubricating fluid (10 to 20 ml total) that allows the heart to move freely within the pericardial sac.

Venous blood returning from the body enters the right atrium through the inferior vena cava from below and the superior vena cava from above (Fig. 1–2). Most venous blood returning from the coronary circulation enters the right atrium via the coronary sinus. Blood from these three sources mixes and enters the right ventricle during diastole, when the tricuspid valve is open. The right ventricle subsequently contracts (systole), closing the tricuspid valve to prevent retrograde blood flow, and ejects blood through the

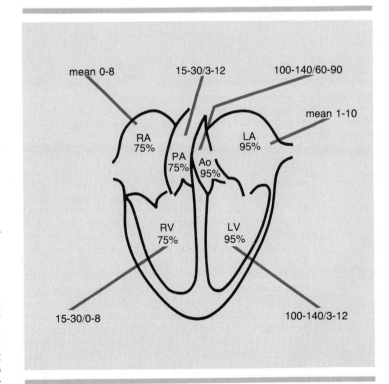

FIGURE 1–1. Orientation of the cardiac chambers and great vessels with normal intracardiac pressures (mm Hg) and oxygen saturations (%).

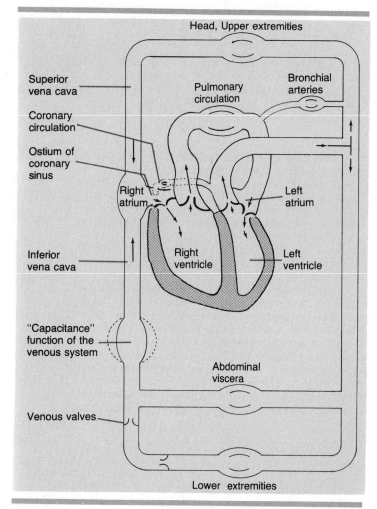

FIGURE 1–2. Schematic representation of the systemic and pulmonary circulatory systems. The venous system contains the greatest amount of blood at any one time and is highly distensible, accommodating a wide range of blood volumes (high capacitance).

pulmonic valve into the pulmonary artery. The right ventricle is anterior to the left ventricle, and the pulmonary artery is anterior to the aorta. The pulmonary artery bifurcates into left and right branches that travel to the left and right lungs. The pulmonary artery has thinner walls than the aorta, and pulmonary arterial pressure is normally much less than aortic pressure. The pulmonary artery progressively divides into smaller and smaller arteries, arterioles, and eventually capillaries, where carbon dioxide is exchanged for oxygen via the pulmonary alveoli. The capillaries lead to pulmonary veins that coalesce to form the four larger pulmonary veins entering the left atrium posteriorly. Oxygenated blood from the pulmonary veins passes from the left atrium through the mitral valve to the left ventricle, which ejects blood during systole across the aortic valve into the aorta. The aorta divides into branches that deliver blood to the entire body (Fig. 1–3). The division continues to form smaller arteries,

arterioles, and eventually capillaries that deliver oxygen and metabolic substrates to the tissues in exchange for CO_2 and other waste products. Blood collected from the peripheral capillaries is returned to the right atrium via the venous system.

The right and left coronary arteries course over the epicardial surface of the heart to distribute blood to the myocardium (Fig. 1–4). The left main coronary artery bifurcates within a few centimeters of its origin into two major vessels. The left anterior descending coronary artery proceeds anteriorly in the anterior interventricular groove (between both ventricles) toward the apex of the heart, supplying the anterior free wall of the left ventricle and the anterior two thirds of the septum. The circumflex coronary artery travels posteriorly in the atrioventricular groove (between left atrium and ventricle) and usually supplies a portion of the posterolateral surface of the heart. The right coronary artery courses in the right atrioventricular groove (between right atrium and ventricle) and distributes several branches to the right ventricle before reaching the left ventricle, where the atrioventricular grooves meet the posterior interventricular groove (the "crux" of the heart). In 90 per cent of patients the right coronary artery reaches the crux of the heart and supplies the branches to the AV node and the inferobasal third of the septum (posterior descending artery). This pattern is termed "right dominant distribution" (even though the left coronary artery supplies the majority of the coronary circulation). In approximately 10 per cent of patients, a relatively large circumflex coronary artery reaches the crux of the heart and gives rise to the posterior descending coronary artery and the branch to the AV node. This situation is termed "left dominant," and the diminutive right coronary artery supplies only the right ventricle. Blood is supplied to the sinus node via a branch of the right coronary artery (55 per cent of cases) or the circumflex coronary artery (45 per cent). Most of the venous network of the heart coalesces to form the coronary sinus. Some of the right ventricular and atrial venous drainage occurs via much smaller anterior cardiac veins and tiny thebesian veins, most of which drain directly into the right atrium.

ELECTRICAL CONDUCTION SYSTEM (Fig. 1–5)

Cardiac electrical impulses originate in the sinus node, a spindle-shaped structure 10 to 20 mm long located near the junction of the superior vena cava and the right atrium. Even though various specialized tissues have been postulated to conduct the electrical impulse from the sinus node to the AV node, electrical transmission is probably cell-to-cell via working atrial muscle. The AV node provides the only normal conduction pathway between the atria and the ventricles. It is situated just beneath the right atrial endocardium above the insertion of the septal leaflet of the tricuspid valve and anterior to the ostium of the coronary sinus. After conduction delay in the AV node, the electrical

FIGURE 1–3. Major components of the systemic vascular tree. Although the capillaries are smallest in diameter, their total cross-sectional area is largest because of their tremendous numbers. The velocity of flow through any portion of the system is inversely proportional to the total cross-sectional area; therefore the flow of blood is slowest in the capillaries, allowing for exchange of fluid and nutrients. The greatest pressure decrease occurs across the arterioles because of their high resistance to flow; this resistance is variable and regulates blood flow to each vascular bed.

		Vessel Diameter	Cross-sectional Area of Entire System (sq cm)	Per Cent of Total Blood Volume in System at Any Time	Mean Pressure (mm Hg)	Resistance
Aorta		25 mm	2.5		100	low
Artery		4 mm	20	15%	96	low
Arteriole		30 μ	40		85→30	high and variable
Capillary		8 μ	2500	5%	30→10	medium
Venule		20 μ	250		10	low
Vein		5 mm	80	59%	5	low
Vena cava		30 mm	8		0	low

impulse travels to the His bundle, which descends posteriorly along the membranous interventricular septum to the top of the muscular septum. The His bundle gives rise to the right and left bundle branches. The right bundle branch is a single group of fibers that travels down the right ventricular side of the muscular interventricular septum. The left bundle branch is a larger, less discrete array of conducting fibers located on the left side of the interventricular septum. The left bundle branch may divide into two somewhat dis-

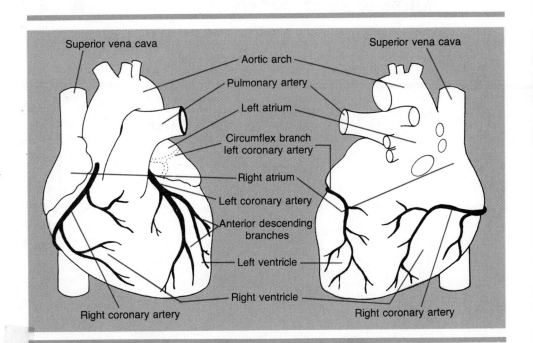

FIGURE 1–4. Major coronary arteries and their branches.

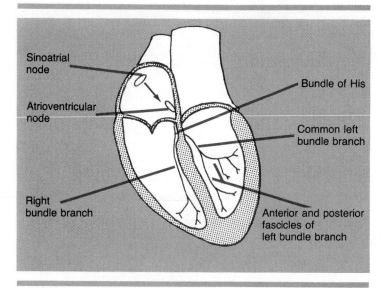

FIGURE 1–5. Schematic representation of the cardiac conduction system.

tinct pathways that travel toward the anterolateral (left anterior fascicle) and posteromedial (left posterior fascicle) papillary muscles. The left posterior fascicle is larger and more diffuse than the anterior fascicle and usually has a more reliable vascular supply than either the left anterior fascicle or the right bundle branch. The left and right bundle branches progressively divide into tiny Purkinje fibers that arborize and finally make intimate contact with ventricular muscle tissue.

MICROSCOPIC ANATOMY

In general, two functional cell types are present in cardiac tissue: those responsible for electrical impulse generation and transmission and those responsible for mechanical contraction. Nodal cells are thought to be the source of normal impulse formation in the sinus node and are richly innervated with adrenergic and cholinergic nerve fibers. Like the sinus node, the AV node and His bundle regions are innervated with a rich supply of cholinergic and adrenergic fibers. Purkinje cells are large clear cells found in the His bundle, bundle branches, and their arborizations. They have particularly well-developed end-to-end connections that may facilitate rapid longitudinal conduction.

Atrial and ventricular myocardial cells, the contractile cells of the heart, contain numerous crossbanded bundles termed myofibrils that traverse the length of the fiber. Myofibrils are composed of longitudinally repeating sarcomeres (Fig. 1–6). Thick filaments composed of myosin constitute the A band, while thin filaments composed primarily of actin extend from the Z line through the I band into the A band, ending at the edges of the central H zone, which is the central area of the A band where thin filaments are absent. Thick and thin filaments overlap in the A

band, and interaction between the thick and thin filaments provides the force for contraction of the heart.

The surface membrane of the cell is termed the sarcolemma, and adjacent myocardial cells are connected end to end by a thickened portion of the sarcolemma termed the intercalated disc. Near the Z lines of the sarcolemma are wide invaginations called the T system that traverse the cell. Not continuous with the T system is the sarcoplasmic reticulum that surrounds each myofibril and participates in the excitation of the muscle. When the sarcolemma is depolarized electrically, the impulse conducts through the T system to cause calcium release from the sarcoplasmic reticulum and therefore activates the myofibrils to contract. The thick fibers in the myofibrils are composed of myosin molecules that have the ability to split ATP and interact with the thin actin filaments when activated by calcium. Regulatory proteins, troponin and tropomyosin, inhibit the interaction of actin and myosin unless a calcium-troponin complex is present, which then allows the actin-

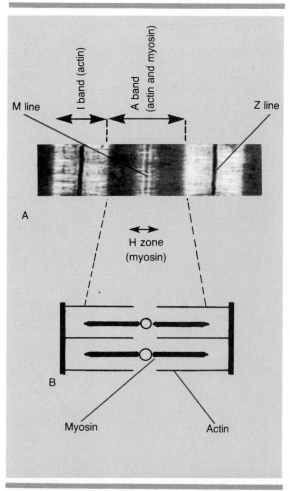

FIGURE 1–6. *A,* A sarcomere as it appears under the electron microscope. *B,* Schematic of the location and interaction of actin and myosin (see text).

myosin interaction to proceed. The sarcolemma possesses the ability to control the flux of various ions (especially sodium, potassium, and calcium) into and out of the cell via specific ionic channels located within the membrane. The selective permeability of the membrane establishes ionic gradients and the electrical forces that create and maintain the resting transmembrane potential and generate the action potential (see Chapter 9).

CARDIAC DEVELOPMENT

Congenital heart disease results from altered embryonic development or failure of the rudimentary portion of a structure ever to be formed. Abnormal development of one structure in turn may hinder the development of another portion of the circulatory system (for example, abnormal development of the mitral valve may lead to abnormal formation of the left ventricle).

The fetus' circulation essentially places the pulmonary and systemic systems in parallel rather than in series as in the adult. Oxygenated blood from the umbilical vein passes into the portal venous system and subsequently into the inferior vena cava and is shunted preferentially across the patent foramen ovale to the left heart to perfuse the coronary arteries, head, and upper trunk. Blood returning from the upper portions of the body arrives at the right atrium via the superior vena cava, and most proceeds through the tricuspid valve to the right ventricle and pulmonary artery. However, only a small proportion of this blood goes into the pulmonary arterial tree; most is shunted via the patent ductus arteriosus to the descending aorta. Note that many congenital lesions that cause intracardiac shunts (for example, tetralogy of Fallot) or markedly abnormal cardiac outflow (for example, transposition of the great arteries) would not cause any difficulty during fetal development.

At birth the pulmonary vascular resistance decreases markedly owing to the inflation of the lungs and the increase in oxygen tension to which the pulmonary vessels are exposed. Systemic vascular resistance rises when the umbilical cord is clamped, removing the low-resistance placental circulation. Left atrial pressure rises, which in turn closes the foramen ovale. The increase in arterial Po_2 along with alterations in prostaglandins causes the ductus arteriosus to close functionally within 10 to 15 hours. Many congenital heart lesions may not become apparent until cyanosis develops after closure of the foramen ovale or ductus arteriosus.

MYOCARDIAL METABOLISM

The heart uses ATP, created by metabolism of carbohydrates or fatty acids, to derive energy for contraction and electrical activity. Energy for electrical activity is minimal compared to that required for contraction. Stored energy reserves are scarce, and the heart must continually have a source of energy in order to function. The principal oxidative substrate for ATP production is fatty acid, but if it is not available, a variety of carbohydrates can be used. Myocardial metabolism is aerobic, and a constant supply of oxygen must be available. The heart, unlike skeletal muscle, is unable to acquire an "oxygen debt" because of its inability to utilize anaerobic metabolism.

CIRCULATORY PHYSIOLOGY

The interaction between myosin and actin, coupled with ATP produced by oxidative phosphorylation, is thought to be the basis for the contraction of each myofibril and therefore the contraction of the whole muscle. Each myofibril exhibits a property called contractility (or inotropic state) that represents the ability of the fiber to develop contractile force. The force exhibited by the fiber is influenced not only by its contractile state but also by its initial length, or preload, according to the Starling curve (Fig. 1–7). This concept can be expanded from the single fiber to describe the function of the entire ventricle. Thus, the abscissa, formerly preload or fiber length, becomes left ventricular filling pressure or volume (i.e., the amount of stretch on the myocardial fibers in diastole); and the ordinate, formerly tension, becomes stroke volume or stroke work (i.e., the ability of the heart to generate tension). Note that as diastolic pressure increases, the normal heart is able to increase its stroke volume, up to a point. This relationship is referred to as a ventricular function curve and, given identical states of contractility and afterload (see below), defines the amount of work that a heart is able to perform. Several factors determine left ventricular filling pressure (Table 1–1).

The term afterload describes the "impedance" or resistance against which the heart must contract. Like preload, afterload also can refer either to a single myofibril or to the heart as a whole. The afterload is approximated by the arterial pressure, the major determinant of the impedance to left ventricular contraction. In the intact heart, the afterload deter-

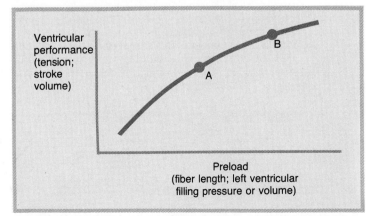

FIGURE 1–7. The normal ventricular function curve. As preload increases from A to B, the curve defines the resultant increase in developed tension or overall cardiac performance.

TABLE 1–1. FACTORS AFFECTING CARDIAC PERFORMANCE

Preload (left ventricular diastolic volume)	Total blood volume Venous tone (sympathetic tone) Body position Intrathoracic and intrapericardial pressure Atrial contraction Pumping action of skeletal muscle
Afterload (impedance against which the left ventricle must eject blood)	Peripheral vascular resistance Left ventricular volume (preload, wall tension) Physical characteristics of the arterial tree (for example, elasticity of vessels or presence of outflow obstruction)
Contractility (cardiac performance independent of preload or afterload)	Sympathetic nerve impulses Circulating catecholamines Digitalis, calcium, other inotropic agents } increased contractility Increased heart rate or post-extrasystolic augmentation Anoxia, acidosis Pharmacological depression } decreased contractility Loss of myocardium Intrinsic depression
Heart Rate	Autonomic nervous system Temperature, metabolic rate

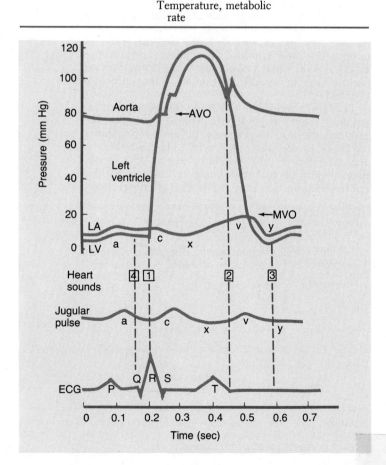

mines the amount of blood the heart can pump given a fixed preload and fixed state of contractility; that is, the higher the workload against which the heart must function, the less blood it can eject, and vice versa. Therefore, the ventricular function curve will be shifted up and to the left with decreasing afterload and shifted down and to the right with increasing afterload. Shifts in ventricular function with changes in afterload are minimal in normal ventricles but prominent in failing ventricles.

Heart rate is another determinant of cardiac performance. Even though an increased demand for cardiac output increases contractility and stroke volume via sympathetic nervous system activation, the most important response to sympathetic stimulation serving to increase cardiac output is the rise in heart rate (cardiac output = stroke volume × heart rate). A decrease in the cardiac output or blood pressure increases sympathetic and decreases parasympathetic discharge via baroreceptor mechanisms to increase heart rate. Likewise, an elevated blood pressure will activate the carotid baroreceptors, augment vagal activity, and slow the heart rate.

Four phases of the cardiac cycle can be identified upon initiation of ventricular myocardial contraction (Fig. 1–8). (1) During "isovolumic contraction," the intramyocardial pressure rises with no ejection of blood or change in ventricular volume. (2) When left ventricular pressure reaches that of the aorta, the aortic valve opens and blood is ejected from the contract-

FIGURE 1–8. Simultaneous ECG, pressures obtained from the left atrium, left ventricle, and aorta, and the jugular pulse during one cardiac cycle. For simplification, right-sided heart pressures have been omitted. Normal right atrial pressure closely parallels that of the left atrium, and right ventricular and pulmonary artery pressures time closely with their corresponding left-sided heart counterparts, only being reduced in magnitude. The normal mitral and aortic valve closure precedes tricuspid and pulmonic closure, respectively, whereas valve opening reverses this order. The jugular venous pulse lags behind the right atrial pressure.

During the course of one cardiac cycle, note that the electrical events (ECG) initiate and therefore precede the mechanical (pressure) events and that the latter precede the auscultatory events (heart sounds) they themselves produce. Shortly after the P wave, the atria contract to produce the a wave; a fourth heart sound may succeed the latter. The QRS complex initiates ventricular systole, followed shortly by left ventricular contraction and the rapid build-up of left ventricular (LV) pressure. Almost immediately LV pressure exceeds left atrial (LA) pressure to close the mitral valve and produces the first heart sounds. When LV pressure exceeds aortic pressure, the aortic valve opens (AVO), and when aortic pressure is once again greater than LV pressure, the aortic valve closes to produce the second heart sound and terminate ventricular ejection. The decreasing LV pressure drops below LA pressure to open the mitral valve (MVO), and a period of rapid ventricular filling commences. During this time a third heart sound may be heard. The jugular pulse is explained under the discussion of the venous pulse.

ing ventricle. (3) As the ventricle relaxes and left ventricular pressure decreases, the aortic valve closes, and "isovolumic relaxation" occurs. (4) Upon sufficient decrease in left ventricular pressure, the mitral valve opens and ventricular filling from the atrium occurs. The ventricle fills most rapidly in early diastole and again in late diastole when the atrium contracts. Loss of atrial contraction (e.g., atrial fibrillation or AV dissociation) can impair ventricular filling, especially into a noncompliant ("stiff") vehicle.

Normal intracardiac pressures are shown in Figure 1–1. Atrial pressure curves are composed of the a wave, which is generated by atrial contraction, and the v wave, which is an early diastolic peak caused by filling of the atrium from the peripheral veins. The x descent follows the a wave and the y descent follows the v wave. A small deflection, the c wave, occurs after the a wave in early systole and probably represents bulging of the tricuspid valve apparatus into the left atrium during early systole. Ventricular pressures are described by a peak systolic pressure and an end-diastolic pressure, which is the ventricular pressure immediately before the onset of systole. Note that the minimum left ventricular pressure occurs in early diastole. Aortic and pulmonary artery pressures are represented by a peak systolic and a minimum diastolic value.

Cardiac output is a measure of the amount of blood flow in liters/minute. The cardiac index is the cardiac output divided by the body surface area and is normally 2.8 to 4.2 L/min/sq m. Cardiac output can be measured by either indicator dilution or the Fick technique (see Chapter 3). The pulmonary and systemic vascular resistances are also important parameters of circulatory function. Resistance is defined as the difference in pressure across a capillary bed divided by the flow across that capillary bed, usually the cardiac output: $[R = (P_1 - P_2)/flow]$ (Fig. 1–3). For example, the pulmonary vascular resistance is the difference between the mean pulmonary arterial pressure and mean pulmonary venous pressure, divided by the pulmonary blood flow. Similarly, systemic vascular resistance is the difference between mean arterial pressure and mean right atrial pressure, divided by the systemic cardiac output. Note that an increase in arterial pressure may occur without necessarily causing an increase in vascular resistance. For example, if both pulmonary arterial and venous pressures are elevated to the same degree, pulmonary vascular resistance will be unchanged; if pulmonary blood flow and pulmonary arterial pressure increase while pulmonary venous pressure remains the same, resistance will be unchanged.

The most widely used parameter for quantitating overall ventricular function is the ejection fraction, defined as the diastolic volume minus the systolic volume (stroke volume), divided by the diastolic volume: $[(DV - SV)/DV]$. These volumes may be estimated from either invasive (e.g., left ventriculography) or noninvasive (e.g., echocardiography or radionuclide ventriculography) tests. The ejection fraction may be a useful gross evaluation of ventricular function, but there are situations (for example, when a large left ventricular aneurysm is present) in which the ejection fraction can give a misleading impression of overall ventricular function.

PHYSIOLOGY OF THE CORONARY CIRCULATION

Three major determinants of myocardial oxygen consumption are contractility, heart rate, and wall tension. Myocardial wall tension is directly proportional to the pressure within the ventricular chamber and the radius of the ventricular chamber (Laplace relationship). The myocardial mass is a determinant of wall tension and therefore myocardial oxygen consumption; the larger the muscle mass, the more oxygen needed.

The coronary vascular bed is able to autoregulate, enabling myocardial oxygen and substrate delivery to equal the demand. Coronary vascular resistance is normally determined by the arterioles and is influenced by neural and metabolic factors. Both the sympathetic and parasympathetic nervous systems innervate the coronary arteries. Alpha receptor stimulation causes vasoconstriction while stimulation of the beta-2 receptor as well as the vagus causes vasodilation. Metabolic factors regulate regional perfusion. Several mediators including oxygen, carbon dioxide, and metabolites such as adenosine are probably important. However, when coronary perfusion pressure falls to below 60 to 70 mm Hg, the vessels become maximally dilated and flow depends on perfusion pressure alone, since capability for further autoregulation is lost. The normal coronary vascular bed has a capacity to increase its blood flow four- to five-fold during maximal exercise. Hemodynamic factors that affect coronary perfusion include arterial pressure (especially diastolic pressure, since coronary flow occurs primarily in diastole), the time spent in diastole, and the intraventricular pressure (which exerts tension on the myocardial walls and diminishes coronary flow).

PHYSIOLOGY OF THE SYSTEMIC CIRCULATION

The aortic wall contains elastic fibers that allow it to expand with the expulsion of blood from the left ventricle, somewhat damping the pulse pressure generated and aiding diastolic flow to the coronary arteries with its recoil. The aorta successively branches into smaller and smaller vessels until arterioles, the major determinants of resistance in the systemic circulation, are reached (see Fig. 1–3). The arterioles contain a vascular sphincter that modulates blood flow dependent on regional metabolic needs; for example, acidosis and decreased oxygen tension increase regional perfusion, and vice versa. The capillaries consist of a single endothelial cell layer and allow diffusion of oxygen, nutrients, CO_2, and waste products. The capillaries lead into the venous system, where blood is eventually delivered back to the right atrium. The flow of blood returning to the heart is aided by the valves in the venous system, which prevent reverse flow, particularly in the larger veins of the legs. The "milking" action of the muscles of the arms and legs and the pressure changes in the thoracic cavity also help to return blood to the heart. The veins have considerably thinner walls than the arteries and can accommodate a larger blood volume under low pressures (capacitance vessels). Vasoconstriction or vasodilation of the venous system can control the amount of blood returning to the heart. More of the total blood volume is located in the venous than in the arterial portion of the circulation. The lymphatic vessels also contribute to the return of fluid from the periphery. The major terminal vessel of the lymphatic system is the thoracic duct, which usually empties into the left brachiocephalic vein.

PHYSIOLOGY OF THE PULMONARY CIRCULATION

The pulmonary circulation has a rich capillary network similar to that of the systemic circulation. The pulmonary alveoli are adjacent to the capillaries, permitting oxygen to diffuse into and carbon dioxide out of the capillary blood. Oxygen is the major mediator of pulmonary autoregulation. In regions where the partial pressure of oxygen is high, pulmonary vasodilation occurs and blood flow is directed preferentially toward well-oxygenated areas of the lung. When the partial pressure of oxygen is low, pulmonary vasoconstriction occurs, preventing the perfusion of areas of the lung that have relatively poor oxygen availability. These vasodilatory effects of oxygen are opposite to those in the systemic circulation. Acidemia potentiates the pulmonary vasoconstrictive effect of hypoxemia, also opposite to its effect on systemic arterioles.

The lungs receive blood through the bronchial arteries as well as the pulmonary arteries (dual blood supply). The bronchial arteries supply arterial blood to the pulmonary tissue and drain into the bronchial veins, some of which drain into the systemic venous bed. Some bronchial veins drain into the pulmonary veins, creating a small physiological right-to-left shunt.

Pulmonary vascular resistance is normally one tenth that of systemic vascular resistance and accounts for the small pressure gradient required to propel blood across the pulmonary vascular bed. Because the pulmonary vasculature is very distensible (compliant), a relatively large left-to-right intracardiac shunt may exist with only a minimal rise in pulmonary arterial pressure.

CARDIOVASCULAR RESPONSE TO EXERCISE

The heart responds to exercise principally by adrenergic stimulation and vagal withdrawal, which increase heart rate and contractility, and by peripheral circulatory alterations (Table 1–2). The increase in heart rate usually accounts for the majority of the increase in cardiac output. Increased contractility contributes to the increase in cardiac output by increasing the stroke volume. Vessels supplying exercising muscles dilate, whereas the remaining vascular beds vasoconstrict. Isometric and isotonic exercises affect the cardiovascular system somewhat differently. The predominant response to isometric exercise (e.g., weight lifting) is an increase in peripheral vasoconstriction with a subsequent increase in arterial pressure. In contrast, isotonic exercise (e.g., jogging) reduces systemic vascular resistance primarily in exercising muscles, which improves cardiac output. Those who exercise regularly obtain a cardiac training effect, with a lower resting heart rate and a greater capacity to increase cardiac output during exercise.

CARDIOVASCULAR PHYSIOLOGY DURING PREGNANCY

See Chapter 13.

ELECTROPHYSIOLOGY

See Chapter 13.

REFERENCE

Berne RM, Levy MN: Cardiovascular Physiology. 5th ed. St. Louis, The CV Mosby Company, 1986.

TABLE 1–2. PHYSIOLOGIC RESPONSES TO EXERCISE

RESPONSE	MECHANISM
↑ Heart rate	↑ Sympathetic stimulation ↓ Parasympathetic stimulation
↑ Stroke volume	
↑ Contractility	↑ Sympathetic stimulation
↑ Venous return	Sympathetic-mediated venoconstriction Pumping action of skeletal muscles ↓ Intrathoracic pressure with deep inspirations Arteriolar vasodilation in exercising muscle
↓ Afterload	Arteriolar vasodilation in exercising muscle (mediated chiefly by local metabolites)
↑ Blood pressure	↑ Cardiac output Vasoconstriction (sympathetic stimulation) of nonexercising vascular beds
↑ O_2 extraction	Shift in oxyhemoglobin dissociation curve due to local acidosis

2

EVALUATION OF THE PATIENT WITH CARDIOVASCULAR DISEASE

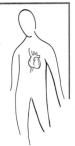

HISTORY

The history is the most important tool in the evaluation of a patient (Table 2–1). *Chest pain* is the most common presenting symptom of cardiovascular disease and must be characterized carefully. Chest pain may be cardiac (myocardial or pericardial) or noncardiac in etiology (Tables 2–2 and 2–3).

Ischemic myocardial pain is a visceral discomfort caused by insufficient oxygen delivery to an area of the heart. A transient oxygen supply/demand mismatch causes angina pectoris, whereas ischemia followed by myocardial necrosis is termed myocardial infarction. Angina pectoris is typically evoked by emotion, exertion, or a heavy meal, but more severe episodes can occur at rest or awaken the patient from sleep. It generally lasts only a few minutes and diminishes after exertion is stopped. When it is due to fixed coronary obstruction, the same degree of activity tends to reliably reproduce the pain. When due to coronary arterial spasm, with or without fixed obstruction, the level of activity that causes pain may vary. Nitroglycerin typically relieves the pain in about 5 minutes. Pain of a prolonged duration (>30 minutes) suggests either myocardial infarction or noncardiac pain. Respiration does not influence ischemic chest pain. The pain of both angina pectoris and myocardial infarction can be atypical in some patients and difficult to diagnose. Many patients describe a chest discomfort or fullness that they do not consider pain. Any patient who has chest discomfort provoked by exertion and relieved by rest and any patient who has chest discomfort similar to the pain of a previous myocardial infarction should be suspected of ischemic myocardial chest pain.

The pain of pericardial inflammation (Table 2–3) may be difficult to differentiate from ischemic pain in a patient with pericarditis following myocardial infarction.

Patients with mitral valve prolapse sometimes present with a chest pain syndrome that may or may not resemble ischemic myocardial pain. The etiology of this chest pain is unclear.

Dyspnea is a subjective sensation of shortness of breath and often is a symptom of cardiac disease, especially in patients with congestive heart failure (Table 2–4). When left ventricular failure occurs, left atrial and subsequently pulmonary venous pressures rise. Pulmonary compliance decreases (stiff lungs) and causes a subjective sensation of air hunger before hypoxia, hypercapnia, or low cardiac output occurs. As congestive heart failure worsens, transudative fluid accumulates in the alveoli and hypoxemia results. Because the supine position compared with the upright position augments venous return, patients with congestive heart failure demonstrate orthopnea, i.e., shortness of breath in the supine position relieved by sitting up. They also may demonstrate paroxysmal nocturnal dyspnea, i.e., awakening with shortness of breath two to three hours after falling asleep. It usually occurs only once nightly, is relieved by sitting or standing, and is probably related to central redistribution of fluid upon assuming the reclining position.

Occasionally, dyspnea can represent the anginal equivalent, a symptom of acute myocardial ischemia. Dyspnea is also a prominent feature of pulmonary disease, and at times the differentiation between pulmonary and cardiac causes of dyspnea are difficult. For example, patients with pulmonary dyspnea can exhibit orthopnea, whereas wheezes may be heard in patients with cardiac dyspnea (e.g., congestive heart failure). Sudden dyspnea is a common presentation of a pulmonary embolus.

Cyanosis is a bluish discoloration of the skin caused by an increased amount of nonoxygenated hemoglobin in the blood. Central cyanosis, often best seen on the oral mucous membranes, is due to right-to-left shunting of blood or impaired pulmonary function. Peripheral cyanosis, best seen in the extremities, may be due to shunting or to local discoloration due to vasoconstriction (e.g., low cardiac output, peripheral vascular disease, or exposure to cold). Cyanosis is more difficult to see in dark-skinned than in light-skinned individuals. Since cyanosis becomes apparent when ≥4 grams/dl of reduced hemoglobin is present, polycythemia tends to accentuate cyanosis and anemia tends to minimize it.

Syncope has multiple origins, including circulatory (e.g., volume depletion from a variety of causes) and neurological (e.g., seizures) as well as cardiac (see Chapter 9).

Palpitation refers to an awareness of heart beat, usually either irregular or rapid (see Chapter 9).

Fatigue is a common cardiac symptom but is extremely nonspecific. Patients who have a reduced cardiac output often complain of fatigue that may be ex-

TABLE 2–1. CARDINAL SYMPTOMS OF CARDIAC DISEASE

Chest pain or discomfort
Symptoms of heart failure
Palpitation
Syncope, presyncope

TABLE 2–2. CARDIOVASCULAR CAUSES OF CHEST PAIN

CONDITION	LOCATION	QUALITY	DURATION	AGGRAVATING OR RELIEVING FACTORS	ASSOCIATED SYMPTOMS OR SIGNS
Angina	Retrosternal region; radiates to or occasionally isolated to neck, jaw, epigastrium, shoulder or arms—left common	Pressure, burning, squeezing, heaviness, indigestion	<10 minutes	Aggravated by exercise, cold weather, or emotional stress, or occurs after meals; relieved by rest or nitroglycerin; atypical (Prinzmetal's) angina may be unrelated to activity and caused by coronary artery spasm	S_4, paradoxical split S_2, or murmur of papillary muscle dysfunction during pain
Rest or crescendo angina	Same as angina	Same as angina	>10 minutes	Same as angina, with gradually decreasing tolerance for exertion	Same as angina
Myocardial infarction	Substernal, and may radiate like angina	Heaviness, pressure, burning, constriction	Sudden onset, 30 minutes or longer but variable; usually goes away in hours	Unrelieved	Shortness of breath, sweating, weakness, nausea, vomiting, severe anxiety
Pericarditis	Usually begins over sternum or toward cardiac apex and may radiate to neck and down left upper extremity; often more localized than the pain of myocardial ischemia	Sharp, stabbing, knifelike	Lasts many hours to days	Aggravated by deep breathing, rotating chest, or supine position; relieved by sitting up and leaning forward	Pericardial friction rub, cardiac tamponade, pulsus paradoxus
Dissecting aortic aneurysm	Anterior chest; radiates to thoracic area of back; may be abdominal; pain may move as dissection progresses	Excruciating, tearing, knifelike	Sudden onset, lasts for hours	Unrelated to anything	Lower blood pressure in one arm, absent pulses, paralysis, murmur of aortic insufficiency, pulsus paradoxus, myocardial infarction

TABLE 2-3. NONCARDIAC CAUSES OF CHEST PAIN

CONDITION	LOCATION	QUALITY	DURATION	AGGRAVATING OR RELIEVING FACTORS	ASSOCIATED SYMPTOMS OR SIGNS
Pulmonary embolism (chest pain often not present)	Substernal or over region of pulmonary infarction	Pleuritic (with pulmonary infarction) or angina-like	Sudden onset; minutes to < hour	May be aggravated by breathing	Dyspnea, tachypnea, tachycardia, hypotension; signs of acute right heart failure and pulmonary hypertension with large emboli; rales, pleural rub, hemoptysis with pulmonary infarction; clinically present in minority of cases
Pulmonary hypertension	Substernal	Pressure; oppressive		Aggravated by effort	Pain usually associated with dyspnea; signs of pulmonary hypertension (Table 5-3)
Pneumonia with pleurisy	Localized over area of consolidation	Pleuritic, well-localized		Painful breathing	Dyspnea, cough, fever, dull to percussion, bronchial breath sounds, rales, occasional pleural rub
Spontaneous pneumothorax	Unilateral	Sharp, well-localized	Sudden onset, lasts many hours	Painful breathing	Dyspnea; hyper-resonance and decreased breath and voice sounds over involved lung
Musculoskeletal disorders	Variable	Aching	Short or long duration	Aggravated by movement; history of muscle exertion	Tender to pressure or movement
Herpes zoster	Dermatomal in distribution		Prolonged	None	Rash appears in area of discomfort
Gastrointestinal disorders (e.g., esophageal reflux, peptic ulcer, cholecystitis)	Lower substernal area, epigastric, right or left upper quadrant	Burning, colic-like, aching		Precipitated by recumbency or meals	Nausea, regurgitation, food intolerance, melena, hematemesis, jaundice
Anxiety states	Often localized to a point	Sharp burning, commonly location of pain moves from place to place	Varies; usually very brief	Situational anger— very brief	Sighing respirations, often chest wall tenderness

TABLE 2–4. SYMPTOMS AND SIGNS OF CARDIAC FAILURE

	SYMPTOMS	SIGNS

Left heart failure	Dyspnea
	Orthopnea
	Paroxysmal nocturnal
	  dyspnea
		Tachypnea
		Left ventricular S₃
		  gallop
		Left ventricular S₄
		  gallop (nonspecific)
		Rales
		Wheezes (cardiac
		  asthma)
		Functional mitral
		  regurgitation
		Pulsus alternans

Right heart failure	Peripheral edema
	Nocturia
	Abdominal fullness
		Jugular venous
		  distention
		Peripheral edema
		Ascites
		Anasarca
		Hepatomegaly
		Splenomegaly
		Hepatojugular reflux
		Right ventricular S₃,
		  S₄ gallops
		Tricuspid regurgitation
		  (holosystolic
		  murmur, pulsatile
		  liver, large jugular V
		  wave)
		Signs of pulmonary
		  hypertension if
		  present (Table 5–3)

Either left or right
  heart failure
	Fatigue
	Weakness
	Anorexia
		Tachycardia
		Blood pressure often
		  elevated
		Narrow pulse pressure
		Sweaty, cool
		  extremities
		Pleural effusion
		  (usually bilateral or
		  isolated right)
		Cardiomegaly
		Cheyne-Stokes
		  (periodic or cyclic)
		  respiration
		Mental confusion

**TABLE 2–5. NEW YORK HEART ASSOCIATION
FUNCTIONAL CLASSIFICATION**

Class I	No limitation	Ordinary physical activity does not cause symptoms
Class II	Slight limitation	Comfortable at rest Ordinary physical activity causes symptoms
Class III	Marked limitation	Comfortable at rest Less than ordinary activity causes symptoms

Class IV	Inability to carry
	  on any physical
	  activity
		Symptoms present at rest

acerbated by drugs (for example, beta-adrenergic blocking drugs).

Edema is common in patients with congestive heart failure. Edema of the lower extremities (or the sacral area in bedridden patients) often is a symptom of right ventricular failure. Other causes of peripheral edema include the nephrotic syndrome, cirrhosis, and venous insufficiency. Peripheral edema may increase at the end of the day and decrease overnight as the dependent part is elevated and the fluid resorbed. Fluid within the peritoneal cavity is referred to as *ascites* and within the chest cavity as *pleural effusion*. Patients who have severe edema secondary to congestive heart failure may develop ascites, and ascites is especially frequent in patients who have constrictive pericarditis. Noncardiac causes of ascites such as cirrhosis, nephrosis, and peritoneal tumor must be excluded.

Cough and *hemoptysis* may be associated with cardiac disease, but it may be difficult to differentiate cardiac from pulmonary disease on the basis of these two symptoms alone. A cough, often orthostatic in nature, may be the primary complaint in some patients with pulmonary congestion. They tend not to bring up thick purulent sputum as do patients with chronic bronchitis. Hemoptysis occurs in congestive heart failure and is especially common in patients with mitral stenosis. Massive hemoptysis is generally not a cardiac symptom.

Nocturia, secondary to resorption of edema at night, is common in patients with congestive heart failure. Anorexia, abdominal fullness, right upper quadrant tenderness (secondary to hepatomegaly), and weight loss are also symptoms of advanced heart failure. Hoarseness may occasionally result from recurrent laryngeal nerve compression by an aortic aneurysm, dilated pulmonary artery, or large left atrium.

A history of rheumatic fever, prolonged febrile illnesses, sore throats, or any rheumatic complaints as a child should be sought. The patient should be asked about any past history of a heart murmur or other cardiac abnormalities noted in a previous examination. Childhood activity levels may be important in evaluating patients suspected of having congenital or rheumatic heart disease. Females should be asked about problems during pregnancy, a state that stresses the cardiovascular system. The presence of risk factors for coronary artery disease (see Chapter 8) should be determined. The New York Heart Association's functional classification of patients with cardiac disease is useful (Table 2–5).

GENERAL PHYSICAL EXAMINATION

The patient's general appearance and vital signs are important in the overall evaluation of suspected cardiac disease (see Table 2–4). In mild to moderately severe heart failure, the blood pressure is usually elevated; hypotension is a sign of advanced myocardial failure. Cheyne-Stokes respirations, thought to be related to a delay in baroreceptor sensing of oxygenation due to poor perfusion of the baroreceptors, may be noted in patients with either advanced heart failure or primary central nervous system disease. Certain distinct syndromes may suggest a congenital anomaly; for example, Down's syndrome is associated with several congenital cardiac malformations (most commonly ventricular septal defect and endocardial cushion defect), and Marfan's syndrome is associated with disease of the aorta and aortic valve.

Examination of the lungs is generally normal in patients with heart disease unless left heart failure with pulmonary congestion is present (see Table 2–4). Pulmonary rales are fine, discrete sounds produced by fluid within alveoli. They occur first at the bases and may be heard toward the pulmonary apices as congestive heart failure worsens; they are not specific for heart failure. Hepatic systolic pulsations along with large jugular venous v waves may occur with tricuspid regurgitation. Hepatojugular reflux, an increase in cervical venous distention when pressure is applied over the liver during normal respiration, is a sign of right heart failure. Ascites and splenomegaly may occur in patients with tricuspid valve disease (especially tricuspid stenosis) or chronic constrictive pericarditis. Splenomegaly may also occur in patients with endocarditis.

EXAMINATION OF THE NECK VEINS

The purpose of neck vein examination is to estimate the right atrial pressure (central venous pressure) and to evaluate abnormalities in the venous pulse waveform. To estimate central venous pressure, the patient's torso should be at an angle so that the top of the internal jugular pulsation can be visualized. The vertical height of this column from the angle of Louis plus 5 cm (the distance from the angle of Louis to the right atrium at most angles is about 5 cm) approximates the actual venous pressure. Normal venous pressure is between 5 and 9 cm H_2O. Therefore, the normal vertical height of the jugular venous column is less than 3 to 5 cm above the sternal angle. Elevated jugular venous pressure occurs in patients who have right ventricular failure or an abnormality of right ventricular filling (e.g., tricuspid valve abnormality, constrictive pericarditis, or tamponade). The normal jugular venous pressure falls with inspiration and increases with expiration. If the opposite occurs (Kussmaul's sign), constrictive pericarditis or restrictive cardiomyopathy should be suspected.

The jugular venous pulse is composed of two large deflections (the a and v waves) and two negative deflections (the x and y descents) (Fig. 2–1). Even though not usually appreciated on physical examination, a second positive deflection after the a wave, the c wave, is recordable. The a wave results from atrial contraction and is accentuated in patients with right ventricular hypertrophy, tricuspid or pulmonic stenosis, or contraction of the atrium against a closed tricuspid valve as occurs in heart block (cannon a

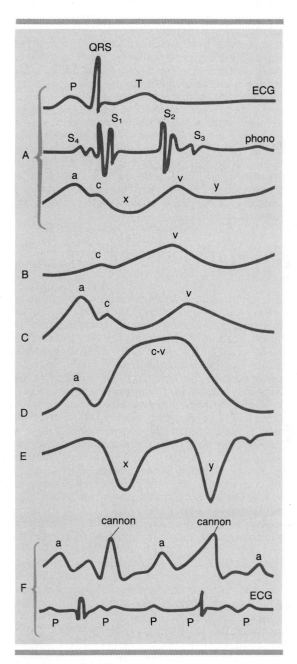

FIGURE 2–1. Normal and abnormal jugular venous pulse tracings. A, Normal jugular pulse tracing with simultaneous electrocardiogram and phonocardiogram. B, Loss of a waves in atrial fibrillation. C, Large a waves in tricuspid stenosis. D, Large c-v waves in tricuspid regurgitation. E, Steep x and y descents in constrictive pericarditis. F, Jugular venous pulse tracing and simultaneous electrocardiogram during complete heart block demonstrating cannon a waves occurring when the atrium contracts against a closed tricuspid valve during ventricular systole.

wave). Irregular cannon a waves occur with AV dissociation. Regular cannon a waves may occur in a junctional or ventricular rhythm that conducts retrogradely to the atrium or during some supraventricular tachycardias (see Chapter 9). The a wave is absent if atrial fibrillation is present. The c wave is due to transmitted pressure from the closed tricuspid valve thrust upward during right ventricular systole. The v wave is normally smaller than the a wave and is due to blood returning from the periphery to the right atrium during ventricular systole when the tricuspid valve is closed. The v wave may be the only visible positive deflection in patients with atrial fibrillation. Tricuspid regurgitation results in a large v wave with attenuation of the x descent. The y descent, representing atrial emptying, is decreased in the presence of tricuspid stenosis. Restricted filling of the right heart (e.g., constrictive pericarditis or restrictive cardiomyopathy) produces a venous pulse with distinctive steep x and y descents.

ARTERIAL PRESSURE AND PULSES

Arterial pressure is measured with a sphygmomanometer. Deflation of the arm cuff previously inflated above the systolic arterial pressure results in the sound of blood intermittently entering the artery (Korotkoff sounds) when cuff pressure falls to less than systolic pressure. As the cuff is progressively deflated to the diastolic pressure, the Korotkoff sounds disappear, signifying that blood is flowing within the artery in both systole and diastole. Spurious blood pressure measurements can be obtained if a cuff of incorrect diameter is used; a narrow blood pressure cuff used on an obese arm gives falsely elevated blood pressure readings, and vice versa. In such a patient, blood pressure can be obtained in the forearm with a regular sized cuff, listening over the radial artery. Blood pressure must be measured in the lower extremities when excluding coarctation of the aorta as a cause for upper extremity hypertension. The normal blood pressure in the leg is approximately 10 mm higher than that in the arm.

Arterial pulses can be palpated over the carotid, axillary, brachial, radial, femoral, popliteal, dorsalis pedis, and posterior tibial arteries. The carotid pulses are most closely related to the aortic pressure in both timing and contour and provide the most information concerning cardiac function. Representative carotid pulse contours are shown in Figure 2–2. Note that the normal upstroke is brisk and that the end of ejection is signified by the dicrotic notch, usually not palpable.

Arterial pulses are symmetrical bilaterally. Inequalities may be explained by chronic atherosclerosis or more acute processes involving regional circulation, for example, dissection of the aorta, peripheral emboli, or vasculitis (e.g., Takayasu's disease). In supravalvular aortic stenosis, there is streaming of the jet toward the right innominate artery, and the carotid and brachial arterial pulses may be stronger on the

right than the left. Strongly palpable pulses in the upper extremities with weakly palpable pulses in the lower extremities may suggest coarctation of the aorta. The amplitude of the carotid pulse increases with anemia, thyrotoxicosis, and aortic insufficiency because of the increased stroke volume and rate of left ventricular ejection. The carotid pulse amplitude is attenuated (pulsus parvus) in conditions associated with decreased left ventricular stroke volume, for example, myocardial failure, tachycardia, hypovolemia, severe mitral stenosis, and constrictive pericarditis. Severe

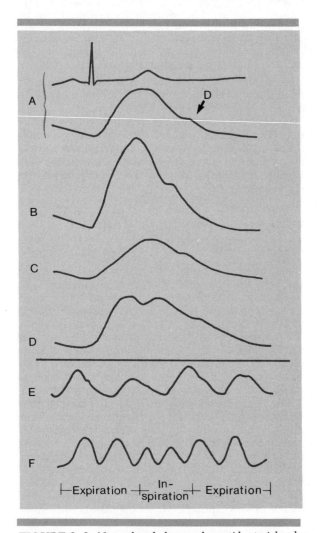

FIGURE 2–2. Normal and abnormal carotid arterial pulse contours. *A,* Normal arterial pulse with simultaneous electrocardiogram. The dicrotic wave (D) occurs just after aortic valve closure. *B,* Wide pulse pressure in aortic insufficiency. *C,* Pulsus parvus et tardus (small amplitude with a slow upstroke) associated with aortic stenosis. *D,* Bisferiens pulse with two systolic peaks, typical of hypertrophic obstructive cardiomyopathy or aortic insufficiency, especially if concomitant aortic stenosis is present. *E,* Pulsus alternans characteristic of severe left ventricular failure. *F,* Paradoxical pulse (systolic pressure decrease of greater than 10 mm Hg with inspiration), most characteristic of cardiac tamponade.

myocardial failure may result in pulsus alternans, an alternating intensity of the arterial pulse. Pulsus parvus et tardus is a slowly rising, low-amplitude, late-peaking arterial pulse due to severe aortic outflow tract obstruction (Fig. 2–2). In addition, severe aortic stenosis may be associated with a carotid shudder, coarse palpable carotid arterial vibrations associated with ejection. Pulsus parvus et tardus may not be present in older patients with aortic stenosis and a stiff, noncompliant arterial system or in patients with concomitant aortic insufficiency. Aortic insufficiency is associated with a high-amplitude pulse with a very rapid upstroke, referred to as a Corrigan or water-hammer pulse. Severe aortic insufficiency with or without aortic stenosis may be associated with a bisferiens pulse, a carotid arterial pressure contour with two palpable systolic peaks. A bisferiens pulse is also associated with hypertrophic obstructive cardiomyopathy (Fig. 2–2). In this condition, a rapid initial upstroke of the carotid artery is attenuated in midsystole and followed by a second late systolic peak, indicative of a late systolic attempt by the ventricle to completely expel its blood. Pulsus paradoxus, a greater than normal decrease (>10 mm Hg) in systolic arterial pressure with inspiration, characteristically occurs in pericardial tamponade but may also be present in other conditions such as airway obstruction (acute exacerbation of chronic obstruction pulmonary disease or asthma). The mechanism of pulsus paradoxus is complex and multifactorial. A pulse of irregular intensity may occur in atrial fibrillation or other irregular arrhythmia.

PRECORDIAL EXAMINATION

Before auscultation, the precordium should be inspected and palpated. With good lighting, the point of maximal cardiac impulse may be visible. Cardiac impulses are not normally observed in any other area. The normal apical impulse occurs in early systole and is located within an area of approximately one square centimeter in the fourth to fifth left intercostal space near the midclavicular line. Inspection of the precordium should reveal any abnormalities of the bony structures (for example, pectus excavatum) that may displace the heart to produce unusual findings on physical examination. Precordial palpation should begin with the point of maximal impulse and progress across the precordium, searching for abnormal impulses, palpable sounds, and thrills.

An abnormally prolonged and diffuse left ventricular impulse with increased amplitude is termed a left ventricular heave and is associated with left ventricular hypertrophy. Displacement of the left ventricular impulse downward and to the left indicates left ventricular dilation, common in left ventricular failure or valvular lesions associated with volume overload, such as aortic or mitral regurgitation. A palpable S_4 gallop is associated with pressure overload states, for example, aortic stenosis or long-standing hypertension. A double systolic apical impulse is characteristic of obstructive hypertrophic cardiomyopathy. A systolic bulge

medial to the point of maximal impulse is sometimes felt after a recent myocardial infarction and probably represents an area of left ventricular asynergy. A left parasternal lift generally indicates right ventricular dilation and/or hypertrophy and is observed in patients with mitral stenosis or other causes of right ventricular stress. Occasionally, late systolic expansion of the left atrium in patients with severe mitral regurgitation can be palpated in the left parasternal area. Vibrations (thrills) associated with the murmurs of valvular or congenital lesions may be palpable, for example, in aortic stenosis or ventricular septal defect. Occasionally, pulmonic closure (P_2) is markedly accentuated and palpable in patients with severe pulmonary hypertension. Systolic retraction of the apical impulse is a characteristic finding in constrictive pericarditis.

CARDIAC AUSCULTATION

Both patient and examiner should be physically comfortable to ensure adequate cardiac auscultation. A good stethoscope has a diaphragm for auscultating relatively high-frequency sounds and a bell for low-frequency sounds. The diaphragm is applied with moderate pressure to the chest, whereas the bell should be applied very lightly, just enough to create a seal. The patient should be auscultated while supine and sitting. Certain sounds (for example, the murmur of aortic insufficiency and the rub of pericarditis) are best heard with the patient sitting upright and leaning forward in end-expiration to bring the heart as close to the chest wall as possible. Gallop rhythms are best heard at the apex with the patient supine or in the left lateral decubitus position. The murmur and opening snap of mitral stenosis are best heard with the patient in the left lateral decubitus position, and sometimes leg or arm exercises are needed to make the murmur audible. The click and late systolic murmur of mitral valve prolapse may be accentuated by standing.

There are four major auscultatory zones. The aortic listening area is the second intercostal space just to the right of the sternum, while the pulmonic area is opposite, at the second intercostal space just to the left of the sternum. The tricuspid area is the fourth intercostal space just to the left of the sternum, and the mitral area is at the point of maximum impulse. These areas provide general guidelines to auscultate pathology for each valve, but exceptions exist.

The normal heart sounds consist of a first heart sound (S_1) and a second heart sound (S_2) (see Fig. 1–8). S_1 occurs at the onset of systole and is generated by mitral and tricuspid valve closure. The closure of the aortic (A_2) and pulmonic (P_2) valves at end-systole generates S_2. A_2 and P_2 occur almost simultaneously at end-expiration. Upon inspiration, venous return increases to the right heart because of decreased intrathoracic pressure and decreases to the left heart because of increased pulmonary vascular capacitance. These changes delay P_2 and slightly advance A_2 so that A_2 and P_2 separate temporally during inspiration, becoming superimposed during expiration. P_2 is normally less intense than A_2 and is best heard at the second intercostal space to the left of the sternum.

An early diastolic gallop rhythm (S_3) is a low-pitched sound heard best with the bell of the stethoscope placed lightly over the point of maximal impulse, especially with the patient in the left lateral decubitus position. It is generated by rapid filling of the left ventricle in early diastole and is a physiologically normal sound in young people into the early twenties. Heard in older age groups, an S_3 signifies left or right ventricular failure. An S_3 must be differentiated from other early diastolic sounds, for example, a widely split S_2, the opening snap of mitral stenosis, a tumor plop from a left atrial myxoma, or the pericardial knock of constrictive pericarditis.

A soft, early-peaking systolic ejection murmur at the second left intercostal space can be a normal finding in some people, especially younger people and patients with high circulatory flow states, for example, anemia, thyrotoxicosis, exercise, and pregnancy. It is probably generated by flow across the pulmonic outflow tract. Diastolic murmurs are never physiological. Systolic and diastolic sounds can sometimes be heard over the cervical venous system (venous hums). These venous hums disappear with a change in position or light pressure over the vein. They are not pathological but must be differentiated from cardiac murmurs or bruits.

ABNORMAL HEART SOUNDS (Fig. 2–3)

Variation in the intensity of S_1 may have diagnostic importance (Table 2–6). After a short PR interval, the mitral and tricuspid valves are wide open at the onset of systole (louder S_1), whereas after a long PR interval they are already almost closed at the onset of systole (softer S_1). S_1 may vary in intensity in patients with atrial fibrillation or some types of heart block, when the mitral and tricuspid valves are in various stages of closure at the onset of ventricular systole. S_1 is loud in patients who have mitral stenosis and a relatively pliable valve (the mitral valve is wide open at the onset of left ventricular ejection). Splitting of S_1 is rarely of any diagnostic significance.

Abnormalities in S_2 may be related to abnormal intensity or abnormal timing (Tables 2–6 and 2–8). A single S_2 is present in any condition in which the intensity of A_2 or P_2 is markedly attenuated. Persistent splitting of S_2 retaining normal respiratory variation occurs when P_2 is delayed, or occasionally when A_2 is early, as in patients with mitral regurgitation or ventricular septal defect. Fixed splitting of S_2 is characteristic of atrial septal defect or lesions in which the right ventricle is unable to augment its stroke volume, for example, severe pulmonic stenosis. Paradoxical splitting of S_2 (P_2 preceding A_2 during expiration and coincident with A_2 on inspiration) is usually caused by conditions that delay A_2.

The fourth heart sound (S_4 gallop) occurs during late diastolic ventricular filling due to atrial contraction. An S_4 is usually abnormal, but occasionally it may be heard in a healthy adult. Inspiration enhances an S_4 originating from the right ventricle but has little effect on a left ventricular S_4. An S_4 gallop is associated with an elevated left ventricular end-diastolic pressure due to decreased left ventricular compliance, second-

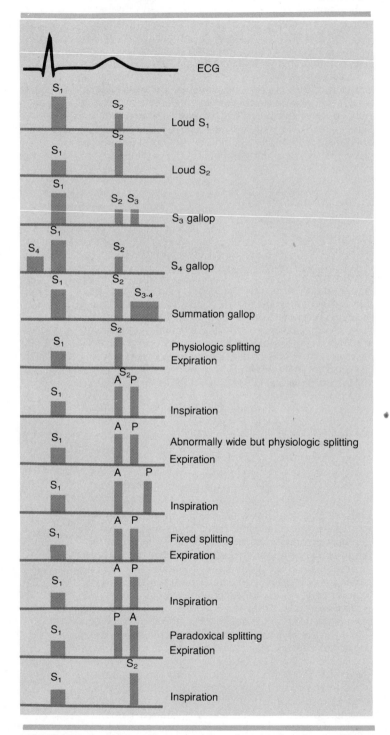

FIGURE 2–3. Abnormal heart sounds can be related to abnormal intensity, abnormal presence of a gallop rhythm, or abnormal splitting of S_2 with respiration.

ary to either left ventricular hypertrophy or ischemia. It is characteristically found in patients with aortic stenosis, hypertrophic cardiomyopathy, acute mitral regurgitation, and myocardial infarction. A right ventricular S_4 is heard in pulmonary hypertension and pulmonic stenosis. An S_4 is not present in atrial fibrillation. A transient S_4 gallop coincident with chest pain may be suggestive of ischemia. The auscultatory rhythm of an S_4 is likened to pronouncing "Tenn´ (S_4) - e (S_1) - see (S_2)."

An early diastolic filling sound (S_3 gallop) may be physiological in older children and young adults (see above), but in adults it occurs with impaired ventricular function of any cause and is the most sensitive and specific physical sign of ventricular dysfunction. It may be heard in chronic aortic or mitral insufficiency, in which it probably also represents some degree of left ventricular dysfunction. Left ventricular gallop sounds are not heard in the presence of significant mitral stenosis. A right ventricular S_3 may be heard at the left lower sternal border or sometimes the epigastrium and is accentuated with inspiration. The auscultatory cadence of an S_3 is likened to pronouncing "Ken (S_1) - tuck´ (S_2) - y (S_3)."

When tachycardia is present and a diastolic gallop cannot be separated into a distinct S_3 and S_4, it often represents the summation of both and is termed a summation gallop. It has a distinct cadence likened to that of a galloping horse.

Normal valves make no sound as they open. However, an abnormal but pliable aortic or pulmonic valve may generate an opening sound called an ejection sound or click (Fig. 2–4, Table 2–7). Ejection sounds are high-pitched and occur early in systole, immediately upon completion of isovolumic contraction. More severe stenosis causes the ejection sound to occur earlier in systole, i.e., closer to S_1. The cause of ejection sounds in pulmonary or systemic hypertension is unclear but probably relates to the dilation of the aortic or pulmonary arterial root.

Mid to late systolic clicks, often followed by a late systolic murmur, occur in patients with mitral valve prolapse. The clicks are thought to result from sudden tensing of the mitral valve apparatus as the valve prolapses. The clicks may be single or multiple and may occur at any time during systole, although they are

generally later than ejection sounds. The behavior of these clicks and associated murmurs during physiological maneuvers is summarized in Table 2–11.

The mitral and tricuspid valves also do not normally make an opening sound. However, with mitral or tricuspid stenosis, an early diastolic opening sound is heard if the valve is still pliable (Fig. 2–4). The opening "snap" (OS) of mitral stenosis is earlier in diastole, is

TABLE 2–6. ABNORMAL INTENSITY OF HEART SOUNDS

	S_1	A_2	P_2
Loud	Short PR interval Mitral stenosis with pliable valve	Systemic hypertension Aortic dilation Coarctation of aorta	Pulmonary hypertension Thin chest wall
Soft	Long PR interval Mitral regurgitation Poor LV function Mitral stenosis with rigid valve Thick chest wall	Calcific aortic stenosis Aortic regurgitation	Valvular or subvalvular pulmonic stenosis
Varying	Atrial fibrillation Heart block		

TABLE 2–7. EJECTION CLICKS

AORTIC	PULMONIC
Noncalcific congenital aortic stenosis Systemic hypertension Dilation of the aorta	Valvular pulmonic stenosis Pulmonary arterial hypertension Idiopathic dilation of the pulmonary artery
No change with respiration Loudest second right intercostal space and apex	Increased intensity with *expiration* (opposite to other right-sided events) Loudest left upper sternal border

TABLE 2–8. ABNORMAL SPLITTING OF S_2

SINGLE S_2	WIDELY SPLIT S_2 WITH NORMAL RESPIRATORY VARIATION	FIXED SPLIT S_2	PARADOXICAL SPLITTING OF S_2
Aortic stenosis Pulmonic stenosis Systemic hypertension Coronary artery disease Any condition that can lead to paradoxical splitting of S_2	Right bundle branch block Left ventricular pacing Pulmonic stenosis Pulmonary embolus Idiopathic dilation of the pulmonary artery Mitral regurgitation Ventricular septal defect	Atrial septal defect Severe RV dysfunction	Left bundle branch block Right ventricular pacemaker Angina, myocardial infarction Aortic stenosis Hypertrophic obstructive cardiomyopathy Aortic regurgitation

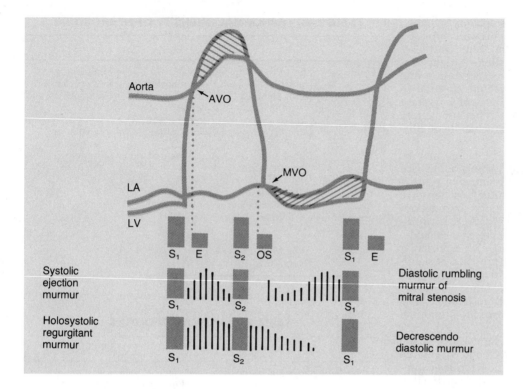

FIGURE 2–4. Abnormal sounds and murmurs associated with valvular dysfunction displayed simultaneously with left atrial (LA), left ventricular (LV), and aortic pressure tracings. AVO = aortic valve opening; MVO = mitral valve opening; E = ejection click of the aortic valve; OS = opening snap of the mitral valve. The shaded areas represent pressure gradients across the aortic valve during systole or mitral valve during diastole, characteristic of aortic stenosis and mitral stenosis, respectively.

of higher pitch than an S_3 gallop, and is located somewhat medial to the point of maximum impulse. More severe stenosis causes the opening snap to occur earlier, i.e., closer to S_2; the higher the left atrial pressure, the earlier the valve opens after the onset of isovolumic relaxation. Opening snaps disappear as the stenotic AV valve calcifies and becomes immobile.

A pericardial knock is an early diastolic sound, sometimes difficult to distinguish from an S_3 gallop, heard in patients with constrictive pericarditis. Another abnormal early diastolic heart sound is the tumor "plop" of an atrial myxoma.

ABNORMAL MURMURS

Heart murmurs are vibrations of longer duration than the heart sounds and represent turbulent flow across abnormal valves caused by congenital or acquired cardiac defects (Fig. 2–4). Murmurs are termed

diastolic or systolic, and their intensity is graded (Table 2–9). The length of the murmur and its radiation (e.g., to the back, neck, axilla, or listening areas other than that of the valve primarily involved) should be described along with the quality of the murmur (e.g., blowing, harsh, rumbling, musical, or high- or low-pitched).

Systolic murmurs are usually divided into ejection and holosystolic types (Table 2–10). Systolic ejection murmurs are generated either by abnormalities within or increased flow across the aortic or pulmonary outflow tracts. The systolic ejection murmur of coarctation of the aorta is late in systole compared to valvular ejection murmurs.

Mitral regurgitation due to the syndrome of mitral valve prolapse may be associated with a late systolic murmur that is often preceded by a systolic click. It may be somewhat atypical for mitral regurgitation in quality as well as timing and is often best heard more toward the left sternal border than at the traditional mitral listening area.

Early diastolic decrescendo murmurs are heard with aortic and pulmonic regurgitation. Aortic regurgitation can be due to valvular leaks or secondary to dilation of the valve ring (for example, after aortic dissection). Pulmonic regurgitation also can be valvular or secondary to dilation of the valve ring associated with pulmonary hypertension (Graham Steell murmur).

In addition to mitral and tricuspid stenosis, rumbles across AV valves can be heard in conditions in which there is increased diastolic flow across a nonstenotic

TABLE 2–9. GRADING SYSTEM FOR INTENSITY OF MURMURS

Grade 1	Barely audible murmur
Grade 2	Murmur of medium intensity
Grade 3	Loud murmur, no thrill
Grade 4	Loud murmur with thrill
Grade 5	Very loud murmur, stethoscope must be on the chest to hear
Grade 6	Murmur audible with stethoscope off the chest

TABLE 2–10. CLASSIFICATION OF HEART MURMURS

CLASS	DESCRIPTION	CHARACTERISTIC LESIONS
Ejection	Systolic Crescendo-decrescendo Often harsh in quality Begin after S_1; end before S_2	Valvular, supravalvular, and subvalvular aortic stenosis Hypertrophic obstructive cardiomyopathy Pulmonic stenosis Aortic or pulmonary artery dilation Malformed but nonobstructive aortic valve ↑ transvalvular flow (e.g., aortic regurgitation, hyperkinetic states, atrial septal defect, physiological flow murmur)
Holosystolic	Extends throughout systole, up to and sometimes past S_2; relatively uniform intensity	Mitral regurgitation Tricuspid regurgitation Ventricular septal defect
Late systolic	Variable onset and duration, often preceded by a nonejection click	Mitral valve prolapse
Diastolic decrescendo	Begins with A_2 or P_2 Decrescendo with varying duration Often high-pitched, "blowing"	Aortic regurgitation Pulmonic regurgitation

Mid-diastolic	Begins after S_2, often after an opening snap
	Low-pitched "rumble" heard best with bell of stethoscope
	With exercise or left lateral decubitus position
	Loudest in early diastole and upon atrial contraction (presystolic accentuation)
		Mitral stenosis
		Tricuspid stenosis
		↑ flow across AV valves:
		  tricuspid regurgitation
		  mitral regurgitation
		  atrial-septal defect
		Atrial myxoma
		Austin Flint murmur

Continuous	Systolic and diastolic components "Machinery murmurs"	Patent ductus arteriosus Coronary AV fistula Ruptured sinus of Valsalva aneurysm into right atrium or ventricle

valve (for example, tricuspid regurgitation or atrial septal defect) or nonvalvular obstruction to flow (for example, atrial myxoma). A diastolic rumbling murmur may be heard in patients with severe chronic aortic insufficiency (Austin-Flint murmur, see Chapter 6).

Continuous murmurs or "machinery murmurs" are caused by lesions that generate turbulent flow in both systole and diastole due to a pressure gradient present throughout the cardiac cycle.

A pericardial friction rub is created when two inflamed layers of pericardium slide over one another. It is a scratchy sound having from one to three components. If all three components are present, one occurs during atrial systole, one during ventricular contraction, and one during rapid early diastolic ventricular filling. Pericardial friction rubs are usually best heard along the left sternal border while the patient is leaning forward in held expiration. Frequently only a single systolic component is audible and may be confused with a systolic murmur. A pleuropericardial friction rub involves not only the pericardial but also the pleural surfaces and varies with respiration.

PROSTHETIC VALVE SOUNDS

Metal valves of the ball and cage variety (e.g., Starr-Edwards valves) demonstrate loud, metallic opening and closing sounds that may be audible without a stethoscope. Tilting disk valves (e.g., the Bjork-Shiley valve) demonstrate a closing metallic sound but only a very soft opening sound. Porcine valves may generate no abnormal sounds; however, a porcine valve in the mitral position sometimes has an opening snap as well as a soft diastolic rumble. Since there is a persistent gradient across any prosthetic valve, there is a systolic murmur across a prosthetic aortic valve and a soft diastolic rumble over a prosthetic mitral or tricuspid valve.

PHYSIOLOGICAL AND PHARMACOLOGICAL MANEUVERS

Various physiological and pharmacological maneuvers are sometimes useful in augmenting the intensity or delineating the etiology of heart sounds and murmurs (Table 2–11). Noting the effects of respiration on murmurs is the simplest test. With inspiration right heart filling is increased, and therefore the intensity of most sounds and murmurs generated from the right heart tends to increase. An exception to this rule is when right ventricular failure is present and the right ventricle is unable to increase its output during inspiration.

TABLE 2–11. EFFECTS OF PHYSIOLOGICAL AND PHARMACOLOGICAL MANEUVERS ON AUSCULTATORY EVENTS

MANEUVER	MAJOR PHYSIOLOGICAL EFFECTS	USEFUL AUSCULTATORY CHANGES*
Respiration	↑ venous return with inspiration	↑ right heart murmurs and gallops with inspiration splitting of S_2 (Table 2–8)
Valsalva (initial ↑ BP, phase I; followed by ↓ BP, phase II)	↓ BP, ↓ venous return, ↓ LV size (phase II)	↑ HOCM ↓ AS, MR MVP click earlier in systole, murmur prolongs
Standing	↓ venous return ↓ LV size	↑ HOCM ↓ AS, MR MVP click earlier in systole, murmur prolongs
Squatting	↑ venous return ↑ systemic vascular resistance ↑ LV size	↑ AS, MR, AI ↓ HOCM MVP click delayed, murmur shortens
Isometric exercise (e.g., hand grip)	↑ arterial pressure ↑ cardiac output	↑ gallops ↑ MR, AI, MS ↓ AS, HOCM
Post PVC or prolonged RR interval	↑ ventricular filling ↑ contractility	↑ AS little change in MR
Amyl nitrate	↓ arterial pressure ↑ cardiac output ↓ LV size	MVP click earlier in systole, murmur prolongs ↑ HOCM, AS, MS ↓ AI, MR, Austin Flint murmur
Phenylephrine	↑ arterial pressure ↓ cardiac output ↑ LV size	↑ MR, AI ↓ AS, HOCM MVP click delayed, murmur shortens

HOCM = hypertrophic obstructive cardiomyopathy AI = aortic insufficiency
AS = aortic stenosis MS = mitral stenosis
MR = mitral regurgitation * ↑ = increased intensity; ↓ = decreased intensity
MVP = mitral valve prolapse

REFERENCES

Perloff JK: Physical Examination of the Heart and Circulation. Philadelphia, WB Saunders Company, 1982.

Perloff JK: The physiologic mechanisms of cardiac and vascular physical signs. J Am Coll Cardiol 1:184, 1983.
Tavel ME: Clinical Phonocardiography and External Pulse Recording. 4th ed. Chicago, Year Book Medical Publishers, 1985.

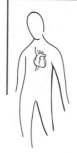

3

SPECIAL TESTS AND PROCEDURES IN THE PATIENT WITH CARDIOVASCULAR DISEASE

CARDIAC RADIOGRAPHY

From the routine PA and lateral chest x-ray, the size of the heart can be estimated. Cardiomegaly is said to be present radiographically if the diameter of the heart exceeds more than half of the thoracic diameter (car-diothoracic ratio). Enlarged hearts not meeting this criterion are not uncommon, however. The structures composing the cardiac borders can be seen in Figure 3–1. Dilation of the right atrium causes bulging of the right heart border, while dilation of the left atrial appendage straightens or bulges the left heart border between the left ventricle and pulmonary artery. In addition, an enlarged left atrium may cause a double density shadow on the right heart border and may elevate the left mainstem bronchus. Dilation of the posteriorly situated left atrium may be highlighted by barium in the esophagus, used to delineate the posterior cardiac border. Dilation of the right ventricle is seen best on the lateral chest radiograph as an encroachment of the anterior clear space between the heart and the sternum. Left ventricular dilation causes prominence of the lower portion of the left heart border. Enlargement of the central pulmonary arteries can be detected by a bulging of the pulmonary artery segment of the left heart border; enlargement of the aorta can be detected by aortic dilation. On many occasions, the particular chambers responsible for cardiomegaly may not be identifiable on routine PA and lateral chest radiographs.

Fluoroscopy or plain films of the chest may be used to detect calcification in valves, pericardium, or aorta. The chest x-ray can be used to identify prosthetic valves. Cardiac fluoroscopy can determine if a ball valve or tilting disk valve opens and closes properly.

Specific radiographic signs of congenital and valvular lesions will be discussed in their respective sections.

The pulmonary vasculature is evaluated from the PA chest radiograph. *Decreased pulmonary blood flow* can be identified by a paucity of vascular shadows throughout the lung and may occur in patients with significant right-to-left shunts such as tetralogy of Fallot. *Increased pulmonary blood flow* can be detected by a generalized increase in pulmonary vascular markings throughout the lung fields and is typical of left-to-right shunts such as atrial septal defect. An *increase in pulmonary vascular resistance* causing pulmonary hypertension may be suspected if the central large pulmonary vessels are dilated but the peripheral pulmonary markings are attenuated. *Pulmonary venous hypertension* can be diagnosed by the radiographic signs of pulmonary edema; interstitial edema causes the small pulmonary vessels to become indistinct; engorged lymphatics cast discrete horizontal shadows in the outer portions of the lung bases called Kerley B lines; redistribution of pulmonary flow from the bases to the apices occurs; as pulmonary congestion worsens, alveolar edema causes confluent bilateral hilar infiltrates with a "butterfly" distribution, usually bilaterally symmetrical but occasionally somewhat atypical in appearance, especially in patients with pre-existing lung disease.

ELECTROCARDIOGRAPHY

It is beyond the scope of this text to provide a comprehensive discussion of electrocardiography; however, some basic principles will be reviewed. Impulses are initiated by the sinus node, travel through the atria initiating atrial contraction, and experience conduction delay through the AV node. The impulse travels from the AV node through the common bundle of His,

down the right and left bundle branches, and through the Purkinje fibers to ventricular myocardium (see Fig. 3–1). The normal electrocardiogram (ECG) is produced by electrical activity of the heart recorded by skin electrodes. The ECG is the sum of all cardiac action potentials of its component cells. The P wave represents atrial depolarization. The PR interval is a measure of the time necessary to travel from the sinus node through the atrium, AV node, and His-Purkinje system up to the point the impulse activates ventricular myocardial cells. The QRS complex represents the sum of all ventricular muscle cell depolarizations (phase 0 of the cardiac action potential); the ST segment represents the plateau phase (phase 2); and the T wave represents the rapid repolarization (phase 3) of the heart as a whole (see Chapter 9). The ventricular septum is activated from left to right before any other part of the ventricle. Subsequently, the bulk of the ventricular muscle is activated simultaneously, followed lastly by activation of the base of the heart superiorly. Myocardial electrical activity can be represented with a vector, a value with both magnitude and direction, at any time during the cardiac cycle. The mean QRS vector during depolarization is termed the electrical axis and can be identified using the surface electrocardiogram.

A diagrammatic representation of an electrocardiographic complex is seen in Figure 3–2. The vertical axis represents amplitude in millivolts (10 mm = 1 millivolt). The horizontal scale represents time (5 mm = 0.20 sec, 1 mm = 0.04 sec). Routine ECG paper speed is 25 mm/sec, and thus one can determine the heart rate by measuring the RR interval in millimeters

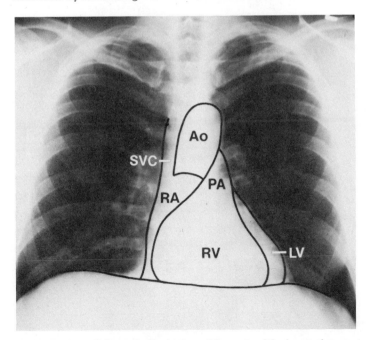

FIGURE 3–1. Schematic illustration of the parts of the heart whose outlines can be identified on a routine chest x-ray. Ao = Aorta; SVC = superior vena cava; RA = right atrium; PA = pulmonary artery; RV = right ventricle; LV = left ventricle.

and dividing that number into 1500, or the RR interval in milliseconds divided into 60,000.

The first relatively low-amplitude and low-frequency deflection of the electrocardiogram, the P wave, represents atrial depolarization. The isoelectric portion of the electrocardiogram between the P wave and the next rapid deflection (QRS complex) is termed the PR segment. The PR interval is measured between the onset of the P wave and the onset of the QRS complex and is normally between 0.12 and 0.20 sec in duration. A PR interval greater than 0.20 sec is termed first-degree AV block. The rapid, high-amplitude deflections following the PR segment are termed the QRS complex and represent ventricular depolarization. Atrial repolarization usually is not visible on the electrocardiogram, since it is a low-amplitude, low-frequency event and occurs simultaneously with ventricular depolarization. An initial negative deflection of the QRS is termed the Q wave; the initial positive deflection is termed the R wave; and if a subsequent negative deflection is present, it is called the S wave. A positive deflection subsequent to the S wave is termed an R′ wave. The duration between the onset and the termination of the QRS complex is called the QRS interval and is normally less than 0.10 sec. Upper and lower case letters are used to indicate the relative size of QRS deflections; for example, qRs refers to a small Q wave, large R wave, and small S wave. The isoelectric portion of the electrocardiogram following the QRS complex is the ST segment, followed by a low-frequency deflection, the T wave, which represents ventricular repolarization. The QT interval is measured from the beginning of the QRS complex to the end of the T wave and represents the time required for ventricular electrical systole. The QT interval is a measure of ventricular muscle refractoriness and varies with heart rate, decreasing as the heart rate increases. The QT interval is usually 0.35 to 0.44 sec for heart rates between 60 and 100 beats per minute, and one can estimate a corrected QT interval (normally less than 0.42 sec in men and 0.43 sec in women) by the Bazett formula, $QT_c = QT / \sqrt{RR}$ interval. In some patients, a broad, low-amplitude deflection follows the T wave and is called a U wave. The genesis of the U wave is not clear. The junction between the QRS and the ST segment is the J point.

Figure 3–3 illustrates the Einthoven triangle and the polarity of each of the six limb leads. Electrodes are connected to the left arm, right arm, and left leg (the right leg lead is a ground). Lead I displays the potential difference between the left and right arms (left arm positive); lead II, the potential difference between the right arm and left leg (left leg positive); and lead III, the potential difference between the left arm and left leg (left leg positive). Likewise, the augmented limb leads aV_L, aV_R, and aV_F are positive toward the left arm, right arm, and left leg, respectively. They are unipolar leads; that is, they measure the potential difference between the limb lead and a central point. When these six leads are taken together, they describe a full circle in the frontal plane at 30-degree intervals. Using this "hexaxial" frontal plane lead reference system, the frontal axis of any cardiac vector can be estimated. The most important axis is that of the mean QRS vector, normally between −30 degrees and +90 degrees. Mean QRS axes more superior than −30 degrees are termed left-axis deviation, and more rightward than +90 degrees, right-axis deviation. The T-wave axis is normally within 30 to 45 degrees of the QRS axis. Leads displaying large positive or negative QRS deflections are generally parallel to the mean QRS axis; leads that are isoelectric, or have equal negative and positive deflections, are perpendicular to the QRS axis.

In addition to the six frontal plane leads, there are six standard precordial leads, V_1 through V_6, which are unipolar leads placed across the anterior chest. The precordial leads are considered positive, and a central reference point serves as the negative pole (unipolar lead). Leads V_1 and to some extent V_2 are close to the right ventricle and interventricular septum of the heart; leads V_4, V_5, and V_6 are close to the lateral wall of the left ventricle. Lead V_1 normally has a small R wave and large S wave, the midprecordial leads have equal R and S waves, and leads V_5 and V_6 have a large R wave and small S wave (often preceded by a small Q wave), reflecting the normal left ventricular predominance in the adult. If the right precordial leads (V_1, V_2) have relatively equal R and S waves with no other abnormality, counterclockwise rotation is said to be present; if V_5 and V_6 have relatively equal R and S waves, clockwise rotation is present. These can be normal variants.

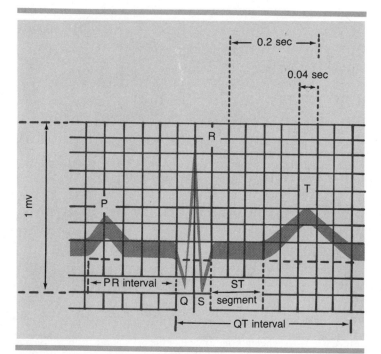

FIGURE 3–2. Normal electrocardiographic complex with labeling of waves and intervals.

A vectorcardiogram is a two-dimensional recording of the vector loop generated by atrial and ventricular depolarization. Vectorcardiograms are infrequently used today.

ABNORMAL ELECTROCARDIOGRAPHIC PATTERNS

The normal P wave vector is positive in leads I, II, and aV_F and negative in aV_R. Criteria for left and right atrial enlargement are described in Table 3–1.

The electrocardiogram can be used to diagnose left ventricular hypertrophy but is relatively insensitive. The hypertrophied ventricle generates increased electrocardiographic voltage that may meet any of several voltage criteria to qualify for left ventricular hypertrophy. However, normal young people may have high ECG voltage, and these criteria are not useful for patients under 35 years of age. At least one additional criterion must be present to diagnose left ventricular hypertrophy (Table 3–1).

The ECG findings in right ventricular hypertrophy are summarized in Table 3–1. The degree of right axis deviation correlates somewhat with the degree of right ventricular hypertrophy, as do certain QRS configurations (e.g., a qR complex in V_1 is associated with right ventricular pressure exceeding left ventricular pressure).

Acute pulmonary embolus may be associated with transient and nonspecific ECG changes. These include right atrial abnormality, right axis deviation with clockwise rotation, incomplete or complete right bundle branch block, S waves in leads I, II, and III ($S_1 S_2 S_3$ pattern), and T-wave inversion in the right precordial leads. Atrial arrhythmias are not uncommon.

Electrocardiographic manifestations of chronic obstructive pulmonary disease are due to both changes in lung volumes and right ventricular hypertrophy. Right atrial abnormality, right axis deviation, and clockwise rotation are often present. An $S_1 S_2 S_3$ pattern may be seen, and QRS voltage may be low. Right ventricular hypertrophy is sometimes present.

The common bundle of His divides into left and right bundle branches. Conduction delay or block in either of these bundle branches results in characteristic electrocardiographic patterns (Fig. 3–4, Table 3–2). In each of these, the QRS duration is 0.12 sec or more. Left bundle branch block often is an indicator of organic heart disease. During left bundle branch block, initial septal activation is abnormal; therefore, the diagnosis of myocardial infarction, dependent upon Q waves in the first 0.04 sec of the QRS, usually cannot be determined. Left ventricular hypertrophy cannot be diagnosed in the presence of left bundle branch block.

Right bundle branch block can be associated with organic heart disease but is sometimes seen in apparently normal hearts. The right ventricle is activated late, and therefore there is a terminal unopposed QRS

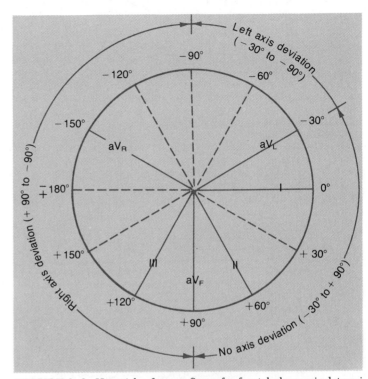

FIGURE 3–3. Hexaxial reference figure for frontal plane axis determination, indicating values for abnormal left and right QRS axis deviation.

TABLE 3–1. ECG MANIFESTATIONS OF CHAMBER ENLARGEMENT

Left atrial enlargement
P wave duration ≥ 0.12 sec
Notched, slurred P wave in leads I and II (P mitrale)
Biphasic P waves in V_1 with a wide, deep, negative terminal component
Mean P wave axis shifted to the left (between $+45$ and -30 degrees)
Right atrial enlargement
P wave duration ≤ 0.11 sec
Tall, peaked P waves of ≥ 2.5 mm in amplitude in leads II, III, or aV_F (P pulmonale)
Mean P wave axis shifted to the right ($\geq +70$ degrees)
Left ventricular enlargement
Voltage criteria:
R or S wave in limb lead ≥ 20 mm
S wave in V_1, V_2, or $V_3 \geq 30$ mm
R wave in V_4, V_5, or $V_6 \geq 30$ mm
Depressed ST segments with inverted T waves in lateral leads ("strain" pattern); more reliable in the absence of digitalis therapy
Left axis of -30 degrees or more
QRS duration ≥ 0.09 sec
Left atrial enlargement
Time of onset of the intrinsicoid deflection (time from beginning of QRS to peak of R wave) ≥ 0.05 sec in lead V_5 or V_6
Right ventricular enlargement
Tall R waves over right precordium and deep S waves over left precordium (R:S ratio in lead $V_1 > 1.0$)
Normal QRS duration (if no right bundle branch block)
Right axis deviation
ST-T "strain" pattern over right precordium
Late intrinsicoid deflection in lead V_1 or V_2

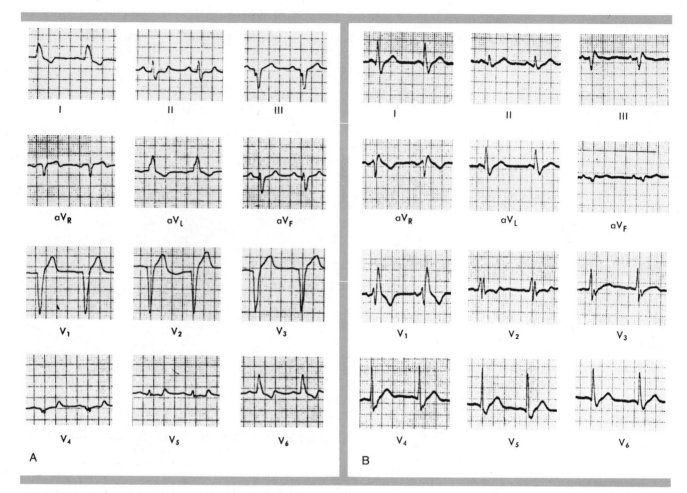

FIGURE 3–4. *A,* Left bundle branch block. *B,* Right bundle branch block. Criteria for bundle branch block are summarized in Table 3–2.

vector directed rightward and anteriorly. Initial ventricular activation is normal (septal activation occurs normally from the left bundle branch), and thus myocardial infarction can be diagnosed in the presence of right bundle branch block.

TABLE 3–2. ECG MANIFESTATIONS OF BUNDLE BRANCH BLOCK

Left bundle branch block
  QRS duration ≥ 0.12 sec
  Broad, slurred, or notched R waves in lateral leads (I, aV_L, V_5-V_6)
  QS or rS pattern in anterior precordium
  Secondary ST-T wave changes (ST and T wave vectors opposite to terminal QRS vectors)
  Late intrinsicoid deflection in leads V_5 and V_6

Right bundle branch block
  QRS duration ≥ 0.12 sec
  Large R′ wave in lead V_1 (rsR′)
  Deep terminal S wave in V_6
  Normal septal Q waves
  Inverted T waves in lead V_1 (secondary T wave change)
  Late intrinsicoid deflection in leads V_1 and V_2

The left bundle branch in many hearts appears to divide into two major divisions (fascicles), the left anterior (superior) fascicle and the left posterior (inferior) fascicle. A delay in conduction in either fascicle is termed a hemiblock or fascicular block and changes the sequence of left ventricular depolarization, reflected in a frontal axis shift. Since the left anterior fascicle is smaller and more discrete than the left posterior fascicle, left anterior hemiblock is much more common than left posterior hemiblock; in fact, the presence of left posterior hemiblock is unusual without concomitant right bundle branch block. The ECG criteria for left fascicular blocks are listed in Table 3–3. The term bifascicular block refers to a right bundle branch block associated with a left anterior or left posterior fascicular block. If evidence of conduction delay or block exists in all three fascicles, trifascicular block is said to be present (e.g., alternating bundle branch block, LBBB with infra-His first-degree AV block or complete infra-His heart block).

Pre-excitation syndromes are discussed in Chapter 9.

The ECG is very useful in evaluating patients with ischemic heart disease. Nontransmural ischemia is manifested by downsloping or horizontally depressed (at least 1 mm) ST segments, which is the classic ischemic ST segment response seen with exercise testing. Symmetrical T wave inversion with or without ST depression may also indicate ischemia. ST depression and T wave changes, however, are nonspecific and must be correlated with the clinical setting. On the other hand, ST segment elevation is more specific and evokes a fairly narrow differential diagnosis. ST elevation may occur with acute transmural myocardial infarction, ventricular aneurysm after myocardial infarction, pericarditis, variant angina (Prinzmetal's an-

TABLE 3–3. ECG MANIFESTATIONS OF FASCICULAR BLOCKS

Left anterior fascicular block
QRS duration ≤ 0.10 sec
Left axis deviation (−45 degrees or greater)
rS pattern in leads II, III, and aV$_F$
qR pattern in leads I and aV$_L$
Left posterior fascicular block
QRS duration ≤ 0.10 sec
Right axis deviation (+90 degrees or greater)
qR pattern in leads II, III, and aV$_F$
rS pattern in leads I and aV$_L$
Exclusion of other causes of right axis deviation (e.g., COPD, RVH, lateral MI)

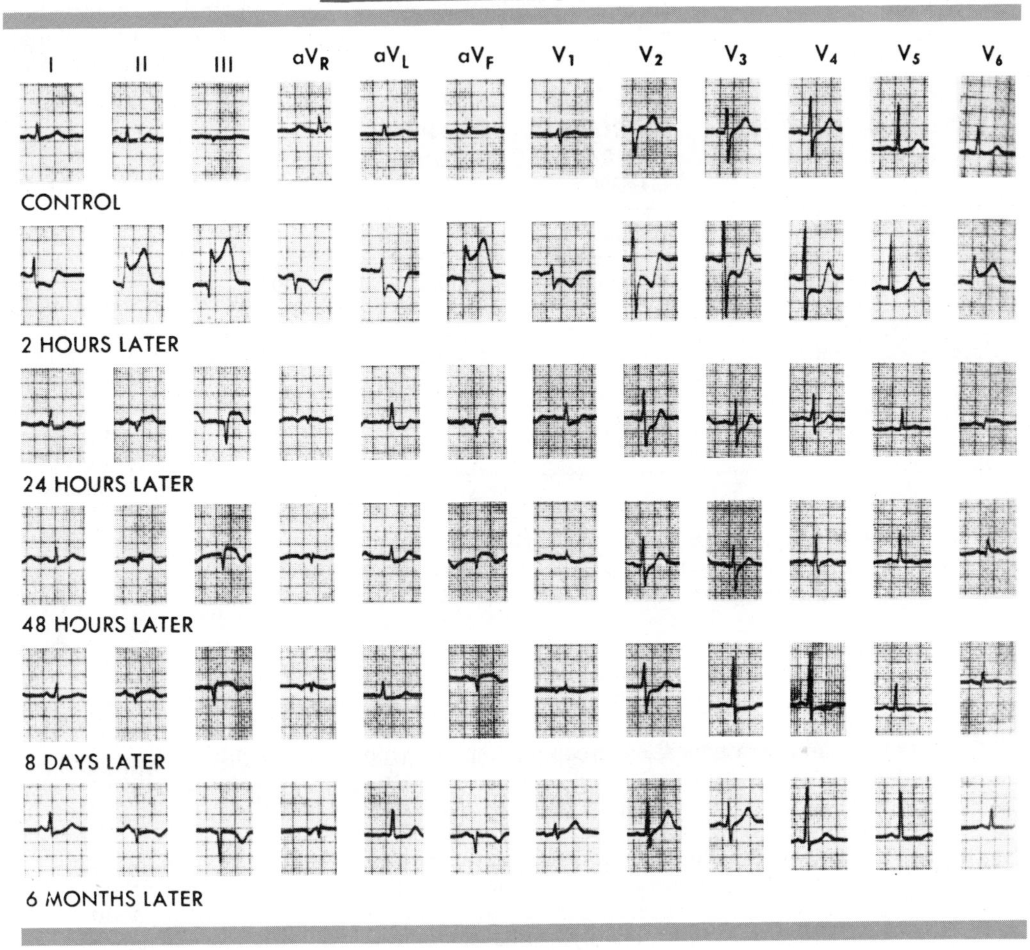

FIGURE 3–5. Evolutionary changes in a posteroinferior myocardial infarction. Control tracing is normal. The tracing recorded 2 hours after onset of chest pain demonstrated development of early Q waves, marked ST segment elevation, and hyperacute T waves in leads II, III, and aV$_F$. In addition, a larger R wave, ST segment depression, and negative T waves have developed in leads V$_1$ and V$_2$. These are early changes indicating acute posteroinferior myocardial infarction. The 24-hour tracing demonstrates evolutionary changes. In leads II, III, and aV$_F$ the Q wave is larger, the ST segments have almost returned to base line, and the T wave has begun to invert. In leads V$_1$ to V$_2$ the duration of the R wave now exceeds 0.04 second, the ST segment is depressed, and the T wave is upright. (In this example, ECG changes of true posterior involvement extend past V$_2$; ordinarily only V$_1$ and V$_2$ may be involved.) Only minor further changes occur through the 8-day tracing. Finally, 6 months later the ECG illustrates large Q waves, isoelectric ST segments, and inverted T waves in leads II, III, and aV$_F$ and large R waves, isoelectric ST segment, and upright T waves in V$_1$ and V$_2$, indicative of an "old" posteroinferior myocardial infarction.

TABLE 3-4. LOCALIZATION OF MYOCARDIAL INFARCTION

AREA OF INFARCTION	ECG CHANGES
Inferior	II, III, aV$_F$
Anteroseptal	V$_1$-V$_3$ ⎫ Q waves
Anterior	V$_3$-V$_4$ ⎬ ST elevation
Anterolateral	V$_4$-V$_6$ ⎭ T wave inversions
Extensive anterior	V$_1$-V$_6$, I, aV$_L$
Posterior	V$_1$-V$_2$: tall broad initial R wave, ST depression, tall upright T wave; usually occurs in association with inferior or lateral MI
Right ventricular	V$_1$ and V$_{4r}$: ST elevation; usually occurs in association with inferior MI

TABLE 3-5. TYPICAL ELECTROCARDIOGRAPHIC EVOLUTION OF A TRANSMURAL MYOCARDIAL INFARCTION

ECG ABNORMALITY	ONSET	DISAPPEARANCE
Hyperacute T waves (tall, peaked T waves in leads facing infarction)	immediately	6–24 hours
ST segment elevation	immediately	1–6 weeks
Q waves > 0.04 sec	immediately or in several days	years to never
T wave inversion	6–24 hours	months to years

gina, secondary to coronary artery spasm), and as a normal variant (early repolarization). ST elevation caused by acute ischemia is referred to as a "current of injury" (Fig. 3–5).

Infarctions are localized electrocardiographically to different areas of the heart (Table 3–4). Transmural myocardial infarction is usually characterized by the development of Q waves of at least 0.04 sec in duration, and by a typical electrocardiographic evolution (Table 3–5), the time course of which is extremely variable. Leads reflecting areas of the heart opposite the infarction will demonstrate ST depression (reciprocal changes). Persistence of ST elevation past the first few weeks implies the development of a ventricular aneurysm. The presence of Q waves and T wave inversion consistent with a myocardial infarction on a single electrocardiogram permits the diagnosis of a myocardial infarction, but of indeterminant age. Electrocardiographic patterns of subendocardial (also called nontransmural, or non-Q wave) myocardial infarctions include ST depression and T wave inversion that are often nonspecific in themselves. Clinical correlation with cardiac isoenzyme determinations is necessary to verify the infarction.

Abnormal Q waves may be present in the absence of myocardial infarction. These situations include myocarditis, cardiac amyloidosis, neuromuscular disorders such as muscular dystrophy, myocardial replacement by tumor, sarcoidosis, chronic obstructive lung disease, hypertrophic cardiomyopathy, and certain varieties of Wolff-Parkinson-White syndrome.

Many patients have electrocardiograms with nonspecific abnormal ST and T wave changes that preclude a definitive diagnosis. These are interpreted as "nonspecific ST and T wave changes" and must be correlated with the clinical status.

Primary T wave changes are those that occur in the absence of depolarization (QRS) abnormalities, whereas secondary T wave changes are those that result from abnormal QRS depolarization. Thus, secondary T wave changes may be due to bundle branch block or ventricular pre-excitation. Various drugs, electrolyte abnormalities, and ischemia may produce primary T wave changes.

Abnormalities of U waves include either increased amplitude of positive U waves or inverted U waves. Prominent positive U waves may be present normally in patients with bradycardia. They may also occur in hypokalemia and with some drugs, particularly digitalis and antiarrhythmic agents such as amiodarone. Negative U waves occur in left ventricular hypertrophy and ischemia. A large U wave may sometimes be a manifestation of the delayed repolarization (prolonged QT) syndrome (see Chapter 9).

Electrical alternans refers to alternation of QRS voltage and sometimes even P wave and T wave voltage. The most common cause of electrical alternans is a large pericardial effusion.

Metabolic and drug influences on the electrocardiogram are enumerated in Figure 3–6. Electrocardiographic manifestations of pericarditis are discussed in Chapter 10.

LONG-TERM AMBULATORY ECG RECORDING

Long-term ambulatory ECG recording (Holter monitor) is used to detect rhythm disturbances in patients with symptoms suggestive of arrhythmia or to document the efficacy of therapy for arrhythmias. Arrhythmia frequency and complexity can be quantitated and correlated with patient symptoms. This test allows documentation of arrhythmias that occur infrequently or occur during a patient's normal daily activities. In addition, long-term ECG recording can document alterations in QRS morphology, ST segment, and T waves, and thus may be useful for evaluation of ischemia that produces ECG changes; however, the efficacy of ambulatory ECG recordings for this purpose is controversial.

Two electrocardiographic leads are usually recorded simultaneously via electrodes attached to the patient's skin. A small box containing the tape recorder is carried for the period of recording, usually 24 hours, and the patient is encouraged to maintain his normal activities and to perform any activity that he feels may precipitate the arrhythmia. The tapes are scanned with a high-speed system with which a technician interacts,

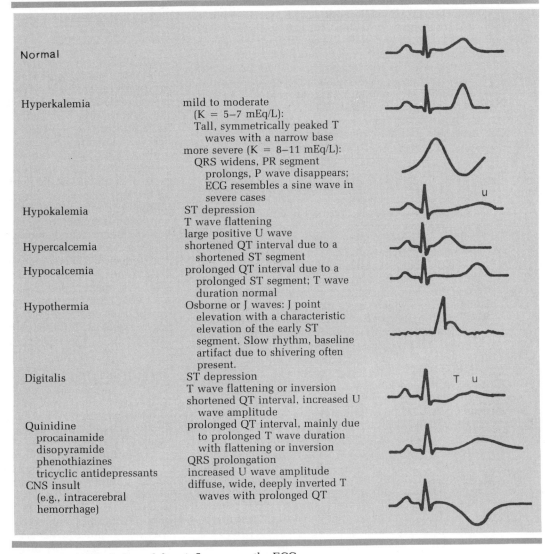

Normal		
Hyperkalemia	mild to moderate (K = 5–7 mEq/L): Tall, symmetrically peaked T waves with a narrow base	
	more severe (K = 8–11 mEq/L): QRS widens, PR segment prolongs, P wave disappears; ECG resembles a sine wave in severe cases	
Hypokalemia	ST depression T wave flattening large positive U wave	u
Hypercalcemia	shortened QT interval due to a shortened ST segment	
Hypocalcemia	prolonged QT interval due to a prolonged ST segment; T wave duration normal	
Hypothermia	Osborne or J waves: J point elevation with a characteristic elevation of the early ST segment. Slow rhythm, baseline artifact due to shivering often present.	
Digitalis	ST depression T wave flattening or inversion shortened QT interval, increased U wave amplitude	T u
Quinidine procainamide disopyramide phenothiazines tricyclic antidepressants	prolonged QT interval, mainly due to prolonged T wave duration with flattening or inversion QRS prolongation increased U wave amplitude	
CNS insult (e.g., intracerebral hemorrhage)	diffuse, wide, deeply inverted T waves with prolonged QT	

FIGURE 3–6. Metabolic and drug influences on the ECG.

and examples are printed on electrocardiographic paper for physician interpretation. In patients whose arrhythmia is infrequent and difficult to document on tape, recording for several days using a patient-activated recorder at the time of symptoms or transtelephonic transmission of the ECG may be useful.

STRESS TESTING

Since symptoms of cardiovascular disease may not be evident in the resting state, exercise stress testing is sometimes necessary to demonstrate an abnormality and assess its severity. The most common type of exercise testing consists of walking on a treadmill at increasing speeds and degrees of incline. The test is continued until the patient has reached 90 per cent of his predicted maximal heart rate, has anginal chest pain that is progressive during exercise, has an excessive degree of ischemic ST segment depression or elevation during exercise, or has various arrhythmias (especially ventricular tachycardia or heart block) precipitated by exercise. The test is stopped if there are any signs of circulatory failure (for example, exhaustion, staggering gait, diminished pulse, or a decrease in systolic blood pressure). In addition to treadmill testing, patients can be stressed with bicycle or arm exercise. Exercise testing results may be enhanced with nuclear (thallium scanning or radionuclide ventriculography) or echocardiographic techniques.

Exercise testing can aid in the differential diagnosis of chest pain. In addition, it can be used to evaluate prognosis and/or functional capacity in patients with known coronary heart disease or following myocardial infarction. In patients with coronary artery disease, an exercise test that is positive (see below) in the first two stages (six minutes) carries a relatively poor prognosis, and further evaluation to include cardiac catheterization may be considered.

The normal response to exercise is an increase in heart rate and both systolic and diastolic blood pressure. The heart rate times maximum blood pressure may be calculated to estimate the work load obtained (double product).

The normal ECG response to exercise is a normal T wave polarity with either no change in the ST segment or mild depression of the J point with a rapidly upsloping ST segment. Abnormal electrocardiographic responses include at least 1 mm depression of the J point and downsloping or horizontal depression of the ST segment similar to the ECG findings of ischemia. ST elevation is a markedly abnormal response to exercise unless it occurs in an area of old transmural infarction, in which case it may be related to regional wall dysfunction rather than ischemia. It may also occur in patients with significant, usually three-vessel, coronary artery disease or with variant angina. The precipitation of negative U waves with exercise is a positive ischemic response and usually indicates disease of the left anterior descending coronary artery. Arrhythmias occurring with exercise may be due to ischemia. In addition to the reproduction of chest pain and ischemic electrocardiographic changes, nonelectrocardiographic signs may be important; for example, the patient may develop an S_4 or S_3 gallop, a systolic murmur of papillary muscle dysfunction, or pulmonary congestion with exercise. A sustained decrease in blood pressure with exercise is a particularly grave finding indicative of extensive coronary artery disease.

The ECG cannot be considered diagnostically reliable in patients with pre-existing nonspecific ST-T wave abnormalities, left ventricular hypertrophy, left bundle branch block, digoxin administration within the past 10 days, electrolyte abnormalities (e.g., hypokalemia), and labile ST-T changes (abnormal ST-T changes occurring with hyperventilation or position changes).

Many physicians perform a limited treadmill test in patients one to two weeks following myocardial infarction. In this situation, the end point is a heart rate of 70 per cent rather than 90 per cent of predicted maximum, or the production of symptoms. The prognosis of patients after infarction who have early exercise symptoms or ECG changes is poorer than it is in those with good exercise capacity. Patients with the following conditions should not be exercised: unstable angina or acute myocardial infarction; severe aortic stenosis; severe hypertension; congestive heart failure; uncontrolled cardiac arrhythmias; acute myocarditis or pericarditis; any acute, noncardiac systemic illness; and known severe coronary artery disease such as left main coronary stenosis.

PHONOCARDIOGRAPHY AND EXTERNAL PULSE RECORDING

Phonocardiography and external pulse recording are techniques for graphically recording heart sounds, murmurs, arterial and venous pulses, and the cardiac apical impulse for careful analysis of timing and quality. Clinical uses include the measurement of systolic time intervals, which can be used as gross indices of left ventricular function; assessment of jugular venous pulse tracings, which can be helpful in the evaluation of right ventricular function or pericardial constriction; quantitation of the interval between the closure of the aortic valve and the opening snap of mitral stenosis to estimate the severity of mitral stenosis; and noninvasive quantitation of aortic stenosis. Except for low-frequency sounds such as gallops, the phonocardiogram does not record cardiac sounds not heard with the stethoscope. The function of prosthetic valves can be examined serially with phonocardiography to assure that opening and closing sounds do not change with time. Simultaneous M-mode echocardiography and phonocardiography can be performed to correlate valve motion with the etiology of specific sounds.

ECHOCARDIOGRAPHY

It is beyond the scope of this text to describe echocardiography in detail. Abnormal echocardiographic findings in specific disease states will be discussed with each disease.

Ultrasound consists of sound frequencies greater than those audible by the human ear which are directed toward the desired structures by a transducer placed on the chest wall. The sound waves are reflected at the interface of structures with differing acoustic densities and return to the transducer where they are recorded. Changes in tissue planes are generally strong reflectors of ultrasound, whereas body fluids such as blood reflect very little ultrasound. The depth of the structure reflecting the ultrasonic signal back to the transducer can be displayed as a one-dimensional "ice-pick" view against time on a strip chart recorder (M-mode) or can be displayed on an oscilloscope in real time as a two-dimensional cross-sectional "slice" of the heart (two-dimensional echocardiography) (Fig. 3–7). Two-dimensional echocardiography is superior to M-mode for most indications, with the exception of certain situations in which higher resolution and careful timing of motion of certain structures are desired.

Echocardiography can be used to diagnose mitral stenosis with high reliability, and two-dimensional echocardiography can quantitate mitral orifice area in most patients. In addition, concomitant lesions (for example, aortic insufficiency or tricuspid stenosis) and hemodynamic aberrations (for example, pulmonary hypertension or right ventricular failure) can be identified in patients with mitral stenosis. Patients with left

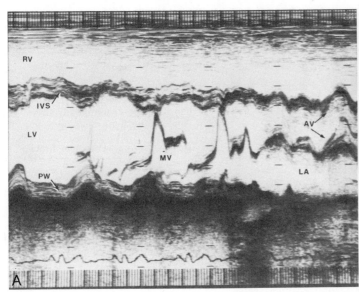

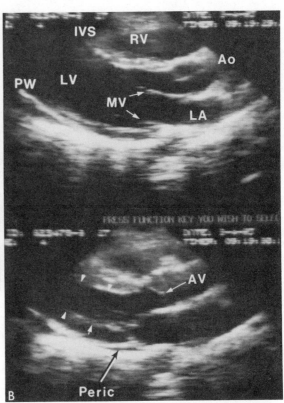

FIGURE 3–7. Portions of normal M-mode (A) and two-dimensional (B) echocardiograms. RV = Right ventricle; LV = left ventricle; MV = mitral valve; IVS = interventricular septum; AV = aortic valve; Ao = aorta; PW = posterior LV wall; Peric = pericardium; LA = left atrium. (Courtesy of William F. Armstrong, M.D.)

ventricular outflow obstruction can be evaluated for either aortic valvular, supravalvular, or subvalvular stenosis. Even though quantitation of aortic stenosis is difficult, echocardiography may be useful to exclude significant aortic stenosis in many patients. Echocardiography is the technique of choice to diagnose mitral valve prolapse, hypertrophic cardiomyopathy, and atrial myxoma. Echocardiography is the most sensitive test for the detection of pericardial effusion, and certain echocardiographic signs are useful clues of hemodynamic compromise (tamponade). Echocardiography may be useful to visualize the vegetations of bacterial endocarditis, but smaller vegetations (<2 mm in diameter) are not usually identified. Even when the vegetations themselves are not seen, echocardiography may detect the structural complications of endocarditis (for example, flail mitral leaflet), the hemodynamic alterations due to valvular dysfunction (for example, the elevated left ventricular end-diastolic pressure in patients with acute aortic regurgitation), or the pre-existing valvular abnormality that predisposed the patient to endocarditis. Echocardiography may help detect pulmonic valve stenosis or pulmonary hypertension via abnormal motion of the pulmonic valve. The internal dimensions of the left atrium and left ventricle can be accurately measured, and an estimate of right ventricular and atrial size can be ascertained. The thickness of the septum and the posterior left ventricular wall can be measured accurately. Certain hemodynamic information can be ascertained, for example, pulmonary

hypertension, decreased flow across the mitral valve, and elevated left ventricular end-diastolic pressure. Conduction abnormalities in left bundle branch block and some cases of the Wolff-Parkinson-White syndrome can be detected. Segmental wall motion abnormalities characteristic of coronary artery disease are detectable. Dilation of the aorta and occasionally an aortic dissection can be noted. The function of prosthetic valves can be evaluated grossly; however, detailed examination of prosthetic valves is often difficult because of their high echogenicity. In patients with congenital heart disease, echocardiography can often establish the diagnosis or complement cardiac catheterization in unraveling complex malformations. Thrombi in the left ventricle and atrium can be detected, but the sensitivity of echocardiography for this purpose is not clear. Mitral and aortic regurgitation are often not detectable directly and are inferred indirectly from their effects on wall motion, chamber size, and motion of other valves.

Contrast echocardiography can be useful in detecting atrial or ventricular intracardiac shunts or tricuspid regurgitation. Contrast agents include agitated saline, indocyanine green dye, and Renografin. Tiny bubbles in agitated solutions are echocardiographically opaque and produce bright echoes. After injection via an antecubital vein, the contrast can be traced through the right atrium and ventricle. The bubbles are absorbed by the pulmonary capillaries and normally do not opacify the left side of the heart. A right-to-left shunt is detected by the appearance of contrast in the left

TABLE 3–6. SELECTED NONINVASIVE CARDIAC LABORATORY TESTS

TEST	REASON FOR TEST	ABNORMAL RESULT	MEANING
Long-term ECG	Palpitations Syncope	Brady- or tachyarrhythmias	Needs correlation with symptoms
Stress testing	Chest pain	ST depression with pain	Ischemia (false-positive and false-negative tests occur)
	Evaluate functional capacity and prognosis in patients with known heart disease	Positive for ischemia within first two stages	High-risk patient, should possibly undergo further evaluation
Radionuclide angiography	LV function	↓ ejection fraction; regional wall motion abnormalities	Abnormal resting ventricular function
	Exercise evaluation of chest pain or ventricular reserve (e.g., aortic regurgitation)	Exercise-induced regional or global wall motion abnormality; inability to ↑ EF with exercise	Ischemia or decreased cardiac reserve
	Intracardiac shunts	Abnormal lung time/activity curve	Left-to-right or right-to-left shunt
Perfusion scintigraphy (exercise)	Chest pain (especially in patients with abnormal baseline ECG); or to evaluate the functional significance of a known coronary lesion	Defect on exercise and reperfusion scans	Myocardial scar
		Defect on exercise scan that reverses on reperfusion scan	Myocardial ischemia
Infarct-avid scintigraphy	Document acute MI, especially if ECG and enzyme evidence are inconclusive	Myocardial uptake of isotope; focal area of uptake is most specific	Acute MI (false-positive scans sometimes occur with older MI's, myocarditis, pericarditis, LV aneurysm, breast lesion, rib fractures, calcified cartilages or valve structures; smaller infarctions can be missed)

atrium or ventricle. A left-to-right shunt is detected by a negative contrast effect in a right-sided chamber. Tricuspid regurgitation is detected by regurgitation of contrast into the inferior vena cava.

Echocardiography during or immediately following exercise may detect regional wall motion abnormalities not present in the resting state.

Doppler ultrasound is a newer technique for the noninvasive detection and quantification of valvular lesions and cardiac shunts. It is based on the principle that blood moving toward or away from an ultrasound transducer alters the frequency of the reflected ultrasound waves in proportion to the velocity of the blood flow. In conjunction with two-dimensional echocardiography, the Doppler probe can be aimed to detect forward or regurgitant flow across valves and through any abnormal intracardiac connection. Doppler ultrasound can help quantitate the severity of aortic or mitral stenosis. The extent of mitral, tricuspid, or aortic regurgitation can be quantitated only roughly. The intracardiac shunts of ventricular septal defect, atrial septal defect, and patent ductus arteriosus can be detected but not adequately quantitated. Doppler flow measurements are useful for detecting serial changes in cardiac output but not for accurately measuring absolute cardiac output.

NUCLEAR CARDIOLOGY

Three techniques using radioactive tracers are useful in clinical cardiology: radionuclide angiography,

perfusion scintigraphy, and infarct-avid scintigraphy (Table 3–6).

The first-pass study and the equilibrium study are two basic techniques employed in radionuclide angiography. In the first-pass study, a high-speed scintillation camera follows the transit of isotope injected into a peripheral vein through the right heart, pulmonary vasculature, and left heart, much as a radiopaque dye injection is recorded during a cardiac catheterization. The equilibrium method involves labeling the "blood pool" by introducing human serum albumin or red cells labeled with technetium-99. Images are acquired with a camera that times or "gates" acquisition according to the electrocardiogram; that is, the cardiac cycle is divided into multiple segments, each of which is counted repeatedly and individually, and the final average is displayed as one cardiac cycle that can be visualized over and over in an endless loop format.

Perfusion scintigraphy, "cold spot scanning," employs a radioactive potassium analogue, thallium-201. Cells must be both perfused and metabolically intact in order to accumulate thallium-201. Therefore, nonperfused or dead myocardium appears as a "cold spot" on the scan. When exercise thallium imaging is performed, the patient is exercised to the usual stress testing end points and a scan is performed immediately after exercise and again four hours later, allowing thallium to redistribute into areas of myocardium that are reperfused after recovery from exercise. An area without thallium uptake (cold) on both exercise and reperfusion scans is considered infarcted, scarred, or irreversibly damaged. An area that is cold on the exercise scan but reperfused four hours later is considered "ischemic," with a reversible lesion.

In infarct-avid scintigraphy or "hot spot scanning," an isotope (usually technetium-99 stannous pyrophosphate) that accumulates in irreversibly damaged myocardial cells is administered intravenously to detect acute myocardial infarction. Technetium pyrophosphate scans are negative during the first few hours after infarction and usually become positive after about 12 hours. The probability of a positive scan decreases the first week after infarction and is low after two weeks. It is most sensitive in patients with transmural myocardial infarctions; however, these are the infarctions that are usually diagnosed with clinical electrocardiographic and enzyme determinations, so the usefulness of infarct-avid scintigraphy for questionable small infarcts is unclear.

NEWER TECHNIQUES

Computerized axial tomography (CAT scanning) is useful to detect dissecting aortic aneurysms and is probably the most sensitive method for detecting the pericardial thickening associated with constrictive pericarditis. CAT scanning may be useful for assessing the patency of saphenous vein grafts used in coronary artery bypass surgery.

Nuclear magnetic resonance can produce high-resolution tomographic images of the heart without employing ionizing radiation. It also has the potential for generating metabolic information about the heart. Future applications may be noninvasive angiocardiography and possibly characterization of diseased tissue.

Digital subtraction angiography is a technique whereby small concentrations of iodinated contrast material introduced in a vascular bed can be detected, analyzed by computer, and displayed as a high-quality angiogram, thus eliminating the need for direct injection of contrast into an artery or cardiac chamber. Venous contrast injections may provide left ventriculograms of good quality. The carotid circulation and coronary bypass grafts may be well visualized by this technique. Venous contrast injection does not usually provide adequate visualization of coronary arteries, but digital subtraction techniques can improve the quality of coronary angiograms obtained by selective coronary catheterization.

CARDIAC CATHETERIZATION

Cardiac catheterization involves introduction of hollow, fluid-filled catheters via the arterial and/or venous system into the heart to measure intracardiac pressures, blood flow, and oxygen saturation, and to inject contrast to perform cardiac angiograms. The complexity of the procedure depends on the particular patient and lesion being investigated and ranges from extensive studies in patients with complex congenital and valvular heart disease to straightforward measurement of left heart pressures, ventriculography, and coronary arteriography in patients with coronary artery disease.

Fluid-filled catheters transmit pressure waves obtained in each chamber entered back to a transducer, and pressure waveforms are displayed on an oscilloscope and recorded. Intracavitary pressures are used to judge the performance of the right and left ventricles, and pressure differences across valves (gradient) are used to evaluate valvular stenosis. The pulmonary capillary wedge pressure is measured by wedging the pulmonary arterial catheter as far into the pulmonary arterial tree as possible or inflating a balloon in a distal pulmonary artery, thus blocking out pulmonary arterial pressure and allowing the catheter to record pulmonary capillary or venous pressure. This pressure, given a patent pulmonary venous system, reflects left atrial pressure, which in turn, given a normal mitral valve, reflects the left ventricular diastolic pressure. This measurement is useful not only in the catheterization laboratory but also during bedside right-heart (Swan-Ganz) catheterization to estimate the left-sided filling pressures.

The cardiac output may be measured during catheterization by one of two basic techniques. Using the *Fick method*, the oxygen consumption of the patient is measured by collecting the expired air over a known period of time and simultaneously measuring arterial and mixed venous (pulmonary artery) oxygen content. The Fick equation states:

$$\text{Cardiac output} = \frac{\text{oxygen consumption (ml/min)}}{\text{arterial } O_2 \text{ content} - \text{mixed venous } O_2 \text{ content (ml/L)}}$$

Cardiac output is expressed in liters/minute and cardiac index in liters/min/m² of body surface. In addition, cardiac output may be measured by an *indicator dilution technique*, using either a dye that is detected by colorimetric methods or temperature (thermodilution) as the indicator. When an indicator is injected into the circulatory system and detected downstream, a curve can be generated. The area under the curve is proportional to the cardiac output.

Intracardiac shunts can be detected by measuring oxygen saturations in various cardiac chambers. For example, an increase in oxygen saturation between the right atrium and right ventricle would occur in a ventricular septal defect in which oxygenated blood is shunted from the left to the right ventricle (oxygen "step-up"). If the cardiac output is known, the shunt can be quantitated. Secondly, indicator dilution methods similar to that used for cardiac output determination may be used to detect shunts. For example, if an indicator is introduced into the right atrium and detected sooner than expected in a systemic artery, a right-to-left shunt is present. In addition, indicator dilution methods can detect valvular regurgitation.

Cardiac catheterization can be used to detect and

quantitate the severity of a stenotic valvular lesion. Valves that are regurgitant can be established (but are difficult to quantitate) by cardiac angiography, which involves injecting radiopaque contrast into various chambers of the heart. Upon coronary injection of contrast, atherosclerotic lesions appear as narrowings of the internal caliber of the vessels and are expressed in terms of per cent diameter narrowing, for example, a 70 per cent diminution in the luminal diameter. Lesions producing narrowings of 70 per cent or greater are definitely hemodynamically significant, and lesions of 50 to 70 per cent diameter narrowing are probably hemodynamically significant.

In congenital or acquired valvular defects, cardiac catheterization may be used to establish the diagnosis, assess the hemodynamic severity of the lesion, and exclude unsuspected additional lesions (for example, concomitant coronary artery disease). A few instances exist in which the value of routine preoperative cardiac catheterization has been questioned; for example, echocardiography is very reliable for diagnosing and quantifying mitral stenosis, and the likelihood of concomitant coronary artery disease in a young patient is small. Therefore, if there is no clinical evidence of significant aortic or tricuspid disease, some physicians would operate on such a patient without catheterization.

In patients suspected of having coronary artery disease, cardiac catheterization is indicated when (1) the etiology of the chest pain remains unclear after noninvasive evaluation; (2) angina is refractory to medical management; (3) patients are at high risk for having left main or severe three-vessel stenosis and may have improved survival with revascularization (see Chapter 8); (4) an acute intervention (i.e., angioplasty or intracoronary thrombosis) is contemplated in the first 4 to 6 hours after infarction. Cardiac catheterization may be indicated to provoke coronary spasm with ergonovine in a patient suspected of having Prinzmetal's angina. Left heart catheterization with coronary arteriography is a relatively safe procedure, with a mortality of between 0.1 and 0.2 per cent. The risk is higher for patients with significant stenosis of the left main coronary artery.

SPECIAL TECHNIQUES

Biopsies of the left or right ventricular endomyocardium can be obtained at the time of catheterization and are useful to diagnose myocardial rejection in patients with cardiac transplants and sometimes useful in the diagnosis of hypertrophic and congestive cardiomyopathies, especially if amyloid or other infiltrative processes are present.

Percutaneous transluminal coronary angioplasty involves passing balloon catheters into the coronary arteries and across stenotic lesions, where the balloon is inflated. This technique is effective in relieving obstruction in patients who have either single vessel disease or in some situations multivessel disease. Left main coronary stenosis is generally not safe to dilate with angioplasty. Long-term results of this technique are still being evaluated (see Chapter 8).

The infusion of thrombolytic agents (e.g., streptokinase), either intravenously or directly into the coronary system, can reopen an acutely occluded coronary artery in patients suffering an acute transmural myocardial infarction. Complications appear to be low from either intravenous or intracoronary administration, although the risk of serious bleeding from any

TABLE 3–7. DIFFERENTIAL DIAGNOSIS USING A BEDSIDE BALLOON FLOW-DIRECTED (SWAN-GANZ) CATHETER

DISEASE STATE	THERMODILUTION CARDIAC OUTPUT	PCW PRESSURE	RA PRESSURE	COMMENTS
Cardiogenic shock	↓	↑	nl or ↑	
Septic shock (early)	↑	↓	↓	↓ systemic vascular resistance; myocardial dysfunction can occur late
Volume overload	nl or ↑	↑	↑	
Volume depletion	↓	↓	↓	
Noncardiac pulmonary edema	nl	nl	nl	
Pulmonary heart disease	nl or ↓	nl	↑	↑ PA pressure
RV infarction	↓	↓ or nl	↑	
Pericardial tamponade	↓	nl or ↑	↑	Equalization of diastolic RA, RV, PA, and PCW pressure
Papillary muscle rupture	↓	↑	nl or ↑	Large v waves in PCW tracing
Ventricular septal rupture	↑ *	↑	nl or ↑	* Artifact due to RA → PA sampling of thermodilution technique. O_2 saturation higher in PA than RA; may have large V waves in PCW tracing

RA = right atrium; PCW = pulmonary capillary wedge; RV = right ventricle; PA = pulmonary artery; nl = normal; ↑ = increased; ↓ = decreased recent arterial punctures or surgical procedures is high (see Chapter 8).

Bedside right heart catheterization with a balloon flow-directed catheter (Swan-Ganz catheter) can be accomplished in an intensive care unit, and the catheter can remain in place from several hours to several days to guide drug therapy or fluid administration. Serial measurements of pulmonary arterial pressure, pulmonary capillary wedge pressure, right atrial pressure, and cardiac output using the thermodilution technique can be obtained. Swan-Ganz catheterization is useful to help manage patients with cardiogenic, septic, and other forms of shock; during or after surgery in patients with significant cardiac disease; in patients with multiorgan failure in whom the fluid and hemodynamic management is complex; and during serial evaluation of pharmacological or other interventions in patients with various cardiopulmonary abnormalities. It is useful in the differential diagnosis of cardiac versus noncardiac pulmonary edema and ventricular septal versus papillary muscle rupture in acute myocardial infarction and in patients with hypotension unresponsive to fluid administration. Swan-Ganz cath-

eterization helps in the diagnosis of right heart abnormalities, such as pericardial tamponade or constriction and right ventricular infarction (Table 3–7).

REFERENCES

Berger HJ, Zaret BL: Nuclear cardiology. N Engl J Med 305:799, 855, 1981.

Davis K, Kennedy JW, Kemp HG, Judkins MP, Gosselin AJ, Killip T: Complications of coronary arteriography from the collaborative study of coronary artery surgery (CASS). Circulation 59:1105, 1979.

Feigenbaum H: Echocardiography. 4th ed. Philadelphia, Lea & Febiger, 1986.

Goldschalager N: Use of the treadmill test in the diagnosis of coronary artery disease in patients with chest pain. Ann Intern Med 97:38, 1982.

Grossman W: Cardiac Catheterization and Angiography. 3rd ed. Philadelphia, Lea & Febiger, 1986.

Lipman BS, Dunn M, Massie E: Clinical Electrocardiography. 7th ed. Chicago, Year Book Medical Publishers, 1984.

Marriott HJL: Practical Electrocardiography. 7th ed. Baltimore, Williams & Wilkins, 1983.

Skorton DJ, Collins SM: New directions in cardiac imaging. Ann Intern Med 102:795, 1985.

4

CIRCULATORY FAILURE

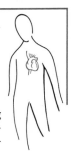

Heart failure refers to a state in which the heart cannot provide sufficient cardiac output to satisfy the metabolic needs of the body. It is commonly termed "congestive" heart failure, since symptoms of increased venous pressure (pulmonary congestion with left heart failure and peripheral edema with right heart failure) are often prominent.

Heart failure can result from several underlying diseases, most commonly in industrialized nations from atherosclerotic coronary artery disease with myocardial infarction. Myocarditis, various cardiomyopathies, and valvular and congenital defects may result in heart failure. Mitral and aortic regurgitation, ventricular and atrial septal defects, and patent ductus arteriosus cause volume overload states; aortic and pulmonic stenosis and systemic hypertension cause pressure overload states. Conditions that restrict ventricular filling, e.g., mitral stenosis, constrictive pericarditis, or restrictive cardiomyopathies, cause heart failure.

Patients with previously compensated heart failure may decompensate as a result of dietary indiscretion (increased sodium intake) or failure to take prescribed medications. Exposure to excess heat or humidity, excess exertion, anemia, pregnancy, hyperthyroidism,

or infection may exacerbate heart failure by increasing the metabolic needs of the body. Systemic hypertension, acute myocardial infarction, pulmonary embolus, and endocarditis should be excluded. Recurrence of the primary etiology, e.g., acute rheumatic fever, must be considered. The sudden onset of an arrhythmia, e.g., atrial fibrillation, may cause decompensation in a previously well-compensated patient.

By adjusting stroke volume and heart rate, the normal heart can increase cardiac output from approximately 5 L/min at rest to as much as 20 L/min during strenuous activity. The stroke volume is dependent upon the inotropic state of the ventricle, the preload (the ventricular filling or end-diastolic pressure), and afterload (the resistance into which the ventricle empties) (see Chapter 1). The inotropic state or contractility does not limit cardiac output in the normal heart but is the limiting parameter in patients with cardiac muscle dysfunction. In heart failure, the resting cardiac output may be normal, but the ability to increase cardiac output with exercise is abnormal. The autonomic nervous system is important in regulating cardiac function in normal hearts. As heart failure ensues, sympathetic nervous system output increases to help maintain cardiac output via positive chronotropic

TABLE 4–1. COMPENSATORY MECHANISMS IN HEART FAILURE

MECHANISM	FAVORABLE EFFECTS	UNFAVORABLE EFFECTS
↑ Sympathetic activity	↑ heart rate ↑ contractility ↑ venoconstriction→ ↑ venous return (preload)	↑ arteriolar constriction → ↑ afterload ↑ O₂ requirements
Cardiac hypertrophy	↑ working muscle mass	↑ wall tension ↓ coronary flow ↑ O₂ requirements abnormal systolic and diastolic properties of hypertrophic muscle
Frank-Starling mechanism	↑ stroke volume for any given amount of venous return	Pulmonary and systemic congestion ↑ LV size → ↑ wall tension and O₂ requirements
Renal salt and water retention	↑ venous return	Pulmonary and systemic congestion ↑ renin-angiotensin → ↑ vasoconstriction (afterload)
Increased peripheral O₂ extraction	↑ O₂ delivery per unit cardiac output	

↑ = increased
↓ = decreased

and inotropic effects (Table 4–1), accounting for some of the clinical features of heart failure (tachycardia, diaphoresis, cool or cyanotic extremities due to peripheral vasoconstriction). However, excessive sympathetic nervous system activity also may be detrimental to cardiac function, most specifically by increasing myocardial oxygen requirements and increasing peripheral vascular resistance (afterload) against which the heart must pump. A downward spiral may occur: increased systemic vascular resistance causes diminished cardiac output which, in turn, leads to increasing sympathetic tone and even higher peripheral vascular resistance. Therefore, the autonomic nervous system plays an important role in both compensatory and decompensatory responses in congestive heart failure.

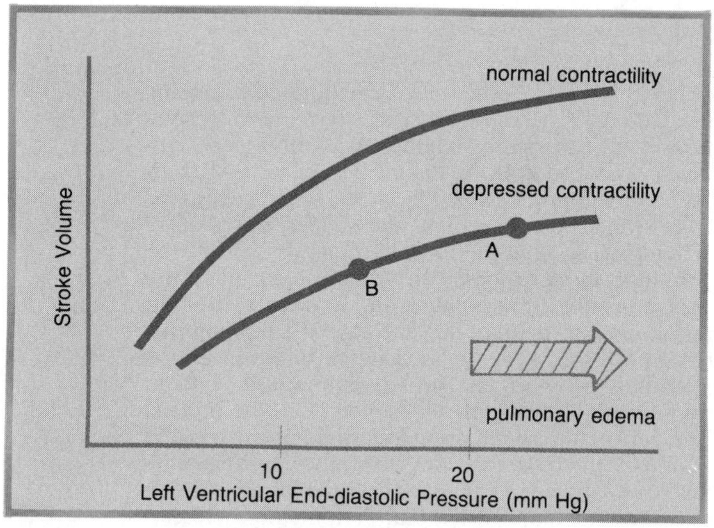

In addition to sympathetic augmentation of heart rate and stroke volume, the failing heart may attempt to compensate by either dilating to increase cardiac output via the Starling mechanism or hypertrophying in patients with pressure overload states. Normal and abnormal ventricular function curves are illustrated in Figure 4–1. The curve is shifted downward to the right and has a flattened contour in the patient with decreased cardiac contractility. In both the normal and decreased inotropic states, an increase in the left ventricular end-diastolic volume or pressure (LVEDP) increases cardiac output. The amount of increase in cardiac output for any given increase in LVEDP is greater in the normal than in the failing heart. In addition, elevation of LVEDP increases pulmonary venous pressures; once the pulmonary capillary wedge pressure exceeds approximately 20 mm Hg, pulmonary edema results. Therefore, augmentation of cardiac output by increasing LVEDP is limited by the relatively flat Starling curve in the failing heart and occurs at the expense of possibly precipitating pulmonary edema. Cardiac dilation increases myocardial oxygen consumption via the increased wall tension.

The mechanism of fluid retention and elevation of LVEDP in patients with heart failure is multifactorial. Two important mechanisms involve (1) sympathetic venoconstriction to decrease the capacitance of the venous system and increase venous return to the heart, and (2) chronic renal salt and water retention because of decreased perfusion.

Cardiac hypertrophy, which is an increase in the number and size of cardiac cells as a compensatory mechanism, also involves trade-offs: the increased muscle mass increases oxygen consumption. The hy-

FIGURE 4–1. Normal and abnormal ventricular function curves. When the left ventricular end-diastolic pressure is greater than 20 mm Hg (A), pulmonary edema often occurs. The effect of diuresis or venodilation is to move leftward along the curve from A to B, with a resultant improvement in pulmonary congestion with minimal decrease in cardiac output. The stroke volume is poor at any point along this depressed contractility curve, and thus therapeutic maneuvers that would raise it more toward the normal curve would be necessary to significantly improve cardiac output (for example, inotropic agents or arterial vasodilators—see Figure 4–3).

pertrophic ventricular muscle is not normal and its contractility is decreased. The hypertrophied ventricle maintains adequate cardiac output for some time via the increase in muscle mass, the Starling relation, and augmented sympathetic stimulation.

Abnormal systolic and diastolic (compliance) function are both features of heart failure due to ischemic heart disease and hypertrophic states. Compliance refers to the pressure required to fill a ventricle to a certain volume. Hypertrophied or ischemic ventricles become "stiff" or relatively noncompliant, requiring a higher LVEDP to achieve diastolic filling adequate to maintain cardiac output. In a patient with congestive heart failure and a relatively noncompliant ventricle, a pulmonary capillary wedge pressure of 15 to 18 mm Hg is usually optimal to maintain adequate left ventricular filling and output but to avoid pulmonary edema.

It is critical to distinguish valvular and congenital etiologies of congestive heart failure from those due to myocardial damage. In the former, corrective or palliative surgery is often possible. In the latter, however, therapy is imperfect and compensates only partly for the decrease in myocardial function. Patients with myocardial dysfunction unrelated to a correctable lesion have a relatively poor long-term prognosis, with a 50 per cent five-year mortality in some studies.

Left heart failure refers to decreased function of the left ventricle with resultant low systemic cardiac output and pulmonary vascular congestion. Right heart failure is characterized by the manifestations of elevated right ventricular end-diastolic pressure, jugular venous distention, hepatomegaly, and peripheral edema. Right heart failure may occur in severe lung disease and congenital or acquired defects involving the right-sided chambers or valves. The most common cause of right ventricular failure is chronic left ventricular failure; this probably occurs both because there is a chronic increase in pulmonary pressures in patients with left ventricular failure and because the failing septum is a structure common to both the left and right ventricle.

Low-output heart failure occurs when myocardial dysfunction prevents normal metabolic requirements from being met. High-output failure refers to inability of the heart to meet elevated circulatory demands in conditions such as arteriovenous fistula, Paget's disease, anemia, hyperthyroidism, and beriberi.

Backward versus forward heart failure are old terms that refer to the more prominent symptoms in any particular patient. The patient who presents with fatigue and weakness due to decreased cardiac output and azotemia due to decreased renal perfusion would be considered to have predominantly forward failure. On the other hand, the patient who presents with pulmonary or systemic congestive symptoms would be considered to have backward failure.

Acute and chronic heart failure are different clinical entities. A patient has acute heart failure when sudden circulatory decompensation occurs, for example, secondary to an acute myocardial infarction or ruptured chordae tendineae. Chronic compensatory mecha-

nisms do not have time to occur, and the patient may experience acute pulmonary edema. A patient with chronic myocardial dysfunction of the same degree may have adequate compensatory mechanisms to make him less symptomatic. Patients with chronic congestive heart failure may develop superimposed acute congestive heart failure if one of the precipitating factors listed above occurs.

The patient's history is important to help establish the diagnosis of congestive heart failure and sometimes to identify its etiology (see Table 2–4). The most common symptoms of left heart failure are respiratory. If heart failure is chronic, dyspnea on exertion occurs before dyspnea at rest, and as the disease progresses, less and less exertion is necessary to provoke dyspnea. Some patients may not complain of shortness of breath but have restricted their activities significantly to avoid it. The patient should be questioned carefully about previous cardiac disease, cardiac medications, and the existence of precipitating factors for congestive heart failure. The physical examination should confirm the physician's suspicion of heart failure (see Table 2–4).

Arterial P_{O_2}, relatively normal in mild heart failure even though pulmonary stiffness due to interstitial edema may cause a sensation of dyspnea, falls as alveolar edema occurs. In early heart failure, the patient hyperventilates and the P_{CO_2} decreases; when pulmonary edema becomes severe, carbon dioxide retention occurs. Hepatic congestion may elevate liver enzymes. Increased sympathetic stimulation may increase slightly the white blood cell count. The blood urea nitrogen and to some extent the creatinine may be elevated owing to low cardiac output (prerenal azotemia) without necessarily indicating intrinsic renal disease. No electrocardiographic changes are specific for heart failure but may reflect underlying cardiac disease (for example, myocardial infarction, left or right ventricular hypertrophy, or rhythm disturbances).

Radiographic signs of left heart failure depend on its severity and chronicity (Fig. 4–2). Manifestations of pulmonary venous hypertension are discussed in Chapter 2. Cardiomegaly is common in patients with chronic heart failure but is often absent in acute forms (for example, acute severe aortic regurgitation). The radiographic manifestations of pulmonary edema resolve 12 to 24 hours after hemodynamic improvement.

Noninvasive tests may be used to estimate ventricular function. Echocardiography demonstrates segmental or global wall motion abnormalities and provides chamber dimensions. Echocardiography may also suggest the etiology of the congestive heart failure. Radionuclide ventriculography reveals chamber size, regional wall motion abnormalities, and ejection fraction. The left ventricular filling pressure and the cardiac output form the two limbs of the ventricular function curve and may be obtained in unstable patients via Swan-Ganz catheterization.

Since many of the clinical manifestations of cardiac failure involve the lungs, the differentiation between heart failure and pulmonary disease is sometimes dif-

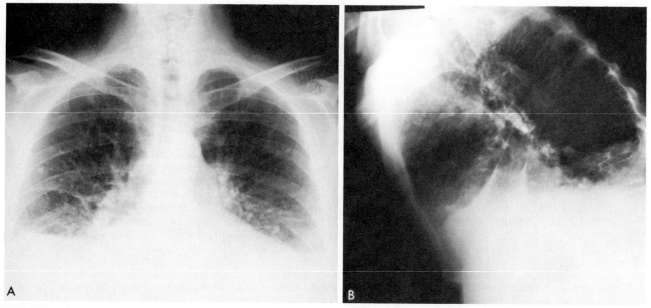

FIGURE 4–2. Posteroanterior (A) and lateral (B) chest x-rays showing cardiomegaly and pulmonary vascular congestion typical of pulmonary edema.

ficult. Noncardiac pulmonary edema (adult respiratory distress syndrome, ARDS) must be distinguished from cardiogenic pulmonary edema. A variety of processes can cause ARDS (for example, infection, shock, neurological injury, and drug toxicity). ARDS results from leakage of plasma into the aveoli because of leaky capillaries; pulmonary venous (capillary wedge) pressures are normal (see Chapter 20).

Chronic congestive heart failure with peripheral edema must be differentiated from other edematous states, for example, the nephrotic syndrome, cirrhosis, and severe peripheral venous disease.

MANAGEMENT OF HEART FAILURE

The ideal treatment of congestive heart failure is to remove or correct the underlying cause, for example, replacing a stenotic aortic valve. Next, removing or correcting any factors exacerbating chronic compensated heart failure should be achieved, for example, correcting anemia. Finally, medical therapy should be aimed at treating the congestive heart failure itself in order to improve the pumping function of the heart, reduce its work load, and reduce excessive salt and water retention (Table 4–2).

ACTIVITY AND DIET

An acute exacerbation of congestive heart failure should be treated with bed rest and adequate oxygenation. Control of excessive salt and water retention can be obtained by salt restriction. The normal American diet contains 10 gm of salt daily. While the usual patient with heart failure does not require rigid salt re-

striction, a 4-gm salt diet can be obtained by avoiding salty foods and not adding salt at the table. For patients with more severe heart failure, a 2-gm salt diet can be prescribed which requires food to be cooked and prepared without salt. In particularly refractory cases, diets of 0.5 to 1 gm can be prescribed, but only the most compliant patients adhere to these diets, and diuretic therapy may be used instead of restricting salt intake so stringently. Salt substitutes are available that contain potassium chloride instead of sodium chloride. It is unusual to have to restrict water intake except when severe congestive heart failure with dilutional hyponatremia occurs. One of the most common causes for exacerbation of congestive heart failure is failure to adhere to a low-salt diet after hospital discharge.

DIGITALIS

Digitalis augments cardiac output in patients with myocardial failure by increasing the inotropic state of the heart, possibly by inhibiting the activity of sodium-potassium ATPase. It may act by altering the membranes of the sarcoplasmic reticulum and the mitochondria so that they release calcium ions more readily. In addition to its inotropic effects, digitalis has significant electrophysiological effects, the most prominent of which at therapeutic doses is an increase in AV nodal conduction time and refractoriness. Sinus rate may slow owing to sympathetic withdrawal as heart failure improves.

Digitalis is available in several different preparations, the most common of which are digitoxin and digoxin (Table 4–3). Digitoxin is less frequently used than is digoxin but is useful in patients with renal insufficiency and appears to control the ventricular response in some patients with atrial fibrillation better than digoxin, possibly because of less fluctuation in plasma drug levels due to the long half-life. The bioavailability of several digoxin preparations appears to differ markedly. Patients with malabsorption syndromes may absorb digoxin poorly, and nonabsorbed substances such as cholestyramine, kaopectate, nonabsorbable antacids, and neomycin may interfere with digoxin absorption. Excretion of digoxin is proportional to the creatinine clearance, and maintenance doses must be reduced in patients with renal failure. Digoxin has a high degree of protein binding and is not removed from the body by dialysis. Digoxin serum concentrations increase when quinidine or amiodarone are added; therefore, the dose of digoxin should be lowered by approximately half when these drugs are added. Digitalis serum concentrations are only guidelines of either adverse or favorable digitalis effects and should be interpreted in the context of the clinical setting. Digoxin serum concentrations should be drawn at least 6 hours after a dose to avoid the peak levels.

Ouabain is a rapidly acting digitalis glycoside with unreliable gastrointestinal absorption that is rarely used today.

The end point of digitalis administration in patients with heart failure is not always clear. Digitalis or any other positive inotropic agent shifts the ventricular function curve (Fig. 4–3) up and to the left; that is, for any given left ventricular end-diastolic pressure, ventricular function is increased. The improvement in ventricular function increases ventricular emptying, promotes a diuresis and, in turn, reduces the filling pressures in the failing ventricle. This shifts the ventricular function along the new curve to the left and reduces pulmonary venous congestion. Even though increased contractility increases oxygen consumption, this may be offset by reducing diastolic pressure and volume, leading to decreased wall tension and decreased net oxygen consumption. Digitalis is useful in myocardial failure due to ischemic, hypertensive, valvular, congenital, or pulmonary heart disease and idiopathic dilated cardiomyopathy. It is not useful in isolated mitral stenosis if normal sinus rhythm and normal right ventricular function are present and is not useful in restrictive states such as pericardial tamponade or constriction. In patients who have dynamic outflow obstruction (obstructive hypertrophic cardiomyopathy), digitalis is contraindicated because the increase in contractility may increase the outflow gradient. A hypertrophied but vigorously functioning ventricle probably does not need digitalis. The need for prophylactic use of digitalis in patients with decreased cardiac reserve about to undergo major surgery is controversial. Use of digitalis in arrhythmias often has a more distinct end point, especially in patients with atrial fibrillation, because the rate of ventricular response reflects the adequacy of digitalization. Digitalis is also useful in many patients with paroxysmal supraventricular tachycardias and atrial flutter.

Digitalis toxicity is one of the most common adverse

TABLE 4–2. MANAGEMENT OF CONGESTIVE HEART FAILURE

OBJECTIVE	THERAPY
Reduce cardiac work load	Physical and psychological rest
	Remove exacerbating factors (e.g., infection, anemia, heat, humidity, obesity)
	Vasodilators
	Intra-aortic balloon pump
Improve cardiac performance	Digitalis
	Other positive inotropic agents
	Correct any rhythm abnormality
	Correct underlying defect if possible (e.g., valve malfunction)
Control excess salt and water	Dietary sodium restriction
	Diuretics
	Mechanical fluid removal (e.g., phlebotomy, dialysis)

drug reactions, encountered in 5 to 15 per cent of hospitalized patients receiving digitalis. Elderly individuals are more prone to digitalis toxicity than younger patients. Manifestations include cardiac arrhythmias of almost any type, commonly ventricular premature complexes and ventricular tachycardia, junctional escape rhythms, nonparoxysmal junctional tachycardia, paroxysmal atrial tachycardia with AV block, and type I (Wenckebach) second-degree atrioventricular block. Digitalis toxic rhythms have in common the combination of increased automaticity of ectopic pacemakers and impaired conduction. Noncardiac manifestations include anorexia, nausea, vomiting, disorientation, confusion, and seizures. Visual symptoms are not uncommon and include scotomas, halos, and changes in color perception (yellow-green halo commonly occurs). Massive overdoses of digitalis can cause a refractory hyperkalemia. Despite digitalis plasma levels, the diagnosis of digitalis toxicity requires clinical and electrocardiographic correlation. Hypokalemia exacerbates digitalis intoxication.

The treatment of digitalis intoxication depends on the degree of intoxication and specific manifestations. Mild rhythm abnormalities (occasional ectopic beats, first- and second-degree AV block, slow ventricular response to atrial fibrillation) require withdrawal of the

TABLE 4–3. THE USE OF DIGOXIN

Intravenous administration	
Initial dose	0.5-1.0 mg
Subsequent dose	0.25 mg every 2-4 hr for total dose ≤ 1.5 mg/24 hr
Onset of action	10-15 min
Peak effect	30 min-4 hr
Elimination half-life ($T_{1/2}$)	36 hr
Oral administration	
Loading dose (in 24 hr)	1.0-1.5 mg
Maintenance dose (in 24 hr)	0.125-0.5 mg
Gastrointestinal absorption	60-85%
Elimination half-life ($T_{1/2}$)	36 hr
Principal route of elimination	Renal
Therapeutic serum levels	0.7-2.0 ng/ml

drug and electrocardiographic monitoring. Ventricular tachycardia and marked bradyarrhythmias must be treated aggressively. Bradyarrhythmias may respond to atropine or if more severe may require temporary pacing. Phenytoin and lidocaine are effective drugs to treat ventricular tachyarrhythmias and have little effect on conduction. Correction of a low serum potassium may suppress ectopic rhythms but must be done cautiously in patients with conduction disturbances, since potassium administration can exacerbate AV block. DC cardioversion is avoided if possible in digitalis intoxication because it may precipitate refractory ventricular fibrillation or cardiac standstill. If a life-threatening ventricular arrhythmia with hemodynamic collapse occurs, cardioversion must be employed with as low an energy level as possible. Since quinidine increases digoxin levels, it probably should be avoided in digitalis intoxication. The use of antibodies specific for digoxin has been reported to be effective for the treatment of severe digitalis intoxication.

DIURETICS (See Chapter 33)

Diuretics are drugs that promote the excretion of sodium and water from the kidney and thus affect predominantly preload. They play a very important role in the treatment of heart failure.

VASODILATORS

Vasodilator therapy was introduced initially to treat refractory, severe heart failure, but it is now often used earlier in the treatment of congestive heart failure. Vasodilating agents can be divided into two broad categories: venodilators decrease preload by increasing venous capacitance, and the arterial dilators reduce systemic arteriolar resistance and decrease afterload. Many vasodilators dilate both venous and arterial beds (Table 4–4).

TABLE 4–4. COMMONLY USED VASODILATING AGENTS

AGENT	PREDOMINANT SITE OF ACTION	ROUTE OF ADMINISTRATION	USUAL DOSE	DURATION OF EFFECT	SIDE EFFECTS
Nitroprusside	A,V	IV	Initially 10 μg/min; titrate upward at 5-min intervals to desired hemodynamic effect	minutes	hypotension thiocyanate toxicity (fatigue, nausea, muscle spasms, psychosis, hypothyroidism)
Nitroglycerin	V	IV	Initially 10 μg/min; titrate upward at 5-min intervals to desired hemodynamic effect	minutes	postural hypotension, dizziness, syncope, headaches, nausea, ischemia upon abrupt withdrawal
		SL	0.3-0.6 mg	minutes	
		topical	1-2 inches of 2% ointment q4-6h; or controlled release topical patch q24h	hours	
Isosorbide dinitrate	V	SL	2.5-10 mg q2-3h	hours	same as nitroglycerin
		oral	10-40 mg q3-6h	hours	
Hydralazine	A	oral	40-400 mg/day in 2-4 divided doses	hours	reflex tachycardia, fluid retention, headache, nausea, lupus erythematosus–like syndrome (usually with doses $\geq$ 200 mg/day)
Prazosin	A,V	oral	1 mg initially; up to 21 mg/day in 2-3 divided doses; small initial test dose	hours	hypotension, especially after first dose; fluid retention, headache, nausea, rash; first dose: impairment of renal function, proteinuria, rash, neutropenia
Captopril	A,V	oral	6.25-25 mg t.i.d. initially; 50-100 mg t.i.d. usual dose	hours	hypotension, especially after first dose; agranulocytosis; proteinuria; hyperkalemia
Enalapril	A,V	oral	5.0 mg q.i.d. initially; 10-40 mg q.i.d. usual dose	hours	hypotension, azotemia, hyperkalemia, neutropenia, angioedema

A = arterial dilator; V = venous dilator; IV = intravenous; SL = sublingual

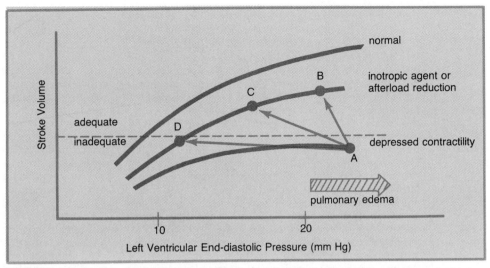

FIGURE 4–3. Ventricular function curve illustrating the effect of inotropic agents or arterial vasodilators. Unlike diuretics, the effect of digitalis or arterial vasodilator therapy in a patient with heart failure is to move onto another ventricular function curve intermediate between the normal and depressed curves. When the patient's ventricular function moves from A to B by the administration of one of these agents, his left ventricular end-diastolic pressure may also decrease because of improved cardiac function; further administration of diuretics or venodilators may shift him further to the left along the same curve from B to C and eliminate the risk of pulmonary edema. A vasodilating agent that has both arteriolar and venous dilating properties (for example, nitroprusside) would shift this patient directly from A to C. If this agent shifts the patient from A to D because of excessive venodilation or administration of diuretics, the cardiac output may fall too low even though the left ventricular end-diastolic pressure would be normal (10 mm Hg) for a normal heart. Thus, left ventricular end-diastolic pressures between 15 and 18 mm are usually optimal in the failing heart to maximize cardiac output but avoid pulmonary edema.

The effect of arteriolar vasodilators on the ventricular function curve is demonstrated in Figure 4–3. Changes in afterload have little effect on normally functioning myocardium, since reflexes adapt the heart rate and stroke volume accordingly. However, elevated afterload can detrimentally affect the failing myocardium, markedly decreasing the ability of the heart to eject blood. The lower the resistance to the outflow of blood, the more blood is ejected with each beat. Since the heart is able to pump more blood with each stroke when afterload is decreased, the ventricular function curve is shifted upward and to the left, just as it is with an increase in contractility. The shift in the curve due to decrease in afterload is not associated with the increased demand for oxygen that an increase in contractility requires. As ventricular function moves from the failing curve to the afterload-reduced curve, the improvement in ventricular emptying subsequently also decreases preload and left ventricular dimensions, shifting down on the new curve to the left. This decrease in left ventricular dimension decreases left ventricular wall tension and myocardial oxygen consumption. Since failing myocardium is more sensitive to changes in afterload than normal myocardium, afterload reduction is particularly effective in patients with poorer myocardial function, whereas therapy to increase contractility depends on the availability of some residual functioning myocardium and is less effective as myocardial function declines.

Pure venodilators, preload-reducing agents, shift ventricular function along the same curve to the left as does diuretic therapy. Thus, preload reduction lowers left ventricular filling pressures; even though it does not directly affect forward cardiac output, the diminished left ventricular size decreases wall tension (one of the determinants of afterload) and oxygen consumption, possibly improving forward cardiac performance somewhat. Since the ventricular function curve for the failing myocardium is relatively flat, decreasing the left ventricular end-diastolic pressure to 15 to 20 mm Hg from higher values does not usually decrease cardiac output significantly.

Note that there are end points beyond which one cannot expect vasodilators to be effective. When agents are administered to reduce preload, the filling pressures must be kept high enough so that cardiac output can be maintained. It is especially important in states associated with decreased ventricular compliance (for example, acute ischemic heart disease and hypertrophic cardiomyopathy) that ventricular filling pressures be maintained higher than normal (15 to 20 mm Hg, normal being approximately 10 mm Hg). When arterial vasodilators are used to attempt to increase forward output, arterial blood pressure may be a limiting factor. In patients whose blood pressure is high, lowering blood pressure by arterial vasodilators may have a beneficial effect. Patients who have relatively low arterial pressure may still benefit from afterload reduction because blood pressure depends not only upon arteriolar resistance, but also upon cardiac output (blood pressure = cardiac output × resistance). Patients may have low normal arterial pressure but still have elevated systemic vascular resistance if the cardiac output is low; therefore, if cardiac output improves as peripheral vascular resistance is decreased by arterial vasodilators, blood pressure may not fall. Once blood pressure falls below acceptable limits (approximately 90 mm systolic) during arteriolar vasodilator therapy, one has reached the limits of such therapy unless the decrease in blood pressure is due to an excessive fall in preload induced either by the afterload decrease or by venodilation from the drug itself. In that case, the hypotension can be corrected by fluid administration or decreasing preload-reducing agents. At times afterload reduction therapy may be tolerated only after the addition of an inotropic agent such as dopamine or dobutamine. Because of these limitations, it is often advisable to employ invasive hemodynamic monitoring in patients who are acutely ill and require intravenous vasodilator therapy. Indications for vasodilator therapy in congestive heart failure are listed in Table 4–5. Chronic administration of vasodilators has not been shown to increase longevity in patients with chronic heart failure. Afterload reduction must be used with caution in patients with aortic or mitral stenosis.

Sodium nitroprusside is a commonly used parenteral, short-acting vasodilator that has a direct smooth muscle relaxant effect on both arteriolar and venous systems. Hypotension, the most common adverse effect, is reversed within 10 minutes after discontinuation of the infusion. A metabolite of nitroprusside, thiocyanate, may accumulate after several days of administration, especially in patients with renal insufficiency. Serum levels of thiocyanate should be measured if the infusion is prolonged and should be kept below 6 mg/dl.

Nitroglycerin preparations are primarily venous dilators with lesser effects on the arterioles. Thus, they relieve pulmonary venous congestion with only a modest increase in cardiac output. An arteriolar dilator such as hydralazine may be combined with nitroglycerin to provide a balanced arteriolar and venous dilation.

Tolerance to the favorable hemodynamic effects of oral vasodilators appears to develop in some patients. The angiotensin-converting enzyme inhibitors (captopril and enalapril) have been reported to be the oral vasodilators to which tolerance is least likely to develop and are the only agents that appear to prolong survival in these patients. Increased fluid retention during chronic vasodilator therapy may respond to an increase in diuretic.

SYMPATHOMIMETIC AMINES

Potent, parenteral inotropic agents other than digitalis are sometimes required in severe heart failure, the two most common being dopamine and dobutamine. These are sympathomimetic agents producing less tachycardia and fewer peripheral vascular effects than the older drugs norepinephrine, epinephrine, and isoproterenol. Dopamine stimulates the myocardium directly by activating beta$_1$-adrenergic receptors and indirectly by releasing norepinephrine from sympathetic nerve terminals. Dopamine at low doses (2 µg/kg/min) activates dopaminergic receptors in the renal, mesenteric, coronary, and cerebral vascular beds and causes vasodilation. This is partially responsible for dopamine-induced diuresis in patients with severe congestive heart failure (renal vasodilator plus inotropic effects). With larger doses of dopamine (5 to 10 µg/kg/min), alpha-adrenergic agonism similar to that of norepinephrine causes peripheral vasoconstriction. Thus, with infusion of 2 to 5 µg/kg/min, renal blood flow, cardiac contractility, and cardiac output all increase with little change in the heart rate and possibly a small decrease in peripheral vascular resistance. Higher doses (5 to 10 µg/kg/min) begin to increase arterial pressure, peripheral vascular resistance, and heart rate. In patients with hypotension, the vasoconstrictor effects of doses up to 20 µg/kg/min may be desired. The elevation of heart rate, contractility, and blood pressure associated with dopamine may increase oxygen demand, but if cardiac performance is improved and cardiac size decreases, the net oxygen consumption may not be adversely affected.

Dobutamine increases cardiac contractility but has less effect on the peripheral vasculature than dopamine. It is useful when the vasoconstrictive effects of higher dopamine doses are to be avoided. Dobutamine

TABLE 4–5. INDICATIONS FOR VASODILATOR THERAPY OF HEART FAILURE

Heart failure refractory to conventional therapy with inotropic agents and diuretics

Treatment of earlier stages of heart failure in:
1. Patients intolerant to digitalis
2. Patients with other indications for vasodilators (e.g., nitrates or nifedipine for angina, hydralazine for hypertension)

Acute severe heart failure after myocardial infarction or transient myocardial contractile depression after cardiac surgery

Aortic or mitral regurgitation (acute or chronic) or ventricular septal defect (afterload reduction decreases regurgitant volume)

PREDOMINANT HEART FAILURE SYMPTOM	CAUSE	VASODILATOR OF CHOICE
Dyspnea	LV filling pressure	preload reduction (e.g., nitrates)
Fatigue	cardiac output	afterload reduction (e.g., hydralazine)
Dyspnea and fatigue	LV filling pressure and cardiac output	balanced vasodilation (e.g., hydralazine plus nitrates; captopril)

does not have the renal vasodilatory effects of dopamine. It is administered intravenously in a dose of 5 to 10 $\mu g/kg/min$.

Amrinone is a noncatecholamine, nondigitalis positive inotropic agent with vasodilator activity. It is available for short-term intravenous use in patients with severe congestive heart failure and is usually infused at 5 to 10 mg/kg/min. Milrinone and enoximone are orally active inotropic agents under investigational use in the United States.

NONPHARMACOLOGICAL MANAGEMENT OF HEART FAILURE

Mechanical support of the failing heart by intra-aortic balloon counterpulsation is sometimes useful. The balloon is inserted either surgically or percutaneously into a femoral artery and advanced to the descending aorta. Timed from the electrocardiogram, the balloon is deflated immediately before ventricular ejection to decrease aortic pressure (afterload) during ventricular systole and inflated in early diastole to increase aortic pressure and to maintain coronary perfusion. Thus, the hemodynamic benefits of balloon counterpulsation are greater than those of vasodilatory drugs alone. Balloon counterpulsation is useful to stabilize patients before an intervention designed to provide long-term benefit (PTCA or surgical revascularization; surgical correction of acute mitral regurgitation or ventricular septal defect). It may be used prophylactically during cardiac catheterization in severely ill patients, as an aid during or after open heart surgery, during treatment of some life-threatening ventricular arrhythmias, and for relieving angina pectoris in patients in whom medical therapy has been unsuccessful.

The role of surgery in patients with congestive heart failure depends on the etiology; surgically correctable lesions should be identified and corrected if possible. In patients with end-stage myocardial dysfunction, the results with cardiac transplantation have recently improved with the introduction of cyclosporine and other improved immunological support. In addition, development of mechanical cardiopulmonary apparatus is promising.

MANAGEMENT OF ACUTE PULMONARY EDEMA

The general management of acute cardiogenic pulmonary edema is summarized in Table 4–6. Furosemide and morphine constitute standard first-line drug therapy. Digitalis is not necessary acutely unless atrial fibrillation or other supraventricular tachyarrhythmia is contributing to the pulmonary edema. Reversible causes or exacerbating factors of pulmonary edema should be sought (e.g., anemia and arrhythmia).

If initial measures fail to correct pulmonary edema, or if drug administration is limited by the development of hypotension, more aggressive management to include invasive hemodynamic monitoring is usually indicated. Parenteral inotropic and vasodilating agents may be administered. If adequate ventilation cannot

TABLE 4–6. MANAGEMENT OF ACUTE PULMONARY EDEMA

INTERVENTION	PURPOSE	COMMENT
Sitting position	Decreases venous return and work of breathing; increases lung volumes	
Oxygen	Increases arterial P_{O_2}; pulmonary vasodilation	Humidify oxygen to prevent drying of secretions; mask may make patient feel like he is suffocating
Furosemide 10-20 mg IV; if no response within 30 minutes, administer progressively larger doses; usual max dose 200 mg, but occasional patient requires more	Decreases pulmonary congestion	Rapid pulmonary vasodilatory effect; diuretic effect onset in 5-10 min, peaks in 30 min
Morphine sulfate 1-4 mg IV q5-10 min as needed	Decreases venous return (venodilator); decreases anxiety	Respiratory depression can be reversed with naloxone
Vasodilators e.g., sublingual or IV nitroglycerin	Decreases venous return; relieves ischemia	
Aminophylline IV	Dilates bronchioles	Relieves "cardiac asthma"; can exacerbate arrhythmias
Phlebotomy	Decreases intravascular volume	Used only if the above fail
Rotating tourniquets applied to three of the four extremities at a time and inflated above venous but below arterial pressure	Reduces venous return from the extremities	Used only if the above fail
Dialysis	Decreases intravascular volume	Useful in renal patients in whom diuretics have been ineffective

TABLE 4–7. ETIOLOGIES OF SHOCK

CATEGORY OF SHOCK	CAUSES
Cardiogenic or vascular obstructive	Arrhythmias Obstructive outflow (valvular and perivalvular) lesions Atrial myxoma Acute myocardial infarction Severe congestive heart failure Cardiac tamponade Massive pulmonary embolism
Hypovolemic	Hemorrhage Vomiting Diarrhea Dehydration Diabetes (mellitus or insipidus) Addison's disease Burns Peritonitis, pancreatitis
Septic	Gram-negative or other overwhelming infections
Miscellaneous	Anaphylactic Neurogenic Drug overdose Hepatic or renal failure Myxedema

TABLE 4–8. CLINICAL MANIFESTATIONS OF SHOCK

FINDING	SIGNIFICANCE
Hypotension	BP is normal in early shock (stage 1) because of effective compensatory mechanisms
Tachycardia	Early manifestation
Increased respiratory rate	May represent compensation for metabolic acidosis or pulmonary congestion; may be an early sign
Fever	Septic shock
Cool, pale, moist skin	Sympathetic-mediated vasoconstriction
Warm skin	Septic shock or late shock of any cause when compensatory mechanisms fail
Elevated neck veins	Cardiogenic shock, cardiac tamponade
Collapsed neck veins	Hypovolemic or septic shock
Rales	Pulmonary edema; adult respiratory distress syndrome
Arrhythmias, murmurs, gallops	Suggest cardiac etiology
Abnormal abdominal exam	Source of sepsis, hemorrhage
Blood on rectal exam	Source of hemorrhage
Abnormal neurological status	Neurogenic shock *or* manifestation of cerebral hypoperfusion
Oliguria	Sign of renal hypoperfusion
Metabolic acidosis (anion gap)	Early sign of hypoperfusion

be maintained, intubation with mechanical ventilation may be required to maintain oxygenation and decrease the work of breathing. In cases refractory to the above measures in whom a reversible process is present, intra-aortic balloon counterpulsation may be employed.

SHOCK

Shock is acute severe circulatory failure. Regardless of etiology, shock is associated with marked reduction of blood flow to vital organs, and therefore profound arterial hypotension, impaired mentation, and diminished urinary output usually occur. The common denominator of all four broad categories of shock (Table 4–7) is eventual cellular damage and death. Shock may be divided into three stages. The first is a stage of "compensated hypotension"; that is, the fall in cardiac output or in delivery of cardiac output to the tissues stimulates a variety of compensatory mechanisms that alter myocardial function and peripheral resistance to maintain circulation to vital organs such as the brain and the heart. The clinical symptoms during this stage are minimal. In stage 2, the compensatory mechanisms for dealing with the low delivery of nutrients to the body are overwhelmed and tissue perfusion is decreased. Early signs of cerebral, renal, and myocardial insufficiency and of excessive sympathetic discharge are present. In stage 3, severe ischemia occurs along with damage to tissues by toxins, antigen-antibody reactions, or complement activation. Especially prone to damage are the capillary endothelia in the kidneys, the liver, and the lungs. Ischemic damage to the gastrointestinal tract allows invasion by bacteria. Renal ischemia may lead to acute renal insufficiency. Damage to capillary endothelia throughout the body allows transudation of fluid and protein into the extracellular space, exacerbating hypotension. The severe acidosis and toxins released into the blood contribute to further myocardial depression.

The etiology of hypoperfusion is evident in cardiogenic and hypovolemic shock. Septic shock is most commonly caused by gram-negative bacterial infections but can occur with infections by other agents. The mechanism of shock appears to be related to the release of an endotoxin (part of the bacterial cell wall) that interacts with substances from the blood and causes increased vascular permeability, intravascular coagulation, depression of myocardial contractility, and other adverse reactions. It is manifest by an abnormality in the distribution of blood flow to the tissues; that is, arteriovenous shunting of blood occurs and causes decreased delivery of nutrients to tissues despite an increase in cardiac output early in the course of the disease. Increased capillary permeability from the toxic products of infection allows fluid to leak into the interstitium, leaving the intravascular space relatively hypovolemic. Therefore, septic shock often involves the therapeutic paradox of needing to administer large quantities of fluid to a patient who is massively edematous in order to maintain adequate filling pressures. The only definitive therapy for this syndrome is control of the infection, but temporizing therapy includes maintaining intravascular volume via fluid administration, often directed by hemodynamic monitoring. One must remember that myocardial dysfunction may be prominent in stage 3 of septic shock. "Leaky" pulmonary capillaries can cause pulmonary edema without myocardial dysfunction (noncardiogenic pulmonary edema or adult respiratory distress syndrome) in which left ventricular filling pressures are normal or low (see Chapter 20).

Signs and symptoms of shock are summarized in Table 4–8 and its management in Table 4–9. Invasive hemodynamic monitoring is often required. Measurement of central venous pressure is sufficient in patients with known hypovolemic shock and good myocardial function; however, in patients with cardiac and lung disease, the central venous pressure may reflect poorly left ventricular filling pressures, and Swan-Ganz catheterization to measure pulmonary arterial and pulmonary capillary wedge pressures should be used in the more critically ill patients.

HIGH-OUTPUT STATES

If the circulatory system cannot meet a heightened demand for oxygen, high-output cardiac failure is said to occur. In high-output states, the heart must pump abnormally large volumes of blood, and the myocardial failure that ensues is similar to that caused by regurgitant valvular lesions. Disease entities associated with high-output heart failure include severe anemia, hyperthyroidism, systemic arteriovenous fistulae and other left-to-right shunts, e.g., patent ductus arteriosus, beriberi heart disease (vitamin B_1 deficiency), and Paget's disease. Increased workloads on the normal heart usually do not result in cardiac failure (e.g., pregnancy, hepatic and renal disease, pulmonary disease, and obesity); however, if superimposed on pre-existing heart disease, high-output failure can occur in these conditions.

Symptoms and signs of pulmonary and systemic congestion are similar to those found in patients with low-output congestive heart failure. Because of the increased stroke volume, decreased peripheral vascular resistance, and increased rate of ejection, the pulses are bounding, with a rapid upstroke and a wide pulse pressure. Physical signs of the underlying process should be sought. Treatment must be aimed at the underlying etiological disorder.

TABLE 4–9. MANAGEMENT OF SHOCK

General Measures
Assure adequate oxygenation
Bladder catheter to monitor urine output
Hemodynamic monitoring to optimize fluid management and cardiac output: indwelling arterial catheter, central venous pressure catheter, and/or Swan-Ganz catheter
Vasopressors as temporizing measures if necessary (e.g., dopamine, norepinephrine)

Specific Types

Cardiogenic	Diuretics
	Inotropic agents
	Vasodilators (if possible)
	Intra-aortic balloon pump
	Correction of underlying lesion (if possible)
Hypovolemic	Fluids/blood products
	Correction of underlying etiology
Septic	Identify source of infection
	Antibiotics
	? Steroids
	Support with fluids (massive edema may develop from leaky capillaries)
Neurogenic	Correct neurological abnormality (if possible)
Anaphylactic	Epinephrine
	Antihistamines
Addisonian	Fluids
	Mineralocorticoids
	Glucocorticoids
	Correct hypoglycemia

REFERENCES

Chatterjee K, Parmley WW: Vasodilator therapy for acute myocardial infarction and chronic congestive heart failure. J Am Coll Cardiol 1:133, 1983.

Colucci WS, Wright RF, Braunwald E: New positive inotropic agents in the treatment of congestive heart failure: Mechanisms of action and recent clinical developments. N Engl J Med 314:290–299, 349–358, 1986.

Consensus Trial Study Group: Effects of enalapril on mortality in severe congestive heart failure: Results of the cooperative north Scandinavian enalapril survival study (Consensus). N Engl J Med 316:1429–1435, 1987.

Goldenheim PD, Kazemi H: Cardiopulmonary monitoring of critically ill patients. N Engl J Med 311:717, 776, 1984.

Gunnar RM, Loeb HS: Shock in acute myocardial infarction: Evaluation of physiologic therapy. J Am Coll Cardiol 1:154, 1983.

Smith TW: Digitalis: Mechanisms of action and clinical use. N Engl J Med 318:358–365, 1988.

Swan HJC, Ganz W: Hemodynamic measurements in clinical practice: A decade in review. J Am Coll Cardiol 1:103, 1983

5

CONGENITAL HEART DISEASE

Congenital heart disease refers to cardiac lesions present at birth. Even though these abnormalities exist before birth, they often become clinically evident at the time of delivery, when profound physiological changes occur in the circulatory system, or months or years after birth. Congenital heart disease (excluding bicuspid aortic valve) occurs in approximately 0.8 per cent of live births and results from both genetic and environmental factors. Congenital heart disease may be familial in some instances, although a distinct pattern of inheritance is usually not recognized. It is more common in children of older mothers. Ventricular septal defect and patent ductus arteriosus are relatively common in premature infants. Environmental factors such as teratogens and maternal rubella are commonly recognized risk factors.

Congenital cardiac defects that are compatible with the fetal circulation (see Chapter 1) may produce symptoms once the child is born. The persistence of normal fetal structures in an infant, such as a patent ductus arteriosus allowing a left-to-right shunt, may be detrimental. However, an abnormal connection may be necessary for an infant to survive in the presence of another congenital anomaly, such as transposition of the great arteries, which must have a connection between the two circuits (e.g., atrial septal defect, patent ductus arteriosus) to allow oxygenation of systemic blood and survival for any period of time after birth. Those at risk for developing endocarditis should receive prophylactic antibiotics at appropriate times.

Congenital defects can be classified generally into acyanotic and cyanotic groups. The acyanotic congenital defects are those either without a shunt or with left-to-right shunts. Cyanosis occurs in the presence of a right-to-left shunt. In addition, it is important to identify whether malformations arise in the left or the right heart, the site of shunts if present, the status of the pulmonary blood flow (increased, normal, or decreased), and the presence of pulmonary hypertension (Tables 5–1, 5–2, and 5–3).

ACYANOTIC LESIONS

SITUS INVERSUS

Situs inversus involves a mirror image reversal of several organs, including the heart, the liver, and the gastrointestinal tract. These patients have normal longevity unless the disorder is associated with chronic sinusitis and bronchiectasis (Kartagener's syndrome). Situs inversus can be identified by physical examination and chest x-ray (cardiac apex and stomach bubble to the right, liver to the left). If the heart is in the right chest but the abdominal viscera are correctly located, dextroversion of the heart is present and, unlike situs inversus, is often associated with other congenital cardiac anomalies.

ATRIAL SEPTAL DEFECT

Atrial septal defects are classified according to their location in the atrial septum. Ostium secundum defects are in the region of the fossa ovalis, ostium primum in the low atrial septum, and sinus venosus in the upper septum near the junction of the vena cava and the right atrium. Ostium primum atrial septal defects are often associated with other endocardial cushion developmental defects, such as a cleft mitral valve or ventricular septal defect. Sinus venosus defects are almost always associated with partial anomalous pulmonary venous return (a pulmonary vein enters the right atrium or vena cava instead of the left atrium, adding to the left-to-right shunt).

In most atrial septal defects, the pressure equilibrates between the left and the right atrium, and the degree of left-to-right shunt depends not on a pressure gradient but instead on the relative compliance of the right ventricle and pulmonary arterial system compared to the left ventricle and systemic arterial system. Pulmonary vascular resistance and pulmonary arterial pressure tend to remain low, and thus pulmonary hypertension and right-to-left shunt (Eisenmenger's syndrome) do not occur commonly.

Atrial septal defects may go undetected in children because there are minimal or no symptoms and the ejection murmur across the pulmonic valve is thought to be functional. Survival into adulthood is expected but longevity is shortened, and death is usually due to cardiac failure. Occasionally, a young adult develops pulmonary hypertension. In addition to findings of congestive heart failure, atrial tachyarrhythmias become more frequent in patients over age 40 and may be the presenting symptom.

Patients with atrial septal defects generally appear normal. However, patients with the Holt-Oram syndrome have upper extremity skeletal abnormalities with a secundum defect, and patients with Down's syndrome have typical features and often a primum defect. The murmur is generated by the increased stroke volume flowing into a dilated pulmonary trunk; a murmur across the atrial septal defect is rare. Echocardiography reveals the dilated right ventricle and abnormal motion of the interventricular septum; these findings are referred to as "right ventricular volume overload" and are also present in pulmonic regurgitation, tricuspid regurgitation, and Ebstein's anomaly. Ostium primum defects and many ostium secundum defects can be visualized directly with two-dimensional echocardiography or indirectly after peripheral venous injection of echocardiographic contrast. However, cardiac catheterization may be required to determine the degree of shunt and evaluate for associated defects. Patients who have uncomplicated atrial septal defects without pulmonary hypertension and shunt ratios exceeding 1.5 should undergo repair electively, preferably during childhood.

TABLE 5–1. COMMON CONGENITAL CARDIAC DEFECTS

TYPE	NATURAL HISTORY	PHYSICAL FINDINGS	ECG	RADIOGRAPH	ECHOCARDIOGRAM	THERAPY
Atrial septal defect	Congestive heart failure, atrial tachyarrhythmias in adulthood; occasionally pulmonary hypertension	Ejection murmur across pulmonic valve Hyperdynamic right ventricle Widely and fixed split S_2 Diastolic flow murmur across tricuspid valve	rSr^1 in V_1 (left axis with primum defect)	Large main pulmonary artery; increased pulmonary vascularity	Dilated RV, abnormal septal motion (right ventricular volume overload); direct or contrast visualization of defect	Surgical repair if shunt ratio exceeds 1.5
Ventricular septal defect	Spontaneous closure of small defects occurs; larger defects lead to heart failure or pulmonary hypertension with reversal of shunt (Eisenmenger's syndrome)	Holosystolic left parasternal murmur, ± thrill Diastolic tricuspid flow murmur; occasionally murmur of associated aortic regurgitation Normal or widely split S_2 Findings of pulmonary hypertension if present (Table 5–3)	Biventricular hypertrophy	Increased pulmonary vasculature, large main pulmonary artery, dilation of both ventricles	Dilated hyperdynamic LV (left ventricular volume overload); direct or contrast visualization of defect	Larger defects repaired surgically unless pulmonary hypertension is present
Patent ductus arteriosus	Heart failure in infancy with larger shunts; eventual pulmonary hypertension	Wide aortic pulse pressure Hyperdynamic LV Continuous "machinery" murmur ± thrill Findings of pulmonary hypertension if present; "differential cyanosis" with right-to-left shunting (see text)	Left and/or right ventricular hypertrophy	Increased pulmonary vasculature; large main pulmonary artery; enlarged LA, LV, aorta; occasionally a calcified ductus is visualized	Left ventricular volume overload, dilated LV, LA, and aorta	Usually requires surgery; may close spontaneously or with indomethacin in premature infants; recent catheter technique for closure
Pulmonic stenosis	May be asymptomatic for a long period of time; symptoms of RV failure when decompensation occurs	Large jugular a waves Pulmonic ejection sound RV lift Systolic ejection murmur ± thrill in second left intercostal space Widely split S_2 with soft (or absent) P_2	Right atrial enlargement Right axis QRS deviation RV hypertrophy	Normal pulmonary vascularity, post-stenotic pulmonary arterial dilation Enlarged RV	Differentiates valvular from nonvalvular	Valvulotomy if gradient > 50 mm Hg
Congenital aortic stenosis (valvular)	Exertional syncope, angina and heart failure depending on severity	Decreased pulse pressure and carotid pulse LV heave, palpable S_4, systolic ejection murmur ± thrill Aortic ejection click, preserved A_2 (noncalcified valve) with single or paradoxical splitting of S_2 S_4 gallop Concomitant aortic regurgitation common	LV hypertrophy	Prominent LV Post-stenotic aortic dilation	Characteristic doming of aortic valve, LV hypertrophy	Aortic valvulotomy or replacement in symptomatic or severe cases
Coarctation of aorta	Most patients live to adulthood but eventually develop heart failure Aorta can dissect or rupture; cerebral hemorrhage occurs	Blood pressure in arms > legs Femoral pulses diminished or late, brisk upper extremity pulses Late systolic or continuous murmur LV lift S_4 gallop Evidence of associated bicuspid aortic valve	LV hypertrophy	Notching of inferior rib surfaces resulting from collateral flow through intercostal arteries Ascending aortic dilation; post-stenotic aortic dilation	Occasionally coarctation can be visualized	Surgical repair of all but mild cases

LV = left ventricle   LA = left atrium   RV = right ventricle   RA = right atrium

Table continues on the following page

TABLE 5–1. *(continued)*

TYPE	NATURAL HISTORY	PHYSICAL FINDINGS	ECG	RADIOGRAPH	ECHOCARDIOGRAM	THERAPY
Ebstein's anomaly	Survival into adulthood but longevity decreased due to RV failure Arrhythmias from accessory bypass tracts	Acyanotic or cyanotic (right-to-left shunt due to increased RA pressure) Increased jugular venous pressure S_4 and/or S_3 gallops Systolic murmur of tricuspid regurgitation; large v waves do not occur due to the large compliant RA	RA enlargement Right bundle branch block PR prolongation Pre-excitation	Enlarged RA Pulmonary vasculature normal or decreased	Abnormal insertion and motion of tricuspid valve	Replace tricuspid valve when RV failure occurs
Tetralogy of Fallot	Usually depends on the degree of pulmonic stenosis: too much leads to right-to-left shunt and cyanosis, too little leads to left-to-right shunt and pulmonary hypertension Pulmonic stenosis tends to gradually increase	Most commonly cyanotic and clubbed but may be acyanotic; underdeveloped Loud pulmonic ejection murmur along left sternal border, softer with more severe stenosis No murmur across ventricular septal defect (equalization of pressure in LV and RV) Soft P_2 (mild stenosis) or absent P_2 (severe stenosis) Normal jugular venous pressure	RV hypertrophy	"Boot-shaped" heart due to RV hypertrophy, small LV, and small pulmonary artery	Pulmonic stenosis, ventricular septal defect, RV hypertrophy, overriding aorta all visualized	Complete surgical repair is usually treatment of choice

TABLE 5–2. CLASSIFICATION OF THE MORE COMMON CYANOTIC CONGENITAL CARDIAC DEFECTS

Increased pulmonary blood flow
    Transposition of the great arteries
    Truncus arteriosus
    Total anomalous pulmonary venous connection
Normal or decreased pulmonary blood flow
    I. Dominant left ventricle
        Tricuspid atresia
        Ebstein's anomaly of the tricuspid valve
    II. Dominant right ventricle
        a. Normal or low pulmonary arterial pressure
            Tetralogy of Fallot
        b. Elevated pulmonary arterial pressure
            Ventricular septal defect with reversed shunt (Eisenmenger's complex)

TABLE 5–3. PHYSICAL FINDINGS OF PULMONARY HYPERTENSION*

Cyanosis or clubbing from right-to-left shunt via congenital defect or propatent foramen ovale
Large jugular a wave (decreased right ventricular compliance)
Large jugular v wave if tricuspid regurgitation occurs
Left parasternal (right ventricular) lift
Palpable pulmonary arterial pulsations (second left intercostal space)
Pulmonic ejection murmur
Pulmonic ejection click
Loud P_2
Diastolic decrescendo murmur of pulmonic insufficiency (Graham Steell)
Holosystolic murmur of tricuspid regurgitation

*Not all manifestations are present in all patients.

Ventricular Septal Defect

Congenital ventricular septal defects are located most commonly in the region of the membranous interventricular septum. There is a tendency as a child grows for the relative size of the defect to diminish, and sometimes spontaneous closure occurs. The hemodynamic consequences of a ventricular septal defect depend on the size of the defect and on the extent of pulmonary vascular resistance. A small defect causes little problem, a moderate defect causes left-to-right shunting with minimal elevation of pulmonary arterial pressure, and a large defect may result in equalization of systolic pressures in the two ventricles with the result that the shunt flow depends on the relative resistance in the pulmonary versus the systemic circulations. As pulmonary vascular resistance increases secondary to the increased pulmonary pressure and flow, the left-to-right shunt may gradually decrease and even become right-to-left (Eisenmenger's complex). There is an increased incidence of aortic insufficiency in patients with large ventricular septal defects, in some patients due to primary aortic valve abnormality and in others due to herniation of a valve leaflet through the septal defect.

Echocardiography reveals left ventricular volume overload (hyperdynamic left ventricle). The defect usually cannot be directly visualized but may be indirectly visualized after a peripheral venous injection of echocardiographic contrast.

Patients with small ventricular septal defects should be watched for gradual closure. Larger defects should be corrected surgically unless the pulmonary vascular resistance has become markedly elevated, at which time operative risk is high and results are poor because pulmonary vascular resistance fails to decrease significantly postoperatively.

Patent Ductus Arteriosus

A patent ductus arteriosus is common in premature infants and is more frequently seen in individuals born at high altitudes. In normal infants, the ductus functionally closes several hours after birth, and after four to eight weeks it closes anatomically. The pathophysiology of patent ductus arteriosus depends on the size of the ductus and the degree of pulmonary vascular resistance. After birth, as the pulmonary vascular resistance falls and the ductus fails to close, a left-to-right shunt occurs. When the ductus is small, pulmonary artery pressure is normal and there is little left-to-right shunting. If the defect is bigger, a large shunt results, and aortic pressure is transmitted to the pulmonary arterial tree. Pulmonary hypertension develops with a sizable left-to-right shunt, along with volume overload of the left heart and pressure overload of the right heart. Eventually, as pulmonary vascular resistance reflexly increases, left-to-right flow disappears, and in late stages the patient may develop a right-to-left shunt. The infant may fail to develop normally and, if the shunt is severe, demonstrates congestive heart failure. If right-to-left shunting occurs,

"differential" cyanosis may be evident owing to nonoxygenated blood entering the aorta distal to the left subclavian artery via the patent ductus arteriosus, preferentially being shunted to the lower extremities, and resulting in cyanotic toes but pink fingers.

Essentially all patients with persistent left-to-right shunt across a ductus should have surgical interruption; interruption also reduces the risk of bacterial endocarditis. Severely elevated pulmonary vascular resistance (Eisenmenger's syndrome) is not reversible and, if present, contraindicates surgery. The operation usually carries low risk, and cardiopulmonary bypass is not required. In older patients with a calcified ductus, ligation is slightly more risky although still indicated. Recently, insertion by catheter technique of an umbrella device into the ductus has been successful in occluding the ductus.

Pulmonic Stenosis

Valvular pulmonic stenosis is more common than isolated subvalvular or supravalvular varieties. The murmur is present at birth, but survival into adulthood is common. Dyspnea and fatigue are the most frequent symptoms, but patients may remain asymptomatic for long periods as long as the right ventricle maintains a normal cardiac output via compensatory mechanisms (hypertrophy); if not, right ventricular failure ensues. Valvular pulmonic stenosis can cause hypertrophy of the right ventricular infundibulum, and secondary infundibular (subvalvular) stenosis can occur.

The longer the duration of the systolic murmur and the earlier the systolic ejection click, the higher the degree of stenosis. As the severity of pulmonic stenosis increases, widened splitting of S_2 occurs with a decrease and eventual disappearance of P_2.

Patients with mild pulmonic stenosis require no treatment other than endocarditis prophylaxis. Those with pulmonic valve gradients exceeding 50 mm Hg should have pulmonary valvulotomy. Balloon dilation techniques via cardiac catheterization are successful in some patients. Pulmonic regurgitation may occur postoperatively but is generally mild and functionally insignificant. Secondary subpulmonic stenosis may require resection that complicates the procedure significantly.

Aortic Stenosis

Congenitally bicuspid aortic valves occur in up to 2 per cent of the population and are the most common congenital cardiac defect manifesting itself in the adult population. Bicuspid valves usually function normally throughout early and mid-life. However, progressive accelerated calcification of the valve can result in significant aortic stenosis during mid-adulthood. Occasionally bicuspid valves are incompetent, either inherently or secondary to damage from infective endocarditis. A short grade I-II/VI systolic murmur loudest at the second right intercostal space is typical and, if accompanied by an ejection sound or a soft murmur of aortic regurgitation, strongly suggests that the systolic murmur is pathological. Bicuspid aortic valve is predominantly a disease of males. The identification of a bicuspid valve can be suggested by echocardiography but is sometimes difficult to make.

In contrast to a bicuspid aortic valve, congenital aortic stenosis refers to an inherently stenotic left ventricular outflow tract. Congenital aortic stenosis is usually valvular but may be subvalvular or supravalvular. It is more common in males, with a ratio of approximately 4:1.

An ejection sound is present in valvular but not in nonvalvular aortic stenosis. It is generated by the sudden tensing upon opening of the abnormal aortic valve, implying good valve motion. In adults the abnormal valve gradually calcifies, and the ejection sound may disappear. In general, the longer and louder the murmur and the later its systolic peak, the greater the obstruction. The intensity of the murmur may decrease when the left ventricle fails, but it usually still peaks late in systole if stenosis is severe. An aortic regurgitation murmur may be present in valvular obstruction or, as the aortic cusps become distorted by the subvalvular jet, in subvalvular obstruction.

Cardiac catheterization is necessary to quantitate the degree of aortic stenosis. Aortic valvulotomy may be employed as a temporizing procedure in younger patients with significant aortic stenosis, but prosthetic aortic valves eventually are required in most severe cases.

Subvalvular stenosis is either dynamic (see Hypertrophic Cardiomyopathy in Chapter 10) or fixed. Two forms of fixed subaortic stenosis are the tunnel (fibromuscular) and the localized (fibromembranous) forms. These are unusual in adults. They can be identified with two-dimensional echocardiography. Surgical excision of an obstructing subvalvular membrane can be curative, but correction of a tunnel deformity is difficult. Supravalvular aortic stenosis often occurs in the presence of mental retardation and peculiar facies. The brachial and carotid arterial pressures may be reduced more on the left than on the right. Aortic regurgitation is rare (cf. subvalvular stenosis). The x-ray shows no post-stenotic dilatation of the ascending aorta, and the aorta is usually small.

COARCTATION OF THE AORTA

Coarctation refers to a narrowing of the aorta usually located immediately distal to the origin of the left subclavian artery and ligamentum arteriosum. It is associated with a bicuspid aortic valve in approximately 25 per cent of patients and occasionally a patent ductus arteriosus. Some patients have an associated aneurysm of the circle of Willis that may rupture. Other than coarctation associated with Turner's syndrome, males are more commonly affected than females. Most patients live to adulthood, but longevity is significantly decreased. Most patients are asymptomatic when the lesion is diagnosed. Discovery of upper extremity arterial hypertension is usually the initial finding. Patients develop one of four complications:

congestive heart failure, rupture of the aorta or dissecting aneurysm, infective endarteritis or endocarditis, or cerebral hemorrhage. Endocarditis is more common on the bicuspid aortic valve than in the region of the coarctation.

Catheterization may be performed to assess the severity of the coarctation and to examine the collaterals. All but mild coarctations warrant surgical repair. In children the optimal age for elective correction is approximately the fifth year. Surgery becomes more difficult in adults.

MISCELLANEOUS NONCYANOTIC ABNORMALITIES

Congenital coronary arteriovenous (AV) fistulae, low resistance connections between the arterial and venous circulations without an intervening capillary bed, may steal blood flow away from a portion of the myocardium. Occasionally a coronary artery may originate from the pulmonary artery and cause myocardial ischemia. A coronary artery may arise from the wrong sinus of Valsalva, most commonly the left circumflex artery arising from the right sinus of Valsalva, and may be subject to compression, especially with exercise. In addition, the odd angle of take-off from the abnormal ostium may limit flow. Congenital aneurysms of a sinus of Valsalva may occasionally rupture into the right atrium or right ventricle, resembling acute aortic regurgitation. Right ventricular dysplasia (Uhl's anomaly) involves a process whereby all or a portion of the right ventricular muscle is replaced with fat and fibrous tissue. It is often associated with ventricular tachycardia.

EBSTEIN'S ANOMALY OF THE TRICUSPID VALVE

In Ebstein's anomaly, the tricuspid valve leaflets are deformed and displaced into the right ventricular cavity, giving rise to a portion of the right ventricle that is functionally right atrium (atrialized right ventricle). Therefore, the pumping action of the right ventricle is decreased and the tricuspid valve is incompetent. Patients may be acyanotic, but a right-to-left shunt through a patent foramen ovale or an atrial septal defect due to elevated right atrial pressure can cause cyanosis. Ebstein's anomaly is compatible with survival into adulthood, but longevity is decreased. The anomaly is associated with right-sided accessory atrioventricular bypass tracts in approximately 10 per cent of cases (see Chapter 9). Patients can usually be managed medically. A tricuspid valve prosthesis is required when significant right ventricular failure occurs.

CYANOTIC LESIONS

TRANSPOSITION OF THE GREAT VESSELS

In complete transposition of the great arteries, the aorta and coronary arteries exit from the right ventricle while the pulmonary artery exits from the left ventricle. The left atrium empties into the left ventricle and the right atrium into the right ventricle. Therefore, the systemic and pulmonary circuits are arranged in parallel instead of in series. For the patient to survive, some means of exchange between the two parallel circuits must exist, for example, an atrial septal defect, ventricular septal defect, or patent ductus arteriosus. Transposition usually produces cyanosis and increased pulmonary blood flow. Bidirectional shunting must be present, and the greater the mixing between the two systems, the more likely the patient's survival. Diagnosis can be established by two-dimensional echocardiography. Palliation may be obtained by atrial septostomy via a balloon or surgery. Corrective surgery involves reversing the atrial input by inserting an atrial baffle that redirects the atrial flow to the opposite ventricle (Mustard procedure) or by transposing the pulmonary artery and aorta.

TOTAL ANOMALOUS PULMONARY VENOUS RETURN

In this condition, oxygenated blood returning from the lungs enters the right atrium instead of the left atrium, usually via a confluence of veins connected to the superior or inferior vena cava, the coronary sinus, or the right atrium directly. Blood from the right atrium enters the left atrium and left ventricle via an obligatory atrial septal defect, but because of the low pulmonary compliance most blood enters the right ventricle and pulmonary artery. Therefore, total anomalous pulmonary venous return is a cyanotic anomaly with increased pulmonary blood flow. Signs and symptoms are somewhat similar to those of an atrial septal defect except that cyanosis and signs of pulmonary hypertension may exist. Echocardiography reveals findings similar to those of an atrial septal defect, but the confluence of veins can often be identified. Surgical correction involves an anastomosis of the confluence to the left atrium.

TRUNCUS ARTERIOSUS

In truncus arteriosus, one great artery with one semilunar valve exits the heart, receives blood from both ventricles, and gives rise to the coronary arteries, aorta, and pulmonary artery. Cyanosis and increased pulmonary blood flow are present. Most patients do not survive childhood. Surgical correction can be performed in which the ventricular septal defect is closed, with the left ventricle communicating with the truncus, and the pulmonary arteries are divided from the truncus and connected to the right ventricle by a valved conduit.

TETRALOGY OF FALLOT

Tetralogy of Fallot is the most common cyanotic congenital anomaly in adults. It includes a ventricular septal defect, pulmonic stenosis, an aorta overriding the ventricular septal defect, and right ventricular hypertrophy as a result of the first two defects. The ventricular septal defect is large and nonrestrictive. Right ventricular pressures are systemic. If the pulmonic stenosis is mild to moderate, the patient is acyanotic. If the pulmonic stenosis is severe, right-to-left shunting occurs across the ventricular septal defect and cyanosis results, the most common situation. Typically the pulmonic stenosis is infundibular, but it can be valvular or located elsewhere in the pulmonary outflow tract.

A large ventricular septal defect with mild pulmonic stenosis results in a left-to-right shunt and physiology similar to that of ventricular septal defect alone, i.e., increased pulmonary blood flow and left ventricular volume overload. With severe pulmonic stenosis, right ventricular pressure does not exceed systemic pressure because of the large ventricular septal defect; thus, right-to-left shunting occurs but right ventricular failure usually does not occur. Exercise increases right-to-left shunting and cyanosis by decreasing systemic vascular resistance. Patients typically have intermittent "spells" associated with hyperpnea, cyanosis, and lightheadedness or syncope thought to be due to an increase in right-to-left shunting. Children achieve relief from dyspnea by squatting, a maneuver that increases both systemic vascular resistance and pulmonary blood flow. Infective endocarditis may occur, and there is a high incidence of brain abscess, presumably because the normal filtering mechanisms of the pulmonary vasculature are bypassed.

The natural history of tetralogy of Fallot is a gradual increase in severity of pulmonic stenosis so that cyanosis increases. Total surgical correction is the treatment of choice and can be performed even in infants; however, the creation of a systemic-to-pulmonary shunt (usually an anastomosis of the subclavian artery to the pulmonary artery, a Blalock-Taussig shunt) is still performed in very young cyanotic infants with complex lesions but adds to the risk of complete repair later. Right bundle branch block occurs after repair, and an increased incidence of ventricular arrhythmias, heart block, and sudden death has been reported years after surgery. Even with only moderate symptoms children should have a complete surgical correction by school age.

TRICUSPID ATRESIA

In tricuspid atresia no tricuspid valve is present, and the right atrium does not connect to the right ventricle. An interatrial connection allows blood to flow to the left heart, and a small ventricular septal defect usually allows some blood flow to the lungs via the rudimentary right ventricle. The patient is usually cyanotic with diminished pulmonary blood flow and has a dominant left ventricle. Transposition of the great arteries is often an associated defect. Systemic arterial to pulmonary arterial shunts and enlargement of the atrial septal defect by balloon septostomy are palliative. The insertion of a prosthetic conduit between the right atrium and pulmonary artery with closure of the atrial septal defect (Fontan procedure) may provide improvement.

GENERAL PROBLEMS DUE TO PROLONGED SURVIVAL

Because of cardiac surgery, more patients with congenital heart disease survive to become adults. Many patients have undergone complete repair of their defects and are asymptomatic. Others, however, may be symptomatic with residual defects or complications from surgery, and some patients may have merely had incomplete correction with palliative surgery. Pregnancy may be complicated in these patients. Infants of patients with cyanotic congenital heart disease tend to be small for their gestational age.

REFERENCES

Adams FH, Emmanouilides GC: Moss' Heart Disease in Infants, Children, and Adolescents. 3rd ed. Baltimore, Williams & Wilkins, 1983.

Perloff JK: The Clinical Recognition of Congenital Heart Disease. 3rd ed. Philadelphia, WB Saunders Company, 1987.

Roberts WC: Adult Congenital Heart Disease. Philadelphia, FA Davis Company, 1987.

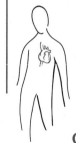

6

ACQUIRED VALVULAR HEART DISEASE

GENERAL CONSIDERATIONS

When an aortic or pulmonic valve is stenotic, the respective ventricle compensates by undergoing hypertrophy; that is, the mass of myocardium increases with little increase in the size of the ventricular cavity. Hypertrophy increases ventricular oxygen consumption and, because of the increased intramural pressure, decreases the diastolic flow of blood to the myocardium from the coronary arteries, resulting in an imbalance of myocardial oxygen demand and delivery. Aortic or pulmonic regurgitation places a diastolic volume overload on the respective ventricle and results in dilation with less hypertrophy. This increase in ventricular volume also leads to increased myocardial oxygen consumption via increased wall tension. Mitral or tricuspid regurgitation also places a diastolic volume overload on the ventricle although not as severe, since the ventricle empties into a lower pressure chamber and systolic pressures are not as high. Mitral regurgitation, therefore, is better tolerated than aortic regurgitation. Mitral and tricuspid stenosis do not overload the ventricle but instead the respective atrium dilates, and either pulmonary or systemic venous pressure may increase markedly. Ventricular myocardial dysfunction eventually occurs in both hypertrophy and dilation. An increase in venous pressure eventually may develop in any valvular lesion when cardiac decompensation occurs. The S_4 gallop correlates with left ventricular hypertrophy and decreased myocardial compliance, and the S_3 gallop correlates with increased blood volume filling the heart in early diastole and is common in volume overload states, usually with some degree of myocardial dysfunction. As left ventricular failure occurs and pulmonary venous pressures increase, right ventricular failure eventually may ensue.

Echocardiography may obviate the need for cardiac catheterization in certain lesions (for example, simple uncomplicated mitral stenosis). However, cardiac catheterization is the standard means to assess the severity or quantitate the degree of most valvular lesions in patients whose clinical status is thought possibly to warrant surgery. Catheterization may be needed to determine the relative severity of multivalvular lesions, to detect significant concomitant lesions, to evaluate the status of the coronary circulation, and to evaluate left ventricular function.

The decision of whether and when to replace an abnormal valve often is difficult, since the natural history of many valvular lesions is chronic and prolonged. In addition, prosthetic valves carry lifelong risks of endocarditis, emboli, and thrombosis, and the lifespan of many prosthetic valves is unknown. The natural history of each valvular lesion is different; some lesions (for example, aortic regurgitation) may be associated with irreversible myocardial damage before symptoms occur, whereas other lesions (for example, mitral stenosis) can await significant progression of symptoms before valve replacement is necessary, since the ventricle is protected by the stenotic valve. In addition, the patient's age, general medical status, and desire to return to previous levels of activity enter into the decision for valve replacement.

MITRAL STENOSIS
(Tables 6–1, 6–2, and 6–3)

Mitral stenosis almost always results from rheumatic fever and is rarely congenital in etiology. It is the most common lesion caused by rheumatic fever. Two thirds of patients with mitral stenosis are female. The valve leaflets become thickened and the commissures fused, and the chordae tendineae may fuse and shorten. Calcium may be deposited in the valve. This process of valve scarring progresses slowly and may take 10 years or more after the episode of rheumatic fever to become hemodynamically significant. Because of the deformation of the mitral valve, mitral regurgitation also may be present. The left atrium enlarges, but the left ventricle remains normal in size unless mitral regurgitation also occurs. The elevated left atrial pressure determines the extent of pulmonary venous congestion that causes the major symptoms in mitral stenosis of dyspnea, orthopnea, and paroxysmal nocturnal dyspnea. Pulmonary arterial hypertension occurs not only secondary to the elevated pulmonary venous pressure but sometimes also secondary to a reactive increase in the pulmonary vascular resistance. Right ventricular failure and functional tricuspid regurgitation may result. Atrial fibrillation is common. Diastolic filling of the left ventricle is determined not only by the pressure gradient across the stenotic mitral valve but also by the amount of time spent in diastole during which the left ventricle can fill. Therefore, when the patient exercises and develops sinus tachycardia or when atrial fibrillation occurs, the rapid ventricular rate diminishes the percentage of the cardiac cycle spent in diastole and ventricular filling is limited. A patient's first episode of pulmonary edema often occurs either with exercise or with the onset of atrial fibrillation.

Even though acute rheumatic fever may have occurred in childhood, the age at the onset of cardiac symptoms is usually between 25 and 45 years. There may be a relatively long period, 5 to 8 years, of mild to moderate pulmonary congestive symptoms before severe compromise occurs. Since reduction in cardiac output is a late finding, fatigue and physical wasting are also late manifestations. Occasionally, hemoptysis may occur due to leaking or rupture of pulmonary vessels. The occurrence of intermittent atrial fibrillation as the left atrium dilates may be associated with peripheral emboli. As pulmonary vascular resistance and reactive pulmonary arterial hypertension increase, flow from the right to the left heart is limited, pulmonary venous hypertension stabilizes, and episodes of pulmonary edema may decrease; however, the complaint of fatigue becomes prominent. Findings of right heart failure with hepatomegaly, ascites, and peripheral edema may occur.

The first heart sound is loud because the mitral valve is maximally open at the onset of systole and the left ventricular pressure is rising rapidly when the valve closes because of the high left atrial pressure. More severe mitral stenosis shortens the interval between S_2 and the opening snap (the higher the left atrial pressure, the sooner the valve will open during isovolumic relaxation). A diastolic, low-pitched, rumbling murmur located near the left ventricular apex immediately follows the opening snap, if present. The rumble is loudest in early diastole during rapid ventricular filling and, if sinus rhythm is present, increases again with atrial contraction (presystolic accentuation). In mild mitral stenosis, as well as severe mitral stenosis with low cardiac output, the murmur may be difficult to hear and may be accentuated with the patient in the left lateral decubitus position, especially after exercise. In addition, a markedly enlarged right ventricle may displace the left ventricle posteriorly, making the murmur even harder to hear. Concomitant rheumatic involvement of the aortic valve may generate murmurs of aortic stenosis or regurgitation.

Echocardiography is diagnostic of mitral stenosis. Cross-sectional echocardiography can be used to es-

TABLE 6–1. ACQUIRED VALVULAR LESIONS: SYMPTOMS AND NATURAL HISTORY

LESION	MAJOR SYMPTOMS	NATURAL HISTORY
Mitral stenosis	Dyspnea, orthopnea, paroxysmal nocturnal dyspnea; later fatigue, wasting, hemoptysis, symptoms of right heart failure Systemic emboli not uncommon Acute decompensation with onset of atrial fibrillation	Onset of symptoms 10+ years after rheumatic fever; slowly progressive
Mitral regurgitation	Pulmonary congestion, fatigue; later right heart failure	Chronic: long asymptomatic phase despite moderately severe regurgitation Acute: if severe, rapid deterioration
Mitral valve prolapse	Chest pain atypical for angina pectoris; palpitations; rarely left heart failure from mitral regurgitation	Usually asymptomatic; endocarditis, rupture of chordae, progressive mitral regurgitation, and sudden death rarely occur
Aortic stenosis	Angina, LV failure; exertional syncope, presyncope	Rapid deterioration once symptoms appear; first manifestation in a rare patient is sudden death
Aortic regurgitation	LV failure Palpitations from arrhythmias or hyperdynamic circulation	Chronic: asymptomatic or minimally symptomatic stage may span years; irreversible myocardial damage may occur in the asymptomatic patient Acute: rapid deterioration
Tricuspid stenosis	Depends on associated mitral valve abnormalities Manifestations of right heart failure	Like mitral stenosis, gradually progressive with onset of symptoms in mid-adulthood
Tricuspid regurgitation	RV failure	Depends on underlying etiology; may improve if associated lesions are corrected

TABLE 6–2. ACQUIRED VALVULAR LESIONS: PHYSICAL AND LABORATORY EXAMINATION

LESION	PHYSICAL FINDINGS	ECG	RADIOGRAPH	ECHOCARDIOGRAM
Mitral stenosis	Decreased pulse pressure Loud S_1 Opening snap if mitral valve is pliable No S_3 or S_4 Diastolic rumble Concomitant murmur of mitral regurgitation or aortic involvement Late features include pulmonary hypertension and RV failure	Atrial fibrillation common Left atrial abnormality RV hypertrophy when pulmonary hypertension develops	Large LA: double density at right heart border, posterior displacement of esophagus, elevation of left mainstem bronchus, straightening of left heart border due to enlarged left atrial appendage Large pulmonary artery Pulmonary venous congestion	M-mode: thickened mitral leaflets, anterior movement of posterior leaflet during systole, decreased mid-diastolic mitral closure (decreased "E to F slope") Two-dimensional: mitral valve doming, visualization of decreased valve area
Mitral regurgitation	Hyperdynamic LV impulse displaced laterally Left parasternal lift from right ventricle or systolic LA expansion S_3, soft S_1, widely split S_2 (early A_2) S_4 absent in chronic, present in acute form Holosystolic murmur radiating to axilla; murmur may be atypical in acute mitral regurgitation, mitral valve prolapse, papillary muscle dysfunction Later features include pulmonary hypertension and RV failure	Atrial fibrillation less common than in mitral stenosis Left atrial enlargement LV hypertrophy	Enlarged LA and LV; pulmonary venous congestion	Large LV and LA with hyperdynamic LV motion (left ventricular volume overload) May reveal underlying cause of mitral regurgitation
Mitral valve prolapse	One or more systolic clicks, often followed by a late systolic murmur High incidence of bony chest abnormalities: straight back syndrome, pectus excavatum, thoracic scoliosis	Usually normal; occasionally ST depression and T wave inversion inferiorly Ventricular or supraventricular ectopy	Usually normal unless significant mitral regurgitation is present; bony abnormalities	Systolic bowing of anterior or posterior mitral leaflets into LA
Aortic stenosis	Pulsus parvus et tardus (may be absent in older patients or those with aortic insufficiency) Carotid "shudder" (thrill) Systolic ejection murmur in aortic area, usually with thrill, harsh quality, radiates to carotids, peaks late in systole if stenosis is severe Sustained, diffuse, but not displaced LV impulse (LV heave or lift) S_4 gallop, often palpable A_2 decreased, S_2 single or paradoxically split S_3 if LV failure is present Aortic ejection click in noncalcified congenital stenosis	LV hypertrophy Left bundle branch block and intraventricular conduction defects common Rare heart block from calcific involvement of the conduction system	LV predominance without dilation Post-stenotic aortic root dilation Calcification in region of aortic valve Cardiomegaly and pulmonary congestion with LV failure	Thick aortic valve leaflets with decreased excursion LV hypertrophy Severity estimated with Doppler techniques
Aortic regurgitation	Chronic: increased pulse pressure (head bobbing), pistol-shot	LV hypertrophy often with "volume overload" pattern (narrow deep Q	LV and aortic dilation	Dilated LV and aorta Left ventricular volume overload

LESION	PHYSICAL FINDINGS	ECG	RADIOGRAPH	ECHOCARDIOGRAM
Aortic regurgitation *continued*	sounds over peripheral arteries, to-and-fro murmur over femoral arteries with light compression by stethoscope (Duroziez's sign), pulsatile blushing of nail beds (Quincke's sign), rapid upstroke with collapsing quality to pulse (water hammer pulse) Bifid pulse contour, especially if stenosis is also present Hyperkinetic, displaced apical impulse Diastolic decrescendo murmur, length correlates with severity Systolic flow murmur Systolic and/or diastolic thrill A_2 decreased or absent S_3 in early LV decompensation Austin Flint murmur Acute: apical impulse not displaced; pulse pressure increased much less Diastolic murmur shorter and softer (high LV diastolic pressure) S_1 decreased (because of early mitral valve closure) Severe LV failure	waves in left precordial leads)		Fluttering of anterior mitral valve leaflet Acute: premature diastolic closure of mitral valve
Tricuspid stenosis	Prominent a wave, attenuated y descent in jugular pulse Jugular venous distention, edema, hepatomegaly Tricuspid opening snap with diastolic rumble loudest in fourth left intercostal space, louder with inspiration	Atrial fibrillation common RA enlargement with RV hypertrophy	Associated valve lesions; large RA	Doming of tricuspid valve; associated lesions
Tricuspid regurgitation	Increased jugular venous pressure with large v waves Hepatomegaly with systolic pulsations Holosystolic murmur along left sternal border ± thrill; increases with inspiration Diastolic flow rumble Right ventricular S_3 (increases with inspiration; loudest along left sternal border) Findings of pulmonary hypertension if tricuspid regurgitation is secondary	RV hypertrophy RA enlargement Atrial fibrillation is common	Enlarged RV and RA; other lesions may be evident	Underlying cause may be identified Contrast echo can establish the diagnosis

TABLE 6–3. ACQUIRED VALVULAR LESIONS: MEDICAL AND SURGICAL MANAGEMENT

LESION	MEDICAL MANAGEMENT	SURGICAL MANAGEMENT
Mitral stenosis	Rheumatic fever and endocarditis prophylaxis Diuretics, salt restriction Control of ventricular rate and anticoagulation in atrial fibrillation	*Indication*: Functional Class III despite medical therapy; severe pulmonary hypertension is not a surgical contraindication *Procedure*: Commissurotomy or valve replacement
Mitral regurgitation	Salt restriction, diuretics, digitalis, afterload reduction Endocarditis prophylaxis	*Indication*: Functional Class III despite medical therapy; patients with lesser symptoms and evidence of myocardial dysfunction; acute severe mitral regurgitation *Procedure*: Mitral valve replacement
Mitral valve prolapse	Endocarditis prophylaxis Beta blockade for chest pain Beta blockade or other antiarrhythmic agents for arrhythmias	Mitral valve replacement for acute and/or severe mitral regurgitation
Aortic stenosis	Endocarditis prophylaxis Avoid strenuous exercise	*Indications*: Symptoms *Procedure*: Valve replacement
Aortic regurgitation	Endocarditis prophylaxis Salt restriction, diuretics, digitalis, afterload reduction	*Indication*: Controversial; greater than mild symptoms, evidence of early LV dysfunction in asymptomatic patients *Procedure*: Aortic valve replacement
Tricuspid stenosis	Endocarditis and rheumatic fever prophylaxis Depends on associated valvular lesions	*Indication*: Severe tricuspid stenosis, usually concomitant with mitral valve surgery *Procedure*: Tricuspid valve replacement
Tricuspid regurgitation	Endocarditis prophylaxis Treatment of associated lesions Diuretics, salt restriction, digitalis	*Indication*: Severe tricuspid regurgitation, often concomitant with mitral valve surgery *Procedure*: Tricuspid annuloplasty or valve replacement

timate accurately the valve orifice area in a high percentage of patients, possibly more accurately than the Gorlin formula at cardiac catheterization, since the presence of mitral regurgitation does not affect the valve area determined echocardiographically.

The patient with significant mitral stenosis has an elevated left atrial or pulmonary capillary wedge pressure with a pressure gradient between the left atrium and left ventricle during diastole. The Gorlin formula is used to calculate the valve area according to the equation:

$$\text{Valve Area} = \frac{\text{Transvalvular Flow}}{\text{Constant} \times \sqrt{\text{Gradient}}}$$

Because the pressure gradient changes with the square of the flow, small increases in cardiac output are associated with relatively large elevations in left atrial pressure. Less severe cases of mitral stenosis have elevated pulmonary arterial pressures without a gradient between pulmonary arterial and venous pressures (passive pulmonary hypertension), whereas more severe cases have reactive pulmonary hypertension due to an increase in pulmonary vascular resistance. The area of a normal mitral valve is about 4 sq cm; severe mitral stenosis occurs when the valve area is less than 1 sq cm. Left ventricular function is generally normal unless complicating lesions are present.

Control of the ventricular rate using digitalis in patients with atrial fibrillation decreases left atrial pressure. Patients with sinus rhythm experiencing exertional dyspnea may benefit from the administration of propranolol to prevent sinus tachycardia. Patients may

be managed for many years medically. Systemic embolization despite anticoagulation is an indication for surgery. Since systolic function of the ventricular myocardium is not impaired in uncomplicated mitral stenosis, the inotropic property of digitalis is not beneficial. When the patient experiences functional Class III or IV symptoms despite medical therapy, surgery should be considered. Surgery is not contraindicated by severe pulmonary hypertension, since the increased pulmonary vascular resistance returns toward normal upon correction of the left atrial hypertension (cf. pulmonary hypertension in patients with left-to-right shunts, e.g., ventricular septal defect).

Mitral commissurotomy can be employed in patients with relatively pliable, noncalcified valves without mitral regurgitation. Commissurotomy spares the patient the risks of a prosthetic valve and anticoagulation for several years. A regurgitant valve is likely to become more regurgitant after commissurotomy, and valve replacement is therefore usually performed in patients with concomitant mitral regurgitation. The average patient experiences 8 to 12 years of symptomatic relief after commissurotomy, but progression of the disease occurs and usually valve replacement is necessary eventually. In older patients with severe mitral stenosis who are not considered good surgical candidates, mitral valvuloplasty can be attempted in the catheterization laboratory using a balloon catheter.

MITRAL REGURGITATION

The most common cause of mitral regurgitation is rheumatic fever, and it occurs more commonly in males. The murmur of mitral regurgitation may appear early after an episode of acute rheumatic fever. Concomitant aortic valve involvement suggests a rheumatic etiology. Other etiologies include congenital mitral regurgitation, which is sometimes associated with other lesions such as an ostium primum atrial septal defect. Mitral valve prolapse, mitral annular calcification, rupture of chordae tendineae from endocarditis, trauma, or degenerative diseases such as Marfan's syndrome may cause mitral regurgitation. Rupture of a papillary muscle after myocardial infarction results in severe, acute mitral regurgitation, while infarction of a papillary muscle can cause chronic papillary muscle dysfunction. Mitral regurgitation is common in patients with hypertrophic cardiomyopathy. It may occur secondary to left ventricular dilation; this "functional" mitral regurgitation probably occurs not so much from dilation of the mitral annulus as from distortion of the normal alignment of the papillary muscles.

Mitral regurgitation is holosystolic; that is, blood flows from the left ventricle to the low-pressure left atrium from the time the mitral valve closes to its opening after S_2. Left ventricular afterload is reduced. The v wave in the left atrial or pulmonary capillary wedge pressure tracing is often increased. However, large v waves can be seen in entities other than mitral regurgitation; if left atrial compliance is increased, v waves may not be present even in severe mitral regurgitation. Left ventricular diastolic volume increases in chronic mitral regurgitation. Because of the low pressure against which the left ventricle ejects blood (i.e., into the left atrium), the clinical course may extend over many years before decompensation occurs. However, as mitral regurgitation becomes severe and long-standing, left ventricular contractility may be irreversibly impaired. The left ventricular systolic as well as diastolic dimensions subsequently increase. Pulmonary hypertension, like that in mitral stenosis, may occur as a result of both increased pulmonary venous pressure and a reactive increase in pulmonary vascular resistance. In chronic mitral regurgitation, the increased volume of blood entering the left atrium is accommodated by dilation of the left atrium with a modest increase in left atrial pressure. However, in acute, severe mitral regurgitation (e.g., secondary to endocarditis or ruptured chordae tendineae), regurgitant blood enters a relatively small, noncompliant left atrium, and left atrial pressure may rise dramatically with very large v waves.

The severity of mitral regurgitation is estimated at catheterization by the amount of contrast regurgitated into the left atrium after injection into the left ventricle. A regurgitant fraction can be calculated but these calculations can be fraught with error. There may be a pressure gradient across the mitral valve in early diastole in the absence of mitral stenosis because of the large volume of blood flowing across the valve. A normal ejection fraction may mask left ventricular dysfunction despite myocardial depression because of the marked afterload reduction afforded by the mitral

regurgitation. Once the valve is replaced, however, the myocardial dysfunction may become evident.

Patients in functional Class III or IV despite medical therapy should be considered for surgery. Patients with lesser symptoms who display early evidence of myocardial dysfunction (e.g., increased systolic left ventricular diameter or decreasing ejection fraction) should be considered for surgery. The mitral valve usually is replaced with a metal or bioprosthetic valve; valvuloplasty usually is not adequate. Acute severe mitral regurgitation generally is not well tolerated and requires emergency valve replacement. Potent afterload reduction, with intravenous nitroprusside, for example, may stabilize the patient until surgery can be performed.

MITRAL VALVE PROLAPSE

Mitral valve prolapse (floppy mitral valve, click murmur syndrome) is common and usually benign, reported to occur in 0.3 to 6 per cent of the population. It derives its clinical significance from its characteristic systolic click and late systolic murmur and the occasional patient who experiences significant mitral regurgitation, chordal rupture, endocarditis, arrhythmias, or sudden death. The severity of mitral regurgitation varies. The mitral valve leaflets are generally redundant, the chordae are elongated, and pathology in more severe cases demonstrates myxomatous degeneration. Mitral regurgitation is occasionally progressive and severe and can occur acutely if a chorda ruptures because of myxomatous degeneration or endocarditis. The cause is unknown, although it is common in Marfan's syndrome and other connective tissue diseases. It has increased incidence in patients with ostium secundum atrial septal defect and hypertrophic cardiomyopathy. It is more common in females than males and occasionally will run in families.

A variety of symptoms has been attributed to mitral valve prolapse, but it is difficult to definitely attribute symptoms to the syndrome, since it is so common. The pathogenesis of the chest pain is not clear but could be related to ischemia or tension on the papillary muscles. Patients may also have a variety of supraventricular or ventricular arrhythmias. Autonomic abnormalities such as orthostatic hypotension have been associated with mitral prolapse.

When the left ventricle contracts, the mitral valve initially closes normally; as ventricular volume decreases, however, the valve leaflets (anterior, posterior, or both) abruptly prolapse into the atrium. This rapid motion generates the midsystolic click and subsequent mitral regurgitation creates the late systolic murmur. Any maneuver that decreases the volume of the left ventricle causes the mitral valve to prolapse earlier during systole (for example, the Valsalva maneuver or standing), also causing the click and murmur to occur earlier in systole. The presence of clicks and the length and intensity of the murmur may vary from time to time in the same patient. There are a few patients who have the characteristic click and murmur on auscultation in whom no mitral valve prolapse is identified on echocardiography. Tricuspid valve prolapse is sometimes associated with mitral valve prolapse.

The natural history of this syndrome is variable, and in most cases the syndrome is benign. The risk of sudden death for any individual patient with mitral valve prolapse is very small unless ventricular tachycardia is demonstrated. Ventricular arrhythmias generally are not treated unless symptoms are present or ventricular tachycardia is demonstrated. These arrhythmias have been reported to respond to propranolol, but many cases are difficult to control with either propranolol or other antiarrhythmic agents. Chest pain often is treated effectively with beta-adrenergic blocking agents.

AORTIC STENOSIS

The most common cause of aortic stenosis is a congenitally bicuspid aortic valve (see Chapter 5) that, although usually not obstructive during childhood, gradually thickens, calcifies, and becomes stenotic by approximately the sixth decade of life. Tricuspid aortic valves may also thicken and calcify from wear and tear, causing aortic stenosis in a few patients. Rheumatic fever may cause aortic stenosis but is almost always accompanied by evidence of mitral valve involvement.

Aortic valve obstruction results in elevation of left ventricular systolic pressure, and the resultant left ventricular hypertrophy maintains cardiac output without dilation of the ventricular cavity. Therefore, the stroke volume is normal until the late stages of the disease. Forceful atrial contraction augments filling of the thick, noncompliant ventricle and generates a prominent S_4 gallop that elevates the left ventricular end-diastolic pressure. The mean left ventricular diastolic pressure is nearly normal unless myocardial decompensation occurs. Left ventricular hypertrophy and high intramyocardial wall tension account for the increased oxygen demand and, along with decreased diastolic coronary blood flow, account for the occurrence of angina pectoris even if coronary anatomy is normal. Compensatory mechanisms may be adequate for many years, although outflow obstruction is severe. However, once congestive heart failure, angina, or syncope occurs the patient experiences a rapid clinical decline. As the myocardium fails, mean left ventricular diastolic pressure increases and symptoms of pulmonary congestion ensue.

Aortic stenosis is three times more common in males than in females. Symptoms occur late, and many patients know of a murmur many years in advance of symptoms. Severe congenital aortic stenosis, however, may present in childhood. In most cases, syncope is due to the inability of the left ventricle to maintain a normal cardiac output with exertion and peripheral vasodilation. A small percentage of patients (3 to 4 per cent) may have sudden death as their only symptom of aortic stenosis. The mechanism of sudden death is not known but is probably similar to that causing syncope or secondary to a ventricular arrhythmia. The onset of symptoms due to aortic stenosis is a grave prognostic sign and an indication for valve replacement.

An ejection murmur may occur across a deformed aortic valve owing to turbulence of flow without necessarily implying aortic stenosis. The murmur of significant aortic stenosis may diminish in the late stages of the disease when left ventricular failure occurs and flow across the stenotic orifice decreases.

Echocardiography can detect thickening of the aortic valve leaflets with decreased systolic separation. However, because of the multiple echoes generated by the calcified valve, the severity of aortic stenosis often cannot be determined. In the adult the presence of thin, pliable aortic valve leaflets virtually excludes the diagnosis of aortic stenosis. However, in children and young adults the congenitally stenotic aortic valve may appear to move well on M-mode echocardiography, but two-dimensional echocardiography reveals the classic doming of the valve diagnostic of congenital aortic stenosis. Identification of a bicuspid valve with echocardiography is difficult. Echocardiographic degree of left ventricular hypertrophy correlates with the severity of aortic stenosis in children but not in adults. Measurement of aortic valve orifice by two-dimensional echocardiography is possible in a few patients but is not very reliable.

Although Doppler echocardiography can be used noninvasively to estimate the sensitivity of aortic stenosis, cardiac catheterization is the more definitive test. The gradient between the left ventricle and aorta is measured simultaneously with the cardiac output, and the valve area is calculated from the Gorlin equation. The pressure gradient alone often does not adequately define the severity of aortic stenosis, since the patient with an increased cardiac output may demonstrate an increased gradient across the aortic valve without necessarily having severe aortic stenosis, and a patient with severe aortic stenosis may demonstrate a decrease in the gradient as his ability to maintain cardiac output decreases. The normal valve area is approximately 2.5 sq cm, and no gradient is present normally. Aortic valvular area of less than 0.7 sq cm defines critical aortic stenosis and is usually associated with a gradient of 50 to 60 mm Hg or more. Right ventricular and pulmonary arterial pressures are normal unless left ventricular failure is present. Ventriculography is performed to assess left ventricular function, and most adult patients require coronary arteriography in case coronary revascularization is required along with aortic valve replacement.

Aortic stenosis can be complicated by the development of aortic insufficiency as the valve calcifies, stiffens, and fails to close properly or by the development of bacterial endocarditis. In younger patients, supravalvular or subvalvular aortic obstruction should be considered.

Patients with known significant aortic stenosis should not participate in strenuous physical exercise to avoid the risk of sudden death. The adult patient should undergo catheterization as soon as angina, syncope, or left ventricular failure appears. Surgical mortality is lowest in patients with good left ventricular function. In patients with poor ejection fraction who survive surgery, the ventricular function tends to improve considerably once the obstruction is relieved; therefore, poor left ventricular function does not contraindicate aortic valve replacement for aortic stenosis. Aortic valve replacement may be performed in children and young adults who have severe congenital aortic stenosis even in the absence of symptoms in order to lower the risk of sudden death. Operative mortality is approximately 3 to 6 per cent, but patients with severe left ventricular dysfunction may have an operative risk as high as 15 per cent. Once symptoms have appeared, survival is improved by surgery. In elderly patients who are poor surgical candidates, a relatively small but often adequate increase in the aortic valve area can be obtained using balloon valvuloplasty at the time of cardiac catheterization.

AORTIC REGURGITATION

Rheumatic fever is the most common cause of aortic regurgitation. Isolated rheumatic aortic valve involvement without mitral valve involvement is unusual. Aortic regurgitation from rheumatic fever may occur with the aortic valvulitis at the time of the acute rheumatic fever or may occur late after the acute attack as the valve becomes thickened and the leaflets retract. Aortic stenosis and regurgitation often occur together in rheumatic heart disease as well as with bicuspid aortic valves. Aortic regurgitation may result from processes that either involve the valve directly or cause dilation of the aortic root. Aortic regurgitation can occur with discrete subvalvular stenosis or ventricular septal defects. Isolated congenital aortic regurgitation is unusual but may occur with a bicuspid aortic valve. Aortic regurgitation may occur after infective endocarditis. The aortic valve leaflets may be affected by rheumatoid arthritis. Conditions that may affect the ascending aorta and cause aortic regurgitation are syphilis, ankylosing spondylitis, Marfan's syndrome, systemic hypertension, aortic dissection, and aortic trauma.

Aortic regurgitation results in a volume overload of the left ventricle. The ventricle compensates by increasing its end-diastolic volume according to the Frank-Starling mechanism. Left ventricular end-diastolic pressure may not be elevated early in the course of the disease as the ventricle dilates and accommodates the increased volume. The amount of blood ejected with each contraction is abnormally increased, consisting of both the blood received from the left atrium and the regurgitant volume. As the ventricular volume increases beyond the capacity of the left ventricle to dilate, however, left ventricular end-diastolic and left atrial pressures may rise. Secondary mitral regurgitation may occur owing to the left ventricular dilation. The physiology of aortic regurgitation is somewhat similar to that of mitral regurgitation, except that

the increased cardiac stroke volume is delivered into the high-pressure aorta instead of the low-pressure left atrium, tending to elevate left ventricular pressures instead of unloading the left ventricle. This, along with decreased aortic pressure during diastole when the majority of coronary flow occurs, may lead to greater oxygen demand than supply and angina may occur, even with normal coronary arteries. The systolic function of the left ventricle is normal in early chronic aortic regurgitation, but as dilation becomes severe, left ventricular function diminishes. Some patients experience an irreversible decrease in left ventricular function before any symptoms occur. The left ventricular dilation is thought to "overstretch" the myofibrils, leading to less actin-myosin interaction and decreased contractility. The mechanisms of compensation for chronic aortic regurgitation are very efficient, and patients with chronic severe aortic regurgitation may remain asymptomatic for years. However, the pathophysiology of acute, severe aortic regurgitation is different because the left ventricle has not had the opportunity to dilate, its compliance is relatively high, and the aortic regurgitation therefore leads to very high left ventricular end-diastolic pressures. The left atrium and pulmonary vasculature may be protected somewhat, since the elevated left ventricular end-diastolic pressure may cause the mitral valve to close early in diastole (mitral preclosure). However, if mitral regurgitation ensues, the elevated left ventricular diastolic pressure is reflected back to the pulmonary vasculature, and acute pulmonary edema may occur. Acute aortic regurgitation is caused most commonly by infective endocarditis, aortic dissection, and trauma. Acute aortic regurgitation results in a lower cardiac output, narrower aortic pulse pressure, and a smaller left ventricle than does chronic aortic regurgitation. Aortic diastolic pressure decreases in chronic aortic regurgitation because of both the regurgitation of blood into the left ventricle and a compensatory decrease in systemic vascular resistance to maintain forward cardiac flow to the periphery. In acute aortic regurgitation, however, left ventricular diastolic pressure is high, systemic vascular resistance is not low, and aortic diastolic pressure does not fall greatly.

The increased pulse pressure in chronic aortic regurgitation is due to the large stroke volume, causing increased systolic and decreased diastolic pressure. This phenomenon determines many of the characteristic physical findings of aortic insufficiency (Table 6–2). Aortic regurgitation murmurs are heard best with the patient upright, leaning forward, and in end-expiration. The murmur of valvular aortic regurgitation is often loudest at the second left intercostal space, whereas the murmur of aortic regurgitation due to aortic dilation may be loudest in the second right intercostal space. Even if concomitant aortic stenosis is not present, a systolic ejection murmur reflecting a large stroke volume across a deformed valve is usually heard in the aortic area and may be transmitted to the carotids. In severe chronic aortic regurgitation, a diastolic low-pitched rumbling murmur may be heard at the apex (Austin Flint murmur), probably owing to flow across the mitral valve, which closes early because of the regurgitant jet from the aortic insufficiency and also the increased left ventricular diastolic pressure.

Echocardiography shows dilation of the left ventricle and sometimes aortic root. Wall motion is hyperdynamic if ventricular function is not impaired. Aortic regurgitation is characterized by diastolic fluttering of the anterior mitral valve leaflet caused by the regurgitant aortic jet striking the open mitral valve during diastole. Acute severe aortic regurgitation with marked elevation of left atrial pressures may result in closure of the mitral valve in diastole before ventricular systole has occurred (mitral preclosure). The cause of the aortic regurgitation may be identified, for example, aortic dissection or endocarditis. The presence of concomitant mitral valvular thickening or stenosis implies a rheumatic etiology.

During cardiac catheterization, supravalvular aortography defines aortic dimensions, and reflux of contrast into the left ventricle grossly quantitates the degree of aortic regurgitation. Left ventriculography is performed to evaluate left ventricular function, and reflux of contrast into the left atrium would reveal mitral regurgitation. Systolic left ventricular and aortic pressures are elevated, and aortic diastolic pressure is low. Left ventricular volume is increased. The left ventricular end-diastolic pressure is normal or only slightly increased until left ventricular failure ensues. Left ventricular dysfunction is demonstrated by decreased cardiac output, decreased ejection fraction, and increased left ventricular end-diastolic pressure. In severe aortic regurgitation, the normally functioning ventricle is hyperdynamic (increased ejection fraction), and even a normal ejection fraction may indicate decreased systolic function. The presence of left ventricular dysfunction markedly increases surgical complications and mortality, and left ventricular function may not be restored after surgery, in contrast to the situation with pure aortic stenosis.

The timing of aortic valve replacement is difficult, since the natural history is prolonged and a long asymptomatic phase occurs. Early replacement of the aortic valve subjects the patient to the immediate surgical risk and the long-term risk created by prosthetic valves. However, if one waits to replace the aortic valve, irreversible left ventricular dysfunction may occur in the absence of symptoms. In these patients with no symptoms, evidence of progressive left ventricular systolic dysfunction may indicate surgery. (Suggested criteria include a left ventricular end-*systolic* diameter of 5.5 cm on M-mode echocardiography or a decrease in radionuclide left ventricular ejection fraction with exercise.) In patients with severe disease of the aortic root, replacement of a portion of the ascending aorta may be required in addition to the aortic valve replacement.

Patients who develop acute severe aortic regurgitation deteriorate rapidly, and aortic valve replacement must be performed emergently. Vasodilators such as nitroprusside can acutely reduce afterload and diminish aortic regurgitation to stabilize the patient for a short period of time until surgery can be performed.

Intra-aortic balloon counterpulsation is not effective in the presence of aortic regurgitation.

TRICUSPID STENOSIS

Tricuspid stenosis is usually rheumatic in etiology and does not occur as an isolated lesion. Like mitral stenosis, it is gradually progressive, is more common in women, and usually becomes symptomatic in mid-adulthood. Tricuspid stenosis can occasionally be caused by carcinoid, endomyocardial fibroelastosis, congenital valvular malformations, or right atrial myxoma.

Because it is such a low-pressure system, relatively small gradients across the tricuspid valve (5 mm) may indicate significant tricuspid stenosis. Echocardiographic diagnosis is probably more accurate than catheterization because of the small gradient involved. Tricuspid stenosis can protect the patient with concomitant mitral stenosis from pulmonary congestion.

TRICUSPID REGURGITATION

Tricuspid regurgitation may occur as a result of rheumatic fever, often associated with tricuspid stenosis. Tricuspid regurgitation is most commonly a functional lesion secondary to right ventricular dilation and pulmonary hypertension, and as in patients with mitral regurgitation, the differentiation of functional from organic valvular regurgitation can be difficult. Functional tricuspid regurgitation can occur with forms of congenital heart disease associated with pulmonary hypertension and with severe pulmonary disease. Tricuspid regurgitation can occur with Ebstein's anomaly, carcinoid syndrome, intracardiac tumors, penetrating or nonpenetrating cardiac trauma, and endocarditis. Normal tricuspid valves may be affected by endocarditis, particularly in drug addicts.

Functional tricuspid regurgitation may regress after associated lesions are corrected and pulmonary hypertension resolves. At times plication of the tricuspid annulus is required to improve functional tricuspid regurgitation. If annuloplasty is unsuccessful or if significant tricuspid stenosis is present, tricuspid valve replacement can be performed.

PULMONIC STENOSIS AND REGURGITATION

Pulmonic stenosis is usually congenital and is discussed in Chapter 5. It can occasionally occur in an acquired form with hypertrophic cardiomyopathy (due to bulging of the septum into the right ventricular outflow tract) or secondary to pericardial tumor involvement in the area.

Acquired pulmonary regurgitation is usually associated with pulmonary hypertension caused by left heart valvular disease (Graham Steell murmur) or pulmonary disease. The murmur sounds similar to that of aortic insufficiency and is heard best at the second left intercostal space. This murmur is high-pitched, early diastolic, and decrescendo in character. In distinction, isolated congenital pulmonic regurgitation results in a lower-pitched murmur that occurs later in diastole, is heard best at the third to fourth left intercostal space, and resembles more the murmur of tricuspid stenosis.

MULTIVALVULAR DISEASE

Combined valvular lesions are common, especially in rheumatic heart disease. In addition to organic lesions, development of mitral and tricuspid regurgitation or pulmonic regurgitation may occur secondary to the hemodynamic disturbance of other valvular lesions. In general, the manifestations of the more proximal valve lesion are the more prominent. For example, in patients with mitral and aortic valvular lesions of similar severity, mitral valve manifestations may predominate and the degree of aortic stenosis may be underestimated. Failure to correct all significant valvular lesions at the time of surgery may lead to an inadequate clinical result and illustrates the importance of excluding concomitant lesions at the time of catheterization. The surgical risk for double valve replacement is greater than that for single valve replacement.

RHEUMATIC FEVER

Rheumatic fever usually occurs in children 5 to 15 years of age. It is caused by group A beta hemolytic streptococcal pharyngitis that occurs one to three weeks prior to the clinical manifestations of rheumatic fever. It is believed that an immune response to the *Streptococcus* is responsible for the disease. Males and females are equally affected. It is more common in patients of lower socioeconomic level. The incidence of rheumatic fever in the United States has declined in recent years.

Aschoff nodules in the myocardium are the characteristic pathological feature of rheumatic fever. The most serious manifestation of rheumatic fever is a pancarditis that may involve the endocardium, myocardium, and pericardium. Usually the mitral valve, less frequently the aortic, and even less frequently the tricuspid valve is involved. Pulmonic valve involvement is extremely rare. Valvulitis is recognized by a new insufficiency murmur. Aortic and mitral stenosis murmurs are not heard acutely. Myocarditis may present with heart failure. Pericarditis may produce a friction rub, and the PR interval may be prolonged. Because of the difficulty in diagnosing rheumatic fever, guidelines (modified Jones criteria) for establishing the diagnosis were developed. Major manifestations include carditis, polyarthritis, chorea, erythema marginatum, and subcutaneous nodules. Minor manifestations include fever, arthralgia, previous rheumatic fever or rheumatic heart disease, elevated acute phase reactants, and a prolonged PR interval. There should also be laboratory evidence of a preceding streptococcal infection (i.e., positive throat culture or increased ASO titer).

Penicillin should be administered to eradicate streptococcal infection. Salicylates are effective rapidly for treating fever and arthritis but probably have no effect on carditis. The usefulness of steroids is unproven. Congestive heart failure is treated traditionally.

The relatively high recurrence rate of rheumatic fever after streptococcal infection continues for at least 5 to 10 years after the initial infection; therefore, rheumatic fever prophylaxis should be discontinued only in adults 5 to 10 years after the acute episode and then only if the risk of the streptococcal infection is low. Adults working with school-age children, those in the military service, those exposed to large numbers of people, and those in the medical or allied health professions should receive prophylaxis indefinitely. Patients who have a significant degree of rheumatic heart disease or a history of repeated occurrences should have prophylaxis indefinitely. The recommended regimen for prophylaxis is 1.2 million units of benzathine penicillin monthly. Oral penicillin, erythromycin, or sulfadiazine can be used but because of noncompliance are somewhat less effective than the parenteral regimen.

PROSTHETIC VALVES

Prosthetic valves may be either mechanical or bioprosthetic. The two basic designs of mechanical valves are the ball and cage and the tilting disk (like a toilet seat cover). Bioprosthetic valves are made from porcine valve tissue mounted on metal struts (Table 6–4).

All prosthetic valves are somewhat stenotic, and residual gradients over both aortic and mitral valves

TABLE 6–4. PROSTHETIC VALVES

TYPE	EXAMPLES	ADVANTAGES	DISADVANTAGES
Ball and cage	Starr-Edwards	Good durability	Anticoagulation required; more hemolysis than other types
Tilting disk	Bjork-Shiley St. Jude	Most favorable hemodynamics (i.e., least residual stenosis for any given valve size); good durability	Anticoagulation required; most thrombogenic type
Bioprosthesis	Hancock, Carpentier-Edwards	Anticoagulation usually not required	Early degeneration, especially in younger patients

occur. Any prosthetic valve can develop a perivalvular leak, that is, a leak exterior to the valve sewing ring, resulting in aortic or mitral regurgitation. In addition to hemodynamic effects, the turbulence from a perivalvular leak can cause red cell hemolysis. Even normally functioning prosthetic valves can cause hemolysis in some patients. The mechanical portion of a prosthetic valve may clot or otherwise malfunction. The long-term durability of mechanical valves has been well documented, but the durability of bioprosthetic porcine valves is not established, and many appear to degenerate, especially in younger patients.

All prosthetic valves carry a risk of thromboembolism. Valves in the aortic position are less likely to cause emboli than valves in the mitral position. Bioprosthetic valves are less likely to cause emboli than mechanical valves; however, a patient with a high embolic risk (for example, atrial fibrillation, markedly dilated left atrium, previous history of peripheral emboli, or documented intracardiac thrombus) requires chronic anticoagulation despite the presence of a porcine valve. All prosthetic valves are prone to develop endocarditis, and vigorous endocarditis prophylaxis should be administered prior to dental, GI, or GU surgery.

REFERENCES

Dalen JE, Alpert JS (eds): Valvular Heart Disease. Boston, Little, Brown and Company, 1981.

Devereau RB, Perloff JK, Reicheck N, Josephson ME: Mitral valve prolapse. Circulation 54:3, 1976.

Morganroth J, Perloff JK, Zeldis SM, Dunkman WB: Acute severe aortic regurgitation. Ann Intern Med 87:223, 1977.

Rahimtoola SH: Valvular heart disease: A perspective. J Am Coll Cardiol 1:199, 1983.

Ross J: Left ventricular function and the timing of surgical treatment in valvular heart disease. Ann Intern Med 94:498, 1981.

Selzer A: Changing aspects of the natural history of valvular aortic stenosis. N Engl J Med 317:91–98, 1987.

Shulman ST, et al: Prevention of rheumatic fever. Circulation 70:1118A, 1984.

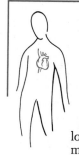

7

PULMONARY HEART DISEASE
(See also Chapter 19)

The normal pulmonary vasculature provides very low resistance to blood flow. However, when pulmonary hypertension occurs, right ventricular hypertrophy, dilation, and failure may develop. Pulmonary arterial hypertension results when there is increased flow in the pulmonary vasculature, when elevated pulmonary venous pressure is reflected back to the pulmonary arteries, or when the caliber of the pulmonary vasculature is decreased by either vasospasm or physical destruction. Pulmonary heart disease (cor pulmonale) occurs when pulmonary arterial pressure is elevated secondary to dysfunction of the lungs and its vasculature and produces right heart failure.

In primary pulmonary hypertension, intimal thickening of the pulmonary arteries and arterioles occurs with a characteristic "onion skin" vascular lesion. It occurs more frequently in women than in men. The pulmonary vascular resistance and pulmonary arterial pressure become markedly elevated. Left atrial and pulmonary capillary wedge pressures are normal, but right ventricular and right atrial pressures increase. The cardiac output may be normal or low, and the heart is unable to increase cardiac output with exercise. Functional tricuspid regurgitation may occur. Most patients become symptomatic late in the course of the disease. Fatigue and weakness are universal. Because of the low, fixed cardiac output, exertional syncope may result, which is an ominous sign; these patients may experience sudden cardiac death.

Secondary pulmonary hypertension can result from several etiologies. Pulmonary venous hypertension secondary to mitral stenosis often results in a "reactive" pulmonary arterial vasoconstriction, increasing pulmonary vascular resistance and causing pulmonary hypertension. The cause of this reactive pulmonary hypertension is unclear, but upon relief of the mitral stenosis and decline of the pulmonary venous pressure, it usually disappears. Various forms of congenital heart disease can result in pulmonary arterial hypertension, and many (for example, ventricular septal defect) are not reversible once present. Pulmonary parenchymal diseases such as chronic obstructive pulmonary disease, restrictive lung disease, pneumoconiosis, and sarcoidosis can lead to pulmonary heart disease. Pulmonary vascular diseases such as recurrent pulmonary embolism and scleroderma can result in pulmonary hypertension. In addition, patients with disorders of their chest wall and muscles of respiration which lead to hypoventilation, such as kyphoscoliosis or sleep apnea syndrome, can develop right heart failure.

Acute pulmonary edema can occur in apparently normal patients exposed to the hypoxia of high altitudes. The precise mechanism is unclear, but these patients tend to have an exaggerated vasoconstrictive response of the pulmonary arterioles to hypoxia. This syndrome responds very quickly to oxygen administration.

Chronic obstructive pulmonary disease (COPD) is the most common cause of pulmonary heart disease. Improvement of oxygenation is the best therapy for right heart failure associated with chronic lung disease. Aggressive treatment of the primary lung disorder with correction of hypoxia and acidosis decreases pulmonary vasoconstriction, and pulmonary hypertension improves.

Patients with pulmonary embolism may present with either dyspnea at rest, manifestations of pulmonary infarction including pleuritic pain, cough, and hemoptysis, circulatory collapse from massive pulmonary embolism, or unexplained exacerbation of known chronic heart failure. Large pulmonary emboli acutely elevate pulmonary arterial pressure and precipitate acute right heart failure.

8
CORONARY HEART DISEASE

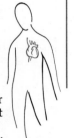

Coronary artery disease is the leading cause of death in the United States and most of the industrialized Western world. In contrast, it is much less common in Asia, the Near East, Africa, and South and Central America. Inexplicably, death from coronary heart disease has declined in the United States since the late 1960's.

ATHEROSCLEROSIS

Atherosclerosis is a thickening and hardening of medium-size and larger arteries with narrowing of the arterial lumen by atherosclerotic plaques. Its cause is multifactorial. Preventable risk factors, genetic susceptibility, local arterial and hemodynamic factors, and sex influence the development of atherosclerosis.

The fatty streak, consisting of lipids and lipoid proteins, located in the intima of the vessel with the overlying endothelium intact, is the earliest form of atherosclerosis. This yellow fatty streak seen in childhood is not necessarily a precursor of adult atherosclerosis and occurs in populations in which atherosclerosis is uncommon; it is presumably reversible at this stage. Around age 25, in populations in which atherosclerosis is common, the fibrous plaque begins to develop. It is white, elevated, and may compromise the arterial lumen. Reversibility is questionable when fibrous tissue and intimal proliferation are present. In more advanced stages, deposition of fibrin and platelets and necrosis of tissue with growth of new vessels may occur. Cholesterol, calcification, and hemorrhage within the atherosclerotic plaque form complicated plaques. The intimal surface may ulcerate, thrombose, and occlude the vessel. Mechanical, chemical, or immunological injury that begins with the fatty streak may cause progression of the atherosclerotic lesion. Different arteries appear to have different degrees of susceptibility to atherosclerotic lesions; the coronary arteries are particularly susceptible, mostly within the first 6 cm of origin. Plaques tend to occur at arterial bifurcations, possibly due to the turbulent flow in these areas.

Atherosclerotic lesions in the coronary arteries may be detected during life by coronary arteriography (Fig. 8–1). When a radiopaque contrast agent is injected into a coronary artery, atherosclerotic plaques appear as narrowings in the column of contrast as it travels down the artery. Narrowing of vessels is described as a per cent diameter narrowing. Lesions >50 per cent are probably hemodynamically significant, causing approximately 75 per cent narrowing of cross-sectional area, while lesions > 75 per cent are definitely significant, producing 95 per cent cross-sectional narrowing. The gradation of obstruction at coronary angiography is approximate and often underestimates the actual degree of obstruction. Complete obstruction of a vessel at angiography is usually represented by a stump, the distal portion of the vessel often opacified via collateral circulation.

RISK FACTORS (Table 8–1)

Several risk factors for the development of coronary artery disease have been identified by epidemiological studies. The more risk factors present in any individual patient, the greater the likelihood that he will develop coronary artery disease. However, there is no absolute correlation between risk factors and incidence of coronary disease. Mortality from coronary artery disease is much higher in males than in females, and females lag behind males in coronary artery disease deaths by approximately 10 years. Coronary disease mortality tends to equalize in men and women at age 50, possibly related to higher risk in women after menopause or the elimination of higher-risk males at an earlier age.

Treatment of even mild hypertension (diastolic pressure 90 to 104 mm Hg) reduces mortality from both stroke and myocardial infarction, implying not only

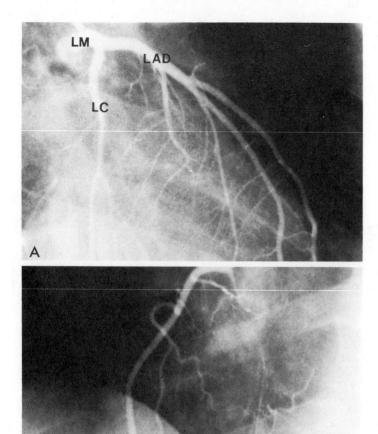

FIGURE 8–1. *A,* Normal left coronary arteriogram in the right anterior oblique projection. LM = Left main coronary artery; LAD = left anterior descending coronary artery; LC = left circumflex coronary artery. *B,* Normal right coronary arteriogram in the left anterior oblique projection. PDA = Posterior descending artery.

TABLE 8–1. RISK FACTORS FOR CORONARY ARTERY DISEASE

Nonmodifiable risk factors
  Older age
  Male sex
  Family history
Modifiable, independent risk factors
  Hypertension
  Hypercholesterolemia (LDL)
  Smoking
  Glucose intolerance
Other possible factors (may not be independent of the above)
  Obesity
  Sedentary lifestyle
  Oral contraceptives

an association but a causative role for hypertension. Elevations in both systolic and diastolic blood pressure are associated with an increased risk. There is no distinct blood pressure value below which risk suddenly becomes low; that is, over a wide range of blood pressures, the higher the blood pressure, the higher the risk.

The higher the serum cholesterol, the higher the risk of coronary disease, even within the usually accepted "normal" cholesterol values of Americans. The low density lipoprotein (LDL) fraction of total cholesterol is directly associated with the risk of atherosclerosis, and the high density lipoprotein (HDL) fraction appears to be inversely related to the incidence of atherosclerosis. HDL levels are higher in women than in men at all age levels. They are increased by regular exercise and are reduced in diabetes mellitus. The serum triglyceride level is a weaker risk factor and may not be independent when adjusted for obesity or glucose intolerance. Recent evidence implies that modifications in serum cholesterol may lead to an improvement in risk. Dietary modification to lower serum cholesterol seems prudent both in asymptomatic patients with an elevated or high normal cholesterol (greater than 200 mg/dl) and in patients with known coronary artery disease. Drug treatment to effect reduction in serum cholesterol should probably be reserved for patients with well-defined hypercholesterolemia. (See Chapter 62.)

NONATHEROSCLEROTIC CAUSES OF CORONARY ARTERY OBSTRUCTION

Although uncommon, there are several nonatherosclerotic causes of coronary artery obstruction. Emboli to coronary arteries can occur in infective endocarditis, from mural thrombi in the left atrium or ventricle, from prosthetic valves, from cardiac myxomas, or associated with cardiopulmonary bypass or coronary arteriography. Trauma to coronary arteries can be associated with both penetrating and nonpenetrating injuries. Various forms of arteritis (syphilis, polyarteritis nodosa, Takayasu's disease, disseminated lupus erythematosus, and rheumatoid arthritis) can affect the coronary arteries. The mucocutaneous lymph node syndrome (Kawasaki's disease) presents as a febrile illness in a child usually below the age of 10. Multiple organ systems can develop vasculitis, but the most significant feature is a vasculitis involving intima, media, and adventitia of the coronary arteries that results in aneurysm and sometimes thrombus formation. Mortality is 1 to 2 per cent secondary to complications from coronary arterial involvement.

Dissection of the aorta involving the coronary arteries or dissection of the coronary arteries themselves may occur in patients with connective tissue abnormalities of the aorta (for example, Marfan's syndrome). In situ thrombosis may occur in certain rare disorders (for example, polycythemia vera, thrombocytosis, or disseminated intravascular coagulation). Spasm of the coronary artery (Prinzmetal's angina, discussed later) is another nonatherosclerotic cause of coronary obstruction.

NONOBSTRUCTIVE CAUSES OF ISCHEMIC HEART DISEASE

Situations associated with increased left ventricular pressure and wall tension, a decrease in diastolic perfusion pressure, and/or an increase in left ventricular mass (for example, aortic stenosis) may cause myocardial ischemia by altering the balance of oxygen supply and demand. In addition, conditions in which substrate delivery is decreased (for example, hypotension, anemia, and carbon monoxide poisoning) may cause myocardial ischemia, especially if pre-existing coronary lesions are present.

A syndrome of myocardial infarction with angiographically normal coronary arteries exists. Approximately 2 per cent of patients with myocardial infarction demonstrate no obstructive lesions on coronary arteriography. These patients tend to be young, have a low incidence of coronary risk factors, and often have no history of angina pectoris prior to infarction. The prognosis for survival after the acute event is usually good. The cause is unknown, but possible etiologies include coronary emboli, coronary artery spasm, coronary artery disease in smaller vessels beyond the resolution of coronary arteriography, and coronary arterial thrombosis with recanalization.

PATHOPHYSIOLOGY OF ISCHEMIC HEART DISEASE

The manifestations of ischemic heart disease occur when the oxygen demand to the heart exceeds the oxygen supply. The most common cause of this imbalance is fixed obstruction within a coronary artery. Normally the arterioles regulate the blood flow to any particular area of the heart, and the more proximal epicardial "conductance" vessels, in the absence of a fixed or dynamic obstruction, do not restrict the flow. Once stenosis of 50 per cent or greater occurs in a conductance coronary artery, the vessel is unable to increase its flow sufficiently to maintain perfusion under conditions of increased demand despite the full dilation of the more distal arterioles. In addition to fixed obstruction, transient or "dynamic" obstruction of the conductance vessels may also occur. The caliber of these larger vessels can be altered by factors that are incompletely understood, and spasm of a localized area may decrease blood supply transiently to an area of the heart (variant or Prinzmetal's angina). Coronary artery spasm with or without the coexistent fixed coronary obstructive lesions may cause angina pectoris because of a temporary decrease in oxygen supply rather than any increase in oxygen demand.

Occasionally oxygen demand can exceed oxygen supply despite normal coronary arteries; the classic example is aortic stenosis when the hypertrophied muscle and increased wall tension increase oxygen demand, but increased intramural pressure and decreased aortic pressure decrease diastolic coronary artery flow and oxygen supply.

Ischemia affects the metabolism of cardiac cells, which can alter contractile and electrical functions. The inability to perform oxidative phosphorylation and generate high-energy compounds results in abnormal systolic myocardial contraction and also defects of diastolic compliance (relaxation). Dysfunction can be transient, for example, only after exercise-induced ischemia, or permanent, such as with myocardial infarction. Decreased compliance requires increased pressure to fill the heart to any given end-diastolic volume and accounts for the need to elevate somewhat the left ventricular filling pressure in order to maintain cardiac filling in patients with ischemic heart disease. The loss of cellular integrity allows release of enzymes (serum glutamic-oxalacetic transaminase, lactate dehydrogenase, and creatine kinase) into the blood that are used clinically to detect the presence of myocardial infarction. Electrical changes occur owing to altered ion transport across the cell membrane. Serious arrhythmias, most frequently ventricular tachycardia and fibrillation, are common.

The time during which ischemia is reversible is clinically important, since interventions exist that may restore flow to myocardium distal to an acute occlusion. Reperfusion after complete occlusion of less than 15 to 20 minutes salvages most if not all of the ischemic tissue. However, longer periods of occlusion cause increased amounts of myocardium to remain irreversibly necrotic. After approximately four to six hours of occlusion, reperfusion salvages very little tissue.

In humans, collateral circulation (small vessels that course from a nonobstructed coronary system to the distal portion of an obstructed system) slowly develops as flow is gradually diminished by fixed coronary obstruction. Collateral flow does provide some perfusion to an ischemic vascular bed, but the adequacy of this perfusion is questionable, especially under periods of increased demand (for example, exercise). Collateral flow does not develop acutely after sudden obstruction of blood flow.

ANGINA PECTORIS

Angina pectoris is chest discomfort caused by transient myocardial ischemia without necrosis, usually resulting from the inability of atherosclerotic arteries to increase myocardial blood flow under conditions of increased demand. Coronary spasm may occur either alone or in the presence of fixed coronary obstruction and reduces flow without an increase in demand. Angina pectoris is considered stable when there exists a chronic course of predictable exertional chest pain and unstable if a change in chronic angina consisting of increased frequency, duration, or severity occurs. The onset of new angina, or angina occurring at rest or with minimal exertion, or angina awakening the patient from sleep is considered unstable. Unstable angina pectoris has also been termed preinfarction angina, crescendo angina, acute coronary insufficiency, and intermediate coronary syndrome and usually requires hospital admission to exclude an acute myocardial infarction (Table 8–2).

The patient's history is crucial in the diagnosis of

TABLE 8–2. ANGINA PECTORIS

TYPE OF ANGINA	TYPICAL PATIENT CHARACTERISTICS	PATTERN	COMPLICATIONS	ECG	ANGIOGRAPHY	THERAPY
Stable	Older Male > female Coronary risk factors	Stable, unchanging pattern of aggravation and relief; exertional, lasts <10 minutes	Usually none	Baseline ECG often demonstrates nonspecific ST-T changes or evidence of old MI but can be normal; ST depression or T wave inversion may occur with pain	Fixed obstructive coronary lesions	Nitrates Beta blockers Calcium blockers
Unstable	Same as above	Markedly increased frequency; prolonged, severe episodes; rest angina, nocturnal angina	Can lead to MI or ischemic arrhythmias	Same as stable angina; ST elevation occasionally occurs with pain	Fixed lesions (although coronary spasm can contribute)	Same as above Hospitalization Consider intra-aortic balloon pump, angiography, revascularization
Variant (atypical or Prinzmetal's)	Younger Male ≅ female Lack of coronary risk factors	Typically severe pain at rest, can be provoked with exertion in a few cases; often early morning pattern	Syncope from tachyarrhythmias, heart block during pain; MI on rare occasions	Baseline ECG often normal; typically ST elevation with pain, although ST depression and T wave inversion also occur	Spontaneous or ergonovine-induced spasm in a normal vessel or at a region of a fixed but often nonstenotic lesion	Calcium blockers Nitrates Avoid beta blockers

angina pectoris (see Table 2–2). Even if coronary artery disease is known to exist anatomically, e.g., by arteriography, the functional significance of these lesions must be assessed from the patient's history of chest pain. The pattern of precipitation by exertion and disappearance with rest is one of the most characteristic features of angina pectoris. The pain or discomfort is often located in the left precordium or midchest directly under the sternum. It is sometimes not considered pain by the patient but described as pressure, burning, tightness, or fullness; the classic gesture is a clenched fist over the chest. The pain may appear over the period of a few seconds or minutes and disappears gradually in the same manner. It is usually not sharp or knifelike and does not occur suddenly at full intensity or leave abruptly. It lasts between one-half minute and approximately 20 minutes. Ischemic pain that lasts longer suggests myocardial necrosis. Typical angina is relieved with nitroglycerin or rest over a period of 30 seconds to several minutes. Immediate relief (within a few seconds), incomplete relief, or relief 20 to 30 minutes after sublingual nitroglycerin is not typical of angina pectoris. The pain may radiate to the neck, jaw, epigastrium, shoulder, and arms, most frequently the left arm. Pain localized to the left inframammary area is less characteristic. Chest wall tenderness is usually not present. Common precipitating factors are brisk walking, climbing stairs, using the hands above the head (for example, shaving, hair combing), emotional upset, exposure to cold, and a large meal. Redistribution of intravascular volume at night may cause angina decubitus, that is, angina occurring with the supine position. Existence of precipitating causes such as anemia, thyrotoxicosis, infection, aortic stenosis, arrhythmias, and hypertension should be excluded. Weakness, dyspnea, nausea,

pallor, and diaphoresis may occur with the pain. Many patients misinterpret the sensation as "gas," and belching is not uncommon.

Findings on physical examination are nonspecific. An S_4 gallop is often present but may only be heard during an episode of acute ischemia (decreased diastolic compliance with ischemia). Likewise, a murmur of papillary muscle dysfunction may occur only with ischemia. When myocardial ischemia is not present at rest, exercise tests may unmask ECG evidence of ischemia (see Stress Testing in Chapter 2). Thallium perfusion scintigraphy or exercise radionuclide ventriculography increases the sensitivity and specificity of exercise testing, particularly in patients with abnormal baseline electrocardiograms because of digitalis, pre-existing nonspecific ST-T wave changes, or left bundle branch block. Exercise echocardiography has become practical with two-dimensional echo techniques and may reveal regional wall motion abnormality during or immediately after exercise. In addition to its diagnostic role, the treadmill exercise test is important to assess the functional capacity and prognosis of patients with known coronary artery disease.

If the patient presents with pain of unknown origin, exercise testing may be useful diagnostically, but only after rest and medication have relieved the pain and an acute myocardial infarction has been excluded. Patients with rest pain or particularly severe anginal syndromes should not undergo exercise testing but instead should proceed directly to coronary angiography after stabilization. Patients who present with unstable angina have a higher percentage of left main and severe three-vessel disease than patients with chronic, stable angina.

The natural history of stable angina pectoris is variable, and several years may pass in some patients without the development of unstable angina or myocardial infarction. The most important factors to judge prognosis are measures of left ventricular function, the number of vessels containing significantly stenotic lesions, and exercise tolerance. Patients with significant left main coronary artery stenoses have a poor prognosis and are considered for surgery on the basis of their anatomy alone.

The indications for coronary angiography are discussed in Chapter 3. For patients in whom the differentiation of coronary artery disease from noncoronary causes of chest pain cannot be made despite a careful history and noninvasive evaluation, coronary arteriography may be the only means to exclude or establish the diagnosis of coronary artery disease. In addition, for patients in whom coronary artery spasm is suspected, the administration of ergonovine at cardiac catheterization may exclude or confirm that diagnosis. When ischemic pain is refractory to medical management, surgery very effectively eliminates pain (Table 8–3). Because specific subgroups of patients may demonstrate increased survival from coronary bypass surgery, some physicians recommend coronary angiography for any patient with known or suspected coronary artery disease in order to exclude left main or certain subsets of three-vessel coronary artery disease. Since this practice subjects many patients to the risk (albeit small) of coronary angiography, most physicians select patients for coronary angiography from subgroups at particularly high risk for having left main or three-vessel coronary artery disease, for example, patients with recurrent chest pain after myocardial infarction (especially subendocardial myocardial infarction), patients with poor exercise performance (positive test in first two stages or 6 minutes of exercise), and patients presenting with an unstable pattern of angina pectoris. Using these high-risk subgroups as a guide to selecting patients for catheterization, few patients with left main coronary artery stenosis would be missed. Many physicians also catheterize any young patient (below age 40) who presents with significant angina or myocardial infarction and any patient resuscitated from cardiac arrest. The ability of coronary artery bypass surgery to prolong life in many other subgroups of patients with coronary artery disease, particularly those patients who are asymptomatic or have mild degrees of angina, is unproven.

Some patients, especially diabetics, may have "silent" ischemia, that is, episodes of ischemia, well-documented by ECG, imaging, or echo techniques, unassociated with chest discomfort. This lack of an anginal "warning system" may result from autonomic nervous system abnormalities and may be dangerous, since severe ischemia can occur without the patient's realizing that he needs to stop his activity. Some patients may manifest symptoms of ischemia as dyspnea rather than chest discomfort (angina-equivalent dyspnea).

Medical Management of Angina

Angina is treated by decreasing myocardial oxygen demand or increasing oxygen supply. Certain general

TABLE 8–3. INDICATIONS FOR CORONARY REVASCULARIZATION

1. Relief of moderate to severe, significantly disabling stable angina in patients refractory or intolerant to medical management
2. Relief of unstable angina in patients refractory or intolerant to medical management; performed preferably after the patient is stable and pain-free, but can be done emergently if necessary
3. Improved survival in less symptomatic patients with left main coronary arterial stenosis and possibly certain subsets of three-vessel disease (for example, those with poor functional capacity or moderate left ventricular dysfunction)
4. Reperfusion during acute myocardial infarction to preserve myocardium (controversial; usually involves angioplasty rather than surgery)

measures may be helpful. Avoiding situations that may increase oxygen demand (for example, cold weather, particularly large meals, and excessive exercise) may be effective. Control of hypertension and correction of other exacerbating conditions such as anemia, infection, hypoxia, and thyrotoxicosis are necessary. Cigarette smoking should be stopped. Treatment of congestive heart failure decreases oxygen consumption and improves oxygen delivery. After physical training under supervised programs the patient may be able to perform tasks with a lower heart rate–blood pressure product and less angina. Whether exercise increases collateral circulation and oxygen delivery is controversial.

The most time-honored antianginal medication is nitroglycerin (Table 8–4), a smooth muscle relaxant of both systemic arteries and veins, although it affects veins predominantly. A decrease in venous return to the heart decreases preload, decreases left ventricular volume, and subsequently reduces wall tension and afterload. These hemodynamic effects are also of value in treating congestive heart failure. In addition, nitroglycerin dilates the larger conductance coronary arteries and probably also the collateral vessels, thus directly increasing blood supply to ischemic myocardium. The reduction in ventricular diastolic pressure brought about by nitrates may lower resistance to coronary blood flow within the myocardium during diastole.

Beta-adrenergic receptor blockade (Tables 8–5 and 8–6) slows the resting heart rate, blunts the increase in heart rate with exercise, and decreases myocardial contractility, all of which decrease oxygen consumption. In addition, beta-blocking drugs are useful antihypertensive agents and may reduce cardiac afterload in such patients. Beta-adrenergic receptors can be divided into beta-1 and beta-2 subgroups. The beta-1 receptors mediate the cardiac actions of the sympathetic nervous system, whereas beta-2 receptors promote the glycogenolysis induced by catecholamines, vasodilation of peripheral blood vessels, and dilation of pulmonary bronchi. Therefore, beta blockers that have predominantly beta-1 rather than beta-2 sympathetic antagonism (e.g., atenolol and metoprolol) may be more useful in treating patients with bronchospastic pulmonary disease, chronic obstructive pulmonary disease, diabetes, and peripheral vascular

TABLE 8–4. NITRATE PREPARATIONS FOR ANGINA

PREPARATION		INDICATION	ONSET*	DURATION*	USUAL DOSE	SIDE EFFECTS
Sublingual nitroglycerin		Acute anginal episodes; prophylaxis before specific activity	2 min	30 min	0.3-0.6 (usually 0.4) mg; can be repeated at 5-min intervals; if pain unrelieved after three doses patient is usually instructed to seek medical attention	Headache (tolerance may develop in 1-2 weeks) Flushing Tachycardia Dizziness Postural hypotension
Topical nitroglycerin 2% nitroglycerin ointment		Angina prophylaxis	15 min	4-6 hr (can be wiped off if side effects occur)	1-2 inches q6h; bedtime doses are useful	Same as above Messy
Sustained release transdermal			—	24 hr	q24h; dose depends on preparation	Variable drug levels and tolerance to nitrate effects have been reported; contact dermatitis
IV nitroglycerin		Unstable, severe angina	Almost immediately	Effects gone 5-10 min after infusion is stopped	Continuous infusion; initially 10 μg/min, titrate upward at 5-min intervals to desired hemodynamic effect	Hypotension
Long-acting (e.g., isosorbide dinitrate)	sublingual	Angina prophylaxis	5-10 min	1-3 hr	2.5-10 mg q2-3h	Same as above Ischemia may occur upon abrupt withdrawal
	oral		15-20 min	4-6 hr	10-40 mg q3-6h (efficacy of long-acting nitrates administered q8-12h is questionable)	

*Varies widely

disease. However, selective beta-1 blockade is only relative, and at higher doses (for example, above 100 mg a day of metoprolol) the selectivity may be lost. Hydrophilic beta blockers, for example atenolol and nadolol, have relatively long half-lives, can be administered once daily, and tend not to penetrate into the central nervous system, which may produce fewer neurological side effects such as mental depression and sleep disturbances. Thus, side effects attributed to one beta blocker may be eliminated by switching to another. Pindolol has mild intrinsic sympathomimetic activity in addition to its beta receptor–blocking activity; that is, it acts as a beta-receptor agonist as well as antagonist. Theoretically, some of the effects at rest of beta-receptor blockade such as slow heart rate or peripheral vasoconstriction may be less prominent even though the sympathetic effects of exercise are blocked. Any clinical advantage to beta-receptor blockers with intrinsic sympathomimetic activity is not clear at present.

Calcium ions play critical roles in myocardial contraction, coronary vascular smooth muscle constriction, and the genesis of the cardiac action potential. Slow channel blocking agents are effective antianginal drugs when used either alone or in combination with beta-receptor adrenergic blockers or nitrates (Table 8–7). All three agents (nifedipine, verapamil, and diltiazem) decrease myocardial contractility and relax coronary and peripheral vascular smooth muscle. Ver-

apamil and diltiazem may decrease the sinus nodal discharge rate and prolong atrioventricular (AV) nodal conduction time. In clinically used doses, nifedipine is the most potent vasodilator of the three and exerts little action on myocardial contractility or on the sinus and AV nodes. Therefore, nifedipine decreases afterload via peripheral vasodilation and increases coronary blood flow via coronary vasodilation. The antianginal effect of verapamil may be related to both coronary artery vasodilation and decreased myocardial contractility, thus decreasing oxygen demand. The effects on contractility and sinus rate are minimized owing to reflex sympathetic stimulation in response to the peripheral vasodilation. Verapamil and the other calcium antagonists enhance left ventricular diastolic filling (increase compliance); this is not an effect of simple beta blockade. In general, the effects of diltiazem are intermediate between those of verapamil and nifedipine.

Since the mechanisms of action of nitrates, beta-receptor blockers, and calcium antagonists differ, combination therapy of two or three of these drugs might be effective. Nitrates can cause reflex tachycardia that beta-receptor blockers can prevent. Therefore, in a patient with no contraindication to beta-receptor blockade, the combination of nitrates and a beta-receptor blocker may be beneficial antianginal therapy. In addition, the combination of beta blockers and calcium channel blockers is often useful if unwanted electrophysiological or inotropic side effects do not become manifest. Patients with particularly severe angina may require one drug from each of the three classes.

A patient experiencing a marked increase in the frequency or severity of angina, the new onset of angina at rest, or nocturnal angina should be admitted to an intensive care unit, placed at bed rest, and sedated if necessary. If not contraindicated, beta blockade should be instituted. Sublingual nitroglycerin and oral and/or cutaneous nitrates should be administered, and if pain recurs, intravenous nitroglycerin can be initiated. In addition, nifedipine may be useful in the patient with no hypotension or with congestive heart failure. Verapamil or diltiazem may be useful in the patient with no heart failure. Most patients having unstable angina experience relief of chest pain with this approach and further evaluation, probably including coronary arteriography, can be undertaken when the patient is stable and pain-free. If angina does not abate with aggressive medical therapy, the patient should be considered for early coronary arteriography and for angioplasty or bypass surgery. An intra-aortic balloon pump may be inserted before cardiac catheterization or surgery to improve diastolic filling of the coronary arteries and to decrease afterload. Many patients experience pain relief once balloon counterpulsation is initiated despite refractoriness to intensive medical antianginal therapy.

NONMEDICAL MANAGEMENT OF ANGINA PECTORIS

Coronary artery bypass surgery is useful to relieve angina unresponsive to medical therapy and, in cer-

TABLE 8–5. BETA BLOCKING AGENTS

DRUG	USUAL DOSAGE	BETA-1 CARDIO-SELECTIVE	INTRINSIC AGONIST ACTIVITY	HYDRO-PHILIC
Propranolol	Oral: 40-480 mg/day in 2-4 doses Intravenous: up to 0.10-0.15 mg/kg given as 1-mg increments at 3-5 minute intervals	–	–	low
Metoprolol	Oral: 50-100 mg twice a day	+	–	moderate
Nadolol	Oral: 40-160 mg once a day	–	–	high
Atenolol	Oral: 50-100 mg once a day	+	–	high
Timolol	Oral: 10-20 mg twice a day	–	–	moderate
Pindolol	Oral: 10-30 mg twice a day	–	+	moderate

+ = present
– = absent

TABLE 8–6. SIDE EFFECTS OF BETA BLOCKERS

Beta-2 blocking effects
  Bronchoconstriction
  Failure to initiate glycogenolysis in insulin-induced hypoglycemia
  Exacerbation of peripheral vascular disease
Other
  Exacerbation of congestive heart failure
  Bradycardia and heart block
  Ischemia upon abrupt withdrawal
  Fatigue, depression, impotence, nightmares

TABLE 8–7. CALCIUM ANTAGONISTS

	SINUS AND AV NODAL EFFECTS	NEGATIVE INOTROPIC EFFECTS	CORONARY AND PERIPHERAL VASODILATION	USUAL DOSE	SIDE EFFECTS
Nifedipine	0	0/+	+ + +	10-20 mg q6-8h	Hypotension Headache Dizziness Nausea Peripheral edema Reflex tachycardia with worsening of angina
Diltiazem	+ +	+	+ +	30-60 mg q6-8h	LV failure Bradycardia, AV block Hypotension Flushing
Verapamil	+ + +	+ +	+ +	80-120 mg q6-8h	LV failure Bradycardia, AV block Nausea Flushing Decreases excretion of digoxin by 30%

0 = none   + + = moderate effect
+ = mild effect   + + + = strong effect

tain subgroups, to prolong life. Coronary artery bypass surgery may be combined with aneurysmectomy in patients with refractory cardiac arrhythmias, congestive heart failure, or recurrent emboli due to a large ventricular aneurysm. Coronary artery bypass alone usually does not improve left ventricular function sufficiently to treat patients in whom congestive heart failure is the major manifestation of ischemic heart disease. Intractable, chronic ventricular arrhythmias also are not usually abolished by revascularization alone and require resection of the tachycardia focus.

Coronary artery bypass grafting most commonly involves harvesting saphenous veins from the legs to anastomose from the ascending aorta to the coronary artery at a site distal to the obstruction. The veins are reversed in direction to permit the flow of blood past the venous valves. As many major arterial branches as possible are grafted beyond significant obstructions. Internal mammary grafts demonstrate a superior long-term patency compared with saphenous grafts. Both the left and right internal mammary arteries may be dissected free and anastomosed to a coronary artery distal to its obstruction. The proximal take-off of the internal mammary artery remains intact from the subclavian artery. Internal mammary grafts are most commonly anastomosed to the left anterior descending coronary artery vessels. The distal coronary vessels must be at least 1 to 2 mm in diameter to accept a bypass graft, and the flow distal to the occlusion, determined at the time of coronary arteriography, should be sufficient to maintain flow in the grafts so that thrombosis is unlikely to occur. Left ventricular dysfunction increases the risk of surgery but does not necessarily contraindicate surgery if chest pain is refractory.

Perioperative mortality is approximately 0.7 per cent for those with normal left ventricular function and 1.8 per cent for those with abnormal ventricular function. Surgical mortality in patients with left main coronary artery disease is approximately 2.5 per cent, and if left ventricular function is abnormal, approaches 4 per cent. Surgical mortality increases with age, reaching 2 per cent in patients older than 65 years. The incidence of perioperative myocardial infarction is reported to be 5 to 10 per cent. Chest pain is completely relieved in approximately 65 per cent of patients, and significant improvement in pain occurs in an additional 25 per cent. The remaining patients are either not improved (5 per cent) or worse (5 per cent) after surgery. Approximately 2 to 4 per cent of patients per year have a recurrence of angina, due either to obstruction of the grafts or to progressive atherosclerosis in the native arteries. If angina recurs either early or late after surgery, repeat catheterization may be indicated if surgery or angioplasty is deemed necessary. Repeat operations carry a higher surgical risk and less successfully relieve pain.

Patients with one- or two-vessel coronary artery disease have relatively good survival with medical or surgical therapy as long as their clinical status is stable, and they usually can be followed medically until refractory angina appears. The role of coronary artery bypass grafting in patients with three-vessel coronary artery disease is more controversial, but a recent study suggests that patients with three-vessel coronary artery disease who have either no symptoms or stable angina pectoris have no higher mortality with medicine than with surgery as their initial therapy. These patients, however, represent a select subgroup of relatively stable patients with three-vessel disease; patients with three-vessel disease and poor functional capacity, judged either on the treadmill or by their inability to perform as much daily activity as they would like, may benefit from bypass grafting. In addition, some studies demonstrate a tendency toward improved survival with surgery in patients with three-vessel disease and moderate ventricular dysfunction.

Graft flow rates at the time of surgery can help predict graft closure. The average flow in a technically successful saphenous bypass graft is about 70 ml/min. Grafts in which the flow is less than 45 ml/min frequently occlude. Causes of poor graft flow include grafting to a vessel with a noncritical stenosis proximal to the graft anastomosis, a technically poor anastomosis, and poor distal run-off secondary to distal vessel disease. Graft patency rates at 6 to 12 months are 75 to 87 per cent; since most patients receive more than one graft, 84 to 95 per cent of patients have at least one patent graft. Internal mammary grafts have a much higher patency rate than saphenous grafts, and over 95 per cent are patent after one year. Low-dose aspirin therapy (325 mg qd or qod) may improve saphenous vein graft patency.

Percutaneous transluminal coronary angioplasty (PTCA) involves passing a balloon catheter into the coronary artery, positioning it across a stenotic lesion, and inflating the balloon with several atmospheres of pressure to dilate the stenosis. This procedure disrupts the intima, splits the atherosclerotic plaque, and often results in a small local dissection with relief of obstruction. Candidates for angioplasty have angina for which surgical revascularization would be recommended and discrete, relatively proximal stenoses in one or more coronary vessels. Studies demonstrate the feasibility of angioplasty on multiple lesions. Patients with left main coronary artery disease are not usually appropriate candidates for coronary angioplasty because a dissection in this vessel would jeopardize the majority of the myocardial blood flow. PTCA is successful (at least 25 to 50 per cent improvement in luminal diameter) in approximately 80 per cent of cases. In about 3 per cent of cases, coronary occlusion occurs and immediate coronary artery bypass grafting must be undertaken. Restenosis occurs in approximately 20 per cent of patients who initially have a good result, usually within the first six months. A second angioplasty is successful in many of these patients. The reported mortality from angioplasty ranges from 0.5 to 1 per cent (Table 8–8).

VARIANT ANGINA

In 1959 Prinzmetal described a syndrome of chest pain occurring unrelated to exertion and associated with ST segment elevation recorded on the ECG (see Table 8–2). The syndrome is often associated with cardiac arrhythmias, including ventricular fibrillation and heart block, and sudden death may occur. These episodes of angina more commonly occur between midnight and 8 a.m. Rarely, acute myocardial infarction results. Prinzmetal's angina appears to be due to spasm in the conductance portion of the coronary arteries, resulting in decreased oxygen delivery to the myocardium. Patients may have concomitant fixed obstructive lesions and therefore also experience angina with exertion. The classic electrocardiographic pattern of coronary spasm is localized ST elevation, although ST depression alone or T wave changes may occur. Coronary angiography during Prinzmetal's angina may reveal spasm at the site of a severe coronary atherosclerotic lesion, a mild atherosclerotic lesion, or a normal coronary artery. Patients with no or mild fixed coronary obstruction tend to have a more benign course than those with severe obstructions. The cause of coronary spasm is unknown. Provocative testing with ergonovine, an ergot alkaloid with alpha-adrenergic and serotoninergic effects, is a relatively sensitive and specific test for coronary artery spasm. Vessels prone to spasm appear to be supersensitive to its vasoconstrictive properties. When administered in incremental doses to a total of 0.05 to 0.4 mg intravenously, coronary artery spasm, chest pain, and ST elevation are provoked in susceptible individuals. Prolonged spasm with significant ischemia and serious arrhythmias is a potential hazard. Nitroglycerin may be injected directly into the coronary vasculature to quickly reverse the spasm if it is severe. Ergonovine testing generally is safe, especially if performed in the catheterization laboratory, but probably should not be done in patients who have flow-restricting coronary obstructions, and the drug should be administered in extremely low starting doses.

In patients with Prinzmetal's angina beta blockade may be detrimental by allowing unopposed alpha-adrenergic vasoconstriction. Calcium channel blockers are very effective in treating vasospastic angina, and their effects may be additive to that of nitrates, since the mechanism of action is different. Coronary artery bypass surgery or angioplasty is not helpful in patients with vasospasm and normal or nearly normal coronary arteries but may be useful in patients who have fixed significant stenoses.

ACUTE MYOCARDIAL INFARCTION

PATHOLOGY AND MECHANISM

Myocardial infarction refers to irreversible necrosis of myocardium. It usually results from thrombosis where there is pre-existing vessel wall injury or ruptured atherosclerotic plaque in a major coronary artery. Initially ischemia occurs and if severe and prolonged, myocardial infarction follows, the extent of which depends on the severity of the ischemia, the

TABLE 8–8. COMPARISON OF CORONARY ARTERY BYPASS GRAFTING (CABG) AND PERCUTANEOUS TRANSLUMINAL CORONARY ANGIOPLASTY (PTCA)

PTCA	CABG
Nonsurgical	Major surgery
Useful for proximal, discrete stenosis. Multiple vessels increase difficulty and risk. Lesions in some vessels (e.g., LAD) are more likely to be successfully dilated than others	Useful for multiple, more distal, and heavily calcified lesions as well as proximal, discrete lesions. Procedure of choice for left main stenosis
Risk of coronary artery dissection and emergency surgery	Risk of elective surgery
Can be done (although with some risk) in patients who are not surgical candidates	Patient must be a surgical candidate
May be faster in an emergency situation (e.g., acute MI)	Associated defects (aneurysm, valve dysfunction) may be addressed
Long-term results appear favorable if early restenosis does not occur	Long-term results good; graft potency better if internal mammary graft is used

area of muscle supplied by the obstructed coronary artery, the extent of collateral blood flow, and the oxygen demands of the tissue supplied by the artery. Myocardial infarction may be transmural, that is, involving the full thickness of the left ventricular wall, or nontransmural, involving only the subendocardium and adjacent myocardium. The electrocardiographic findings of "transmural" versus "subendocardial" infarction do not correlate well with the pathological extent of infarction. No gross pathological changes occur in the myocardium until approximately six hours after myocardial infarction, and even light microscopic findings until that time are subtle. The myocardium initially appears pale and slightly edematous and over the next few days changes color as exudate and neutrophil infiltration occur. Eight to ten days after infarction the myocardium in the region of the infarction thins as debris is removed by mononuclear cells, and granulation tissue forms that by three to four weeks extends through the necrotic tissue. Subsequently, a thin scar develops that becomes firm over a six-week interval.

Ninety per cent of transmural myocardial infarctions are associated with complete obstruction of a coronary artery, consisting of fresh thrombus superimposed on a critically stenotic lesion. Nontransmural myocardial infarctions frequently occur distal to severely stenotic but still patent arteries. Mechanisms by which thrombosis occurs in the region of atherosclerotic plaques may include changes in the atherosclerotic intima promoting thrombosis, hemorrhage into the atherosclerotic plaque, ulceration of the plaque with activation of clotting factors, platelet thrombi, or coronary spasm at the site of a plaque causing sludging of blood flow and deposition of platelets and fibrin. Reperfusion can be achieved in many cases using intracoronary or intravenous fibrinolytic agents; however, residual high-grade atherosclerotic lesions are usually present at the site of occlusion after thrombus dissolution.

CLINICAL PRESENTATION

Signs and symptoms of acute myocardial infarction are summarized in Tables 8–9 and 2–2. The usual patient with myocardial infarction has severe chest pain that lasts until treated. Some patients are discovered to have suffered a myocardial infarction by electrocardiography or noninvasive evaluation of left ventricular function without any clinical history of infarction. In many of these patients, when a very careful history is obtained, an episode can be identified that probably represents the myocardial infarction. However, some people, especially diabetics, have true "silent" myocardial infarctions.

The electrocardiogram in acute myocardial infarction is discussed in Chapter 3 (see Tables 3–4 and 3–5 and Fig. 3–5). The diagnosis of subendocardial infarction may be suspected from electrocardiographic ST and T wave changes but must be confirmed by enzyme determinations. There are no chest x-ray findings characteristic of myocardial infarction. The white blood cell count rises the first day after a myocardial infarction and returns to normal within a week; it usually peaks between 12,000 and 15,000 cells/cu mm. Acute phase reactants, such as the erythrocyte sedimentation rate, may be elevated. Several cardiac enzymes released into the blood (Fig. 8–2) are used to diagnose myocardial infarction. Creatine kinase MB (the fraction characteristic of cardiac muscle) is the

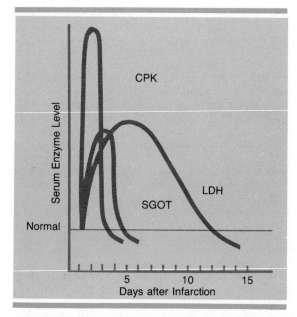

FIGURE 8–2. Typical time course for detection of enzymes released from the myocardium upon necrosis. CPK = Creatine kinase; SGOT = serum glutamic oxaloacetic transaminase; LDH = lactic dehydrogenase.

most sensitive and specific marker of myocardial necrosis, and an MB fraction exceeding 7 to 8 per cent is indicative of myocardial infarction even if the total CK is not greater than normal. Injury to skeletal muscle causes the skeletal muscle fraction (MM) of CK to rise. Other forms of injury to cardiac muscle, such as myocarditis, trauma, and cardiac surgery, may release significant amounts of creatine kinase MB fraction. Cardioversion and CPR usually do not elevate the MB function. Serum lactate dehydrogenase (LDH) may be fractionated into five isozymes. LDH_1 is principally from the heart, and if LDH_1 exceeds LDH_2, myocardial infarction is likely. LDH is sometimes useful in diagnosing myocardial infarction in a patient who presents several days after the event, when the creatine kinase has normalized. Hemolysis can raise LDH_1 activity, but LDH_2 also elevates and exceeds LDH_1. Liver and skeletal muscle contain mainly LDH_4 and LDH_5.

The use of infarct-avid scintigraphy has been discussed in Chapter 3. Echocardiography may demonstrate a segmental wall motion abnormality but cannot distinguish whether it is old or new.

MANAGEMENT OF MYOCARDIAL INFARCTION

Since approximately 50 per cent of patients who die from myocardial infarction do so within the first four hours after the onset of chest pain, often before they ever arrive at the hospital, the prehospital manage-

---

TABLE 8–9. SYMPTOMS AND SIGNS OF ACUTE MYOCARDIAL INFARCTION

Symptoms (see Table 2–2)
  Severe, prolonged chest pain, similar in quality to angina pectoris
  Nausea, vomiting
  Diaphoresis
  Shortness of breath
  Weakness
Signs
  Anxiety
  Elevated blood pressure (if shock not present)
  Tachycardia (may have bradycardia with inferior MI)
  Dyskinetic left ventricular impulse
  Small amplitude carotid pulses
  Soft heart sounds
  S_4 gallop
  Fixed or paradoxically split S_2
  Systolic murmur of papillary muscle dysfunction
  Loud systolic murmur with papillary muscle or ventricular septal rupture
  S_3 gallop and/or rales (congestive heart failure)
  Right ventricular S_3 gallop with jugular venous distention (right ventricular infarction)
  Signs of cardiogenic shock if > 40% of myocardium is infarcted
  Low-grade fever
  Pericardial friction rub (3rd-4th day, with transmural infarctions)
  Atrial or ventricular tachyarrhythmias, heart block

ment of myocardial infarction is important. Many large cities employ emergency medical technicians who can recognize the symptoms of myocardial infarction, initiate electrocardiographic monitoring, and treat ventricular tachyarrhythmias, terminating them with electrical defibrillation if necessary. Airway management, intravenous drug delivery, and cardiopulmonary resuscitation may be administered, if needed. Prehospital emergency cardiac care, especially the rapid treatment of life-threatening ventricular arrhythmias, improves both early and late survival from myocardial infarction.

The coronary intensive care unit allows continuous electrocardiographic and hemodynamic monitoring, delivery of intensive nursing care, and immediate treatment of arrhythmias or other problems. The advent of the coronary care unit has improved survival of patients with myocardial infarction mainly by reducing mortality from arrhythmias. Death from hemodynamic deterioration has been less preventable and accounts for most of the mortality in coronary care units. Future progress in this area will probably come from thrombolysis of acute coronary obstructions.

Any intervention to limit the size of evolving infarction must be performed within the first four to six hours of infarction, before cells become irreversibly damaged. The most promising techniques involve early reperfusion by either thrombolysis or coronary angioplasty or both. Most patients (85 to 90 per cent) with acute transmural myocardial infarction have complete obstruction of a coronary artery due to thrombosis in a region of high-grade atherosclerotic narrowing. Streptokinase and urokinase interact with plasminogen to produce plasmin, a proteolytic enzyme that degrades fibrin clots, producing systemic fibrinolytic effects. Tissue plasminogen activator is an enzyme that causes only limited conversion of plasminogen in the absence of fibrin, but when exposed to fibrin in a thrombus converts the entrapped plasminogen to plasmin, initiating local fibrinolysis with limited systemic effects. When a patient presents with ST segment elevation unresponsive to nitroglycerin (to rule out coronary spasm) within six hours after the onset of chest pain, streptokinase can be administered intravenously in a dose of 1.5 million units over 30 to 60 minutes. Tissue plasminogen activator dosage is not as clearly defined but consists of a total intravenous dose of 100 mg administered over three hours. Each is followed by heparin for two to five days. Tissue plasminogen activator may be somewhat more effective in lysing clots (65 to 70 per cent of patients) than IV streptokinase, and streptokinase can be given only once to any individual patient because of subsequent immune reactions. Intracoronary streptokinase administration results in increased thrombolytic efficacy. Both agents are associated with approximately the same incidence of bleeding complications (for example, approximately 0.5 per cent incidence of intracranial bleeding) and therefore should not be given to patients having any condition in which bleeding is likely to occur or would be particularly difficult to manage because of its lo-

TABLE 8–10. RELATIVE CONTRAINDICATIONS TO THROMBOLYTIC THERAPY IN ACUTE MYOCARDIAL INFARCTION

Recent (within 10 days) major surgery
Recent puncture of noncompressible vessels
Cerebrovascular disease
Recent gastrointestinal or genitourinary bleeding
Recent trauma
Prolonged cardiopulmonary resuscitation
Hypertension (systolic BP ≥180, diastolic BP ≥110 mm Hg)
Acute pericarditis
Subacute bacterial endocarditis
High likelihood of left heart thrombus, e.g., mitral stenosis with atrial fibrillation
Hemostatic defects, including those from severe renal or hepatic disease
Pregnancy
Diabetic hemorrhagic retinopathy
Oral anticoagulation
Advanced age

cation (Table 8–10). Coronary thrombolysis may be associated with reperfusion arrhythmias that include ventricular tachycardia or fibrillation. It is not known whether thrombolysis is more effective in salvaging myocardium than immediate coronary angioplasty, but administration of intravenous medications can be performed more quickly and does not require access to a cardiac catheterization laboratory. Electrocardiographic evidence of infarction usually still evolves. The time course of cardiac enzyme elevation is accelerated, thought to be evidence of wash-out of enzymes from the heart by reperfusion. Thus, even if reperfusion does not prevent infarction, it may salvage a portion of the myocardium in jeopardy. Any residual high-grade stenosis in the area of thrombosis can be dilated with coronary angioplasty at the time of thrombolytic infusion or approached with angioplasty or bypass surgery at a later date to prevent reocclusion (Fig. 8–3).

Some general principles in treating patients with uncomplicated myocardial infarction include sedation if necessary, a calm, quiet coronary care unit atmosphere, and control of pain to decrease patient anxiety, sympathetic drive, and myocardial oxygen demand. Morphine can be administered intravenously in doses of 2 to 8 mg repeated at intervals of 5 to 15 minutes until pain is relieved or drug side effects (e.g., hypotension, respiratory depression, nausea, vomiting, or vagal side effects such as bradycardia) appear. Small IV doses of atropine treat the vagomimetic side effects of morphine, and naloxone, 0.4 mg IV at 5-minute intervals to a maximal dosage of 1.2 mg, reverses respiratory depression if needed. After the acute severe pain is relieved, nitroglycerin can be used cautiously for recurrent angina, and chronic nitrate therapy may be initiated if angina persists. Oxygen can be omitted if the patient is not hypoxemic.

The patient with *uncomplicated* acute myocardial infarction should be confined to bed for the first 24 to 36 hours except for the use of a bedside commode. He

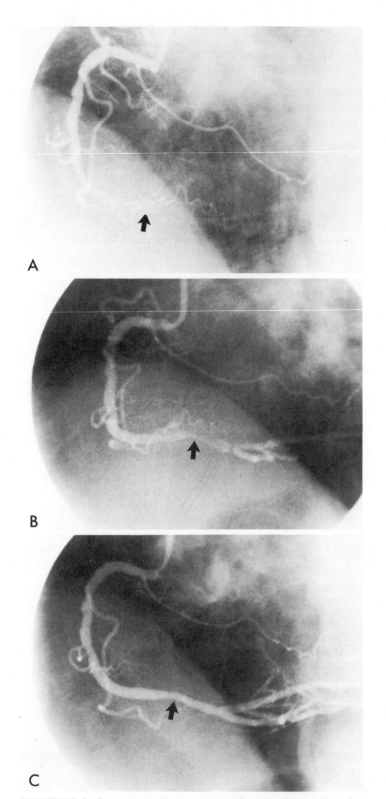

should then be allowed to sit up out of bed for short periods of time and can be transferred out of the coronary care unit after three days, since life-threatening arrhythmias are uncommon after 36 to 48 hours. Ambulation is usually begun on the fourth to fifth day and is increased progressively so that at discharge the patient is able to walk up a flight of stairs. Early mobilization increases the patient's psychological well-being, prevents deconditioning, and decreases the incidence of thromboembolism. Many patients require stool softeners or laxatives to avoid constipation and straining at stool. Nausea and vomiting either from the infarction or from drugs can be treated with a clear liquid diet. A gentle rectal examination in patients with acute myocardial infarction is not contraindicated.

The use of anticoagulation in acute myocardial infarction is controversial. If no contraindication exists, "minidose" heparin (5000 units subcutaneously every 8 to 12 hours) may decrease the incidence of deep vein thrombosis and possibly systemic embolization. In patients who have a high risk of embolization, such as those who have a ventricular aneurysm with thrombus, past or present thrombophlebitis, or previous systemic or pulmonary embolism, full systemic anticoagulation may be reasonable in the absence of contraindications. Systemic anticoagulation is contraindicated in patients with postinfarction pericarditis because of the risk of hemorrhage into the pericardium. Minidose heparin is stopped once the patient is ambulating, usually two to three days prior to hospital discharge. Continuation of systemic anticoagulation depends upon the original indication for therapy. Patients with left ventricular thrombi after myocardial infarction are at high risk of embolization, and this risk may be decreased by prophylactic systemic anticoagulation for about six months.

In patients with known or suspected acute myocardial infarction, lidocaine effectively prevents many ventricular tachyarrhythmias. If it is administered appropriately, side effects such as confusion, dizziness, and paresthesias can be minimized. Both the loading and maintenance doses of lidocaine should be decreased in elderly patients, patients with congestive heart failure, and patients with liver disease. Although ventricular fibrillation should be easily treatable in the coronary care unit, many physicians feel that, given the safety of lidocaine, it is advisable to attempt to prevent ventricular fibrillation rather than have to electrically defibrillate it should it occur. However, the prophylactic administration of lidocaine in this situation is still somewhat controversial. The dose of lidocaine should be increased if ventricular tachycardia occurs. Suppression of premature ventricular contractions (PVC's) is questionable, since their value (including "R on T" PVC's) as prognostic indicators or precipitators of the onset of more severe arrhythmias has not been proved. Prophylactic lidocaine is continued for approximately 48 hours, after which the risk of ventricular tachyarrhythmias is reduced.

Patients with uncomplicated courses are usually discharged from the hospital between 7 and 12 days following infarction. The patient should gradually in-

FIGURE 8–3. Restoration of coronary blood flow after thrombolytic therapy and coronary angioplasty. *A,* Complete occlusion of the distal right coronary artery (*arrow*). *B,* Same view of the right coronary artery after thrombolysis with streptokinase, showing reperfusion but persistence of a high-grade lesion. *C,* Improvement on the luminal diameter after coronary angioplasty of the persistent lesion. (Courtesy of James C. Dillon, M.D.)

crease his activity but avoid isometric exercise (for example, lifting weights) and get adequate rest. He should be instructed in the use of sublingual nitroglycerin even if he requires no antianginal therapy on discharge. Many centers have formal rehabilitation programs in which the patient is supervised during activity and his electrocardiogram monitored. Exercise testing in patients after acute myocardial infarction helps determine what level of activity can be performed safely at home and is useful to identify those patients at high risk for recurrent events by finding a positive ST response and/or chest pain within the first two stages of exercise. Some physicians perform a limited treadmill test (the heart rate achieved is only 70 per cent of predicted maximum) just prior to hospital discharge, whereas others prefer a more normal stress test protocol six weeks after infarction. Patients who are considered at high risk on the basis of their clinical course and/or treadmill exercise test results may subsequently undergo coronary arteriography.

Large studies with timolol, propranolol, and metoprolol have shown that these agents reduce overall mortality, sudden death, and/or reinfarction if administered to patients after their first infarction. This outcome may be related to anti-ischemic effects, antianginal effects, or some other unknown effect of these drugs. Patients with contraindications to beta-adrenergic receptor blockers, especially heart failure, cannot receive these drugs; unfortunately, these patients are at the highest risk for a recurrent event. In addition, the mortality in the group of patients that can tolerate these drugs is relatively small, and thus even a 50 per cent reduction in sudden death or reinfarction does not represent a large proportion of the total patients. Despite these reservations, many physicians feel that it is advisable to administer beta-adrenergic receptor blocking drugs in doses sufficient to blunt the heart rate response to exercise in postinfarction patients who have no contraindication, and the drug should be continued for approximately two years. The administration of aspirin, 325 mg qd or qod, appears to decrease the incidence of reinfarction (and also possibly the occurrence of a first myocardial infarction).

Early ventricular tachyarrhythmias during acute myocardial infarction (i.e., first 24 to 48 hours) do not warrant chronic antiarrhythmic drug therapy. Patients with chronic complex ventricular ectopy, especially ventricular tachycardia, are at particularly high risk for sudden death in the first six months to a year after myocardial infarction. However, chronic antiarrhythmic therapy has not been shown to decrease mortality in patients with premature ventricular contractions (PVC's) or ventricular tachycardia after infarction. Therefore, at the present time there appears to be no compelling evidence to support treating patients with uniform or multiform PVC's or pairs of PVC's after infarction. In patients with episodes of nonsustained ventricular tachycardia after infarction, it seems prudent to treat with a type I antiarrhythmic agent (i.e., quinidine) to eliminate the spontaneous tachycardia, although there are no objective data to support this approach.

COMPLICATIONS OF MYOCARDIAL INFARCTION AND THEIR MANAGEMENT (Table 8–11)

In patients who develop mild congestive heart failure with pulmonary congestion during acute myocardial infarction, administration of a diuretic may be sufficient therapy. Indications for hemodynamic monitoring are listed in Table 8–12. Hemodynamic monitoring allows measurement of left ventricular filling pressures (pulmonary capillary wedge pressure) and cardiac output, and the calculation of systemic vascular resistance. Patients with myocardial infarction may be grouped into subsets based on these measurements (Table 8–13). When the normal cardiac index (approximately 2.5 to 3.6 L/min/sq m) is reduced to 1.8 to 2.2 L/min/sq m, hypoperfusion occurs; shock occurs at levels less than 1.8 L/min/sq m. The normal pulmonary capillary wedge pressure is 10 to 12 mm Hg, but the optimum wedge pressure in a patient with acute myocardial infarction and a relatively noncompliant ventricle is usually 14 to 18 mm Hg.

Even if pharmacological therapy or intra-aortic balloon counterpulsation provides temporary improvement, patients with cardiogenic shock due to cardiac muscle destruction have a poor prognosis. However, patients who have cardiogenic shock secondary to surgically correctable mechanical factors—for example, acute mitral regurgitation or acquired ventricular septal defect—have a somewhat more favorable outlook. Myocardial revascularization improves an occasional patient with episodes of profound but reversible myocardial ischemia producing hypotension and shock.

Patients with right ventricular infarction may present with hypotension or shock (due to decreased cardiac output) and signs of right ventricular failure. The lungs are clear if left ventricular failure or pre-existing pulmonary disease is not present. Tricuspid insufficiency may occur. Fluid administration to raise right ventricular filling pressures and augment left ventricular filling reverses the shock and hypotension, even when jugular venous distention and other manifestations of systemic congestion exist. Right ventricular infarction is relatively common in patients with inferior myocardial infarction and is sometimes difficult to differentiate from cardiac tamponade. Most patients with right ventricular infarction do well, and their long-term prognosis depends on the extent of left ventricular infarction.

Approximately 20 per cent of patients extend their myocardial infarction within the first five days after infarction. The extension may be associated with recurrent chest pain that is sometimes difficult to distinguish from post–myocardial infarction pericarditis or recurrent angina. Continued angina and extension of myocardial infarction are usually unfavorable signs and may be indications for catheterization.

Many patients upon presentation with an acute myocardial infarction have mild to moderate hypertension because of pain, anxiety, and sometimes mild congestive heart failure. With relief of pain and treatment of heart failure, hypertension usually disappears

TABLE 8–11. COMPLICATIONS OF ACUTE MYOCARDIAL INFARCTION

COMPLICATION	CLINICAL PRESENTATION	PROGNOSIS/NATURAL HISTORY	THERAPY
Congestive heart failure	Symptoms and signs of heart failure (Table 2–4) or cardiogenic shock (Table 4–8)	Severe heart failure carries a poor prognosis unless a surgically correctable condition (e.g., ruptured ventricular septum or papillary muscle) is present	See Table 4–6 See Table 4–9
Right ventricular infarction	Usually accompanies inferior MI; hypotension with clear lungs, distended jugular veins; cardiac output low, left ventricular filling pressure low; ST elevation in leads V_1 and V_{4R}	Depends on extent of LV infarction	Fluid administration
Extension of infarction	Recurrent chest pain after initial stabilization; further ECG changes and enzyme increases	Guarded prognosis	Pain relief Antianginal therapy Consider early catheterization and revascularization
Hypertension	Often related to pain or early heart failure May exacerbate angina	Usually responds to therapy	Pain relief Sedation Treat heart failure Antianginal vasodilators If BP elevation remains significant, may need to use IV nitroprusside
Papillary muscle rupture	Acute onset of congestive heart failure, usually 1-7 days after infarction; loud systolic murmur along left sternal border; echo may show flail mitral valve; Swan-Ganz shows no left-to-right shunt, often large v waves in wedge position	If patient can be stabilized, surgery can be postponed 4-6 weeks to allow healing of infarct; if not, early surgery may be life-saving although risky	Afterload reduction Diuretics Digitalis Intra-aortic balloon pump Surgery
Ventricular septal rupture	Same presentation and murmur as above; contrast echo may demonstrate defect; Swan-Ganz shows left-to-right shunt	Same as above	Same as above
Ventricular aneurysm	Often no symptoms, but may be associated with congestive heart failure, arrhythmias, or emboli; persistent ST elevation on ECG; visualized on two-dimensional echo	Does not rupture; prognosis depends on amount of remaining myocardium and complications (heart failure, arrhythmias, emboli)	Anticoagulation if mural thrombus is detected on echo or angiography Antiarrhythmic therapy as needed Treat heart failure Surgery if symptoms persist
Cardiac rupture	Acute onset of cardiogenic shock, usually within first week after infarction; occasional patient will wall off the rupture within the pericardial space (pseudoaneurysm) and survive; pseudoaneurysm detectable on echocardiography	Usually rapid death	Emergency surgery if possible
Deep venous thrombosis, pulmonary embolism	Warm, tender edematous extremity; with pulmonary embolus dyspnea, tachycardia, hypoxia, pleuritic chest pain, hemoptysis; cardiovascular collapse with massive pulmonary embolus; diagnosis via venogram, lung scan, and/or pulmonary angiogram	Recurrent emboli if therapy is not instituted	Anticoagulation with heparin, then warfarin

TABLE 8–11. COMPLICATIONS OF ACUTE MYOCARDIAL INFARCTION (*continued*)

COMPLICATION	CLINICAL PRESENTATION	PROGNOSIS/NATURAL HISTORY	THERAPY
Pericarditis early after MI	Chest pain sharper than that of infarction, usually located to the left of sternum toward the apex, not responsive to nitrates, better when sitting up and leaning forward, occurs within a week after a transmural infarction; causes sinus tachycardia, diffuse ST elevation on ECG	Self-limited	Aspirin Nonsteroidal anti-inflammatory agents Avoid anticoagulation
Postinfarction (Dressler's) syndrome	Occurs 2 weeks to 9 months after MI; pericarditis, pericardial effusion, pleural effusion, pneumonitis, fever	Self-limited, but multiple recurrences may occur	Aspirin Nonsteroidal anti-inflammatory agents If above unsuccessful, short course of steroids
Arrhythmias (see also Chapter 9) a. Ventricular tachycardia or fibrillation	Syncope, cardiac arrest; dizziness, palpitations	Immediate prognosis depends on prompt termination; long-term prognosis depends on LV function and chronic recurrences	Cardioversion/defibrillation of sustained arrhythmias Lidocaine or other antiarrhythmic agent
b. Atrial fibrillation/flutter	Increased angina, heart failure, palpitations Associated with pericarditis, pulmonary embolus, and heart failure	Prognosis depends on underlying condition	Digitalis ± quinidine Cardioversion
c. Heart block and conduction disturbances	Dizziness, syncope, increased angina, or heart failure if symptoms occur	Natural history depends on type of block present (see text); long-term prognosis depends on LV function	Indications for pacing in text

within a few hours. However, sustained or severe blood pressure elevation should be treated vigorously to decrease myocardial oxygen consumption. Intravenous nitroprusside may be employed, and oral agents can be substituted as needed.

Rupture of an entire papillary muscle due to myocardial infarction is usually rapidly fatal owing to massive mitral regurgitation. However, rupture of one head of a papillary muscle may be tolerated for a period of time, allowing for diagnostic evaluation and surgical correction. Some form of papillary muscle rupture occurs in less than 5 per cent of patients with acute infarction. Papillary muscle dysfunction is more common than rupture and occurs when ischemia interferes with contraction of the papillary muscles and normal coaptation of the mitral valve leaflets. The degree of mitral regurgitation from papillary muscle dysfunction is usually less than that caused by papillary muscle rupture. Acute medical therapy for papillary muscle rupture may require inotropic agents, diuretics, vasodilators, or intra-aortic balloon counterpulsation. If the patient can be stabilized and weaned from balloon counterpulsation, surgical mitral valve replacement may be attempted four to six weeks after infarction when infarct scar formation is advanced. However, if hemodynamic stabilization cannot be obtained or requires intra-aortic balloon counterpulsation, early mitral valve replacement should be done.

Rupture of the ventricular septum develops in about 1 per cent of myocardial infarctions and results in marked biventricular failure. It may occur with both inferior and anterior infarctions. It is associated with a holosystolic murmur along the left sternal border and is often difficult to differentiate from acute mitral insufficiency. A thrill is more common with ventricular septal defects than with acute mitral regurgitation. Right heart (Swan-Ganz) catheterization may be necessary to distinguish acute ventricular septal rupture from mitral regurgitation by detecting an oxygen step-up between the right atrium and right ventricle. Increased pulmonary vascularity due to the left-to-right shunt may be seen on chest x-ray. Two-dimensional echocardiography can occasionally visualize the ven-

TABLE 8–12. INDICATIONS FOR HEMODYNAMIC MONITORING IN ACUTE MYOCARDIAL INFARCTION

Hypotension unresponsive to simple measures such as treatment of bradycardia or fluid administration

Moderate or severe LV failure despite diuretic therapy, especially if blood pressure is unstable

Unexplained features such as persistent sinus tachycardia, cyanosis, hypoxia, or acidosis

Suspicion of ventricular septal defect, rupture of papillary muscle, or cardiac tamponade

TABLE 8–13. HEMODYNAMIC INDICES IN ACUTE MYOCARDIAL INFARCTION

CLINICAL STATE	CARDIAC OUTPUT	PULMONIC CAPILLARY WEDGE	LIKELY CAUSE	THERAPY
No pulmonary congestion, normal systemic perfusion	normal	normal	Uncomplicated MI	None
Pulmonary congestion, normal perfusion	normal	↑	Mild to moderate heart failure	Diuretics, preload reduction
Hypoperfusion but no pulmonary congestion	↓	↓	Volume depletion RV infarction	Fluids
Hypoperfusion and pulmonary congestion	↓	↑	Severe heart failure, cardiogenic shock	Diuretics, preload and afterload reduction, inotropic agents, intra-aortic balloon pump

tricular septal defect, but more often a septal aneurysm is demonstrated, with the ventricular septal defect presumably located in the apex of the aneurysm. Contrast echocardiography may define the defect. Surgical mortality is highest within the first month after infarction, but if ventricular failure is severe, surgery must be undertaken early.

A ventricular aneurysm is a localized area of thin, scarred myocardium that protrudes beyond and distorts the ventricular cavity. Ventricular aneurysms may develop within days of myocardial infarction and gradually stretch, thin, and enlarge over weeks to months. The wall motion of an aneurysm on ventriculography may be akinetic or dyskinetic. Large aneurysms may contribute to congestive heart failure by expanding during systole, decreasing the efficiency of blood expulsion. Most patients with ventricular aneurysms are asymptomatic. True ventricular aneurysms do not rupture. Mural thrombi commonly form in the ventricular aneurysms and appear less likely to embolize in patients who are systemically anticoagulated. Ventricular aneurysms often are associated with ventricular tachyarrhythmias originating from the edge of the aneurysm. Patients with ventricular aneurysms usually demonstrate electrocardiographic evidence of transmural myocardial infarction, and in many cases there is persistent ST segment elevation in the ECG leads with vectors pointing toward the aneurysm. Occasionally, the aneurysm can distort the cardiac silhouette enough to be visible on chest x-ray, appearing as a localized bulge on the surface of the left ventricle, sometimes with calcium in the wall. Two-dimensional echocardiography reliably delineates ventricular aneurysms. Refractory congestive heart failure or recurrent systemic emboli despite anticoagulation warrant aneurysmectomy. Aneurysmectomy alone is usually in-

sufficient to control recurrent refractory ventricular tachyarrhythmias, which require combined aneurysmectomy and resection.

Rupture of the ventricular free wall is usually rapidly fatal. Rupture usually occurs within the first five days following transmural infarction. The patient's initial course may be uneventful until the abrupt occurrence of cardiogenic shock and rapid progression to death. Rare patients have survived after successful pericardiocentesis and emergency surgical repair. Occasionally, the course is less acute and blood is walled off within the pericardial space, giving rise to a pseudoaneurysm. In contrast to true aneurysms, pseudoaneurysms may rupture and require immediate intervention. The diagnosis of pseudoaneurysm is usually made by echocardiography, showing a narrow-based communication between the ventricular cavity and pseudoaneurysm, whereas the communication between a true aneurysm and the ventricular cavity is wide.

Early ambulation and the use of prophylactic subcutaneous minidose heparin have decreased the risk of venous thrombosis and pulmonary embolism after myocardial infarction. If deep vein thrombophlebitis or pulmonary embolism is documented, intravenous heparin should be administered for at least seven days and followed by two to six months of oral warfarin. Patients who have systemic emboli also should be treated with intravenous heparin followed by two to six months of oral warfarin. Consideration should be given to removal of peripheral emboli by surgical embolectomy.

Pericarditis occurs in 7 to 15 per cent of patients within the first week after acute infarction, most frequently in those with transmural infarction of at least moderate size. If a pericardial friction rub is heard, the diagnosis is confirmed, but many patients do not have audible rubs. It is sometimes difficult to distinguish the pain of pericarditis from that of angina pectoris. Anticoagulation should be avoided in patients with active pericarditis because of the risk of developing hemorrhagic tamponade. Sinus tachycardia occurring with pericarditis must be differentiated from other causes of sinus tachycardia, for example, hemodynamic deterioration.

A small number of patients, probably less than 5 per cent, develop a late postinfarction syndrome (Dressler's syndrome) consisting of pericarditis, pericardial effusion, pleural effusion, and sometimes fever. The etiology is unknown but may be immunological. Multiple recurrences sometimes occur. If salicylates or nonsteroidal anti-inflammatory agents are not sufficient, short courses of high-dose corticosteroids provide relief.

ARRHYTHMIAS IN ACUTE MYOCARDIAL INFARCTION

Arrhythmias occurring in patients with acute myocardial infarction should be treated if they cause hemodynamic compromise, augment myocardial oxygen requirements, or predispose to more malignant arrhythmias such as sustained ventricular tachycardia or fibrillation. Some rhythms not ordinarily deleterious may decrease cardiac output in patients who have stiff, noncompliant ventricles by the loss of atrioventricular synchrony. Reversible causes of ventricular ectopy—for example, digitalis excess or metabolic abnormalities—should be considered.

Ventricular premature complexes (PVC's) are very common following acute myocardial infarction. Unless very frequent, they usually cause no problem in themselves but may be forerunners of more serious sustained ventricular tachyarrhythmias. The danger of "R on T" PVC's (a ventricular premature complex occurring during the T wave of a previous complex) has probably been overestimated in the past and probably does not carry any worse prognosis than any other PVC. Even though PVC's are sometimes considered a warning arrhythmia for the subsequent development of ventricular tachycardia or fibrillation, many episodes of ventricular fibrillation occur without any warning arrhythmia. Approximately half of those patients who develop ventricular fibrillation have no warning PVC's, while half of those with warning PVC's do not develop a sustained ventricular tachyarrhythmia. If ventricular tachycardia is not suppressed by lidocaine, intravenous procainamide can be substituted or added to lidocaine. Intravenous bretylium may also be useful to prevent recurrence of sustained or symptomatic ventricular tachyarrhythmias. High-dose or multiple antiarrhythmic drug therapy in patients with simple ventricular ectopy is not warranted. If sustained ventricular tachycardia occurs, it should be cardioverted immediately if hemodynamic compromise occurs. If it is well-tolerated for a short period of time, a limited trial of lidocaine for termi-

nation may be tried. The patient with acute infarction should not be allowed to continue having sustained ventricular tachycardia for a prolonged period of time. Ventricular fibrillation occurs in 2 to 3 per cent of hospitalized patients with acute myocardial infarction and should be promptly defibrillated with 200 to 400 joules.

Ventricular tachycardia and fibrillation during the first 36 to 48 hours of acute myocardial infarction do not carry the same prognosis as when they occur later in the recovery period. These early ventricular arrhythmias appear to be due to acute ischemia and do not necessitate long-term, chronic antiarrhythmic therapy. On the other hand, ventricular tachycardia and fibrillation occurring more than 48 hours after infarction are probably due to different electrophysiological mechanisms and may be forerunners of severe, chronic arrhythmias.

Accelerated idioventricular rhythm with rates of 60 to 100 beats/minute occurs commonly during the acute infarction period. This arrhythmia probably does not increase the incidence of more rapid ventricular tachyarrhythmias. It usually does not cause hemodynamic deterioration unless cardiovascular compensation is tenuous and dependent upon normal atrioventricular synchrony. If the rhythm appears to be affecting hemodynamics adversely or increasing the incidence of ventricular ectopy, it can be treated by lidocaine or in some instances by accelerating the sinus rate slightly with atropine or atrial pacing.

Sinus tachycardia that persists in a patient with acute infarction after relief of pain and anxiety is often due to inability of the ventricle to maintain an adequate stroke volume. It is not only a sign of hemodynamic impairment in some patients but also is detrimental by increasing oxygen demand. Pericarditis, pulmonary embolus, and fever commonly cause sinus tachycardia. The treatment of sinus tachycardia is directed at the underlying cause.

Sinus bradycardia often occurs early after acute inferior myocardial infarction and may be related to ischemia of the sinus node or abnormally elevated vagal tone. If asymptomatic and hemodynamically tolerated, it should not be treated. If it creates symptoms, atropine or temporary pacing may be required.

A rapid ventricular response caused by atrial flutter or fibrillation should be treated vigorously because of the increase in myocardial oxygen consumption. If the ventricular rate cannot be slowed pharmacologically, early electrical cardioversion should be considered. The treatment of atrial tachyarrhythmias is discussed in Chapter 9. Atrial tachyarrhythmias also may be features of pericarditis or pulmonary embolus.

First-degree AV block requires no therapy; if digitalis is thought to be the etiology, it should be discontinued. Second-degree AV block of the Mobitz type I (Wenckebach) type (see Chapter 9) is common in patients with inferior myocardial infarction due to increased vagal tone and/or ischemic involvement of the AV node. It is usually temporary and, if asymptomatic, requires no therapy. If hemodynamic compromise occurs, atropine is effective; if sustained improvement does not occur, temporary pacing may be needed. Type I AV block usually does not lead to high-degree AV block; if it does, the ventricular escape is junctional and usually reliable at reasonable rates (40 to 60 per minute). Mobitz type II second-degree AV block is an indication for prophylactic pacing. Type I second-degree AV block is more common with inferior and type II more common with anterior myocardial infarctions.

A prophylactic temporary pacemaker is usually recommended for any patient who has developed complete heart block with an acute myocardial infarction, especially if the infarction is anterior and the site of the heart block likely to be in the His-Purkinje system. Complete AV block should be differentiated from AV dissociation, common in inferior myocardial infarction due to sinus bradycardia with junctional escape or accelerated junctional rhythms (see Chapter 9).

The occurrence of new intraventricular conduction defects (left or right bundle branch block, or right bundle branch block with left anterior or posterior fascicular block) is associated with anterior more often than inferior infarction. The prognosis of these patients, as of those with Mobitz II second-degree heart block, is poor, reflecting the extensive infarction rather than the conduction disturbance itself. Even though temporary pacing in these patients has not been shown definitely to increase survival, it is still reasonable to insert a temporary pacemaker if heart block is deemed likely. Therefore, temporary prophylactic pacing is indicated in patients who develop new bifascicular block. Temporary prophylactic pacing in patients who have a new right bundle branch block and a normal axis or a new left bundle branch block with a normal PR interval is more controversial. Patients who have pre-existing left or right bundle branch block with or without axis deviation probably do not require prophylactic pacing with acute infarction (see Table 9–6).

REFERENCES

CASS principal investigators and their associates: Coronary artery surgery study (CASS): A randomized trial of coronary artery bypass surgery. Survival data. Circulation 68:939, 1983.

Cohn PF: The role of noninvasive cardiac testing after an uncomplicated myocardial infarction. N Engl J Med 309:90, 1983.

DeBusk RF, Blomqvist CG, Kouchoukos NT, et al: Identification and treatment of low-risk patients after acute myocardial infarction and coronary-artery bypass graft surgery. N Engl J Med 314:161–166, 1986.

Detre K, Holubkov R, Kelsey S, et al: Percutaneous transluminal coronary angioplasty in 1985–1986 and 1977–1981: The National Heart, Lung, and Blood Institute Registry. N Engl J Med 5:265–270, 1988.

Forrester JS, Diamond G, Chatterjee K, Swan HJC: Medical therapy of acute myocardial infarction by application of hemodynamic subsets. N Engl J Med 295:1356, 1404, 1976.

Gruentzig AR, King III SB, Schlumpf M, Siegenthaler W: Long-term follow-up after percutaneous transluminal coronary angioplasty: The early Zurich experience. N Engl J Med 316:1127–1135, 1987.

Hillis LD, Braunwald E: Coronary artery spasm. N Engl J Med 299:695, 1978.

Hillis LD, Braunwald E: Myocardial ischemia. N Engl J Med 296:971, 1977.

Koch-Weser J: β-adrenergic blockade for survivors of acute myocardial infarction. N Engl J Med 310:830, 1984.

National Cholesterol Education Program Expert Panel: Report of the National Cholesterol Education Program Expert Panel on detection, evaluation, and treatment of high blood cholesterol in adults. Arch Intern Med 148:36–69, 1988.

Parker JO: Drug therapy: Nitrate therapy in stable angina pectoris. N Engl J Med 316:1635–1642, 1987.

Rahimtoola SH: Coronary bypass surgery for chronic angina 1981. Circulation 65:225, 1982.

Ross R: The pathogenesis of atherosclerosis—an update. N Engl J Med 314:488–500, 1986.

Silverman KJ, Grossman W: Angina pectoris: Natural history and strategies for evaluation and management. N Engl J Med 310:1712, 1984.

Smith B, Kennety JW: Thrombolysis in the treatment of acute transmural myocardial infarction. Ann Intern Med 106:414, 1987.

Topol EJ, Califf RM, George BS, et al: A randomized trial of immediate versus delayed elective angioplasty after intravenous tissue plasminogen activator in acute myocardial infarction. N Engl J Med 317:581–588, 1987.

9

ARRHYTHMIAS

MECHANISMS OF ARRHYTHMOGENESIS

If a microelectrode is introduced into a single myocardial cell, an action potential (Fig. 9–1) can be recorded by measuring the potential difference between the inside and the outside of the cell (inside negative). The resting membrane potential of a normal Purkinje cell is approximately −90 millivolts (mv) with respect to the outside of the cell. When the membrane potential is depolarized to a certain threshold level, an action potential occurs with a rapid upstroke (phase 0); a return toward zero from the initial overshoot or early rapid repolarization (phase 1); a plateau

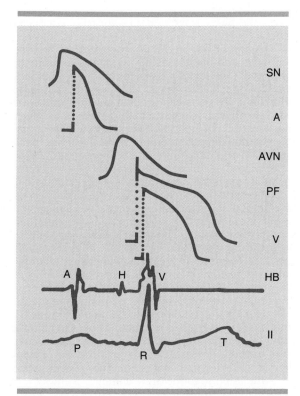

FIGURE 9–1. Action potentials recorded from different tissues in the heart remounted with a His bundle recording and scalar ECG from a patient to illustrate the timing during a single cardiac cycle. SN = Sinus nodal potential; A = atrial muscle potential; AVN = atrioventricular nodal potential; PF = Purkinje fiber potential; V = ventricular muscle potential; HB = His bundle recording; II = lead II. The A-H interval measured in the His bundle recording approximates AV nodal conduction time, and the H-V interval approximates His-Purkinje system conduction time.

(phase 2); final rapid repolarization (phase 3); and resting membrane potential and diastolic depolarization (phase 4). The normal resting potential is maintained by the active (i.e., energy-requiring) exclusion of sodium and the accumulation of potassium inside the cell. Phase 0 or rapid depolarization is due chiefly to the opening of the sarcolemmal channels to sodium entrance in atrial and ventricular muscle and cells in the His-Purkinje system. Calcium is important in the maintenance of the action potential plateau of fast sodium channel–dependent cells and in the generation of the action potential upstroke in slow calcium channel–dependent cells such as those of the sinus and AV nodes. Phase 3 is mediated chiefly by an outward potassium current, and the membrane returns to its negative resting potential during electrical diastole.

Automaticity is a property of some cardiac tissues to undergo gradual phase 4 depolarization spontaneously until threshold potential is reached and the cell initiates an action potential that is propagated from one cell to another. Normal automaticity is present in sinus nodal tissue, some atrial and junc-

tional tissues, the bundle branches, and Purkinje fibers. The sinus node discharges more rapidly than the other cells and is the normal pacemaker of the heart. *Conduction* is the propagation of a cardiac impulse and is most closely influenced by the amplitude and upstroke velocity of phase 0 of the action potential. *Refractoriness* is a property of cardiac tissue during which a stimulus occurring soon after a previous action potential fails to elicit another normal action potential; it is most closely related to the duration of phase 3 of the cardiac action potential in most cardiac tissues.

Although the autonomic nervous system may affect atrial and ventricular tissue to a small extent, the most prominent autonomic effects are observed on the sinus and the AV nodes. Sympathetic stimulation increases the rate of automaticity and increases conduction velocity, whereas parasympathetic (vagal) activation does the opposite. Baroreceptors in the carotid sinus, located at the bifurcation of the internal and external carotid arteries, activate the vagus nerve when blood pressure increases and reflexively decrease heart rate and AV nodal conduction velocity.

The genesis of cardiac arrhythmias is divided into disorders of impulse formation, disorders of impulse conduction, and combinations of the two (Table 9–1). One cannot unequivocally determine the mechanism for most clinical arrhythmias, but each arrhythmia may be most consistent with or best explained by a particular electrophysiological mechanism. Disorders of impulse formation are defined as an inappropriate discharge rate of the normal pacemaker (the sinus node) or abnormal discharge from an ectopic pacemaker that usurps control of the atrial or ventricular rhythm. An appropriate discharge rate of a subsidiary pacemaker that takes control of the cardiac rhythm upon sinus slowing is termed an escape beat or rhythm, whereas an inappropriately rapid discharge rate of an ectopic pacemaker (abnormally increased automaticity) that usurps control of the cardiac rhythm from the normal sinus mechanism is termed

TABLE 9–1. GENESIS OF ARRHYTHMIAS

DISORDERS OF IMPULSE FORMATION	DISORDERS OF IMPULSE CONDUCTION
Atrial tachycardia with or without block	Heart block
Accelerated junctional rhythm	Re-entry:
Nonparoxysmal AV junctional tachycardia	Paroxysmal supraventricular tachycardia
Accelerated idioventricular rhythm	Reciprocating tachycardia using an accessory pathway (Wolff-Parkinson-White syndrome)
Parasystole	Atrial flutter
	Atrial fibrillation
	Ventricular tachycardia
	Ventricular flutter
	Ventricular fibrillation
EITHER OR BOTH	
Atrial, junctional, or ventricular extrasystoles	
Flutter and fibrillation	
Ventricular tachycardia	

a premature complex or, when they occur in a series, an ectopic tachycardia.

Parasystole may be due to abnormal automaticity and refers to an ectopic atrial or ventricular pacemaker that discharges regularly and appears to be protected from the dominant cardiac rhythm by entrance block into the area of abnormal automaticity. Therefore, it may depolarize the myocardium intermittently whenever the myocardium is excitable, but it is not discharged by the dominant rhythm. In addition, the abnormal focus may demonstrate variable degrees of exit block, and thus it may intermittently fail to depolarize the myocardium at a time when it would be expected. Characteristic features of ventricular parasystole are (1) premature ventricular parasystolic complexes that are a multiple of a common integer, (2) coupling of premature ventricular complexes to preceding normally conducted complexes that is not fixed, as it often is in patients with nonparasystolic premature ventricular complexes, and (3) periodic fusion complexes be-

tween the parasystolic and the normally conducted beat.

Disorders of impulse conduction include conduction delay and block that can result in bradyarrhythmias and provide the basis for re-entry, the most common mechanism responsible for arrhythmia development. Re-entry can occur at any level of the cardiac electrical system, including the sinus node, the atria, the AV node, the His-Purkinje system, and the ventricular myocardium. Normal cardiac tissue has relative homogeneity of conduction and refractoriness so that an impulse starts at the sinus node, travels through the atrium, the AV node, and the His-Purkinje system, and terminates with organized depolarization of ventricular muscle. Once all tissues are depolarized, the impulse is extinguished because there is no further tissue to activate. However, a re-entrant or reciprocating rhythm can occur within various tissues if certain criteria are met, giving rise to a continuous reactivation of tissue and generating a tachycardia. For re-entry to occur (Fig. 9–2) there must be two functionally dissociated pathways, permitting the impulse to travel in one direction down one pathway but blocking it in the other pathway. Thus, the pathway with longer refractoriness may block a premature impulse traveling antegradely. The first pathway, having shorter refractoriness but slower conduction, conducts the impulse to the distal common pathway with a delay that permits it to travel retrogradely up the second pathway and find the proximal tissue re-excitable. If this circus movement continues, a tachycardia occurs.

APPROACH TO THE PATIENT WITH SUSPECTED OR CONFIRMED ARRHYTHMIAS

History-taking in patients with suspected or confirmed rhythm abnormalities should be aimed at detecting the presence of cardiac or noncardiac disease that may be linked causally to the genesis of a rhythm abnormality. Common symptoms that prompt patients with rhythm disturbances to consult a physician are palpitations, syncope, presyncope, and congestive heart failure. The ability of a patient to sense an irregular, slow, or rapid heart rhythm varies greatly; some patients are completely unaware of a marked arrhythmia whereas others feel every premature impulse. In addition, some patients may complain of palpitations when they have no detectable rhythm disturbance or merely sinus tachycardia. Dizziness is a common complaint in people with tachy- or bradyarrhythmias but also may be due to nonarrhythmic causes. Syncope refers to complete but transient loss of consciousness and also has a variety of causes (see Table 9–9). Exacerbation of congestive heart failure may occur with arrhythmias. If a patient senses palpitations, the physician should determine whether the patient senses a slow heart beat, a rapid heart beat, a regular or irregular heart beat, its rate, and whether the onset and termination of the palpitations are sudden or gradual.

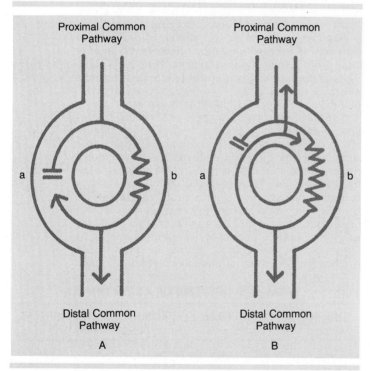

FIGURE 9–2. Mechanism of re-entry. Re-entry requires the presence of two separate pathways that join proximally and distally. Panel A illustrates a premature impulse that blocks antegradely in pathway a (double bars) but conducts down pathway b, albeit with a moderate conduction delay (serpentine arrow). The impulse attempts to return up pathway a but meets refractory tissue. In Panel B, a more premature impulse blocks earlier in pathway a and experiences more conduction delay in pathway b. This impulse finds pathway a recovered from its previous activation and returns retrogradely to the proximal common pathway. If able to again travel antegradely over pathway b, it would activate the distal common pathway prematurely. If this cycle were to continue, a circus movement or re-entrant tachycardia would result. For example, in AV nodal re-entrant tachycardia, the atrium represents the proximal common pathway and the His bundle represents the distal common pathway, with the re-entrant circuit located within the AV node.

The physical examination is useful to detect evidence of underlying cardiac disease. In addition, abnormalities of the pulse may be noted, and clues regarding AV dissociation during an arrhythmia may be detected (for example, intermittent cannon a waves in the jugular venous pulse or varying intensity of S_1 during a regular tachyarrhythmia).

The resting electrocardiogram may reveal the specific arrhythmia responsible for symptoms or give clues regarding a tachyarrhythmia; for example, short episodes of nonsustained ventricular tachycardia may be recorded in a patient who has presented with syncope or cardiac arrest due to a sustained ventricular tachycardia. In addition, indirect evidence may be obtained from the electrocardiogram which may suggest the etiology of the arrhythmia; for example, the presence of a delta wave should alert the physician to the possibility that a tachycardia due to Wolff-Parkinson-White syndrome may be present. The electrocardiogram may also provide evidence as to the etiology of the arrhythmia, such as the presence of ischemic heart disease documented by ECG evidence of myocardial infarction.

Long-term ambulatory electrocardiography (Holter monitoring) is an important tool for evaluating patients with suspected arrhythmias. It permits quantitation of arrhythmia frequency and complexity, correlation with the patient's symptoms, potential diagnosis of an unknown arrhythmia, and evaluation of the effect of antiarrhythmic therapy. It can record arrhythmias while patients are engaged in their normal daily activities. It can also document alterations in the QRS, ST, and T waves and may be useful in documenting pacemaker function or malfunction. Certain arrhythmias are common during prolonged ECG monitoring in normal patients and may be of no clinical significance. In many patients symptoms are very infrequent and difficult to detect even with prolonged electrocardiographic monitoring. Exercise testing can be used to precipitate arrhythmias in some patients. Patients with no demonstrable structural heart disease may have an increase in premature ventricular or atrial complexes with exercise. However, patients who have ischemic heart disease are more likely to have ventricular ectopy at lower heart rates and in the early recovery period.

Invasive electrophysiological procedures are useful and involve introducing catheter electrodes into the heart to record electrical activity from the atria, ventricles, and the His bundle, and to stimulate the atria or ventricles electrically. Supraventricular or ventricular tachycardias may be induced by programmed electrical stimulation. The test may be used diagnostically to determine whether a particular rhythm disorder exists or to determine the mechanism of a known arrhythmia. The test may also be used therapeutically to terminate a tachycardia or to determine the efficacy of drug or other therapy. Electrophysiological testing is important in patients with resistant tachyarrhythmias undergoing either surgical resection or ablation of a tachycardia focus or accessory pathway. Patients considered candidates for antitachycardia pacemaker devices or implantable cardioverter-defibrillator devices require electrophysiological study to confirm the mechanism and origin of the arrhythmia and the efficacy and safety of this mode of therapy. Electrophysiological study may be helpful in identifying patients with sinus nodal dysfunction or atrioventricular block.

Esophageal electrocardiography is sometimes a useful noninvasive technique to diagnose arrhythmias. An electrode introduced approximately 40 cm from the patient's nares into the esophagus can record an atrial electrogram and often can be used to pace the atrium.

Autonomic and pharmacological manipulations sometimes aid in diagnosing arrhythmias. Most commonly, vagal maneuvers (e.g., carotid sinus massage), edrophonium, or administration of verapamil to slow AV nodal conduction is used. Carotid sinus massage is performed with the patient in the supine position. With the neck hyperextended and the head turned away from the side being tested, light pressure is applied to the carotid impulse at the angle of the jaw. If no change occurs, pressure is more firmly applied with a gentle rotating motion for approximately 5 seconds on one side and then on the other; both sides are not stimulated simultaneously. Prior to carotid sinus massage, the carotid artery should be auscultated; massage should not be performed in patients who have carotid bruits.

MANAGEMENT OF CARDIAC ARRHYTHMIAS

Before initiating antiarrhythmic therapy, one must determine whether the arrhythmia should be treated. Any arrhythmia that causes symptomatic hypotension or sudden death should be suppressed. However, the situation in which the arrhythmia occurs dictates whether chronic, long-term therapy is necessary. For example, an episode of ventricular fibrillation in a patient at the onset of an acute myocardial infarction does not necessarily require long-term drug therapy because of the low likelihood of recurrence. However, ventricular fibrillation in a patient without an acute myocardial infarction carries a high risk of recurrence. Some patients may have arrhythmias that, while not life-threatening, produce disabling symptoms of dizziness or palpitations and require therapy. Rhythms that are tolerated well in patients with structurally normal hearts (for example, paroxysms of supraventricular tachycardia) may not be tolerated in patients with diseased hearts (for example, ischemic heart disease or mitral stenosis) and may require therapy. The decision to treat a patient with an asymptomatic tachyarrhythmia is more difficult. Certain arrhythmias, such as short episodes of asymptomatic nonsustained ventricular tachycardia, are in themselves harmless but may be forerunners of more serious sustained ventricular tachyarrhythmias. The decision to treat is complicated by the side effects, occasionally life-threatening, of antiarrhythmic drugs, such as exacerbation of ventricular arrhythmias in 5 to 15 per cent of cases. Even though patients with premature ventricular complexes and complex ventricular ectopy after myocardial infarction are at increased risk of subsequent sudden death, it is not clear that antiarrhythmic treatment reduces the increased mortality.

Before beginning chronic antiarrhythmic therapy, factors contributing to the occurrence of the arrhythmia should be considered. These include digitalis excess, hypokalemia, hypomagnesemia, hypoxia, thyrotoxicosis, and other severe metabolic derangements. Congestive heart failure, anemia, or infection should be corrected. Smoking, excessive alcohol intake, caffeine- or theophylline-containing beverages or foods, fatigue, emotional upset, and some over-the-counter drugs (for example, nasal decongestants) may exacerbate arrhythmias.

DRUGS

"Therapeutic" serum concentrations of antiarrhythmic drugs are those that usually exert therapeutic effects without adverse effects in most patients. However, dosage and blood concentrations must be adjusted for any particular patient, and the measured serum concentration is of secondary importance if the response to the drug is appropriate and side effects are absent. The therapeutic-to-toxic ratio of most antiarrhythmic drugs is relatively narrow, and knowledge of drug pharmacokinetics is important to avoid toxic peak and subtherapeutic trough concentrations. Most antiarrhythmic drugs can be administered at intervals equal to the elimination half-life of the drug after an initial loading dose. At a constant dosing interval without a loading dose, the time required to reach steady state is a function of the elimination half-life of the drug. Ninety-four per cent of steady-state level is achieved after four half-lives and 99 per cent after seven half-lives. The same principle applies to the decrease in drug levels after discontinuation of the drug.

TABLE 9–2. VAUGHN WILLIAMS (MODIFIED) CLASSIFICATION OF ANTIARRHYTHMIC DRUGS

Class I	Predominantly reduce the maximum velocity of the upstroke of the action potential (phase 0): IA: quinidine 　　procainamide 　　disopyramide IB: lidocaine 　　phenytoin 　　tocainide 　　mexiletine IC: flecainide 　　encainide
Class II	Inhibit sympathetic activity: propranolol and other beta blockers
Class III	Predominantly prolong action potential duration: amiodarone bretylium
Class IV	Block the slow inward current: verapamil and other calcium antagonists

Therefore, a drug with a longer half-life takes longer to reach steady state and longer to be eliminated than does one with a shorter half-life. Drugs with shorter half-lives are inconvenient to administer orally because of more frequent dosing requirements. Some medications with relatively short half-lives can be given in long-acting forms that release the drug gradually and result in adequate blood concentrations for a longer period of time without a high peak level immediately upon administration of the drug. The pharmacokinetics of drug distribution and elimination are often important; for example, lidocaine blood concentrations may be high after an intravenous bolus but drop very quickly as the drug is redistributed throughout the body. Once this early redistribution phase occurs, blood concentrations fall much less precipitously during the elimination phase, at which time the lidocaine is metabolized by the liver. Therefore, to avoid very high serum concentrations within the first 10 minutes and a subtherapeutic nadir after redistribution has occurred, lidocaine therapy may be initiated in two or more boluses, 5 to 10 minutes apart, instead of as one larger bolus. The organ responsible for elimination of a particular drug, usually the kidneys or liver, must be known, and dosage adjustments must be made in patients with organ dysfunction. The per cent gastrointestinal absorption of some drugs is important to estimate intravenous versus oral dosages; for example, digoxin is only about 80 per cent absorbed orally, compared to 100 per cent availability of an intravenous dose. Some drugs are metabolized to compounds that also demonstrate antiarrhythmic activity, such as N-acetyl procainamide, which is the active metabolite of procainamide. Drug interactions may necessitate dosage adjustments. For example, quinidine increases digoxin serum concentrations. Changes in pharmacokinetics may occur in some groups of patients, such as decreased lidocaine requirements in elderly patients or those with congestive heart failure. Disparity in drug absorption and metabolism may occur in different patients owing to genetically controlled enzyme systems that allow some patients to metabolize drugs such as procainamide quickly (rapid acetylators). The amount of drug bound to serum proteins affects the activity and metabolism of a drug and also may affect the interpretation of serum drug concentrations, since many assays measure both free and protein-bound drug.

Although in vitro electrophysiological properties are known for each drug and certain drugs are known to be more useful for one type of arrhythmia than another, much of antiarrhythmic drug therapy is trial and error. Even drugs grouped within the same class (Table 9–2) may vary in their clinical electrophysiological effects, and when one is unsuccessful in a particular patient, another drug from the same class may be effective. It is important to remember that this classification serves a useful communication purpose but cannot be applied rigidly for several reasons. Not all drugs assigned to a single group exhibit entirely similar actions, and some drugs have properties of more than one class. The classification is based on in vitro electrophysiological effects on normal Purkinje fibers; drug effects on diseased in vivo tissues may be different, or its mechanism of action may even have nothing to do with its direct electrophysiological actions. Tables 9–3, 9–4, and 9–5 summarize the currently available antiarrhythmic agents. It is important to remember that a potential adverse effect of any antiarrhythmic agent is arrhythmia exacerbation.

TABLE 9–3. ANTIARRHYTHMIC DRUGS: DOSAGE AND PHARMACOKINETICS*

DRUG	USUAL DOSE RANGES (mg)				EFFECTIVE SERUM OR PLASMA CONCENTRA-TION (µg/ml)	ELIMINATION HALF-LIFE AFTER ORAL DOSE (hr)	MAJOR ROUTE OF ELIMINATION
	INTRAVENOUS		ORAL				
	Loading	*Maintenance*	*Loading*	*Maintenance*			
Lidocaine	1 to 3 mg/kg at 20 to 50 mg/min	1 to 4 mg/min			1 to 5	1 to 2	Liver
Quinidine	6 to 10 mg/kg at 0.3 to 0.5 mg/kg/min		600 to 1000	300 to 600 g6h	3 to 6	5 to 9	Liver
Procainamide	6 to 13 mg/kg at 0.2 to 0.5 mg/kg/min	2 to 6 mg/min	500 to 1000	2000 to 6000 qd (q3-4h doses for procainamide, q6h doses for sustained-release form)	4 to 10	3 to 5	Kidneys
Disopyramide			300 to 400	100 to 400 q6-8h	2 to 5	8 to 9	Kidneys
Phenytoin	100 mg q5min for ≤1000 mg		1000	100 to 400 q12-24h	10 to 20	18 to 36	Liver
Propranolol	0.25 to 0.5 mg q5min for ≤0.15 to 0.20 mg/kg			10 to 200 q6-8h		3 to 6	Liver
Bretylium	5 to 10 mg/kg at 1 to 2 mg/kg/min	0.5 to 2 mg/min			0.5 to 1.5	8 to 14	Kidneys
Verapamil	10 mg over 1 to 2 min	0.005 mg/kg/min		80 to 120 q6-8h	0.10 to 0.15	3 to 8	Liver
Amiodarone	5 to 10 mg/kg over 20-30 min; then 1 gm/24 hr		800 to 1600 qd for 1 to 3 weeks	200 to 400 qd	1 to 2.5	30 to 50 days	Liver
Tocainide			400 to 600	400 to 600 q8-12h	4 to 10	11	Liver
Mexiletine			400 to 600	150 to 300 q6-8h	0.75 to 2	10 to 17	Liver
Flecainide				100 to 200 q12h	0.2 to 1.0	20	Liver
Encainide				25 to 75 q6-8hr	0.5 to 1.0	3 to 4 (active metabolites: 12 hr)	Liver

* Results presented may vary according to doses, disease state, and IV or oral administration.

TABLE 9–4. ANTIARRHYTHMIC DRUGS: ELECTROCARDIOGRAPHIC EFFECTS

DRUG	SINUS RATE	P-R	QRS	Q-T
Lidocaine	0	0	0	0
Quinidine	0 ↑	↓ 0 ↑	↑	↑
Procainamide	0	0 ↑	↑	↑
Disopyramide	0 ↑	0	↑	↑
Phenytoin	0	0	0	0 ↓
Propranolol	↓	0 ↑	0	0 ↓
Bretylium	0 ↓	0 ↑	0	0 ↑
Verapamil	0 ↓	↑	0	0
Amiodarone	↓	0 ↑	0	↑
Tocainide	0 ↓	0	0	0 ↓
Mexiletine	0	0	0	0 ↓
Flecainide	0 ↓	↑	↑	↑
Encainide	0	↑	↑	↑

TABLE 9–5. ANTIARRHYTHMIC DRUGS: SIDE EFFECTS

DRUG	MAJOR SIDE EFFECTS
Lidocaine	CNS: dizziness, paresthesias, confusion, delirium, stupor, coma, seizures
Quinidine	Hypotension
	GI: nausea, vomiting, diarrhea, anorexia, abdominal pain
	"Cinchonism": tinnitus, hearing loss, visual disturbances, confusion, psychosis
	Rash, fever, anemia, thrombocytopenia
	"Quinidine syncope"
Procainamide	Drug-induced lupus erythematosus
	Nausea, vomiting
	Hypotension
	Giddiness, psychosis
Disopyramide	Anticholinergic: urinary retention, constipation, blurred vision, closed-angle glaucoma
	Congestive heart failure
Phenytoin	CNS: nystagmus, ataxia, drowsiness, stupor
	Nausea, anorexia
	Rash, gingival hypertrophy, megaloblastic anemia, lymph node hyperplasia, peripheral neuropathy, hyperglycemia, hypocalcemia
Propranolol	See Table 8–6
Bretylium	Orthostatic hypotension
	Transient hypertension, tachycardia and worsening of arrhythmias (initial catecholamine release)
	Nausea, vomiting
Verapamil	See Table 8–7
Tocainide	CNS: dizziness, tremor, paresthesias, ataxia, confusion
	GI: nausea, vomiting
Amiodarone	Agranulocytosis, pulmonary fibrosis, elevation of hepatic enzymes, corneal microdeposits, bluish-gray skin discoloration, hyper- or hypothyroidism, nausea, constipation, anorexia, bradycardia, exacerbation of heart failure; elevates plasma levels of digoxin, quinidine, procainamide; potentiates effects of warfarin
Mexiletine	CNS: dizziness, tremor, paresthesias, ataxia, confusion
	GI: nausea, vomiting
Flecainide	Congestive heart failure, sinus node dysfunction, dizziness, blurred vision, incessant ventricular tachycardia
Encainide	Dizziness, blurred vision, headaches, incessant ventricular tachycardia

LIDOCAINE

Lidocaine has minimal effects on automaticity or conduction in vitro unless marked abnormalities are pre-existent. Lidocaine affects fast channel–dependent tissues (atrial and ventricular muscle and His-Purkinje tissue) but usually not slow channel–dependent tissues (sinus and AV nodes). It appears to be particularly potent at altering electrophysiological parameters in ischemic tissue. Lidocaine rarely causes clinically significant hemodynamic effects. It is used only parenterally because of extensive first-pass hepatic metabolism upon oral administration. Its metabolism is decreased in elderly patients and those with hepatic disease, heart failure, and shock. Maintenance doses should be reduced by one third to one half in patients with low cardiac output. Prolonged infusion of lidocaine can reduce its clearance, and dosage may have to be decreased after a day or so. Intramuscular administration has been advocated for use by emergency medical technicians when caring for a patient with an acute myocardial infarction before reaching the hospital, but lidocaine is usually administered intravenously. The ability to achieve rapid effective plasma concentrations and a fairly wide toxic-to-therapeutic ratio with a low incidence of hemodynamic complications make lidocaine a very useful antiarrhythmic drug. It is effective against a variety of ventricular arrhythmias but is generally ineffective against supraventricular arrhythmias. The use of lidocaine prophylactically in patients with acute myocardial infarction is controversial (see Chapter 8). Lidocaine is usually the parenteral drug of first choice in patients with ventricular arrhythmias. Even though lidocaine may decrease ventricular response in some patients with Wolff-Parkinson-White syndrome and atrial fibrillation, it usually has no effect or can even accelerate the ventricular response in patients with rapid ventricular responses.

QUINIDINE

Quinidine is useful for long-term oral treatment of both atrial and ventricular arrhythmias. Quinidine has little effect on normal automaticity but depresses automaticity from abnormal cells. It prolongs conduction time and refractoriness in most cardiac tissues, and it increases the threshold of excitability in atrial and ventricular tissue. Although the direct effect of quinidine is to prolong conduction time in the AV node, its vagolytic actions may shorten conduction time, and the overall result is a balance between the two effects. Quinidine has alpha-adrenergic blocking effects that may cause significant hypotension, especially if vasodilators are administered concomitantly. If given slowly, quinidine may be administered intravenously. Intramuscular quinidine is incompletely absorbed and may cause tissue necrosis.

Quinidine prolongs the effective refractory period of atrial and ventricular muscle and accessory pathways. It may be effective in treating patients with AV nodal re-entry and tachycardias in Wolff-Parkinson-White syndrome. Quinidine may prevent supraventricular tachycardias not only by its effects on tissue refractoriness but also by preventing the atrial or ventricular premature complexes that may trigger the arrhythmia. Quinidine can terminate existing atrial flutter or fibrillation in about 10 to 20 per cent of patients, especially if the arrhythmia is recent in onset and the atria are of normal size. Because quinidine slows the rate of atrial flutter and also exerts a vagolytic effect on AV nodal conduction, it may increase the ventricular response in patients with atrial flutter. Therefore, the patient should be treated with digitalis, propranolol, or verapamil to control the ventricular rate before administering quinidine. Prior to electrical cardioversion, quinidine may be administered to attempt chemical conversion of atrial fibrillation or atrial flutter and may also help maintain sinus rhythm once it is achieved, either chemically or electrically.

Quinidine may produce syncope in 0.5 to 2 per cent of patients, thought most often to result from a polymorphic ventricular tachyarrhythmia termed torsades de pointes when associated with a long Q-T interval. Many patients with quinidine syncope have significantly prolonged Q-T intervals and are also receiving digitalis. Treatment for quinidine syncope entails discontinuation of the drug and avoidance of similar antiarrhythmic agents. Drugs that do not prolong the Q-T interval, such as lidocaine, tocainide, or phenytoin, may be tried. Phenobarbital or phenytoin and related drugs that induce hepatic enzyme production shorten the duration of quinidine's action by increasing its elimination. Quinidine elevates serum digoxin and digitoxin concentrations.

PROCAINAMIDE

Electrophysiological effects of procainamide resemble those of quinidine. Procainamide exerts less intense anticholinergic effects than disopyramide and quinidine. It has a major metabolite, N-acetyl procainamide (NAPA), that exhibits much weaker electrophysiological effects than does procainamide. In patients with renal failure, NAPA levels increase more than procainamide levels and must be monitored to prevent toxicity. A sustained-release form is available that can be administered every 6 hours instead of every 3 to 4 hours; the total daily dose of both procainamide and the sustained release form of procainamide should be the same. Procainamide depresses myocardial contractility only in high doses. It may produce peripheral vasodilation, probably via a mild ganglionic blocking action. The clinical indications for procainamide are very similar to those for quinidine. Although the effects of both drugs are similar, an arrhythmia not suppressed by one drug may be suppressed by the other. Conduction disturbances and ventricular tachyarrhythmias similar to those caused by quinidine can occur.

Procainamide does not increase serum digoxin levels. A systemic lupus erythematosus–like syndrome including arthralgia, fever, pleuropericarditis, hepatomegaly, and hemorrhagic pericardial effusion with tamponade has been described. The brain and kidneys are usually spared and hematologic complications are unusual. Sixty to 70 per cent of patients who receive procainamide develop antinuclear antibodies (ANA), but clinical symptoms occur in only 20 to 30 per cent and are reversible when the drug is stopped. A positive ANA is not necessarily a reason to stop procainamide therapy.

DISOPYRAMIDE

Disopyramide has electrophysiological actions similar to those of quinidine and procainamide but exerts greater anticholinergic effects than either, without antiadrenergic effects. Disopyramide has prominent negative inotropic effects, and patients who have evidence of abnormal ventricular function should receive the drug either not at all or only with extreme caution.

The role of disopyramide in the treatment of atrial and ventricular arrhythmias is similar to that of quinidine. Like quinidine, it can cause a 1:1 conduction during atrial flutter if the patient is not adequately digitalized. Disopyramide does not alter digitalis metabolism.

PHENYTOIN

Phenytoin is a potent medication to treat central nervous system seizures, but its antiarrhythmic actions are limited. It effectively abolishes abnormal automaticity caused by digitalis toxicity. Sinus nodal automaticity and AV conduction are only minimally affected by phenytoin. Phenytoin's electrophysiological effects in vitro appear similar to those of lidocaine. It exerts minimal hemodynamic effects. Phenytoin may be successful in treating atrial and ventricular arrhythmias due to digitalis toxicity but is much less effective in treating arrhythmias of other etiologies.

TOCAINIDE

Tocainide is an analogue of lidocaine that undergoes negligible hepatic first-pass metabolism and therefore approaches 100 per cent oral bioavailability. It is effective for ventricular tachyarrhythmias, but its efficacy appears to be less than that of lidocaine. Currently, its use has been curtailed owing to the occasional occurrence of granulocytosis.

BETA BLOCKERS

Propranolol will be discussed as a prototype beta-adrenergic receptor blocker. Differences in the pharmacokinetics, beta-adrenergic receptor selectivity, and antagonist/agonist actions have been discussed in Chapter 8.

Propranolol slows the sinus nodal discharge rate and lengthens AV nodal conduction time (P-R interval increases) and refractoriness. These effects may be marked if the heart rate or AV conduction is particularly dependent on sympathetic tone or if sinus or AV nodal dysfunction is present. There is no effect on refractoriness or conduction in the His-Purkinje system at usual doses, and the QRS complex and Q-T interval do not change. It appears that the beta-blocking activity of propranolol is responsible for its antiarrhythmic effects, since a local anesthetic (or quinidine-like) effect of propranolol is present only at doses ten times those causing the beta-blocking effect. There is variability in serum concentrations from patient to patient, and the appropriate dose is determined by the patient's physiological response, such as changes in resting heart rate or prevention of an increase in heart rate with exercise. If one beta blocker is ineffective against arrhythmias, the other beta blockers are usually also ineffective.

Propranolol is used most commonly to treat supraventricular tachyarrhythmias. Sinus tachycardia due to thyrotoxicosis, anxiety, and exercise may be slowed by propranolol. Propranolol does not usually terminate atrial flutter or fibrillation but may, by itself or combined with digitalis, control the ventricular response by prolonging AV nodal conduction time or refractoriness. Re-entrant supraventricular tachycardias using the AV node as one limb of the pathway (e.g., AV nodal re-entrant tachycardia and reciprocating tachycardias associated with the Wolff-Parkinson-White syndrome) may be prevented by propranolol alone or combined with other drugs. Propranolol is useful in treating ventricular arrhythmias associated with the prolonged Q-T syndrome and mitral valve prolapse. It usually does not prevent chronic recurrent ventricular tachycardia in patients with ischemic heart disease if the tachyarrhythmia occurs without acute ischemia. A new short-acting beta blocker, esmolol, has a half-life of only 9 minutes after intravenous infusion and may be useful for the acute termination of supraventricular tachycardias such as AV nodal re-entry.

BRETYLIUM TOSYLATE

Bretylium tosylate initially releases norepinephrine stores from adrenergic nerve terminals but subsequently prevents further norepinephrine release. This initial catecholamine release may aggravate some arrhythmias and produce transient hypertension. Although the chemical sympathectomy-like state may be antiarrhythmic, other electrophysiological properties may also contribute to the antiarrhythmic properties of bretylium. Bretylium does not depress myocardial contractility or affect vagal reflexes. After the initial increase in blood pressure, the drug may subsequently cause hypotension, usually orthostatic and controlled if the patient is supine. Bretylium is poorly absorbed orally and is commonly administered intravenously. Bretylium has been reported to induce spontaneous termination of ventricular fibrillation. Bretylium is indicated in patients with life-threatening ventricular arrhythmias that have not responded to lidocaine and possibly to other drugs.

VERAPAMIL

The calcium antagonists have been discussed in Chapter 8. Verapamil has the most potent antiarrhythmic actions (although diltiazem is also useful).

It does not affect cells with normal fast response characteristics (atrial and ventricular muscle, His-Purkinje system), but in fast channel–dependent cells rendered abnormal by disease, verapamil may suppress electrical activity. Slow channel–dependent tissue (sinus and AV nodes) exhibits an increase in conduction time and refractoriness after verapamil administration. Therefore, verapamil prolongs the A-H interval without affecting His-Purkinje conduction or the QRS interval. Sinus rate may decrease, but in intact animals it often does not change significantly because of counteraction by sympathetic reflexes activated by peripheral vasodilation. Verapamil does not affect directly refractoriness of atrial or ventricular muscle or the accessory pathway. Combined therapy with propranolol and verapamil can be attempted in patients with normal cardiac contractility, but the patient should be observed for the development of heart failure and/or symptomatic bradycardias because the compensatory sympathetic response to slow channel blockade is blocked. Calcium infusion or isoproterenol may counteract some of the adverse effects of verapamil until temporary pacing can be initiated.

Intravenous verapamil is the drug of choice for terminating sustained paroxysmal supraventricular tachycardias that are not terminated by vagal maneuvers, such as those reciprocating tachycardias employing the AV node or SA node in the tachycardia circuit. Verapamil can decrease the ventricular response in patients with atrial fibrillation or flutter but converts only a small number of these rhythms to sinus rhythm. Verapamil may be used in patients with congestive heart failure and supraventricular tachycardia if it is thought that termination of the arrhythmia will relieve the heart failure. Verapamil may increase the ventricular response in patients with atrial fibrillation and Wolff-Parkinson-White syndrome, and the drug is relatively contraindicated in that situation. Verapamil is usually not effective in patients with recurrent ventricular tachyarrhythmias.

AMIODARONE

Amiodarone is an antiarrhythmic agent initially introduced as an antianginal coronary vasodilator. It has a broad spectrum of antiarrhythmic efficacy against supraventricular and ventricular arrhythmias. Even though it prolongs the Q-T interval, it may suppress arrhythmias in patients with the long Q-T syndrome. It is effective in AV nodal re-entry, reciprocating tachycardias associated with the Wolff-Parkinson-White syndrome, atrial flutter, and atrial fibrillation, as well as ventricular tachyarrhythmias. Antiarrhythmic efficacy develops after several days of oral administration but may occur earlier with intravenous administration. Amiodarone prolongs action potential duration and refractoriness in all cardiac tissues, slows sinus discharge, and prolongs AV nodal conduction time. Because of a variety of adverse effects, amiodarone should be administered only to patients with highly symptomatic or life-threatening arrhythmias and only if conventional drug therapy has failed.

MEXILETINE

Mexiletine is similar to lidocaine in many of its electrophysiological actions. It is effective for ventricular but not supraventricular tachyarrhythmias and may be useful when combined with type IA antiarrhythmic agents such as quinidine. Adverse effects and efficacy are similar to those of tocainide. Like tocainide, the toxic effects occur at plasma concentrations only slightly higher than therapeutic levels, and therefore effective use of this drug requires careful titration of dosage. A patient's response to intravenous lidocaine may help predict his response to oral mexiletine.

FLECAINIDE

Flecainide profoundly slows conduction in all cardiac fibers but only minimally increases refractoriness. It modestly depresses the cardiac inotropic state and should be used with caution in patients with heart failure. It is useful for ventricular tachyarrhythmias and is especially effective at suppressing PVC's or runs of nonsustained ventricular tachycardia. In patients with ventricular tachyarrhythmias, therapy should begin in the hospital while the ECG is monitored because of the high incidence of aggravation of existing ventricular arrhythmias or onset of new ventricular arrhythmias (5 to 25 per cent of patients). This proarrhythmic effect is especially prominent in patients who have sustained ventricular tachycardia and poor left ventricular function and receive higher doses of the drug. Dose increases should not be made more frequently than every four days. Although not approved for these indications, flecainide may be very useful in patients with AV nodal re-entry, tachycardias involving accessory pathways, and atrial fibrillation.

ENCAINIDE

Encainide resembles flecainide electrophysiologically. Encainide has several active metabolites, one of which is more potent than the parent compound and contributes to its antiarrhythmic efficacy. Variation in the conversion of encainide to its active metabolites may be a source of interpatient differences in drug response. Encainide has little effect on myocardial contractility. Because of the long half-life of its active metabolites, it can be administered three times a day. It is effective for ventricular as well as supraventricular tachyarrhythmias, including AV nodal re-entry, Wolff-Parkinson-White syndrome, and atrial fibrillation. Like flecainide, encainide also has a high incidence of ventricular tachycardia exacerbation. Dose increases should not be made more frequently than every four days owing to the long half-life of the metabolites.

DC CARDIOVERSION AND DEFIBRILLATION

Direct current (DC) electrical cardioversion or defibrillation is the method of choice for terminating ˜ tachyarrhythmias that result in hemodynamic deterioration and those unresponsive to pharmacological termination. Cardioversion refers to the delivery of a DC shock, usually of relatively low energy, synchronized with the QRS complex of an organized tachyarrhythmia. QRS synchronization is important to avoid delivering a shock during ventricular repolarization (T wave) that may precipitate ventricular fibrillation. Defibrillation refers to an asynchronously delivered, relatively high energy shock to terminate ventricular fibrillation. Most supraventricular and ventricular tachyarrhythmias terminate with DC shock, although rhythms due to abnormally increased automaticity, especially if associated with digitalis intoxication, may not.

Prior to elective cardioversion the procedure should be explained to the patient and a physical examination, including palpation of all pulses, performed. Metabolic parameters (i.e., blood gases, electrolytes) should be normal, and ideally the patient should have fasted for six to eight hours prior to the procedure. Digitalis should be withheld on the morning of cardioversion. Patients receiving digitalis without clinical evidence of toxicity are at very low risk for digitalis-induced complications. A short-acting barbiturate or diazepam can be used for anesthesia. Intravenous access should be available and resuscitation equipment at hand. Paddles should be lubricated with an electrolyte jelly and placed firmly to contact with the chest wall, either one paddle in the left infrascapular region and the other over the upper sternum at the third interspace, or one paddle to the right of the sternum at the first or second interspace and the other in the left midclavicular line at the fourth or fifth interspace. Shocks of 25 to 50 joules terminate most tachyarrhythmias except for atrial fibrillation, which may require 100 to 200 joules, and ventricular fibrillation, which may require 100 to 400 joules. If the first low-energy shock fails to terminate the arrhythmia, the energy should be titrated upward.

Tachycardia that produces complications of hypotension, congestive heart failure, or angina and does not respond promptly to medical management should be terminated electrically. DC shock should be avoided if possible in patients with tachyarrhythmias caused by digitalis toxicity because of the risk of precipitating life-threatening refractory ventricular tachyarrhythmias. The administration of an antiarrhythmic drug prior to electrical termination of the arrhythmia may help maintain sinus rhythm after cardioversion. Many arrhythmias, especially chronic atrial fibrillation, commonly recur, and maintenance of sinus rhythm is sometimes a difficult problem.

Ventricular fibrillation due to an improperly synchronized or at times a properly synchronized shock is a complication of DC cardioversion. Immediate electrical defibrillation is mandatory. Systemic emboli occur, and patients with atrial fibrillation, especially those with a high risk for emboli (e.g., mitral stenosis, atrial fibrillation of recent onset, a history of emboli, a prosthetic mitral valve, enlarged left ventricle or left atrium, or congestive heart failure) may require an-

TABLE 9–6. INDICATIONS FOR TEMPORARY AND PERMANENT PACING

	DEFINITELY INDICATED	PROBABLY INDICATED	PROBABLY NOT INDICATED	DEFINITELY NOT INDICATED
Complete AV Block				
Congenital (AV nodal)				
Asymptomatic				X
Symptomatic	T,P			
Acquired (His-Purkinje)				
Asymptomatic		T,P		
Symptomatic	T,P			
Surgical (persistent)				
Asymptomatic	T	P		
Symptomatic	T,P			
Second-degree AV block				
Type I (AV nodal)				
Asymptomatic				X
Symptomatic	T,P			
Type II (His-Purkinje)				
Asymptomatic		T,P		
Symptomatic	T,P			
First-degree AV block				
AV nodal				
Asymptomatic				X
Symptomatic			X	
His-Purkinje				
Asymptomatic				X
Symptomatic			X	
Bundle Branch Block (BBB)				
Asymptomatic				X
Symptomatic		P†		
LBBB during right heart catheterization	T			
Acute Myocardial Infarction				
Newly acquired bifascicular BBB	T			
Pre-existing BBB				X
Newly acquired BBB plus transient complete AV block	T	P		
Second-degree AV block				
Type I (asymptomatic)				X
Type II	T	P		
Complete AV block	T	P		
Atrial Fibrillation with Slow Ventricular Response				
Asymptomatic				X
Symptomatic	T,P			
Sick Sinus Syndrome (bradytachy syndrome)				
Asymptomatic			X	
Symptomatic	T,P			
Hypersensitive Carotid Sinus Syndrome				
Asymptomatic			X	
Symptomatic	T,P			

T = temporary
P = permanent
X = not indicated
† = no other cause found for symptoms

ticoagulation for two weeks before cardioversion to lower the risk of emboli. Anticoagulation should be continued for several weeks after cardioversion. Elevation of myocardial enzyme fractions after cardioversion is not common.

CARDIAC PACEMAKERS

Cardiac pacemakers are devices either implanted permanently or inserted temporarily, consisting of a pulse generator and an electrode that is either placed transvenously into the right ventricle and/or atrium or sutured directly into the epicardium at the time of surgery. Small electrical impulses, generated by the pulse generator and delivered via the electrode catheter, depolarize local cells to threshold potential and cause the entire chamber to depolarize. Pacemakers are widely used for treating bradyarrhythmias but can also be useful for treatment of some tachyarrhythmias. Indicators for temporary and permanent pacing are summarized in Table 9–6.

A five-position pacemaker code has been developed to describe the pacing modalities available in any particular pacemaker. The first three letters of the code are used commonly and the last two are optional. The first letter is the chamber paced (V=ventricle, A=atrium, and D=atrium and ventricle). The second letter is the chamber in which sensing occurs (V=ventricle, A=atrium, D=atrium and ventricle, and O=none). The third letter indicates the mode of response: sensed spontaneous activity inhibiting pacemaker output (I), trigger discharge into the refractory period (T), or trigger ventricular pacing in response to a sensed atrial event as well as inhibition of ventricular pacing during a sensed ventricular event (D). The fourth letter codes programmability of the pacemaker, and the fifth codes antitachyarrhythmia functions. Some examples are illustrated in Table 9–7. The main advantages of dual-chamber pacing modes are the preservation of AV synchrony and/or the ability to increase ventricular paced rate with an increase in atrial rate. Safeguards are built into the VDD and DDD modes so that the ventricular response cannot exceed a predetermined upper rate should an atrial tachyarrhythmia occur. A problem unique to dual-chamber pacing modes (DDD or VDD) that trigger ventricular depolarization from sensed atrial activity is pacemaker-mediated tachycardia. During pacemaker-mediated tachycardia, the pacemaker senses a retrograde P wave conducted after a paced ventricular beat or a premature ventricular complex and triggers a subsequent ventricular depolarization after the programmed AV delay. This paced ventricular complex can again conduct retrogradely to the atrium, creating a sensed P wave that generates another paced ventricular complex. If this continues, a sustained "reciprocating" tachycardia that utilizes the pacemaker as the antegrade limb may occur. Extensive programmability of the newer pacemaker models, particularly that of atrial refractoriness, avoids pacemaker-mediated tachycardia in most cases.

For patients in whom a pacemaker is implanted only for an occasional symptomatic bradycardia or in

TABLE 9–7. COMMON PACEMAKERS

PACEMAKER TYPE	CODE	CHAMBER PACED	CHAMBER SENSED	MODE
Ventricular Asynchronous	VOO	V	None	Continuous pacing
Ventricular Demand	VVI	V	V	Ventricular pacing inhibited by spontaneous QRS
Atrial Demand	AAI	A	A	Atrial pacing inhibited by spontaneous P wave
Atrial Synchronous, Ventricular Inhibited	VDD	V	A,V	Ventricular pacing follows a sensed P wave after a preset AV delay; ventricular pacing inhibited by spontaneous QRS; no atrial pacing
AV Sequential	DVI	A,V	V	Ventricular pacing follows atrial pacing after a preset AV delay; ventricular and atrial pacing inhibited by spontaneous QRS; no P wave sensing
Optimal Sequential	DDD	A,V	A,V	Ventricular pacing follows sensed P waves or atrial pacing after a preset AV delay; ventricular pacing inhibited by spontaneous QRS, atrial pacing inhibited by spontaneous P wave

TABLE 9–8. NONPHARMACOLOGICAL THERAPY OF TACHYARRHYTHMIAS

THERAPY	INDICATION	ADVANTAGES	DISADVANTAGES
Pacing	Prevention of drug-refractory tachyarrhythmias (for example, VT associated with bradycardia or prolonged Q-T syndrome)	Avoids drug side effects; may be the only effective therapy in some patients	Effective only for very narrow indications
	Termination of tachyarrhythmias (especially paroxysmal supraventricular tachycardia, atrial flutter)	Same as above	Requires electrophysiology study to determine efficacy Not effective for rapid VT or VF; may accelerate rather than terminate arrhythmia
Implantable cardioverter-defibrillator	Ventricular tachycardia or fibrillation unresponsive to drug therapy	Failsafe to abort cardiac arrest or need for transthoracic DC shock	Does not prevent arrhythmia; drug therapy may still be required and syncope may occur before arrhythmia is terminated Can accelerate or precipitate arrhythmias Shock is uncomfortable Requires surgery, usually thoracotomy
Catheter ablation of arrhythmia focus or pathway	Drug-resistant ventricular or supraventricular tachycardias in which the focus of origin or pathway can be located and is accessible to a catheter	Nonsurgical Avoids drug side effects AV nodal/His bundle ablation is safe and effective	Successful suppression of ventricular tachycardia disappointing AV nodal ablation leaves patient pacemaker dependent
Surgery	Cut accessory pathway in Wolff-Parkinson-White patients with markedly symptomatic or life-threatening arrhythmias; usually young or drug-refractory patients	Avoids drug side effects Definitive therapy	Surgical risk (small)
	Electrophysiologically guided aneurysmectomy for VT, usually drug-refractory	Avoids or decreases drug therapy Concomitant coronary bypass and aneurysmectomy	Surgical risk Not all patients are good candidates Not universally effective

whom optimal hemodynamic function is of no consequence, a simple VVI pacemaker may be sufficient. However, there are some patients in whom maintenance of physiological AV synchrony may be advantageous. The normal increase in heart rate with exercise may be preserved either by dual-chamber, atrial-synchronous pacing (for example, DDD mode) or by a VVI pacemaker that is able to sense a physiological event such as activity and increase its discharge rate appropriately. Pacemaker malfunction may be manifested by (1) failure to capture (activate myocardium), (2) abnormal sensing (oversensing or undersensing), or (3) abnormal discharge rate. Malfunction may be intermittent. Many pacemakers alter their discharge rate when the battery approaches depletion.

NONPHARMACOLOGICAL THERAPY OF TACHYARRHYTHMIAS

Electrical or surgical therapy may be useful in some patients with supraventricular or ventricular tachyar-

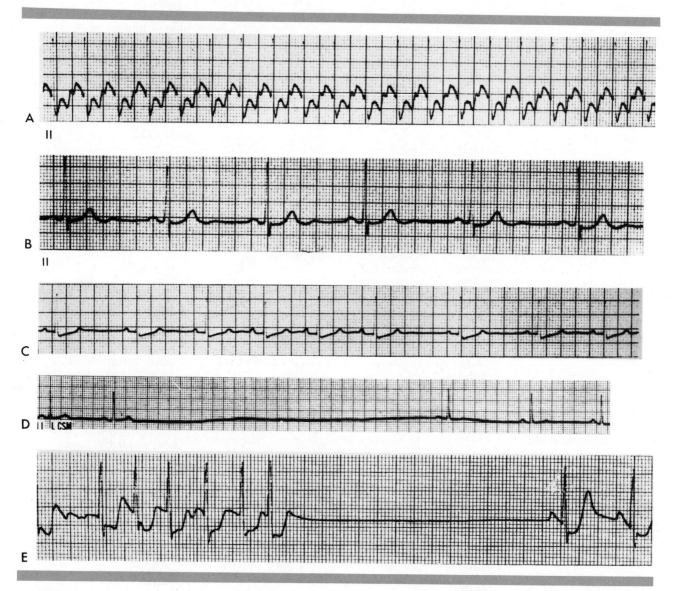

FIGURE 9–3. A, Sinus tachycardia (rate 150 beats/min) in a patient during acute myocardial ischemia; note ST segment depression. B, Sinus bradycardia (rate 46 beats/min) in a patient receiving propranolol. C, Respiratory sinus arrhythmia. The phasic variation in heart rate corresponds to a respiratory rate of approximately 12/min. D, Hypersensitive carotid sinus syndrome. Gentle left carotid sinus massage produced a prolonged period of asystole. E, Bradycardia-tachycardia syndrome. A fairly long period of asystole results before restoration of sinus rhythm upon termination of an episode of atrial fibrillation.

rhythmias (Table 9–8). Pacemakers activated by the patient or automatically when the pacemaker senses tachycardia can deliver timed single or multiple extrastimuli to the atrium, ventricle, or both chambers to interrupt the tachycardia circuit and terminate the arrhythmia. Before implantation, detailed electrophysiological evaluation should be performed to determine the pacing protocol that most safely and reliably terminates the tachycardia.

SPECIFIC ARRHYTHMIAS

SINUS NODAL RHYTHM DISTURBANCES (Fig. 9–3)

Normal sinus rhythm refers to impulse formation beginning in the sinus node and, in adults, having a rate of between 60 and 100 beats per minute. The P wave is upright in leads 1, 2, and aV_F and negative in lead aV_R. The rate of sinus nodal discharge is under autonomic control and increases with sympathetic and decreases with parasympathetic stimulation. Sinus tachycardia refers to a tachycardia of sinus origin with a rate exceeding 100 beats per minute. *Sinus tachycardia* occurs with stresses such as fever, hypotension, thyrotoxicosis, anemia, anxiety, exertion, hypovolemia, pulmonary emboli, myocardial ischemia, congestive heart failure, shock, drugs (e.g., atropine, catecholamines, thyroid, alcohol, caffeine), or inflammation. Therapy should be focused on the cause of the tachycardia. If the sinus tachycardia must be treated directly, propranolol may be used. *Sinus bradycardia* refers to sinus node discharge at a rate less than 60 beats per minute. The P wave contour is normal, but sinus arrhythmia is often present. Sinus bradycardia frequently occurs in young adults, especially well-trained athletes, and is common at night. Sinus bradycardia can be produced by a variety of conditions, including eye manipulation, increased intracranial pressure, myxedema, hypothermia, sepsis, fibrodegenerative changes, vagal stimulation, or vomiting, and the administration of parasympathomimetic drugs, beta-adrenergic blocking drugs, or amiodarone. It occurs commonly in the acute phase of myocardial infarction, especially inferior myocardial infarction. Treatment of asymptomatic sinus bradycardia is usually not necessary. If cardiac output is low or tachyarrhythmias occur owing to the slow heart rate, atropine or, if necessary, isoproterenol may be effective. There is no drug that effectively and safely increases the heart rate over a long period of time, and therefore electrical pacing is the treatment of choice chronically if symptomatic sinus bradycardia is present.

Sinus arrhythmia refers to phasic variation in the sinus cycle length by greater than 10 per cent. P wave morphology is normal. Respiratory sinus arrhythmia occurs when the P-P interval shortens during inspiration as a result of reflex inhibition of vagal tone and lengthens during expiration. Nonrespiratory sinus arrhythmia refers to sinus arrhythmia not associated with the respiratory cycle. Symptoms are unusual and treatment not necessary.

In *sinus pause (sinus arrest)* and *sinoatrial exit block*, a sudden unexpected failure of a P wave occurs. In sinoatrial exit block, the P-P interval surrounding the absent P wave is a multiple of the P to P intervals, implying that the sinus impulse was generated but did not propagate through the perinodal tissue to the atrium. If no such cycle relationship can be found, the term sinus pause or sinus arrest is employed. Acute myocardial infarction, degenerative fibrotic changes, digitalis toxicity, or excessive vagal tone can produce sinus arrest or exit block. Therapy involves searching for the underlying etiology. Patients are not treated if they are asymptomatic. If they are symptomatic and the arrhythmia is not reversed by correcting the underlying etiologies, pacing is employed.

Wandering atrial pacemaker involves a transfer of the dominant pacemaker from the sinus node to latent pacemakers in other atrial sites or in the AV junction. The change from one pacemaker focus to another occurs gradually, associated with a change in the R-R interval, P-R interval, and P wave morphology. Treatment is usually not necessary except if symptoms occur from bradyarrhythmias.

The *hypersensitive carotid sinus syndrome* is characterized by cessation of atrial activity due to sinus arrest or sinoatrial exit block with light pressure over the carotid baroreceptors. In addition, AV block may be observed. Adequate junctional or ventricular escape complexes may not occur. Cardioinhibitory carotid sinus hypersensitivity is arbitrarily defined as ventricular asystole exceeding 3 seconds during carotid sinus stimulation. Vasodepressor carotid sinus hypersensitivity is defined as a fall in systolic blood pressure of 30 to 50 mm Hg without cardiac slowing, usually with reproduction of a patient's symptoms. The treatment in symptomatic patients is pacemaker implantation (to include at least a ventricular lead, since the sinus node slowing is usually also associated with AV block). Neither atropine nor pacing prevents the vasodepressor manifestations of carotid sinus hypersensitivity. Severe vasodepressor carotid sinus hypersensitivity occasionally requires denervation of the carotid sinus.

The *sick sinus syndrome* is applied to a variety of sinus nodal and AV nodal abnormalities that occur alone or in combination. They include (1) persistent spontaneous sinus bradycardia not caused by drugs and inappropriate to the physiological circumstances, (2) sinus arrest or exit block, (3) combinations of sinus and AV conduction disturbances, and (4) alternation of paroxysms of atrial tachyarrhythmias with periods of slow atrial and ventricular rates (bradycardia/tachycardia syndrome). The sick sinus syndrome may be associated with AV nodal or His-Purkinje conduction disturbances. If symptoms are present from bradyarrhythmias, pacemaker implantation is appropriate. Pacing for the symptomatic bradyarrhythmia combined with drug therapy for the tachyarrhythmia is often needed.

Sinus nodal re-entrant tachycardia accounts for 5 to 10 per cent of paroxysmal supraventricular tachycardias. Its mechanism is presumed to be re-entry within

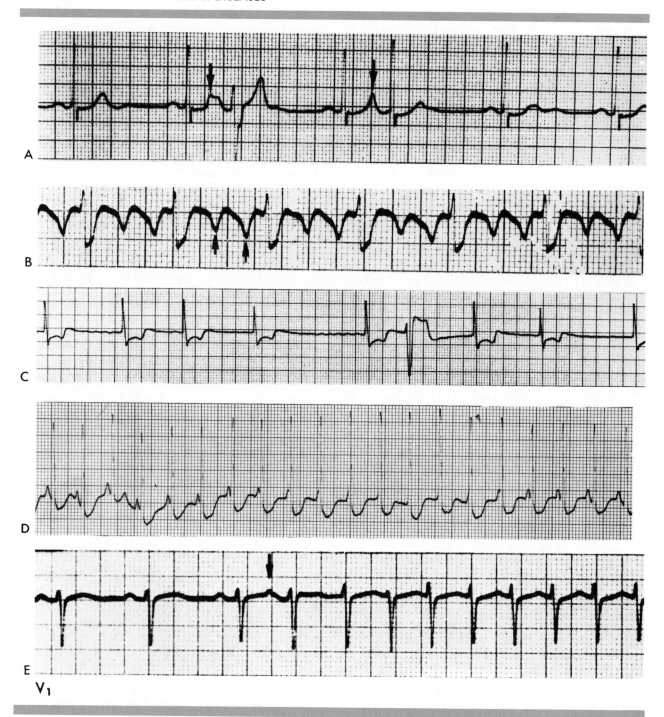

FIGURE 9–4. *A,* Premature atrial systoles with and without aberrancy. The first premature atrial systole (*arrow*) occurs at a shorter P-R interval than does the second premature atrial systole (*arrow*) and conducts with a bundle branch block contour. The first premature atrial systole conducts with aberrancy, while the second does not because the first reaches the bundle branch system before complete recovery of repolarization. *B,* Atrial flutter. Flutter waves are indicated by arrows. The conduction ratio is 3:1, that is, three flutter waves to one QRS complex, and is a less common conduction ratio. *C,* Atrial fibrillation. Atrial ac-

tivity is present as the undulating wavy base line seen in the midportion of the ECG strip. The premature ventricular complex must be differentiated from aberrant supraventricular conduction. *D,* Nonparoxysmal junctional tachycardia with AV dissociation. *E,* Paroxysmal supraventricular tachycardia. Three sinus beats are interrupted by a premature atrial systole (*arrow*), which conducts with P-R prolongation and initiates the supraventricular tachycardia. The most common mechanisms of this arrhythmia are AV nodal re-entry and atrioventricular re-entry using an accessory pathway as the retrograde limb.

the sinus node and the perinodal tissues, giving rise to a tachycardia, usually with a rate of 130 to 140 beats per minute and containing P waves very similar to sinus P waves. AV block may occur without affecting the tachycardia. Vagal activation may slow and then abruptly terminate the tachycardia by its action on sinus nodal tissue. Tachycardia may be induced and terminated at electrophysiological study with premature atrial stimulation. Treatment with propranolol, verapamil, or digitalis is effective therapy.

ATRIAL RHYTHM DISTURBANCES
(Fig. 9–4)

Premature atrial complexes (PAC's) are characterized by a premature P wave, usually of differing morphology from the sinus P wave. PAC's occurring very early in diastole may be followed by either aberrantly conducted QRS complexes or no QRS complexes (nonconducted PAC). In general, the shorter the interval from the last QRS to the P wave, the longer the P-R interval after the PAC. PAC's are less likely to be followed by a fully compensatory pause than are PVC's (see discussion later). PAC's are common in normal people but may occur in a variety of situations, for example, infection, inflammation, myocardial ischemia, psychological stress, tobacco or alcohol use, or caffeine ingestion. PAC's can be the forerunner of a sustained supraventricular tachyarrhythmia. They do not require therapy unless they produce symptoms or precipitate tachyarrhythmias.

In *atrial flutter*, the atrial rate is usually 250 to 350 per minute. Ordinarily, the ventricular rate is half of the atrial rate. If AV block is greater than 2:1 in the absence of drugs, abnormal AV conduction is suggested. In children, patients with pre-excitation syndrome, or patients with hyperthyroidism, 1:1 AV conduction can occasionally occur. Drugs such as quinidine, procainamide, or disopyramide may reduce the atrial rate to the range of 200 per minute, raising the danger of 1:1 AV conduction. The atrial activity appears as regular sawtooth waves without an isoelectric interval between flutter waves. Flutter waves are commonly inverted in leads 2, 3, and aV$_F$. Ventricular response to atrial flutter may be irregular, generally of a Wenckebach nature, or regular. Chronic atrial flutter is usually associated with underlying heart disease, but paroxysmal atrial flutter may occur in patients without organic heart disease. Toxic and metabolic conditions such as thyrotoxicosis, alcoholism, or pericarditis may be associated with atrial flutter. There are fewer systemic emboli in patients with atrial flutter than in patients with atrial fibrillation, presumably because of the atrial contraction. Carotid sinus massage may decrease the ventricular response but does not terminate the arrhythmia. Cardioversion (less than 50 joules) usually restores sinus rhythm. If atrial fibrillation ensues, a second shock of higher energy may be necessary. Rapid atrial pacing also terminates atrial flutter, although some patients develop atrial fibril-

lation instead of sinus rhythm; however, atrial fibrillation is usually an easier arrhythmia in which to control the ventricular response.

Intravenous verapamil, beta blockers, or digitalis may slow the ventricular response to atrial flutter, and in a few patients may restore sinus rhythm. Type 1 antiarrhythmic drugs such as quinidine, procainamide, or disopyramide may terminate atrial flutter in some patients and are often useful to prevent recurrences. These drugs should not be administered unless AV nodal block has been previously achieved, since slowing the atrial flutter rate combined with the vagolytic effects of disopyramide or quinidine may lead to 1:1 AV conduction.

Atrial fibrillation is characterized by totally disorganized atrial activation without effective atrial contraction. The electrocardiogram shows small, irregular baseline undulations of variable amplitude. The ventricular response is irregularly irregular, usually between 100 and 160 beats per minute in the untreated patient with normal AV conduction. It is easier to slow the ventricular response with drugs in patients with atrial fibrillation than in patients with atrial flutter because of the greater number of atrial impulses reaching the AV node and decreasing the overall number of impulses that conduct to the ventricles. Chronic atrial fibrillation is usually associated with underlying heart disease, whereas paroxysmal atrial fibrillation may occur in apparently normal hearts. Atrial fibrillation commonly results from rheumatic heart disease (especially with mitral valve involvement), cardiomyopathy, hypertensive heart disease, pulmonary emboli, pericarditis, coronary heart disease, thyrotoxicosis, or heart failure from any cause. Episodes of atrial fibrillation may cause decompensation of patients with borderline cardiac function, especially those with mitral or aortic stenosis. Patients with chronic atrial fibrillation are at a greatly increased risk of developing systemic emboli, particularly if mitral valve disease is also present. Left atrial diameter tends to be smaller in patients with paroxysmal atrial fibrillation or in patients whose atrial fibrillation is easily terminated with cardioversion. Physical findings in patients with atrial fibrillation include a variation in the intensity of the first heart sound, absence of a waves in the jugular venous pulse, and an irregular ventricular rhythm. A pulse deficit may appear with faster ventricular rates; that is, the auscultated apical rate exceeds the palpable radial rate owing to failure of many of the ventricular contractions to generate a palpable peripheral pulse. Although atrial fibrillation with a very rapid ventricular response can sometimes seem regular, it is always irregular upon careful measurement, and true regularization of the ventricular rhythm in patients with atrial fibrillation should suggest development of sinus rhythm, atrial flutter, junctional rhythm, or ventricular tachycardia (the latter two may be manifestations of digitalis intoxication).

It is important to correct any precipitating causes of atrial fibrillation such as thyrotoxicosis, mitral stenosis, pulmonary emboli, or pericarditis. If the onset of atrial fibrillation is associated with acute hemodynamic decompensation, DC cardioversion should be employed (usually requires 100 to 200 joules). In the absence of decompensation, the patient should be treated with digitalis to maintain a resting apical rate of 60 to 80 beats per minute that does not exceed 100 beats per minute after mild exercise. At times, the addition of a beta- or calcium-blocker may be useful to slow the ventricular rate. Quinidine or other type 1 antiarrhythmic drugs may be useful either to convert atrial fibrillation to sinus rhythm or to maintain sinus rhythm once it is restored with electrical cardioversion. Patients with atrial fibrillation of less than 12 months' duration or without markedly enlarged left atria are more likely to remain in sinus rhythm after cardioversion. The role of anticoagulation is controversial, but anticoagulation prior to drug or electrical cardioversion is definitely indicated in patients at high risk of emboli, i.e., those with mitral stenosis, previous emboli, a prosthetic mitral valve, or cardiomegaly. Anticoagulation therapy should be administered two weeks prior to cardioversion and continued for about two weeks afterward. Rapid atrial pacing does not terminate atrial fibrillation.

In *atrial tachycardia with AV block*, the atrial rate is usually 150 to 200 beats per minute, and variable degrees of AV conduction are present. This rhythm is often associated with digitalis excess and occurs most commonly in patients with significant organic heart disease, such as coronary heart disease, cor pulmonale, and digitalis intoxication. Isoelectric intervals are present between P waves in contrast to atrial flutter. Carotid sinus massage should be performed with caution in patients suspected of having digitalis toxicity. If the patient is not receiving digitalis, the rhythm may be treated with digitalis to slow the ventricular response, and subsequently quinidine, disopyramide, or procainamide may be added. If atrial tachycardia occurs in a patient receiving digitalis, digitalis toxicity should be suspected. Usually the ventricular response is not rapid and withholding digitalis is sufficient therapy.

Chaotic or *multifocal atrial tachycardia* is characterized by atrial rates between 100 and 130 beats per minute with marked variation in P wave morphology and irregular P-P intervals. It occurs commonly in patients with pulmonary disease and in diabetics or older patients who eventually may develop atrial fibrillation. Digitalis is usually not helpful in this arrhythmia. Therapy is directed toward the underlying disease.

AV JUNCTIONAL RHYTHM DISTURBANCES

If suprajunctional pacemakers fail, a *junctional escape rhythm* may emerge at a rate of 35 to 60 beats per minute. The junctional escape rhythm is usually fairly regular, but the rate may increase gradually when the escape rhythm first begins (warm-up phenomenon). A junctional rhythm may be associated with retrograde P waves for each QRS complex, or AV dissociation may be present.

Premature junctional complexes arise from the AV junction. A retrograde P wave is usually present but may be prevented by a sinus P wave. They usually do not require therapy.

A regular junctional rhythm with a rate exceeding 60 beats per minute (usually between 70 and 130 per minute) is considered an accelerated junctional rhythm or *nonparoxysmal AV junctional tachycardia*. The gradual onset and termination account for the term nonparoxysmal and may imply that the mechanism of the tachycardia is increased automaticity. Retrograde activation of the atria or AV dissociation may be present. Nonparoxysmal AV junctional tachycardia occurs most commonly in patients with underlying heart disease, such as inferior myocardial infarction, myocarditis, and acute rheumatic fever, or after open heart surgery. The most common cause is digitalis excess. Therapy is directed toward the underlying etiological factor.

Paroxysmal supraventricular tachycardias (PSVT's) are regular tachycardias that occur and terminate suddenly. They are due to a variety of mechanisms, the most common of which are atrioventricular (AV) nodal re-entry (approximately 60 per cent of cases) and AV re-entry using a concealed accessory bypass tract (approximately 30 per cent of cases). Sinus nodal re-entry, intra-atrial re-entry, and automatic atrial tachycardias account for the remaining PSVT's.

AV nodal re-entry is characterized by narrow QRS complexes (unless functional aberration has occurred), sudden onset and termination, and regular rates, usually between 150 and 250 beats per minute. Carotid sinus massage may slow the tachycardia slightly, and if termination occurs, it is abrupt. AV nodal re-entry commonly occurs in patients with no organic heart disease. Symptoms vary according to the rate of the tachycardia and the presence of organic heart disease. In some patients, rest, reassurance, and sedation may abort an attack. Vagal maneuvers including Valsalva, carotid sinus massage, and gagging may terminate the tachycardias and should be repeated after each pharmacological intervention. Intravenous verapamil, 5 to 10 mg, terminates AV nodal re-entry after about two minutes in over 90 per cent of cases and is the treatment of choice should vagal maneuvers fail. Edrophonium chloride, a short-acting cholinesterase inhibitor, may also terminate AV nodal re-entry and is administered in a total dose of 10 mg IV after a 1-mg test dose. Edrophonium should be used cautiously in patients who have hypotension or bronchospastic lung disease. Intravenous propranolol may be given (see Table 9–3) but must be used cautiously in patients with heart failure or chronic lung disease. Intravenous digoxin may also be used, but its onset of action is longer. If the patient is experiencing hemodynamic compromise, DC cardioversion with low energies is effective. Atrial or ventricular pacing also may restore sinus rhythm. In some patients, type I antiarrhythmic agents such as procainamide, quinidine, and disopyramide may be required to terminate AV nodal re-entry, but these drugs are used more often to prevent recurrences. Vasopressors (e.g., phenylephrine or metaraminol) may terminate AV nodal re-entry by inducing reflex vagal stimulation but are not commonly used. Digitalis is usually the initial drug choice for chronic therapy. If unsuccessful, verapamil, propranolol, quinidine, or flecainide may be tried. In some hard-to-control cases, antitachycardia pacemaker implantation or surgery may be considered.

PSVT may be caused by re-entry utilizing a retrograde concealed accessory pathway. The presence of the accessory pathway is not evident during sinus rhythm because antegrade conduction is not present, and therefore the ECG manifestations of the Wolff-Parkinson-White syndrome are not evident. However, the mechanism of tachycardia is the same as that in most patients with the Wolff-Parkinson-White syndrome, that is, antegrade conduction over the AV node and retrograde conduction over the accessory pathway. Since it takes a relatively long time for the impulse to travel through the ventricular tissue to the accessory pathway and back to the atrium, the retrograde P wave during this form of tachycardia occurs after completion of the QRS complex, usually in the ST segment or early T wave. In distinction, patients with AV nodal re-entrant tachycardias usually have their retrograde P wave inscribed during or just after the QRS complex, although longer retrograde conduction intervals can occur in AV nodal re-entry. Tachycardia rates tend to be somewhat faster than those in AV nodal re-entry (≥200 per minute), but a great deal of overlap exists. Vagal maneuvers, verapamil, digitalis, and propranolol are acceptable choices for prompt termination. Chronic therapy often involves combinations of drugs that prolong accessory pathway conduction time and refractoriness (for example, quinidine or flecainide) and drugs affecting AV nodal conduction.

PRE-EXCITATION SYNDROMES (Fig. 9–5)

Pre-excitation syndromes occur when ventricular activation occurs earlier than would be expected using the normal AV conduction system. There are several varieties of anomalous AV connections; the most common is the Wolff-Parkinson-White syndrome, in which an accessory atrioventricular pathway (Kent bundle) connects atrium with ventricle, short-circuiting the normal AV conduction system. A portion of the ventricle is activated via conduction over the accessory pathway before the remainder of the ventricle is activated via the normal AV conduction system, and the resultant QRS is a fusion of activation initiated by each of the two (normal and abnormal) AV pathways. Therefore, the P-R interval is usually shortened (<0.12 sec) and the duration of the QRS is increased (>0.12 sec). The initial slurring of the QRS secondary to ventricular pre-excitation is referred to as the delta wave. Although the Wolff-Parkinson-White syndrome has been divided into Type A (positive delta wave in V_1 and V_6) and Type B (negative delta wave in V_1 and positive delta wave in V_6), this classification system is a gross oversimplification of the many ECG varieties produced by AV connections at different sites and is not very useful clinically. Accessory AV pathways may

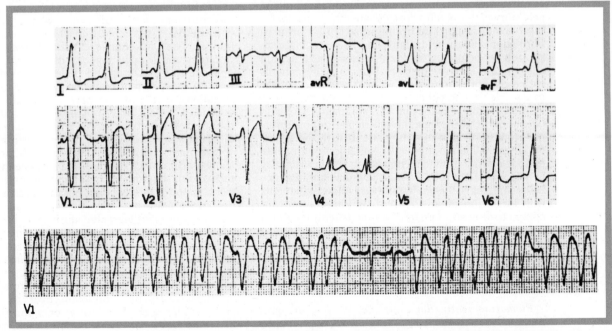

FIGURE 9–5. Pre-excitation syndrome is apparent in the 12-lead ECG (short P-R interval, wide QRS, delta wave). During atrial fibrillation the ventricular rate is extremely rapid, at times approaching 350 beats/min. The gross irregularity of the cycle lengths, wide QRS complexes interspersed with normal QRS complexes, and very rapid rate should suggest the diagnosis of atrial fibrillation and an atrioventricular bypass tract.

be located anywhere along the AV ring on either the left or right side or along the septum and are occasionally multiple.

The most common arrhythmia caused by an abnormal AV (Kent) connection is termed *orthodromic* reciprocating tachycardia: the antegrade limb of the re-entrant circuit is the AV node and the retrograde limb is the accessory pathway. *Antidromic* tachycardia utilizes the accessory pathway for the antegrade limb and the AV node as the retrograde limb. In the orthodromic variety, the QRS complexes either are normal or exhibit functional left or right bundle branch block. In the antidromic variety, the QRS complexes are totally pre-excited and consist of a wide, bizarre QRS. Similar pre-excited QRS complexes can occur when an atrial tachyarrhythmia (for example, atrial fibrillation) results in an extremely rapid ventricular response via the accessory AV connection. Most adults with pre-excitation have normal hearts, although Ebstein's anomaly has an increased incidence of pre-excitation. Sudden death occurs rarely but may be a threat in patients with atrial fibrillation and rapid ventricular responses or in patients with associated congenital anomalies.

Patients who have frequent episodes of tachyarrhythmias and/or in whom the arrhythmias cause significant symptoms should receive therapy. Drugs that prolong refractoriness of the accessory pathway (e.g., quinidine, procainamide, disopyramide, flecainide, and encainide) or the AV node (e.g., digitalis, verapamil, and propranolol) may be effective in treating the reciprocating tachycardia; long-term therapy may require one drug from each group. Drugs that prolong accessory pathway refractoriness are effective in slowing the ventricular rate during atrial flutter or atrial fibrillation. Because digitalis has been reported to shorten refractoriness in the accessory pathway and accelerate the ventricular response in some patients with atrial fibrillation, it is advisable not to use digitalis as a single drug in patients with the Wolff-Parkinson-White syndrome. Lidocaine and verapamil have also been reported to increase the ventricular response during atrial fibrillation in some patients with the Wolff-Parkinson-White syndrome. Termination of an acute episode of orthodromic reciprocating tachycardia may be approached as for AV nodal re-entry, but digitalis, verapamil, and lidocaine should be avoided in patients with atrial fibrillation or flutter. In patients with incomplete drug response or in young patients who wish not to take drugs for the rest of their lives, surgical ablation of the accessory pathway is safe and effective.

VENTRICULAR RHYTHM DISTURBANCES (Fig. 9–6)

Premature ventricular complexes (PVC's) are premature, bizarrely shaped QRS complexes of prolonged duration differing in contour from the dominant QRS complex. The T wave is large and oriented in the opposite direction from the major QRS deflection. The sinus node and atria are usually not activated prematurely by retrograde conduction from the PVC, and

therefore a "compensatory pause" results; that is, the pause after the PVC is sufficiently long that the interval between the two normally conducted QRS complexes flanking the PVC equals two sinus cycle lengths. A PVC that does not produce a pause is termed interpolated. Two successive premature PVC's are termed a pair or couplet, while three or more successive PVC's are arbitrarily termed ventricular tachycardia. If PVC's have different contours, they are called multifocal, multiform, polymorphic, or pleomorphic. If PVC's are not coupled to the previous QRS, parasystole should be considered; however, many nonparasystolic PVC's do not exhibit fixed coupling. The prevalence of PVC's increases with age. They are often asymptomatic but can give rise to palpitations, or if present in long runs of bigeminy, may produce hypotension, since they are premature and relatively ineffective at ejecting blood. The number of PVC's may increase during infection, ischemia, anesthesia, psychological stress, and excessive use of tobacco, caffeine, or alcohol. In the absence of underlying heart disease, the presence of PVC's probably has no significance regarding longevity or limitation of activity, and antiarrhythmic therapy is not indicated. The presence of PVC's identifies patients at an increased risk of cardiac death if they have coronary artery disease, hypertrophic cardiomyopathy, or mitral valve prolapse; however, treatment of PVC's has not been demonstrated to decrease sudden death. If drug therapy is indicated (usually only in patients with symptoms), lidocaine can be used acutely and procainamide, quinidine, or disopyramide may be considered for chronic therapy.

Ventricular tachycardia occurs when three or more consecutive PVC's occur with a rate exceeding 100 per minute. The QRS complexes usually have a prolonged duration and bizarre shape, with ST and T vectors opposite to the major QRS deflection. Atrial activity may be independent of ventricular activity (AV dissociation), or the atrium may be depolarized by the ventricles retrogradely (VA association). QRS contours may be unchanging (uniform) or may vary. The differentiation between sustained and nonsustained ventricular tachycardia is somewhat arbitrary but clinically useful; one guideline is that sustained ventricular tachycardia lasts at least 30 seconds or requires termination prior to 30 seconds because of hemodynamic decompensation.

The electrocardiographic distinction between supraventricular tachycardia with abnormal intraventricular conduction and ventricular tachycardia can be difficult. Supraventricular tachycardia may be associated with prolonged QRS complexes when pre-existing bundle branch block is present, functional aberration exists, or conduction over an accessory pathway is present. When fusion or capture QRS complexes occur during a wide-complex tachycardia (that is, early, narrow complexes that are either partially [fusion] or completely [capture] caused by activation from a supraventricular source), ventricular origin of the tachycardia can be assumed. The identification of AV dissociation, sometimes requiring esophageal or

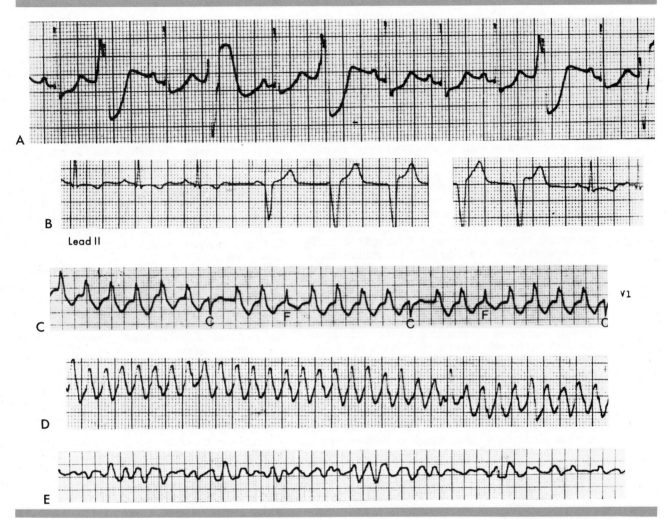

FIGURE 9–6. *A,* Multiform premature ventricular systoles. Each sinus beat is followed by premature ventricular complexes that have two contours, one predominantly upright and the other predominantly negative. *B,* Accelerated idioventricular rhythm. The sinus rate slows slightly and allows the escape of an idioventricular rhythm. A fusion beat with a short P-R interval results. Subsequently the sinus node once again regains control of the ventricular rhythm. *C,* Ventricular tachycardia. A regular wide complex tachycardia is present. Atrial activity is not readily apparent. The complexes marked C and F most likely represent capture and fusion complexes that confirm the ventricular origin of the arrhythmia. *D,* Ventricular flutter. Ventricular depolarization and repolarization appear as a sine wave with regular oscillations. The QRS complex cannot be distinguished from the ST segment or T wave. *E,* Ventricular fibrillation. The baseline is irregular and undulating without any electrical evidence of organized ventricular activity.

intracardiac recordings to determine atrial activity, is much more characteristic of ventricular than supraventricular tachycardia. However, only about 50 per cent of ventricular tachycardias demonstrate complete AV dissociation. In addition, the following characteristics favor a supraventricular origin: slowing or termination of the tachycardia by increased vagal tone, onset after a premature P wave; R-P interval ≤100 msec, more atrial impulses than ventricular impulses (for example, 2:1 AV conduction), initiation of wide complexes after a long/short cycle sequence; and rsR′

in V_1. With preceding normal QRS conduction, if left axis deviation or QRS duration of 140 msec or more is present during tachycardia, ventricular tachycardia is likely.

Ventricular tachycardia occurs in patients with ischemic heart disease, congestive and hypertrophic cardiomyopathy, mitral valve prolapse, valvular heart disease, and primary electrical disease (no identifiable structural heart disease). Even short runs of ventricular tachycardia may be important when detected in the late hospital phase of acute myocardial infarction, since the one-year mortality rate of this group appears to be much greater than for patients without tachycardia.

Deciding when to treat patients with ventricular tachycardia is sometimes difficult. Patients with chronic recurrent sustained ventricular tachycardia and those with symptomatic nonsustained ventricular tachycardia are treated. Treatment of patients with asymptomatic nonsustained ventricular tachycardia is controversial; we tend to treat those with structural heart disease, especially left ventricular dysfunction, and not treat those with no structural heart disease. Acute therapy of ventricular tachycardia is achieved with intravenous lidocaine; if unsuccessful, intravenous procainamide or bretylium may be used. If hypotension, shock, angina, congestive heart failure, or symptoms of cerebral hypoperfusion are present, the rhythm should be terminated promptly with DC cardioversion, beginning with very low energies (10 to 50 joules) synchronized with the QRS. DC cardioversion of digitalis-induced ventricular tachycardia may be hazardous but is sometimes necessary. If ventricular tachycardia is recurrent despite drug therapy, pacing may occasionally be useful for termination. Before embarking on chronic drug therapy, a search for reversible conditions contributing to the arrhythmia should be initiated; for example, metabolic abnormalities, hypoxia, digitalis excess, and congestive heart failure should be corrected. Effective drugs for chronic therapy include quinidine, procainamide, disopyramide, and tocainide. Phenytoin is usually not successful unless digitalis toxicity is present, and propranolol is usually unsuccessful unless the ventricular tachycardia is related to ischemia or catecholamine stimulation. Amiodarone is very effective in patients in whom conventional agents have failed. Combinations of drugs are sometimes necessary. Surgery or implantable electrical devices may be considered in patients with ventricular tachycardia refractory to drug therapy.

Accelerated idioventricular rhythm refers to impulse formation originating in the ventricle with a rate of approximately 60 to 110 per minute. It often competes with the sinus node for control of the heart, and fusion and capture complexes occur commonly. The onset of the arrhythmia is often gradual (nonparoxysmal), and enhanced automaticity is presumed to be the mechanism. Precipitation of more rapid ventricular arrhythmias is not common. The arrhythmia usually occurs in patients with acute myocardial infarction or digitalis toxicity, and suppressive therapy is usually not necessary. If symptoms occur or if more malignant tachyarrhythmias result, therapy as noted above is indicated. Often simply increasing the sinus rate with atropine or atrial pacing suppresses the accelerated idioventricular rhythm.

The term *torsades de pointes* refers to a ventricular tachyarrhythmia characterized by QRS complexes of changing amplitude that appear to twist around the isoelectric line, occurring in the setting of a prolonged Q-T interval. Episodes of torsades de pointes often terminate spontaneously, but ventricular fibrillation may supervene. The syndrome may be either congenital or acquired. Acquired forms may be caused by any antiarrhythmic drug that prolongs the Q-T interval (for example, quinidine, procainamide, or disopyramide) or by psychoactive drugs such as phenothiazines and tricyclic antidepressants. In addition, potassium depletion, liquid protein diet, and other metabolic abnormalities may be associated with the long Q-T syndrome. Acute therapy involves withdrawing the offending drug and correcting metabolic abnormalities. Antiarrhythmic agents that prolong the Q-T interval may worsen the arrhythmia. Temporary ventricular or atrial pacing is the most effective therapy for suppressing the bursts of polymorphic tachycardia. Isoproterenol has been reported to be effective until pacing is instituted. Magnesium or bretylium therapy may be useful. If a polymorphic ventricular tachycardia resembling torsades de pointes is present but the Q-T interval is normal, standard antiarrhythmic drugs may be given.

Patients with congenital prolonged Q-T syndrome who are at increased risk for sudden death include those who have family members who died suddenly at an early age and those who have experienced syncope or torsades de pointes. Electrocardiograms should be obtained from all family members when a patient presents with suspected congenital long Q-T syndrome. Auditory stimuli, psychological stress, and exercise may provoke an arrhythmia in susceptible patients. For patients who have idiopathic long Q-T syndrome but no syncope, complex ventricular arrhythmias, or family history of sudden cardiac death, no therapy is recommended. In asymptomatic patients with long Q-T syndrome who have complex ventricular arrhythmias or a family history of premature sudden cardiac death, beta blockers at maximally tolerated doses are recommended. In patients with syncope, beta blockers at maximally tolerated doses, combined with phenytoin or phenobarbital if necessary, are suggested. For patients who continue to have syncope despite drug therapy, left-sided cervicothoracic sympathetic ganglionectomy has been effective, since sympathetic imbalance appears to be important in the pathogenesis of this syndrome.

Ventricular fibrillation generates little or no blood flow and is usually fatal within three to five minutes unless terminated. Ventricular fibrillation is recognized by the presence of irregular undulations of varying contour and amplitude without distinct QRS complexes, ST segments, or T waves. *Ventricular flutter* appears as a sine wave with regular, large oscillations occurring at a rate of 150 to 300 per minute. Ventricular fibrillation occurs in a variety of situations, including coronary artery disease, antiarrhythmic drug administration, hypoxia, ischemia, atrial fibrillation with rapid ventricular rates in the pre-excitation syndromes, accidental electrical shock, and poorly timed cardioversion. Most patients resuscitated from out-of-hospital cardiac arrest have ventricular fibrillation as their arrhythmia, often without acute myocardial infarction. Treatment is an immediate nonsynchronized DC shock using 200 to 400 joules. If ventricular fibrillation has been present for more than a few minutes, correction of metabolic abnormalities may aid in electrically converting the rhythm, although DC shock should not be delayed to await correction of hypoxia or acidosis. Once ventricular fibrillation has been terminated, medications to prevent recurrence of ventricular fibrillation should be initiated (e.g., lidocaine). Ventricular fibrillation rarely, if ever, terminates on its own and is lethal unless DC shock is applied.

HEART BLOCK (Fig. 9–7)

Heart block refers to a disturbance of impulse conduction and should be distinguished from interference, a normal phenomenon in which impulse conduction is blocked owing to physiological refractoriness in the wake of a preceding impulse. Heart block may occur anywhere in the heart but is commonly recognized electrocardiographically in the AV node, His bundle, or bundle branches. In *first-degree AV heart block*, AV conduction time is prolonged (P-R interval ≥0.20 sec), but all impulses are conducted. *Second-degree heart block* occurs in two forms: *type I second-degree heart block (Wenckebach)* is characterized by a progressive lengthening of the PR interval until a P wave is not conducted. *Type II second-degree AV heart block* denotes occasional or repetitive sudden block of a P wave without prior measurable lengthening of the P-R interval. Type II AV block often antedates the development of Stokes-Adams syncope and complete AV block, while type I AV block with a normal QRS complex is usually more benign and does not progress to advanced forms of AV conduction disturbances. In the patient with acute myocardial infarction, type I AV block usually accompanies inferior infarction, is transient, and does not require temporary pacing, whereas type II AV block usually accompanies anterior myocardial infarction, may require temporary or permanent pacing, and is associated with a high mortality, mostly due to pump failure. First-degree or type I second-degree AV block can occur in healthy young people, especially well-trained athletes. Any medication that affects AV nodal conduction (for

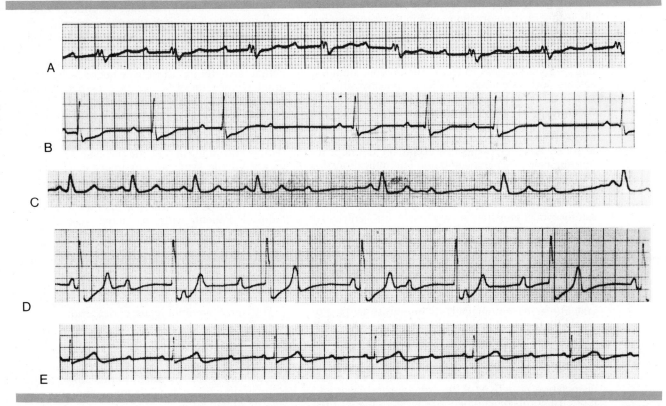

FIGURE 9–7. *A,* First-degree AV block. The P-R interval is prolonged. *B,* Second-degree AV block (type I, Wenckebach), characterized by progressive P-R prolongation preceding the nonconducted P wave. In the setting of a normal QRS complex, Wenckebach almost always occurs at the level of the AV node. *C,* Second-degree AV block, type II. Left bundle branch block is present in this recording of lead I. Sudden failure of AV conduction results, without antecedent P-R prolongation. *D,* Acquired third-degree (complete) AV block. Complete AV dissociation is present owing to complete AV heart block. Atria and ventricles are under control of separate pacemakers, the sinus node and an idioventricular escape rhythm, respectively. *E,* Congenital third-degree (complete) AV block in a young adult at the level of the AV node. The QRS complex is normal.

example, digitalis, beta blockers, or verapamil) may cause first- or second-degree AV block.

Type I AV block with a normal QRS complex is usually at the level of the AV node proximal to the His bundle. Type II AV block usually occurs in association with a bundle branch block and is localized to the His-Purkinje system. Type I AV block in a patient with a bundle branch block may represent block in either the AV node or the His-Purkinje system. Type II AV block in a patient with a normal QRS complex may be due to intra-His block but is more likely to be type I AV nodal block that exhibits small increments in AV conduction time. Note that 2:1 AV block may represent either AV nodal or His-Purkinje block.

Complete AV block occurs when no atrial activity conducts to the ventricles. The atria and ventricles are controlled by independent pacemakers, and thus complete AV block is one cause of AV dissociation. The ventricular rhythm is usually regular. If the AV block is at the level of the AV node (for example, congenital AV block), the QRS complexes are normal in morphology and duration, with rates of 40 to 60 per minute, and respond to autonomic influences. If the AV block is in the His-Purkinje system (usually acquired), the escape rhythm originates within the ventricle, has a wide QRS and a slower rate, and is less reliable and under less autonomic influence. Causes of AV block include surgery, electrolyte disturbances, endocarditis, tumor, Chagas' disease, rheumatoid nodules, calcific aortic stenosis, myxedema, polymyositis, infiltrative processes such as amyloid, sarcoid, or scleroderma, drug toxicity, coronary disease, and degenerative processes. In children the most common cause of AV block is congenital and is usually asymptomatic; in some, however, symptoms eventually develop, requiring pacemaker implantation. The indications for pacemaker therapy in heart block are summarized in Table 9–6. Atropine (for AV nodal block) and isoproterenol (for heart block at any site) may be used transiently while preparations are made for ventricular pacing. Drugs cannot be relied on to increase the heart rate for more than several hours to a few days without producing significant side effects.

The term AV *dissociation* describes independent depolarization of the atria and ventricles. AV dissociation is not a primary disturbance of rhythm but is a "symptom" of an underlying rhythm disturbance produced by one or a combination of three causes that prevent the normal transmission of impulses from atrium to ventricle: (1) Slowing of the dominant pacemaker of the heart (usually the sinus node), allowing escape of a subsidiary or latent pacemaker. This is AV dissociation by default of the primary pacemaker and is often a normal phenomenon, e.g., sinus bradycardia and a junctional escape rhythm. (2) Acceleration of a latent pacemaker that usurps control of the ventricles. This abnormally enhanced discharge rate of a usually slower subsidiary pacemaker is pathological, e.g., junctional or ventricular tachycardia. (3) Block at the AV junction that prevents impulses formed at a normal rate in a dominant pacemaker from reaching the ventricles so that the ventricles beat under the control

of a subsidiary pacemaker, e.g., complete AV block with a ventricular escape rhythm. It is important to remember that complete AV dissociation is not synonymous with complete AV block.

SYNCOPE (See Also Chapter 116)

Syncope refers to sudden transient loss of consciousness, usually due to transient cerebral hypoperfusion. Presyncope is described as a lightheaded spell that, if more prolonged, would cause loss of consciousness. Both may occur in the same patient and have similar etiologies. The causes of syncope are summarized in Table 9–9.

Cardiac syncope is due either to lesions that obstruct outflow of blood from the heart or to arrhythmias. In patients with severe aortic stenosis or other causes of obstructive syncope, when the systemic vascular resistance decreases upon exercise, the heart is unable to augment cardiac output sufficiently to maintain perfusion and syncope results. Both tachyarrhythmias and bradyarrhythmias that result in cerebral hypoperfusion can cause cardiac syncope. The hypersensitive carotid sinus syndrome, described earlier, is a well-recognized cause of syncope.

The history and physical examination are valuable in excluding many causes of syncope (Table 9–9). Even though the electrocardiogram may not reveal the actual arrhythmia causing syncope, electrocardiographic clues (for example, the presence of simple or complex ventricular ectopy, evidence of a previous myocardial infarction, or the delta wave of the Wolff-Parkinson-White syndrome) may suggest potential arrhythmic causes. Prolonged electrocardiographic (Holter) recording may be the cornerstone of diagnosis in arrhythmic syncope. On many occasions, more than 24 hours of recording are required to detect the responsible arrhythmia. Exercise testing is also valuable in some patients whose arrhythmias are exercise-induced. Patients with obstructive syncope such as aortic stenosis should not undergo exercise testing. In selected patients invasive electrophysiological studies may be useful to delineate the etiology of the syncope.

SUDDEN CARDIAC DEATH

The most commonly used definition of sudden death is unexpected, nontraumatic death occurring within an hour after the onset of symptoms; some studies have included death occurring within 24 hours of the onset of symptoms. Sudden cardiac death claims approximately 1200 lives daily in the United States and is the leading cause of death among men between the ages of 20 and 60. By far the most common cause of sudden death is cardiac, and within that group, the most common cause is ventricular tachyarrhythmias.

Nonarrhythmic causes of sudden death are listed in Table 9–10.

Ventricular tachyarrhythmias, generally related to ischemic heart disease, are the most common cause of sudden cardiac death. Although 75 per cent of patients resuscitated from ventricular fibrillation have extensive coronary artery disease, only 20 per cent have evidence of acute transmural myocardial infarction. Approximately 75 per cent of patients with sudden death have a previous history of cardiac disease; sudden death is the first manifestation of cardiac disease in the remainder. The difference in occurrence of sudden death in patients with (2 per cent at one year) and without (22 per cent at one year) acute myocardial infarction may be due to different arrhythmia mechanisms. Patients with ventricular fibrillation at the time of an acute myocardial infarction probably do not need long-term antiarrhythmic therapy unless chronic late ventricular tachycardia is documented. The risk of recurrent ventricular fibrillation is higher if there is evidence of left ventricular dysfunction or evidence of previous myocardial infarction. Non-atherosclerotic etiologies of ventricular tachyarrhythmias associated with sudden death are mitral valve prolapse, hypertrophic or other cardiomyopathies, antiarrhythmic drugs, myocarditis, prolonged Q-T syndrome, and Wolff-Parkinson-White syndrome with rapid antegrade conduction over an accessory pathway.

The identification of patients at high risk for sudden cardiac death can be difficult. The occurrence of complex ventricular ectopy including multiform PVC's, pairs, and ventricular tachycardia in survivors of myocardial infarction is associated with a two- to three-fold increase in subsequent sudden death; however, suppression of ventricular ectopy with antiarrhythmic agents has not been proven to decrease the incidence of sudden death, and the necessity of suppressing less complex forms of ventricular ectopy is unclear. The risk of sudden cardiac death and the incidence of complex ectopy are greater in patients with poor left ventricular function.

The patient who has suffered sudden cardiac arrest in the absence of acute myocardial infarction and the patient with recurrent symptomatic ventricular tachyarrhythmias must be treated with antiarrhythmic therapy. The end point of antiarrhythmic therapy to be used to judge efficacy is often unclear. The mere attainment of "therapeutic" serum levels of an antiarrhythmic agent is not usually sufficient to guard against recurrent ventricular tachyarrhythmias. Prolonged electrocardiographic monitoring is noninvasive, simple, and widely available. However, many patients with sudden death demonstrate very little spontaneous ectopy between episodes; therefore, suppression of spontaneous ectopy cannot be used as an end point in these patients. In addition, even in patients with spontaneous ectopy, it is not clear whether an appropriate end point would be elimination of all ventricular tachycardia, all complex ectopy, or all PVC's. Drug evaluation using exercise testing and prolonged ambulatory recording to judge efficacy has been reported to decrease the incidence of recurrent malignant tachyarrhythmias but can only be used in patients with spontaneous high-grade ventricular ectopy between episodes of sustained tachyarrhythmia. Most investigators feel that patients experiencing sudden cardiac arrest in the absence of acute myo-

cardial infarction should undergo serial electrophysiological testing to guide antiarrhythmic therapy. The suppression with a drug of ventricular tachycardia inducible by electrical stimulation appears to provide a

TABLE 9–9. CAUSES OF SYNCOPE

CAUSE	FEATURES
Peripheral Vascular or Circulatory Causes	
Vasovagal syncope	Prodrome of pallor, yawning, nausea, diaphoresis. Precipitated by stress or pain. Occurs when patient is upright, aborted by recumbency. Fall in blood pressure without appropriate rise in heart rate
Micturition syncope	Syncope with urination (probably vagal)
Post-tussive syncope	Syncope after paroxysm of coughing
Hypersensitive carotid sinus syndrome	Vasodepressor and/or cardio-inhibitory responses with light carotid sinus massage (see text)
Drugs	Orthostasis Occurs with antihypertensive drugs, tricyclic antidepressants, phenothiazines
Volume depletion	Orthostasis Occurs with hemorrhage, excessive vomiting or diarrhea, Addison's disease
Autonomic dysfunction	Orthostasis Occurs in diabetes, alcoholism, Parkinson's disease, deconditioning after a prolonged illness
Central Nervous System	
Cerebrovascular	Transient ischemic attacks and strokes are unusual causes of syncope. Associated neurologic abnormalities are usually present
Seizures	Warning aura sometimes present, jerking of extremities, tongue biting, urinary incontinence, postictal confusion
Metabolic	
Hypoglycemia	Confusion, tachycardia, jitteriness prior to syncope. Patient may be taking insulin
Cardiac	
Obstructive	Syncope is often exertional. Physical findings consistent with aortic stenosis, hypertrophic obstructive cardiomyopathy, cardiac tamponade, atrial myxoma, prosthetic valve malfunction, Eisenmenger's syndrome, tetralogy of Fallot, primary pulmonary hypertension, pulmonic stenosis, massive pulmonary embolism
Arrhythmias	Syncope may be sudden; occurs in any position. Episodes of dizziness or palpitations. May be a history of heart disease. Brady- or tachyarrhythmias may be responsible; check for hypersensitive carotid sinus

TABLE 9–10. SELECTED CAUSES OF SUDDEN DEATH

Noncardiac
  Central nervous system hemorrhage
  Massive pulmonary embolus
  Drug overdose
  Hypoxia secondary to lung disease
  Aortic dissection or rupture
Cardiac
  Ventricular tachycardia
  Bradyarrhythmias, sick sinus syndrome
  Aortic stenosis
  Tetralogy of Fallot
  Pericardial tamponade
  Cardiac tumors
  Complications of infective endocarditis
  Hypertrophic cardiomyopathy (arrhythmia or obstruction)
  Myocardial ischemia
    Atherosclerosis
    Prinzmetal's angina
    Kawasaki's arteritis

better indicator of drug success than suppression of spontaneous ectopy and can be used in patients with little or no spontaneous ectopy. If arrhythmias cannot be controlled with drugs, the implantable cardioverter-defibrillator and/or cardiac surgery are options. Coronary artery revascularization alone is usually not sufficient to prevent recurrent ventricular tachyarrhythmias.

Antiarrhythmic therapy in patients after myocardial infarction as prophylaxis for malignant cardiac arrhythmias has not been proven effective. However, in certain high-risk patients antiarrhythmic therapy may be warranted, for example, those with nonsustained ventricular tachycardia after infarction. Several large multicenter studies have demonstrated a decrease in the incidence of sudden death in patients treated with beta-adrenergic receptor blocking agents after myocardial infarction, and these drugs probably should be considered if no contraindication to their administration exists.

PRINCIPLES OF CARDIOPULMONARY RESUSCITATION

Cardiopulmonary resuscitation consists of basic and advanced life support. Upon evaluating a patient with suspected cardiac arrest, one should first quickly establish that the patient is truly unresponsive and not breathing. If a pulse is not present, a precordial thump to the midsternum may be tried. Subsequently, the "ABC's" of basic life support should be observed: Airway, Breathing, and Circulation. The mouth and pharynx should be examined to assure that no obstruction is present. The tongue should be removed from the posterior pharynx by tilting the head backward and hyperextending the neck. This maneuver can sometimes cause resumption of spontaneous respiration. If no breathing is noted, mouth-to-mouth or mouth-to-nose breathing should be initiated in four quick breaths. Time is often wasted trying to intubate a patient when adequate ventilation could be accomplished immediately via mouth or mask ventilation. One should check to see that the chest rises with each ventilation. If a carotid pulse is not present after the initial ventilations, external cardiac compression over the lower half of the sternum (not over the xiphoid process) should be initiated. The sternum should be depressed 3 to 5 cm, with the patient lying on a hard surface. Compressions should be approximately 60 per minute, with a ratio of 5 compressions to 1 ventilation if two rescuers are present. A single rescuer must give 15 chest compressions alternating with two ventilations every 15 seconds.

Advanced life support should be initiated while basic life support continues. Defibrillation should be applied if indicated as soon as possible and *is the single most definitive treatment available for most cardiac arrests*. Oxygen should be administered and an adequate intravenous access should be established. If circulation has not been restored quickly, sodium bicarbonate (1 mEq/kg IV) is given to treat metabolic acidosis and is repeated after 10 minutes; further administration of sodium bicarbonate should be guided by blood gas and pH measurements once effective circulation is restored. Epinephrine (5 to 10 ml of a 1:10,000 solution administered via an intravenous, intracardiac, or endotracheal route every 5 minutes as needed) is useful in treating asystole and also in aiding defibrillation of fine (low-amplitude) ventricular fibrillation. Atropine (boluses of 0.5 mg IV at 5-minute intervals to a total dose of approximately 2 to 4 mg) can be administered for profound bradycardia. Isoproterenol given as a constant infusion (2 to 20 µg/min) and titrated according to response may be used to treat bradyarrhythmias if atropine is ineffective. Emergency cardiac pacing may be attempted for bradyarrhythmias if atropine and isoproterenol are unsuccessful.

Lidocaine, procainamide, or bretylium tosylate can be administered to help terminate ventricular tachyarrhythmias and prevent their recurrence. Intravenous furosemide and/or morphine may be used to relieve pulmonary edema. Calcium chloride (2.5 to 5 ml of a 10 per cent solution repeated if necessary in 10 minutes) is given to increase myocardial contractility, especially if electromechanical dissociation is present. Calcium should be used with caution in a patient with known digitalis excess. Calcium chloride will precipitate if given in the same intravenous line with sodium bicarbonate.

Electromechanical dissociation refers to the presence of cardiac electrical activity without appropriate mechanical activity. It may be caused by decreased filling of the heart (e.g., hypovolemia, cardiac tamponade, pulmonary embolus) or severe myocardial pump depression that may respond to calcium. Emergency pericardiocentesis may be attempted if cardiac tamponade is suspected.

The widespread application of cardiopulmonary resuscitation via education of the public and extensive emergency care systems in many cities has increased both the number of cardiac arrest victims who reach the hospital and the number who survive to be discharged. Survival critically depends on the time from arrest to the initiation of resuscitation and is best if basic life support can be initiated within 3 to 4 minutes and more definitive therapy (i.e., defibrillation) shortly thereafter.

REFERENCES

Benditt DG, Benson DW (eds): Cardiac preexcitation syndrome: Origins, evaluation, and treatment. Boston, Martinus Nijhoff, 1986.

Bigger JT, Fleiss JL, Kleiger R, Miller JP, Rolnitzky L, et al: The relationships among ventricular arrhythmias, left ventricular dysfunction, and mortality in the 2 years after myocardial infarction. Circulation 69:250, 1984.

Cobb LA, Werner JA, Trobaugh GB: Sudden cardiac death. I. A decade's experience with out-of-hospital resuscitation. II. Outcome of resuscitation; management, and future directions. Mod Concepts Cardiovasc Dis 19:31, 37, 1980.

Gallagher JJ, Pritchett ELC, Sealy WC, Kasell J, Wallace AG: The preexcitation syndromes. Prog Cardiovasc Dis 20:285, 1978.

Health and Public Policy Committee, American College of Physicians: Diagnostic endocardial electrical recording and stimulation. Ann Intern Med 100:452, 1984.

Josephson ME, Kastor JA: Supraventricular tachycardia: Mechanisms and management. Ann Intern Med 87:346, 1977.

Ludmer PL, Goldschlager N: Cardiac pacing in the 1980's. N Engl J Med 311:1671, 1984.

Mason JW: Drug therapy: Amiodarone. N Engl J Med 316:455–466, 1987.

Mitchell LB, Duff HJ, Manyari DE, Wyse DG: A randomized clinical trial of the noninvasive and invasive approaches to drug therapy of ventricular tachycardia. N Engl J Med 317:1681–1687, 1987.

Morganroth J: Ambulatory Holter electrocardiography: Choice of technologies and clinical uses. Ann Intern Med 102:73, 1985.

Scheinman MM, Morady F: Invasive cardiac electrophysiologic testing: The current state of the art. Circulation 67:1169, 1983.

Smith WM, Gallagher JJ: "Les torsades de pointes": An unusual ventricular arrhythmia. Ann Intern Med 93:578, 1980.

Standards and guidelines for cardiopulmonary resuscitation (CPR) and emergency cardiac care (ECC). JAMA 255:2905, 1986.

Zipes DP: Cardiac Arrhythmias. In Braunwald E (ed): Heart Disease. A Textbook of Cardiovascular Medicine. 3rd ed. Philadelphia, W. B. Saunders Company, 1988.

Zipes DP (ed): An Update on Cardiac Arrhythmias I & II. Progress in Cardiology, 1988.

10

MYOCARDIAL AND PERICARDIAL DISEASE

MYOCARDIAL DISEASE

MYOCARDITIS

Acute myocardial inflammation is termed myocarditis and may be associated with fever, dyspnea, edema, fatigue, palpitations, and pleuropericardial pain. Myocarditis is frequently not clinically apparent and is suspected only on the basis of ST and T wave changes or a transient conduction defect on electrocardiography in a patient with a systemic illness. Physical examination may reveal signs of pericarditis or biventricular cardiac failure. Intraventricular or atrioventricular conduction disturbances or arrhythmias may occur.

Therapy is usually supportive. Congestive heart failure responds to routine management with digitalis, diuresis, and afterload reduction. Significant arrhythmias should be treated with antiarrhythmic agents. Steroids may be of benefit in acute rheumatic carditis but should be avoided in suspected infectious myocarditis. Immunosuppressive therapy may be helpful in selected patients.

Most patients recover completely. An unknown percentage of patients, probably small, develop a chronic process leading to a dilated cardiomyopathy after a varying latency period.

Infectious agents cause myocarditis by three basic mechanisms: (1) invasion of the myocardium, (2) production of a myocardial toxin, for example, diphtheria, and (3) autoimmunity, as in acute rheumatic fever. The infectious agents are multiple, most commonly thought to be viral, especially Coxsackie group B. Primary bacterial myocarditis is a rare but grave complication of bacterial endocarditis, most commonly caused by streptococci or staphylococci. *Mycoplasma pneumoniae* infections, toxoplasmosis, trichinosis, and rickettsial diseases such as Rocky Mountain spotted fever are associated with myocarditis. Protozoal myocarditis from trypanosomiasis (Chagas' disease) is common in Central and South America where it is a frequent cause of chronic congestive cardiomyopathy, heart block, and ventricular arrhythmias. Hypersensitivity reactions to various agents and radiation therapy can result in inflammation of the myocardium. A myocarditis associated with the acquired immunodeficiency syndrome has been described.

CARDIOMYOPATHY

Cardiomyopathy, a disease involving the heart muscle itself, is classified into three basic categories (Table 10–1). This classification is not rigid, and some cardiomyopathies may demonstrate characteristics that overlap among the three groups.

Dilated Cardiomyopathy

In dilated cardiomyopathy, ventricular enlargement occurs and systolic dysfunction results in symptoms of congestive heart failure. The cause of dilated cardiomyopathy is often not apparent but appears to be the end result of myocardial damage produced by a variety of toxic, metabolic, and infectious agents (Table 10–2). Clinical symptoms usually develop slowly, and patients may have ventricular dysfunction for some time before symptoms, usually of both left and right ventricular failure, appear. Q waves may be present on ECG without infarction when extensive left ventricular fibrosis has occurred. Echocardiography is important to exclude other causes of congestive heart failure. A pericardial effusion is sometimes present. Ventriculography shows enlargement of the left ventricle with diffuse wall motion reduction and sometimes left ventricular thrombi. Functional mitral regurgitation may be present, and occasionally it is difficult to distinguish from primary mitral regurgitation. The coronary arteries are normal or incidentally involved. Endomyocardial biopsy may sometimes be useful in diagnosing patients with cardiomyopathy.

Peripartum cardiomyopathy refers to congestive cardiomyopathy occurring in the last month of pregnancy or within five months of delivery in the absence of pre-existing heart disease. It occurs most frequently in multiparous blacks and is more common in older women and those with poor nutrition, poor prenatal care, or toxemia. Doxorubicin (Adriamycin) is an effective antitumor drug that commonly produces congestive cardiomyopathy. The risk of toxicity appears to be related to the cumulative dose, increasing as the dose increases but with a relatively abrupt increase in risk after approximately 450 to 550 mg/sq m. The prognosis after development of symptoms is extremely poor.

TABLE 10–1. CLASSIFICATION OF CARDIOMYOPATHY

TYPE	CHARACTERISTICS	SYMPTOMS AND SIGNS	LABORATORY DIAGNOSIS
Dilated (congestive)	Cardiac dilation, generalized hypocontractility	Left and right ventricular failure (see Table 2–4)	X-ray: cardiomegaly with pulmonary congestion ECG: sinus tachycardia, nonspecific ST-T changes, arrhythmias, conduction disturbances, Q waves Echo: dilated LV, generalized decreased wall motion, mitral valve motion consistent with low flow Catheterization: dilated hypocontractile ventricle; mitral regurgitation
Hypertrophic	Ventricular hypertrophy, especially the septum, with or without outflow tract obstruction Typically good systolic but poor diastolic (compliance) ventricular function	Dyspnea, angina, presyncope, syncope, palpitations Large jugular a wave, bifid carotid pulse, palpable S_4 gallop, prominent apical impulse; "dynamic" systolic murmur and thrill, mitral regurgitation murmur	X-ray: LV predominance, dilated left atrium ECG: left ventricular hypertrophy, Q waves, nonspecific ST-T waves; ventricular arrhythmias Echo: hypertrophy, usually asymmetric (septum > free wall); systolic anterior motion of mitral valve; midsystolic closure of aortic valve Catheterization: provokable outflow tract gradient; hypertrophy with vigorous systolic function and cavity obliteration; mitral regurgitation
Restrictive	Reduced diastolic compliance impeding ventricular filling; normal systolic function	Dyspnea, exercise intolerance, weakness Elevated jugular venous pressure, edema, hepatomegaly, ascites, S_4 and S_3 gallops, Kussmaul's sign	X-ray: mild cardiomegaly; pulmonary congestion ECG: low voltage, conduction disturbances, Q waves Echo: characteristic myocardial texture in amyloidosis with thickening of all cardiac structures Catheterization: square root sign; M-shaped atrial waveform, elevated left- and right-sided filling pressures

Hypertrophic Cardiomyopathy

Hypertrophic cardiomyopathy is characterized by myocardial hypertrophy, especially involving the interventricular septum. In many patients a dynamic pressure gradient can be detected in the subvalvular left ventricular outflow tract (hypertrophic obstructive cardiomyopathy or idiopathic hypertrophic subaortic stenosis). This gradient demonstrates wide fluctuations in severity and often is not present at rest, requiring physiological or pharmacological maneuvers to be precipitated. Even though much attention has been focused on the systolic gradient, the most characteristic pathophysiological abnormality in this syndrome is not systolic but rather diastolic dysfunction, characterized by abnormal stiffness of the left ventricle with impaired filling. Therefore, pulmonary venous pressures are elevated, and dyspnea is the most common symptom despite a typically hypercontractile left ventricle. In many patients the disease appears to be transmitted genetically as an autosomal dominant disorder with a high degree of penetrance, but sporadic cases do occur. Hypertrophy can involve predominantly the septum (asymmetric septal hypertrophy) or the septum and free wall equally (concentric left ventricular hypertrophy). Hypertrophied and bizarrely arranged myocardial cells are commonly but not always visualized pathologically, especially in the septum.

Signs and symptoms in hypertrophic cardiomyopathy are summarized in Table 10–1. A large jugular venous a wave may be present on physical examination owing to reduced compliance of the right ventricle. The carotid arterial upstroke is brisk and bifid in character with a rapid initial rise, a midsystolic dip, and a second late systolic rise characteristic of the dynamic outflow tract obstruction (see Fig. 2–2). The systolic outflow murmur typically is harsh, is crescendo-decrescendo, is often heard best between the apex and left sternal border, and radiates to the lower sternum, axilla, and base of the heart but often not into the neck. A murmur of concomitant mitral regurgitation is not uncommon. The systolic outflow murmur is said to be "dynamic" because its intensity varies inversely with the dimensions of the outflow tract. The outflow tract becomes larger with an increase in ventricular diastolic volume, an increase in systolic pressure against which the heart must pump, or a decrease in myocardial inotropic state. The outflow tract narrows with reversal of these factors (Table 10–3).

Left ventricular hypertrophy is common on ECG, and large Q waves, probably related to abnormal septal depolarization, may simulate septal myocardial infarction. Atrial fibrillation and other tachyarrhythmias are poorly tolerated owing to the hemodynamic abnormalities.

Echocardiography is the best technique for visualizing the hypertrophic myocardium and asymmetric septal hypertrophy. It is useful for screening family members of patients with hypertrophic cardiomyopathy. Narrowing of the left ventricular outflow tract by systolic anterior motion of the anterior leaflet of

TABLE 10–2. CAUSES OF DILATED CARDIOMYOPATHY

Idiopathic
Infectious
  viral
  parasitic (e.g., Chagas' disease)
Toxins
  alcohol
  cobalt
  doxorubicin
Radiation
Systemic diseases
  connective tissue diseases (e.g., systemic lupus erythematosus)
  sarcoidosis
  hemochromatosis
Metabolic disorders
  thyrotoxicosis
  myxedema
  beriberi
  starvation
  glycogen storage diseases
  mucopolysaccharidoses
Neuromuscular disorders (e.g., certain muscular dystrophies)
Peripartum cardiomyopathy

TABLE 10–3. BEHAVIOR OF THE DYNAMIC OUTFLOW MURMUR IN HYPERTROPHIC OBSTRUCTIVE CARDIOMYOPATHY

MANEUVERS	PHYSIOLOGY	INTENSITY OF MURMUR
Valsalva Standing Amyl nitrate	Decrease LV cavity size	↑
Isoproterenol	Increase contractility	↑
Squatting Phenylephrine Elevation of legs Isometric exercise (handgrip)	Increase LV cavity size	↓

the mitral valve is characteristic of patients with obstructive cardiomyopathy, and the degree of systolic anterior motion appears to correlate with the degree of obstruction. The aortic valve may close partially in midsystole owing to the dynamic outflow obstruction; this finding, in addition to the systolic anterior motion, may be provoked with pharmacological manipulations (e.g., amyl nitrate, nitroglycerin, or isoproterenol). Mitral valve prolapse is sometimes observed along with evidence of a small left ventricular cavity and poor left ventricular compliance.

At cardiac catheterization, the systolic subvalvular gradient may or may not be present at rest, and provocative maneuvers such as nitroglycerin, amyl nitrate, isoproterenol infusion, and induced PVC's may provoke a gradient. The left ventricular end-diastolic pressure and a wave are elevated. Angiography demonstrates marked thickening of the ventricular septum and left ventricular free wall, with large papillary muscles distorting the ventricular shape and producing a characteristic hourglass configuration. The left ventricular cavity is usually small and systolic function vigorous, resulting in virtual obliteration of the ventricular cavity with systole. Mitral regurgitation is common.

The clinical course is variable, although symptoms may remain stable over a period of several years. Symptoms are often unrelated to the presence or severity of a gradient. Ventricular arrhythmias are common and sudden death may occur even in previously asymptomatic individuals. Any protective effect of medical therapy against arrhythmias is unproven.

Interventions that decrease ventricular contractility, increase ventricular volume, increase systemic arterial pressure, increase the dimensions of the outflow tract, or increase ventricular compliance decrease symptoms and the converse. Digitalis should not be used unless atrial fibrillation with a rapid ventricular response or left ventricular dilation and dysfunction without a gradient occur. Diuretics should be used with caution as hypovolemia increases obstruction and symptoms. Beta-adrenergic receptor blockade can prevent the increase in outflow tract gradient that may occur with exercise; its efficacy at preventing sudden death has not been established. It also has antianginal effects. It can be used in large doses (propranolol ≥ 320 mg/day) if not limited by contraindications, but the overall efficacy of beta blockers is disappointing. Calcium channel blockers such as verapamil decrease myocardial contractility and probably decrease the outflow gradient. More importantly, both verapamil and nifedipine appear to improve the diastolic function (i.e., compliance) of the hypertrophic myocardium. Verapamil can exacerbate poor left ventricular contractility if present. Nifedipine has less negative inotropic effect but is a more potent vasodilator, which may be disadvantageous. Combined administration of a beta blocker and calcium antagonist may be effective in some patients. Patients with hypertrophic cardiomyopathy should receive endocarditis prophylaxis, since infection may occur on the aortic or mitral valves or on the endocardium at the site of septal contact of the anterior mitral leaflet. In the patient who is markedly symptomatic due to an outflow gradient and has not responded to medical management, septal myotomy-myectomy may be performed. This procedure usually relieves obstruction as well as mitral regurgitation.

Restrictive Cardiomyopathy

Restrictive cardiomyopathies are less common than the dilated and hypertrophic varieties. They are caused by a variety of infiltrative processes, including amyloidosis, hemochromatosis, sarcoidosis, endomyocardial fibrosis, Löffler's endocarditis, and Fabry's disease. Restrictive cardiomyopathy is characterized by abnormal diastolic function that impedes ventricular filling. Contractile function is usually relatively normal. Restrictive cardiomyopathy is often difficult to distinguish from constrictive pericarditis, and endomyocardial biopsy may sometimes be necessary to

make the distinction. Ventricular pressure recordings reveal a deep nadir in early diastole with a rapid rise to a plateau, termed the "square root" sign. The atrial pressure tracing demonstrates a corresponding prominent "y" descent with a rapid rise and plateau. The "x" descent and "a" wave are also often prominent, resulting in a characteristic M-shaped waveform. The left-sided filling pressures are often higher than the right-sided pressures, in distinction to the equalization of pressures in constrictive pericarditis.

Signs and symptoms are listed in Table 10–1. Kussmaul's sign (an inspiratory increase in central venous pressure) may be present. The apical impulse is usually palpable, in distinction to constrictive pericarditis.

Amyloidosis is characterized by deposition in many tissues of an amorphous, hyalin-like substance and is the most common cause of restrictive cardiomyopathy. In addition, it sometimes may cause systolic dysfunction and symptoms more typical of a dilated cardiomyopathy. Arrhythmias and conduction disturbances are common. The electrocardiogram in cardiac amyloidosis is usually abnormal and often demonstrates generalized decreased voltage. Q waves from myocardial infiltration may simulate myocardial infarction. Echocardiography reveals increased thickness of all cardiac structures, including the ventricular walls, the atrial septum, and the cardiac valves. A characteristic sparkling texture of the myocardium is typical on echocardiography. Diagnosis is made by biopsy of various tissues; if necessary, endomyocardial left or right ventricular biopsies may be performed. There is no treatment for the cardiac manifestations of amyloidosis, and the disease is slowly progressive. Digoxin must be used with caution because patients are particularly sensitive to its toxic effects. Pacemaker implantation may be necessary in patients who develop atrioventricular block. Death from congestive heart failure as well as sudden death, presumably due to arrhythmias, occurs.

PERICARDIAL DISEASES

Acute Pericarditis

Inflammation of the pericardial lining around the heart from a variety of causes (Table 10–4) is termed acute pericarditis. Its typical manifestations include chest pain, a pericardial friction rub, and characteristic electrocardiographic changes. Chest pain, often localized substernally or to the left of the sternum, is usually worsened by lying down, coughing, and deep inspiration, and is relieved somewhat by sitting up and leaning forward. There is often adjacent pleural involvement. The pericardial friction rub, diagnostic of pericarditis, is a scratchy, high-pitched sound that has from one to three components corresponding to atrial systole, ventricular systole, and early diastolic ventricular filling. The ventricular systolic component is present most consistently. The rub is often transient; its absence does not exclude the diagnosis of pericar-

TABLE 10–4. CAUSES OF PERICARDITIS

CAUSE	FEATURES	THERAPY
Idiopathic	Specific etiology not identified Common; symptoms and natural history resemble viral pericarditis	Symptomatic: aspirin, nonsteroidal anti-inflammatory agents; short course of steroids if pain persists
Viral Coxsackie B, echovirus, measles, mumps, influenza, infectious mononucleosis, poliomyelitis, varicella, hepatitis B, cytomegalovirus	Prodromal syndrome resembling a "cold" Typical pericardial pain, rub, ECG changes Usually self-limited, lasts 1–3 weeks Associated myocarditis, recurrent pericarditis, tamponade, or later development of constrictive pericarditis occur infrequently	Symptomatic
Purlent Pericarditis Staphylococcus, streptococcus, pneumococcus	Associated with postoperative infection, endocarditis, hematogenous or contiguous spread High mortality; patients appear acutely ill: fever, chills, sweats, dyspnea; typical pericardial chest pain is unusual If suspected, pericardial fluid must be obtained immediately for examination	Surgical drainage, antibiotics
Tuberculosis	Develops slowly; low-grade fever, malaise, anorexia, weight loss, dyspnea; typical pericardial chest pain is unusual X-ray findings of tuberculosis are usually absent; tuberculin skin test is positive if patient not anergic Constrictive pericarditis common; pericardium may be calcified on x-ray Diagnostic yield is much higher if pericardial tissue as well as fluid is examined and cultured	Antituberculosis agents; pericardiectomy for constriction
Histoplasmosis	Usually occurs with a self-limited pulmonary infection Large pericardial effusions with tamponade common; constriction uncommon Difficult to culture; serologic tests usually positive Hilar adenopathy common on x-ray	Usually not treated with antifungal agents
Pericarditis after Myocardial Infarction (see Chapter 8)	Early form (usually 1–4 days after transmural infarction) probably due to local irritation and is self-limited Later form (>10 days after infarction, Dressler's syndrome) probably immunological in etiology and tends to recur	Symptomatic
Post-pericardiectomy Syndrome	Similar to Dressler's, usually occurs 1–4 weeks after cardiac surgery	
Cardiac Trauma	Penetrating or nonpenetrating trauma Pericarditis can occur early owing to direct pericardial injury or late analogous to Dressler's syndrome	
Uremia	Large effusions with tamponade common	May respond to vigorous dialysis but pericardiectomy is sometimes necessary
Neoplasm	Large effusions with tamponade common Most commonly due to metastatic lung and breast carcinoma, leukemia, lymphoma, and melanoma Tumor cells often detectable in pericardial fluid	Needle or surgical drainage; systemic or local chemotherapy
Radiation	Usually doses >4000 rads to the heart May appear early or several months after radiation; constriction may eventually occur	Symptomatic; pericardiectomy if constrictive
Myxedema	Large pericardial effusions without tamponade are characteristic	Thyroid replacement
Connective Tissue Diseases, Hypersensitivity Syndromes	For example, systemic lupus erythematosus, rheumatoid arthritis, scleroderma, polyarteritis nodosa, drug reactions (e.g., procainamide)	Anti-inflammatory therapy

ditis and its presence does not exclude the existence of a large pericardial effusion. The rub often is best heard with the diaphragm of the stethoscope as the patient sits forward at forced end-expiration. Single-component friction rubs must be differentiated from systolic cardiac murmurs, skin rubbing against the diaphragm of the stethoscope, and the crunching sound of mediastinal air.

The electrocardiogram may be diagnostic, especially if obtained serially, and reveals ST segment elevation with upright T waves at the onset of chest pain (Fig. 10–1). The ST elevation is characteristic in all leads except aV_R and V_1. The ST segments are often concave upward in distinction to those of acute myocardial infarction, but this distinction is often difficult or impossible to make. Reciprocal ST segment depression as in acute myocardial infarction generally does not occur. Several days later the ST segments characteristically return to normal, and the T waves begin to flatten. Subsequently, diffuse T wave inversion develops, usually after the ST segments return to normal, in contrast to the typical pattern of myocardial infarction. Weeks to months later the T waves usually return to normal but may remain abnormal indefinitely. The P-R segment may be depressed, reflecting atrial injury. The ECG changes of acute pericarditis must be distinguished from early repolarization. Early repolarization is common in young patients, usually without P-R segment depression, more often associated with sinus bradycardia than the sinus tachycardia of acute pericarditis, and without a characteristic evolution as described earlier for pericarditis. Atrial rhythm disturbances during pericarditis are common, especially intermittent atrial fibrillation; AV conduction disturbances and ventricular tachyarrhythmias are unusual and should suggest myocardial infarction. If a large pericardial effusion is present, low QRS voltage and electrical alternans may occur.

The chest x-ray is of little value in the diagnosis of acute pericarditis, but an enlarged cardiac silhouette may be noted if a pericardial effusion is present. Calcification of the pericardium may be detected in patients with long-standing pericarditis, especially secondary to tuberculosis. The echocardiogram is extremely accurate for detection and quantitation of pericardial fluid and is also useful to evaluate suspected hemodynamic compromise (tamponade).

Nonspecific indicators of inflammation such as elevated erythrocyte sedimentation rate and leukocytosis are usually present. Cardiac isoenzymes are usually normal. Other laboratory tests that may exclude specific diagnoses include blood cultures, acute and convalescent viral serologies, fungal serology (e.g., histoplasmosis), ASO titer (rheumatic fever), cold

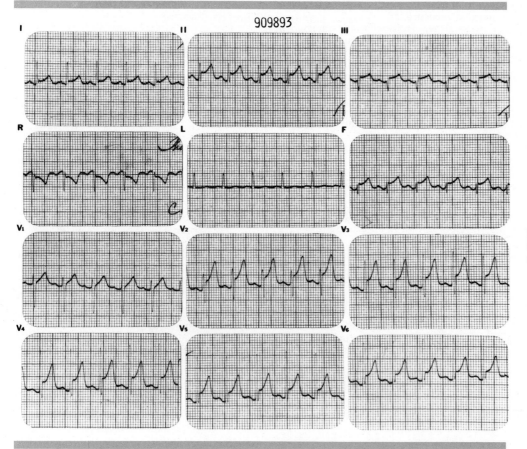

909893

FIGURE 10–1. Typical electrocardiogram in pericarditis showing diffuse ST elevation.

agglutinins (mycoplasma), heterophile test (mononucleosis), thyroid function tests (hypothyroidism), BUN and creatinine (uremia), and connective tissue disease screens such as ANA, rheumatoid factor, and complement.

Management of the patient with acute pericarditis involves treating its etiology. Patients are usually hospitalized to make sure that myocardial infarction is not present and to watch carefully for the occurrence of cardiac tamponade. Salicylates or nonsteroidal anti-inflammatory agents are often effective to relieve pain. Corticosteroids may be used if necessary, but long-term administration should be avoided. Anticoagulants should not be administered because of the risk of hemopericardium. In rare cases, pericardiectomy may be indicated to relieve recurrent symptoms. Most causes of pericarditis are self-limited, and inflammation abates after two to six weeks. Recurrent episodes of pericarditis occur in some patients. Rarely, pericarditis eventually results in pericardial constriction or a combination of effusion and constriction (effusive-constrictive pericarditis).

PERICARDIAL EFFUSION

The hemodynamic effects of fluid in the pericardial cavity depend on the volume and rate of fluid accumulation. Because the pericardium is not compliant, an increase in pericardial effusion that occurs acutely may cause a rapid rise in intrapericardial pressure. If the accumulation of fluid is more gradual, the pericardium may accommodate, and the intrapericardial pressure increase is not as great for any given amount of pericardial fluid. Small increases in the volume of pericardial fluid may have little hemodynamic effect at first, but subsequent small increases may result in a rapid rise in intrapericardial pressure, accounting for the rapid clinical deterioration of patients with stable pericardial effusion.

The patient with pericardial effusion and hemodynamic compromise has dyspnea, tachycardia, distended jugular veins, and a rapid thready pulse. Rales typical of pulmonary edema are absent. Dullness, increased fremitus, and bronchial breath sounds posteriorly below the angle of the left scapula due to compression of the left lower lung by the pericardium (Ewart's sign) may be present. The precordium often is quiet to auscultation, and the apical impulse frequently is not palpable. Kussmaul's sign, an increase in jugular venous pressure with inspiration, is unusual in pericardial effusion or tamponade. When cardiac tamponade results, pulsus paradoxus, characterized by a decrease in the systolic blood pressure of more than 10 mm Hg with normal inspiration, frequently is present. The paradoxical pulse often can be noted by marked weakening or disappearance of a peripheral pulse during inspiration. Paradoxical pulse is not diagnostic of pericardial tamponade and can occur in chronic lung disease, acute asthma, and severe congestive heart failure.

Any cause of acute pericarditis can lead to pericardial effusion. The electrocardiogram may be normal, may demonstrate low voltage, or may reveal ST and T wave changes typical of pericarditis. Electrical alternans, a variation in voltage of P, QRS, and T waves in alternate beats, may occur in patients with large effusions. The chest x-ray may show an enlarged "water bottle" cardiac silhouette, but if the pericardial effusion has developed rapidly, the chest x-ray may show a normal heart size. Definitive diagnosis of pericardial effusion is usually obtained by echocardiography. Cardiac catheterization shows pulsus paradoxus, equalization of diastolic pressures throughout the heart, elevated systemic venous pressure, and normal or reduced cardiac output with reduced stroke volume.

The management of pericardial effusion without tamponade is similar to that of acute pericarditis. Patients with acute significant pericardial effusions should be hospitalized to monitor for impending tamponade. If tamponade occurs, the pericardium should be drained by pericardiocentesis or surgery. Patients with cardiac tamponade and hypotension should receive intravenous volume (and possibly isoproterenol) to optimize cardiac performance until pericardial drainage can be performed. Diuresis is contraindicated.

The pericardial fluid should be examined microscopically for bacteria, cells, glucose, and protein content. An indwelling catheter or drain is sometimes left in place for subsequent drainage of pericardial fluid or chemotherapy instillation.

CONSTRICTIVE PERICARDITIS

Constrictive pericarditis results from pericardial thickening and fibrosis occurring long after acute episodes of pericarditis. It is less common since the advent of antituberculous therapy but can occur after bacterial, fungal, viral, neoplastic, or uremic pericarditis. The fundamental hemodynamic abnormality is abnormal diastolic filling. Eventually the underlying myocardial tissue may atrophy and decreased systolic function may result. Pericardial effusion and constriction may occur together (effusive-constrictive pericarditis), in which case pericardiocentesis may only partially relieve the symptoms. Occasionally constriction can be localized to only certain chambers of the heart.

Symptoms of dyspnea, peripheral edema, abdominal swelling, and fatigue usually develop gradually. On physical examination, the jugular veins are distended with a prominent y descent (corresponding to early rapid ventricular filling). Tachycardia, hepatomegaly, ascites, and peripheral edema are common. Splenomegaly may occur. The pulse pressure is usually normal, and pulsus paradoxus is usually not present. Kussmaul's sign may be present. The apical impulse sometimes is not palpable or may retract with systole. An early diastolic apical sound termed a pericardial knock is often present and can be confused with an S_3 gallop.

Electrocardiographic findings include low voltage and nonspecific T wave changes. The chest x-ray reveals clear lungs and normal or only slightly increased heart size. Pericardial calcification is most common in tuberculous constriction. Echocardiography sometimes can suggest constrictive pericarditis but is usually not diagnostic. At cardiac catheterization the right and left ventricular pressures may demonstrate an early diastolic dip with a subsequent rise termed a square root sign. The right atrial pressure tracings may show sharp x and y descents, generating a typical M-shaped contour. There is equalization of end-diastolic pressures in all four chambers and the pulmonary artery. Occasionally these findings become evident only after an infusion of saline (occult constriction).

It is sometimes difficult to distinguish constrictive pericarditis from restrictive cardiomyopathy. Left ventricular ejection fraction is more likely to be decreased in patients with restrictive cardiomyopathy than constrictive pericarditis. Computed tomography is the procedure of choice to demonstrate the thickened pericardium. Endocardial biopsy or even surgical exploration is sometimes necessary.

Constrictive pericarditis is slowly progressive. Patients may be managed conservatively with mild sodium restriction and diuretics; however, the mortality and morbidity of pericardiectomy are less when it is performed early than after progressive calcification and fibrosis have occurred. Therefore, pericardiectomy should probably not be performed in patients with very mild, early disease or in elderly patients with severe disease and a fibrotic, calcified pericardium. Improvement occurs in about 75 per cent of patients who survive the operation but may be delayed for several weeks or months postoperatively. Cardiac function may not normalize after pericardiectomy either because of inability to completely remove the pericardium or because of fibrosis and atrophy of the underlying myocardium.

REFERENCES

Fowles RE, Mason JW: Endomyocardial biopsy. Ann Intern Med 97:885, 1982.

Fuster V, Gersh BJ, Giuliani ER, Tajik AJ, Brandenberg RO, Frye RL: The natural history of idiopathic dilated cardiomyopathy. Am J Cardiol 47:525, 1981.

Maron BJ, Bonow RO, Cannon RO III, Leon MB, Epstein SE: Hypertrophic cardiomyopathy: Interrelations of clinical manifestations, pathophysiology, and therapy. N Engl J Med 316:780–789, 844–852, 1987.

Shabetai R: Cardiomyopathy: How far have we come in 25 years, how far yet to go? J Am Coll Cardiol 1:252, 1983.

Spodick DH: The normal and diseased pericardium: Current concepts of pericardial physiology, diagnosis, and treatment. J Am Coll Cardiol 1:240, 1983.

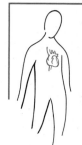

11

CARDIAC TUMORS AND TRAUMA

CARDIAC TUMORS

Tumors involving the heart may be primary or metastatic; both are rare. Although a variety of metastatic tumors has been described in the heart, the most common are malignant melanomas, leukemia, and lymphomas. The treatment of metastatic tumors is treatment of the primary malignancy.

Primary cardiac tumors may be benign or malignant. Myxoma is the most common primary tumor of the heart and is usually benign. Almost all malignant cardiac tumors are sarcomas, angiosarcoma and rhabdomyosarcoma being the most frequent. It is impossible prior to histologic examination to distinguish benign from malignant tumors, but malignant tumors are more likely to present with evidence of metastases, invasion, or rapid growth. Tumor type may be identified occasionally from tissue at the time of peripheral embolectomy. Malignant primary tumors of the heart have a very poor prognosis.

Myxomas may arise from the endocardial surface of any cardiac chamber, but the majority arise from the left atrium, most commonly in the region of the fossa ovalis. They are usually pedunculated. As a general rule, 10 per cent of cardiac myxomas manifest malignant characteristics and 10 per cent arise in locations other than the left atrium. Occasionally they can be bilateral and usually present in one of three general ways: (1) progressive interference with mitral valve function that causes decreased exercise tolerance, dyspnea on exertion, and pulmonary edema; syncope or presyncope may occur; (2) stroke or occlusion of a major systemic artery due to an embolus; (3) systemic manifestations that include fever, wasting, arthralgias, malaise, anemia, or Raynaud's phenomenon.

If the left atrial myxoma interferes with mitral valve

function, a regurgitant valvular murmur may occur. A murmur resembling mitral stenosis may be present owing to obstruction of the valve orifice during diastole. The intensity of the murmur may change with changes in body position. An early diastolic sound termed a "tumor plop" may occur secondary to movement of the tumor toward the left ventricle in early diastole. The erythrocyte sedimentation rate, gamma globulins, and white blood cell count may be elevated. The cause of the systemic manifestations is not clear but may result from products secreted by the tumor, necrotic tumor debris, or an immunologic reaction.

Cardiac myxoma is usually diagnosed by echocardiography. Two-dimensional echocardiography shows the tumor location and movement with the cardiac cycle. Cardiac catheterization with angiocardiography usually is not necessary when the diagnosis has been established noninvasively and is associated with risk of tumor embolus.

Cardiac myxomas should be excised surgically once identified. A recurrent or second myxoma occurs following resection in a small number of patients. Atrial myxoma occasionally may behave as a malignant tumor and demonstrate metastases.

NONPENETRATING TRAUMA

Blunt chest trauma is especially common after steering wheel impact from an automobile accident. It may produce myocardial contusion, resulting in myocardial hemorrhage and at times some degree of necrosis. Often there is little or no residual myocardial scar once healing is complete. Large contusions may lead to myocardial scars, cardiac or septal rupture, congestive heart failure, or formation of true or false aneurysms. Necrosis or hemorrhage involving the cardiac conduction system can produce intraventricular or atrioventricular block. Coronary artery laceration, valvular damage, or pericardial tears may occasionally occur after blunt trauma. The chest pain of myocardial contusion is similar to that of myocardial infarction and is often confused with musculoskeletal pain from the chest trauma. The electrocardiogram at the time of injury may show a diffuse injury pattern similar to that of pericarditis. Later, the electrocardiogram may reveal serial development of Q waves similar to that of acute myocardial infarction if significant necrosis has occurred. Bradyarrhythmias and tachyarrhythmias are common. Contractile abnormalities are usually not severe unless concomitant injury to a valve or the septum has occurred. The MB fraction of creatine kinase is elevated. Myocardial contusion is usually treated similarly to myocardial infarction with initial monitoring and subsequent progressive ambulation. Anticoagulants should not be administered to patients with myocardial contusion. If the patient survives the acute episode, his long-term prognosis is usually good, although late complications such as ventricular arrhythmias occasionally occur.

Rupture of the aorta is a common consequence of blunt trauma. It most commonly occurs just distal to the take-off of the left subclavian artery. The patient may complain of pain in the back or chest similar to that of aortic dissection. The chest x-ray usually reveals widening of the mediastinum. Many patients demonstrate increased arterial pressure in the upper extremities and decreased arterial pressure and pulse pressure in the lower extremities. Signs of decreased renal or spinal cord perfusion may become evident. The diagnosis is usually confirmed by aortography, and the treatment is surgical.

PENETRATING TRAUMA

Penetrating cardiac injuries may be due to external objects such as bullets or knives and also bony fragments occurring from chest injury. Because of its anterior location, the right ventricle is most commonly involved. Iatrogenic causes of cardiac penetrating injury include perforation of the heart during catheterization or cardiac trauma from cardiopulmonary resuscitation.

Penetrating injury to the heart may present as exsanguinating hemorrhage with hemothorax or cardiac tamponade if hemorrhage has been limited to within the pericardial sac. Immediate pericardiocentesis and administration of large volumes of fluids may be performed as preparations are being made for emergency surgery. A "post-pericardiotomy" type of pericarditis, infection, arrhythmias, aneurysm formation, and ventricular septal defects are late complications of penetrating cardiac injury. The risk of bacterial endocarditis, infection from a retained foreign body, and foreign body embolus are complications peculiar to penetrating as opposed to nonpenetrating injuries.

REFERENCES

Peters MN, Hall RJ, Cooley DA, Leachman RD, Garcia E: The clinical syndrome of atrial myxoma. JAMA 230:695, 1974.

Sutton M, Mercier L, Guiliani E, Lie J: Atrial myxomas. A review of clinical experience in 40 patients. Mayo Clin Proc 55:371, 1980.

Symbas PN: Trauma to the Heart and Great Vessels. New York, Grune & Stratton, 1978.

12

AORTIC AND PERIPHERAL VASCULAR DISEASE

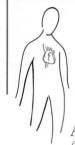

AORTIC ANEURYSMS
(Table 12–1)

Aortic aneurysms, localized areas of increased aortic diameter, may occur in the ascending aorta, aortic arch, descending thoracic aorta, or abdominal aorta, depending on the etiology. For example, aneurysms of the sinuses of Valsalva may occur in Marfan's syndrome or syphilis, as a complication of infective endocarditis, or as a congenital lesion, while aneurysms of the ascending aorta or aortic arch occur in syphilis, aortic dissection, or cystic medial necrosis with or without Marfan's syndrome. Aneurysms of the de-scending thoracic aorta occur from syphilis, atherosclerosis, or dissection. Aneurysms just distal to the take-off of the left subclavian artery are commonly due to trauma. Abdominal aortic aneurysms are usually atherosclerotic but can be secondary to syphilis or extension of a dissection from above. Connective tissue diseases such as Takayasu's arteritis can lead to aneurysm formation anywhere in the aorta, most commonly the proximal portion.

Arteriosclerotic aneurysms are characterized in Table 12–1. A prominent abdominal aortic pulsation may be felt in normally thin people and mistakenly diagnosed as an abdominal aortic aneurysm; on the other hand, an abdominal aortic aneurysm may not

TABLE 12–1. AORTIC ANEURYSMS

ANEURYSM TYPE	ETIOLOGY	LOCATION	CLINICAL FEATURES	PHYSICAL FINDINGS	LABORATORY FINDINGS	TREATMENT
Arterosclerotic	Atherosclerosis	Usually abdominal (between renal arteries and aortic bifurcation)	Older males Often asymptomatic until rupture Abdominal fullness or pulsations; back or epigastric pain, worse prior to rupture	Palpable, pulsatile abdominal mass Peripheral emboli Abdominal bruit Associated peripheral vascular disease	Size measured by abdominal ultrasound Angiography less accurate at estimating size but necessary to define surgical anatomy	Rupture or >6 cm diameter: surgery <4 cm diameter: observe
Dissecting	Hypertension Marfan's syndrome Cystic medial necrosis Aortic coarctation Trauma	Type I: proximal ascending aorta to descending aorta Type II: confined to ascending aorta Type III: begins in descending aorta and extends distally	Severe, sudden, tearing chest pain radiating to abdomen and back (occasional patient will have no pain) Aortic branch occlusions causing myocardial infarction, stroke, spinal infarction with paraplegia, renal impairment Aortic root involvement causing acute aortic insufficiency, rupture into pericardium with pericardial friction rub or tamponade	Hypertension Asymmetric pulses Signs of aortic insufficiency, neurologic involvement, or tamponade if present	ECG may show myocardial infarction Wide medi-astinum on chest x-ray (not always present) CT scan usually diagnostic Angiography necessary to define surgical anatomy	Surgical indications: Ascending aortic involvement Impairment of vital organs Etiology not hypertensive Hemodynamic impairment Medical therapy may be tried in older patient with distal hypertensive dissection: control hypertension and lessen force of contraction (nitroprusside + beta blocker)

be palpable in patients who are obese or who have muscular abdominal walls. Aneurysms may rupture into the inferior vena cava producing an arteriovenous fistula, into the duodenum with acute massive gastrointestinal hemorrhage, into the retroperitoneal space manifested by flank or groin hematomas, or into the abdominal cavity causing abdominal distention. Half of all aneurysms exceeding 6 cm in diameter rupture within one year, and surgical resection with prosthetic graft replacement is usually recommended. Aneurysms less than 6 cm also may rupture. In patients with relatively high surgical risk, aneurysms of 4 to 6 cm should be followed closely and surgery undertaken upon signs of expansion or impending rupture.

A dissecting aneurysm (Table 12–1) is caused by a tear of the aortic intima with formation of a false channel within the aortic media. Blood in the false channel may re-enter the true aortic channel via a second intimal tear or rupture through the adventitia into the periaortic tissues. Most dissections arise either in the ascending aorta within several centimeters of the aortic valve or in the descending thoracic aorta just beyond the origin of the left subclavian artery in the region of the ligamentum arteriosum. Patients with proximal dissections tend to be younger and to have a higher incidence of Marfan's syndrome and cystic medial necrosis; distal dissections more commonly involve older patients with hypertension. Surgery generally is indicated in proximal (type I and type II) dissections, whereas medical therapy may be the treatment of choice for uncomplicated distal dissection (type III). Medical therapy must be administered to surgical patients both during the preoperative stabilization period and chronically postoperatively to prevent progression or repeat dissection.

AORTIC ARTERITIS

Aortitis is an inflammatory process of the aortic wall that may be caused by several disease processes. When it involves the origin of various aortic branches (e.g., the innominate artery, the left common carotid artery, and the left subclavian artery), it is termed the "aortic arch syndrome" and is characteristically produced by Takayasu's syndrome but also by syphilis, arteriosclerosis, or dissecting aneurysm. Takayasu's arteritis or pulseless disease appears to be most common in Japanese females and is an aortic panarteritis that leads to eventual luminal obliteration from the thickened walls and superimposed thrombus. Localized aneurysm formation may occur. The process may involve the coronary ostia or any of the branches of the aortic arch. Tertiary syphilis causes an aortic arteritis that may lead to an ascending aortic aneurysm, aortic valvulitis with insufficiency, and/or coronary ostial stenosis. It is a late manifestation of syphilis, usually occurring 10 to 30 years after the primary infection. Routine serological tests may be negative, but the *Treponema pallidum* immobilization or the fluorescent Treponema antibody absorption test are almost always positive.

The media of the aorta is destroyed from necrosis of smooth muscle and elastic tissue. The intima assumes a wrinkled appearance referred to as "tree barking." Involvement is much more prominent in the aortic root than in the distal aorta, in contrast to atherosclerotic aortic aneurysms. This whole process is often asymptomatic and detected by eggshell calcification of the ascending aorta on chest x-ray.

MISCELLANEOUS AORTIC DISEASE

Large peripheral arterial emboli may obstruct the abdominal aortic bifurcation, resulting in so-called saddle emboli. These usually originate from the left heart but rarely may originate from the aorta itself in the area of an atherosclerotic lesion. Other, rarer causes are "paradoxical emboli" (from the right heart or venous system in patients with right-to-left shunts), atrial myxomas, or infective endocarditis (very large emboli can occur in acute endocarditis and fungal endocarditis). Obstruction at the aortic bifurcation is characterized by the sudden onset of severe pain in both legs, peripheral neurological abnormalities, and evidence of decreased perfusion bilaterally. It must be differentiated from acute atherosclerotic aortic thrombosis and dissecting aneurysm. The diagnosis is confirmed by angiography. Surgical removal of the clot with subsequent anticoagulation and/or treatment of the underlying cause is necessary.

Infected aortic aneurysms are rare. The most common congenital aortic anomaly is coarctation of the aorta (see Chapter 5). Congenital aortic aneurysms of the sinus of Valsalva may rupture into the right atrium or ventricle, producing a continuous murmur. Sinus of Valsalva aneurysms can occasionally produce coronary occlusion, conduction disturbances, or valvular malfunction.

PERIPHERAL VASCULAR DISEASE (Table 12–2)

Arteriosclerosis obliterans refers to atherosclerotic narrowing of large and medium-sized arteries, usually those supplying the lower extremities (the superficial femoral artery, the aortoiliac area, and the popliteal artery). The symptoms of claudication may remain stable over a very long time period. Many of these patients eventually die from other complications. Pentoxifylline, a drug that improves the flow properties of blood, may be useful to relieve symptoms in patients with chronic peripheral arterial disease. The mechanism by which pentoxifylline decreases blood viscosity is unclear but may be related to improving erythrocyte flexibility.

Thromboangiitis obliterans, or Buerger's disease, is an inflammatory process causing obliteration of peripheral arteries and veins. In its later stages, it may be difficult to differentiate from arteriosclerosis obliterans. Patients may do well for long periods of time,

TABLE 12–2. PERIPHERAL VASCULAR DISEASES

DISEASE	PATHOLOGY	CLINICAL FEATURES	PHYSICAL FINDINGS	LABORATORY FINDINGS	TREATMENT
Arteriosclerosis obliterans	Atherosclerotic narrowing of large and medium-sized arteries of lower extremities; segmental with skip areas. Occasionally involves upper extremities (subclavian steal syndrome)	Male > female Common in diabetics Exertional leg pain relieved with rest (claudication); rest pain implies severe compromise Cold, numb legs Buttock claudication and impotence with aortoiliac obstruction (Leriche's syndrome)	Decreased or absent lower extremity pulses Aortic, iliac, or femoral bruit Limb ischemia: cool, pale, cyanotic; shiny dry skin without hair; nail changes, ulcerations, gangrene	Doppler and arteriography locate obstructions	Intermittent claudication: —exercise (stop when claudication occurs) —stop smoking —avoid peripheral vasoconstricting drugs, e.g., propranolol —meticulous skin and nail care —pentoxifylline Severe claudication or rest ischemia: —percutaneous transluminal angioplasty or surgical bypass; amputation if gangrenous
Thromboangiitis obliterans	Intimal proliferation and thrombi in small to medium-sized vessels with inflammatory infiltrates Segmental involvement of arteries and veins Upper and lower extremity involvement	Male > female Usually occurs before age 30 Etiology not understood but related to smoking Cool extremities Raynaud's phenomenon Distal limb claudication (e.g., instep or hand)	Cool extremities Digital ulcers Migrating thrombophlebitis	Biopsy of artery diagnostic	Stop smoking Sympathectomy to prevent vasospasm Amputation of distal extremities for gangrene
Arterial embolism	Emboli tend to lodge at arterial bifurcations with subsequent thrombus formation (e.g., "saddle embolus" at aortic bifurcation)	Sudden onset of painful extremity (occasionally more gradual)	Cold, pale extremity with absent pulses distal to embolus	Pathologic examination of embolus may reveal etiology Doppler examination helps localize embolus	Heparin Surgical embolectomy for larger vessels Chronic anticoagulation if embolic source cannot be eliminated
Raynaud's phenomenon	Vasospasm of digital vessels precipitated by cold and relieved by heat	Underlying causes: Arterial occlusive diseases Connective tissue diseases Neurologic diseases Ingestion of vasoconstricting drugs Nerve compression syndromes Cryoglobulinemia or cold agglutinins Post-frostbite or trench foot Raynaud's disease (female > male)	White, cyanotic digit upon exposure to cold or emotional upset; hyperemic upon resumption of circulation Normal pulses Chronic nail and skin changes (sclerodactyly) in severe cases; small areas of distal gangrene but digital amputation rare		Limitation of cold exposure Stop smoking Vasodilators Regional sympathectomy

but the need for amputation of distal extremities is common if patients continue to smoke. No medication has been shown to be helpful.

Peripheral arterial emboli usually originate from thrombi in either the left atrium or left ventricle or, uncommonly, from atheromatous emboli located in atherosclerotic plaques in the aorta. A "paradoxical embolus" refers to an embolus originating from the venous system, passing through a right-to-left intracardiac shunt, and lodging in the systemic arterial tree. Septic emboli may occur with endocarditis and tumor emboli with cardiac myxoma. Acute thrombosis of a vessel is sometimes difficult to distinguish from embolism but should be suspected if no source for emboli is present and if concomitant severe atherosclerotic disease is present.

Raynaud's phenomenon involves bilateral paroxysmal ischemia of fingers or toes, usually precipitated by cold and relieved by heat. The entire hand or foot is usually not affected. Raynaud's phenomenon may be secondary to a variety of underlying diseases; if no underlying disease can be found, the patient is said to have Raynaud's disease.

ENVIRONMENTAL DAMAGE OF THE EXTREMITIES

Both freezing (frostbite) and nonfreezing injuries may damage the extremities. The presence of dampness or peripheral vascular disease enhances the tissue loss for any given temperature reduction or duration of exposure. Tissue damage is probably due to a combination of direct freezing and marked vasoconstriction. Cold produces numbness in tissues that may allow freezing without warning, so that the first indication of frostbite may be a prickling feeling. The affected area initially looks pale or waxy yellow and may be anesthetic. In severe frostbite, edema and bulla formation occur with thawing, and gangrene may result. Frostbite should be treated immediately by rewarming, but excessive warming, massage, and exercise should be avoided. Infection is the greatest danger and the affected areas must be handled with aseptic technique.

Prolonged immersion of extremities in water leads to a syndrome known as immersion foot or trench foot. Wetness plus cold produces the most serious form of the syndrome. It does not necessarily require freezing temperatures and is due in part to direct and reflex vasoconstriction.

PERIPHERAL ANEURYSMS AND FISTULAE

Occasionally true or false aneurysms may occur in peripheral vessels. True aneurysms are usually secondary to atherosclerosis; false aneurysms (i.e., a tear in the arterial wall allowing accumulation of blood in the perivascular tissues) may be associated with trauma or rupture of a true aneurysm. True aneurysms of peripheral vessels are located most commonly in the popliteal artery but can occur in the femoral artery, iliac artery, arteries of the upper extremities, and occasionally visceral arteries such as renal or splenic arteries. Aneurysms of the popliteal and femoral arteries are often palpable. Aneurysms may occasionally be infected (mycotic). Symptoms result from arterial occlusion, rupture, distal embolization, or local pressure on adjacent structures such as nerves or veins. Surgery for renal or splenic artery aneurysms is usually recommended in patients who are pregnant (increased incidence of rupture) or whose aneurysm is symptomatic, enlarging, or more than 1.5 to 2.0 cm in diameter. Femoral and popliteal aneurysms should be treated surgically if the patient's condition allows.

Arteriovenous fistulae are acquired or congenital abnormal communications between arteries and veins without an intervening capillary network. Acquired fistulae may be created to facilitate hemodialysis or may occur after trauma such as a gunshot or stab wound. Increased blood flow leads to venous dilation and makes the region of the fistula abnormally warm; the area distal to the fistula may be cool. If the fistula is large, a high cardiac output state may occur and may produce heart failure. Because of the low resistance pathway, diastolic blood pressure tends to decrease, and systolic blood pressure and pulse pressure increase. A bruit and thrill may be present over the fistula. If the artery serving the fistula is compressed, shunting via the low resistance circuit is prevented, and a prompt decrease in the pulse rate may occur (Branham's sign). Acquired fistulae are best treated surgically. Congenital AV fistulae are usually multiple, small, and often accompanied by cutaneous birthmarks. Enlargement of the entire involved limb may occur, since the fistulae are present during the period of rapid bone growth. Bruits and pulsatile masses are uncommon, since the fistulae are small and multiple. Treatment is less satisfactory than that of large acquired AV fistulae.

ARTERIAL TRAUMA

Arterial trauma is usually a surgical emergency. It occurs with penetrating or blunt trauma, including fractures and dislocations. Swelling within a compartment of an extremity after blunt trauma can cause both arterial and neurological damage and responds to decompression of that compartment. Direct arterial injury from trauma requires acute surgical repair. Arterial injury may be iatrogenic from catheterization of brachial or femoral arteries. Loss of local pulse after a catheterization procedure should be approached surgically with early thrombectomy and/or repair, since waiting may necessitate more complicated procedures.

PERIPHERAL VENOUS DISEASE

The most common disorder involving the peripheral veins is venous thrombosis with thrombophlebitis.

Thrombophlebitis refers to inflammation of the vein, usually from thrombus but occasionally from trauma or infection. Predisposing factors to thrombophlebitis are venous stasis, local venous injury, and hypercoagulable states. Particular risk factors for thrombophlebitis include oral contraceptives, trauma or fractures of the extremities, pregnancy, major surgery, prolonged immobilization, heart disease, varicose veins, and myeloproliferative syndromes. Local thrombophlebitis may occur from administration of irritating drugs such as chemotherapeutic agents or from indwelling intravenous catheters, especially if infection has supervened (septic phlebitis). Patients with malignancies appear to be prone to migrating, recurrent thrombophlebitis. Thrombophlebitis can occur with thromboangiitis obliterans or processes causing extrinsic obstruction of venous flow. In some patients no predisposing factors can be found. Low-dose subcutaneous heparin appears to be effective prophylaxis against deep vein thrombosis in patients with a variety of medical or surgical conditions.

Symptoms and signs of venous thrombosis and thrombophlebitis in the leg vary. The onset may be inapparent until pulmonary embolism occurs. Warmth and edema may occur, and the affected leg may become larger than the other. Tenderness over the deep vein upon palpation or inflation of a blood pressure cuff may be noted. Pain upon dorsiflexion of the foot (Homans' sign) is neither sensitive nor specific. Skin changes such as mottling or cyanosis may be present. A palpable venous "cord" occurs in only about 20 per cent of patients. When thrombophlebitis is superficial, red, tender, indurated areas occur just beneath the skin, often corresponding to the distribution of the superficial veins. The distinction, usually requiring laboratory evaluation, between deep and superficial thrombophlebitis is critical because the former is prone to embolization whereas the latter is not.

The clinical presentation of iliofemoral thrombosis is characterized by unilateral leg swelling, and the diagnosis usually can be confirmed by Doppler examination. The main differential diagnosis of this syndrome is extrinsic venous obstruction by tumor or adenopathy. Deep venous thrombosis in calf veins is more difficult to diagnose clinically. Doppler studies and impedance plethysmography may be helpful, but a venogram is usually necessary. Venograms are usually reliable diagnostically; however, inadequate opacification of the deep venous system may occur, and areas of previous thrombophlebitis may be difficult to distinguish from new thrombophlebitis. Phlebitis may occur as a complication of venography in a small number of patients.

Management of deep venous thombosis includes heat, elevation of the extremity, and administration of anti-inflammatory agents. Anticoagulation is required to prevent additional thrombus formation and pulmonary embolism. Heparin should be used for immediate anticoagulation to keep the activated partial thromboplastin time 2 to 2.5 times normal. Heparin is continued for seven to ten days. Warfarin should be given for several days before heparin is discontinued, and its effect may be estimated using the prothrombin time. Bed rest is necessary for several days until pain and swelling have improved. Upon ambulation, an elastic support stocking should be worn. The duration of anticoagulation therapy is controversial but is usually between six weeks and six months. If risk factors for thrombophlebitis cannot be corrected or if recurrent thrombophlebitis occurs, chronic anticoagulation may be necessary. In patients with deep vein thrombosis who have contraindications to anticoagulation or in whom pulmonary embolism recurs despite anticoagulation, surgical plication of the inferior vena cava or insertion of an inferior vena caval umbrella is indicated to prevent pulmonary embolism. Fibrinolytic agents such as urokinase or streptokinase may be useful to treat deep venous thrombosis but should be used only in patients with serious iliofemoral thrombophlebitis.

Superficial thrombophlebitis caused by intravenous indwelling catheters is treated by removal of the catheter and warm heat. Because of this potential complication, IV lines should not be inserted in the leg. If infection is present, appropriate antibiotics should be given. Anticoagulation is not used unless lower extremity deep venous involvement is present. Heat and elevation should be applied. Ambulation with elastic stockings is possible. Anti-inflammatory drugs may aid in alleviating the symptoms.

Varicose veins (distended, tortuous superficial veins with incompetent valves) can result from thrombophlebitis but may also occur congenitally or in conditions associated with increased venous pressure such as pregnancy, prolonged standing, and ascites. In most people the edema resolves overnight. Many people complain of aching discomfort from the superficial varicosities, relieved by elastic stockings and leg elevation. Occasionally stripping or sclerosing of the saphenous veins may be necessary. Chronic deep venous insufficiency is more serious and gives rise to more edema, darkening and induration of the skin and sometimes indolent skin ulcers (stasis dermatitis). Arterial pulses are normal. The post-phlebitic syndrome refers to chronic swelling and skin changes in extremities due to chronic venous insufficiency, often caused by a previous episode of thrombophlebitis.

Swelling of an extremity can also occur from obstruction of the lymphatic outflow (lymphedema). Lymphedema may be idiopathic (primary) or more commonly secondary (for example, due to lymphangitis, neoplasms, adenopathy, or surgical removal of lymph nodes). Venous distention, stasis dermatitis, and ulcers are usually not present, but lymphangiography and/or venography may be necessary to differentiate lymphedema from venous obstruction.

REFERENCES

Bergan JJ, Flinn WR, Yao JST: Operative therapy of peripheral vascular disease. Prog Cardiovasc Dis 26:273, 1984.
Coffman JD, Davies WT: Vasospastic diseases: a review. Prog Cardiovasc Dis 18:123, 1975.

Coffman JD: Intermittent claudication and rest pain; physiologic concepts and therapeutic approaches. Prog Cardiovasc Dis 22:53, 1979.

DeSanctis RW, Doroghazi RM, Austen WG, Buckley MJ: Aortic dissection. N Engl J Med 317:1060–1067, 1987.

Moser KM, Fedullo PF: Venous thromboembolism. Three simple decisions. Chest 83:117, 256, 1983.

Roberts W: Aortic dissection: Anatomy, consequences, and causes. Am Heart J 101:195, 1981.

Sabiston DC (ed): Textbook of Surgery. 13th ed. Philadelphia, WB Saunders Company, 1986.

Schwartz SI, Shives GT, Spencer FC, Storer EH (eds): Principles of Surgery. 4th ed. New York, McGraw-Hill Book Company, 1984, pp 873–1002.

13

CARDIAC TRANSPLANTATION; SURGERY IN PATIENTS WITH CARDIOVASCULAR DISEASE; PREGNANCY AND CARDIAC DISEASE

CARDIAC TRANSPLANTATION

Cardiac transplantation was first performed in humans in 1967 but met with a high graft rejection rate. The development of cyclosporine immunosuppression sharply reduced the number of patients with graft rejection so that now the one-, three-, and five-year survival rates are about 80 per cent, 70 per cent, and 55 per cent, respectively.

Candidates are usually less than 55 years old, are free of other illnesses such as diabetes mellitus requiring insulin and co-existent liver or renal disease, and suffer from end-stage heart disease with a life expectancy of less than one year. Most patients have coronary disease, with idiopathic viral or rheumatic cardiomyopathies affecting the rest of the group. Combined heart/lung transplantation may be considered in patients with severe irreversible pulmonary hypertension. Sequential transplantation has been performed in which a patient with severe pulmonary disease but a normal heart receives a heart/lung transplantation from one patient and donates his/her heart to another. Donors generally have sustained irreversible cerebral damage due to trauma or intracranial hemorrhage.

For orthotopic transplantation, the patient's heart is removed, leaving the posterior walls of the atria with their venous connections to suture to the donor atria. The great vessels are then anastomosed. Heterotopic heart transplantation involves leaving the recipient's heart in situ and attaching the donor heart in parallel, with anastomoses between the atria, pulmonary arteries, and aortae. Immunosuppression is accomplished with combinations of cyclosporine, azathioprine, prednisone, and antithymocyte globulin. Acute rejection is monitored by histologic analysis of repeated right ventricular endomyocardial biopsies. Accelerated coronary atherosclerosis, possibly due to rejection-induced injury to the coronary arterial intima, is a potential hazard, as is the development of hypertension, renal disease, and infections.

GENERAL SURGERY IN THE PATIENT WITH HEART DISEASE

Noncardiac surgery is particularly stressful in patients with pre-existing heart disease. The burdens of anesthesia, surgical trauma, wound healing, infection, hemorrhage, and pulmonary insufficiency may overwhelm the diseased heart. The internist is often asked to assess cardiovascular risk in patients undergoing noncardiac surgery and to aid in their preoperative and postoperative management.

General anesthetics reduce myocardial contractility and also have autonomic nervous system effects that may cause either hypotension or hypertension. Regional, spinal, or epidural anesthesia minimizes myocardial depression, but sympathetic blockade and hypotension still may result. In general, there appears to be no difference in risk between general anesthesia and spinal anesthesia in cardiac patients. The anesthesiologist must maintain adequate ventilation, oxygenation, and blood pH throughout the procedure. The ECG is routinely monitored throughout surgery. If cardiac disease is significant, arterial blood pressure, central venous pressure, and/or pulmonary arterial wedge pressure may need to be monitored throughout the procedure. Cardiac arrhythmias are particularly likely in patients with heart disease and occur most commonly during induction of anesthesia and intubation. Excessive vagal tone can cause bradyarrhythmias and usually responds to adjusting the depth of anesthesia or administering atropine. Antiarrhythmic agents may be administered if needed.

Some patients have life-threatening indications for surgery, and cardiac risk does not affect whether or not the surgery should be performed. In elective surgery, however, the timing of the operation or even whether the operation should be done may depend upon a preoperative estimation of surgical risk. Cardiac risk is strongly associated with the type of surgical procedure. Herniorrhaphy and transurethral resection of the prostate carry relatively low risk, whereas chest, abdominal, and retroperitoneal surgery have a relatively high risk. Emergency surgery is associated with greater risk than nonemergent surgery because there is no time to optimize the patient's cardiac status.

Ischemic heart disease is one of the major determinants of cardiac risk. The incidence of perioperative myocardial infarction is 4 to 8 per cent in patients who have had remote prior infarctions. In addition, the mortality from perioperative myocardial infarction is two to three times greater in patients with previous infarction than in those without previous infarction. Particularly high risk of reinfarction occurs if surgery is performed early after infarction but levels off if surgery is delayed until six months after infarction. The surgical risk in patients with stable angina pectoris is about the same as that in patients with remote myocardial infarction. Patients with unstable angina pectoris should not have elective surgery until the angina is stabilized and possibly invasive evaluation of the coronary arteries obtained.

Decompensated congestive heart failure is another major operative risk factor and should be treated vigorously prior to noncardiac surgery. Patients with congestive heart failure or atrial tachyarrhythmias should probably receive digitalis prior to surgery.

Patients with symptomatic heart block may need prophylactic pacing prior to surgery. Patients with chronic bifascicular block or asymptomatic type I second-degree AV block probably do not require prophylactic pacemaker placement prior to anesthesia. Patients with frequent or symptomatic atrial or ventricular tachyarrhythmias should be treated prior to surgery.

Patients with valvular heart disease tend to tolerate the operation according to their pre-existing functional status. Patients with critical aortic or mitral stenosis are at particularly high risk. Treatment of heart failure should be optimized preoperatively, and those with severe valvular lesions should be considered for corrective surgery prior to elective noncardiac operation. In patients with valvular disease or prosthetic heart valves, endocarditis prophylaxis should be administered if appropriate. In patients with prosthetic heart valves, anticoagulation can usually be stopped temporarily immediately preoperatively and in the early postoperative period in order to prevent bleeding complications.

Mild to moderate hypertension does not alter surgical risk. Severe hypertension should be controlled prior to surgery, as should heart failure or angina associated with it.

Patients with congenital heart disease are at increased risk according to their functional disability. Patients with cyanotic congenital heart disease and polycythemia have an increased risk of hemorrhage due to coagulation defects and thrombocytopenia, and they may tolerate hypotension and hypoxia poorly. Appropriate endocarditis prophylaxis should be administered. Patients with right-to-left shunts are at risk for paradoxical emboli.

In addition to evaluating and optimizing the patient's cardiac status, the general medical status should also be optimized. Pulmonary function is especially important; cessation of smoking and treatment of chronic bronchitis may improve risk.

HEART DISEASE AND PREGNANCY

Marked changes in normal circulatory physiology occur during pregnancy. The cardiac output rises by the end of the first trimester, peaking at a level (30 to 50 per cent rise) in the twentieth to twenty-fourth week that is maintained until after delivery. Increases in stroke volume, heart rate (10 beats per minute), and blood volume (40 to 50 per cent) and decreases in systolic blood pressure and the systemic and pulmonary vascular resistances result. Oxygen consumption and minute ventilation increase. Easy fatigability, decreased exercise tolerance, dyspnea, peripheral edema, a third heart sound, and a midsystolic murmur may be normal in pregnancy. The mechanical pressure of a gravid uterus on the inferior vena cava may decrease venous return and reduce cardiac output. The hemodynamic stresses of pregnancy can exacerbate any pre-existing cardiac abnormality.

Most rheumatic valvular disease in young women involves mitral stenosis. Mitral stenosis is aggravated by the increased cardiac output and heart rate required during pregnancy. The incidence of heart failure increases as pregnancy progresses. These patients have an increased risk of complications from atrial fibrillation, emboli, or endocarditis during pregnancy. Nevertheless, most of these patients can be managed carefully through a relatively uneventful pregnancy. Right ventricular failure may increase the peripheral edema, venous stasis, and risk of pulmonary embolism.

Women with significant mitral or aortic valvular disease who desire children may require surgical correction of the lesion before conception. Cardiac surgical intervention *during* pregnancy carries an increased risk for both mother and fetus. If a valve is inserted, one should consider a porcine valve so that anticoagulation may be avoided. Warfarin crosses the placenta but heparin does not. Warfarin may produce fetal developmental abnormalities if administered in the first trimester. The use of heparin versus warfarin during various stages of pregnancy is controversial, but it is clear that warfarin should be replaced by heparin during the last two to three weeks of pregnancy. Heparin is discontinued and if necessary protamine administered upon the onset of labor. Patients given warfarin should not breast feed, since it is excreted in breast milk. Patients with prosthetic valves probably should receive peripartum endocarditis prophylaxis.

Survival to reproductive age in patients with congenital heart disease has become more common since the advent of surgical intervention. The risk of pregnancy in patients after surgical correction of congenital heart lesions depends on the completeness of their repair and residual defects such as left ventricular dysfunction or pulmonary hypertension. Patients with uncomplicated cardiac lesions such as ostium secundum atrial septal defects usually tolerate pregnancy without any problem. Patients with uncorrected cyanotic heart disease such as tetralogy of Fallot may have difficulty carrying a pregnancy to term. The infants often have low birth weights. Adverse hemodynamics may result in increased right-to-left shunt and increasing maternal cyanosis, magnifying the risk to both mother and child. In patients with severe pulmonary vascular obstruction (for example, Eisenmenger's syndrome), the fixed resistance allows little circulatory reserve, and fluctuations in systemic vascular resistance, cardiac output, and blood volume are very poorly tolerated, especially during labor and the puerperium. Severe aortic stenosis also limits cardiac reserve, and the risk of exertional syncope may increase during pregnancy. Patients with Marfan's syndrome are at markedly increased risk of aortic dissection during pregnancy. Women with coarctation of the aorta also have an increased risk of aortic dissection during pregnancy. Women with persistent cardiomegaly following peripartum cardiomyopathy are at high risk during subsequent pregnancies.

Maternal and fetal complications and mortality are directly related to functional class, and therapy should be optimized throughout pregnancy. Heart failure should be treated by decreased activity, decreased salt intake, and administration of digitalis and diuretics. If heart failure is refractory to medical therapy, termination of pregnancy should be considered. Patients with heart failure may need to be hospitalized during the final weeks of pregnancy. Serious arrhythmias are managed with conventional therapy. Chest x-rays and cardiac catheterization should be avoided if possible because of the radiation risks to the fetus. Factors that may exacerbate heart failure should be eliminated. Most women with heart disease should undergo a spontaneous term vaginal delivery, although cesarean section may be necessary in selected seriously ill patients.

REFERENCES

Goldman L: Cardiac risks and complications of noncardiac surgery. Ann Intern Med 98:504, 1983.
Sullivan JM, Ramanathan KB: Current concepts: Management of medical problems in pregnancy—severe cardiac disease. N Engl J Med 313:304–309, 1985.

GENERAL REFERENCES

Braunwald E (ed): Heart Disease. A Textbook of Cardiovascular Medicine. 3rd ed. Philadelphia, WB Saunders Company, 1988.
Hurst JW (ed): The Heart. Arteries and Veins. 6th ed. New York, McGraw-Hill Book Company, 1986.

Wallace AG (ed): Cardiovascular diseases. *In* Wyngaarden JB, Smith LH Jr (eds): Cecil Textbook of Medicine. 17th ed. Philadelphia, WB Saunders Company, 1985.

SECTION

II

RESPIRATORY DISEASES

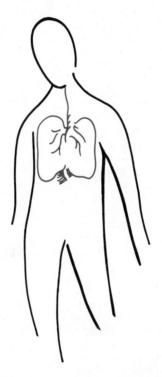

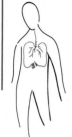

14

APPROACH TO THE PATIENT WITH RESPIRATORY DISEASE

The lungs are the major organs of gas exchange and are affected by a wide variety of acute and chronic diseases. The correct diagnosis of respiratory illness requires careful attention to both the history and the physical examination as well as the use of carefully chosen diagnostic studies.

COMMON PRESENTING COMPLAINTS

Cough is "the watch dog of the lungs." It is provoked by mechanical or chemical stimulation of the airways. The cough is preceded by a deep breath followed by glottic closure. Then active compression causes a rapid rise in intrathoracic pressure until sudden opening of the glottis allows rapid decompression. The high flow velocity achieved serves to clear the airway of secretions or foreign bodies. Cough has a number of causes, including the presence of secretions, viral infection of the airway epithelium, stimulation of parenchymal receptors by pulmonary edema, and fibrotic lung disease. It may be the sole manifestation of bronchospasm, and up to 45 per cent of patients presenting with chronic cough as a sole complaint have asthma. Chronic cough at night can often be ascribed to the presence of postnasal drip, reflux esophagitis, or aspiration. Recent alteration in the character of a chronic cough may be due to bronchial carcinoma. The cause of chronic isolated cough can usually be elucidated without recourse to invasive measures.

Hemoptysis requires immediate evaluation. A bleeding site in the upper airway should be excluded. Blood-streaked sputum is commonly seen in bronchitis, bronchiectasis, pneumonia, and tuberculosis, but in the absence of infection, persistent or intermittent hemoptysis usually indicates the presence of tumor. Massive hemoptysis (>600 ml in 24 hr) is a medical emergency; unless it is promptly treated, the patient may asphyxiate. Unexplained hemoptysis requires a complete evaluation, including a chest x-ray, and fiberoptic bronchoscopy may eventually be required.

Breathing is an automatic, unconscious act. Dyspnea indicates an awareness of increased difficulty in breathing. Its pathophysiology is unclear but may be due to a disproportion between the perceptive demand for ventilation and the level achieved. This may result from a change in the relationship between respiratory center drive and minute ventilation or the work of breathing. Clarification of the predisposing factors is important in the diagnosis of its origin. Episodic dyspnea associated with wheezing at rest or following exercise may indicate bronchospasm. Dyspnea causing arousal from sleep may be due to nocturnal asthma, pulmonary edema, sleep apnea syndrome, or aspiration. Dyspnea on exertion may be cardiac or pulmonary in origin, and differentiation often requires exercise testing.

Chest pain originates in the chest wall, the parietal pleura, the large airways, and the structures located within the mediastinum, since the lung parenchyma and visceral pleura are insensitive to painful stimuli. Pleuritic pain is distinctive, being sharp, knifelike, and exacerbated by breathing and coughing. It must be differentiated from pericardial pain, involvement of the intercostal nerves by herpes zoster, and inflammation of the costochondral junctions (Tietze's syndrome). Disease involvement of the diaphragmatic pleura may cause referred pain to the shoulder because the phrenic nerve supply arises from the cervical roots (C3 to C5).

Careful review of the remainder of the history is important. Prior episodes of respiratory infections may indicate acquired or congenital abnormalities of pulmonary clearance mechanisms. Similar findings in family members may suggest an inherited disorder such as immotile cilia syndrome. Attention should be paid to occupation, travel, habits (smoking), and hobbies (pets).

PHYSICAL EXAMINATION

The physical examination of the chest remains a cornerstone of the diagnostic process. It is wise to follow a set system to avoid inadvertently neglecting some aspects of the examination (Table 14–1). Unobtrusive observation of the patient as he breathes quietly is important. A respiratory rate above 22 breaths per minute suggests underlying lung disease. Normally the rib cage and abdomen move synchronously on respiration, both moving out on inspiration and in on expiration. Movement of the rib cage and abdomen in opposite directions is termed paradoxical breathing. This is observed in the presence of an increased respiratory load, diaphragmatic paralysis, and intercostal muscle paralysis (quadriplegia). Retraction of the intercostal, supraclavicular, and suprasternal spaces reflects the generation of increased negative intrathoracic pressure in the presence of lung disease. Downward pull of the trachea, called tracheal tug, is commonly observed in obstructive lung disease. The distance between the cricoid cartilage and the sternal notch is less than the usual three to four finger breadths in patients with hyperinflation.

Cyanosis is a bluish discoloration of the skin which becomes detectable when the O_2 saturation falls to about 80 to 90 per cent. Accuracy diminishes in the presence of inadequate capillary blood flow or anemia. Finger clubbing is recognized by loss of the angle between the nail and the nail bed. It may be associated with painless swelling of tissues of the terminal phalanx and/or arthralgias of the wrist and ankles (hypertrophic pulmonary osteoarthropathy). Common causes include chronic suppurative diseases, chronic interstitial lung disease, pulmonary malignancy, cyanotic congenital heart disease, endocarditis, and chronic liver and bowel disease, as well as a congenital idiopathic form.

Contraction of the sternomastoid muscles during resting breathing is an important indicator of respiratory distress. Patients with obstructive lung disease often derive symptomatic benefit from pursed-lip breathing, but the mechanism of this improvement is unknown. A "barrel-shaped" chest wall is seen in emphysema, while deformity of the chest wall may explain a restrictive pattern on pulmonary function testing.

Decreased movement of one side of the chest on palpation indicates the presence of ipsilateral lung disease. Deviation of the trachea from the midline may reflect a shift in the mediastinum and is helpful in the diagnosis of a pneumothorax (Table 14–2). Vocal fremitus is the palpable vibration associated with transmission of the spoken word to the chest wall. It is increased with consolidation and decreased if fluid or air is present in the pleural space. Its absence helps to differentiate pleural effusion from a dense parenchymal infiltrate seen on radiographs.

Percussion helps in detecting the interface between the aerated lung and solid structures (liver, pleural

fluid, or consolidation). Determination of heart and mediastinal size and probably also the extent of diaphragmatic movement is better done radiographically.

During auscultation, the observer needs to compare the two sides of the chest at equidistant points from

TABLE 14–1. SYSTEMATIC APPROACH TO PHYSICAL EXAMINATION OF THE CHEST

I. Inspection
Initial impression—distress, wheeze, malnourished, etc.
Respiratory rate, depth, and pattern
Asynchronous motion of the rib cage and abdomen
Recession of the intercostal, supraclavicular, or suprasternal spaces
Tracheal tug
Cyanosis
Finger clubbing or nicotine stains
Accessory muscle employment
Pursed-lip breathing
Chest wall shape and deformity

II. Palpation
Tracheal deviation
Chest expansion (globally/locally)
Vocal fremitus
Pleural rub
Lymphadenopathy
Subcutaneous emphysema

III. Percussion
Normal, dull, or increased

IV. Auscultation
Breath sounds—can only be normal, reduced, or bronchial (latter associated with increased vocal resonance, whispering pectoriloquy, and egophony)
Added sounds—can only be absent, wheezes, crackles, or pleural rub

TABLE 14–2. PHYSICAL FINDINGS IN COMMON PULMONARY DISORDERS

DISORDER	MEDIASTINAL DISPLACEMENT	CHEST WALL MOVEMENT	VOCAL FREMITUS	PERCUSSION NOTE	BREATH SOUNDS	ADDED SOUNDS	VOICE SOUNDS
Pleural effusion	Heart displaced to opposite side	Reduced over affected area	Absent or markedly decreased	Stony dull	Absent over fluid; bronchial at upper border	Absent; pleural rub may be found above effusion	Absent over effusion; increased with egophony at upper border
Consolidation	None	Reduced over affected area	Increased	Dull	Bronchial	Crackles	Increased with egophony and whispering pectoriloquy
Pneumothorax	Tracheal deviation to opposite side if under tension	Decreased over affected area	Absent	Resonant	Absent	Absent	Absent
Atelectasis	Ipsilateral shift	Decreased over affected area	Absent	Dull	Absent or diminished	Absent	Absent
Bronchospasm	None	Decreased symmetrically	Normal or decreased	Normal or decreased	Normal	Wheeze	Normal or decreased
Interstitial fibrosis	None	Decreased symmetrically	Normal or increased	Normal	Normal	Coarse crackles unaffected by cough or posture	Normal

the midline and while listening answer only two questions: (1) What is the character of the breath sounds? (2) Are added sounds present, and if so what is their nature?

Breath sounds are caused by turbulent air flow, with the intensity depending on the flow rate. They are produced entirely in the trachea and large airways and transmitted to the chest wall initially by the smaller airways and finally through the lung parenchyma. The passage through the lung filters out the high frequencies and accounts for the differences in normal breath sounds heard at different places. As we move away from the central airways to the periphery of the lung, the filtering effect serves to diminish the inspiration and almost eliminate the expiratory noise. This is the normal vesicular breath sound. Bronchial breath sounds are essentially unfiltered, and both inspiration and expiration are clearly heard. These are heard normally over the trachea and the central airways in the back.

The breath sounds can only be normal, decreased, or increased. Decreased intensity of the breath sounds is due to either (1) impaired movement of air that normally generates the breath sounds, such as in emphysema, diaphragmatic paralysis, or bronchial obstruction, or (2) impaired transmission from the lung to the chest wall due to pneumothorax, pleural effusion, or pleural thickening. An increased transmission of the breath sounds is characterized by the finding of bronchial breath sounds (similar to the sound normally heard over the trachea) over the peripheral lung fields. Bronchial breathing is most commonly found with consolidation but also occurs at the interface with a pleural effusion where the lung is compressed. Upon completion of initial auscultation, the examiner can verify the presence of bronchial breathing by demonstrating the presence of the associated features: increased vocal resonance, whispering pectoriloquy (whispered sounds are heard more clearly), and egophony (the phonated e is heard as a).

Added sounds can be only of three types: wheezes, crackles, and pleural sounds. Wheezes are continuous, musical sounds thought to occur as air passes through a narrowed airway, setting up oscillations in the walls. They are more common during expiration, since dynamic compression exaggerates the constriction. Wheezes may be diffuse (asthma or chronic bronchitis) or localized in the case of a partially obstructed bronchus (tumor, secretions, or foreign body).

Crackles, formerly called rales or crepitations, are short sequences of discontinuous sounds which may be heard in inspiration or expiration. Very coarse crackles heard over the large airways are thought to result from air moving through secretions. However, most crackles are generated further out in the lung field as a result of the popping open of small airways that were closed during the previous expiration owing to low lung volumes, alterations in lung compliance, or increases in interstitial pressure. These factors are magnified in the bases, and they are more common there even if the underlying process is diffuse. When fine, a crackle is mimicked by rubbing hair close to the ear between the thumb and finger, whereas the coarse crackle is like the sound of a Velcro fastener opening. The finding of crackles is a nonspecific indicator of pulmonary parenchymal disease, and the crackles of congestive failure cannot be differentiated from those of pulmonary infection or fibrosis.

Pleural sounds may be a rub, like the creaking of leather, found with pleural inflammation, or the mediastinal crunching sound synchronous with systole found with a pneumomediastinum and likened to the sound created by walking through snow.

The typical physical findings in the major pulmonary disorders are outlined in Table 14–2.

REFERENCE

Bramsen SS (ed): Pulmonary signs and symptoms. Clin Chest Med 8:177–334, 1987.

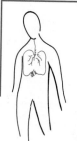

15

ANATOMICAL AND PHYSIOLOGICAL CONSIDERATIONS

The major function of the lungs is to deliver to the tissues sufficient oxygen (O_2) to meet their energy demands and to remove the carbon dioxide (CO_2) formed as a by-product of metabolism. This demand varies dramatically from basal levels of 3 to 4 ml of O_2 or CO_2 kg^{-1} · min^{-1} to as much as 60 ml of O_2 or CO_2 kg^{-1} · min^{-1} at maximum exercise capacity. To accomplish this, sufficient blood and gas must be brought together at a sufficiently large surface area to allow for rapid and adequate gas exchange.

THE AIRWAY

STRUCTURE

The inspired air travels through a complex pathway on its way to the alveoli. Most people (85 per cent) breathe through the nose, although the mouth is an additional route of air passage when ventilatory requirements are high (in excess of 35 to 40 L/min). The nose and pharynx serve to heat, humidify, and filter the air. Air then passes through the larynx, a complex group of muscles and cartilages, which remains patent during inspiration and closes during swallowing and maneuvers that require an increase in intrathoracic pressure, such as defecation and vomiting.

Beyond the larynx is the trachea, a 10- to 12-cm tube supported by U-shaped cartilages and a fibrous posterior membrane. The trachea divides into two mainstem bronchi at the carina. The right mainstem bronchus is a more direct continuation of the trachea, and thus aspirated foreign bodies tend to lodge on the right side. Moving further out, the airways branch in an irregular dichotomous pattern. In the smaller airways, the cartilage becomes less complete and disappears when the airways are 1 to 2 mm in diameter. The first 19 branches, ending at the terminal bronchioles, provide a rapid and enormous expansion of the total airway cross-sectional area, increasing from 2.5 sq cm in the trachea to approximately 900 sq cm (Fig. 15–1). Beyond this are three generations of respiratory bronchioles with their walls made up of increasing proportions of alveoli. This progresses into the alveolar

ducts and culminates in the alveolar sacs. At this point, the cross-sectional area of the alveolar capillary membrane has increased to an incredible 50 to 100 sq meters.

The epithelial surface of the alveolar capillary membrane, the site of gas exchange, consists of type I and type II pneumonocytes, the latter thought to be the progenitor of the former. The type II cell is responsible for the production of surfactant and possibly for other metabolic activities within the lung. Following a significant injury to the alveolar-capillary membrane, this cell proliferates and is probably responsible for the repair.

VENTILATION

During inspiration, respiratory muscle contraction increases intrathoracic volume, which in turn decreases airway pressure below atmospheric and causes air to enter the lungs. Expiration is passive, as the intrinsic elasticity of the lungs and chest wall return the volume of the system back to its resting position. With increased ventilatory requirements, the expiratory muscles may be enlisted to assist in lung emptying.

The respiratory muscles include the diaphragm, the intercostal and accessory muscles, and the abdominal muscles. The diaphragm, the major muscle of inspiration, arises from the lower ribs and inserts into the central tendon under the heart. When the diaphragm contracts, it pushes down against the abdominal contents, causing the thoracic cage to expand by moving

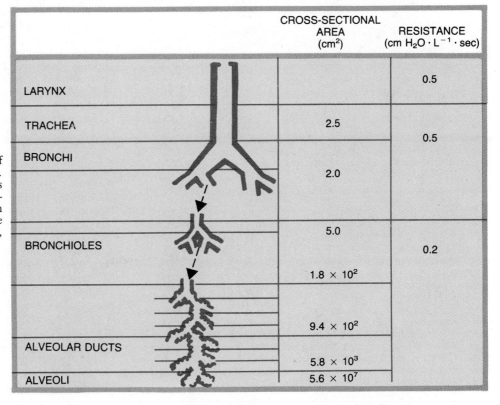

FIGURE 15–1. The subdivision of the airways and their nomenclature. The cross-sectional area increases dramatically as we reach the peripheral, small airways. (Adapted from Weibel ER: Morphometry of the Human Lung. Berlin, Springer, 1963.)

	CROSS-SECTIONAL AREA (cm²)	RESISTANCE (cm H₂O · L⁻¹ · sec)
LARYNX		0.5
TRACHEA	2.5	0.5
BRONCHI	2.0	
BRONCHIOLES	5.0	0.2
	1.8×10^2	
	9.4×10^2	
ALVEOLAR DUCTS	5.8×10^3	
ALVEOLI	5.6×10^7	

the chest wall in a cephalad direction. The increase in abdominal pressure causes an outward motion of the abdominal wall, the clinical hallmark of diaphragmatic contraction. The external and internal intercostal muscles serve inspiratory and expiratory functions, respectively. The accessory muscles, primarily the sternocleidomastoid and the scalene muscles, facilitate inspiration by directly elevating the chest wall. The abdominal muscles increase abdominal pressure and drive the relaxed diaphragm upward during ex-

piration and other situations requiring increases in intrathoracic pressure, such as coughing. As expiration is normally passive, abdominal muscle activity does not normally commence until minute ventilation increases to 40 L/min.

The respiratory muscles are much like other skeletal muscles in terms of their physiological behavior. If stressed they may fatigue, and proper training can induce a small but significant increase in their strength and endurance. The typical relations between resting length and the amount of tension developed also exist. For the respiratory muscles, length can be translated into lung volume, and when increased, as in emphysema, inspiratory muscle efficiency is decreased (Fig. 15–2).

The major work of the respiratory muscles is expended in overcoming the elastic and resistive forces encountered in breathing. If the lungs of a normal individual were removed from the chest, they would collapse until the airways closed (minimal volume). Concurrently, the elastic forces of the chest wall would increase the thoracic cage volume to about 80 per cent of the total capacity of the thoracic space. Thus, when combined, the lungs and chest wall pull in opposite directions, with the resting volume of the system, the functional residual capacity (FRC), occurring at the volume at which the outward pull of the chest wall equals the inward pull of the lungs, which is normally less than 50 per cent of total lung capacity (TLC).

Changes in elasticity are commonly considered in terms of its inverse function: compliance = change in volume/change in pressure. In normal lungs, near FRC, it takes an average of 1 cm H_2O to inflate the lungs by 200 ml (Fig. 15–3); i.e., compliance at this volume is 200 ml/cm H_2O. However, near TLC the lung and chest wall get stiffer, requiring greater inflationary pressure. Compliance decreases with pulmonary fibrosis or pulmonary edema and increases with emphysema. The normal compliance of the chest wall is also 200 ml/cm H_2O, and this may be decreased by skeletal abnormalities such as scoliosis or increased by the loss of respiratory muscle tone in neuromuscular disease.

The second force that must be overcome during breathing is airway resistance, defined as the driving pressure divided by air flow, normally 1 to 2 cm H_2O $L^{-1} \cdot sec^{-1}$. It is greatly dependent on the total cross-sectional areas of the airways and thus, even though the individual peripheral airways are narrow, their contribution to overall airway resistance is small because of the increase in total cross-sectional area (see Fig. 15–1). Because of their small contribution to overall resistance, disease in the small airways, an early manifestation in some patients with obstructive lung disease, is often difficult to detect by routine spirometry. Many factors influence airway resistance. An increase in lung volume decreases resistance because of the tethering effect of the alveoli on the airways. Thus, resistance should be referred to the lung volume at which it is measured. Other factors that influence airway resistance include bronchial smooth muscle

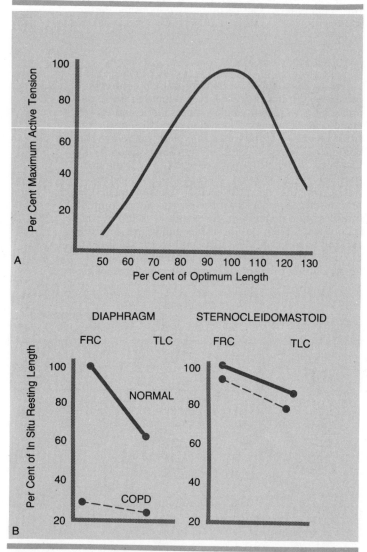

FIGURE 15–2. A, The length-tension curve for the diaphragm. At lengths above or below the optimal in situ resting length, the amount of tension generated decreases. B, The change in the length of the diaphragm and sternocleidomastoid muscles at functional residual capacity (FRC) and total lung capacity (TLC) in a normal subject and a patient with chronic obstructive lung disease (COPD) and hyperinflation. Increased FRC shortens the resting length of the diaphragm so that contraction during inspiration becomes inefficient. Consequently, rib cage expansion becomes more dependent on accessory muscle contraction. (From Druz et al: Am Rev Disp Dis 119:145, 1979.)

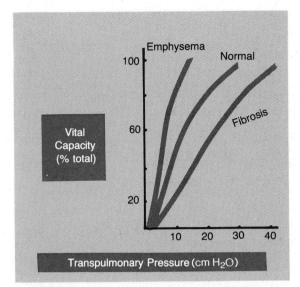

FIGURE 15–3. The compliance curves for normal subjects and patients with emphysema and pulmonary fibrosis. An increase in the transpulmonary pressure required to achieve a given lung volume increases the work of breathing.

contraction (bronchospasm), intrinsic or extrinsic airway compression, and the dynamic compression of a forced expiration.

The work of breathing is the product of the pressure generated and the change in volume. In normal subjects, this represents a tiny fraction of the overall energy utilized by the body (4 to 5 per cent), even with high ventilatory requirements such as exercise. However, in the presence of lung disease, as the work of breathing increases, the O_2 requirements of the respiratory muscles can become inordinately high, greater than 25 per cent of total. Under these circumstances any improvement in gas exchange achieved by increasing ventilation may be offset, or even exceeded, by the increased O_2 consumption and CO_2 production of the respiratory muscles.

Gas entering the lungs is divided into that entering the gas-exchanging regions of the lung, the alveolar volume (V_A), and that remaining in the conducting airways, the dead space (V_D). At end expiration, V_D is filled with gas that has already equilibrated with pulmonary capillary blood, and thus on the subsequent inspiration the amount of fresh gas reaching the alveoli is equal to the tidal volume (V_T) minus V_D. V_D makes up 20 to 40 per cent of a normal V_T.

Distribution of V_A within the lung depends on the regional pleural pressure. Normally, pleural pressure is most negative at the apex of the lung and becomes less negative as we move toward the lung base. This gradient is caused by a combination of gravity due to the weight of the lung and the different stresses imposed by the shape of the lung and chest wall. As a result of this gradient, the lung bases are better ventilated than the apices, since during tidal breathing they are on a steeper portion of the compliance curve at FRC.

CONTROL OF VENTILATION

The precise adjustment in ventilation necessary to meet changing metabolic demands is performed by balancing tidal volume and respiratory frequency through the integrative function of the three components of the respiratory control system: respiratory control centers, respiratory sensors, and respiratory effectors (Fig. 15–4).

RESPIRATORY CONTROL CENTERS

The neurons controlling respiration are located at several levels in the brain stem. The most important network resides in the medulla oblongata, where respiratory rhythm originates. The pons contains an apneustic center, uninhibited activity of which results in sustained inspiratory spasm (apneusis), and a pneumotactic center, which regulates respiratory timing, thus determining the relative duration of inspiration and expiration. While these brain stem centers are responsible for the automatic control of ventilation, the cerebral cortex can override them during wakefulness to permit speech and other actions requiring voluntary control of ventilation.

RESPIRATORY SENSORS

The respiratory sensors consist of the central and peripheral chemoreceptors and the chest wall and intrapulmonary sensory receptors. The central chemoreceptors, located on the ventral surface of the medulla oblongata, rapidly respond to any increase in

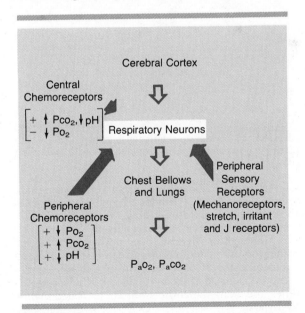

FIGURE 15–4. Schematic representation of the respiratory control system. The respiratory neurons in the brain stem receive information from the chemoreceptors, peripheral sensory receptors, and cerebral cortex. This information is integrated, and the resulting neural output is transmitted to the chest bellows and lungs.

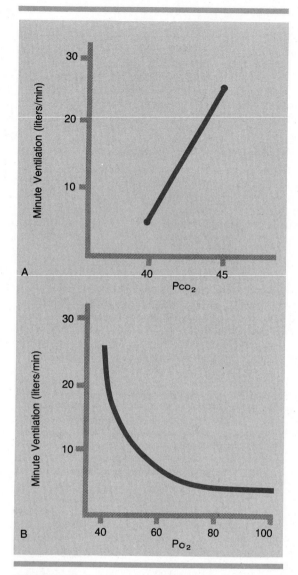

FIGURE 15–5. Minute ventilation increases linearly with rising P_{CO_2} (A) and decreases exponentially with falling P_{O_2} (B).

CO_2 or hydrogen ion concentration by increasing ventilation (Fig. 15–5A). Under normal circumstances these receptors are very sensitive, keeping the $PaCO_2$ constant despite marked variability in CO_2 production. In contrast, hypoxia does not act as a central respiratory stimulant but instead depresses the central chemoreceptors. Conversely, the peripheral chemoreceptors, located at the bifurcation of the carotid arteries and along the aortic arch, are activated mainly by hypoxia and less so by CO_2 and hydrogen ions. They are also sensitive to a fall in blood pressure, which may partly account for hyperventilation seen in shock. Unlike the central chemoreceptors, which have a linear response to P_{CO_2}, the peripheral chemoreceptors cause little increase in ventilation until there

is significant hypoxemia (P_{O_2} less than 60 mm Hg) (Fig. 15–5B). Mechanoreceptors in the chest wall respond to stretch of the intercostal muscles and reflexly modulate the rate and depth of breathing. Tidal volume and respiratory frequency may also be reflexly affected by stimuli arising in (1) airway irritant receptors, which respond to physical or chemical stimulation, (2) pulmonary stretch receptors, which respond to marked increases in lung volume (Hering-Breuer reflex), or (3) J receptors found in the juxtacapillary junctions, which respond to vascular engorgement and congestion.

EFFECTORS OF THE RESPIRATORY SYSTEM

Signals are transmitted from the respiratory center to the respiratory muscles by (1) the phrenic nerves, which supply the diaphragm, (2) the intercostal nerves, which innervate the intercostal and abdominal muscles, (3) the accessory cranial nerves, which supply the sternomastoid muscles, and (4) the lower cervical nerves, which supply the scalene muscles. In addition, a variety of muscles acting on the soft palate, tongue, and hyoid bone maintain upper airway patency and offset the collapsing effect of the negative pressures generated by the respiratory muscles. During wakefulness, both the upper airway and chest wall muscles display rhythmic inspiratory activity. During sleep, upper airway muscle activity wanes, whereas diaphragmatic activation changes little.

THE BLOOD VESSELS

STRUCTURE

The lung receives its blood supply from two vascular systems—the bronchial and pulmonary circulations. The nutritive blood flow to all but the alveolar structures comes from the bronchial circulation. About one third of the venous effluent of the bronchial circulation drains into the systemic veins and back to the right ventricle. The remainder drains into the pulmonary veins and, along with the contribution from the thebesian veins in the heart, represents a component of the 1 to 2 per cent right-to-left shunt found in normal subjects.

The pulmonary arterial system runs alongside the airways from the hila to the periphery. The arteries down to the level of the subsegmental airways (2 mm diameter) are thin-walled, predominantly elastic vessels. Beyond this, the arteries become muscularized until they reach diameters of 30 μm, where the muscular coat disappears. Most of the arterial pressure drop takes place in these small muscular arteries, which are responsible for the active control of blood flow distribution in the lung. The pulmonary arterioles empty into an extensive capillary network and drain into thin-walled pulmonary veins, which eventually join with the arteries and bronchi at the hilum and exit the lung to enter the left atrium.

PERFUSION

The pulmonary vascular bed serves as a source of nutritive blood to the alveolar membrane, but its most important role is in pulmonary gas exchange. It delivers the entire systemic venous return to the pulmonary capillary bed, where exchange of O_2 and CO_2 occurs. While it receives the same blood flow per minute as the systemic circulation, there are differences between the vascular beds. First, since the pulmonary vascular resistance, calculated as pulmonary artery pressure–left atrial pressure/cardiac output, is only about one tenth of systemic vascular resistance, the pressure in the pulmonary vascular bed is only one tenth of that in the systemic circulation. Second, all structures within the thorax, including the pulmonary vascular bed, the heart, and the great vessels, are exposed to the surrounding pressures, both pleural and alveolar, which vary during respiration.

Blood entering the lung at the hilum must either be pumped upward toward the lung apex or flow down with the help of gravity toward the base. Thus, pulmonary arterial pressures display great variation from the apex to the lung base, whereas the alveolar pressure is the same throughout the lung. The blood flows through any alveolus and therefore the distribution of blood in the lung depends on the interaction of the vascular pressure across the capillary bed (arterial-venous difference) and the surrounding alveolar pressures (Fig. 15–6). At the apex, pulmonary artery pressure is usually just able to overcome alveolar pressure. However, a fall in arterial pressure or any rise in alveolar pressure (positive pressure breathing) may cause alveolar pressure to exceed arterial pressure, with cessation of flow. This is known as zone 1 conditions. Below this lies zone 2, where the alveolar pressure is less than arterial pressure but greater than venous pressure. Blood flow in zone 2 depends on the difference between arterial pressure and the surrounding alveolar pressure. Blood flow continues to increase with increasing arterial pressure and eventually reaches a point, zone 3, at which venous pressure exceeds alveolar pressure and flow becomes dependent on arterial-venous pressure difference.

Many factors affect the pressure-flow relations in the pulmonary circulation. When blood flow increases in normal upright man, as during exercise, pulmonary vascular resistance actually falls owing to the ability to recruit new vessels and distend the ones already open. This allows large increases in blood flow with lesser increases in pressure, thus preventing the transudation of fluid into the lungs owing to a higher microvascular pressure. Pulmonary vascular resistance is also affected by lung volume. It is lowest at FRC and increases at lower lung volumes because there is less distention of extra-alveolar vessels and at higher lung volumes owing to compression of the intra-alveolar vessels.

In addition to these passive influences, a number of factors actively affect pulmonary vascular tone. The most important is alveolar hypoxia, which results in constriction of the perfusing artery by as-yet-unknown

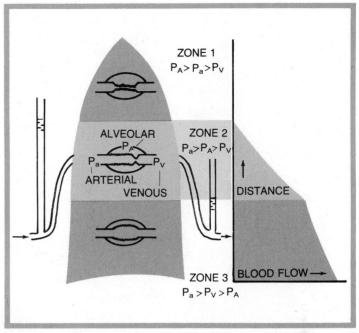

FIGURE 15–6. The zonal model of blood flow in the lung. Because of the interrelationship of vascular and alveolar pressures, the lung base receives the most flow (see text for explanation). (From West et al: J Appl Physiol 19:713, 1964.)

mechanisms. This may be a conservation mechanism when alveolar hypoxia is localized, since reduction in perfusion to poorly ventilated alveoli reduces the abnormality of gas exchange, which is otherwise inevitable. During generalized hypoxia, its beneficial nature is not always apparent, as in sojourners at high altitude, in whom it may be a major cause of pulmonary edema. Acidosis causes a vasoconstrictor response of lesser magnitude. Other vasoactive compounds produced in the body, such as prostaglandins and adrenergic substances, may also alter pulmonary vascular tone.

GAS TRANSFER

CO_2 and O_2 are transported between the environment and the tissues by convection and diffusion (Fig. 15–7). In the blood, O_2 combines with hemoglobin, and the resulting O_2 saturation is determined by the oxyhemoglobin dissociation curve (Fig. 15–8A). More than 98 per cent of the O_2 in the blood is combined with hemoglobin; the remainder is dissolved in the plasma. Above a PaO_2 of 150 mm Hg, hemoglobin is totally saturated and carries 1.34 ml O_2/gm hemoglobin; further rises in PaO_2 increase only the amount of O_2 dissolved in the plasma at the rate of 0.003 ml O_2/100 ml blood/mm Hg PO_2. CO_2 is carried in the blood in three forms: bicarbonate (90 per cent), dissolved in plasma, or combined with protein, predominantly hemoglobin. The relation between the PCO_2 and the CO_2 content is described by the carbon dioxide dissociation

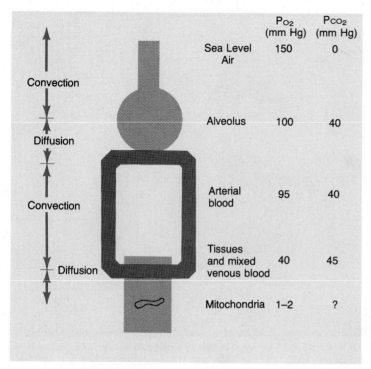

		P_{O_2} (mm Hg)	P_{CO_2} (mm Hg)
	Sea Level Air	150	0
	Alveolus	100	40
	Arterial blood	95	40
	Tissues and mixed venous blood	40	45
	Mitochondria	1–2	?

FIGURE 15–7. The transfer of O_2 and CO_2 from the atmosphere to the mitochrondria.

curve (Fig. 15–8B), which is steeper and more linear than the oxyhemoglobin dissociation curve.

A number of factors influence the relations between P_{O_2} and P_{CO_2} and their contents, which can be described as changes in the position of the respective dissociation curves. Increased P_{CO_2} and temperature and decreased pH shift the oxyhemoglobin dissociation curve to the right, decreasing affinity of hemoglobin for O_2 and expediting its release to the tissues. Converse changes in the above factors have the opposite effect. Increased levels of 2,3-DPG, produced during chronic hypoxemia or anemia, also shift the curve to the right, whereas carbon monoxide shifts it to the left and also reduces the O_2 content by competitively binding to hemoglobin. The most important influence on the carbon dioxide dissociation curve is P_{O_2}; increased P_{O_2} shifts the curve to the right, thus reducing the affinity of hemoglobin for CO_2 and assisting in the unloading of CO_2 in the lungs.

PULMONARY GAS EXCHANGE

The arterial blood gas values are determined by the gas composition in the alveoli and its successful equilibration with the blood in the pulmonary capillaries. In turn, the P_{O_2} and P_{CO_2} in the alveoli are determined by the inspired gas tensions, the mixed venous P_{O_2} and P_{CO_2}, the total ventilation, the blood flow, and, most important, the success with which the lung is able to match ventilation and blood flow. Abnormality of any

of these factors leads to hypoxemia and/or hypercapnia. For convenience they are grouped into four basic mechanisms.

Hypoventilation. Hypoventilation is characterized by a minute ventilation insufficient to maintain a normal Pa_{CO_2} for the level of metabolic activity, as measured by CO_2 production ($\dot{V}_{CO_2}$). If the lung is considered as a simple homogeneous system, the alveolar P_{CO_2} (Pa_{CO_2}) and thus the arterial P_{CO_2}

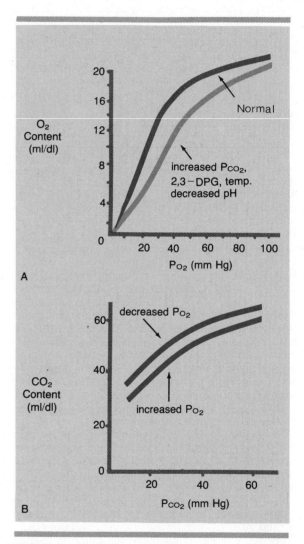

FIGURE 15–8. *A*, The oxyhemoglobin dissociation curve. The bulk of the O_2 is carried combined with hemoglobin. The various factors that decrease the hemoglobin O_2 affinity are shown. Opposite changes increase hemoglobin O_2 affinity, shifting the curve to the left. *B*, The carbon dioxide dissociation curve. It is more linear than the oxyhemoglobin curve throughout the physiological range. Increased P_{O_2} shifts the curve to the right, which decreases CO_2 content for any given P_{CO_2} and thus facilitates CO_2 off-loading in the lungs. The shift to the left at a lower P_{O_2} facilitates CO_2 onloading at the tissues.

(Pa_{CO_2}) depend on the alveolar ventilation ($\dot{V}_A$) and V_{CO_2}, as

$$P_{A_{CO_2}} = \frac{V_{CO_2}}{V_A} \times K$$

where K is a constant. Any decrease in ventilation will lead to a concomitant rise in $P_{A_{CO_2}}$, provided that $\dot{V}_{CO_2}$ remains unchanged. The effect of this on alveolar P_{O_2} ($P_{A_{O_2}}$) can be appreciated using the alveolar air equation

$$P_{A_{O_2}} = (P_B - P_{H_2O}) F_{I_{O_2}} - \frac{Pa_{CO_2}}{R}$$

where $P_{A_{O_2}}$ is alveolar P_{O_2}, P_B is atmospheric pressure (usually 760 mm Hg), P_{H_2O} is the partial pressure of water vapor (47 mm Hg), $F_{I_{O_2}}$ is the fractional concentration of inspired O_2, and R is the respiratory exchange ratio (which can be estimated at 0.8). We see that any rise in Pa_{CO_2} leads to a concomitant fall in $P_{A_{O_2}}$ and thus in Pa_{O_2}. The presence of hypoventilation should direct attention to abnormalities of the chest wall, respiratory muscles, or respiratory center drive.

Abnormal Diffusion.   Under normal conditions, blood spends about 0.75 sec in the pulmonary capillaries. Since it ordinarily takes only about one third of this time for the blood to equilibrate with alveolar gas, there is a wide safety margin before abnormal pathology results in nonequilibration, i.e., a diffusion impairment. It has been estimated that the diffusing capacity of the lung must fall to less than 10 per cent of normal before it affects Pa_{O_2} at rest. Three factors may stress the system sufficiently to interfere with complete equilibration: increased diffusion distance due to a thickening of the alveolar capillary membrane; increased rate of blood flow, or a reduction in the number of open capillaries, decreasing the time the blood spends in the process of equilibration; and reduced driving pressure from alveolus to blood, as seen at extreme altitudes. Diffusion impairment almost never plays a role in the hypoxemia of disease unless at least two of the above factors are in force. Even when abnormal diffusion is present, it usually accounts for only a minimal amount of the observed disturbance in gas exchange.

Ventilation-Perfusion Inequality.   The proper matching of ventilation and blood flow within the lung is necessary for the adequate uptake of O_2 and elimination of CO_2. While the lung is sometimes regarded as a single gas-exchanging unit, it really contains units that differ in their relative amounts of blood flow and ventilation. In normals, the span of ventilation-perfusion ($\dot{V}_A/\dot{Q}$) ratios is very small, varying from about 0.5 to 3.0, with an average of 0.8. As lung disease develops, the range increasingly widens, with some units receiving very little ventilation relative to perfusion while others are excessively ventilated. If $\dot{V}_A/\dot{Q}$ inequality is imposed on a lung, the arterial P_{O_2} will fall and the Pc_{O_2} will rise (Fig. 15–9). In patients with normal chemosensitivity and without severe limitation in ventilatory capacity, the increasing Pc_{O_2} leads to a pro-

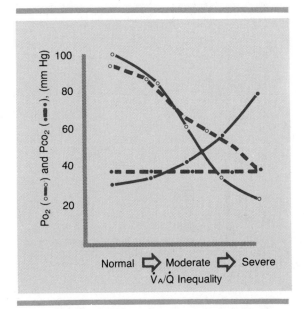

FIGURE 15–9. The effect of increasing ventilation-perfusion ($\dot{V}_A/\dot{Q}$) inequality on arterial P_{O_2} and Pc_{O_2}. The solid lines show the change in gas tensions when cardiac output and minute ventilation are held constant. The change in gas tensions when ventilation is allowed to increase is shown by the dotted lines. Increased ventilation can maintain a normal Pc_{O_2} but can only partially correct the hypoxemia. (From Dantzker DR: Gas exchange abnormalities. *In* Montenegro H [ed]: Chronic Obstructive Pulmonary Disease. New York, Churchill Livingstone, 1984, pp 141–160.)

gressive increase in ventilation. This increase in ventilation is capable of bringing the Pc_{O_2} back toward normal but only minimally attenuates the fall in the P_{O_2} because of the different shapes of the oxy- and carboxyhemoglobin dissociation curves. The oxyhemoglobin dissociation curve plateaus at a high P_{O_2}, and thus the increased P_{O_2} in alveoli receiving increased ventilation fails to increase the O_2 content of blood leaving that unit. The carboxyhemoglobin dissociation curve, on the other hand, is linear throughout the physiological range. Any decrease in Pc_{O_2} is accompanied by a fall in CO_2 content, allowing the overventilated alveoli to compensate for the failure of poorly ventilated lung units to eliminate CO_2. As $\dot{V}_A/\dot{Q}$ inequality worsens with progression of the underlying disease, further increases in ventilation eventually become impossible, and both hypoxemia and hypercapnia result. $\dot{V}_A/\dot{Q}$ inequality is the characteristic abnormality of gas exchange in chronic obstructive and restrictive lung diseases.

Shunt.   Intrapulmonary or intracardiac shunt, where blood bypasses ventilated lung units, is a most potent source of hypoxemia, but hypercapnia is not seen (Fig. 15–10). In fact, as the hypoxemia progresses, hypocapnia is usually found owing to the stimulatory effects of the low Pa_{O_2} on ventilatory drive. Shunting is the major mechanism of hypoxemia in pulmonary edema, pneumonia, and atelectasis.

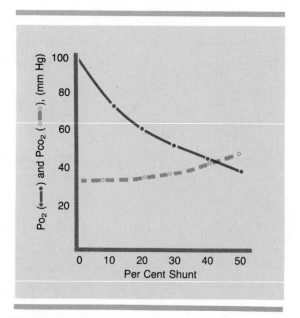

FIGURE 15–10. The effect of increasing shunt on the arterial P_{O_2} and P_{CO_2}. The minute ventilation has been held constant in this example. Under normal circumstances, the hypoxemia would lead to an increased minute ventilation and a fall in the P_{CO_2} as the shunt increases. (From Dantzker DR: Gas exchange abnormalities. *In* Montenegro H [ed]: Chronic Obstructive Pulmonary Disease. New York, Churchill Livingstone, 1984, pp 141–160.)

NONPULMONARY FACTORS

Abnormalities other than alterations in lung function may influence the Pa_{O_2} through their effect on the mixed venous P_{O_2} (Pv_{O_2}). The Pv_{O_2} is decreased when cardiac output is inappropriately low, when O_2 consumption ($\dot{V}_{O_2}$) is increased (as with exercise or fever), or when the hemoglobin concentration or O_2 saturation is low. For any lung unit, the resultant end-capillary P_{O_2} is influenced by the Pv_{O_2}, although the magnitude of this effect on the arterial O_2 content will be greatest in lungs with $\dot{V}_A/\dot{Q}$ inequality or shunt (Fig. 15–11). The importance of this phenomenon is the recognition that a fall in Pa_{O_2} in a patient with lung disease may be due to one of these nonpulmonary factors rather than to deterioration in lung function, thus requiring a very different intervention.

TISSUE GAS EXCHANGE

As in the lung, gas exchange in the tissues is accomplished by passive diffusion, which requires, for optimal functioning, that an adequate amount of blood be brought into proximity with the actively metabolizing cells. Unfortunately, much less is known about the factors that control this process than is understood about gas exchange in the lung. It is likely, however, that under pathological conditions similar

pathophysiological abnormalities are present. A reduction of total O_2 delivery to the tissues (analogous to hypoventilation) leads to a reduction of tissue P_{O_2} and acidosis. Abnormal diffusion resulting from a shortened residence time of blood in the capillaries or increased distance from the capillary to the cell is likely under conditions of tissue inflammation or abnormal microvascular control. Maldistribution of blood flow with regard to tissue O_2 requirements or even shunting of blood around capillary beds has been postulated in gram-negative sepsis. Confirmation of the role of any of these proposed mechanisms in disease states awaits further technological advances that will allow measurement of gas exchange at the tissue level.

NONRESPIRATORY FUNCTIONS OF THE LUNG

In addition to its central role in gas exchange, the lung is active in both the metabolism and the degradation of many substances. Surfactant production by the alveolar type II cell is an important metabolic function of the lungs. This phospholipid minimizes surface tension and thus confers stability on the alveoli and small airways, preventing atelectasis and decreasing the work of breathing. The failure of the immature lung to produce sufficient surfactant leads to the respiratory distress syndrome (RDS) of the newborn. The lung is also involved in the biosynthesis of arachidonic

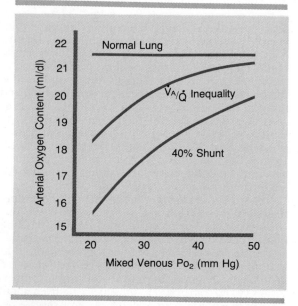

FIGURE 15–11. The effect of altering mixed venous P_{O_2} (Pv_{O_2}) on the arterial oxygen content under three assumed conditions: a normal lung, severe ventilation-perfusion ($\dot{V}_A/\dot{Q}$) inequality, and the presence of a 40 per cent shunt. For each situation the patient is breathing 50 per cent O_2 and the Pv_{O_2} is altered, keeping all other variables constant. (From Dantzker DR: Gas exchange in the adult respiratory distress syndrome. Clin Chest Med 3:57, 1982.)

acid into products of both the lipoxygenase and cyclo-oxygenase pathways. While a myriad of physiological functions have been ascribed to these agents, a clear relation to pulmonary function is still lacking. Additionally, the lung is capable of removing or inactivating a large number of biologically active substances, including serotonin, bradykinin, and prostaglandins. It is also the principal site of the conversion of angiotensin I to angiotensin II.

REFERENCES

Dantzker DR: Cardiopulmonary Critical Care. Orlando, FL, Grune & Stratton, 1986.

Murray JF: The Normal Lung, 2nd ed. Philadelphia. WB Saunders Company, 1986.

Weibel ER: The Pathway for Oxygen. Cambridge, MA, Harvard University Press, 1984.

West JB: Respiratory Physiology—The Essentials, 3rd ed. Baltimore, Williams & Wilkins, 1985.

16

DIAGNOSTIC TECHNIQUES AND THEIR INDICATIONS

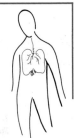

IMAGING PROCEDURES

The standard chest roentgenogram complements the history and physical examination as the starting point for the diagnosis of pulmonary disorders. The chest x-ray may demonstrate a density that only physical examination can differentiate between consolidation and loculated fluid. Conversely, the chest x-ray may show dramatic involvement of the lung by tuberculosis while the physical findings are not remarkable. Standard views include the posteroanterior (PA) and the left lateral projections; they reduce disproportionate magnification of the heart and anterior mediastinal structures. These films allow visualization of the air-containing lung, vascular markings, heart and mediastinal structures, pleura, lymph nodes, ribs, spine, and soft tissues of the thorax. Correct interpretation requires that the film be taken as close to total lung capacity as possible. A correctly exposed film allows the vertebral bodies to be barely visible behind the heart. A number of specialized views and procedures can be added to the standard PA and lateral films (Table 16–1).

Significant improvement in visualization of chest structures has occurred with the use of computed tomography (CT), which provides excellent visibility of areas previously difficult to see and has ten times the contrast resolution of conventional radiography. Excellent evaluation of the mediastinum makes it valuable in the work-up of bronchogenic neoplasms. Differentiating pleural from parenchymal densities, a common problem on the routine film, has been improved. CT has virtually replaced the standard tomograms for evaluating the presence of early metastatic spread to the lung parenchyma. Unfortunately, specificity is low, and 20 to 60 per cent of nodules visualized on CT scan but not on x-ray are benign. In addition, CT is useful for detecting calcification in pulmonary nodules.

Ultrasound is useful in helping to differentiate between solids and fluids in pleural opacities and to localize loculated pleural effusions. Other imaging methods such as nuclear magnetic resonance and digital subtraction angiography are not generally available, and their superiority over available methods has yet to be proven.

PULMONARY FUNCTION EVALUATION

Routine studies performed in the pulmonary function laboratory can be grouped into four categories: lung volumes, air flow, diffusing capacity, and maximal pressures. Additional studies, such as measurement of lung compliance, rarely provide information beyond that obtained by more easily performed measurements.

The lung is conveniently divided into four volumes and three capacities (Fig. 16–1). The components of the vital capacity can be obtained with routine spirometry. The residual volume (RV), however, must be measured indirectly, since it represents air left in the lungs at completion of a full expiration. In fact, we actually measure functional residual capacity (FRC) rather than RV, since the former, i.e., the volume at the end of a normal expiration, is a more reproducible point. The expiratory reserve volume (ERV) is then subtracted from FRC to obtain the residual volume.

Three techniques are commonly used to measure FRC: nitrogen washout, helium dilution, and body plethysmography. The first two techniques are limited by the ability of the test gas to either wash out or equil-

TABLE 16–1. SPECIALIZED RADIOGRAPHIC TECHNIQUES

STUDY OR VIEW	INDICATION	COMMENT
Oblique	Visualization of hilum and pleural plaques. Contralateral oblique is best view for apical disease.	Better done with CT
Lordotic	Right middle lobe and lingular disease	
Lateral decubitus	Identification of pleural effusions, air-fluid levels, and fungus balls	Both left and right should always be done
Upright-supine	Differentiation of pleural from parenchymal disease in critically ill patients requiring portable radiography	
Inspiratory-expiratory	Obstruction of bronchus or air-trapping in enclosed pleural or lung spaces	
Tomograms	Visualization of lesions obscured by overlying tissue; visualization of bronchi, pulmonary vessels, and hili; demonstration of parenchymal calcifications	Better done with CT
Bronchograms	Diagnosis of bronchiectasis	Indicated only in the rare situation when surgery is contemplated; can now be diagnosed by CT
Pulmonary angiogram	Detection of congenital anomalies of the pulmonary vasculature. Diagnosis of pulmonary emboli	
Fluoroscopy	Diaphragmatic movement. Differentiation between chest wall lesions and lung parenchymal lesions	

ibrate completely with all portions of the lung. In the presence of significant airway obstruction, this will not occur and the FRC will be significantly underestimated. Body plethysmography eliminates this problem and measures the total thoracic gas volume, whether it is located in a bulla or in direct communication with the airway, and thus provides a truer reflection of the FRC.

The dynamics of airflow can be evaluated during a forced expiratory maneuver by recording the change in volume against time to calculate flow rate or by directly measuring volume and flow (Figs. 16–2 and 16–3). The flow-volume loop is particularly useful in demonstrating the presence of upper airway obstruc-

tion, which, by affecting primarily the peak inspiratory and expiratory flows, gives a characteristic loop (Fig. 16–3). An estimate of total airway resistance can be determined by the body plethysmography.

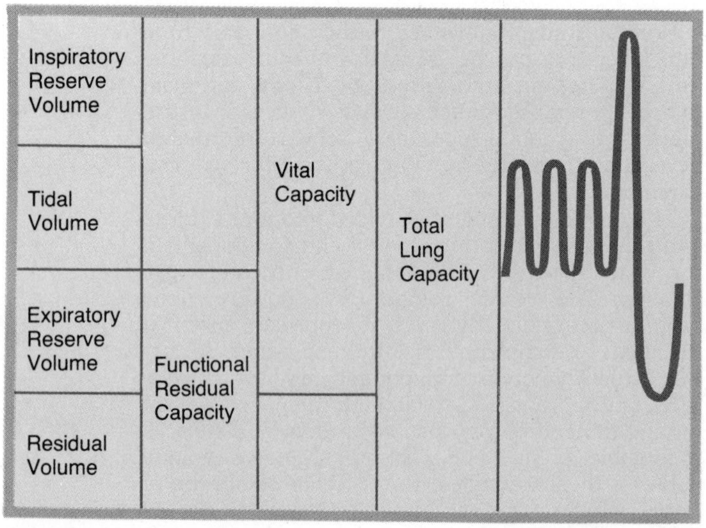

The measurement of the diffusing capacity for carbon monoxide (D_LCO) is an indicator of the adequacy of the alveolar-capillary membrane and so is reduced when the latter is decreased, as in pulmonary fibrosis, emphysema, and pulmonary vascular disease. In patients with a restrictive physiological defect, diffusing capacity helps to differentiate chest bellows (D_LCO normal) from parenchymal disease (D_LCO decreased).

Measurement of maximal static respiratory pressures is probably the most sensitive and specific method of diagnosing respiratory dysfunction in patients with neuromuscular disease. Maximal inspiratory pressure is obtained by recording mouth pressure during a maximal inspiratory effort from residual volume, and maximal expiratory pressure is recorded during a maximum expiratory effort at total lung capacity.

Interpretation of pulmonary function studies requires consideration of the technical quality of the tracings and a knowledge of the degree of variation for a particular index. Small deviations in vital capacity may be abnormal, whereas larger deviations in D_LCO are required to confidently diagnose abnormality. Fixed percentages of a normal value should not be considered to indicate disease.

Measurement of lung volumes and flow rates after certain challenges such as methacholine, exercise, cold air, or exposure to organic or inorganic substances helps in the diagnosis of bronchospasm. Acute reversibility is determined by their repetition after bronchodilator administration. However, failure of flow to improve following a single dose of a broncholidator does not necessarily indicate irreversible disease and does not exclude the possibility of a clinical response to bronchodilator treatment.

More complex testing is occasionally required to an-

FIGURE 16–1. Lung volumes and capacities. While vital capacity and its subdivision can be measured by spirometry, calculation of residual volume requires measurement of functional residual capacity by body plethysmography, helium dilution technique, or nitrogen washout.

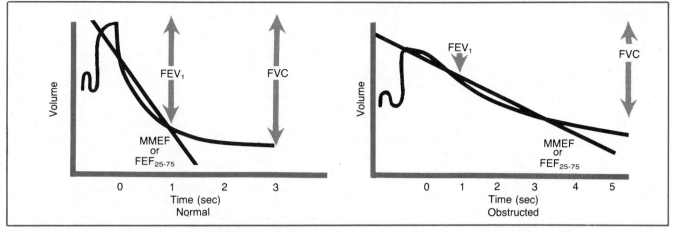

FIGURE 16–2. Spirometry in a normal subject and a patient with obstructive lung disease. FEV_1 represents the forced expired volume in 1 sec and FVC represents the forced vital capacity. The slope of the line connecting the points at 25 per cent and 75 per cent of the FVC represents the forced expired flow, FEF_{25-75}, or maximum mid-expiratory flow (MMEF). The FEF_{25-75} is less reproducible and less specific than the FEV_1.

swer specific questions. Exercise studies are valuable in judging the degree of disability as well as in elucidating the cause of dyspnea on exertion. Expired gas, minute ventilation, heart rate, and arterial oxygenation are measured during increased workloads. The degree of limitation and the relative contribution of ventilatory and cardiovascular factors can be assessed. Polysomnography is an essential tool in the diagnosis of sleep apnea (Chapter 22), and measurement of CO_2 sensitivity is used to assess the regulation of breathing.

CLINICAL ASSESSMENT OF THE REGULATION OF VENTILATION

Clinical assessment is currently limited to the chemical control of ventilation, as the precise role of sensory receptor influences is unknown and satisfactory techniques for their assessment do not exist. Depressed chemosensitivity should be suspected when one of the conditions listed in Table 16–2 is present, and formal assessment of respiratory center function should be considered.

The rebreathing test is the most common clinical method of assessing CO_2 sensitivity. Normally, minute ventilation increases by an average of 2 L/min/mm Hg CO_2 (range $1–8$ $L^{-1} \cdot min^{-1} \cdot mm^{-1}$ Hg CO_2) (see Fig. 15–5A). Blunting of the CO_2 response occurs in idiopathic hypoventilation, obesity-hypoventilation syndrome, narcotic or sedative ingestion, hypothyroidism, metabolic alkalosis, and primary neurological disorders. The reduced response in patients with COPD and CO_2 retention is discussed later. Chemosensitivity to hypoxia is technically more difficult

FIGURE 16–3. *A,* The maximum expired flow-volume curve in a normal subject. The peak expiratory flow (PEF) and forced expiratory flows at 50 per cent and 75 per cent of the exhaled vital capacity are indicated. *B,* In obstructive lung disease (OLD) hyperinflation pushes the position of the curve to the left, and there is characteristic scalloping on expiration. In restrictive lung disease (RLD), lung volumes are reduced but flow for any one point in volume is normal. The flow-volume curve displays different patterns with various forms of upper airway obstruction (UAO), with reduction in respiratory flow if the obstruction is outside the thoracic cavity and, additionally, in expiratory flow if the obstruction is due to a fixed deformity.

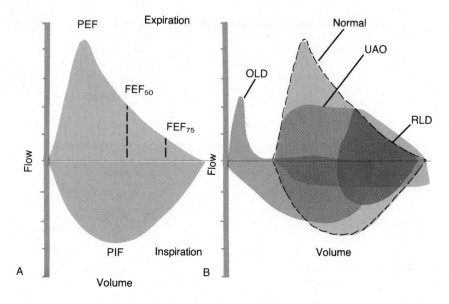

TABLE 16–2. SUSPECT IMPAIRED CHEMOSENSITIVITY IN THE PRESENCE OF HYPERCAPNIA AND THE FOLLOWING

1. Disproportionately small reduction in FEV_1
2. Normal alveolar-arterial Po_2 gradient
3. Ability to achieve normocapnia with voluntary hyperventilation
4. Ability to generate a negative inspiratory pressure of at least minus 30 torr, which eliminates muscle weakness as a cause of hypercapnia

to measure, and generally there is a good relationship between reduced chemosensitivity to O_2 and that to CO_2.

ASSESSING THE EFFICIENCY OF PULMONARY GAS EXCHANGE

A number of indices are used to assess the efficiency of pulmonary gas exchange. The simplest are the arterial blood gases. While extremely useful in patient management, they are neither sensitive nor specific to changes in the efficiency of gas exchange because they are influenced not only by changes in overall minute ventilation but also by nonpulmonary factors that alter the mixed venous Po_2. When the patient breathes enriched O_2 mixtures, arterial blood gases become an even less accurate guide to impairment of gas exchange. With normal lungs, or in patients with small shunts or minor degress of $\dot{V}_A/\dot{Q}$ inequality, the Pa_{O_2} increases almost linearly as the FI_{O_2} is increased. However, with progressive lung disease, the response is less predictable. Measurement of the arterial blood gases requires an arterial puncture, which is uncomfortable for the patient and occasionally difficult or dangerous to perform. When multiple samples are required over a relatively short period of time, an indwelling arterial catheter may be useful. When the patient is breathing room air and 100 per cent O_2, arterial blood gases and derived indices can be very useful in diagnosing the mechanism of abnormal gas exchange (Table 16–3).

The alveolar-arterial O_2 difference (A-a Do_2) is a derived measure of gas exchange efficiency that is not influenced by changes in overall minute ventilation. The ideal PA_{O_2} is calculated from the alveolar gas equation (see Chapter 15). If gas exchange is optimal, then calculated PA_{O_2} should be close to measured Pa_{O_2}. Any factor making gas exchange less efficient will widen

the A-a Do_2. In normals, this is usually less than 10 mm Hg, increasing to as much as 20 mm Hg in older normal subjects. When hypoxemia is due to hypoventilation, the A-a Do_2 remains normal, since the fall in Po_2 is due to the rise in Pco_2, and the calculated PA_{O_2} should fall to the same degree as the Pa_{O_2}. Thus, the A-a Do_2 is a practical way of differentiating hypoventilation from the other causes of hypoxemia.

The second derived index of gas exchange efficiency is the calculation of venous admixture ($\dot{Q}s/\dot{Q}t$). The model on which this index is based assumes that the lung has two compartments: one is a shunt, and so blood flowing through this compartment ($\dot{Q}s$) has a Po_2 equal to that of mixed venous blood (Pv_{O_2}); the second is well ventilated and receives the remainder of the cardiac output ($\dot{Q}t$) (i.e., $\dot{Q}t - \dot{Q}s$) and has a Po_2 equal to that of alveolar gas (PA_{O_2}). Thus, O_2 content of systemic arterial blood (Ca_{O_2}) is the weighted contribution of blood from these compartments:

$$\dot{Q}t \times Ca_{O_2} = \dot{Q}s \times Cv_{O_2} + \dot{Q}(t - s) \times Cc_{O_2}$$

and solving for venous admixture, we obtain:

$$\dot{Q}s/\dot{Q}t = (Cc_{O_2} - Ca_{O_2})/(Cc_{O_2} - Cv_{O_2})$$

The Ca_{O_2} and the Cv_{O_2} are calculated from measurements of partial pressures and saturations of the arterial and mixed venous blood. The O_2 content of end-capillary blood (Cc_{O_2}) cannot be measured and is derived from the calculated PA_{O_2}, assuming that Pc_{O_2} equals PA_{O_2}. If PA_{O_2} is greater than 150 mm Hg, then the saturation of end-capillary blood can be assumed to be 100 per cent. If PA_{O_2} is lower, then the saturation must be calculated from one of the many algorithms for the oxyhemoglobin dissociation curve. Although modifications of the shunt equation have been suggested in order to make the calculations easier, they should be avoided. They assume either that there is a standard arterial–mixed venous O_2 difference or that both the Pa_{O_2} and Pc_{O_2} are fully saturated, an unlikely situation in patients with lung disease. An increased $\dot{Q}s/\dot{Q}t$ in a patient breathing room air is usually due to $\dot{V}_A/\dot{Q}$ inequality or shunt. When the patient is breathing 100 per cent O_2, the $\dot{Q}s/\dot{Q}t$ quantitates the amount of the shunt that is present, as the contribution of $\dot{V}_A/\dot{Q}$ inequality is abolished at an FI_{O_2} of 1.0.

A third commonly calculated index is the dead space–tidal volume ratio (V_D/V_T). It is measured using the Bohr equations

$$V_D/V_T = \frac{Pa_{CO_2} - Pe_{CO_2}}{Pa_{CO_2}}$$

where Pa_{CO_2} and Pe_{CO_2} are the arterial and mixed expired Pco_2, respectively. In normal individuals, V_D is 20 to 40 per cent of V_T and consists almost entirely of the additional component of alveolar dead space due to the presence of ventilation-perfusion inequality.

TABLE 16–3. DIFFERENTIAL DIAGNOSIS OF HYPOXEMIA

	Pa_{O_2}	Pa_{CO_2}	A-a Do_2 RA	A-a Do_2 100% O_2	$\dot{Q}s/\dot{Q}t$ RA	$\dot{Q}s/\dot{Q}t$ 100% O_2
Hypoventilation	↓	↑	N	N	N	N
Abnormal diffusion	↓	N	↑	N	↑	N
Shunt	↓	N or ↓	↑	↑	↑	↑
$\dot{V}_A/\dot{Q}$ inequality	↓	N or ↑	↑	N	↑	N

Abbreviations: ↓ = decreased; ↑ = increased; N = normal.

Noninvasive Oximetry

The use of oximeters with lightweight sensors that clip on the ear or fingertip has become commonplace. These devices measure O_2 saturation (Sa_{O_2}) on the basis of the different absorption spectra of oxyhemoglobin and deoxyhemoglobin. User calibration is not required, since the instruments automatically compensate for variations in skin thickness and slight differences in pigmentation and vascular perfusion. Accuracy of the various commercial oximeters differs but is generally about ±4 per cent for Sa_{O_2} levels above 80 per cent; falsely high readings are common below this level. Oximetry is not a sensitive guide to gas exchange in patients with high baseline Pa_{O_2} values because of the peculiar shape of the O_2 dissociation curve (see Fig. 15–8), whereby large changes in Pa_{O_2} may result in little change in Sa_{O_2}.

Invasive Diagnostic Techniques

Bronchoscopy. This is used to visualize the airways, to sample secretions, and to perform forceps biopsy. The rigid scope remains the instrument of choice when a wide channel is required, such as in massive hemoptysis or removal of large foreign bodies. Otherwise, the flexible scope is preferable because it is easy to maneuver. The latter is invaluable in the evaluation and biopsy of endobronchial lesions or in localizing the site of hemoptysis, since it allows visual access out to the segmental airways. Together with fluoroscopy, peripheral lung lesions can be biopsied. In the immunocompromised host, it is the standard approach to the diagnosis of fungal or *Pneumocystis* pneumonia. It is also effective in the diagnosis of tuberculosis in a patient not producing sputum. Its indication in the diagnosis of common bacterial infections is less clear, although the development of special protective brushes has reduced the problem of contamination with upper airway flora. In most patients requiring bronchial toilet and drainage, physical therapy is sufficient, but when that fails, especially in patients on mechanical ventilation, bronchoscopy may be effective in re-expanding atelectatic areas.

While generally a benign procedure, bronchoscopy has a number of complications. Worsening hypoxemia is almost inevitable, and supplemental O_2 should be used in hypoxemic patients. Laryngospasm, bronchospasm, fever, and new pulmonary infiltrates may occur. Significant bleeding and pneumothorax infrequently follow lung biopsy.

Transthoracic Needle Aspiration. Aspiration of lung tissue through a skinny needle inserted percutaneously is most useful with peripheral lesions, with which the bronchoscope has its least success. It provides material for cytological examination or microbial studies rather than histological examinations. The major complication is pneumothorax, which occurs in 20 to 30 per cent of cases; chest tube drainage is required in only 1 to 15 per cent of cases. Hemoptysis may occur but is rarely of clinical significance.

Thoracentesis and Pleural Biopsy. Pleural fluid examination and interpretation are covered in Chapter 23. Parietal pleural biopsy can be accomplished if sufficient fluid separates the lung from the chest wall. Histological examination reveals granulomas in greater than 60 per cent of cases of suspected tuberculosis effusion, and when histology is combined with culture of the tissue sample the yield may be 90 per cent. Biopsy is positive in 39 to 75 per cent of cases of suspected malignancy, which is a lower rate than for cytological examination of the fluid. Thorascopy with biopsy of pleural lesions under direct vision can be performed when the pleural effusion remains undiagnosed after thoracentesis and biopsy.

Mediastinoscopy. A small tube is passed into the mediastinum through an incision in the sternal notch. Lymph nodes in the anterior mediastinum and the right peritracheal region can be biopsied.

Open Lung Biopsy. When the above procedures are negative, an open lung biopsy may be indicated. In the immunocompromised host, it has a greater diagnostic yield than transbronchial biopsy using a fiberoptic bronchoscope, but still a proportion of patients display nonspecific findings. Despite the critical nature of the patients' illness, the mortality rate in large series of open lung biopsy is less than 0.5 per cent, with a complication rate of 11 per cent.

REFERENCES

Clausen JL: Pulmonary Function Testing. Guidelines and Controversies. New York, Academic Press, 1984.
Murray JF: The Normal Lung, 2nd ed. Philadelphia, WB Saunders Company, 1986.
Shure D: Diagnostic techniques. Clin Chest Med 8:1–171, 1987.

17

OBSTRUCTIVE LUNG DISEASE

The obstructive lung diseases are characterized by reduction of expiratory flow rates and include common disorders such as asthma and chronic obstructive pulmonary disease (COPD) and less common ones such as bronchiectasis and cystic fibrosis. Controversy and confusion reign over the definition of even the common ones because of the marked overlap of clinical and pathophysiological features. Some have even suggested the abandonment of the traditional names and the substitution of groupings based on signs and symptoms. Chronic mucus hypersecretion, with or without obstruction, and chronic airway obstruction, reversible or nonreversible, are probably more useful designations than debating whether a patient has COPD or asthma. Nevertheless, we will try to define each of the diseases as currently understood, pointing out overlap where it exists (Table 17–1).

PATHOPHYSIOLOGY OF AIRWAY OBSTRUCTION

The mechanism of airway obstruction in these disorders is always multifactorial, although in any individual patient one mechanism may play a dominant role. Air flow in the lungs is directly proportional to the driving pressure and inversely related to the airway resistance. During most of a forced expiration, the effective driving pressure is the elastic recoil pressure of the lung. Thus, reduction in elasticity, as in emphysema, decreases the maximum expiratory flow. Decreased elasticity also increases airway resistance, since the elastic recoil pressure exerts radial traction on the airways, which limits their dynamic compression during expiration.

A second cause of increased airway resistance is bronchoconstriction. The airways are lined by smooth muscle that is innervated by both adrenergic (bronchodilating) and cholinergic (bronchoconstricting) pathways. Cholinergic control is mediated by a vagal reflex, via irritant receptors lying just beneath the mucosa of the large aiways, trachea, and upper respiratory tract. Stimulation of these receptors by inhaled irritants or inflammation produces bronchoconstriction. In addition, endogenous mediators such as histamine and prostaglandins may dilate or constrict bronchial smooth muscle directly or reflexly by exciting the irritant receptors. Such mechanisms function to protect the lungs of normal subjects from noxious agents, but hyperreactivity of these pathways exists in patients with obstructive lung disease.

A third cause of increased airway resistance is chronic inflammation. In response to irritation in the form of external pollutants, recurrent infection, or chronic immunological stimulation, there is inflammatory goblet cell metaplasia of the bronchiolar epithelium, narrowing of the airways, and the production of excessive, thick secretions. If this process is allowed to continue it often results in the loss of ciliated epithelium, squamous metaplasia, and eventual peribronchial fibrosis.

Airway obstruction leads to characteristic changes in lung volumes (Table 17–2), with an increase in residual volume (RV) and functional residual capacity (FRC) and a normal or increased total lung capacity (TLC). The vital capacity (VC) is decreased as the RV takes up more and more of the thoracic gas volume. The mechanism of the increase in RV and FRC is not completely understood, although several factors are likely to contribute to a variable degree depending on the specific etiology involved. Decrease in the elastic

TABLE 17–1. OBSTRUCTIVE LUNG DISEASES

DISORDER	MAJOR CLINICAL CRITERIA	DISTINCTIVE LABORATORY FINDINGS
Chronic obstructive lung disease	Chronic progressive dyspnea	Decreased expiratory flow rates, hypoxemia ± hypercapnia
Emphysema	Little or no sputum, cachexia	Hyperinflation, increased lung compliance, and low carbon monoxide diffusing capacity
Chronic bronchitis	Cough and sputum production, history of chronic irritant exposure (mostly smoking, occasionally industrial exposure)	By itself, no significant physiological impairment
Asthma	Episodic dyspnea; may be associated with allergy to environmental agents	Marked airway hyperreactivity
Bronchiectasis	Large volume sputum production, clubbing	Chest x-ray findings of dilated bronchi with thickened walls, decreased lung volumes, and decreased expiratory flow
Immotile cilia syndrome	Associated with situs inversus or dextrocardia, sinusitis, and infertility	Abnormal sperm anatomy
Hypogammaglobulinemia		Abnormal decrease in one or more immunoglobulins
Cystic fibrosis	Bronchiectasis associated with GI disease, sinusitis, and infertility	Increased sweat Cl and Na, abnormal pancreatic function

recoil of the lungs moves the FRC closer to the relaxed volume of the chest wall (about two thirds of TLC). The greater tendency of abnormal airways, particularly at the lung base, to collapse during expiration traps air behind the closed airways. The marked resistance to expiratory flow may not permit complete exhalation during the time available for expiration. Finally, certain patients with asthma have persistent activity of the inspiratory muscles during expiration, which actively maintains a high FRC.

There are three major consequences of these changes in lung volume. Because of the nonlinear nature of the pressure-volume relationship of the lung, breathing at high lung volumes along the flat portion of the curve requires a greater pressure for the same change in volume (see Fig. 15–3), further increasing the work of breathing, which is already high owing to the abnormal airway resistance. In addition, the higher the resting lung volume, the shorter the inspiratory muscles are at the beginning of the breath (see Fig. 15–2). This places them at a disadvantaged position on their length-tension curve, diminishing their ability to alter transpulmonary pressure, and predisposes them to fatigue. Hyperinflation, however, has one beneficial effect. Owing to the tethering effect of the lung parenchyma on the airways, there is an inverse relationship between lung volume and airway resistance. Thus, hyperinflation is the one strategy immediately available in asthmatics to minimize sudden changes in airway caliber.

Abnormal pulmonary gas exchange is an inevitable consequence of obstructive lung disease. Airway obstruction and the breakdown of alveolar walls produce ventilation-perfusion mismatch that interferes with the efficient transfer of both O_2 and CO_2. Up to a certain point, patients with obstructive lung disease can increase their minute ventilation sufficiently to prevent the development of hypercapnia despite worsening hypoxemia (see Fig. 15–9). However, with continued progression of the disease, a point is reached beyond which further increase in ventilation is impractical because of the high energy requirements or the development of muscle fatigue. At that point, it is more efficient, physiologically, to allow the Pa_{CO_2} to rise, eliminating it at a higher concentration but lower minute ventilation and metabolic cost. The onset of hypercapnia is not always clearly related to the degree of mechanical impairment, and it appears that some patients prefer to work harder to maintain normocapnia, while others with the same degree of impairment are satisfied to breathe less and allow worse gas exchange (see Chapter 22).

Acute exacerbations of the chronic process brought on by increased bronchospasm, infection, or congestive heart failure may lead to worsening ventilation-perfusion inequality or the development of intrapulmonary shunt and further worsen gas exchange. During sleep, gas exchange is also usually worse owing to a characteristic reduction in minute ventilation. A patient with adequate arterial blood gases during the day may develop significant hypercapnia and arterial desaturation at night.

TABLE 17–2. ABNORMALITIES OF LUNG VOLUME

LUNG VOLUME	PULMONARY DISORDER		
	OBSTRUCTIVE DISEASE	RESTRICTIVE DISEASE	NEUROMUSCULAR DISEASE
Vital capacity	D	D	D
Functional residual capacity	I	D	N
Residual volume	I	D	I
Total lung capacity	N or I	D	D

Abbreviations: D = decreased; I = increased; N = normal.

ASTHMA

Asthma has been defined as a disease in which there is an increased responsiveness of the airways to various stimuli, causing widespread narrowing of the airways which varies over time. The stimulus may be immunological in origin, as in classic extrinsic asthma, in which mast cells, sensitized by IgE antibodies, degranulate and release bronchoactive mediators following exposure to a specific antigen. The cause may also be unclear, as in adult-onset asthma, in which the patients frequently show no evidence of allergy. The airway obstruction may be due to bronchoconstriction alone or may involve mucosal inflammation and excessive mucus production. Symptoms may be intermittent, or they may gradually become persistent. The recognized categories of asthma are listed in Table 17–3. Clinical differentiation is important only in situations in which there are clear-cut, easily identifiable, and avoidable extrinsic factors, such as drugs or industrial substances.

The diagnosis of asthma is based on the presence of

TABLE 17–3. TYPES OF ASTHMA

CLASSIFICATION	INITIATING FACTORS
Extrinsic	IgE-mediated external allergens
Intrinsic	?
Adult onset	?
Exercise induced	Alteration in airway temperature and humidity; mediator release
Aspirin sensitive (associated with nasal polyps)	Aspirin and other nonsteroidal anti-inflammatory drugs
Allergic bronchopulmonary aspergillosis	Hypersensitivity to *Aspergillus* species (not infection)
Occupational	Metal salts (platinum, chrome, and nickel)
	Antibiotic powder (penicillin, sulfathiazole, tetracycline)
	Toluene diisocyanate (TDI)
	Flour
	Wood dusts
	Cotton dust (byssinosis)
	Animal proteins

TABLE 17–4. DIAGNOSTIC STUDIES IN ASTHMA

1. Routine pulmonary function test	Decreased FEV_1; hyperinflation; improvement with bronchodilator
2. Special pulmonary function test	
a. methacholine, histamine or cold-air challenge	Indicate the presence of nonspecific bronchial hyper-reactivity; bronchoconstriction occurs at lower dose in asthma
b. challenge with specific agents: occupational, drugs, etc.	Occasionally performed
c. portable peak flow measurements	Helpful in diagnosis of occupational asthma and managment of brittle asthmatic
3. Chest x-ray	Fleeting infiltrates and central bronchiectasis in ABPA
4. Skin tests	Demonstrate atopy; little value except prick test to *Aspergillus fumigatus* positive in ABPA
5. Blood tests	Eosinophils and IgE usually increased in atopy; levels may be very high in ABPA. *Aspergillus* precipitins increased in many but not all patients with ABPA

Abbreviation: ABPA = allergic bronchopulmonary aspergillosis.

episodic dyspnea associated with wheezing. Intermittent cough, probably due to stimulation of the irritant receptors, is commonly seen and may be the sole presenting symptom in some patients. Typically, symptoms are worse at night, following exercise, after going out in the cold, while exposed to irritating gases, etc.

Laboratory studies may be required to determine the presence of specific types of asthma (Table 17–4). The chest x-ray demonstrates hyperinflation in the symptomatic patient, whereas in patients with allergic bronchopulmonary aspergillosis serial films may show infiltrates that change location or features suggestive of central bronchiectasis. Pulmonary function studies show the findings of obstruction, which improve significantly following the acute administration of bronchodilators. During the asymptomatic phase, the diagnosis can often be made by initiating bronchospasm by the inhalation of histamine, methacholine, or cold air.

Acute severe asthma (status asthmaticus) refers to an attack of increased severity that is unresponsive to routine therapy. While the attack is sometimes prolonged, fatal episodes may occur unexpectedly with overwhelming suddenness. A history of increasing bronchodilator use with little benefit is expected, but clinical signs, including pulsus paradoxus, are extremely unreliable in judging the severity. The degree of physiological disturbance can best be appreciated by a measure of expiratory flow rates. In the emergency room management of these patients, such indices are helpful in assessing the response to therapy, as they provide immediate quantitative information and can be obtained at frequent intervals without discomfort. Complementary information can be ob-

tained by measurement of arterial blood gases, and this may be the only measurement possible in the critically ill asthmatic. Hypoxemia is usually, but not invariably, present and does not correlate closely with airway obstruction. Pa_{CO_2} is typically reduced early in an attack. With increasing severity Pa_{O_2} falls and Pa_{CO_2} returns to normal and then rises, accompanied by a mixed respiratory and metabolic acidosis, such that intubation and mechanical ventilation may become necessary. Hypercapnia at presentation is not an indication for intubation, as most patients improve with vigorous treatment, but careful monitoring is essential. In general, arterial blood gas measurements are less sensitive and specific than assessment of airway obstruction in judging the response to therapy.

CHRONIC OBSTRUCTIVE LUNG DISEASE (COPD)

Patients with chronic obstructive lung disease have slowly progressive airway obstruction. The course of the disease is punctuated by periodic exacerbations resulting in an increase in dyspnea and sputum production or, occasionally, the precipitation of acute respiratory failure. These exacerbations are often due to pulmonary infection, the development of heart failure, or poor patient compliance with prescribed therapy. Until recently, an episode of acute respiratory failure was associated with a poor long-term prognosis, but with modern management such an episode does not appear to alter overall prognosis.

COPD generally affects middle-aged and older individuals. Patients usually present with dyspnea and exercise intolerance. Cough and sputum production are other common complaints but may be absent in many patients. Physical examination reveals signs of lung overinflation, prominent use of accessory respiratory muscles, diminished breath sounds, and diffuse wheezing especially during a forced expiration. Patients may vary in their appearance from thin and even cachectic-looking to edematous and cyanotic. In the past these two extremes of clinical presentation have been associated with specific pathological entities, emphysema and bronchitis. However, recent clinical-pathological correlations have not supported this impression. In its early stages, the physical examination may be normal, and the diagnosis will depend on laboratory studies documenting reduced expiratory flow rates.

Pulmonary function studies generally show decreased VC and expiratory flow rates, and increased RV, FRC, and TLC. Unlike asthma, COPD is not characterized by marked temporal variability in the degree of airway obstruction. However, like asthma, bronchospasm is present and expiratory flow can often be increased acutely by bronchodilators. The usual improvement in patients with COPD, on the order of 15 to 20 per cent of the prebronchodilator value, is less than that observed in asthma. Arterial blood gases generally evidence hypoxemia of varying severity and, in the advanced stage of the disease, hypercapnia. The degree of hypoxemia may not correlate very well with either the severity of the airflow obstruction or the degree of dyspnea, and some severely limited patients have relatively well-preserved blood gases. During sleep, pulmonary gas exchange may further worsen. When the degree of hypoxemia becomes severe (Pa_{O_2} less than 60 mm Hg), hypoxic vasoconstriction of the pulmonary arteries leads to the development of pulmonary hypertension and subsequent right heart failure (cor pulmonale). It may also result in significant polycythemia.

There are three pathophysiological disorders recognized as a part of the syndrome of COPD. These include emphysema, small airways disease, and chronic bronchitis. In any given patient, one or more of these manifestations may predominate.

Emphysema

Emphysema is characterized by two features. Anatomically, it is defined as an abnormal enlargement of the air spaces distal to the terminal bronchioles, accompanied by destructive changes in the alveolar walls. Physiologically, it is characterized by a loss of elastic recoil and thus an increased lung compliance. The degree of airway obstruction in patients with COPD correlates most closely with the severity of emphysema, and patients who have significant functional impairment usually have at least a moderate degree of emphysema.

The pathogenesis of emphysema has yet to be determined with certainty, although most workers favor an imbalance of proteases and antiproteases in the lung, with resultant lung destruction. This theory is based on the discovery of a small number of patients with an inherited deficiency of alpha-1-antiprotease, the major antiprotease, who develop emphysema even without other risk factors. Cigarette smoke, the major etiological factor in the development of emphysema, has been shown to increase the numbers of alveolar macrophages and neutrophils in the lung, enhance protease release, and impair the activity of antiproteases. However, other factors must determine susceptibility to emphysema, as less than 10 to 15 per cent of smokers develop clinical evidence of airway obstruction.

The diagnosis of emphysema is usually inferred from the clinical and laboratory findings. Chest roentgenograms demonstrate hyperinflation with depressed diaphragms, increased anteroposterior diameter, and widened retrosternal air space. These findings, however, are seen whenever hyperinflation is present, and more specific features in emphysema include attenuation of the pulmonary vasculature and the presence of hyperlucent areas. The one finding that correlates well with the anatomical presence of emphysema is a reduction in diffusing capacity because of the loss of alveolar capillary surface area.

Small Airways Disease

The earliest manifestation of COPD appears to be in the peripheral airways. Abnormalities that have been identified include inflammation of the terminal and respiratory bronchioles, fibrosis of the airway walls leading to narrowing, and goblet cell metaplasia. These lesions undoubtedly contribute to airway obstruction, although the correlation is not as close as with the degree of emphysema. Furthermore, only a small proportion of cigarette smokers with these pathological abnormalities go on to develop symptomatic COPD.

Chronic Bronchitis

Chronic bronchitis is defined as a persistent cough resulting in sputum production for more than three months in each year over the previous three years. Diagnosis requires exclusion of other conditions associated with cough and sputum production, such as bronchiectasis. As with emphysema, cigarette smoke is the major etiological factor, although exposure to other pollutants such as dusts may play a role by causing chronic irritation. Cough and sputum production do not appear to have an independent effect on the development of airway obstruction. The airway obstruction seen in the setting of chronic bronchitis is due to associated emphysema, bronchospasm, and obstruction of the peripheral airways. The findings on physical examination, pulmonary function assessment, and x-ray depend on the degree of associated airway obstruction.

Bronchiectasis

Bronchiectasis is an abnormal and persistent dilatation of the bronchi due to destructive changes in the elastic and muscular layers of the walls. It may be widespread or localized to a single lung segment. It is usually a consequence of a severe necrotizing lung infection. In the past, it was often seen as a sequal to measles or pertussis pneumonia, whereas today it is more likely to be a residual from a gram-negative infection. Immune deficiency states such as hypogammaglobulinemia predispose to frequent respiratory tract infections and the development of bronchiectasis. Exposure to corrosive gases is an additional inflammatory injury that may result in permanent airway damage. Interference with the normal clearance mechanisms may also cause chronic inflammation and bronchiectasis. An unusual congenital cause of decreased lung clearance and bronchiectasis is the immotile cilia syndrome, which is due to structural abnormalities in the microtubular system. This is often associated with sinusitis, situs inversus or dextrocardia, and infertility.

The diagnosis is made by a history of long-standing chronic cough and the production of large quantities of foul sputum, occasionally blood tinged, and physical findings of persistent crackles over the affected lung regions. With severe, long-standing disease, clubbing and cor pulmonale are frequent and massive hemoptysis may occasionally occur. The chest x-ray may be normal or may display minor nonspecific features, such as increased markings or linear atelectasis. On

TABLE 17–5. CYSTIC FIBROSIS—ORGAN INVOLVEMENT

I. **Pulmonary**
   Cough and sputum production
   Recurrent pneumonias
   Bronchial hyperreactivity
   Hemoptysis
   Pneumothorax
   Marked digital clubbing
   Cor pulmonale
II. **Upper Respiratory Tract**
   Nasal polyps
   Chronic sinusitis
III. **Gastrointestinal**
   Meconium ileus in the neonate
   Meconium ileus equivalent (childhood, adult)
   Rectal prolapse
   Hernias
   Chronic pancreatic dysfunction causing steatorrhea,
      malnutrition, and vitamin deficiency
   Acute pancreatitis (rare)
   Diabetes mellitus
   Cirrhosis and portal hypertension
   Salivary gland inflammation
IV. **Genitourinary**
   Sterility in men
   Low fertility rate in women

occasion, the x-ray is very suggestive of bronchiectasis, demonstrating thickening of the bronchial walls well out to the lung periphery and even cystic lesions. Definitive diagnosis usually requires contrast bronchography, but this is rarely indicated. More recently, CT scanning has been able to resolve the presence of bronchiectasis with a reasonable degree of specificity, although it is not as sensitive as bronchography. Pulmonary function studies invariably show obstruction and occasionally significant hyperinflation, although restricted lung volumes may be present with severe disease.

Cystic Fibrosis

Cystic fibrosis is a common generalized disorder of exocrine gland function, which impairs clearance of secretions in a variety of organs (Table 17–5). This autosomal recessive disorder occurs in about 1 in every 200 white births. While the gene has now been localized to a small part of chromosome 7, the underlying defect is unknown. Recent studies point to an abnormality of electrolyte transport in epithelial tissue, perhaps a blockage of the chloride channel. The pulmonary pathophysiology is similar to that of other causes of bronchiectasis, with tenacious mucus and impaired ciliary function resulting in recurrent infections, chronic inflammation, and bronchial wall destruction.

The disease is usually manifest in childhood, often with gastrointestinal symptoms, particularly steatorrhea and bowel obstruction (Table 17–5). However, the pulmonary features pose the biggest problem. Classically, *Staphylococcus aureus* in childhood and the mucoid strain of *Pseudomonas aeruginosa* in later years cause recurrent respiratory infections that are particularly difficult to treat because of chronic colonization of the airways. Definitive diagnosis requires the finding of an elevated concentration of sodium or chloride in the sweat. When correctly collected and analyzed, levels above 60 mEq/L in children or 80 mEq/L in adults are diagnostic in the proper clinical setting. The course is usually one of gradual but progressive respiratory failure. Most patients are diagnosed in childhood, even occasionally at birth. Some patients with milder disease escape diagnosis until their late teens or even early 20's. These patients usually have minimal extrapulmonary problems and have often been labeled with a diagnosis of asthma or even just recurrent bronchitis. The true diagnosis is usually made when the disease worsens or when problems with another organ system, such as the discovery of infertility, lead to a more complete evaluation. Recent improvements in antibiotics, nutritional therapy, and supportive care, however, have improved the prognosis such that the median survival has increased from less than two years in the 1940's up to more than 20 years today.

Treatment

For the most part, our current knowledge of the etiology of the various obstructive lung diseases prevents specific therapy aimed at basic pathophysiological mechanisms. Specific replacement therapy with alpha-1-antiprotease is available for patients with a homozygous absence of the required gene, but the efficacy of such treatment is not yet known. Thus, the treatment of all forms of obstructive lung disease is symptomatic and directed toward the reduction of abnormal airway tone and specific complications such as infection, excessive bronchial secretions, hypoxemia, and cor pulmonale.

Bronchodilators

Drugs that relax bronchial smooth muscle can be divided into four groups (Table 17–6). The sympa-

TABLE 17–6. BRONCHODILATORS

Sympathomimetics
   Epinephrine
   Isoproterenol
   Beta-2–specific agents:
      metaproterenol,
      terbutaline, albuterol
Xanthines
   Theophylline
   Aminophylline
Anticholinergics
   Atropine
   Ipratropium bromide
Corticosteroids
   Hydrocortisone
   Prednisone
   Beclomethasone

TABLE 17–7. FACTORS AFFECTING THEOPHYLLINE CLEARANCE

Clearance increased by	Cigarette smoking
	Marijuana smoking
	Charcoal-broiled meat
	Phenobarbital
Clearance decreased	
by 25%	Erythromycin
	Propranolol
	Allopurinol
	Oral contraceptives
by 50%	Cimetidine
	Phenytoin
	Influenza vaccine
	Infection
by 100% or more	Heart failure
	Hepatic cirrhosis

thomimetics are the most potent bronchodilators. Subcutaneous epinephrine and nebulized isoproterenol have a relatively short duration of action and act on both beta-1 and beta-2 receptors, whereas epinephrine has additional, undesirable alpha effects. The development of noncatecholamine, beta-2–specific agents has improved the specificity of the sympathomimetic agents for the adrenergic receptor found in airway smooth muscle, but more importantly it has increased the duration of action from 60 to 90 minutes to more than 4 hours and permits oral administration. Aerosol therapy is the preferred route of administration, because the lower total dose reduces side effects. Oral use often leads to muscle twitching, and parenteral administration appears to markedly reduce their apppparent beta-2 specificity. Tolerance to these agents does not occur, and a failure to respond usually indicates an insufficient dose or ineffective use of the metered dose device or nebulizer.

Methylxanthines such as theophylline are about 50 per cent as potent as the sympathomimetics. Effectiveness is related to the blood level and is optimal between 8 and 20 μg/ml. Above these concentrations, the incidence of gastrointestinal, cardiac, and neurological toxicity is unacceptable. The usual adult dose is 10 to 12 mg/kg/day but may vary widely, depending on the presence of factors that alter the metabolism of theophylline (Table 17–7). In patients with COPD it is difficult to demonstrate that the addition of theophylline provides additional bronchodilation to that achieved by optimal doses of beta-2–specific sympathomimetics. However, many patients obtain symptomatic improvement that may relate, in part, to the additional small beneficial effects theophylline has on cardiac and respiratory muscle function. In asthma, theophylline functions mainly to reduce the wide swings in airway smooth muscle tone seen especially in the early morning hours. Its addition, when sympathomimetics are not sufficient, theophylline decreases symptomatic complaints.

Anticholinergic agents were the first clinically available bronchodilators, but their usage declined because of concerns about their side effects, specifically the purported inhibition of lower airway secretions, which is no longer considered to be a problem. As the importance of vagally mediated bronchospasm has been elucidated, these agents have received renewed interest. They are particularly effective in patients with COPD and in selected patients with asthma. A new anticholinergic agent, ipratropium bromide, has been developed; unlike atropine, its systemic absorption is poor, and therefore it has fewer extrapulmonary effects.

Corticosteroids are invaluable, although they do not work acutely to relieve airway obstruction. Their usage early and in sufficient doses in the treatment of acute asthma or the acute exacerbation of COPD has been shown to lessen the degree of airway obstruction (over 12 to 24 hours), to decrease the total time of hospitalization, and to reduce recurrence. The complications of chronic administration limit their usefulness, although the introduction of potent, inhaled corticosteroids (beclomethasone) has significantly reduced this problem. Unfortunately, an alternate-day regimen, to minimize steroid complications, is usually ineffective in patients with bronchospastic lung disease.

Inhaled sodium cromolyn prevents bronchospasm in some asthmatics but is not helpful in the management of an acute asthmatic attack. While stabilization of the mast cell membrane and the prevention of mediator release are the major proposed mechanisms of action, it is also effective in forms of asthma without an atopic association. In asthmatics who are difficult to control, it is a useful drug to try before turning to chronic oral steroid therapy. The drug should be used for three to four weeks before deciding on its efficacy. It may also be used intranasally to relieve the symptoms of allergic rhinitis.

A suggested scheme for the administration of the bronchodilators is shown in Figure 17–1.

OXYGEN

The hypoxemia seen in obstructive lung disease has two major deleterious consequences: decreased O_2 delivery to the tissues and hypoxic pulmonary vasoconstriction with resultant cor pulmonale. Oxygen therapy is thus an integral part of the treatment of patients with obstructive lung disease and should be used whenever the arterial saturation falls below 90 per cent. In some patients O_2 may be required only with acute exacerbations, but in those with chronic disease it may be needed during sleep, with exercise, or continuously, depending on when desaturation occurs. Because of the mechanism of the hypoxemia, namely ventilation-perfusion inequality, the desaturation can be corrected by small increases in the inspired fractional O_2 concentrations, achieved with less than 4 L/min of nasal flow. It has been clearly demonstrated in COPD patients having a resting Pa_{O_2} below 55 torr that

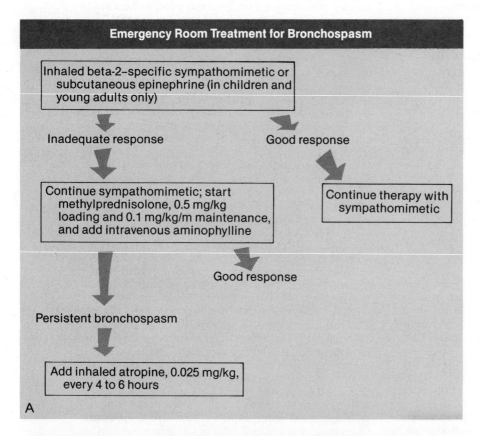

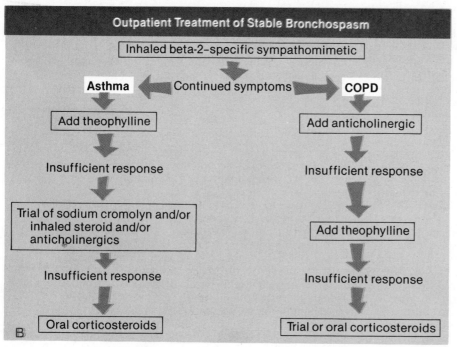

FIGURE 17–1. Scheme for treatment of bronchospasm in the emergency room (*A*) and in patients with stable disease (*B*).

long-term O_2 therapy markedly improves survival, and maximal benefit is achieved when it is delivered throughout the 24 hours of the day.

ANTIBIOTICS AND VACCINES

Some exacerbations of airway obstruction are secondary to acute infections. In patients with obstructive airway diseases airway colonization with putative bacterial pathogens is common. However, in the absence of systemic signs of infection or a clear-cut change in the quality and quantity of sputum there is no indication for antibiotics. In patients with bronchiectasis or cystic fibrosis, the specific organism responsible, usually *S. aureus* or *Pseudomonas*, is easily identifiable. However, in patients with COPD or asthma, a specific agent is not usually isolated. In the first case, the appropriate antibiotic can be chosen, while in the latter case it is often more cost-efficient to administer a broad-spectrum antibiotic such as ampicillin, trimethoprim-sulfamethoxazole, or tetracycline. The route of administration, oral or intravenous, depends on the specific agent and the acuteness of the process.

Influenza vaccines directed at specific epidemic strains are effective in reducing morbidity and mortality. Pneumococcal vaccine is effective in preventing infection in young healthy individuals but has not proved to be similarly effective in patients with chronic lung diseases.

IPPB AND NEBULIZATION THERAPY

Intermittent positive-pressure breathing (IPPB) has been shown to have no specific value in the management of patients with airway obstruction. Thinning of secretions is a controversial topic. While a normal state of hydration is probably important to maintain normal bronchial secretions, there is no evidence that additional fluids have any effect. Neither is there evidence for the efficacy of nebulized saline, mucolytics, enzymes, detergents, or iodides, and side effects may be significant. Probably the most important measures to improve airway secretions are to control the primary irritants by eliminating smoking, maximizing bronchodilation, and utilizing antibiotics when indicated.

SMOKING CESSATION

One of the most important factors in the management of patients with COPD is the cessation of cigarette smoking. Susceptible smokers who develop COPD have an increased rate of decline in lung function measured as FEV_1 (80 ml/yr) compared with nonsusceptible smokers and nonsmokers (30 ml/yr) FEV_1 (Fig. 20–2). Following cessation of smoking, the rate of decline in the susceptible smoker is reduced to that in the nonsmoker (30 ml/yr).

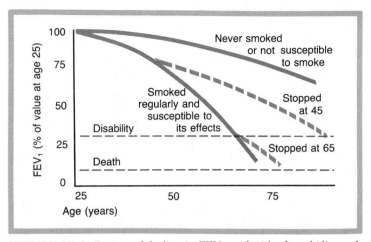

FIGURE 17–2. Pattern of decline in FEV_1, with risk of morbidity and mortality from respiratory disease in a susceptible smoker compared with a normal subject or nonsusceptible smoker. While cessation of smoking does not replenish the lung function already lost in a susceptible smoker, it decreases the further rate of decline. (Adapted from Fletcher and Peto: Br Med J 1:1645, 1977.)

PHYSICAL THERAPY AND REHABILITATION

Chest physiotherapy (percussion and postural drainage) is employed on the assumption that sputum retention has undesirable consequences. While this is a reasonable although unproved assumption, and while physiotherapy increases the immediate volume of sputum cleared, there is no evidence that it affects the natural history of any disease. Similarly, breathing training and exercise rehabilitation lack a clear scientific basis. However, patients with pulmonary disease of sufficient severity to prevent normal daily living commonly demonstrate an improved quality of life when enrolled in a properly run rehabilitation program. Finally, nutritional needs in these patients must be addressed. This is important in cystic fibrosis, as supplemental pancreatic enzymes and vitamins are necessary. However, the debilitated patient with emphysema must also be considered for nutritional support, since poor nutrition may render him susceptible to respiratory failure through decreased muscle strength.

REFERENCES

Snider GL: Emphysema. Clin Chest Med 4:329–499, 1983.
Standards for the diagnosis and care of patients with chronic obstructive pulmonary disease (COPD) and asthma. Am Rev Resp Dis 136:225–244, 1987.
Ziment I, Popa V: Respiratory Pharmacology. Clin Chest Med 7:313–518, 1986.

18

DIFFUSE INFILTRATIVE
DISEASES OF THE LUNG

A large number of lung diseases are characterized by the replacement or infiltration of normal lung by abnormal tissue (Fig. 18–1). On rare occasions, the insulting agent may be well recognized, as in silicosis. More often, the causative process is unknown and only the response is obvious. The insult may cause injury by direct toxicity, as a result of an inflammatory response, or through an immunologically mediated reaction. Regardless of the mechanism of injury, the influx of inflammatory cells into the lung interstitium, perivascular space, and alveolar space results in the development of an alveolitis or vasculitis and, if carried to completion, lung fibrosis.

CLINICAL MANIFESTATIONS

The spectrum of clinical presentation in this group of disorders is as varied as the conditions themselves. The majority of patients present with an insidious onset of dyspnea, exercise limitation, and dry nonproductive cough. Certain historical features may suggest a specific diagnosis as detailed in the discussion of each entity. Examination of the chest characteristically reveals mid to late inspiratory crackles and tachypnea. Physical findings of pulmonary hypertension, cor pulmonale, and cyanosis are usually late manifestations. Evidence of extrathoracic disease is valuable in suggesting a specific diagnosis, such as the skin lesions of sarcoidosis or the arthritis of a collagen vascular disease. The chest x-ray may confirm the presence of diffuse infiltrative disease but is rarely diagnostic on its own.

The physiological consequences depend on the proportion of lung involved and the speed with which the infiltration develops. As fibrosis replaces normal lung structures, there is a decrease in all lung volumes (see Table 17–2), a fall in lung compliance, and a decline in the diffusing capacity. The loss of alveolar space and airway abnormalities produce ventilation-perfusion inequality, but hypoxemia is usually mild until the disease progresses to a significant degree, and hypercapnia is uncommon.

A specific diagnosis, when not clear from the presentation, depends on lung biopsy findings. In certain diseases, such as sarcoidosis, sufficient tissue can be obtained using a fiberoptic bronchoscope and a transbronchial biopsy, but this may be insufficient in others, such as idiopathic pulmonary fibrosis, and an open lung biopsy may be required.

SPECIFIC ENTITIES

DISEASES WITH KNOWN ETIOLOGIES
PNEUMOCONIOSES

Pneumoconioses are lung diseases produced by the inhalation of inorganic dust. These dusts may be fibrous minerals, such as asbestos, or nonfibrous minerals, such as silica or metals. The clinical spectrum varies widely according to the nature of the inhaled substance and the type of response it evokes in the lung. Some substances such as asbestos lead to progressive fibrosis, whereas others such as iron dust produce little or no reaction even when deposited in large amounts. The common organic dusts are listed in Table 18–1, and are divided according to their structure and fibrogenic potential.

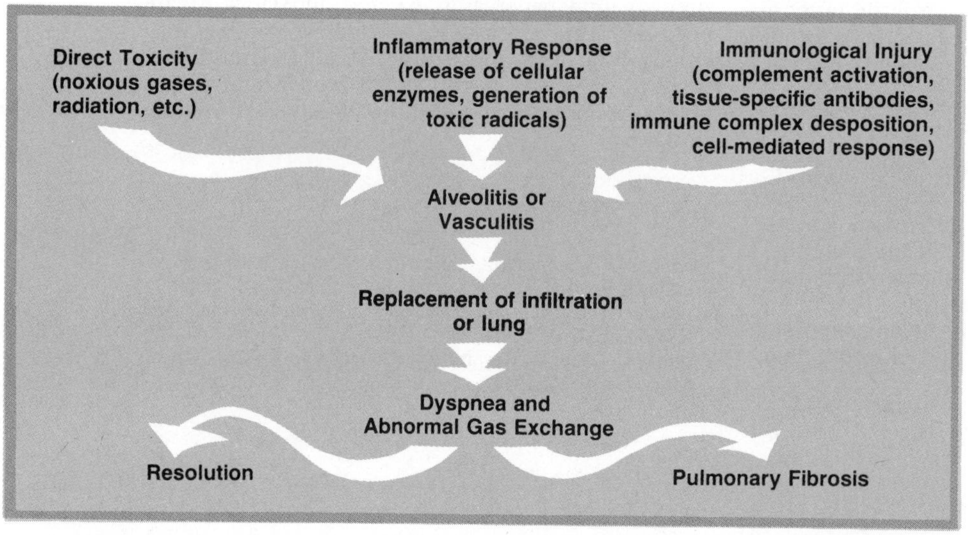

Direct Toxicity (noxious gases, radiation, etc.)	Inflammatory Response (release of cellular enzymes, generation of toxic radicals)	Immunological Injury (complement activation, tissue-specific antibodies, immune complex desposition, cell-mediated response)

Alveolitis or Vasculitis

Replacement of infiltration or lung

Dyspnea and Abnormal Gas Exchange

Resolution   Pulmonary Fibrosis

FIGURE 18–1. Pathophysiology and outcome of diffuse infiltrative lung disease.

Among the fibrous minerals, asbestos is the most important health hazard (Table 18–2). The pulmonary fibrosis (asbestosis) is dose-dependent, whereas diseases in the pleural space do not seem to be related to the intensity of exposure. In addition to pulmonary fibrosis and benign pleural disease, there is a fivefold increase in the rate of bronchogenic carcinoma among nonsmoking asbestos workers compared with a nonsmoking control population. Among smoking asbestos workers the risk is 60- to 90-fold. Malignant mesotheliomas of the pleura and peritoneum are also associated with asbestos exposure but bear no apparent relationship to smoking. There is a prolonged latency period between the exposure and the tumors, usually at least 20 years and sometimes as long as 30 to 40 years.

Deposition of coal dust around the first- and second-order respiratory bronchioles causes coal workers' pneumoconiosis, or "black lung." This may be accompanied by minimal inflammation but is insufficiently severe to cause symptoms or measurable physiological derangement in most workers. Simple pneumoconiosis consisting of a fine, diffuse, reticulonodular pattern seen on chest roentgenogram and the development of a productive cough develops in 5 per cent of coal workers. Physiological impairment when present is slight. In a smaller number of miners, perhaps 0.4 per cent, nodular densities of 1 cm or greater may be visible on chest x-ray, representing dense collagenous nodules (complicated coal workers' pneumoconiosis). Unlike the simple form, this can eventually result in progressive massive fibrosis and restrictive lung disease.

The pulmonary response to a more fibrogenic dust, such as silica, is dramatically magnified. Silica exposure occurs in most mining operations, sandblasting, pottery working, brick making, and foundry work. In most cases, silicosis develops after at least 20 years of exposure, although it can develop in 5 years or less with intense exposure to a high concentration of dust. Roentgenographic gradation of disease ranges from small diffuse nodules with minimal hilar node enlargement to large nodules, predominantly in the upper lobes, which vary from about 1 cm to conglomerate masses occupying most of a lobe (progressive massive fibrosis). Eggshell calcification of the hilar nodes is characteristic. The chest x-ray findings do not correlate well with the symptomatology and physiological impairment in silicosis. The course of the disease may be modified by other factors such as coexisting smoking or superinfection with mycobacterial disease, either *M. tuberculosis*, *M. intracellulare*, or *M. kansasii*. The more acute the silicosis, the more likely it will be complicated by tuberculosis.

No specific treatment exists for any pneumoconiosis, and only removal from the offending environment may modify the eventual progression to respiratory failure. A careful and repeated search for mycobacterial disease is mandatory in silicosis, especially with sudden worsening of the condition. Cessation of smoking, aggressive treatment of routine bacterial infections, and the use of oxygen to treat

TABLE 18–1. PNEUMOCONIOSES

SUBSTANCE	FIBRO-GENICITY	OCCUPATION
I. Fibrous minerals		
Asbestos	High	Asbestos mining, shipyard and boiler workers, insulators
Talc	High	Talc mining and milling
Fiberglass	Low	Insulation
II. Nonfibrous minerals		
Silica	High	Mining, sandblasting, etc.
Coal	Low	Mining
III. Metals		
Iron	Low	Mining, refining, and fabricating
Aluminum	Uncertain	Mining, refining, and fabricating
Beryllium	High	Mining and fabricating

TABLE 18–2. ASBESTOS-RELATED RESPIRATORY DISEASE

FORM	COMMENT
Asbestosis	Interstitial fibrosis; long latent period; clubbing; crackles
Pleural thickening	Calcified plaques; intensity proportional to exposure; only significant in that it indicates prior exposure
Benign effusions	Hemorrhagic; asymptomatic; spontaneous remission and recurrence
Pleural mesothelioma	Latent interval 20 to 40 years; not dose-related; probably unrelated to smoking; median survival 12 months
Bronchogenic carcinoma	Fivefold increased risk in exposed nonsmoker and 60- to 90-fold risk in exposed smoker

complicating cor pulmonale may improve function and prolong life.

HYPERSENSITIVITY PNEUMONITIS

Hypersensitivity pneumonitis or extrinsic allergic alveolitis occurs in individuals who have developed an abnormal sensitivity to some organic agent. Four to six hours following exposure in a sensitized subject, there is the onset of cough, dyspnea, fever, and malaise; wheezing is usually absent. Diffuse crackles are heard on auscultation and the x-ray reveals nodular or reticulonodular infiltrates with relative sparing of the apices. In most cases these symptoms gradually resolve but recur on subsequent exposure. The duration of symptoms may gradually increase with repeated exposure and eventually result in the development of pulmonary fibrosis and restrictive lung disease.

A vast array of substances can cause this disorder

TABLE 18–3. HYPERSENSITIVITY PNEUMONITIS

ANTIGEN	SOURCE	DISEASE EXAMPLES
Thermophilic bacteria	Moldy hay and other organic material, heated humidifiers	Farmer's lung, bagassosis, humidifier lung
Other bacteria, particularly *Bacillus subtilis*	Water	Detergent worker's and humidifer lung
Fungi	Moldy organic material, water	Maple bark–stripper's lung, suberosis, sequoiosis
Animal protein	Bird droppings, animal dander	Pigeon breeder's lung, rodent handler's disease
Amoeba	Water	Humidifier lung

(Table 18–3), the prototype being farmer's lung, a hypersensitivity to thermophilic *Actinomyces*, a funguslike organism found in moldy hay. Patients with these disorders have serum precipitins to specific proteins, although the presence of precipitins does not, by itself, define the disease, since 50 per cent of similarly exposed subjects develop precipitins but remain asymptomatic.

The treatment is to remove or avoid the offending agent. Occasionally in the acute situation corticosteroids are required. The efficacy of corticosteroids in the chronic phase, once fibrosis has set in, however, is less clear, although a trial in symptomatic patients is usually worthwhile.

TABLE 18–4. COMMON DRUG-INDUCED LUNG DISEASES

DRUG	DOSE RELATION	PATHOLOGICAL AND CLINICAL APPEARANCE
I. Cancer chemotherapeutic agents		
Bleomycin	Both acute and dose-dependent	Pulmonary fibrosis
Busulfan	Greater than 600 mg	Pulmonary fibrosis
Chlorambucil	Greater than 2 g	Pulmonary fibrosis
Methotrexate	None	Pneumonitis
II. Analgesics and hypnotics		
Aspirin	Serum level greater than 45 mg/dl	Pulmonary edema
Ethchlorvynol, propoxyphene hydrochloride, heroin	Overdose	Pulmonary edema
Opiates and other psychotropic drugs	Chronic intravenous abuse	Pulmonary fibrosis and vasculitis
III. Antibiotics		
Nitrofurantoin	Acute	Hypersensitivity pneumonitis
Sulfonamides	Chronic	Pulmonary fibrosis, Löffler's syndrome

OTHER CLEARLY EXTRINSIC CAUSES OF DIFFUSE INFILTRATIVE LUNG DISEASE

External radiation in doses in excess of 5000 rads over a 4- to 6-week period frequently produces radiation pneumonitis within the first 6 months following exposure, and almost always by 13 months after exposure. Many drugs cause diffuse lung disease (Table 18–4). Some cancer chemotherapeutic agents, such as chlorambucil, produce dose-related toxicity, while others, like methotrexate, produce hypersensitivity reactions. Both phenomena occur with bleomycin in an acute syndrome; chronic illness is almost inevitable when more than 400 to 500 units are used. Synergism between bleomycin and other causes of lung injury, such as radiation and high concentrations of oxygen, has been suspected. Antibiotics, especially nitrofurantoin and sulfonamides, may cause hypersensitivity lung disease, while a number of sedatives and hypnotics have been implicated in noncardiogenic pulmonary edema, especially with intravenous abuse. Exposure to noxious gases such as chlorine, ammonia, phosgene, ozone, hydrogen sulfide, and nitrogen dioxide can cause severe lung injury. The nature of the injury depends upon the reactivity of the gas, its concentration, and the length of exposure and ranges from tracheobronchitis to adult respiratory disease syndrome.

DIFFUSE LUNG DISEASE OF UNKNOWN ETIOLOGY

COLLAGEN-VASCULAR DISEASES

Rheumatoid arthritis is associated with five different pulmonary manifestations present in a high percentage of seropositive cases: exudative pleural effusion characterized by a very low glucose concentration; pulmonary nodules varying from a few millimeters to more than 5 cm in diameter; rheumatoid nodules in association with coal workers' pneumoconiosis (Caplan's syndrome); diffuse interstitial fibrosis; and pulmonary vasculitis. With the exception of the nodules and the low glucose in the pleural fluid, patients with systemic lupus erythematosus (SLE) may have many of the same manifestations. Pleuritis and pneumonitis have also been described in Sjøgren's syndrome, polymyositis, and dermatomyositis. The lung is commonly involved in scleroderma presenting as pulmonary fibrosis and/or pulmonary hypertension.

PULMONARY VASCULITIS

Pulmonary vasculitis may occur as a part of one of the aforementioned connective tissue disorders or in the course of a systemic granulomatous or hypersensitivity vasculitis.

The granulomatous vasculitides include classic Wegener's granulomatosis, limited Wegener's granulomatosis, and lymphomatoid granulomatosis. Classic Wegener's is a necrotizing vasculitis initially described as involving three organ systems: the lung, the upper respiratory tract, and the kidneys. However, many other organs in the body may be affected. Lung involvement usually takes the form of single or multiple nodular lesions that have a propensity to cavitate. In the limited form of Wegener's granulomatosis, patients have a similar pathology but are free of renal disease. Both diseases respond well to cyclophosphamide. Lymphomatoid granulomatosis resembles Wegener's but differs in three important features: there is frequent central nervous system involvement; more than 15 per cent develop malignant lymphoma; and although cyclophosphamide may achieve remission, relapses are very common.

In hypersensitivity vasculitis, pulmonary involvement is a less prominent part of a systemic disease. The disorders in which this is most commonly seen are anaphylactoid purpura, essential mixed cryoglobulinemia, and the vasculitis associated with malignancy, infection, or drugs.

PULMONARY INFILTRATES WITH EOSINOPHILIA (PIE)

The combination of pulmonary infiltrates and peripheral eosinophilia occurs in five relatively well-characterized disorders. Löffler's syndrome is a benign condition characterized by fleeting pulmonary infiltrates and eosinophilia, probably related to an immune response to some external agent. It is often asymptomatic, but fever and cough may occur. Although recurrent, it usually clears within four to six weeks, and it also displays a rapid response to steroids. Chronic eosinophilic pneumonia is a more symptomatic form of PIE, often persistent or recurrent in nature. Because of its tendency to involve the periphery of the lung, its roentgenographic appearance is called the inverse of pulmonary edema. Despite a rapid response to corticosteroids, relapse may occur once treatment is discontinued, so that therapy may be required for a year or more. PIE in asthma is most commonly due to allergic bronchopulmonary aspergillosis, which may result in a central destructive bronchiectasis. Topical eosinophilia consists of symptoms of wheeze, fever, and a diffuse reticulonodular pattern on the x-ray that is thought to result from an infestation with microfilariae of *Wuchereria bancrofti*. Finally, it may be associated with a collagen-vascular disease, in which case the underlying disorder determines the overall presentation.

SARCOIDOSIS

Sarcoidosis is a systemic disease of unknown etiology characterized by abnormal T-cell function and noncaseating granulomas found diffusely throughout the body. It occurs most commonly in the third and fourth decade, is slightly more likely in women, and is roughly ten times more frequent in black people in the United States.

Most of the dysfunction associated with sarcoidosis results from the physical presence of the granulomas in the tissues, although systemic signs of inflammation may also be present. Organs commonly involved include the lungs, skin, lymph nodes, liver, spleen, eyes, joints, central nervous system, and muscles (Table 18–5). The presenting symptoms are quite variable, although in the United States 50 per cent of patients will present with pulmonary disease, 25 per cent with constitutional symptoms, and 7 per cent with extrapulmonary involvement; the remainder are asymptomatic and are discovered during routine examination.

Diagnosis depends on the finding of noncaseating granuloma in the setting of a characteristic clinical picture with typical radiographic findings, in the absence of another specific cause of granulomatous disease, such as tuberculosis, fungal disease, carcinoma, and lymphoma. Histological confirmation is most commonly obtained by a transbronchial biopsy during bronchoscopy. Conventional chest x-ray staging is as follows; stage 0, normal film; stage 1, bilateral hilary adenopathy; stage 2, adenopathy plus pulmonary infiltrates; and, stage 3, pulmonary infiltrates alone. There is no evidence that staging has any relationship to the natural progression of disease. Rarely, the x-ray may show multiple nodules similar to those seen with metastatic tumor or a pleural effusion. Nonspecific laboratory abnormalities include hypercalcemia (up to 20 per cent of patients), anemia, hypergammaglobulinemia, and an elevated angiotensin-converting enzyme level. Skin test anergy is usually present (two thirds of patients) in association with lymphopenia and decreased number and function of peripheral blood T cells.

The disorder is usually self-limited with complete resolution of symptoms and chest x-ray changes within a year or two. A minority have a persistent mild abnormality with some fibrotic changes visible on chest x-ray. Approximately 10 per cent develop severe progressive disease with progressive pulmonary fibrosis or significant extrapulmonary involvement.

TABLE 18–5. CLINICAL MANIFESTATIONS OF SARCOIDOSIS

Pulmonary
  Asymptomatic with abnormal chest x-ray
  Gradually progressive cough and shortness of breath
  Pulmonary fibrosis with pulmonary insufficiency
  Laryngeal and endobronchial obstruction
Extrapulmonary
  Löfgren's syndrome—fever, arthralgias, bilateral hilar adenopathy, erythema nodosum
  Heerfordt's syndrome (uveoparotid fever)—fever, swelling of parotid gland and uveal tracts, VII nerve palsy
  Skin—lupus pernio or skin plaques
  Central nervous system—cranial nerve palsies, subacute meningitis, diabetes insipidus
  Joints—polyarticular and monoarticular arthritis
  Erythema nodosum
  Punched-out cystic lesions in phalangeal and metacarpal bones
  Peripheral lymphadenopathy and/or splenomegaly
  Heart—paroxysmal arrhythmias, conduction disturbances
  Eye—chorioretinitis, anterior uveitis, keratoconjunctivitis
  Hypercalcemia with nephrocalcinosis or nephrolithiasis
  Granulomatous hepatitis

TABLE 18–6. INDICATIONS FOR USE OF CORTICOSTEROIDS IN SARCOIDOSIS

Iridocyclitis	Corticosteroid eye drops
	Local subconjunctival depot of cortisone
Posterior uveitis	Oral prednisone
Pulmonary involvement	Steroids rarely recommended for Stage I; usually employed if infiltrate remains static or worsens over three-month period, or the patient is symptomatic
Upper airway obstruction	Rare indication for IV steroids
Lupus pernio	Oral prednisone shrinks the disfiguring lesions
Hypercalcemia	Responds well to corticosteroids
Cardiac involvement	Corticosteroids usually recommended if patient has arrhythmias or conduction disturbances
CNS involvement	Response is best in patients with acute symptoms
Lacrimal/salivary gland involvement	Corticosteroids recommended for disordered function, *not* gland swelling
Bone cysts	Corticosteroids recommended if symptomatic

Corticosteroids are quite effective in ameliorating the acute granulomatous inflammation, but their efficacy in altering the long-term prognosis is unproven. The usual indications for corticosteroid therapy are listed in Table 18–6. Other agents, such as chloroquine, indomethacin, azathioprine, and methotrexate, are occasionally employed, especially for symptomatic skin involvement; satisfactory studies of their efficacy have not been undertaken.

PULMONARY HEMORRHAGIC DISORDER

The combination of hemoptysis, anemia, and diffuse pulmonary infiltrates along with the development of glomerulonephritis is known as Goodpasture's syndrome. This is predominantly a disease of young white males. The etiology is unknown, but the presence of antiglomerular basement membrane antibodies lining both the glomerulus and the alveolus suggests an autoimmune mechanism. While the lung disease may be intermittent, the kidney disease rapidly progresses to renal failure. On occasion, hemoptysis by itself may be life-threatening. Bilateral nephrectomy results in cessation of the hemoptysis, but present therapy is directed at the presumed immunological basis for the disease. Plasmapheresis is used to remove the antibodies, immunosuppressive drugs are used to decrease antibody production, and steroids are given empirically to decrease the pulmonary hemorrhage. Untreated patients usually die within two years.

Idiopathic pulmonary hemosiderosis can present similarly to Goodpasture's syndrome, although it predominantly affects young girls and does not involve the kidneys. The etiology is unknown, and there are no clear-cut immunological markers. Despite this, treatment similar to Goodpasture's syndrome is usually attempted, although the efficacy in this disease is much less clear and average survival is about two to three years.

Finally, pulmonary hemorrhage, with or without renal disease, may accompany one of the collagen-vascular diseases, particularly SLE and periarteritis nodosa. It may also be seen with systemic vasculitis, in particular Wegener's granulomatosis, hypersensitivity vasculitis, mixed cryoglobulinemia, and Behcet's syndrome.

MISCELLANEOUS

Pulmonary histiocytosis X, or eosinophilic granuloma of the lung, is a relatively benign disease presenting wiith dyspnea and radiographic evidence of diffuse nodular or reticulonodular infiltrates with relative sparing of the lung bases. It should be suspected in patients in the third and fourth decades presenting with diffusely abnormal chest x-rays. It is easy to confuse with sarcoidosis, although pneumothorax or honeycombing on the chest x-ray and the rarity of hilar adenopathy favor histiocytosis X. Diagnosis is made pathologically, treatment is uncertain, and spontaneous remissions are common.

The lymphocytic infiltrative disorders include lymphocytic interstitial pneumonia and immunoblastic lymphadenopathy among other specific entities. They differ from other interstitial lung diseases in their common association with dysproteinemia and frequent progression to lymphoid malignancy.

Pulmonary alveolar proteinosis is a rare, idiopathic disease in which the alveoli become filled with a proteinaceous material rich in lipids. Most cases recover spontaneously, but total lung lavage is necessary when diffuse involvement causes severe hypoxemia. These patients are particularly prone to infection with *Nocardia*, and less so to *Aspergillus* and *Cryptococcus*.

IDIOPATHIC PULMONARY FIBROSIS

A large number of patients with diffuse interstitial lung disease will not fit into any of the previously mentioned categories. These patients, usually middle-aged with no sex predominance, present with dyspnea and radiographic evidence of interstitial disease. Rarely, the disease progresses very rapidly from respiratory failure to death within six months of the onset of symptoms (Hamman-Rich syndrome). When the disease is more slowly progressive, it is termed idiopathic pulmonary fibrosis or cryptogenic fibrosing alveolitis.

TREATMENT

While the treatment of these disorders depends on the particular one being discussed, certain general statements can be made. The most rational decisions can be made only if a clear diagnosis has been obtained. If the offending substance is identified, as in the pneumoconiosis and hypersensitivity pneumonitis, avoidance is the best solution. When there is an active alveolitis component, corticosteroids may be of benefit. Dosage should be high (60 to 100 mg prednisone) initially and then reduced to the lowest possible dose that successfully suppresses the inflammatory response. Immunosuppressive agents are added to effect remission in certain types of vasculitis, such as Wegener's granulomatosis, but are of questionable value in Goodpasture's syndrome and have little efficacy in idiopathic pulmonary fibrosis. Plasmapheresis should be reserved for illnesses in which circulating antibody is known to be the etiological factor, as in Goodpasture's syndrome.

The decision to initiate therapy with one of these relatively high-risk agents and the determination of how long to maintain treatment depend on the ability to evaluate the presence of active alveolitis and to judge the effectiveness of the therapeutic regimen. The chest roentgenogram does not ordinarily determine the acuteness of the process, although a diffuse honeycomb pattern usually suggests severe fibrosis. It is useful, however, to follow the course of the disease, although in itself it may not accurately predict the course or response to therapy. Like the chest x-ray, the pulmonary function studies give an indication of the degree of involvement but are not reliable in separating reversible phases of inflammation from far-advanced fibrosis. They are used predominantly to follow the course of the disease and the response to therapy. Depending on the initial abnormalities, any of a number of studies may be used, including the measurement of lung volumes, diffusing capacity, arterial blood gases at rest or during exercise, and maximum exercise tolerance. Gallium lung scanning and bronchoalveolar lavage are providing interesting insights into the mechanisms of these disorders but have no proven clinical utility.

REFERENCES

Crystal RG, Bitterman PB, Rennard SE, Hance AJ, Keogh BA: Interstitial lung diseases of unknown cause. N Engl J Med 310:154–166, 235–244, 1984.

DeRemee RA: Diffuse interstitial pulmonary disease from the perspective of the clinician. Chest 92:1068–1073, 1987.

Hunninghake GW, Fauci AS: Pulmonary involvement in the collagen vascular diseases, state of the art. Am Rev Resp Dis 119:471–501, 1979.

Morgan WKC, Seaton A: Occupational Lung Disease, 2nd ed. Philadelphia, WB Saunders Company, 1984.

19

PULMONARY VASCULAR DISEASE

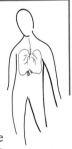

The pulmonary vascular bed is normally a low-pressure, low-resistance system. When it is involved in disease, either through obliteration of cross-sectional area or less commonly through an increase in tone, the resulting pulmonary hypertension and redistribution of pulmonary blood flow lead to profound changes in cardiac function and pulmonary gas exchange.

PHYSIOLOGICAL EFFECTS OF PULMONARY HYPERTENSION

CARDIAC FUNCTION

The right and left sides of the heart are functionally integrated by their anatomical contiguity. There is continuity between their free walls, they share a common wall (the intraventricular septum), and they are covered by the pericardium. When pulmonary vascular resistance is normal, the right ventricle serves as a capacitance chamber, performing only minimal con-

tractile work. It compensates ineffectually for acute rises in pulmonary artery pressure and acutely can only generate a mean pressure of 40 mm Hg. Acute elevations of right ventricular pressure also interfere with left ventricular performance, presumably owing to a shift in the intraventricular septum to the left which decreases left ventricular compliance. Chronic elevations of pulmonary artery pressure cause gradual hypertrophy of the right ventricle, which eventually allows it to generate pressures equal to those in the left ventricle.

PULMONARY FUNCTION

Abnormalities of pulmonary function in patients with pulmonary vascular disease are usually a consequence of the underlying lung disease rather than an intrinsic effect of the pulmonary vascular disease. An exception is the decreased diffusing capacity due to capillary obliteration. In addition, pulmonary vascular occlusion and obliteration cause shunt and ventilation-perfusion inequality by undefined mechanisms. The resulting hypoxemia is further exaggerated by the associated reduction of cardiac output and low mixed venous P_{O_2}.

CAUSES OF PULMONARY HYPERTENSION

Table 19–1 categorizes the causes of pulmonary hypertension by the underlying pathophysiological mechanism. Hyperkinetic and postcapillary disorders cause increased pulmonary pressures indirectly when cardiac abnormalities produce an increase in pulmonary blood flow and outflow pressure, respectively. These disorders are further discussed in Chapters 7 and 8. Reactive pulmonary hypertension is due predominantly to hypoxic vasoconstriction. The most common etiology is chronic obstructive lung disease, discussed in Chapter 17. This chapter will focus on two disorders that typify primary involvement of the pulmonary vessels—one acute, pulmonary embolism, and one chronic, primary pulmonary hypertension.

PULMONARY EMBOLISM

A great variety of substances may embolize to the pulmonary vascular bed with the resulting clinical presentation dependent on the composition of the embolic material. Talc granules and cotton fibers injected along with illicit drugs, sickled red blood cells, and blood-borne parasites like schistosomes lead to slowly progressive disease clinically similar to primary pulmonary hypertension. Embolization of fat, air, or amniotic fluid, however, alters alveolar capillary membrane integrity and presents as the adult respiratory distress syndrome (see Chapter 20). The consequences of the most common embolic material, thromboemboli, depend on the amount of clot reaching the lung and the cardiopulmonary status of the patient. It may

vary from a persistent tachycardia or mild dyspnea to cardiopulmonary arrest. Thromboemboli directly or indirectly cause 200,000 deaths per year.

Most thromboemboli originate in the iliofemoral deep veins. Less common sources include the vessels below the knee, pelvic veins, upper extremities, and mural thrombi in the right side of the heart. Stasis and intimal injury are important factors in the development of thrombosis. The clinical diagnosis of deep venous thrombosis is highly inaccurate, as physical examination is often misleading, and specialized diagnostic techniques should be utilized whenever it is suspected (Table 19–2).

The diagnosis of pulmonary embolism is often missed in sick hospitalized patients, while in the healthy outpatient population it is overdiagnosed. Predisposing situations are listed in Table 19–3. Clinical findings suggestive of pulmonary embolism are nonspecific and are often more commonly indicative of other acute cardiopulmonary disorders. Typical symptoms include dyspnea (80 per cent), pleuritic chest pain (70 per cent), and hemoptysis (20 to 30 per cent). Physical findings include tachypnea (invariable), obvious thrombophlebitis (unusual), acute right ventricular strain (right ventricular heave, increased P_2, gallop) in less than 40 per cent of cases, and occasionally rubs, crackles, or wheezing. Patients who present without dyspnea, pleuritic chest pain, or tachypnea are unlikely to have acute pulmonary embolism. A low-grade fever is common, but persistent high fever and marked leukocytosis are unusual in embolic disease and suggest, as a more likely diagnosis, an infectious etiology such as pneumonia or pleurisy.

Abnormal chest x-ray findings are common but nonspecific: atelectasis, infiltrates, pleural effusions, and an elevated diaphragm. Clear-cut hypovascularity is difficult to detect. The chest roentgenogram is most useful in ruling out other causes of dyspnea and chest pain such as pneumothorax and lung abscess. The electrocardiograph (EKG) helps to exclude myocardial infarction and pericarditis and may show right ventricular strain, but nonspecific ST and T wave changes are more common, and often sinus tachycardia is the only abnormality. Hypoxemia and hypocapnia are typical, but arterial P_{O_2} is greater than 80 mm Hg in 13 per cent of patients without prior cardiopulmonary disease. The hypoxemia is due to the development of ventilation-perfusion inequality and a low mixed venous P_{O_2} secondary to reduced cardiac output. In summary, the clinical presentation and routine laboratory studies may suggest diagnosis, but confirmation requires specific investigations.

Absence of activity on the perfusion lung scan, which visualizes the gross distribution of blood flow in the lung, may be due to anatomical blockage of the vessels or to vasoconstriction. A normal perfusion scan excludes pulmonary embolism. Lobar or multiple segmental defects that do not correspond to abnormalities on chest x-ray are consistent with pulmonary emboli. A ventilation scan helps to differentiate anatomical from functional blockage of blood flow. Inhalation of radioactive gas defines the distribution of ventilation,

TABLE 19–1. PULMONARY HYPERTENSION

Hyperkinetic Pulmonary Hypertension
  Atrial and ventricular septal defects
  Patent ductus arteriosus
  Peripheral arteriovenous shunts
Postcapillary Pulmonary Hypertension
  Left ventricular failure
  Mitral valve disease
  Left atrial myxoma
Obliterative or Obstructive Hypertension
  Embolic
  Parenchymal lung disease
  Arteritis
  Pulmonary artery stenosis
  Primary
Reactive Hypertension
  High altitude
  Chronic obstructive lung disease
  Persistent or intermittent hypoventilation
    Neuromuscular disease
    Sleep apnea syndrome

and delayed clearance during washout of the gas suggests that airway disease may have caused the decreased perfusion secondary to hypoxic vasoconstriction. A normal ventilation scan with a perfusion scan showing segmental or larger defects is considered a high-probability ventilation-perfusion scan and is highly successful at diagnosing pulmonary embolism. Anything other than normal or high-probability ventilation-perfusion scan is an indeterminate scan and is nondiagnostic and cannot confirm or exclude pulmonary embolism. Pulmonary emboli have been found in 13 to 46 per cent of patients with indeterminate scans.

When the lung scan is not diagnostic, or the patient is at high risk for the complications of anticoagulation, or there is an indication for other than standard anticoagulation, the anatomy of the pulmonary vessels must be visualized by angiography. With a markedly abnormal chest x-ray or severe cardiopulmonary disease, the lung scan is not likely to be useful, and immediate angiography is appropriate. Angiography has a sufficiently low risk to make it practical in routine diagnosis, and it is almost always positive even 10 to 14 days following the embolic event. Definitive diagnosis of pulmonary emboli is vital, as both missed diagnosis and unwarranted anticoagulation have high morbidity and mortality rates. A diagnostic decision tree is shown in Figure 19–1.

Treatment of deep venous thrombosis and pulmonary embolism consists of anticoagulation with heparin by continuous infusion for 7 to 10 days at a dosage to prolong the partial thromboplastin time (PTT) 1.5 to 2 times control. As an alternative, heparin can be given by intermittent boluses or subcutaneous doses adjusted to achieve similar prolongation of the PTT. During heparin therapy, the platelet count should be monitored to prevent the development of thrombocytopenia. The indications for treatment of deep calf vein thrombosis are controversial, but patients with symptomatic occlusion of the calf veins proven by venography should probably be anticoagulated. Oral anticoagulation (warfarin) should be started after three to four days in a dose sufficient to maintain the prothrombin time (PT) at 1.3 to 1.5 times baseline. A further prolongation of the PT increases the risk of bleeding without improving the therapeutic outcome. Heparin at a dose adjusted to prolong the PTT to 1.5 times baseline can be used as an alternative for long-term maintenance anticoagulation and should always be used in pregnant women, since warfarin may be injurious to the fetus. Long-term anticoagulation should be continued for three months in patients whose risk factor has resolved, or indefinitely if the predisposing condition persists. Patients who have recurrences of thromboembolic disease may also require prolonged therapy. Most emboli completely resolve, and chronic persistent pulmonary hypertension develops in less than 2 per cent of patients.

Rarely additional therapy may be required (Table 19–4), but it should be undertaken only when clear indications are present because of significant added risks. Fibrinolytic drugs (streptokinase and urokinase)

TABLE 19–2. METHODS OF DIAGNOSING DEEP VENOUS THROMBOSIS

METHOD	USEFULNESS
Contrast venography	The "gold standard"; low incidence of post-study phlebitis.
Impedance plethysmography (IPG)	Most sensitive noninvasive technique for detecting thrombi above the knee. Detects only 30% of thrombi confined to calf veins. False positives with heart failure, ascites, and prior deep venous thrombosis.
Doppler ultrasound	May add to diagnostic accuracy of IPG.
Radioiodine fibrinogen scanning	Most sensitive of all but not as specific as IPG; better for calf vein thrombosis.
Nuclide venography	Functional study; high incidence of false-positive studies.

TABLE 19–3. FACTORS PREDISPOSING TO PULMONARY THROMBOEMBOLI

Medical
  Cancer
  Stroke
  Myocardial infarction
  Congestive heart failure
  Sepsis
  Pregnancy
Surgical
  Orthopedic surgery and lower extremity fractures
  Major surgical procedures (general anesthesia > 30 min)
  Urological, gynecological, and neurosurgical procedures
Acquired
  Lupus anticoagulant
  Paroxysmal nocturnal hemoglobinemia
  Nephrotic syndrome
  Polycythemia vera
Inherited
  Antithrombin III, protein S, and protein C deficiency
  Dysfibrinogenemia
  Plasminogen and plasminogen activation disorders

TABLE 19–4. TREATMENT OF PULMONARY EMBOLI

TREATMENT	INDICATION
Anticoagulation with heparin and warfarin	All patients with pulmonary emboli unless risk of bleeding is unacceptable
Fibrinolytic drugs—streptokinase, urokinase, tissue plasminogen activator	Patients with massive emboli and hemodynamic instability
Vena caval interruption with vena cava filters	When anticoagulants are contraindicated or have failed
Acute embolectomy	Rarely, if ever, useful because of high mortality

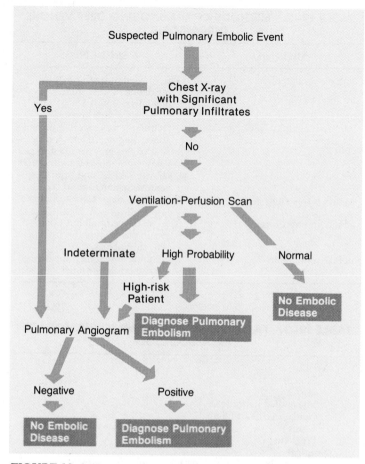

FIGURE 19–1. Diagnostic approach to pulmonary embolism.

are capable of augmenting the dissolution of fresh emboli and have been shown to increase resolution of pulmonary perfusion abnormalities in the first 24 hours when compared with heparin. Based on this, it is often recommended that they be used in patients with marked hemodynamic instability following acute pulmonary embolization. They have not, however, been demonstrated to alter overall mortality or morbidity, and since their use is accompanied by a significantly increased incidence of bleeding, routine employment is unwarranted. Tissue plasminogen activator (TPA) is currently being evaluated for the thrombolysis of pulmonary emboli. It is unclear at this time whether or not the benefits or risks of TPA are significantly better than those of currently available thrombolytic agents, and thus their place in standard therapy of acute pulmonary embolism is unknown.

Vena caval interruption should be considered when the thrombus originates in the lower extremities and there has been proven recurrence after at least 24 hours of heparin therapy. It should also be used when anticoagulation is contraindicated. The preferred technique is the transvenous placement of a Greenfield vena caval filter.

The best way to treat thromboembolic disease is to prevent its occurrence. Appropriate prophylaxis of high-risk patients is safe and efficient. Most can be treated with low-dose subcutaneous heparin, 5000 units every 12 hours. Patients undergoing orthopedic procedures on the lower extremity, especially the hip, are not protected by this regimen and require either heparin adjusted to therapeutic PTT levels or therapeutic doses of warfarin. In patients in whom postoperative bleeding represents an unacceptable risk, as in neurosurgical procedures, intermittent pneumatic compression of the lower extremities is recommended.

PRIMARY PULMONARY HYPERTENSION

Primary pulmonary hypertension can occur at any age but is most common in the third and fourth decades. In children, there is no apparent sexual predominance, but the female-to-male ratio is about 2:1 in the older patients. The etiology is unknown but is possibly related to increased vasoconstrictors or a vascular bed abnormally responsive to vasoconstrictor substances. Occasional clinical associations include chronic portal hypertension, ingestions of an appetite suppressant (aminorex), and a family history.

Patients present with progressive dyspnea and marked exercise limitation. With time, fatigue, chest pain, cor pulmonale, and syncopal episodes on exertion (decreased left ventricular output) develop. Physical examination may be normal or may reveal evidence of pulmonary hypertension. The chest x-ray shows an enlarged right ventricle and main pulmonary arteries, with oligemia in the outer lung fields. EKG evidence of right ventricular hypertrophy is invariable when the mean pulmonary artery pressures are chronically elevated above 40 mm Hg. Pulmonary function studies are often normal except for a small reduction in total lung capacity and diffusing capacity. Mild hypoxemia and hypocapnia are almost always found. Diagnosis is made by catheterization and by excluding other causes of pulmonary hypertension. Prognosis is dreadful, with only 20 per cent surviving three years.

Drug therapy is actively being investigated. Nitroglycerine, hydralazine, and calcium blockers, among other agents, reduce pulmonary vascular resistance in 30 to 50 per cent of patients, but it is not known if they alter the natural course of the disease. Chronic anticoagulation is often recommended, since thrombosis in the small pulmonary arteries is thought to contribute to progressive deterioration of right heart function.

REFERENCES

Hyers TM: Antithrombotic therapy for venous thromboembolism. Clin Chest Med 5:479–486, 1984.

Hyers TM, Hull RD, Weg JG: Antithrombotic therapy for venous thromboembolic disease. Chest 89:26S–35S, 1986.

Rich S, Dantzker DR, Ayres SM, et al: Primary pulmonary hypertension. Ann Intern Med 107:216–223, 1987.

Will JA, Dawson CA, Wein EK, Buckner CK: The pulmonary circulation in health and disease. New York, Academic Press, 1987.

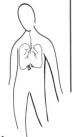

20

THE ADULT RESPIRATORY DISTRESS SYNDROME

In 1967 a syndrome of acute respiratory failure characterized by severe hypoxemia, bilateral pulmonary infiltrates, and decreased lung compliance, usually occurring without preceding lung disease, was dubbed the adult respiratory distress syndrome (ARDS). Since that time, its incidence has increased as improvements in intensive care allow more patients to survive the catastrophic illnesses that act as the initiating events, but its mortality rate remains unacceptably high.

PATHOPHYSIOLOGY

The physiological abnormalities in ARDS, regardless of the predisposing event, are associated with an increase in extravascular lung water. Water movement in the lung is governed by vascular permeability and the balance of the hydrostatic and oncotic pressures across the capillary endothelium as described in the Starling equation (Fig. 20–1). Hydrostatic forces favor fluid filtration, while oncotic pressure promotes reabsorption. Normally, filtration forces dominate and fluid continuously moves from the vascular space into the interstitium. Despite this, extravascular water does not accumulate because the lung lymphatics effectively remove the filtered fluid and return it to the circulation. However, the capacity of the lymphatic system is limited, and if the rate of fluid filtration exceeds its functional capabilities, water accumulates. Initially, it accumulates in the loose interstitial tissues around the airways, pulmonary arteries, and later the alveolar walls (interstitial edema). This causes increased lung stiffness and dyspnea but rarely produces significant abnormalities in the arterial blood gases. If the process continues the excess fluid accumulates in the alveolar space with two consequences: Alveolar surface forces are altered, leading to a further reduction in compliance and a decreased lung volume, and the flooded alveoli can no longer be ventilated, thus converting their blood supply into intrapulmonary shunt. Shunt is the major cause of the severe hypoxemia characteristic of ARDS (see Chapter 15).

Two alterations of the Starling equation are of clinical importance. Patients with cardiogenic pulmonary edema and fluid overload have an increase in pulmonary capillary hydrostatic pressure. Edema fluid in this setting has a low protein content and is essentially an ultrafiltrate of plasma. In ARDS, the hydrostatic pressure is usually normal and fluid accumulation is due to an alteration in alveolar-capillary membrane permeability, which may result from either endothelial or epithelial cell injury (Fig. 20–2). The etiology of the injury is occasionally clear-cut, as in gastric aspiration or viral pneumonia, but is more commonly elusive and

ascribed to complex immunological or biochemical events involving complement activation, arachidonic acid metabolites, leukocyte trapping in the lung, and O_2 radical release. The resulting edema has a high protein content similar to that of plasma. While alterations in oncotic pressure are unusual as the sole cause of pulmonary edema, the presence of low intravascular oncotic pressure increases the rate of fluid transudation in both low- and high-pressure pulmonary edema. Similarly, any increase in microvascular hydrostatic pressure in the setting of increased capillary permeability dramatically increases the rate of fluid filtration.

In addition to the obvious lung injury, ARDS is associated with additional systemic manifestations. These alterations in tissue function are often difficult to separate clearly from abnormalities due to the condition which incited the development of the ARDS. Irrespective of the inciting agent, some of these alterations are so characteristic of ARDS as to consti-

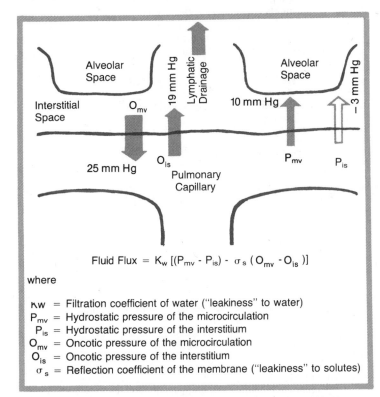

Fluid Flux $= K_w [(P_{mv} - P_{is}) - \sigma_s (O_{mv} - O_{is})]$

where

K_w = Filtration coefficient of water ("leakiness" to water)
P_{mv} = Hydrostatic pressure of the microcirculation
P_{is} = Hydrostatic pressure of the interstitium
O_{mv} = Oncotic pressure of the microcirculation
O_{is} = Oncotic pressure of the interstitium
σ_s = Reflection coefficient of the membrane ("leakiness" to solutes)

FIGURE 20–1. Factors affecting fluid filtration in the lung. The filtration is from the pulmonary microcirculation into the interstitium of the lung. Normally excessive accumulation of fluid is prevented by the capacity of the lymphatics to drain it back into the systemic circulation.

tute, at least in part, an intrinsic component of the syndrome. The most characteristic alteration is an inability of tissues to increase the extraction of oxygen in response to a decrease in oxygen delivery. The second is the progressive development of multiorgan failure. Either abnormality is an indication of a poor prognosis.

CLINICAL PRESENTATION AND DIAGNOSIS

As with any clinically defined syndrome, the diagnosis of ARDS is made by finding the appropriate signs and symptoms (Table 20–1) in the proper clinical setting (Table 20–2). Some predisposing conditions are more likely than others to result in ARDS, such as lung injury secondary to aspiration of gastric contents, pneumonias and sepsis requiring admission to the intensive care unit, and disseminated intravascular coagulopathy.

The clinical presentation is relatively uniform regardless of etiology. Initially the signs and symptoms are limited to those of the primary disorder. Within the first 12 to 24 hours, however, early accumulation of lung water causes dyspnea, hyperventilation, and the appearance of a fine diffuse reticular infiltrate on chest x-ray. Unless the underlying disease is reversed rapidly, as in some instances of sepsis, the patient quickly progresses to the full-blown syndrome with the development of progressive bilateral pulmonary infiltrates, severe hypoxemia, and a dramatic fall in lung compliance. Most patients manifest respiratory failure

TABLE 20–1. DIAGNOSIS OF ARDS

1. Proper clinical setting (Table 20–2) and the exclusion of left ventricular failure or chronic lung disease
2. Diffuse pulmonary infiltrates on chest x-ray
3. $Pa_{O_2} < 50$ mm Hg on $F_{I_{O_2}} > 0.60$
4. Decreased respiratory compliance <50 ml/cm H_2O

TABLE 20–2. CONDITIONS ASSOCIATED WITH ARDS

Inhalant injuries
  aspiration
  smoke and toxic gases
  near drowning
  oxygen toxicity
Infections
  gram-negative sepsis
  viral, bacterial, and *Pneumocystis carinii* pneumonia
  miliary tuberculosis
Drug overdose—heroin, methadone, propoxyphene, aspirin
Disseminated intravascular coagulopathy
Burns
Pancreatitis
Multiple transfusions
Trauma—lung contusion, fat emboli
Uremia
Head injury
Amniotic fluid and air emboli

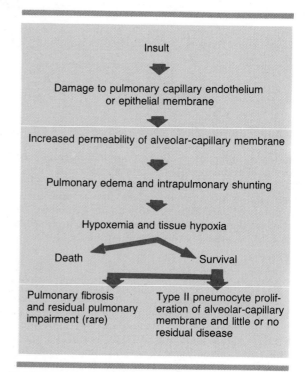

FIGURE 20–2. Pathogenesis and outcome of the adult respiratory distress syndrome.

within 24 hours of the onset of the predisposing event, and almost 90 per cent of those who eventually develop ARDS will do so by 72 hours. Treatment is generally supportive and directed at maintaining an adequate delivery of O_2 to the tissues while minimizing iatrogenic complications. Therapy directed at the predisposing condition, when known, is imperative, since its continued presence prevents resolution of the ARDS.

OXYGEN THERAPY AND MECHANICAL VENTILATION

Correction of the severe hypoxemia by increasing the fractional concentration of the inspired O_2 ($F_{I_{O_2}}$) is useful early in the disease. However, because the hypoxemia is due to shunt, this is less effective than in patients with obstructive or restrictive lung disease in which ventilation-perfusion inequality is the major underlying mechanism. Figure 20–3 plots the relationship between the $F_{I_{O_2}}$ and arterial P_{O_2} (Pa_{O_2}) and O_2 content for different levels of shunt. Increasing the $F_{I_{O_2}}$ may significantly increase O_2 content and thus the O_2 delivery despite the negligible increase in Pa_{O_2}. While O_2 content can be increased substantially, a high $F_{I_{O_2}}$ by itself is toxic to the lung, and thus this strategy has distinct limitations. Oxygen toxicity depends on a number of factors, including $F_{I_{O_2}}$, duration of treatment, and the underlying condition of the lung. The $F_{I_{O_2}}$ likely to induce toxicity in man is un-

FIGURE 20–3. The effect of changing the inspired oxygen concentration on the arterial Po_2 and O_2 content for lungs having shunts of 10 to 50 per cent. When the shunt is small, as may be seen early in the course of ARDS, increasing the inspired oxygen to 40 to 50 per cent will effectively increase the Pa_{O_2}. As the shunt increases and approaches 30 to 50 per cent, the levels commonly seen in ARDS, only small increases in arterial Po_2 will be achieved even when 100 per cent O_2 is administered. Although Po_2 increases very little (*left panel*), this occurs at a steep portion of the O_2 dissociation curve so that O_2 saturation increases disproportionately, resulting in a considerable increase in O_2 content (*right panel*). (From Dantzker D: Gas exchange in the adult respiratory distress syndrome. Clin Chest Med 3:57–67, 1982.)

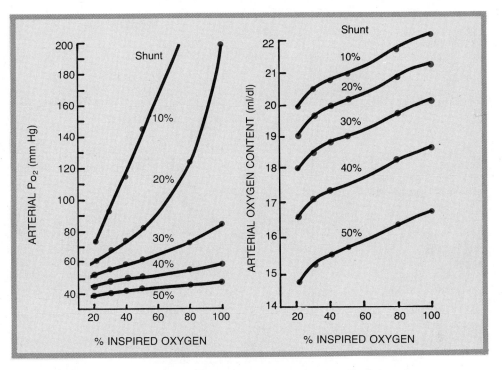

known, although it is probable that a continuum rather than a threshold exists. As a general rule, an $F_{I_{O_2}}$ above 0.60 can be tolerated for short periods such as 24 hours, but after 72 hours O_2 toxicity may contribute to further lung damage.

When adequate oxygenation cannot be maintained by O_2 therapy alone, or if hypercapnia develops, mechanical ventilation is essential. The positive pressure generated by the ventilator increases mean airway pressure, which in turn increases lung volume. This results in an increase in alveolar size, spreading the fluid that is present over a greater surface area as well as redistributing fluid from the alveolar to interstitial space, allowing gas exchange to take place. Mechanical ventilation also reduces the O_2 demands caused by increased O_2 consumption by the respiratory muscles as patients try to cope with the increased work of breathing.

An oral or nasal endotracheal tube is necessary for mechanical ventilation. While nasal tubes often seem to be more comfortable to the patient, they usually are smaller in diameter than an oral tube and tend to cause difficulties in suctioning and to increase the work of breathing during the weaning period. In addition, a tube in the nasopharynx may lead to the development of a purulent otitis media, as it interferes with eustachian tube drainage. With proper care, low-compliance cuffed tubes can be left in place for at least three to four weeks. The major complication from endotracheal tubes is damage to the larynx resulting from tube motion as the patient moves about, a complication that can be minimized by adequate fixation of the tube at the mouth or nose. The decision to proceed to a tracheostomy should not be made on the basis of any arbitrary time limit. Tracheostomy has its own complications, e.g., tracheal stenosis, which may exceed the morbidity associated with endotracheal tubes. Thus a tracheostomy should be performed only if it is necessary for adequate care or if it is clear that continued mechanical ventilation will be required for a prolonged time.

Mechanical ventilators are classified on the basis of what terminates inspiratory flow. Pressure-cycled ventilators terminate flow when a present pressure is reached in the airway. Consequently, tidal volume and minute ventilation vary with changes in airway resistance and lung compliance. These are no longer used for ventilatory support of patients. Volume-cycled ventilators provide a present volume to the patient over a range of airway pressures. A pressure limit is set to prevent trauma to the lung in the event of a sudden change in pulmonary mechanics when airway pressure increases in an attempt to achieve the required tidal volume. Although the precise volume delivered to the patient may vary somewhat with changes in lung mechanics and compliance of the ventilator circuit, volume-cycled ventilators allow greater control of the patient's ventilation. Time-cycled ventilators set tidal volume by fixing the inspiratory time and flow rate. They accomplish the same goal as volume ventilators but are smaller and more easily manufactured. This is the principle used in many of the new generation of mechanical ventilators.

Mechanical ventilators can be set to operate in a variety of modes (Fig. 20–4). Controlled ventilation, in which both tidal volume and rate are determined by the machine, are used only when the patient is unable to initiate a spontaneous breath, e.g., drug overdose, severe neuromuscular disease, muscle relaxants, or excessive sedation. The modes most com-

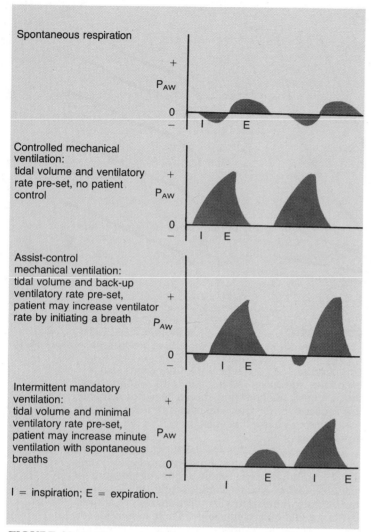

Spontaneous respiration

P_{AW}

I E

Controlled mechanical ventilation:
tidal volume and ventilatory rate pre-set, no patient control

P_{AW}

I E

Assist-control mechanical ventilation:
tidal volume and back-up ventilatory rate pre-set, patient may increase ventilator rate by initiating a breath

P_{AW}

I E

Intermittent mandatory ventilation:
tidal volume and minimal ventilatory rate pre-set, patient may increase minute ventilation with spontaneous breaths

P_{AW}

I E I E

I = inspiration; E = expiration.

FIGURE 20–4. Changes in airway pressure during spontaneous respiration and various modes of mechanical ventilation.

lung. Thus, these ventilatory techniques should be used only to the degree that they may help in achieving an adequate O_2 saturation (90 per cent) at a relatively nontoxic F_{IO_2} (<0.60). However, improvement in arterial oxygenation by itself is an insufficient guide to ventilatory therapy, as the increase in airway pressure may cause a fall in cardiac output with an overall reduction in O_2 delivery to the tissues. This is a serious problem for tissues unable to increase oxygen extraction. Pulmonary barotrauma, manifested as subcutaneous emphysema, pneumodiastinum, and pneumothorax, is an additional serious complication.

The mechanism by which high intrathoracic pressure interferes with cardiac output is complex, with a reduction in venous return to the heart playing a major role. With small increases in intrathoracic pressure (5 to 10 cm of PEEP), impairment of cardiac output may be minimal as long as cardiac filling pressures are adequate. With higher levels of PEEP, cardiac output is invariably reduced unless filling pressures are increased above normal. The increase in filling pressure required to maintain cardiac output in the face of large increases in PEEP also elevates pulmonary hydrostatic pressure and thus is likely to increase the accumulation of extravascular lung water. To monitor these important variables, especially in patients with a questionable cardiovascular status or those in whom high levels of PEEP are required, a flow-directed pulmonary artery catheter is often useful. The catheter is inserted at the bedside, preferably through an internal jugular vein, and is carried by the flow of blood through the right heart until its balloon occludes a pulmonary artery. In this position both pulmonary artery and occlusion pressure (an index of left arterial pressure) can be monitored, as well as cardiac output measured by thermodilution. In addition to evaluating the adequacy of cardiac filling pressure, the catheter is often required to distinguish between ARDS and congestive heart failure, a distinction that is difficult to make by physical examination alone in many sick patients. The insertion and maintenance of the pulmonary artery catheter must be accomplished with great care to limit the risk of complications, including pneumothorax, myocardial or vascular perforation, bleeding, air embolism, arrhythmias, valve trauma or endocarditis, sepsis, and pulmonary infarction.

Care must be taken in interpreting readings obtained from the pulmonary artery catethers in patients on mechanical ventilation, since a variable amount of the positive pressure applied to the lungs is transmitted to the heart and pulmonary vessels. This leads to an apparent rise in vascular pressures during inspiration. The amount of the pressure transmitted depends on a number of complex factors, including the compliance of the lungs and the cardiovascular system and the intravascular volume. The vascular pressures should be read at the same point in the breathing cycle, preferably at end-expiration, when the effect of positive pressure ventilation is minimized. This requires reading the pressure from a continuous recording, since digital displays record mean pressures throughout the respiratory cycle.

monly used in the treatment of ARDS are intermittent mandatory ventilation (IMV) and assist-control ventilation (ACV). While controversy exists as to which of these modes is more effective, no good comparison has been made, and for most patients it probably makes very little difference as long as sufficient support is provided.

The goal of increased lung volume is achieved by two strategies regardless of the ventilatory mode: (1) high tidal volume, such as 10 or even 15 ml/kg rather than the normal 6 ml/kg; (2) positive end-expiratory pressure (PEEP), which prevents the airway pressure from falling back to atmospheric at end-expiration. While these strategies allow inspired gas to enter previously unventilated alveoli, there is no convincing evidence that increasing lung volume alters the primary pathological process or reverses the transudation of fluid from the blood vessels into the lung. In fact, very high inflation pressures may further damage the

Since hypoxemia in ARDS is due to shunting of systemic venous blood through the lung, any alteration in mixed venous P_{O_2} (Pv_{O_2}) proportionally alters the Pa_{O_2} resulting from a given amount of shunt. Increase in the O_2 consumption, decrease in cardiac output, and fall in the hemoglobin concentration may all necessitate increased O_2 extraction by the tissues and thus decrease Pv_{O_2}. Unless this is kept in mind, it is possible that a fall in Pa_{O_2} due to one of these factors may be misinterpreted as a worsening of ARDS and corrective therapy may be aimed in the wrong direction.

Assessing the adequacy of O_2 and ventilatory therapy in these complex conditions is a major challenge. Clearly, Pa_{O_2} is an adequate index, since it reflects only one facet of O_2 delivery (O_2 Del), which is defined as:

$$O_2 \text{ Del} = \text{Cardiac output} \times \text{Arterial } O_2 \text{ content}$$

Thus, O_2 Del also includes a convection term, cardiac output, and a capacitance term, O_2 content, which, in addition to Pa_{O_2}, includes O_2 saturation and hemoglobin concentration. All components must be adequate to ensure sufficient peripheral delivery of O_2. In addition to O_2 Del, tissue oxygenation depends on the distribution of blood flow within various tissues, about which little is known.

Is there a useful parameter to monitor which will reflect the adequacy of O_2 Del? The Pv_{O_2} has been suggested, but this represents the weighted means from all the tissues and thus is markedly influenced by the distribution of blood flow and the ability of individual tissue to extract the oxygen that is delivered. For example, in septic shock, because blood flow is redistributed to tissues with a low O_2 extraction, the Pv_{O_2} may actually rise *pari passu* with the development of systemic acidosis. In this instance, Pv_{O_2} misrepresents the true status of O_2 delivery. Lactic acidosis is a sure sign of inadequate tissue O_2 Del, but since lactic acid is rapidly cleared by a well-perfused and functioning liver while its washout is delayed from poorly perfused tissues, the appearance of lactic acidosis is a late indicator of O_2 deficiency. The best current indicators are the performance of the end-organs (heart, kidney, and liver) although even this may be insensitive in the early, correctable stage of inadequate O_2 delivery.

OTHER THERAPEUTIC MODALITIES

The development of pharmacological agents to treat or, more important, to prevent ARDS would represent a major advancement. Administration of high-dose corticosteroids is of no value in gram-negative sepsis and has no proven efficacy in ARDS due to other etiologies. Some prostaglandins (PGI and PGE) as well as antiprostaglandin agents, e.g., ibuprofen, affect the course of experimental disease leading to ARDS but have yet to be shown effective in patients.

Antibiotics are the most important group of agents, since correct treatment of infection may be lifesaving while the failure to recognize infection ensures the continuation of the pulmonary capillary leak. As far as possible, antibiotics should be selected on the basis of reliable microbial studies, but until the results are known empirical therapy is not only appropriate but necessary. Continued bacteremia in the face of appropriate antibiotics raises the possibility of an abscess and should lead to an aggressive diagnostic search, as this is a common cause of persistent ARDS and a fatal outcome. The lungs and the peritoneal cavity are the most common sites of undiagnosed infection.

Appropriate fluid management is important to ensure adequate cardiac output and thus O_2 delivery. Fluid loading to maintain adequate cardiac filling pressures in the face of the high intrathoracic pressures generated during mechanical ventilation must be balanced against the resultant increase in microvascular pressure and its tendency to increase the extravascular lung water accumulation. The controversy over the use of colloid vs. crystalloid therapy is moot in the presence of such marked alterations in microvascular permeability. Until more is known concerning the dynamics of fluid movement in this disease, a good rule of thumb is to maintain filling pressures in a normal range (pulmonary artery wedge pressures of about 10 cm H_2O).

PROGNOSIS

The mortality rate in ARDS is 50 to 80 per cent. In any particular patient this is strongly influenced by the presence of other acute or chronic disorders. The cause of death is often unclear. Infection, particularly when associated with bacteremia of unknown origin, is a major determinant of mortality. Inadequate tissue oxygenation and organ failure are also likely to play significant roles.

Of those patients who survive the acute event, the prognosis depends primarily on the presence of other underlying disease. For most patients who began with normal lungs, pulmonary function returns slowly toward normal. A small number of patients will be left with residual fibrosis, rarely of a severe nature.

REFERENCES

Dantzker R: Cardiopulmonary Critical Care. Orlando, FL, Grune and Stratton, 1986.

Wiedemann HP, Matthay MA, Matthay RA: Acute lung injury. Crit Care Clin Vol 2, 1986.

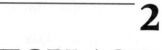

21
NEOPLASTIC DISEASES
OF THE LUNG

Lung cancer causes over 120,000 deaths per year in the United States and is the leading cause of cancer deaths in men and women. Carcinoma of the lung is most common in the fifth and sixth decades and is rarely seen before the age of 35.

Cigarette smoking is the most important causative factor, with lung cancer being 10 to 30 times more common among smokers; approximately 4 per cent of those who have smoked for 40 years develop lung cancer. While there is still some controversy, most experts feel that there is a small but significant risk to the development of lung cancer from environmental or passive smoke exposure. All cell types except bronchoalveolar carcinoma are associated with smoking. Of the other causative agents, asbestos is the most important, especially when combined with cigarette smoking, and up to 14 per cent of smokers with asbestosis develop lung cancer. Other industrial risks include uranium, arsenic, chromium, chloromethyl, methylethers, polycylic aromatic hydrocarbons, nickel, and possibly beryllium. Lung cancer may rarely develop in pre-existing scars due to old granulomatous disease, diffuse interstitial fibrosis, or scleroderma.

PATHOLOGY

Benign tumors, composing 5 per cent of the total, are usually diagnosed on routine chest x-rays, and symptoms, if present, are usually related to bronchial obstruction. The most common central tumor is the bronchial adenoma, which usually appears benign but is potentially malignant and rarely produces features of the carcinoid syndrome. The most common peripheral tumor is the pulmonary hamartoma, which has a characteristic "popcorn" pattern of calcification.

Primary malignant neoplasms of the lung can be classified on the basis of their cell type, as summarized in Table 21–1. The relative incidence of each cell type varies from study to study. Adenocarcinoma is the most common cell type (33 to 35 per cent), followed by squamous cell (30 to 32 per cent), small cell (20 to 25 per cent), and large cell (15 to 20 per cent). Bronchoalveolar carcinoma is considered a variant of adenocarcinoma. Squamous cell carcinoma spreads mainly by local invasion, whereas adenocarcinoma and large cell tumors metastasize early, especially to the central nervous system, skeleton, and adrenal glands. Small cell undifferentiated carcinoma, or oat cell carcinoma, has the greatest propensity to metastasize early in its course, leading most clinicians to assume disseminated disease at diagnosis even without objective evidence.

Starting as a single malignant cell (10 μ size), 30 volume doublings are required to produce a tumor of 1 cm diameter, the smallest size detectable on a chest x-ray (Table 21–1). Ten further doublings produce a tumor 10 cm in diameter, but most patients die before the tumor reaches this size. Small cell carcinoma has the fastest doubling time and the worst prognosis. While adenocarcinoma has the longest doubling time, it has a worse prognosis than squamous cancers because of early extrathoracic spread.

Metastatic spread of neoplasms to the lung is common, involving the parenchyma, endobronchial mucosa, chest wall, pleural space, or mediastinum. Direct extension is the least common mode of spread, occurring with breast, liver, and pancreatic tumors. Hematogenous spread is common with renal, thyroid, and testicular tumors and bone sarcomas and presents with asymptomatic discrete nodules on chest x-ray. Lymphangitic spread presents as an infiltrate or diffuse reticulonodular pattern on chest x-ray and causes severe dyspnea, usually out of proportion to the x-ray

TABLE 21–1. FEATURES OF MALIGNANT NEOPLASMS

CELL TYPE	PATHOLOGICAL FEATURES	COMMON CHEST X-RAY FINDING	VOLUME DOUBLING TIME (DAYS)
Squamous cell carcinoma	Keratin production, intercellular bridges	Central lesion with hilar involvement, cavitation frequent	90
Adenocarcinoma	Gland formation, mucin production	Peripheral lesion, cavitation may occur	180
Bronchoalveolar carcinoma	Distinction from adenocarcinoma imprecise	Usually peripheral lesion, pneumonic-like infiltrate, occasionally multifocal	
Large cell carcinoma	Probably represents poorly differentiated adenocarcinoma	Usually peripheral lesion, larger than adenocarcinoma with tendency to cavitate	90
Small cell carcinoma	Involvement by cells twice the size of lymphocytes	Central lesion, hilar mass common, early mediastinal involvement, no cavitation	30

findings. This pattern is typical of spread from aden-ocarcinoma of the breast, stomach, pancreas, ovary, prostate, and lung.

CLINICAL PRESENTATION

Clinical presentation may be related to tumor location within the chest, metastatic spread, or extrapulmonary paraneoplastic manifestations. Most patients present with weight loss and symptoms related to local involvement such as cough (75 per cent) that has changed in character, hemoptysis (50 per cent) that is rarely life-threatening, dyspnea (60 per cent), chest pain (40 per cent), and a marked increase in sputum production with bronchoalveolar carcinoma. Pancoast's syndrome refers to apical tumors that involve the brachial plexus and often lead to Horner's syndrome resulting from invasion of the inferior cervical ganglion. Compression and obstruction of the superior vena cava, usually by small cell tumor, cause facial and upper extremity edema, dyspnea, stridor, and symptoms related to increased intracranial pressure. Partial obstruction of a bronchus may lead to unilateral, persistent wheezing, whereas complete obstruction causes postobstructive pneumonia. Recurrent laryngeal nerve involvement, typical of a left hilar mass, causes hoarseness. Phrenic nerve entrapment by a mediastinal mass causes diaphragmatic paralysis. Finally, direct spread of the tumor to the pleural or pericardial space will result in effusions. Bronchogenic carcinoma is frequently discovered only after it metastasizes to other organs. The brain, liver, bone, and lymph nodes are common sites, and the evaluation of tumor found in these locations, in a smoker, should include a search for a primary lung neoplasm. In 10 to 50 per cent of patients, bronchogenic carcinoma produces one or more paraneoplastic syndromes. These may manifest themselves as neuromuscular, skeletal, endocrine, hematologic, cutaneous, or cardiovascular abnormalities (Table 21–2).

DIAGNOSIS AND EVALUATION

A careful history and physical examination are crucial in patient evaluation, and availability of a previous chest x-ray is of tremendous value. Certain generalizations regarding the relations of the chest x-ray to the tissue type can be made: (1) A hilar mass as the only abnormal finding is most common in small cell carcinoma and almost never seen in adenocarcinoma. (2) A peripheral mass 4 cm or less in diameter is most likely an adenocarcinoma, while one greater than 4 cm may be any of the cell types except small cell carcinoma. (3) Multiple masses are very rare in primary lung cancer. (4) Apical tumors are usually squamous cell carcinoma. (5) Atelectasis strongly suggests squamous cell carcinoma. (6) Consolidation is a rare finding in all cell types. (7) Cavitation is most common in squamous cell, is less common with large cell and adenocarcinoma, and is never seen in small cell carcinoma. (8)

TABLE 21–2. COMMON PARANEOPLASTIC SYNDROMES ASSOCIATED WITH BRONCHOGENIC CARCINOMA

SYNDROME	CELL TYPE USUALLY IMPLICATED	MECHANISM
Hypertrophic pulmonary osteoarthropathy	All types except small cell	Unknown
Gynecomastia	Large cell	Chronic gonadotropin production
Syndrome of inappropriate ADH (SIADH) secretion	Usually small cell (may be associated with any cell type)	Inappropriate ADH release
Hypercalcemia	Usually squamous cell	Direct involvement of bone, prostaglandins, osteoclast-activating factor, PTH-like action
Cushing's syndrome	Usually small cell	Ectopic ACTH production
Eaton-Lambert myasthenic syndrome	Usually small cell	Unknown
Other neuromyopathic disorders (see appropriate chapter)	Frequently small cell but reported with most types	Unknown
Thrombophlebitis	All types	Unknown

Mediastinal widening usually signifies spread from small cell carcinoma (after Fraser and Paré).

Routine laboratory studies are rarely helpful in the diagnosis of bronchogenic carcinoma but can be invaluable in evaluating extrathoracic spread of the disease, especially liver function studies and serum calcium and alkaline phosphatase, which screen for bone metastases.

Therapeutic decisions are based on a correct tissue diagnosis. Cytological examination of expectorated sputum is the easiest and least invasive approach. False-positive results are rare, but false-negative results are relatively common (40 to 50 per cent), especially with peripheral lesions. When cytological examination of expectorated sputum is negative, bronchoscopy should be the next procedure in patients with central lesions, lung infiltrates, hoarseness, or hemoptysis. Positive yield ranges from 90 per cent for central, endobronchially visible tumors to 50 per cent for peripheral lesions. Small peripheral lung nodules should probably be approached by percutaneous needle aspiration performed under fluoroscopic guidance, which provides material for cytological examination. Diagnostic accuracy is greater than 80 per cent for malignant disease but is disturbingly less accurate with benign lesions.

Once bronchogenic carcinoma is diagnosed, therapeutic decisions depend on both physiological and anatomical considerations (Fig. 21–1). Since successful surgery offers the only change of cure, clinical evaluation is directed toward determining suitability for

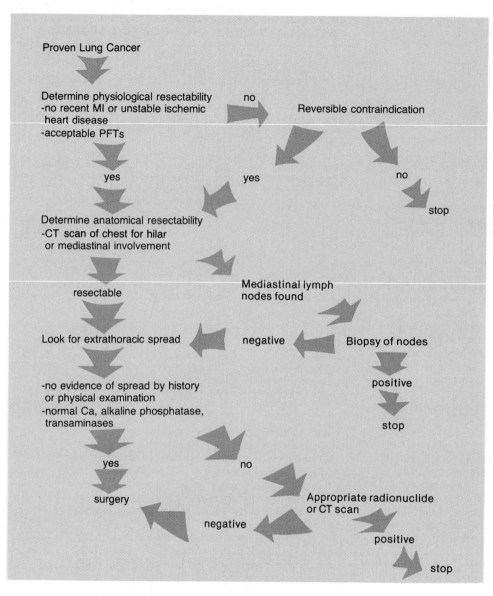

FIGURE 21–1. Decision regarding operability in the presence of proven lung cancer.

resection. Spirometric measurement of the forced expired volume in one second (FEV_1) is sufficient for screening. Patients whose FEV_1 is greater than 2.0 liters will have acceptable pulmonary function following a pneumonectomy. When the FEV_1 is less, a quantitative perfusion scan can be used to estimate the postoperative value by multiplying the preoperative value by the per cent of counts in the lung that will remain. A predicted postoperative FEV_1 of greater than 0.8 L is necessary to permit surgery.

Determination of anatomical operability is the next step. Endobronchial lesions within 2 cm of the carina on bronchoscopy are inoperable. Intrathoracic spread to the lungs and to the hilar or mediastinal lymph nodes can often be determined from the plain radiograph, but computed tomography (CT) may be required. Visualization of mediastinal adenopathy by CT must be corroborated by biopsy before a patient

is denied surgery, since there is a significant incidence of false-positive studies.

Once intrathoracic spread is excluded, a negative history and physical examination combined with a normal routine laboratory evaluation are usually adequate to exclude metastatic spread. Multiple imaging techniques in the absence of symptoms or signs suggesting specific organ involvement are cost-inefficient and are frequently misleading.

SOLITARY PULMONARY NODULE

A solitary pulmonary nodule is defined as a rounded lesion with well-demarcated margins. Between 5 and 40 per cent are malignant. Benign lesions are usually smaller (less than 2 cm), have sharp borders and no satellite lesions, and are present in younger people (less than 40 years). Three characteristics help to separate benign from malignant nodules. Nodules with doubling times of less than 10 to 20 or more than 450 days are most likely benign. The presence of calcification with a central, speckled, diffuse, laminar, or "popcorn" pattern, but not eccentric calcification, is also evidence of its benign nature. On rare occasions the clinical picture is clearly benign, e.g., a patient with a previously normal chest x-ray who develops well-documented histoplasmosis that resolves, leaving a single histoplasmoma. A suggested decision tree for the approach to the solitary nodule is shown in Figure 21–2.

TREATMENT AND PROGNOSIS

Surgery is the therapy of choice for patients with non–small cell carcinoma who meet both physiological and anatomical criteria and have no evidence of extrathoracic spread. There has been renewed interest in surgical treatment of limited small cell carcinoma, but proof of efficacy has not been established yet. There is no evidence that postoperative radiation therapy or chemotherapy improves survival.

For those patients with small cell carcinoma or nonoperable non–small cell tumors, radiation therapy and chemotherapy are the only other modalities. Chemotherapy in various combinations has improved the median survival of patients with small carcinoma limited to the thorax from 3 months untreated to 16 to 17 months. For non–small cell carcinoma, chemotherapy has not significantly altered the outcome (Fig. 21–3) and because of the significant toxicity involved, it should not be used except in controlled experimental settings.

Radiation therapy is often used in small cell carcinoma, both to treat the primary lung lesion and as prophylaxis against cerebral metastases. However, there is no evidence that this prolongs survival. Radiation therapy is not beneficial in non–small cell carcinoma and is limited to the palliative management of pain, recurrent hemoptysis, effusions, or obstruction of airways or the superior vena cava.

The five-year survival rate for all patients with bronchogenic carcinoma is 8 to 12 per cent and has improved only slightly over the past few years despite the introduction of multiple new chemotherapeutic agents. Large trials of routine screening of high-risk people with sputum cytology and chest roentgenographs have not improved survival.

REFERENCES

Filderman AE, Shaw C, Matthay RA: Lung cancer. Invest Radiol 21:80–90, 173–185, 1986.

Fraser RG, Paré JAP: Diagnosis of Diseases of the Chest, 2nd ed. Philadelphia, WB Saunders Company, 1986.

Iannuzzi MC, Scoggin CH: Small cell lung cancer. Am Rev Respir Dis 134:593–608, 1986.

Loeb LA, Ernster VL, Warner KC, et al: Smoking and lung cancer: An overview. Cancer Res 44:5940–5958, 1984.

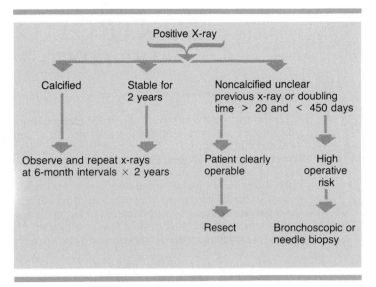

FIGURE 21–2. Decision tree for management of a solitary pulmonary nodule.

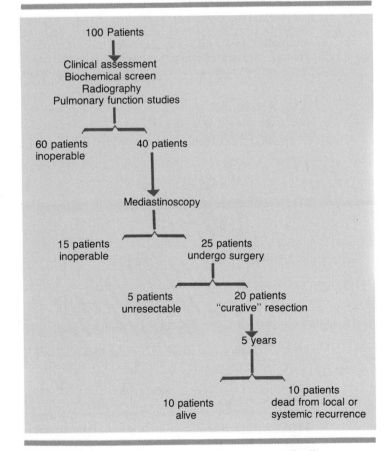

FIGURE 21–3. Outcome in 100 patients with non–small cell carcinoma.

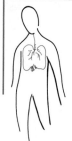

22

CONTROL OF BREATHING IN DISEASE STATES

Disordered respiratory control usually accompanies other states and rarely in itself constitutes an independent clinical disorder. In the past, most attention has been focused on decreased respiratory center output, but increased respiratory drive is a more common phenomenon. Increased respiratory drive may contribute to the development of dyspnea in patients with lung disease, whereas the combination of hypercapnia and excessive somnolence should lead one to suspect disorders associated with decreased respiratory drive.

CHRONIC OBSTRUCTIVE PULMONARY DISEASE (COPD)

Patients with physiologically significant COPD have a reduced ventilatory response to hypoxia and hypercapnia. This was formerly thought to be due entirely to decreased chemosensitivity of the respiratory centers; however, most of these patients display an *increased* resting respiratory center drive. In hypercapnic patients, this heightened respiratory drive fails to translate into a sufficiently increased minute ventilation to maintain a normal Pco_2 owing to the increased work of breathing and marked ventilation-perfusion

mismatch. The level of hypercapnia is related in general to the degree of obstruction, although lung mechanics, resting respiratory drive, and the pattern of breathing are often similar in patients with and without CO_2 retention (Fig. 22–1). The development of hypercapnia depends on poorly understood interactions of inherited respiratory drive, peripheral sensory receptor stimulation, associated hypoxemia, degree of ventilation-perfusion mismatching, and the metabolic milieu.

ASTHMA

Patients with acute asthma display hyperventilation and hypocapnia, presumably due to stimulation of lung sensory receptors. CO_2 retention is a late finding in the progression of a severe asthmatic attack. Indeed, eucapnia, rather than the expected hypocapnia, is a warning sign of impending deterioration.

Other disorders in which abnormal peripheral sensory receptor stimulation is thought to result in an increased respiratory drive with resultant dyspnea, tachypnea, and hypocapnia include restrictive lung disease, pulmonary vascular disease, and abnormalities of the chest wall.

CENTRAL HYPOVENTILATION

This may occur secondary to brain stem involvement by tumor, ischemia, or inflammatory disease; a primary, idiopathic form has also been described. Patients display decreased chemosensitivity, often with resting hypercapnia and cor pulmonale. Rarely, the impairment of chemosensitivity may be so severe that the patient breathes adequately only when stimulated by wakefulness, but hypoventilates and becomes apneic during sleep, when rostral neural influences are removed.

OBESITY HYPOVENTILATION SYNDROME

Some patients with obesity display chronic hypoventilation with hypoxia, hypercapnia, reduced chemosensitivity, and cor pulmonale. The hypoventilation may partly reflect the response to the increased load of fatty tissue on the chest wall, although hypoventilation is not directly related to the degree of obesity. Independent neural factors, yet undefined, are probably important. A subgroup of patients, often de-

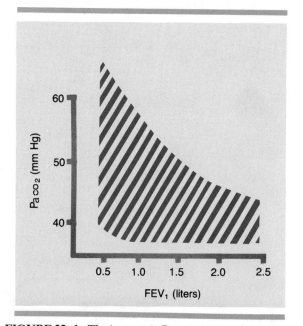

FIGURE 22–1. The increase in Pa_{CO_2} as airway obstruction becomes more severe, as reflected by decreasing FEV_1. Note the large scatter of Pco_2 values for any level of obstruction.

noted as having the pickwickian syndrome, have obesity, daytime hypoventilation, hypersomnolence, polycythemia, and cor pulmonale. Most patients with the pickwickian syndrome probably have sleep apnea.

BREATHING PATTERN ABNORMALITIES ASSOCIATED WITH NEUROLOGICAL DISEASE

Central neurogenic hyperventilation has been considered a characteristic feature of lower brain stem and upper pontine disease. Rarely, it is an isolated finding as most patients display associated pulmonary complications that could reflexly stimulate the respiratory center through hypoxia or activation of intrapulmonary sensory receptors. Apneustic breathing consists of sustained inspiratory pauses localizing damage to the mid pons, most commonly due to a basilar artery infarct. Biot's or ataxic breathing, a haphazard random distribution of deep and shallow breaths, is caused by disruption of the respiratory rhythm generator in the medulla.

Cheyne-Stokes respiration is characterized by regular cycles of crescendo-decrescendo changes in tidal volume separated by apneic or hypopneic pauses. Many affected patients have evidence of cardiac or neurological disease. In patients with cardiac disease, the disturbance arises because of prolongation of the circulation time, which delays transmission of information concerning arterial Po_2 and Pco_2 to the respiratory centers, thus leading to system instability with resulting oscillations in tidal volume. It has no localizing value in patients with neurological disease but has generally been considered to indicate an ominous prognosis. While this is sometimes the case, many patients display subtle evidence of Cheyne-Stokes respiration, especially during sleep, without serious consequences; it is also not an uncommon pattern of breathing in otherwise normal elderly subjects.

NEUROMUSCULAR DISEASE

Respiratory center function is poorly defined in neuromuscular disease. Decreased ventilatory capacity may result from impaired neural output or poor translation of this neural output into respiratory muscle contraction. Typically, the patients display an increased respiratory rate and inability to take deep breaths, with consequent tendency to atelectasis. Characteristic changes in lung volume result from an inability to adequately inspire above or expire below functional residual capacity (see Table 17–2). Paradoxical motion of the rib cage and abdomen is commonly observed. Typical causes include inflammatory polyneuropathy, amyotrophic lateral sclerosis, myasthenia gravis, and poliomyelitis. The features of diaphragmatic paralysis are discussed in Chapter 23.

THE SLEEP APNEA SYNDROME

The sleep apnea syndrome is characterized by daytime hypersomnia in patients who display at least 30 apneic episodes of 10 seconds or longer during 6 hours of nocturnal sleep. The apneic episodes are of two types: (1) central apnea due to decreased respiratory center output and manifested by cessation of breathing efforts (Fig. 22–2A), and (2) obstructive apnea due to upper airway obstruction and characterized by continued respiratory efforts, indicated by paradoxical motion of the rib cage and abdomen, during the period of absent airflow (Fig. 22–2B). Commonly both types combine to give mixed apnea. The less common central type usually causes little physiological disturbance, whereas the obstructive variety is accompanied by severe O_2 desaturation with occasional values below 50 per cent (Po_2, 27 torr). Arrhythmias are common and may rarely result in sudden death.

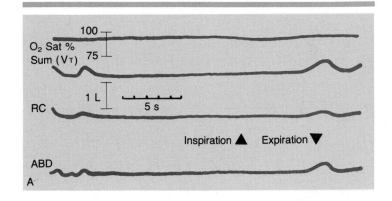

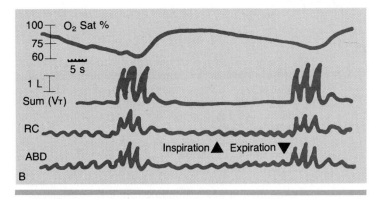

FIGURE 22–2. A, Central sleep apnea. There is absence of abdominal (ABD) and rib cage (RC) movement, and their sum (V_T), during central apnea associated with a small fall of arterial oxygen saturation (O_2 Sat %) measured by ear oximetry. B, Obstructive sleep apnea. This depicts obstructive apnea terminated by deep breaths. Apnea in midportion of recording is marked by absence of sum movements (V_T) despite respiratory efforts indicated by paradoxical movement of rib cage (RC) (movement downward) and abdominal (ABD) (movement upward) compartments that is associated with marked fall in arterial oxygen saturation (O_2 Sat%) measured by ear oximetry. (Reproduced with permission from Tobin MJ, et al: Breathing abnormalities during sleep. Arch Intern Med 143:1221, 1983.)

The prevalence of this syndrome is unknown, but it probably affects more than 1 per cent of the general population. The major predisposing conditions can be grouped as: (1) neurological states associated with impaired respiratory drive (previously discussed) and (2) conditions associated with upper airway obstruction such as enlarged tonsils and adenoids, retrognathia, fat deposition in obesity, macroglossia associated with acromegaly, myxedema, and Down's syndrome, and nasal packing for nosebleeds or nasal surgery.

Characteristically, these patients have a long history of loud sonorous snoring, often combined with thrashing movements of the limbs. Repetitive arousals produce sleep deprivation and lead to excessive daytime sleepiness. Many patients are obese, but this is not invariable, and only a small fraction can be classified as pickwickian. Other features of the sleep apnea syndrome include hypertension, morning headache, intellectual deterioration, and reduced libido.

Polysomnography including the monitoring of the electroencephalograph (EEG), electro-oculogram, motion of the rib cage and abdomen, and arterial O_2 saturation is required to make a definite diagnosis.

The most common mode of therapy is the application of continuous positive airway pressure (CPAP) via a nose mask. This acts as a pneumatic splint and prevents upper airway obstruction. Surgical approaches include tracheostomy to bypass the site of upper airway obstruction and uvulopalatopharyngoplasty (UPP) to remove redundant tissue from the upper airway. Rarely, respiratory stimulants, such as medroxyprogesterone, may be helpful. In some obese patients, marked weight loss has led to an improvement in the obstruction.

REFERENCES

Saunders NA, Sullivan CE: Sleep and Breathing. New York, Marcel Dekker, Inc, 1984.

Tobin MJ, Cohn MA, Sackner MA: Breathing abnormalities during sleep. Arch Intern Med 143:1221–1228, 1983.

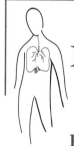

23

DISORDERS OF THE PLEURAL SPACE, MEDIASTINUM, AND CHEST WALL

PLEURAL DISEASE

The pleural spaces are defined by the visceral pleura of the lungs and the parietal pleura of the rib cage, diaphragm, and mediastinum. The spaces themselves are potential rather than real, since the visceral and parietal pleurae are normally separated by only a thin film of fluid.

The lung's elastic recoil pulls the visceral pleura inward and the chest wall's recoil pulls the parietal pleura outward. The net pressure in the pleural space at functional residual capacity is below atmospheric pressure. In the pleural space fluid flows from the parietal surface into the pleural space, with subsequent reabsorption by the capillaries of the visceral pleura (Fig. 23–1). This system is remarkably well balanced and ordinarily prevents the collection of significant amounts of fluid despite the formation and absorption of 5 to 10 liters of pleural fluid each day. In addition, fluid and leakage of protein are drained by lymphatics, which can increase their absorptive capacity severalfold.

Fluid accumulates with abnormalities in the hydrostatic and osmotic pressure, increased permeability of the capillaries, or lymphatic dysfunction. Pleural inflammation, either infectious or noninfectious, increases permeability and results in the collection of a high-protein pleural fluid. Alterations in the pulmonary venous pressures, as in heart failure, increase fluid transudation from the parietal capillaries and disease reabsorption on the visceral side. Decreasing the osmotic pressure (hypoalbuminemia) may also result in more rapid fluid transudation. Finally, lymphatic dysfunction due to anatomical or functional obstruction also facilitates the accumulation of pleural fluid.

PLEURAL EFFUSIONS

The causes of pleural effusions are best considered in terms of the underlying pathophysiology: transudates due to abnormalities of hydrostatic or osmotic pressures and exudates resulting from increased permeability or trauma (Table 23–1).

Patients present with dyspnea, nonspecific discomfort, or pleuritic chest pain—a sharp, stabbing pain exacerbated by coughing or breathing. Such pain must be carefully differentiated from pericardial or musculoskeletal pain. Rarely, the effusion will be asymptomatic and discovered only on chest x-ray.

Physical examination reveals decreased vocal fremitus, dullness on percussion, and decreased breath sounds over the effusion, with bronchial breathing and egophony at its upper limit. Greater than 250 ml of fluid can be seen on the upright chest x-ray as blunting of the costophrenic angle. Increasing amounts cause dense opacification of the lung fields with a concave meniscus. In certain situations the initial x-ray is misleading and further studies are required: (1) a subpulmonic effusion presenting as an elevated hemodiaphragm can be confirmed on lateral decubitus x-ray; (2) a hazy diffuse density on the supine film in a seriously ill patient will disappear on an upright x-ray; and (3) a loculated effusion, especially with coexisting parenchymal disease, may require ultrasound or CT scan for diagnosis.

Thoracentesis is essential in the differential diagnosis. The gross appearance of the fluid is rarely helpful except when frank blood or the milky fluid of a chylous effusion is encountered. The criteria for separation of the fluid into transudate and exudate (Table 23–2) are not rigid, and an effusion due to congestive heart failure may occasionally be exudative while a transudate may occur with malignancy. Pleural fluid glucose concentrations less than 10 to 20 mg/dl are usually diagnostic of rheumatoid arthritis but may be seen in cancer and infection. Pleural fluid amylase is about twice normal in effusions due to pancreatitis and esophageal perforation, whereas smaller elevations may be seen with malignancy. The presence of a high rheumatoid factor or LE cells in the fluid is strong evidence that the effusion is due to rheumatoid arthritis and systemic lupus erythematosus, respectively. Measurement of pleural fluid pH in the diagnosis and management of empyema usually does not add to other more routine measurements.

Surprisingly few red blood cells are required to impart a red color to the fluid, but a hemothorax should be diagnosed only when the pleural fluid hematocrit is greater than 20 per cent. Bloody fluid should arouse suspicion of malignancy, trauma, or pulmonary embolus but may also occur with other disease entities. The number of polymorphonuclear neutrophils is of little or no specific diagnostic value. A high eosinophil count is usually due to air or blood in the pleural space. There is a high probability that an exudate is due to tuberculosis or malignancy if small lymphocytes constitute more than 50 per cent of the white cells. Cytological examinations for malignant cells are positive in about 60 per cent of patients on first thoracentesis, rising to about 80 per cent if three separate samples are obtained. Gram's stain and routine culture should always be obtained and special stains and cultures added when tuberculosis or fungal disease is suspected.

Transcutaneous needle biopsy of the pleura at the bedside with subsequent histology and culture is positive in over 90 per cent of tuberculous effusions, whereas fluid culture is positive in only 25 per cent.

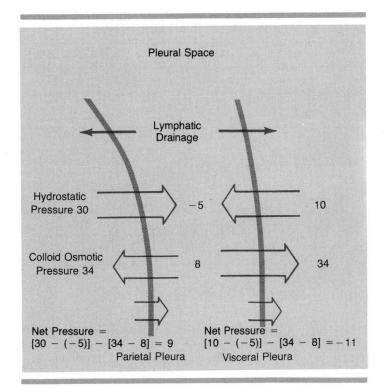

FIGURE 23–1. Factors affecting fluid and solute movement in the pleural space. The blood supply of the parietal pleura is from the intercostal arteries (branches of the systemic circulation), while the visceral pleura is predominantly supplied by the pulmonary circulation, a low-pressure system. Taking into account the osmotic pressure in the parietal and visceral vessels, which are roughly equal, and the changes in intrapleural pressure, fluid flows from the parietal surface into the pleural space and is subsequently reabsorbed by the visceral pleura (indicated pressures are in cm H_2O).

TABLE 23–1. PLEURAL EFFUSIONS

Transudates
  Congestive heart failure
  Hypoalbuminemia—nephrotic syndrome, starvation, cirrhosis
  Abdominal fluid collection—ascites, peritoneal dialysis
Exudates
  Infection
    Empyema
    Bacterial—Gram-positive and -negative, *Actinomyces*, *Mycobacterium tuberculosis*
    Viral—Coxsackie virus, *Mycoplasma*
    Fungal—*Nocardia*, *Coccidioides* (rarely)
    Parasitic—*Amoeba*, *Echinococcus*
    Parapneumonic
  Malignancy—bronchogenic Ca, mesothelioma, lymphoma
            metastatic Ca—breast, ovary, kidney, pancreas, GI tract
  Pulmonary embolism and infarction
  Collagen vascular disease—systemic lupus erythematosus, rheumatoid arthritis
  Intra-abdominal processes—pancreatitis, subphrenic abscess, Meigs' syndrome, postabdominal surgery
  Trauma—hemothorax, chylothorax, ruptured esophagus
  Miscellaneous—myxedema, uremia, asbestosis, lymphedema (yellow nail syndrome), drug sensitivity, Dressler's syndrome

TABLE 23–2. DIFFERENTIATION OF EXUDATIVE AND TRANSUDATIVE PLEURAL EFFUSION

	EXUDATE	TRANSUDATE
Protein	>3 g/dl	<3 g/dl
Pleural/serum protein	>0.5	<0.5
LDH	>200 IU/L	<200 IU/L
Pleural/serum LDH	>0.6	<0.6

Although less frequently positive (40 per cent) than cytological examination, biopsy occasionally makes a diagnosis of malignant effusions when cytology is negative.

Treatment depends on the underlying etiology and the degree of physiological impairment. Specific therapy to control the underlying etiology is the only successful approach. Although removal of fluid results in symptomatic improvement, lung volumes and gas exchange improve very little. Parapneumonic effusions resolve with antibiotic therapy (90 per cent), but empyemas, i.e., fluid with positive smear or culture, should be drained by repeated aspirations or tube thoracostomy; otherwise the fluid may spontaneously drain through the chest wall (*empyema necessitans*) or lead to subpleural lung necrosis with resultant bronchopleural fistula and endobronchial spread of infection. Palliative therapy should be considered for a malignant effusion only if the patient is symptomatic and displays benefit from thoracentesis. Repeated thoracentesis should be avoided, as significant protein loss results and the fluid reaccumulates within one to three days. Chemical pleurodesis with intrapleural tetracycline obliterates the pleural space and is helpful in about 80 per cent of malignant effusions.

PNEUMOTHORAX

The most common causes of air in the pleural space are listed in Table 23–3. Idiopathic spontaneous pneumothorax typically causes dyspnea, chest pain, and few abnormalities on physical examination. On chest x-ray, the one-dimensional view grossly underestimates its true volume. Without surgery, 50 per cent develop a recurrence, usually within two years. Unlike

TABLE 23–3. CAUSES OF PNEUMOTHORAX

Spontaneous
  Idiopathic
  Emphysema
  Interstitial lung disease
  Eosinophilic granuloma/histiocytosis X
  Cystic fibrosis
  Asthma
  Malignancy
Traumatic
  Penetrating and nonpenetrating chest trauma
  Transbronchoscopic or transthoracic lung biopsy
  Thoracentesis
  Mechanical ventilation
  Esophageal perforation

the low mortality with idiopathic pneumothorax, that due to underlying lung disease has a 15 per cent mortality rate. Under certain circumstances, particularly in patients on mechanical ventilators, the rent in the pleura forms a one-way valve that permits air to enter but not to escape, causing positive pressure to build up in the chest (tension pneumothorax).

Treatment depends on the amount of air and the underlying status of the patient. Spontaneous pneumothorax in a healthy asymptomatic patient may require no treatment, whereas treatment is required for the same size pneumothorax in a patient with cardiopulmonary insufficiency. Treatment is almost always required for pneumothoraces greater than 50 per cent in size or for a pneumothorax of any size in patients on mechanical ventilation or with diffuse lung disease. Drainage by tube thoracostomy is successful in most instances, and instillation of tetracycline to produce pleurodesis may prevent recurrence. Sometimes open thoracotomy with partial pleurectomy and oversewing of apical blebs or abrasion of the pleural surface is required.

TUMORS OF THE PLEURAL SPACE

Mesotheliomas may be localized benign growths curable by surgical resection or aggressive, untreatable malignancies spreading extensively in the pleural space and beyond. Malignant mesotheliomas are almost always associated with asbestos exposure. More commonly, neoplasms of the pleural space are due to adjacent spread (bronchogenic carcinoma) or metastatic disease (carcinoma of the breast, ovary, and kidney and lymphoma). They produce bloody pleural effusions, although chylous effusions resulting from lymphatic obstruction are also seen.

MEDIASTINAL DISEASE

The mediastinum is bounded by the thoracic outlet, the diaphragm, the sternum, the vertebral column, and the medial borders of the lungs. It contains the heart, esophagus, trachea, lymphatics, thymus gland, and a large number of nerves and blood vessels. Generally, benign mediastinal masses grow slowly, displace surrounding structures, and are painless, whereas malignant lesions invade and compress the important mediastinal structures, giving rise to earlier symptoms such as pain, dysphagia, hoarseness, stridor, cough, dyspnea, and features of Horner's and superior vena cava syndromes. Myasthenia gravis is associated with thymomas, while neurogenic tumors cause spinal cord or nerve compression.

The chest x-ray localized the process and often suggests the correct diagnosis. CT is invaluable because it separates vascular from nonvascular lesions and cystic from solid structures and identifies local invasion. Definitive diagnosis often depends on obtaining tissue.

MEDIASTINITIS

Acute mediastinitis is usually due to esophageal perforation or traumatic rupture of the airway, or, rarely, spread of infection from the neck or abdomen. Features are usually typical of mediastinal disease along with fever, leukocytosis, pneumomediastinum, pneumothorax, and often a pleural effusion. Distinctive features include a high pleural fluid amylase with esophageal perforation and fracture of the first three ribs seen with bronchial rupture. Treatment includes antibiotics, surgical drainage, and closure of the perforated viscus.

Chronic mediastinitis is usually a granulomatous process, most often histoplasmosis and less frequently other fungal infections, tuberculosis, and syphilis. Noninfectious causes include sarcoidosis and, in the past, the use of methysergide. An idiopathic cause should be considered only when specific disorders are ruled out. Treatment other than that specifically directed at the underlying disorder, such as surgery, is usually unsuccessful.

MEDIASTINAL MASSES

These are mostly tumors but also include glandular lesions, vascular abnormalities, and esophageal disease. They are conveniently divided by anatomic location (Fig. 23–2).

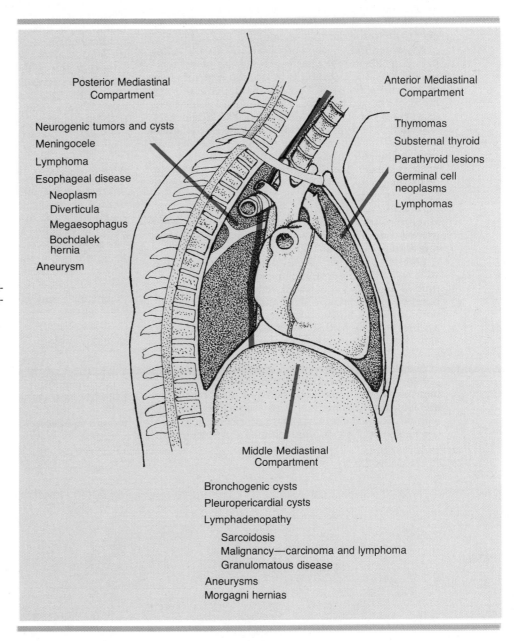

FIGURE 23–2. Masses of the mediastinum indicated by their anatomical location.

Posterior Mediastinal Compartment

Neurogenic tumors and cysts
Meningocele
Lymphoma
Esophageal disease
   Neoplasm
   Diverticula
   Megaesophagus
   Bochdalek hernia
Aneurysm

Anterior Mediastinal Compartment

Thymomas
Substernal thyroid
Parathyroid lesions
Germinal cell neoplasms
Lymphomas

Middle Mediastinal Compartment

Bronchogenic cysts
Pleuropericardial cysts
Lymphadenopathy
   Sarcoidosis
   Malignancy—carcinoma and lymphoma
   Granulomatous disease
Aneurysms
Morgagni hernias

CHEST WALL DISEASE

Adequate ventilation depends on efficient movement of the chest wall in response to neural stimulation. Interference with this may result in increased work of breathing, restricted lung volumes, exercise limitation, and gradual progression to respiratory failure. Total lung capacity and vital capacity are decreased, but unlike parenchymal restrictive lung disease the residual volume is usually normal or even increased. Hypoventilation is the predominant mechanism of abnormal gas exchange, and thus hypercapnia is found at much higher levels of arterial Po_2 than in parenchymal lung disease. In addition, progressive ventilation-perfusion inequality, resulting from basilar atelectasis, causes gradual widening of the alveolar-arterial gradient. Continued, prolonged hypoxemia eventually causes cor pulmonale.

Kyphoscoliosis. Kyphoscoliosis is usually idiopathic or may be associated with Marfan's syndrome or poliomyelitis. The severity of scoliosis is quantitated by measuring the angle between the upper and lower limbs of the spinal curve. Mild scoliosis (angle >35 degrees) is common (incidence, 1/1,000); respiratory dysfunction becomes detectable only when the angle is greater than 70 degrees (incidence 1/10,000), and early cardiopulmonary failure is expected when the angle is greater than 120 degrees. Surgical correction of the deformity in adults does not influence the incidence of respiratory complications.

Ankylosing Spondylitis. Respiratory failure in the absence of additional parenchymal lung disease is extremely rare. Apical fibrocavitary disease develops in rare instances.

Obesity. Patients have a small expiratory reserve volume (ERV) and thus breathe close to residual volume. This leads to decreased ventilation of the lung bases and hypoxemia. This is magnified in the supine position, which further decreases ERV. These abnormalities may be further complicated by disorders of ventilatory control and upper airway obstruction (see Chapter 22).

Diaphragmatic Paralysis. Causes of unilateral diaphragmatic paralysis include phrenic nerve involvement by tumor, trauma, or herpes zoster, but many are idiopathic in origin. Patients are asymptomatic with an elevated hemidiaphragm on chest x-ray, a 25 per cent reduction in lung volume, and evidence of hypoxemia on recumbency. Fluoroscopic examination shows paradoxical upward motion of the diaphragm during sniffing. Bilateral diaphragmatic paralysis is rare and may be due to chest trauma, cervical surgery, neuromuscular disease, or (rarely) phrenic nerve injury during topical cardiac hypothermia employed in cardiopulmonary bypass. Severe orthopnea and paradoxical inward motion of the abdomen during inspiration are the clinical hallmarks. Assumption of the supine posture is associated with hypoxemia and 50 per cent fall in vital capacity, and the ERV may be become undetectable.

Respiratory Muscle Fatigue. Increasing attention is being focused on the role of respiratory muscle fatigue as a cause of respiratory failure. Respiratory muscle dysfunction may arise as a result of excessive demands (increased work of breathing or ventilatory requirements) or decreased energy supplies (malnutrition, metabolic disturbance, decreased O_2 supply). Unfortunately, none of the techniques used to investigate fatigue in experimental settings is satisfactory for the clinical diagnosis of fatigue. In addition, while many disease states affect respiratory muscle function, the importance of respiratory muscle fatigue as a primary determinant of ventilatory failure has not been established.

TREATMENT

Treatment is directed at correcting reversible abnormalities and minimizing the development of parenchymal lung disease. Respiratory failure develops in some patients and mechanical ventilation is required. Initially, this is particularly valuable during sleep at night; in many patients, it may be possible to deliver mechanical ventilation via a nose mask, circumventing the need for tracheostomy. Eventually, mechanical ventilation may be required on a continuous basis.

REFERENCES

Heitzman ER: The Mediastinum, Radiologic Correlations with Anatomy and Pathology. St. Louis, CV Mosby Company, 1977.

Light RW: Pleural Diseases. Philadelphia, Lea and Febiger, 1983.

Roussos C, Macklem PT: The Thorax (Parts A and B). New York, Marcel Dekker, 1985.

24
INHALATIONAL INJURY

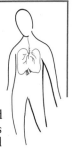

DROWNING AND NEAR-DROWNING

The pathophysiology of near-drowning in both fresh water and salt water is similar. Survival depends on the pulmonary insult, the amount of hypoxemic brain damage, and the degree of acidosis. A drowning victim responds initially by closing his glottis, and 10 per cent of drowned victims aspirate no fluid but die from asphyxia. The remainder aspirate fluid, develop pulmonary edema and intrapulmonary shunt, and may progress to profound hypoxemia accompanied by a clinical picture identical to the adult respiratory distress syndrome (ARDS). The quantity of aspirated fluid is rarely sufficient to produce significant change in blood volume. Occasionally, however, near-drowning in hypotonic fresh water can cause transient hypervolemia, whereas hypovolemia may follow hypertonic saltwater aspiration. Alterations in hematocrit or serum electrolytes are rarely life-threatening and are the same with both salt- and freshwater near-drowning. Metabolic acidosis develops in 70 per cent of victims. Renal function remains normal in most, but some develop hemoglobinuria, albuminuria, or oliguria and acute tubular necrosis. The cardiovascular system displays remarkable stability, and alterations are primarily a consequence of hypoxemia or acidosis. The likelihood of neurological impairment depends on the duration of immersion and possibly the temperature of the water. Recovery has been reported after submersion in very cold water for up to 40 minutes. This may be due partly to the diving reflex, which is initiated by facial immersion in cold water (<20°C) and results in severe bradycardia and the shunting of blood to the heart and brain in an attempt to limit hypoxic damage. Additionally, hypothermia lowers O_2 requirements and prolongs the brain's and heart's tolerance to severe hypoxemia.

The most decisive factor in the management of near-drowning victims is resumption of ventilation using mouth-to-mouth resuscitation. Even in victims with evident aspiration of fluid, time should not be wasted in attempting to drain liquid from the lungs, as large volumes are rarely aspirated. In the absence of an effective pulse, closed-chest cardiac resuscitation is required. Hospital admission for all surviving victims is imperative because the patient's clinical status may belie life-threatening hypoxemia, and supplemental O_2 should be continued until the measurement of Pa_{O_2} indicates a satisfactory level. Intubation, mechanical ventilation, and hemodynamic monitoring (as described in Chapter 20) will be required in patients who subsequently develop ARDS. Brochodilators counteract bronchospasm, and bicarbonate administration may be necessary to correct metabolic acidosis. Electrolyte disturbances, hemolysis, and renal failure should be treated appropriately. Prophylactic steroid or antibiotic therapy is not indicated. The prognosis is good for patients who are alert or who have a blunted level of consciousness on admission to the emergency room but poor for those in coma.

SMOKE INHALATION INJURY

Pulmonary injury due to inhalation of the thermal, gaseous, or particulate products of combustion is the most common cause of death in fire injury victims. Two major types of lung injury are observed: thermal injury of the airways and inhalation of gaseous or particulate matter.

Thermal injury is usually limited to structures above the vocal cords because the airways possess a very efficient cooling system. Combustion (flame) and pyrolysis (smolder) of materials release a complex array of organic acids, aldehydes, and gases that may induce a chemical injury of the airway mucosa with resultant peribronchial edema and bronchoconstriction. Asphyxia may also occur, since the ambient $F_{I_{O_2}}$ in the area of a fire usually falls to about 0.10 because combustion uses O_2. Impairment of mucociliary and phagocytic function predisposes to subsequent lung infection, and alveolar damage may result in ARDS. The presence of a body burn markedly aggravates the lung injury. ARDS is uncommon, possibly because the degree of exposure required for its development is likely to result in fatal carbon monoxide poisoning. Carbon monoxide is an odorless, tasteless, and colorless gas that does not produce lung injury but has a dual effect on tissue oxygenation. Its marked affinity for hemoglobin (Hb) (210 times that of O_2) limits the O_2 carrying capacity of blood. In addition, it shifts the O_2 dissociation curve to the left, which impairs O_2 release to the tissues.

The clinical presentation depends on the predominant form of injury. Facial burns and singed nasal hairs should arouse suspicion of lung injury, although pulmonary involvement occurs in only a small proportion of such patients. Thermal injury may produce upper airway obstruction with stridor, hoarseness, and phonation difficulties, necessitating further evaluation (with possible bronchoscopy) and intubation to maintain a patent airway. Lower airway involvement may be associated with the production of carbonaceous sputum, wheezes, and crackles. The chest x-ray is insensitive in the early stages, although pulmonary infiltrates or edema may subsequently develop. Features associated with carbon monoxide intoxication include headache, nausea, fatigue, behavioral change, ataxia, and hypoxic damage of the heart or brain. Cherry-red coloration of the lips is usually absent unless the carboxyhemoglobin (COHb) concentration is above 40 per cent. An intoxicated patient displays a normal

173

TABLE 24–1. TOXIC GASES AND FUMES

MECHANISM OF INJURY	AGENT	OCCUPATIONAL EXPOSURE
Asphyxia	Carbon dioxide	Mining, foundry work
	Nitrogen	Mining, underwater work
	Carbon monoxide	Mining, petroleum refining, air pollution
	Methane	Mining
Local irritation	Ammonia	Fertilizer, refrigerator, cleaning agents
	Nitrogen dioxide	Farming (silo), fertilizer, welding
	Chlorine	Bleaching, disinfectant
	Sulfur dioxide	Smelting, air pollution
Toxic absorption	Carbon monoxide	Mining, petroleum refining
	Cyanide	Electroplating, fumigants
	"Metal fume fever" (metal oxides)	Welding, galvanizing, smelting
Allergy	Isocyanates	Plastics, paint
	Platinum	Electroplating, photography
	Formalin	Insulation, textiles, chemical manufacturing

Pa_{O_2} and *calculated* O_2 saturation, but there is a severe reduction in *measured* O_2 saturation. Despite the severe O_2 desaturation, minute ventilation is not increased in carbon monoxide intoxication, since the carotid body responds to Pa_{O_2}. Confirmation is made by measurement of blood COHb: less than 2 per cent in healthy subjects, 5 to 10 per cent in cigarette smokers, and 30 to 50 per cent in fire injury victims.

Management includes removing the victim from exposure, checking vital signs, and establishing a patent airway. Administration of supplemental O_2 relieves hypoxemia and enhances the dissociation of carbon monoxide from Hb, decreasing the half-time for elimination from 300 min on room air, to 60 min, with an $F_{I_{O_2}}$ of 1.0. In order to achieve an adequate $F_{I_{O_2}}$, intubation and mechanical ventilation may be required. The use of hyperbaric O_2 has been suggested for patients with severe CO intoxication, although its advantage over breathing 100 per cent O_2 is unproven. Bronchospasm usually responds to bronchodilators. Corticosteroids are no longer recommended in the management of smoke-inhalation injury. Antibiotics should be prescribed only if there is evidence of infection. In the rare cases in which ARDS supervenes, the management is identical to that described in Chapter 20. Patients surviving the acute clinical course usually recover completely. Long-term complications of tracheal stenosis, bronchiolitis obliterans, or bronchiectasis are rare.

NOXIOUS GASES AND FUMES

Exposure to toxic gases and fumes is an increasing problem in modern industrial society and may cause harm by four basic mechanisms (Table 24–1). Asphyxia occurs when the O_2 in inspired air is displaced by another gas. The most common mechanism of injury is local irritation, the form and extent of which depend on the concentration, solubility, and duration of exposure to the toxic gas. Highly soluble gases, such as *ammonia*, rapidly injure the mucous membranes of the eye and upper airway, causing an intense burning pain in the eyes, nose, and throat with lacrimation, rhinorrhea, and a sense of suffocation. This, combined with the strong pungent odor of ammonia, causes the victim to flee from the site of exposure. Lower airway injury is not observed unless the victim is trapped or a massive spill occurs, in which case laryngeal or pulmonary edema may ensue. In contrast, insoluble gases, such as nitrogen dioxide, are distributed to the peripheral airways and usually cause a diffuse lung injury. Exposure to *nitrogen dioxide* is classically encountered in farmers, as large quantities of this gas are formed by fermentation during the first week after filling a silo. The victim typically presents with cough, dyspnea, bronchospasm, and weakness, with little evidence of ocular or upper airway irritation. After a lag of one or more hours there may be progression to frank pulmonary edema. Following recovery from the acute illness the patient may develop bronchiolitis obliterans, characterized by progressive dyspnea. Absorption of a toxic gas with systemic consequences is best characterized by carbon monoxide, as discussed under smoke inhalation. Exposure to isocyanate, platinum compounds, or formalin vapors may cause asthma, either immediate or delayed in onset, and is more fully discussed in Chapter 17.

Management of exposure to a toxic gas is generally supportive in nature. The victim should be removed from the source of exposure and a patent airway with adequate ventilation should be ensured. Correction of hypoxemia may be possible with supplemental O_2, or intubation and mechanical ventilation may be necessary. The patient should be carefully monitored for a delayed reaction to the agent. Additional measures that may be required include bronchodilators and correction of acid-base disturbance or shock. The role of prophylactic antibiotics or steroids remains undetermined, although a trial of steroids is usually employed in patients with bronchiolitis obliterans.

REFERENCES

Haponik EF, Summer WR: Respiratory complications in burned patients: Pathogenesis and spectrum of inhalation injury. J Crit Care 2:49–74, 1987.

Modell JH: Biology of drowning. Annu Rev Med 29:1–8, 1978.

Morgan WKC, Seaton A: Occupational Lung Diseases, 2nd ed. Philadelphia, WB Saunders Company, 1984.

SECTION III

RENAL DISEASE

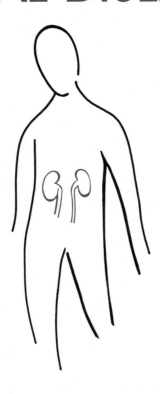

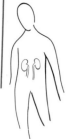

25

APPROACH TO THE PATIENT WITH RENAL DISEASE

The patient with renal disease often presents to the physician with mild, nonspecific signs and symptoms but may also appear with severe, life-threatening manifestations of renal dysfunction. Certain signs and symptoms should alert the physician to the possibility that renal disease is present. Complaints of flank pain, dysuria, gross hematuria, and the passage of a renal stone are directly referable to the urinary tract. Other findings such as hypertension, edema, congestive heart failure, or constitutional symptoms of lethargy, anorexia, or pruritus are nonspecific but may reflect the impact of reduced renal function on other organ systems. The approach to the patient with suspected renal disease begins with a careful history and physical examination which focus on features outlined in Table 25–1. A particular renal syndrome such as chronic renal failure, glomerulonephritis, urinary tract infection, or urinary tract obstruction is often suggested by the constellation of presenting signs and symptoms. This initial impression can then be used in the formulation of a differential diagnosis and in the design of a diagnostic evaluation.

ASSESSMENT OF RENAL FUNCTION AND STRUCTURE

Specific laboratory tests and renal imaging studies are often indicated in patients with suspected renal disease. These studies help to define the renal disease, the extent of functional and anatomical impairment, and the rate of progression.

URINALYSIS

A complete analysis of the urine is a simple, noninvasive, and inexpensive means of detecting renal pathology. A first morning voided urine specimen obtained by a clean catch technique yields the most information. The urine should be examined promptly by both chemical and microscopic means.

Normal urine color ranges from almost colorless to deep yellow, depending on the concentration of urochrome pigment. Abnormal urine colors may be a sign of disease or may indicate the presence of a pigmented drug or dye (Table 25–2). The presence of red blood cells in the urine or large amounts of free hemoglobin or myoglobin will often result in red or smoke-colored urine. Cloudiness of the urine may occur when a high concentration of white blood cells is present (pyuria) or when amorphous phosphates precipitate in alkaline urine.

A chemical assessment of the urine is performed with the "dipstick," a plastic strip impregnated with various reagents that detect the presence of protein, occult blood, glucose, and ketones in the urine. These assays are semiquantitative and are graded on the basis of color changes in the various reagent strips. The dipstick method for the detection of urinary protein is very sensitive to albumin but will not detect immunoglobulins or tubular proteins (Tamm-Horsfall mucoprotein). The urine sulfosalicylic acid test is an alternate test that detects all urinary proteins by a process of precipitation. A very concentrated urine may show trace to 1+ protein (10 to 30 mg/dl) in a normal individual. The finding of occult blood in the urine is abnormal and indicates the presence of either

TABLE 25–1. IMPORTANT FEATURES OF THE HISTORY AND PHYSICAL EXAMINATION IN THE PATIENT WITH RENAL DISEASE

Historical Data
Familial Renal Disease—polycystic kidney disease, hereditary nephritis, renal calculi
Systemic Disease—systemic lupus erythematosus, diabetes mellitus, hypertension, sickle cell anemia
Toxic Exposure—heavy metals, radiographic contrast material, drugs: analgesics, antibiotics, nonsteroidal anti-inflammatory agents
Associated Symptoms
General: fever, weight loss, fatigue, skin rash, pruritus, sore throat
Cardiovascular: dyspnea, chest pain, edema
Gastrointestinal: anorexia, nausea, vomiting
Genitourinary: polyuria, dysuria, flank pain, hematuria, passage of a renal stone
Physical Examination
Cardiovascular: hypertension, cardiac failure, pericardial rub, edema
Genitourinary: palpable kidneys or bladder, prostatic enlargement
Neurological: peripheral neuropathy, asterixis, encephalopathy
Funduscopic: diabetic retinopathy, hypertensive retinopathy

TABLE 25–2. URINE COLORS

COLOR	ASSOCIATION
colorless	dilute urine, diabetes mellitus, diabetes insipidus
yellow	normal, riboflavin, quinacrine
amber	concentrated urine, Pyridium, sulfasalazine
blue, blue-green	biliverdin, methylene blue, amitriptyline, triamterene
red	hematuria, hemoglobinuria, myoglobinuria, phenytoin, phenolphthalein, rifampin, Adriamycin, anthrocyanin (pigment in beets and blackberries)
red-brown	porphyria, urobilinogen, bilirubin, nitrofurantoin, primaquine, chloroquine, metronidazole
brown-black	acidification of hemoglobin pigment, melanin, alkaptonuria, senna, cascara, rhubarb
milky white	chyluria, pyuria

intact red blood cells or free hemoglobin or myoglobin molecules.

The microscopic examination of the urine sediment confirms the presence of cellular elements, casts, crystals, and microorganisms (Table 25–3). Microscopic hematuria is defined as more than two red blood cells per high-power field on a centrifuged urine specimen in the absence of contamination by menstrual blood. Pyuria is defined as the presence of more than four white blood cells per high-power field. Epithelial cells are commonly found in the urinary sediment and may derive from any site along the urinary tract from the renal pelvis to the urethra. Renal tubular cells that contain absorbed lipids are termed oval fat bodies. Free fat droplets, composed primarily of cholesterol esters, may also be observed in the urine, particularly in association with heavy proteinuria. Both the oval fat bodies and free fat droplets have doubly refractile characteristics under the polarizing microscope and share the characteristic "Maltese cross" appearance. Urinary casts are cylindrical structures derived from the intratubular precipitation of mucoprotein and cellular debris. Hyaline casts, composed of tubular mucoprotein, are frequently observed in concentrated urine and are of little significance. Casts that contain cellular elements in addition to protein are named according to the predominant cell type. The presence of red or white blood cell casts provides presumptive evidence of inflammatory parenchymal renal disease. Granular, waxy, and broad casts represent successive stages in the degeneration of cellular casts.

Crystals of calcium oxalate (envelope-shaped) and uric acid (rhomboid) are often identified in acidic urine depending on the degree of supersaturation, but in the absence of specific symptoms they are of little clinical significance. The presence of cystine crystals in the urine indicates the rare disease cystinuria. Triple phosphate crystals ("coffin-lid"–shaped) may be identified in alkaline urine. Bacteria in the urine are almost always recognized in a centrifuged specimen but do not necessarily imply significant bacteriuria. The presence of bacteria in an unspun specimen, however, is significant and provides presumptive evidence for a urinary tract infection.

RENAL FUNCTION TESTS

Specific tests of renal function are used to assess both the glomerular and tubular functions of the kidney. The glomerular filtration rate is most accurately determined by measurement of the clearance of a marker that is completely filtered by the glomerulus and neither reabsorbed, secreted, nor metabolized by the renal tubule. The sugar inulin is an ideal marker for such a study, but because inulin is not an endogenous substance, performance of an inulin clearance study is not practical in the routine clinical setting. Determination of the clearance of endogenous creatinine is a more convenient test and provides a reasonable estimate of the glomerular filtration rate. Because 10 per cent of creatinine is excreted by the process of tubular secretion, however, the creatinine

TABLE 25–3. MICROSCOPIC EXAMINATION OF THE URINE

	FINDING	ASSOCIATIONS
Casts	Red blood cell	glomerulonephritis, vasculitis
	White blood cell	interstitial nephritis, pyelonephritis
	Epithelial cell	acute tubular necrosis, interstitial nephritis, glomerulonephritis
	Granular	renal parenchymal disease (nonspecific)
	Waxy, broad	advanced renal failure
	Hyaline	normal finding in concentrated urine
	Fatty	heavy proteinuria
Cells	Red blood cell	urinary tract infection, urinary tract inflammation
	White blood cell	urinary tract infection, urinary tract inflammation
	Eosinophil	drug-induced interstitial nephritis
	(Squamous) epithelial cell	contaminants
Crystals	Uric acid	acid urine, acute uric acid nephropathy, hyperuricosuria
	Calcium phosphate	alkaline urine
	Calcium oxalate	acid urine, hyperoxaluria, ethylene glycol poisoning
	Cystine	cystinuria
	Sulfur	sulfadiazine antibiotics

clearance overestimates the true glomerular filtration rate. The creatinine clearance (C_{cr}) is calculated as $C_{cr} = U_{cr} \times V/P_{cr}$. P_{cr} is the plasma creatinine in mg/dl, U_{cr} is the urine creatinine in mg/dl, and V is the volume of urine excreted over a specific time interval in ml/min. Normal values of C_{cr} range from 75 to 160 ml/min or 95 to 105 ml/min/1.75 sq m when normalized to body surface area (Table 25–4). The creatinine clearance is elevated 30 to 50 per cent over baseline values in pregnancy because of the increase in renal plasma flow during gestation. Protein loading is also associated with a transient rise in creatinine clearance due to changes in glomerular hemodynamics. The renal response to an acute increase in the dietary intake of protein can be used as a measure of the functional reserve capacity of the kidney.

An approximate assessment of glomerular filtration

TABLE 25–4. CALCULATION OF THE CREATININE CLEARANCE

$$C_{cr} = U_{cr} \times V/P_{cr}$$

C_{cr} = clearance of creatinine (ml/min)
U_{cr} = urine creatinine (mg/dl)
V = volume of urine (ml/min) (for 24 hour volume: divide by 1440)
P_{cr} = plasma creatinine (mg/dl)
Normal range: 95 to 105 ml/min/1.75 sq m

TABLE 25–5. CAUSES OF ALTERED UREA NITROGEN–TO–CREATININE RATIO

Increased Ratio (>10:1)
  Increased urea input
    Increased dietary protein intake
    Gastrointestinal hemorrhage
    Hemolysis
    Sepsis/catabolic states
    Drugs that inhibit anabolism
      Corticosteroids
      Tetracyclines
  Decreased effective circulating volume
    Volume depletion
    Congestive heart failure
    Cirrhosis/ascites
    Nephrotic syndrome
  Obstructive uropathy
Decreased Ratio (<10:1)
  Decreased urea input
    Starvation
    Liver disease
  Increased creatinine production
    Rhabdomyolysis
  Volume expansion
    SIADH
    Iatrogenic
  Chronic renal failure with dialysis

is most easily obtained by the measurement of the concentration of creatinine and urea nitrogen in the serum. Creatinine is a metabolite of creatine, a major muscle constituent. In a given individual, the daily rate of production of creatinine is constant and determined by the mass of skeletal muscle. Because body creatinine is disposed of almost entirely by glomerular filtration, its steady-state concentration in the serum has been used as a marker of glomerular function. The "normal" range for serum creatinine concentration is 0.5 to 1.5 mg/dl. In any individual, however, a value in this range does not necessarily imply normal renal function. A more accurate assessment of renal function is obtained by determining the creatinine clear-

TABLE 25–6. CALCULATION OF THE FRACTIONAL EXCRETION OF SODIUM

Fractional excretion of sodium (FE_{Na}) = fraction of sodium filtered at the glomerulus which is ultimately excreted in the urine

$$FE_{Na} = \frac{\text{amount Na}^+ \text{ excreted/volume}}{\text{amount Na}^+ \text{ filtered/volume}} = \frac{U_{Na} \times V}{P_{Na} \times GFR}$$

$$GFR = C_{cr} = \frac{U_{cr} \times V}{P_{cr}}$$

$$FE_{Na} = \frac{U_{Na} \times V}{P_{Na}} \times \frac{1}{U_{cr} \times V/P_{cr}} = \frac{U_{Na} \times P_{cr}}{U_{cr} \times P_{Na}} \times 100$$

P_{Na} = plasma sodium (mEq/L)

P_{cr} = plasma creatinine (mg/dl)

U_{Na} = urine sodium (mEq/L)

U_{cr} = urine creatinine (mg/dl)

ance. However, once the relationship between the serum creatinine and the creatinine clearance is established for a given patient, the serum creatinine can be followed as a reliable indicator of renal function.

The blood urea nitrogen concentration (BUN) in the serum is often used in conjunction with the serum creatinine concentration as a measure of renal function. Urea is the major end product of protein metabolism, and its production reflects the dietary intake of protein as well as the protein catabolic rate. Urea is excreted by glomerular filtration, but significant amounts of urea are reabsorbed along the renal tubule, particularly in sodium-avid states such as extracellular volume contraction. Consequently, the BUN may vary in relation to the extracellular fluid volume, whereas the serum concentration of creatinine does not. The usual ratio of urea nitrogen to creatinine concentration in the serum is 10:1. This ratio is altered in a number of clinical settings and the BUN/creatinine ratio may be helpful in suggesting a specific diagnosis (Table 25–5).

Renal tubular function is evaluated by tests that examine the ability of the kidney to maintain salt and water balance as well as acid-base homeostasis. Maximal urinary concentrating ability can be assessed by restriction of fluid intake for 18 to 24 hours. The urinary osmolality should be in excess of 90 mOsm/kg water, with a specific gravity of greater than 1.023. In the polyuric patient suspected of a defect in urinary concentrating ability, the administration of five units of aqueous vasopressin once the urinary osmolality reaches steady state distinguishes patients with either central or nephrogenic diabetes insipidus. While the patient with central diabetes insipidus will have a doubling of the urinary osmolality with aqueous vasopressin, the individual with nephrogenic diabetes insipidus will not respond with further urinary concentration.

The fractional excretion of various solutes in the urine provides useful information about the tubular handling of a solute relative to its rate of glomerular filtration. Determination of fractional rates of solute clearance is accomplished by measuring the urinary excretion of the solute in question relative to the excretion of creatinine. The fractional excretion is calculated as the clearance of the solute divided by the clearance of creatinine × 100 and is expressed as a per cent. The fractional excretion of sodium, for example, is the fraction of sodium filtered at the glomerulus which is ultimately excreted in the urine (Table 25–6). Determination of the fractional excretion of sodium is most useful in the differential diagnosis of a patient with acute renal insufficiency as outlined in Chapter 29. Determination of the fractional excretion of calcium, phosphate, uric acid, and amino acids is useful in the evaluation of patients with suspected disorders of renal tubular function and in the evaluation of renal stone disease.

Acidification of the urine is an important tubular function that can be assessed by the measurement of the urine pH. In the presence of systemic acidosis (arterial pH <7.3), the urine pH should be 5.3 or less.

A timed urine collection for the determination of protein excretion is an important study in the evaluation of glomerular and tubular diseases of the kidney. Normal individuals excrete less than 150 mg/24 hr of urinary protein. Patients with various glomerular or tubular diseases typically have increased excretion of protein in the urine. On all timed urine samples for protein, a simultaneous determination of urine creatinine is useful as a means of assuring the accuracy of collection. The daily excretion of creatinine in the urine is relatively constant and averages 15 to 20 mg/kg in women and 20 to 25 mg/kg in men. If the creatinine excretion deviates significantly from these values, the collection may not be accurate.

ANATOMIC IMAGING OF THE URINARY TRACT (Table 25–7)

The plain film of the abdomen, or KUB, is a simple way of determining renal size and shape. The normal kidney shadow will approximate the length of three and one-half vertebral bodies, or about 12 cm. Bilaterally small kidneys in a patient with renal insufficiency implies a chronic, irreversible process, whereas the presence of enlarged kidneys suggests obstructive, inflammatory infiltrative, or cystic disease. Radiopaque renal calculi composed of calcium, magnesium ammonium phosphate (struvite), or cystine are often apparent on a plain film of the abdomen.

Renal ultrasonography is another noninvasive method of obtaining an anatomical image of the kidney and the collecting system. This technique is particularly useful for the detection of renal masses, cysts, and dilation of portions of the collecting system (hydronephrosis). Ultrasonography can also be used to assess the patency of the renal veins in cases of suspected renal vein thrombosis.

The radioisotopic renal scan provides important information about renal blood flow and tubular function. The test involves the intravenous administration of radiolabeled compounds that are excreted by the kidney. An external scintillation camera provides an image of the kidneys and calculates the rate of uptake and excretion of the labeled compound. Technetium-99 DPTA is the compound used to assess renal vascular perfusion qualitatively. Impaired renal perfusion, as in the setting of unilateral renal artery stenosis or renal infarction, is characterized by asymmetrical uptake of technetium. Generalized renal hypoperfusion, as in the setting of acute glomerulonephritis or renal transplant rejection, can be recognized also. An evaluation of renal tubular function may be obtained by the use of hippuran I-131, a compound eliminated by tubular secretion. Impaired hippuran excretion in association with normal technetium perfusion is commonly observed in acute tubular necrosis or chronic renal disease.

The intravenous urogram involves the intravenous administration of iodinated radiographic contrast medium that is excreted through the kidney by glomerular filtration. The contrast medium concentrates in the renal tubules and produces a nephrogram image

TABLE 25–7. IMAGING STUDIES OF THE URINARY TRACT: COMPARATIVE ASPECTS

STUDY	INFORMATION	CONSIDERATIONS
KUB	Renal size, opaque calculi	Inexpensive
Ultrasound	Renal size, cysts, hydronephrosis, renal arterial/venous flow by Doppler	Noninvasive
Renal scan	Renal blood flow, tubular function	Functional study
Intravenous urogram	Renal size, shape, cysts, tumors, stones, obstruction	Requires IV contrast
Computerized tomography (CT)	Renal size, shape, cysts, tumors, stones, obstruction, retroperitoneal space	Requires IV contrast
Retrograde pyelography	Ureteral obstruction	Invasive
Renal arteriography	Renal vasculature, tumors	Invasive
Renal venography	Renal vein thrombosis, renal vein blood sampling	Invasive

within the first few minutes after injection. As the medium passes into the collecting system, the calyces, renal pelvis, ureters, and bladder are visualized. This study is useful in the identification of renal calculi, pyelonephritic scars, cysts, or renal tumors and in defining various congenital anomalies of the urinary tract. The computed tomographic (CT) scan of the kidney provides more precise information regarding renal masses as well as a definition of the perinephric space and other retroperitoneal structures. In both studies, the uptake and excretion of contrast by the kidney are prolonged in patients with renal insufficiency. Delayed views obtained 24 to 48 hours after injection of contrast may provide useful information. However, the risk of contrast medium–induced nephrotoxicity limits the utility of these studies in certain high-risk patients (see Chapter 33). CT scanning of the kidney can be performed without intravenous contrast material in selected cases. The role of magnetic resonance imaging (MRI), the newest imaging technique in radiology, is uncertain at present.

Retrograde pyelography is performed by the injection of radiocontrast material directly into the ureters at the time of cystoscopy. This technique is useful in the definition of obstructing lesions within the ureter or renal pelvis, particularly in the setting of a nonvisualizing kidney on intravenous pyelography. If an obstruction is identified, it can often be removed or bypassed by the placement of a ureteral catheter at the time of the procedure. Cystoscopy is often indicated in the evaluation of unexplained hematuria when bladder lesions are suspected.

Renal arteriography involves the direct injection of radiographic contrast medium into the aorta and renal arteries and is used to assess the renal vasculature.

Renal arteriography is particularly useful in the evaluation of patients with suspected renal artery stenosis or thrombosis and in those with a renal mass. Because renal arteriography is a more invasive test, its use has been limited to those situations in which a strong clinical indication exists and the patient is considered a candidate for surgical intervention. Renal vein catheterization is used to confirm the diagnosis of renal vein thrombosis or to obtain blood samples from the renal vein, particularly in the setting of suspected renovascular hypertension.

RENAL BIOPSY

A renal biopsy should be considered in a patient with parenchymal renal disease when the diagnosis or extent of disease cannot be ascertained by the studies outlined earlier. Most renal biopsies are performed when a glomerular lesion is suspected. These diseases often require accurate diagnosis prior to initiating treatment with potent drugs such as corticosteroids or immunosuppressive agents. The percutaneous biopsy is the most commonly employed technique and is a relatively safe procedure. An open renal biopsy is considered in the patient with a solitary functioning kidney or a bleeding diathesis. The biopsy specimen should be submitted for light, immunofluorescent, and electron microscopy. Potential complications of a renal biopsy include hematuria, renal hematoma, vascular laceration with the development of arteriovenous fistulae, and the inadvertent biopsy of liver, spleen, or bowel.

SPECIFIC MANIFESTATIONS OF RENAL DISEASE

This section reviews the approach to the patient with specific manifestations of renal disease such as proteinuria, hematuria, pyuria, and azotemia. The evaluation of all such patients includes a detailed history and physical examination, a urinalysis, and determination of the serum concentration of creatinine, urea nitrogen, and electrolytes. A timed collection of urine for calculation of the creatinine clearance and total protein excretion is often helpful. Other studies, including anatomical imaging of the urinary tract or renal biopsy, may be indicated.

PROTEINURIA

A normal individual excretes less than 150 mg of low molecular weight tubular protein in the urine on a daily basis. The glomerular basement membrane serves as an effective barrier to the passage of high molecular weight proteins such as albumin, and the renal tubules have the capacity to reabsorb the small amount of protein that is filtered through the glomerulus. Abnormal proteinuria may occur as a transient phenomenon in individuals with febrile illnesses or congestive heart failure or after vigorous exercise.

Persistent proteinuria, however, is almost always indicative of renal disease.

Nephrotic range proteinuria (>3 to 3.5 gm/24 hr) is indicative of glomerular disease and is commonly associated with features of the nephrotic syndrome such as edema, hypoalbuminemia, and hyperlipidemia (see Chapter 31). Lesser amounts of protein may be excreted in various tubulointerstitial diseases, in glomerular diseases, and in some cases of acute or chronic renal failure. When proteinuria of any magnitude is associated with red blood cell casts, glomerulonephritis should be suspected. Tubulointerstitial pathology is suggested by the association of proteinuria with alterations in tubular function such as the inability to concentrate the urine or to maintain acid-base homeostasis.

The laboratory evaluation of the patient with proteinuria includes a quantitation of protein excretion in a 24-hour urine specimen. The majority of patients with nephrotic-range proteinuria will have a primary glomerulopathy. In these cases, a renal biopsy may be necessary to establish an accurate diagnosis. However, the nephrotic syndrome may result from a secondary glomerular lesion related to systemic diseases such as diabetes mellitus, various collagen vascular diseases, amyloidosis, occult malignancy, or drug reaction. In these settings, a careful review of the clinical presentation will often provide a clue to the presence of underlying systemic disease with renal involvement. Individuals with non–nephrotic-range proteinuria may have a variety of glomerular or interstitial renal diseases. When proteinuria is associated with either hypertension or renal insufficiency, the renal prognosis is less favorable.

HEMATURIA

The presence of red blood cells in the urine, as detected by gross visual or microscopic examination, should be regarded as a significant finding. Hematuria is a nonspecific sign of genitourinary tract inflammation and occurs in a number of disorders, including glomerulonephritis, acute and chronic renal failure, urinary tract infection, urinary tract obstruction, neoplasia, and nephrolithiasis. Although the source of the bleeding may not be localized on the basis of the presenting signs and symptoms or the urinalysis, certain findings are helpful. The presence of red blood cell casts and associated proteinuria is good evidence for a glomerular inflammatory lesion. Smoke-colored urine is also considered a sign of glomerular bleeding. The passage of gross clots in the urine is suggestive of bleeding distal to the renal tubule.

The evaluation of the patient with hematuria will often require anatomical imaging of the urinary tract to exclude a lesion such as tumor or renal stone. Cystoscopy may be indicated to exclude an inflammatory lesion of the bladder. A urine culture should be obtained to rule out the possibility of hemorrhagic bacterial cystitis. If the bleeding is of glomerular or tubular origin and a specific diagnosis cannot be made by other means, a renal biopsy may be helpful.

PYURIA

The finding of more than four white blood cells per high-power field on a urine specimen is suggestive of urinary tract inflammation, although, as with hematuria, the precise site cannot be identified. Pyuria as an isolated finding is most commonly associated with bacterial urinary tract infection. When associated with hematuria or proteinuria, pyuria is suggestive of parenchymal renal disease such as glomerulonephritis or interstitial nephritis.

The presence of pyuria should initiate a search for urinary tract infection, particularly when the patient complains of dysuria, flank pain, or fever. Renal imaging studies are often indicated to exclude the presence of renal parenchymal scarring, obstruction, or abscess formation, particularly when accompanied by signs of renal dysfunction such as azotemia. Sterile pyuria associated with frequency and urgency may indicate nongonococcal urethritis. Occult renal tuberculosis may also present with sterile pyuria. A Wright's or Hanson's stain of the urine for eosinophils is often helpful in the patient with pyuria who is suspected of having acute allergic interstitial nephritis.

AZOTEMIA

The patient with azotemia often comes to the attention of a physician because of signs or symptoms referable to impaired renal function. Occasionally, an elevation of the plasma concentration of urea nitrogen or creatinine is an incidental finding on a screening laboratory profile in an asymptomatic patient. In either case, the major clinical questions are the following: (1) Is the renal dysfunction acute or chronic? (2) Are there any reversible features to the azotemia? (3) What is the rate of progression of the renal disease?

The history of the patient and prior blood chemistry determinations, if available, provide important information in distinguishing acute from chronic renal disease. The presence of small kidneys assessed by renal imaging studies is suggestive of chronic disease. The presence of normal-sized or enlarged kidneys, however, does not exclude the diagnosis of chronic renal insufficiency. Patients with chronic renal failure tend to be more anemic and to have higher plasma concentrations of phosphate than those with acute renal failure. Neither of these determinations, however, is sufficiently discriminating to differentiate acute from chronic disease. The patient must be evaluated for the presence of any potentially reversible coexisting insults to the kidney, such as partial urinary tract obstruction, infection, depletion of the extracellular fluid volume, congestive heart failure, hypercalcemia, and drug-induced renal insufficiency.

Evaluation of the rate of progression of renal dysfunction can provide important information for management and therapy of patients with renal disease. Most patients with chronic renal failure, regardless of the underlying etiology, have an unrelenting progres-

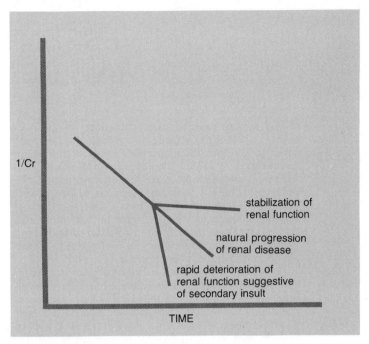

FIGURE 25–1. Evaluation of the rate of progression of renal insufficiency by graphing the reciprocal of the serum creatinine concentration (1/Cr) versus time.

sive deterioration in renal function over time. Secondary insults may accelerate the rate of deterioration in renal function in a patient with chronic renal disease. A valuable method of evaluating such individuals is to graph the reciprocal of the serum creatinine concentration (1/Cr) versus time (Fig. 25–1). Such a graph describes a straight line with a negative slope in patients with progressive renal failure. Secondary insults would be indicated by a relatively abrupt increase in the slope of this relationship. In addition, such a graph can be used to evaluate the response to therapy in a patient with renal disease. A decrease in the slope of 1/Cr versus time indicates a slowing in the rate of deterioration of renal function. A graph of 1/Cr versus time is also of value in predicting when a given patient will require dialysis treatment or consideration for renal transplantation.

REFERENCES

Fine E, Axelrod M, Blaufox MD: Physiologic aspects of diagnostic renal imaging. Semin Nephrol 5:188, 1985.

Pru C, Kjellstrand C: Urinary indices and chemistries in the differential diagnosis of prerenal failure and acute tubular necrosis. Semin Nephrol 5:224, 1985.

Schumann GB: Cytodiagnostic urinalysis for the nephrology practice. Semin Nephrol 6:308–345.

Thompson C: Hematuria: A clinical approach. Am Fam Physician 33:194, 1986.

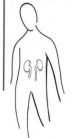

26
ESSENTIALS OF NORMAL RENAL FUNCTION

The kidney has one major function: to maintain nearly constant the volume and composition of body fluids in the face of fluctuations in the volume and composition of daily intake, thus permitting safe habitation in a wide range of external environments. The renal contribution to the homeostasis of body fluids involves a number of individual, specialized renal functions; these include the excretion of metabolic end products and toxins, the regulation of body fluid volume and solute composition, and additional metabolic and hormonal functions.

Body fluids are confined to discrete "compartments" that are separated by semipermeable barriers. The volume and composition of these individual fluid compartments can be approximated as indicated in Figure 26-1. Water constitutes from 50 to 70 per cent of total body weight, being in greatest proportion in lean individuals and in decreasing proportion as body fat increases.

The intracellular fluid (ICF) and extracellular fluid (ECF) compartments are separated by cell membranes that are, with few exceptions, freely permeable to water but impermeable to most solutes. This free mobility of water helps to maintain equality of osmolar concentration among all body fluid compartments. Although the osmolalities of the ICF and ECF are identical, the compositions of the two compartments differ substantially. The ECF, including the vascular space (VS), is predominantly a solution of sodium salts. The kidney operates directly on the fluid of the vascular space of the ECF to alter its volume and composition. The appropriate movement of water and/or solutes across the compartmental barriers maintains equilibrium among body fluid compartments and allows the kidney to regulate the volume, content, and composition of *all* body fluids.

THE NEPHRON

The nephron is the basic organizational unit of the kidney and consists of a specialized capillary bed (the

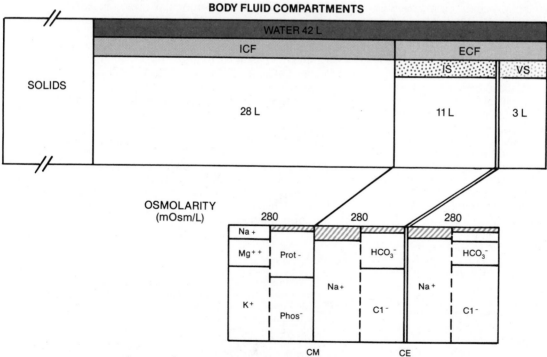

FIGURE 26–1. The body fluid compartments created by cell membranes (CM) and capillary endothelium (CE) with representative volumes for a 70-kg man. Note equality of osmolar concentration among compartments despite wide variation in cation and anion composition. ICF = Intracellular fluid; ECF = extracellular fluid; IS = interstitial space; VS = vascular space; hatched areas = minor constituents.

glomerulus) enveloped by urinary epithelium (Bowman's capsule) and connected to a continuum of specialized epithelial segments (the tubule). Each human kidney has about 1 million individual nephrons. The tubule has three functional divisions, each of which is composed of a number of discrete anatomical segments as depicted in Figure 26–2. The nephron conducts two serial processes: glomerular ultrafiltration and tubular resorption/secretion. Regulated by feedback loops, the cooperative actions of glomerular and tubular function cause the kidney to process up to 12 times the volume of the extracellular fluid each day in order to excrete a small volume (1 to 2 L) of urine in which wastes and excess solutes are concentrated 100- to 200-fold above the concentrations normally present in plasma water.

The juxtaglomerular apparatus (JGA) is a distinctive region of the nephron composed of both tubular and vascular elements. The macula densa is a cluster of specialized epithelial cells located at the end of the thick ascending limb and lying in contact with the vascular pole of the glomerulus from which that tubule originated. Cells of the afferent and efferent arterioles and distinctive extraglomerular mesangial cells compose the remainder of the JGA.

The JGA is the site of renin synthesis and secretion within the kidney. Three sets of stimuli, operating independently or jointly, may contribute to renin release by the JGA: the composition of tubular fluid (Na^+, Cl^-, or osmolar content) passing the macula densa, the degree of volume- or pressure-mediated stretch of the glomerular arterioles, and direct adrenergic stimulation. The secreted renin leads ultimately to the generation of angiotensin II (AII), which participates in regulation of renal function through effects on systemic and intrarenal hemodynamics and aldosterone release.

The work of the nephron can be considered in relation to the functional anatomy of the nephron. The glomerulus, by delivering a pure ultrafiltrate of plasma to the tubule, supplies the substrate for urine formation. The proximal tubule reclaims the bulk, about two thirds, of the volume of the ultrafiltrate by a process that does not alter the tonicity of the intratubular fluid but does change its composition. The loop of Henle absorbs less than one fifth of the ultrafiltrate volume but does so by separating the absorption of salt from water. This differential absorption sets the stage for urinary dilution and concentration. Finally, the distal tubule, which handles less than 15 per cent of the ultrafiltrate volume, performs the final adjustments to urine composition and volume.

THE GLOMERULUS

The glomerular capillaries receive blood through afferent arterioles that, in turn, originate from terminal interlobular arteries in the renal cortex. The glomerular capillary bed is drained by a second muscular vessel, the efferent arteriole. This unique suspension of a capillary network between two resistance vessels, as opposed to the arteriole-capillary-venule arrangement

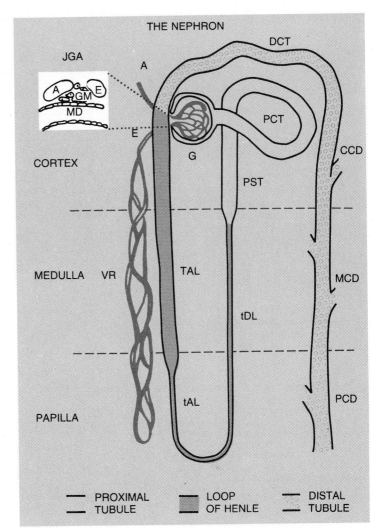

FIGURE 26–2. Functional and anatomical divisions of the nephron. PCT = proximal convoluted tubule; PST = proximal straight tubule; tDL = thin descending limb; tAl = thin ascending limb; TAL = thick ascending limb; DCT = distal convoluted tubule; CCD/M CP/PCD = cortical/medullary/papillary collecting ducts; JGA = juxtaglomerular apparatus; A = afferent arteriole; E = efferent arteriole; G = glomerulus; GM = extraglomerular matrix; MD = macula densa; VR = vasa recta.

of other tissues, makes possible the regulation of blood flow and high intracapillary hydrostatic pressure that drives ultrafiltration across the glomerular capillary wall.

Renal blood flow and glomerular filtration are maintained nearly constant over a wide range of mean aortic pressure. This autoregulatory response includes the action of the intrinsic renal vasoconstrictor angiotensin II; the effect of opposing vasodilating renal prostaglandins, PGE_2 and PGI_2; and the contractile response of vascular myoepithelium and the glomerular mesangium.

Glomerular ultrafiltration occurs as a result of an outwardly directed net pressure that moves fluid across the semipermeable capillary wall. The glomerular filtration rate (GFR) can be expressed as

$$GFR = K_f(\Delta P)$$

where ΔP is the net ultrafiltration pressure that represents the sum of Starling forces across the capillary wall and K_f is a factor that expresses both the permeability of the glomerular capillary wall and the surface area of the capillary bed available for ultrafiltration. Clinically important alterations in GFR may follow changes in the hydrostatic pressure gradient (ΔP) across the glomerular capillary wall. Changes in hydrostatic pressure in the capillary lumen result from alterations in the tone in the afferent and/or efferent arterioles. Afferent and efferent arteriolar tone is regulated, in part, by the opposing influences of vasoconstrictors (AII) and vasodilators (PGE_2, PGI_2). In some circumstances, a rise in tubular hydrostatic pressure, opposing glomerular capillary pressure, may retard ultrafiltration. In addition, changes in the permeability or surface area of the glomerular capillary bed will affect the GFR.

The glomerular filtration barrier consists of the glomerular endothelial cell, the glomerular basement membrane (GBM), and the urinary epithelial cell. This barrier allows free entry of water and small molecular weight solutes into the urinary space yet totally excludes passage of cells and proteins. The GBM appears to be a hydrated gel of intertwined collagen fibers which can be pictured as having water-filled channels that restrict passage of solutes of greater than 40° radius. Clusters of anion-rich macromolecules both within the GBM and along the surface of epithelial and endothelial cells further restrict filtration of large serum proteins that carry a net negative charge. The negative charge of the filtration barrier explains the fact that anionic albumin, which has a molecular radius (3.6 nm) less than the limiting pore size of 4.0 to 4.2 nm, does not normally enter the urinary space.

THE PROXIMAL TUBULE

The primary function of the proximal tubule is bulk, isosmotic reabsorption of ultrafiltrate. Under normal, euvolemic conditions, about two thirds of ultrafiltrate volume is absorbed in the proximal tubule. Alterations in ECF volume may change the rate of ultrafiltrate absorption in the proximal tubule and result in delivery of greater or lesser volumes of isotonic fluid to more distal nephron segments. Such a change in fluid delivery out of the proximal tubule can alter the separation of salt and water absorption in the loop of Henle and the fine adjustment of urine composition in more distal nephron segments.

A number of solutes undergo nearly complete reabsorption in the proximal tubule. Active H^+ secretion leads to reclamation of the vast majority of the filtered bicarbonate (Fig. 26–3). The rates of H^+ secretion and bicarbonate reabsorption vary directly with changes in P_{CO_2} and inversely with changes in body potassium. Thus, hypercapnia and hypokalemia both augment the rate of bicarbonate reabsorption. By a mechanism coupled to active sodium absorption, glucose, amino acids, and other organic solutes are completely reabsorbed and phosphate is substantially reclaimed in this segment. Calcium is absorbed in parallel with sodium in the proximal tubule. In the more distal, straight portion of the proximal tubule, secretion of organic acids, including uric acid and drugs such as penicillins, occurs.

THE LOOP OF HENLE

The loop of Henle begins at the corticomedullary junction with the thin descending limb, continues around a hairpin turn as the thin ascending limb, becomes the thick ascending limb in the outer medulla, and ends in the macula densa of the level of the glomerulus from which it originated. Each segment of the loop has different permeabilities to sodium chloride and water, so that about 15 per cent of the volume of the isosmotic ultrafiltrate is absorbed, but about 25 per cent of the sodium chloride is absorbed. This differential absorption converts the isotonic fluid entering from the proximal tubule into a dilute (hypotonic to plasma) fluid delivered to the distal tubule. In addition, a major portion of calcium absorption occurs in the loop of Henle. Calcium absorption in the medullary portion of the thick ascending limb varies with the magnitude of the lumen-positive transepithelial voltage that accompanies active salt absorption but is not regulated by parathyroid hormone (PTH). In contrast, PTH stimulates the rate of calcium absorption in the cortical thick ascending limb while sodium absorption is not changed by the hormone.

Passive water absorption and salt absorption in the thin limbs of the loop occur as a result of the selective permeability of these segments. The thick ascending limb absorbs NaCl by an active, energy-dependent process. Since this segment is impermeable to water, the luminal fluid leaving the thick ascending limb is made hypotonic with respect to plasma by the active salt absorption, a vital step in urinary dilution. The NaCl addition to the medullary interstitium is the primary step that allows a multiplication process to build and maintain the interstitial hypertonicity necessary to absorb water from the terminal nephron and represents a major contribution to maximum urinary concentrating ability.

The hairpin arrangement and countercurrent flow of the loop minimize the work needed to maintain a papillary osmolality of 1200 mOsm/kg H_2O compared to the 300 mOsm/kg H_2O osmolality of the cortex. A similar organization of the vasa recta, capillaries that branch from efferent arterioles of deep glomeruli, allows the sodium chloride absorbed from the loop of Henle and urea absorbed from the papillary collecting duct to be trapped within the interstitium at increasing concentrations. The integrity of these anatomical relationships is essential to the concentrating ability of the kidney.

THE DISTAL NEPHRON

Two distinct functional segments make up the distal portion of the nephron. The distal convoluted tubule

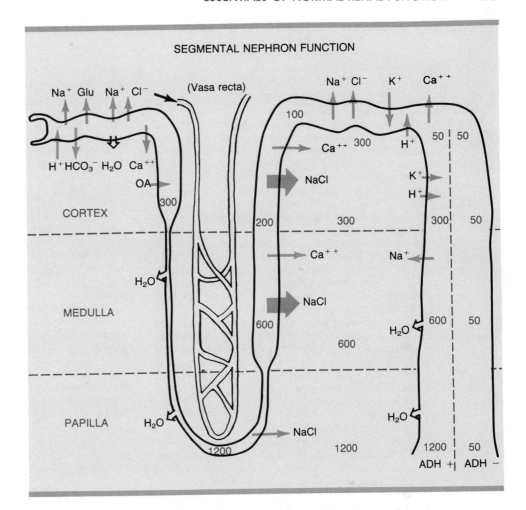

FIGURE 26–3. Major transport functions of each nephron segment, including representative osmolalities (color) in vasa recta, interstitium, and tubule at different levels within kidney. Glu = glucose; OA = organic acid.

is a water-impermeable cortical structure that continues the dilution of luminal fluid through active sodium chloride absorption. Since the cortical interstitium remains isotonic to plasma, salt absorption from these segments affects urinary dilution but not urinary concentration. Potassium secretion and H⁺ secretion are also seen in the distal convolution. As in the cortical thick ascending limb, PTH increases calcium absorption in the distal convoluted tubule so as to separate the absorption of calcium from sodium.

The collecting ducts (cortical, medullary, and papillary) are the primary sites of antidiuretic hormone (ADH) action (Fig. 26–3). They are minimally permeable to water in the absence of ADH and, in that circumstance, can deliver the hypotonic (50 to 100 mOsm/kg H_2O) fluid issuing from the distal convoluted tubule unchanged into the urine. When ADH is present, water passes across the tubule wall readily, and the luminal fluid tonicity approaches that of the interstitium at any level. Maximal urinary concentrating ability thus depends on the availability of ADH plus the degree of medullary hypertonicity generated from thick ascending limb NaCl absorption and trapping of salt and urea by the countercurrent flow of the

loop of Henle and the vasa recta. The intrinsic renal prostaglandin PGE_2 may reduce the ADH-induced increase in collecting duct water permeability and thereby limit maximal urinary concentration.

Distal nephron segments reabsorb sodium and secrete protons (H⁺) and potassium. All three processes are stimulated by aldosterone. In states of volume depletion and maximal aldosterone production, the urine can be rendered virtually free of sodium.

Potassium secretion begins in the late distal convoluted tubule and continues through the collecting ducts. Virtually all of the filtered potassium is reabsorbed in more proximal nephron segments so that the potassium appearing in the urine is secreted distally. Potassium secretion proceeds by diffusion of the intracellular cation down both concentration and electrical gradients into the tubule lumen. Table 26–1 lists factors that augment distal tubule potassium secretion.

Proton (H⁺) secretion in the distal nephron allows absorption of any bicarbonate present in these segments, thereby completing reclamation of filtered bicarbonate. However, the major contribution of the distal nephron to acid-base homeostasis is the gener-

TABLE 26–1. FACTORS THAT INCREASE POTASSIUM EXCRETION

Increased cell potassium content
Increased plasma potassium concentration
Systemic alkalosis
Aldosterone secretion
Increased fluid flow rate in distal tubule
Increased sodium delivery to distal tubule
Increased nonchloride anion delivery to distal tubule

ation of new bicarbonate. Within tubule cells, the reaction

$$CO_2 + H_2O \rightleftarrows H_2CO_3 \rightleftarrows H^+ + HCO_3^-$$

takes place. The protons (H^+) are secreted into the tubular fluid either to be buffered by phosphate ($Na_2HPO_4 + H^+ \rightleftarrows NaH_2PO_4 + Na^+$) or excreted as free H^+. The collecting duct can maintain an intraluminal free H^+ concentration 1000 times that of blood, i.e., a urine pH of 4.4 versus a plasma pH of 7.4. The bicarbonate generated within the cell diffuses into the blood to replenish bicarbonate consumed during buffering of nonvolatile acids. The quantity of new bicarbonate added to body fluids is about 1 mEq HCO_3/kg body wt/day under usual conditions of dietary intake and metabolism.

SUMMARY

The kidney regulates the volume and composition of the extracellular fluids by modifying an ultrafiltrate of plasma water. The majority of this ultrafiltrate is returned to the circulation by selective tubular reabsorption. A very small portion of the ultrafiltrate is excreted as urine, carrying with it the undesirable or excess solutes that threaten the homeostatic balance of body fluids.

The proximal tubule absorbs the bulk of the ultrafiltrate volume, and almost all of the filtered glucose, amino acids, and bicarbonate, by a process that leaves the tubular fluid isotonic to plasma. The volume of proximal tubular absorption is influenced by changes in GFR and ECF volume. The loop of Henle, through its unique structure, separates the absorption of salt and water and sets the conditions for urinary dilution or concentration. The distal nephron is regulated by specific hormones and establishes the final composition of the urine. ADH activity determines the osmotic concentration of urine by governing H_2O absorption in the collecting ducts. PTH regulates calcium absorption, and aldosterone regulates sodium, potassium, and hydrogen concentrations in the urine.

RENAL HOMEOSTATIC FUNCTIONS

The contribution of the kidney to maintaining a constant internal environment can be categorized in a number of ways. Table 26–2 presents one such list.

It is evident that a given renal function may overlap these homeostatic categories. For instance, salt and water absorption contribute to both volume and blood pressure regulation. This section will describe these homeostatic functions.

Renal homeostasis operates to maintain each component of body fluid composition within a narrow range of values. In order to achieve this end, the kidney must match urinary output of any substance to total intake, regardless of the rate of glomerular filtration. This principle can be applied to body water homeostasis, which is reflected in the plasma osmolality. The plasma osmolality is maintained nearly invariant (<2 per cent variation) by the excretion of a small volume of highly concentrated urine when water intake is curtailed or by the excretion of large volumes of maximally dilute urine when water intake is great. The kidney rapidly adjusts renal water excretion so that the volume of solute-free water in urine is equal to the volume of water ingested over any short time period.

When renal function (GFR plus tubular function) is totally normal, the kidney can maintain homeostasis despite a wide range of intake. For the case of water regulation, the kidney accommodates ingestion of as much as 16 to 18 L daily or as little as 0.5 L daily without perturbation of body water balance. However, as renal function decreases, the kidney's ability to excrete excess ingested water or to conserve water when intake is reduced is diminished. Thus, the *range* of tolerable intake is progressively narrowed and approaches a fixed value. At minimally tolerable levels of renal function, body homeostasis is maintained only by regulating intake at some nearly invariant level.

WASTE/TOXIN EXCRETION

One of the most obvious functions of the kidney is to eliminate endogenous end products of metabolism as well as exogenous toxins and drugs from the circulation. The nitrogenous metabolic products, urea and creatinine, are the most familiar clinical markers for intact renal waste elimination.

As indicated above, glomerular filtration is the first step in the elimination of most substances by the kidney. Since homeostatic requirements necessitate the maintenance of low concentrations of most metabolic end products and toxins within the circulation, very large volumes of ultrafiltrate formation are needed to deliver into the urine the absolute quantity of material requiring excretion. The production of up to 180 L/24

TABLE 26–2. HOMEOSTATIC FUNCTIONS OF THE KIDNEY

Waste/toxin excretion
Extracellular fluid volume regulation
Body fluid osmolar regulation
Blood pressure regulation
Acid-base regulation
Mineral regulation
Metabolic and hormonal regulation

hr of glomerular ultrafiltrate makes possible such mass elimination after the bulk of ultrafiltrate volume (99 to 99.5 per cent) is reclaimed. By this means, a daily urine output of 900 to 1800 ml can contain waste products concentrated 100- to 200-fold above their concentration in plasma.

A second means of solute entry into the urine is via tubular secretion of both organic acids (such as urate, citrate, and lactate) and organic bases (such as creatinine). A large number of drugs, including antibiotics and diuretics, are also eliminated via this mechanism. For substances that are protein bound and have a low free-solution concentration for ultrafiltration, the secretory process is the major route of elimination.

EXTRACELLULAR FLUID VOLUME REGULATION

Approximately one third of the volume of body water (Fig. 26–1) is contained in the extracellular fluid (ECF) compartment. Close regulation of the volume of the vascular space (VS) of the ECF is critical for stability of cardiovascular function. Since sodium salts account for almost 90 per cent of the solute in this compartment, the ECF volume can be considered, for practical purposes, to be composed of isotonic saline. Operationally, the kidney regulates NaCl absorption as the primary adjustment to ECF volume. The requisite water absorption needed to maintain an isotonic state is controlled by osmotic regulatory influences.

Renal NaCl absorption is controlled by the volume regulatory scheme depicted in Figure 26–4. Both extrarenal and intrarenal systems act to regulate salt absorption from proximal and distal nephron sites.

Baroreceptors in the atria, pulmonary vessels, aortic arch, and carotid bifurcations sense volume changes in the vascular compartment of the ECF. Sending signals to the CNS via cranial nerves IX and X, these receptors influence peripheral sympathetic nerve activity. Sympathetic tone, in turn, regulates renal perfusion pressure, renal vascular tone, glomerular blood flow, and proximal tubular fluid absorption. In addition, vasoactive hormones that affect renal hemodynamics, such as vasopressin and angiotensin II, are released into the circulation. The net effect of all these influences is to increase salt absorption in the proximal tubule and loop of Henle.

Through increased sympathetic tone, the direct influence of efferent arteriolar pressure, and the composition of tubular fluid leaving the loop of Henle, the juxtaglomerular apparatus (JGA) secretes renin. Intrarenal angiotensin II, generated from this renin, further regulates renal and glomerular hemodynamics and stimulates aldosterone secretion by the adrenal gland. Aldosterone makes possible the almost complete reclamation of sodium from the distal tubular fluid.

In conditions in which the intake of sodium is negligible or in the repair of ECF volume losses (hemorrhage, emesis), the renal excretion of sodium is nearly zero and the defense of ECF volume is maximal. This is accomplished by an increase in NaCl and water absorption by proximal nephron segments, resulting in delivery of a reduced volume to the distal nephron. This decreased distal delivery, coupled to the aldosterone-dependent increase in distal nephron sodium avidity, makes possible the complete recovery of sodium from the urine.

When ECF volume is expanded, proximal tubular

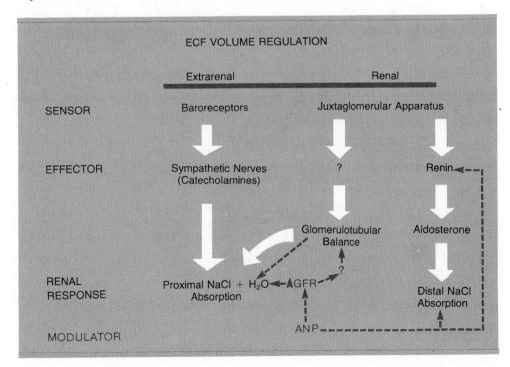

FIGURE 26–4. Scheme of renal regulation of ECF volume. Factors favoring NaCl conservation are shown in black, factors favoring NaCl excretion in color.

absorption of sodium and water is decreased and aldosterone secretion is suppressed. In addition, a polypeptide natriuretic factor that originates from the right atrium may augment renal sodium excretion in certain volume-expanded and hypertensive states. A major action of atrial natriuretic peptide (ANP) appears to be an alteration of renal hemodynamics, which leads to an increase in the filtered load and distal delivery of NaCl. In addition, ANP can reduce renin secretion and, thereby, aldosterone secretion. Thus, the greater delivery of NaCl to the distal nephron is coupled to a hormonal environment that does not favor sodium absorption. Finally, ANP may directly hinder sodium absorption in terminal collecting ducts. As a result, more sodium is lost in the urine, and the excess ECF volume is eliminated.

BODY FLUID OSMOLAR REGULATION

Body fluid osmolality, the ratio of solute to water in all fluid compartments, is maintained within a very narrow range. Unlike volume regulation, which is keyed to renal handling of sodium, osmolar balance depends on close renal regulation of ECF water. Since water moves freely across most cell membranes, the osmolality of intracellular fluid is dictated by water balance in extracellular fluids. Therefore, the kidney is able to regulate the osmolality of all body fluids via adjustments of water balance in the ECF.

ECF osmolality is regulated by dual pathways in the water repletion reaction, as shown in Figure 26–5. Os-

moreceptor cells in the CNS, located in the wall of the third ventricle, sense as little as 1 to 2 per cent change in the osmolality of blood in the internal carotid circulation. Neuronal signals from osmoreceptors stimulate the release of ADH from the posterior pituitary gland and simultaneously stimulate the sensation of thirst. The former action, ADH release, causes water conservation in the kidney by increasing water permeability and water absorption in collecting ducts. The latter response, thirst, leads to an increase in water intake. An excess of body water has the opposite effect. ADH release and thirst are suppressed, dilute fluid from the loop of Henle passes through the collecting ducts unchanged, and the excess water is excreted. There is evidence that ANP, perhaps of CNS origin, may participate in the feedback inhibition of ADH release when body water is in excess. Because of the high sensitivity of the osmotic regulation of renal water absorption, the sodium chloride absorbed in operation of the ECF volume regulatory scheme is accompanied by a volume of water sufficient to maintain isotonicity of the extracellular fluid.

When the ECF volume is reduced by about 10 per cent (Fig. 26–5), water repletion is activated as a means of replenishing ECF volume irrespective of ECF osmolality. In this case, baroreceptors in the venous and arterial circulations stimulate ADH release through neuronal pathways. This nonosmotic stimulation of ADH release occurs independently of osmoreceptor function. Thirst is also stimulated, probably by increased generation of angiotensin II. The

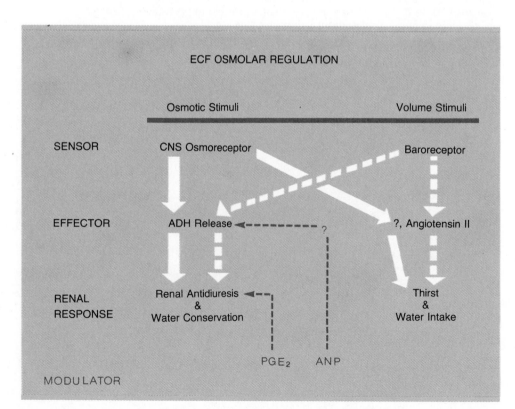

FIGURE 26–5. Scheme of renal regulation of ECF osmolality. Factors favoring H$_2$O conservation are shown in black, factors favoring H$_2$O excretion in color.

volume stimulus to ADH secretion can override osmoregulation via osmoreceptors, and water will be resorbed by the kidney even in the face of continuing dilution of body fluids.

Successful osmoregulation depends on the normal function of nephron segments proximal to the collecting ducts, regardless of the level of circulating ADH. Adequate volumes of filtrate must be delivered to the loop of Henle to form the quantity of solute-free water needed for excretion in states of body water excess. Excess filtrate delivery may hinder the ability of the loop of Henle to dilute the tubular fluid. The loop of Henle itself must be intact to dilute the luminal fluid maximally when water excretion is required or to set medullary hypertonicity at a maximum when water resorption is needed. The highly ordered medullary structure of countercurrent tubular fluid and blood flow must also be intact in order to maintain medullary hypertonicity.

BLOOD PRESSURE REGULATION

The two major renal inputs into the complex scheme of blood pressure regulation are through control of ECF volume and generation of vasoactive compounds. Because most types of hypertension are ultimately responsive to changes in ECF volume, there appears to be some degree of impairment in ECF volume regulation in many types of hypertension. In these cases, the maintenance of salt balance appears to depend on a "resetting" of the mean arterial pressure to a higher level. The role of the kidney in setting total systemic vascular resistance through the control of vasoactive substances, particularly angiotensin II, is well documented in some forms of hypertension.

The renal response to hypotension, sensed either at central vascular baroreceptors or at the renal efferent arteriole, is the generation and release of renin. Renin enzymatically converts plasma angiotensinogen into angiotensin I, which is converted into the potent vasoconstrictor angiotensin II (AII). AII increases systemic vascular resistance and blood pressure. AII stimulation of aldosterone secretion ultimately complements the vasoconstrictor effect through aldosterone-dependent augmentation of sodium absorption and an increase in ECF volume. Restoration of blood pressure may allow relaxation of this response, or maintenance of blood pressure may become dependent on its continuation.

The role of the kidney in decreasing systemic vascular tone is far less certain. Two potent vasodepressor substances, prostaglandins and kinins, are produced in the kidney. These compounds, however, probably act only as intrarenal vasodilators and have little or no systemic effect.

ACID-BASE REGULATION

The kidney contributes to acid-base homeostasis by the reclamation in the proximal tubule of the bulk of the filtered load of bicarbonate and by the generation in the distal tubule of new bicarbonate that replenishes the body buffer stores. Both bicarbonate reclamation and generation depend on the active secretion of hy-

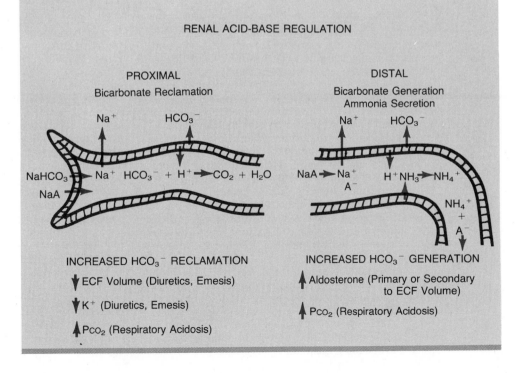

FIGURE 26–6. Scheme of renal acid-base regulation with representative reactions in both proximal and distal tubules.

drogen ion by the respective tubule segments (Fig. 26–6).

The filtered load of bicarbonate buffer amounts to about 4500 mEq daily. The proximal tubule has an apparent maximal reabsorptive rate for bicarbonate which can be increased by ECF volume depletion. Rates of bicarbonate reabsorption in the proximal tubule are also increased by an increase in P_{CO_2}, as occurs in chronic respiratory acidosis, or by hypokalemia. Conversely, ECF volume expansion or a lowering of P_{CO_2}, as seen in respiratory alkalosis, lowers the proximal tubular resorptive rate for bicarbonate. ECF volume contraction, an elevation of P_{CO_2}, and hypokalemia permit the maintenance of increased serum bicarbonate concentrations by increasing the rate of proximal tubular bicarbonate absorption. In contrast, BCF volume expansion and a lowered P_{CO_2} cause a reduction in the serum bicarbonate concentration.

As nonvolatile acid is formed from metabolic processes, bicarbonate is consumed in buffering the acid in the ECF. The acid anion is filtered at the glomerulus as a sodium salt. In the distal nephron, H^+ is excreted in an amount equal to the quantity of filtered acid anion. This H^+ is excreted in phosphate or ammonium buffer or as free proton. Bicarbonate, equivalent in amount to the H^+ secreted in the distal tubule, is added to blood, thereby replenishing the bicarbonate consumed in the original buffering reaction. About 50 to 70 mEq of acid is processed daily in this manner. Factors that increase H^+ secretion in the distal nephron, such as aldosterone or an elevated P_{CO_2}, may lead to the addition to blood of new bicarbonate that is in excess of that consumed in buffering metabolic acids.

MINERAL REGULATION

The kidney maintains the composition of the ECF with respect to a number of minerals. This section will consider the three most important of these: potassium, calcium, and magnesium. *Potassium*, the major intracellular cation, is freely filtered at the glomerulus and undergoes resorption along the length of the proximal nephron. In the distal nephron, potassium is secreted under the control of several influences. As noted above, aldosterone promotes potassium secretion in association with sodium absorption. Two other factors are also important determinants of the rate of potassium secretion. Distal nephron potassium secretion increases as the rate of fluid flow through the distal nephron increases and as the absolute amount of sodium delivered to the distal tubule increases. Thus, it is not surprising that the administration of diuretics that inhibit the absorption of sodium in the loop of Henle is associated with an increase in potassium secretion.

Conservation of potassium is less well regulated. While sodium can be virtually eliminated from the urine when aldosterone is present, the minimum urinary concentration of K^+ is seldom less than 10 to 12 mEq/L. Only when body and cellular potassium stores are severely depleted does the renal conservation of potassium become maximum.

Calcium reabsorption from the glomerular ultrafiltrate helps to regulate body calcium balance. The bulk of filtered calcium, about 60 per cent, is absorbed in the proximal tubule in parallel with sodium. Factors that change fractional proximal tubular reabsorption greatly influence calcium excretion. The separation of calcium from sodium absorption occurs in the cortical thick ascending limb and the distal convoluted tubule, where parathyroid hormone (PTH) uniquely governs the rate of calcium absorption.

While PTH-dependent calcium absorption acts efficiently to correct hypocalcemia, the renal response to hypercalcemia is less satisfactory. When PTH is suppressed, calcium excretion is increased as sodium excretion rises. However, hypovolemia, which often is associated with hypercalcemic states, usually causes renal sodium conservation and further increases in the tubular reabsorption of calcium. In addition, elevations of serum calcium to 12 to 15 mg/dl may suppress GFR by decreasing renal blood flow and further limit the urinary excretion of calcium.

Magnesium is absorbed in the proximal tubule at a rate less than that of sodium absorption, and the majority of magnesium absorption occurs in the loop of Henle. Both decreases in fractional proximal tubular absorption (ECF expansion) and decreases in NaCl absorption in the loop of Henle (diuretics) increase the excretion of magnesium. Renal loss of magnesium is a common cause of hypomagnesemia, and hypermagnesemia is almost always the result of severe decreases in GFR.

RENAL METABOLIC AND HORMONAL REGULATION

The kidney contributes to the metabolic degradation of a number of peptide hormones, including most pituitary hormones, glucagon, and insulin. Decreased renal catabolism of insulin in diabetics with renal insufficiency may be manifest as a prolongation of the effect of exogenous insulin.

Aside from regulation of calcium excretion, the kidney plays a major role in total calcium metabolism. Vitamin D, cholecalciferol, requires two in vivo hydroxylations to become the potent hormone that regulates intestinal calcium absorption. After hydroxylation in the liver at position 25 of the molecule, renal proximal tubular cells may add a second hydroxyl ion at the 1- or 24-position of the molecule. In the face of low serum ionized calcium, elevated PTH levels, and lowered cellular phosphorus, renal hydroxylation yields 1,25-dihydroxycholecalciferol, the potent hormonal form of the vitamin. Renal hydroxylation at all other sites on the molecule yields metabolites whose biological activities are less well defined.

The kidney is the major site for production of an erythrocyte-promoting factor, erythropoietin. This hormone is a highly glycosylated protein of 39,000 daltons which has at least two major actions in erythroid-producing tissue. Erythropoietin acts as a differentiating factor to promote transition of the erythrocyte colony–forming unit to the proerythroblast stage and as a growth factor to promote mitosis in the series of cells leading to the reticulocyte. Erythropoietin production increases in states of decreased tissue O_2 delivery. This may occur as a result of chronic hypoxemia, as seen in persons living at high altitudes or in patients with lung disease, or as a result of decreased O_2-carrying capacity of blood, as is seen in anemic individuals. The decline in erythropoietin production which accompanies the loss of renal mass in most forms of chronic renal disease accounts, in large part, for the chronic anemia of patients with chronic renal failure. Erythrocyte production in anephric individuals is apparently supported by the small amount of erythropoietin made in the liver (10 to 15 per cent of total under normal conditions).

REFERENCES

Ballerman BJ, et al: Atrial natriuretic peptide and the kidney. Am J Kidney Dis 10(S1):7–12, 1987.

Brenner BM, Stein JH (eds): Body Fluid Homeostasis. Contemporary Issues in Nephrology, Vol. 16. Edinburgh, Churchill Livingstone, 1987.

de Rouffignac C, and Jamison RL (eds): Symposium on the urinary concentrating mechanism. Kidney Int, Vol 31, No 2, 1987, pp 501–689.

Fried TA, Stein JH: Glomerular dynamics. Arch Intern Med 143:787–791, 1983.

Klahr S: Structure and function of the kidneys. *In* Wyngaarden JB, Smith LH Jr (eds): Cecil Textbook of Medicine, 18th ed. Philadelphia, WB Saunders Co, 1988, pp 508–520.

Knepper M, Burg M: Organization of nephron function. Am J Physiol 244:F579–589, 1983.

27

ELECTROLYTE AND VOLUME DISORDERS

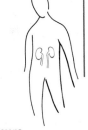

In health, the functional capacities of the mechanisms regulating water and electrolyte balance are so large that one can vary the intake of solutes and water over a wide range without developing perceptible metabolic disturbances. But when these mechanisms are impaired, the limits between which solute and water intake can be varied become narrower. This chapter considers four major derangements of fluid and electrolyte balance: volume disturbances, osmolality derangements, abnormalities of potassium balance, and acid-base disorders.

VOLUME DISORDERS

Protection of extracellular fluid volume is the most fundamental characteristic of fluid and electrolyte homeostasis. The mechanisms regulating volume balance respond primarily to changes in the effective circulating volume, that is, an arterial flow rate sufficient to maintain adequate perfusion of body tissues.

In healthy adults, body water comprises approximately 60 per cent of body weight and exists in two compartments: The intracellular compartment (ICF) contains two thirds of body water, or 40 per cent of body weight; the extracellular compartment (ECF) contains the remaining one third of total body water. Total blood volume, that is, plasma plus formed elements, constitutes one third of the total ECF volume. The transfer of fluid between vascular and interstitial compartments occurs at the capillary level and is governed by the balance between hydrostatic pressure gradients and plasma oncotic pressure gradients. Under normal circumstances, interstitial tissue pressure is low, and interstitial fluid is protein-poor. The oncotic pressure of plasma proteins is due principally to albumin. Details of the comparison of the body fluid compartments are considered in Chapter 26.

Two cardinal mechanisms protect extracellular fluid volume. These are alterations in systemic hemodynamic variables and alterations in external sodium and water balance. Table 27–1 summarizes some of the characteristics of the response to volume contraction.

TABLE 27–1. RESPONSE TO VOLUME CONTRACTION

	SYSTEMIC HEMODYNAMIC CHANGES	EXTERNAL SALT AND WATER BALANCE
Response	Tachycardia ↑ Peripheral resistance ↓ Venous capacitance	Thirst Renal Na^+, water retention
Onset	Minutes	Hours
Major activators	Catecholamines Angiotensin II ADH	Catecholamines Aldosterone ADH
Major inactivators	Prostaglandins Atriopeptin	Prostaglandins Atriopeptin

From Andreoli TE: Disorders of fluid volume, electrolyte, and acid-base balance. *In* Wyngaarden JB, Smith LH Jr (eds): Cecil Textbook of Medicine, 18th ed. Philadelphia, WB Saunders Co, 1988, p 529.

Chapter 26 provides a summary of the renal factors regulating volume homeostasis.

VOLUME DEPLETION

Volume depletion is the consequence of renal or extrarenal fluid losses. Table 27–2 lists the major groups of diseases which account for most states of true volume contraction.

Volume contraction can occur whenever there is loss of ADH or aldosterone. Untreated *diabetes insipidus*, either pituitary or nephrogenic, produces profound volume contraction and hypertonic encephalopathy in patients denied free access to water. Approximately 10 per cent of the glomerular filtrate, or about 18 L daily, reaches the early distal convoluted tubule. In diabetes insipidus, a large fraction of hypotonic tubular fluid may escape reabsorption, and the obligatory loss of solute-free water may be as high as 10 to 18 L daily. *Addison's disease* may impair aldosterone production and hence lead to renal sodium wasting. A second major cause of aldosterone lack occurs in *hyporeninemic hypoaldosteronism*, which may accompany interstitial renal disease. Other disorders that also impair renal tubular sodium or water conservation also lead to volume contraction. These include various tubular nephropathies, osmotic diuresis, and chronic renal failure.

The major extrarenal losses include *hemorrhage*, insensible water loss in *excessive sweating*, *burns*, which cause the loss of large amounts of plasma and interstitial fluid through burn areas, and *gastrointestinal* volume losses.

CLINICAL MANIFESTATIONS

The clinical findings in states of true volume contraction are referable both to underfilling of the arterial tree and to the renal and hemodynamic responses to this underfilling. In mild or partially compensated volume contraction, the patient may exhibit nothing more than mild postural giddiness, postural tachycardia, and weakness. In advanced stages of volume depletion, particularly those occurring acutely, there is recumbent hypotension, tachycardia, and a reduced urine volume. Finally, when volume contraction is severe, the combination of profound fluid loss and increased sympathetic activity produces circulatory collapse, recumbent tachycardia, and cold extremities.

The pulse, blood pressure, and changes of these variables with position, together with a clinical estimate of the venous pressure and skin temperature, provide an initial assessment of circulatory dynamics. Because these findings may be inconclusive in moderate degrees of volume contraction, invasive hemodynamic monitoring may be required in critically ill patients who are hemodynamically unstable. In such patients, the central venous pressure may correlate poorly with cardiac output and with pulmonary vascular volume. Measurement of the pulmonary capillary wedge pressure with a Swan-Ganz (flow-directed) catheter may therefore be required.

However, even the pulmonary capillary wedge pressure may remain within normal limits when blood volume has been reduced by 5 to 10 per cent. Consequently, a fluid challenge is useful in the evaluation of critically ill patients in whom a volume deficit is thought to be a contributory factor to a reduced cardiac output. A convenient way of achieving this goal is to administer 500 ml of normal saline over one to three hours and to measure the change in the pulmonary capillary wedge pressure of the cardiac output, as estimated by thermal dilution.

The initial renal responses to a decrease in effective circulating blood volume result in a fall in urine volume and a reduction in sodium excretion. Severe degrees of volume contraction also produce filtration rate reductions and prerenal azotemia. The urinary sodium concentration and the fraction of filtered sodium excreted in the urine are clinically useful indices to renal sodium avidity (see Chapter 26). In the volume-contracted state, the urinary sodium concentration is generally less than 10 mEq/L and the FE_{Na} is less than 1 per cent, whereas in acute tubular necrosis, the urinary sodium concentration is greater than 40 mEq/L and the FE_{Na} is greater than 1 per cent.

TREATMENT

The major goal of the treatment of volume contraction is to expand the effective circulating volume by replacing fluid deficits. The degree to which a given volume of crystalloid solution expands the effective circulating volume depends on solution composition. The infusion of 5 per cent glucose in water (D_5W) is equivalent to administering solute-free water that distributes uniformly in total body water. Since less than 10 per cent of total body water is in the intravascular compartment, infusion of 1 L D_5W expands the intravascular volume by 75 to 100 ml, that is, by about 2 per cent. Infusion of 1 L of a normal saline solution increases blood volume by about 300 ml, or about 6

TABLE 27–2. MAJOR CAUSES OF VOLUME DEPLETION

RENAL LOSSES	EXTRARENAL LOSSES
Hormone Deficit	**Hemorrhage**
Pituitary diabetes insipidus	**Cutaneous Losses**
Aldosterone insufficiency	Sweating
Addison's disease	Burns
Interstitial nephritis	**Gastrointestinal Losses**
Renal Deficit	Vomiting
Tubular nephropathies	Diarrhea
Renal tubular acidosis	Gastrointestinal fistulae
Bartter's syndrome	Tube drainage
Nephrogenic diabetes	
insipidus	
Diuretic abuse	
Post-obstructive diuresis	
Osmotic diuresis	
Chronic renal failure	

Adapted from Andreoli TE: Disorders of fluid volume, electrolyte, and acid-base balance. *In* Wyngaarden JB, Smith LH Jr (eds): Cecil Textbook of Medicine. 18th ed. Philadelphia, WB Saunders Co, 1988, p 531.

per cent; the remaining portion is distributed in the interstitial compartment. Colloid-containing solutions, such as iso-oncotic albumin solutions and plasma, preferentially expand the intravascular compartment, since large molecules like albumin are restricted mainly to the intravascular space. Finally, blood, which contains formed elements, is the most potent expander of the intravascular space. A unit of packed red blood cells will remain entirely in the vascular bed.

CIRCULATORY COMPROMISE WITHOUT TRUE VOLUME CONTRACTION

Table 27–3 lists some disorders in which inadequate arterial filling occurs in the absence of external fluid losses. A profound collapse of *cardiac output* may result in circulatory collapse because the heart fails to translocate blood adequately from venous to arterial beds. Circulatory collapse will also occur when there is a sudden *capacitance increase* in the venous part of the circulation. This occurs most commonly in sepsis. Finally, profound hypotension occurs when there are rapid *fluid shifts* from vascular to interstitial compartments, as in infarction of the small or large intestine, acute pancreatitis, and rhabdomyolysis.

VOLUME EXCESS

A convenient way of considering volume-expanded states is to view them in the context of three different classes of physiological explanations (Table 27–4).

The most common diseases encountered in which both volume expansion and edema occur are those disorders in which *derangements in the Starling forces* promote expansion of the interstitial compartment at the expense of the effective circulating volume. Consequently, renal sodium retention and edema occur. This group of disorders is characterized by increases in capillary hydrostatic pressure, decreases in capillary oncotic pressure, or a combination of these two factors. The plasma renin activity and aldosterone concentrations in these disorders tend to be elevated, although the results are variable.

The second category in Table 27–4 includes those disturbances in which there is *unregulated production of mineralocorticoids or ADH*. The volume expansion that occurs in primary hyperaldosteronism or in Cushing's syndrome is due to sodium retention and is accompanied by preferential expansion of the ECF and by hypertension. The serum sodium is generally normal or minimally elevated. In the syndrome of inappropriate ADH production (SIADH), primary water retention occurs with dilutional hyponatremia; hypertension is uncommon. Edema is not characteristic of either of these disorders.

Finally, acute glomerulonephritis is an example of unidentified *primary renal mechanisms* responsible for edema formation. Patients with acute glomerulonephritis retain salt and water and become hypertensive without reductions in glomerular filtration rate, when

TABLE 27–3. CIRCULATORY COMPROMISE WITHOUT EXTERNAL FLUID LOSSES

Impaired Cardiac Output
  Acute myocardial infarction
  Pericardial tamponade
Increased Vascular Capacitance
  Septic shock
Vascular → Interstitial Fluid Shifts
  Acute pancreatitis
  Bowel infarction
  Rhabdomyolysis
  Noncardiogenic pulmonary edema

From Andreoli TE: Disorders of fluid volume, electrolyte, and acid-base balance. *In* Wyngaarden JB, Smith LH Jr (eds): Cecil Textbook of Medicine. 18th ed. Philadelphia, WB Saunders Co, 1988, p 534.

TABLE 27–4. DISORDERS OF VOLUME EXCESS

I. Disturbed Starling Forces (Reduced effective circulating volume; edema formation)	II. Primary Hormone Excess (Increased effective circulating volume)
Systemic venous pressure increases	Primary aldosteronism
Right heart failure	Cushing's syndrome
Constrictive pericarditis	SIADH
Local venous pressure increases	
Left heart failure	III. Primary Renal Sodium Retention (Increased effective circulating volume)
Vena cava obstruction	
Portal vein obstruction	Acute glomerulonephritis
Reduced oncotic pressure	
Nephrotic syndrome	
Combined disorders	
Cirrhosis	

From Andreoli TE: Disorders of fluid volume, electrolyte, and acid-base balance. *In* Wyngaarden JB, Smith LH Jr (eds): Cecil Textbook of Medicine, 18th ed. Philadelphia, WB Saunders Co, 1988, p 535.

plasma renin activity and aldosterone concentration are normal or reduced, and when the serum albumin concentration is normal.

DIURETICS

Table 27–5 provides a summary of some of the major commonly used diuretics and certain of their properties. For convenience, the drugs are classified according to their sites of action in the nephron. Acetazolamide is a carbonic anhydrase inhibitor that blocks proximal reabsorption of sodium bicarbonate. Prolonged use of acetazolamide may lead to hyperchloremic acidosis. Metolazone is a congener of the thiazide class of diuretics which blocks sodium chloride absorption in two nephron sites.

Loop diuretics such as ethacrynic acid and furosemide produce diuresis by inhibiting the coupled entry of Na^+, K^+, and Cl^- across apical plasma membranes in the thick ascending limb of Henle. Loop diuretics are, for practical purposes, the most potent diuretics currently available and are therefore com-

TABLE 27–5. DIURETICS

	PRIMARY EFFECT	SECONDARY EFFECT	COMPLICATIONS
Proximal Diuretics			
Acetazolamide	↓ Na$^+$/H$^+$ exchange	↑ K$^+$ loss, ↑ HCO$_3^-$ loss	Hypokalemic, hyperchloremic acidosis
Metolazone	↓ Na$^+$ absorption	↑ K$^+$ loss, ↑ Cl$^-$ loss	Hypokalemic alkalosis
Loop Diuretics			
Furosemide } Ethacrynic acid }	↓ Na$^+$:K$^+$:2Cl$^-$ absorption	↑ K$^+$ loss, ↑ H$^+$ secretion	Hypokalemic alkalosis
Early Distal Diuretics			
Thiazide } Metolazone }	↓ Na$^+$ absorption	↑ K$^+$ loss, ↑ H$^+$ secretion	Hypokalemic alkalosis
Late Distal Diuretics			
Aldosterone antagonists Spironolactone Nonaldosterone antagonists Triamterene Amiloride }	↓ Na$^+$ absorption	↓ K$^+$ loss, ↓ H$^+$ secretion	Hyperkalemic acidosis

Adapted from Andreoli TE: Disorders of fluid volume, electrolyte, and acid-base balance. In Wyngaarden JB, Smith LH Jr (eds): Cecil Textbook of Medicine. 18th ed. Philadelphia, WB Saunders Co, 1988, p 536.

monly referred to as "high-ceiling" diuretics. Early distal tubule diuretics, such as thiazide and metolazone, interfere primarily with sodium chloride absorption in the earliest segments of the distal convoluted tubule.

Finally, Table 27–5 lists agents that inhibit sodium absorption in terminal regions of the distal tubule and therefore indirectly suppress potassium secretion and proton secretion. Spironolactone competes with aldosterone, whereas both triamterene and amiloride operate independently of aldosterone. Hyperkalemic, hyperchloremic metabolic acidosis may complicate the injudicious use of any of these three diuretics.

OSMOLALITY DISTURBANCES

In normal individuals, the serum osmolality is virtually constant. The mechanisms that adjust water balance in normal individuals are determined by changes in cell volume that result from variations in effective ECF osmolality. If the ECF osmolality is increased by solutes such as urea, which penetrate cell membranes readily, osmoregulatory mechanisms are not activated.

Since cell membranes are freely permeable to water, intracellular and extracellular osmolalities are identical. Cell membranes are partially permeable to sodium and potassium. Therefore there are leakages of sodium and potassium into and out of cells, respectively. These ionic leakages are counterbalanced exactly by active outward sodium transport coupled to inactive inward potassium transport, mediated by membrane-bound (Na$^+$ + K$^+$)-ATPase.

When the effective ECF osmolality is increased or decreased, there is a tendency for change in cell volume, and additional processes are called into play to maintain the constancy of cell volume. In hypotonic disorders, cell swelling is offset by the loss of potassium chloride from cells, activated by small increases in cell

volume produced by ECF dilution. In chronic hypernatremia, brain shrinkage is minimized by the accumulation of amino acids and other unidentified solutes, often called "idiogenic osmoles," within brain cells.

HYPOTONIC DISORDERS

A hypotonic disorder is one in which the serum osmolality and serum sodium are both reduced in parallel. True hypotonicity must be distinguished from disorders in which the *measured* serum sodium is low while the measured serum osmolality is either normal or increased. Hyperglycemia draws water from the cellular compartment. The serum sodium is therefore reduced even though the serum osmolality may be increased. When a small, nonsodium solute is distributed in total body water, as in ethanol intoxication or azotemia, the serum osmolality rises but the serum sodium concentration remains normal, resulting in an "osmolar gap."

Hyponatremia occurs because the ability of the kidney to excrete a maximally dilute urine is reduced. This inability to dilute urine occurs (1) because of reductions in the rate of salt absorption by the diluting segment, that is, the thick ascending limb of Henle; (2) because of sustained nonosmotic release of ADH; and (3) because of a combination of these factors. Table 27–6 summarizes these disorders. Profound hyponatremia is rare in primary polydipsia because the ability of the kidney to excrete large volumes of maximally dilute urine is not impaired.

Reduced sodium delivery to diluting segments occurs when a reduced sodium intake, without significant sodium depletion or ECF volume contraction, decreases the rate of sodium delivery to the diluting segment. Because sodium and urea are the major urinary solutes, dietary restriction of these solutes, particularly sodium, increases the fractional rate of proximal sodium absorption, diminishes the rate of salt delivery to diluting segments, and limits the daily rate of formation of dilute urine.

SIADH

The syndrome of inappropriate ADH production (SIADH) is the prototype disorder in which hyponatremia occurs as a result of *sustained endogenous production and release of ADH* or ADH-like substances. Table 27–7 lists the major causes of SIADH and Table 27–8 lists the typical features of SIADH. The cardinal results of the sustained water conservation in SIADH are hyponatremia and volume expansion. Patients with SIADH generally gain about 3 kg in water weight, or about 10 per cent of body water, but do not develop edema. The urine osmolality in patients with SIADH may be either inappropriately high for the level of serum osmolality or maximally dilute.

Finally, hyponatremia occurs commonly in conditions in which there is *reduced filling of the arterial tree.* These disorders include true volume depletion as well as edematous states. In both sets of disorders, two factors contribute to the pathogenesis of hyponatremia: nonosmotic, volume-mediated ADH release and reductions in the rate of sodium delivery to the diluting segment.

DIAGNOSIS

The clinical manifestations of hyponatremia are produced by the brain swelling that accompanies acute dilution of total body water and generally become manifest when the serum sodium concentration falls to 120 mEq/L or less. Early symptoms include lethargy, weakness, and somnolence, which proceed rapidly to seizures, coma, and death as hyponatremia worsens. Untreated acute water intoxication therefore represents a medical emergency. In chronic hyponatremia, central nervous system manifestations are far less common, even when the serum sodium concentration is as low as 110 mEq/L, because the loss of brain solutes minimizes brain cell swelling for a given reduction in body water osmolality.

The most difficult differential diagnosis among hyponatremic disorders involves the distinction between patients who are modestly volume contracted and those who have SIADH. When volume losses are due to extrarenal causes, the urinary sodium concentration is less than 10 to 15 mEq/L and the FE$_{Na}$ is generally less than 1 per cent. The presence of hyperuricemia may also be a useful index to the possibility of EFC volume contraction. Prerenal azotemia may also occur if the volume contraction is severe. In patients with SIADH, the BUN and creatinine are normal, the serum uric acid is generally reduced, the urinary sodium concentration usually exceeds 30 mEq/L, and the FE$_{Na}$ is greater than 1 per cent. Tests of adrenal function are normal. Importantly, the urine osmolality in SIADH need not be hypertonic; in fact, with significant hyponatremia, the urine osmolality in SIADH may become maximally dilute.

A useful diagnostic and therapeutic maneuver in

TABLE 27–6. HYPONATREMIA DUE TO IMPAIRED RENAL WATER EXCRETION

Reduced Sodium Delivery to the Diluting Segment
 Starvation
 Beer potomania
 ? Myxedema
Primary Excess of ADH
 SIADH
 Drug-induced ADH production
 Drug potentiation of ADH action
 Trauma
 Potassium depletion
 ? Myxedema
 ? Acute intermittent porphyria
Mixed Disorders
 Volume contraction (Addison's disease)
 Advanced edema states (congestive heart failure, constrictive pericarditis, and cirrhosis)

Adapted from Andreoli TE: Disorders of fluid volume, electrolyte, and acid-base balance. In Wyngaarden JB, Smith LH Jr (eds): Cecil Textbook of Medicine. 18th ed. Philadelphia, WB Saunders Co, 1988, p 538.

SIADH is to observe the results of water restriction. When water intake is restricted to 600 to 800 ml daily, patients with SIADH exhibit a 2- to 3-kg weight loss accompanied by correction of hyponatremia and cessation of salt wasting. If weight loss fails to correct hyponatremia and urinary sodium wasting simultaneously, the diagnosis of SIADH is doubtful.

TABLE 27–7. MAJOR CAUSES OF SIADH

Malignant Neoplasia
 Carcinoma: bronchogenic, duodenal, pancreatic, ureteral, prostatic, bladder
 Lymphoma and leukemia
 Thymoma and mesothelioma
CNS Disorders
 Trauma
 Infection
 Tumors
 Porphyria
Pulmonary Disorders
 Tuberculosis
 Pneumonia
 Ventilators with positive pressure

From Andreoli TE: Disorders of fluid volume, electrolyte, and acid-base balance. In Wyngaarden JB, Smith LH Jr (eds): Cecil Textbook of Medicine, 18th ed. Philadelphia, WB Saunders Co, 1988, p 539.

TABLE 27–8. MAJOR CHARACTERISTICS OF SIADH

Hyponatremia
Volume expansion without edema
Natriuresis
Hypouricemia
Normal or reduced serum creatinine
Normal thyroid and adrenal function

From Andreoli TE: Disorders of fluid volume, electrolyte, and acid-base balance. In Wyngaarden JB, Smith LH Jr (eds): Cecil Textbook of Medicine, 18th ed. Philadelphia, WB Saunders Co, 1988, p 539.

TREATMENT

The goal of treatment in hyponatremia is to correct body water osmolality and therefore restore cell volume to normal by raising the ratio of sodium to water in extracellular fluid. Acute hyponatremia associated with a serum sodium concentration below 120 mEq/L and central nervous system manifestations requires immediate therapy. The goal of therapy is to raise the serum sodium to 120 to 125 mEq/L acutely, with subsequent correction of the serum sodium to 140 mEq/liter gradually, over a 48- to 72-hour interval. One should not raise the serum sodium acutely to levels greater than 120 to 125 mEq/L because of the danger of CNS damage.

The choice of therapy varies with the condition. In volume-contracted states, the treatment of choice is to raise the serum sodium to 125 mEq/L over a six-hour interval by administering hypertonic 3 to 5 per cent saline. Hypertonic saline solutions are hazardous in volume-expanded, salt-retaining states such as congestive heart failure. Moreover, in SIADH associated with volume expansion and sodium wasting, hypertonic saline alone is ineffective in correcting hyponatremia because the administered salt is excreted promptly in a relatively concentrated urine. A preferable alternative in these instances is to use normal saline in combination with furosemide administration. The diuresis induced by furosemide is characterized by urine having a sodium concentration appreciably lower than that in plasma. Consequently, the combination of intravenously administered normal saline coupled with furosemide-induced diuresis provides an effective way of raising the serum sodium in SIADH or other volume-expanded states.

Chronic hyponatremia in SIADH may be corrected by restricting water intake. An alternative approach involves the use of agents such as lithium or demethylchlortetracycline, which interfere with the renal tubular effects of ADH.

TABLE 27–9. MAJOR CAUSES OF HYPERNATREMIA

Impaired Thirst
Coma
Essential hypernatremia

Solute Diuresis
Osmotic diuresis: diabetic ketoacidosis, nonketotic
    hyperosmolar coma, mannitol administration

Excessive Water Losses
Renal
    Pituitary diabetes insipidus
    Nephrogenic diabetes insipidus
Extrarenal
    Sweating

Combined Disorders
Coma plus hypertonic nasogastric feeding

From Andreoli TE: Disorders of fluid volume, electrolyte, and acid-base balance. *In* Wyngaarden JB, Smith LH Jr (eds): Cecil Textbook of Medicine. 18th ed. Philadelphia, WB Saunders Co, 1988, p 542.

HYPERTONIC DISORDERS

The most common causes of clinically significant hyponatremia occur as a consequence of three pathogenic mechanisms: *impaired thirst; osmotic diuresis;* and *excessive losses of free water*, either via the kidneys or extrarenally; and combinations of these derangements. These disorders are grouped in Table 27–9.

Inadequate intake of water occurs in patients who are comatose or otherwise unable to communicate thirst. Osmotic diuresis produces renal water losses in excess of sodium losses and therefore hypertonicity. This occurs commonly in uncontrolled glycosuria. Excessive water losses in pituitary or nephrogenic diabetes insipidus lead to profound water deficits and hyponatremia. The urine volumes are large, the urine osmolality is low, and the net rate of solute excretion is low. Finally, striking water losses also occur with excessive sweating.

DIAGNOSIS AND TREATMENT

Primary water losses tend to have modest effects on circulating volume unless fluid losses are profound. Rather, the clinical manifestations are produced by brain shrinkage and range from somnolence and confusion to coma, respiratory paralysis, and death. In acute hypertonicity, symptoms generally appear when the effective ECF osmolality exceeds 320 to 330 mOsm/kg H_2O. Chronic hypertonicity produces fewer central nervous system manifestations, because brain cells accumulate solutes that minimize the tendency to brain shrinkage.

The treatment of acute hypernatremia requires the administration of saline solutions by an intravenous route. In the severely volume-contracted patient with severe hypernatremia, the administration of isotonic saline solutions provides fluid resuscitation. The isotonic salt solution, which is hypotonic with respect to the hypertonic patient, also avoids an unnecessarily rapid fall in the serum sodium. In patients who are hypernatremic but not significantly volume contracted, more dilute salt solutions, such as half-normal saline, are appropriate for correcting hypernatremia.

The rapid correction of hypertonicity to a normal serum osmolality is hazardous, since a normal serum osmolality may be relatively hypotonic to brain cells that have accumulated solutes. A useful guide is to reduce the serum sodium by no more than 1 mEq/L during every two hours of the first two days of treatment.

POTASSIUM DERANGEMENTS

The total body potassium content is approximately 3500 mEq, of which only 60 mEq, or about 2 per cent of the total, is extracellular. Therefore the intracellular compartment acts as a large potassium reservoir in series with the small ECF potassium pool. The cardinal transport process regulating K^+ distribution between ICF and ECF is cell membrane–bound (Na^+ + K^+)-ATPase, which actively transports potassium into cells and therefore counterbalances the passive leak of potassium from cells into interstitial fluid. Insulin and beta-adrenergic agents such as epinephrine and isoproterenol also promote cellular uptake of potassium.

A number of passive processes also regulate the partition of potassium between the ICF and the ECF. Alterations in ECF pH reproducibly shift potassium between the ICF and the ECF. As a general rule, a plasma pH reduction of 0.1 unit raises the serum potassium by 0.6 mEq/L, while a plasma pH increase of 0.1 unit produces a similar reduction in serum potassium. Second, cellular shrinkage produced by increases in effective ECF osmolality raises the intracellular potassium concentration and thereby increases the driving force for passive potassium leakage from the ICF to the ECF. Finally, brain cells and other cells lose potassium chloride when exposed to chronic ECF hypotonicity.

The renal handling of potassium is discussed in Chapter 26. Virtually all dietary potassium, ordinarily about 50 to 200 mEq per day, appears in the urine because of tubular secretion of potassium by terminal nephron segments. The major factors enhancing distal nephron potassium excretion include increased distal tubular sodium delivery, increased dietary potassium intake, increased plasma pH, aldosterone, and excretion of impermeant anions.

The clinical consequences of hypokalemia and hyperkalemia are generally referable to changes in the excitable characteristics of heart, skeletal muscle, and smooth muscle. At rest, excitable tissues are far more permeable to potassium than to sodium. When excitable tissues are suddenly depolarized, there is a profound increase in sodium permeability. The accompanying rapid sodium entry into cells produces the initial spike of the action potential, and the cell interior becomes electropositive.

Hyperkalemia reduces the K_i/K_o ratio and consequently partially depolarizes electrical tissues at rest. Hyperkalemia also increases the potassium permeability of excitable cells and decreases the rate of sodium entry into cells during excitation. The net effect of progressive hyperkalemia is therefore to make the heart progressively refractory to excitation.

The effects of hypokalemia on excitable tissues are more complex. Because the K_i/K_o ratio rises in hypokalemia, excitable cells at rest should be hyperpolarized. This occurs initially, but resting depolarization eventually follows because the high K_i/K_o ratio, by itself, reduces the potassium permeability of excitable cells. The net effect of these changes in cardiac tissue is to increase the likelihood of sinus bradycardia, and, because of a prolonged relative refractory period, the risk of arrhythmia formation.

Figure 27–1 shows the typical electrocardiographic effects of hypokalemia and hyperkalemia. In hypokalemia, the V wave produced prolongation of the ST segment. In progressive hyperkalemia, the T waves peak first. Then there is loss of the P wave followed by QRS prolongation, resulting in the classic "sine wave" appearance.

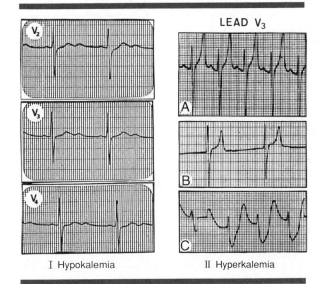

I Hypokalemia   II Hyperkalemia

FIGURE 27–1. Effects of hypokalemia and hyperkalemia on the electrocardiogram. I. The electrocardiographic manifestations of hypokalemia. The serum potassium was 2.2 mEq/L. Note that the ST segment is prolonged, primarily because of a V wave following the T wave, and that the T wave is flattened. II. The effects of progressive hyperkalemia on the electrocardiogram. All of the illustrations are from lead V_3. A, Serum K^+ = 6.8 mEq/L; note the peaked T waves together with normal sinus rhythm. B, Serum K^+ = 7.7 mEq/L; note the peaked T waves and absent P waves. C, Serum K^+ = 8.9 mEq/L; the classic sine wave with absent P waves, marked prolongation of the QRS complex, and peaked T waves. (From Andreoli TE: Disorders of fluid volume, electrolyte and acid-base balance. *In* Wyngaarden JB, Smith LH Jr (eds): Cecil Textbook of Medicine, 18th ed. Philadelphia, WB Saunders Co, 1988, pp 547–548.)

HYPOKALEMIA

Chronic hypokalemia indicates a reduction in total body potassium. A 1 mEq reduction in serum potassium generally implies the net loss of 100 to 200 mEq of potassium from the body. In extreme body potassium depletion, the serum potassium may be as low as 1.5 to 2.0 mEq/L. Acute reductions in serum potassium without parallel reductions in total body potassium occur when potassium is shifted from extracellular to intracellular compartments.

The four major causes of hypokalemia are given in Table 27–10. Reduced potassium intake may result in potassium depletion and hypokalemia because maximal renal conservation of potassium requires, as indicated above, 7 to 10 days. During this interval, the net renal potassium loss may be as much as 150 to 200 mEq.

Excessive renal losses of potassium may occur in states of mineralocorticoid excess, with diuretic excess, and during metabolic alkalosis. In fact, the hypokalemia associated with upper gastrointestinal fluid losses, as in vomiting or nasogastric suction, is primarily the result of the renal potassium losses pro-

TABLE 27–10. MAJOR CAUSES OF HYPOKALEMIA

Inadequate Intake
Excess Renal Loss
   Mineralocorticoid excess
   Bartter's syndrome
   Diuresis
      Diuretics with a pre-late distal locus
      Osmotic diuresis
   Chronic metabolic alkalosis
   Impermeant anion antibiotics
      Carbenicillin
   Renal tubular acidosis
Gastrointestinal Losses
   Vomiting
   Diarrhea, particularly secretory diarrheas
   Villous adenoma
ECF → ICF Shifts
   Acute alkalosis
   Hypokalemic periodic paralysis
   Insulin therapy
   Vitamin B_{12} therapy

Adapted from Andreoli TE: Disorders of fluid volume, electrolyte, and acid-base balance. In Wyngaarden JB, Smith LH Jr (eds): Cecil Textbook of Medicine. 18th ed. Philadelphia, WB Saunders Co, 1988, p 546.

duced by secondary hyperaldosteronism and/or bicarbonaturia. The potassium losses from the upper gastrointestinal tract are small, since upper gastrointestinal tract fluid contains only about 10 mEq/L of potassium.

Gastrointestinal losses provide the other major route for potassium depletion. Diarrhea produces significant potassium losses, since diarrheal fluid contains 30 mEq/L of potassium. The most striking diarrheal potassium losses occur in secretory diarrheas and

TABLE 27–11. HYPERKALEMIC SYNDROMES

Diminished Renal Excretion
   Reduced GFR
      Acute oliguric renal failure
      Chronic renal failure
   Reduced tubular secretion
      Addison's disease
      Hyporeninemic hypoaldosteronism
      Potassium-sparing diuretics
Transcellular Shifts
   Acidosis
   Cell destruction
      Trauma, burns
      Rhabdomyolysis
      Hemolysis
      Tumor lysis
   Hyperkalemic periodic paralysis
   Diabetic hyperglycemia
      Insulin dependence plus aldosterone lack
   Depolarizing muscle paralysis
      Succinylcholine

Adapted from Andreoli TE: Disorders of fluid volume, electrolyte, and acid-base balance. In Wyngaarden JB, Smith LH Jr (eds): Cecil Textbook of Medicine. 18th ed. Philadelphia, WB Saunders Co, 1988, p 547.

laxative abuse. Hypokalemia is uncommonly seen in inflammatory bowel disease.

Finally, acute hypokalemia with a normal total body potassium may occur because of *potassium shifts* from the ECF to the ICF. These shifts occur in *hypokalemic periodic paralysis* and with *insulin therapy*.

DIAGNOSIS AND TREATMENT

The most serious disturbances in hypokalemia are those affecting the neuromuscular system. At serum potassium concentrations in the range of 2 to 2.5 mEq/L, muscular weakness is likely to occur; with more severe hypokalemia, the patient may develop areflexic paralysis, in which case respiratory insufficiency is an immediate threat to survival. The severity of the neuromuscular disturbance tends to be proportional to the speed with which the potassium level has declined. Losses of large amounts of potassium from skeletal muscle may be accompanied by rhabdomyolysis and myoglobinuria. The electrocardiographic findings in hypokalemia are shown in Figure 27–1.

The treatment of hypokalemia involves replacement therapy with potassium salts and attempts to correct the underlying disorder. Except in extreme circumstances, oral rather than parenteral potassium replacement is prudent. In parenteral therapy, it is prudent to add potassium chloride to intravenous solutions at a final concentration of 40 to 60 mEq/L, and to administer no more than 10 to 20 mEq of potassium per hour. The serum potassium should be monitored at appropriate intervals. Parenteral potassium should be avoided in azotemic patients.

HYPERKALEMIA

Acute or chronic hyperkalemia occurs most commonly either because of diminished *renal excretion* or because there is a sudden *transcellular shift* of potassium from the ICF to the ECF. The major causes of hyperkalemia are listed in Table 27–11.

Hyperkalemia may occur in *acute oliguric renal failure* of any cause. In *chronic renal failure*, hyperkalemia generally does not occur until the glomerular filtration rate has reached markedly low levels. Hyperkalemia also occurs with small to modest reductions in the glomerular filtration rate, if there is impairment of potassium secretion by terminal nephron regions, as in *Addison's disease, hyporeninemic hypoaldosteronism*, and with the injudicious administration of *potassium-sparing diuretics*.

The second class of disorders causing acute hyperkalemia includes situations in which there is an abrupt shift of potassium from the ICF to the ECF. This occurs in acidosis or in circumstances that result in *cell destruction*.

Pseudohyperkalemia may occur in thrombocytosis or leukocytosis, because clotting of blood promotes potassium release from these cells. The *serum* potassium is elevated while the *plasma* potassium is normal. This kind of artifact occurs most commonly in patients with myeloproliferative disorders.

DIAGNOSIS AND TREATMENT

The most important clinical manifestations of hyperkalemia relate to alterations in cardiac excitability. For this reason, the electrocardiogram is the single most important guide in appraising the threat posed by hyperkalemia and in determining how aggressive a therapeutic approach is necessary. The electrocardiographic manifestations of hyperkalemia are shown in Figure 27-1.

Three kinds of maneuvers are used in the treatment of hyperkalemia: agents such as glucose plus insulin or sodium bicarbonate, which promote the transfer of potassium from the ECF to the ICF; maneuvers that enhance potassium elimination from the body, such as diuretics, exchange resins, or dialysis; and the use of calcium, which does not alter serum potassium concentrations but counteracts the effects of hyperkalemia on cardiac excitability.

The administration of 25 gm of glucose, together with 10 units of regular insulin, is an effective way of reducing the serum potassium rapidly. The administration of 40 to 150 mEq of sodium bicarbonate intravenously over a 30- to 60-minute interval also promotes potassium entry into cells.

Gastrointestinal potassium losses may be produced by the use of cation exchange resins in the sodium cycle, such as sodium polystyrene sulfonate (Kayexalate). Each gram of the resin contains approximately 1 mEq of sodium and exchanges for about 1 mEq of potassium. Sorbitol is used to suspend the resin. The sorbitol creates an osmotic diarrhea and enhances resin passage through the gastrointestinal tract. Acute hemodialysis or peritoneal dialysis provides another mechanism for potassium removal from the body.

In settings of extreme hyperkalemic cardiotoxicity, when P waves are absent and the QRS complexes are widened, the administration of calcium gluconate, 10 to 30 ml of a 10 per cent solution over a 10- to 20-minute interval, may be life-saving. The calcium salt does not reduce the serum potassium but counteracts the membrane effects of hyperkalemia.

ACID-BASE DISORDERS

The pH of arterial blood and interstitial fluid normally ranges between 7.38 and 7.42. The widest range of pH values compatible with life is from 6.8 to 7.8.

The major buffer system in extracellular fluid is the bicarbonate–carbonic acid pair. A convenient way to consider the total body buffering capacity is as follows: Bicarbonate is predominantly an extracellular anion, and the total ECF bicarbonate content in a 70-kg man having 15 liters of ECF is (24 mEq/L × 15 L), or 360 mEq HCO_3^-. However, about two thirds of a given acid or alkali load is buffered within cells. Consequently, the total body buffering capacity, often referred to as the "bicarbonate space," is calculated as:

$$\text{arterial } HCO_3^- \times 0.6 \text{ body weight}$$

that is, using total body water as an index to total buffering capacity.

ACID PRODUCTION AND ELIMINATION

The largest source of endogenous acid production is from combustion of glucose and fatty acids to carbon dioxide and water or, in other words, to a volatile acid. The average rate of metabolic water production, about 400 ml daily, yields 22,000 mmol of water and an equal number of carbon dioxide molecules. Thus, the rate of volatile acid production amounts to about 22,000 mEq of hydrogen ion daily.

Pulmonary ventilation excretes the carbon dioxide formed by cellular respiration. The primary factors normally regulating alterations in the rate of minute ventilation are subtle changes in cerebrospinal fluid (CSF) pH or arterial pH. On an average, for every 1 mEq/L reduction in plasma bicarbonate produced by metabolic acidosis, increased minute ventilation will produce a 1.2 mm Hg fall in the Pa_{CO_2}. Hyperventilation to Pa_{CO_2} values less than 10 mm Hg in metabolic acidosis almost never occurs. An increase in arterial pH reduces the rate of minute ventilation and therefore results in CO_2 retention. For increases in plasma bicarbonate concentrations to 35 mEq/L, the Pa_{CO_2} usually remains 50 mm Hg. When profound metabolic alkalosis occurs, the Pa_{CO_2} may rise further but virtually never exceeds 65 mm Hg.

In addition to volatile acid production, cellular metabolism also results in the formation of a number of nonvolatile acids. The major source for nonvolatile acid production is the metabolism of sulfur-containing amino acids such as cysteine and methionine. Nonvolatile acids also derive from oxidation of phosphoproteins and phospholipids, from nucleoprotein degradation, and from incomplete combustion of carbohydrates and fatty acids. The daily rate of nonvolatile acid production under normal conditions is about 1 mEq/kg of body weight.

Renal hydrogen ion excretion, which is equivalent to renal bicarbonate regeneration, occurs mainly as protons trapped in an undissociated form by urinary buffers.

The kidneys also filter large quantities of bicarbonate daily, and virtually all filtered bicarbonate is absorbed together with sodium by the proximal tubule. These renal mechanisms are discussed in Chapter 26.

pH DISEQUILIBRIA BETWEEN PLASMA AND CSF

Because central rather than arterial chemoreceptors are the prime sensors for pH-mediated changes in respiration, the ventilatory responses to pH changes mediated by respiratory processes or metabolic processes differ. The blood-brain barrier is freely permeable to carbon dioxide. Consequently, pH changes produced exclusively by hyperventilation or hypoventilation occur almost simultaneously in arterial plasma and in the CSF, and the respiratory response to primary increases or decreases in the Pa_{CO_2} occurs almost instantaneously. However, the blood-brain barrier imposes a lag in the rate at which arterial bicarbonate equilibrates with the CSF. Thus in metabolic acidosis, the arterial pH and bicarbonate concentrations fall more rapidly than that in the CSF; and in metabolic alkalosis, the CSF pH and bicarbonate concentrations rise more slowly than that in arterial plasma. Consequently, in the early stages of acute metabolic acidosis, there may be a one- to three-hour delay in the development of a maximal hyperventilatory response. Conversely, when metabolic acidosis is corrected rapidly, hyperventilation may persist for a few hours because of a delay in the rise of cerebrospinal fluid pH.

The Anion Gap. A convenient formula for calculating the anion gap is:

$$\text{anion gap} = Na - (Cl + HCO_3)$$

where Na, Cl, and HCO$_3$ are the serum sodium, chloride, and bicarbonate concentrations, respectively. The anion gap includes primarily phosphates and sulfates derived from tissue metabolism; lactate and ketoacids arising from incomplete combustion of carbohydrates and fatty acids; and negatively charged protein molecules, principally albumin. The normal value for unmeasured anions, or the anion gap, is 10 to 12 mEq/L; albumin and other proteins normally account for about half of the anion gap.

An *increased* anion gap generally indicates the presence of metabolic acidosis. The anion gap will be *reduced* if the sodium concentration falls while the chloride plus bicarbonate concentrations are unchanged. This may occur in multiple myeloma of the IgG variety, if the myeloma proteins are cationic at pH 7.4. Hyperviscosity syndromes may also result in a reduced anion gap because of a laboratory artifact. Rarely, lithium intoxication, hypermagnesemia, and hypercalcemia raise nonsodium cation concentrations sufficiently high to reduce the anion gap. The anion gap will also be decreased if the serum sodium concentration remains normal while the serum chloride plus bicarbonate concentrations are increased. This occurs in hypoalbuminemia and in bromide intoxication.

METABOLIC ACIDOSIS

A convenient way to consider the metabolic acidoses is to divide them into normal anion gap and increased anion gap acidoses. Table 27–12 presents a classification according to this format.

Normal Anion Gap Metabolic Acidosis

The metabolic acidoses have a *normal anion gap* result whenever there are abnormally high net bicarbonate losses. This may occur because the kidneys fail to reabsorb or regenerate bicarbonate, because there are extrarenal losses of bicarbonate, or because excessive amounts of substances yielding hydrochloric acid have been administered.

Bicarbonate losses occur either when the proximal tubule fails to absorb filtered bicarbonate or when there are losses of bicarbonate from the gastrointestinal tract. Renal bicarbonate wasting occurs in *proximal renal tubular acidosis*, with the administration of *carbonic anhydrase inhibitors*, and in primary *hyperparathyroidism*. *Diarrheal states* and *ileal drainage* also result in significant bicarbonate losses.

Hyperchloremic acidosis occurs in those disorders in which the ability of the distal nephron to regenerate bicarbonate is impaired, for example, *gradient-limited renal tubular acidosis* and chronic interstitial renal disease with *hyporeninemic hypoaldosteronism*. Finally, chloremic acidosis occurs with the administration of *acidifying salts*.

Increased Anion Gap Metabolic Acidosis

Metabolic acidoses characterized by an increased anion gap occur either because the kidneys fail to excrete inorganic acids, such as phosphate or sulfate, or because there is net accumulation of organic acids. Thus renal failure, either acute or chronic, results in metabolic acidosis with an increased anion gap due to retention of sulfates and phosphates. In chronic renal failure, metabolic acidosis occurs because the net amount of ammonium excreted daily falls as functional renal mass diminishes. In acute tubular necrosis, acidosis occurs because of impaired net acid excretion.

Organic acid accumulation represents the second major cause for metabolic acidosis with an increased anion gap. Normally, combustion of carbohydrates and fatty acids to carbon dioxide and water is highly efficient. Processes that impair cellular respiration therefore lead to profound metabolic acidosis.

Under these circumstances, the interplay of three cardinal factors determines the magnitude of the anion gap acidosis. One of these is the rate of lipolysis, regulated by insulin, and the rate of glycolysis. The second is the rate of cellular respiration, which in practical terms is determined by the rate of tissue perfusion

TABLE 27–12. MAJOR CAUSES OF METABOLIC ACIDOSIS

NORMAL ANION GAP	INCREASED ANION GAP
Bicarbonate Loss	**Reduced Excretion of Inorganic Acids**
Proximal renal tubular acidosis	Renal failure
Diarrheal states	**Accumulation of Organic Acids**
Small bowel drainage	Lactic acidosis
Ureterosigmoidostomy	Ketoacidosis: alcoholic
Failure of Bicarbonate Regeneration	diabetic
Distal, gradient-limited renal tubular acidosis	starvation
Hyporeninemic hypoaldosteronism	Ingestion: salicylates
Diuretics: triamterene, spironolactone	paraldehyde
Acidifying Salts	methanol
Ammonium chloride	ethylene glycol
Lysine hydrochloride	
Arginine hydrochloride	
Hyperalimentation	

Adapted from Andreoli TE: Disorders of fluid volume, electrolyte, and acid-base balance. *In* Wyngaarden JB, Smith LH Jr (eds): Cecil Textbook of Medicine. 18th ed. Philadelphia, WB Saunders Co, 1988, p 552.

with oxygen, and the functional state of mitochondria. The last factor is the extent of renal perfusion, which in turn regulates the proximal renal tubular threshold for organic acid excretion.

The syndrome of *lactic acidosis* results from impaired cellular respiration. Lactic acid is produced in muscle, red blood cells, and other tissues as a consequence of anaerobic glycolysis. Since lactic acidosis occurs because of impaired cellular respiration, the lactate to pyruvate ratio (L/P) rises. Lactic acidosis is also characterized by negative serum nitroprusside (Acetest) reactions, since Acetest tablets react with acetoacetic acid and acetone but not with beta-hydroxybutyric acid. Lactic acidosis occurs most commonly in disorders characterized by inadequate oxygen delivery to tissues, such as shock, septicemia, and profound hypoxemia.

A second cause of anion gap metabolic acidosis includes disorders in which accelerated rates of organic acid production, particularly from lipolysis, result in an increased anion gap. These include alcoholic ketoacidosis, *diabetic ketoacidosis*, and starvation. *Alcoholic ketoacidosis* occurs in patients with chronic alcoholism and a recent history of binge drinking, little or no food intake, and recurrent vomiting. Hypoglycemia may be present. These illnesses share at least one common feature: accelerated lipolysis and ketogenesis due to insulin lack.

Finally, a number of ingested substances result in severe metabolic acidosis. These agents are listed in Table 27–12.

DIAGNOSIS AND TREATMENT

The diagnosis of metabolic acidosis requires analysis of serum electrolytes and, when indicated, measurement of arterial pH and Pa_{CO_2}. A cardinal clinical manifestation of metabolic acidosis is hyperventilation, which, when severe, is manifest as Kussmaul respiration. Severe metabolic acidosis exerts a negative inotropic effect on the heart, which depends, at least in part, on the fact that acidosis diminishes tissue responsiveness to catecholamines. Acidosis shifts the oxyhemoglobin dissociation curve to the right. However, acidosis also tends to reduce red blood cell 2,3–DPG; this may offset partially the compensatory Bohr effect and aggravate inadequate tissue oxygenation in acidosis.

The treatment of metabolic acidosis varies depending on the underlying process and on acuteness and severity. In chronic renal failure, alkali therapy is generally not required unless the plasma bicarbonate falls below 16 to 18 mEq/L. In distal tubular acidosis, 30 to 60 mEq of bicarbonate daily usually corrects the acidosis.

The therapy of patients with *external bicarbonate loss* varies with the disorder. In gastrointestinal losses, bicarbonate therapy should be instituted when the arterial pH falls below 7.1.

The treatment of acidoses due to *accumulation of organic acids* varies with the disorder. In *lactic aci-*

TABLE 27–13. MAJOR MECHANISMS FOR METABOLIC ALKALOSIS

ECF volume contraction
Potassium depletion
Increased distal salt delivery
Mineralocorticoid excess
Liddle's syndrome
Bicarbonate loading (post-hypercapneic alkalosis)
Delayed conversion of administered organic acids

From Andreoli TE: Disorders of fluid volume, electrolyte, and acid-base balance. *In* Wyngaarden JB, Smith LH Jr: Cecil Textbook of Medicine. 18th ed. Philadelphia, WB Saunders Co, 1988, p 555.

dosis, therapy should be directed toward improving tissue perfusion. The response to alkali therapy is not predictable. In experimental lactic acidosis, bicarbonate therapy worsens the disorder by increasing the rate of splanchnic lactate production. The treatment of *alcoholic ketoacidosis* generally requires only the administration of saline solutions and glucose. In *diabetic ketoacidosis*, insulin therapy promotes glucose utilization and oxidation of ketoacids, and alkali therapy is ordinarily not required. Sodium bicarbonate therapy in diabetic ketoacidosis should be reserved for cases in which the arterial pH is below 7.0 to 7.1 and cardiac contractility is impaired.

METABOLIC ALKALOSIS

While metabolic alkalosis may be *initiated* by the loss of hydrogen ion from the body, the *maintenance* of a sustained metabolic alkalosis requires that the net rate of renal bicarbonate generation be greater than normal. Table 27–13 lists the major clinical causes of metabolic alkalosis.

The most common cause is hydrochloric acid loss because of vomiting or gastric suction. Volume con-

TABLE 27–14. ANION PATTERNS IN METABOLIC ACID-BASE DISORDERS

CONDITION	SERUM ANION CONCENTRATIONS		
	HCO₃⁻	Cl⁻	ANION GAP
Simple Disorders			
Hyperchloremic acidosis	↓	↑	nl
Anion gap acidosis	↓	nl	↑
Metabolic alkalosis	↑	↓	nl
Mixed Disorders			
Metabolic alkalosis + anion gap acidosis	nl, ↑ or ↓	↓	↑
Anion gap acidosis + hyperchloremic acidosis	↓	↑	↑
Metabolic alkalosis + hyperchloremic acidosis	nl	nl	nl

From Andreoli TE: Disorders of fluid volume, electrolyte, and acid-base balance. *In* Wyngaarden JB, Smith LH Jr (eds): Cecil Textbook of Medicine, 18th ed. Philadelphia, WB Saunders Co, 1988, p 556.

traction maintains the alkalosis by increasing the apparent proximal tubular threshold for bicarbonate. *Potassium depletion*, when sufficiently severe, can raise the rate of renal tubular bicarbonate reabsorption and hence maintain a metabolic alkalosis. When serum potassium concentrations are reduced to about 2 mEq/L, metabolic alkalosis due to gastric fluid loss becomes saline resistant but responsive to potassium chloride administration.

Situations in which there occurs *enhanced delivery of sodium chloride* to terminal nephron segments lead to metabolic alkalosis by increasing the rate of renal bicarbonate generation. This occurs with loop diuretics such as furosemide.

Mineralocorticoid excess, either primary or secondary, can result in metabolic alkalosis because of increased generation of bicarbonate by terminal nephron segments and is accentuated by potassium depletion.

Patients with chronic hypercapnia develop compensatory increases in plasma bicarbonate. If ventilatory status is improved acutely, the Pa_{CO_2} will fall quickly but the plasma bicarbonate will remain transiently elevated. Delayed conversion of *accumulated organic acids* is a second mechanism for producing transient metabolic alkalosis. This may occur after insulin therapy for diabetic ketoacidosis, during the recovery phase of lactic acidosis, and following high-efficiency hemodialysis.

DIAGNOSIS AND TREATMENT

Relatively severe metabolic alkalosis can result in cardiac arrhythmias. Severe metabolic alkalosis can also result in severe hypoventilation, especially in patients with reduced renal function.

The diagnosis is inferred in most cases from routine measurements of serum electrolytes and can be confirmed by arterial blood gas analysis. Hypokalemia is generally present. In volume-contracted states with alkalosis, the urinary chloride concentration is generally less than 10 mEq/L.

In metabolic alkalosis associated with hypokalemia and volume contraction, therapy consists of volume expansion with saline solutions and potassium replacement. If the metabolic alkalosis is sufficiently severe that significant hypoventilation is present, dilute hydrochloric acid or other acidifying salts may be required.

MIXED METABOLIC DISORDERS

Table 27–14 indicates the pattern of serum anion concentrations in single and mixed acid-base disorders. In the single acid-base disturbances, the change in the concentration of one anion is usually balanced by a reciprocal change in one other anion. In mixed disorders, the anion patterns are more complex. In a mixed metabolic alkalosis combined with an anion gap acidosis, the pattern is an increased anion gap offset partially or entirely by a reduction in chloride. In an anion gap acidosis with hyperchloremic acidosis, the reduction in bicarbonate is offset by increases in both chloride and the anion gap. In metabolic alkalosis combined with hyperchloremic acidosis, offsetting changes in serum bicarbonate and chloride concentrations may result in normal anion concentrations.

RESPIRATORY ACIDOSIS

Respiratory acidosis occurs whenever there is impairment in the rate of alveolar ventilation. *Acute respiratory acidosis* occurs when there is a sudden depression of the medullary respiratory center, as in narcotic overdose, with paralysis of the respiratory muscles, and when there is airway obstruction. *Chronic respiratory acidosis* generally occurs in individuals with chronic bronchitis, emphysema, and bullous lung disease; in patients with extreme kyphoscoliosis; and in individuals with extreme obesity (pickwickian syndrome).

The arterial pH and plasma bicarbonate concentrations differ in acute and chronic respiratory acidosis. The compensatory response to carbon dioxide retention is to increase the renal bicarbonate reabsorption. Since this compensatory increase in plasma bicarbonate concentration requires two to three days, the plasma bicarbonate is not increased in acute hypoventilation. A compensatory polycythemia also occurs commonly in chronic hypercapneic states.

DIAGNOSIS AND TREATMENT

Acute increases in Pa_{CO_2} values result in somnolence, confusion, and ultimately in CO_2 *narcosis*. Asterixis may also be present. Because carbon dioxide is a cerebral vasodilator, the blood vessels in the optic fundi are often dilated, engorged, and tortuous; in severe hypercapneic states, frank papilledema may occur.

The only practical treatment for acute respiratory acidosis involves treatment of the underlying disorder and ventilatory support. Drug abuse should always be considered in patients who suddenly develop acute respiratory depression. In patients with chronic hypercapnia who develop sudden Pa_{CO_2} increases, attention should be directed toward identifying factors that may have aggravated the disorder. Alkalinizing salts have no place in the management of chronic respiratory acidosis.

RESPIRATORY ALKALOSIS

Respiratory alkalosis occurs when hyperventilation reduces the arterial Pa_{CO_2} and consequently increases arterial pH. Acute respiratory alkalosis is most commonly the result of the hyperventilation syndrome. It may also occur because of damage to the respiratory centers; in acute salicylism; in fever and septic states; and in association with pneumonia, pulmonary emboli, or congestive heart failure. The disorder may also be produced iatrogenically by injudicious mechanical ventilatory support. Chronic hyperventilation occurs in the acclimation response to high altitudes (a low ambient oxygen tension), in advanced hepatic insufficiency, and in pregnancy.

MANIFESTATIONS AND TREATMENT

Acute hyperventilation is characterized by light-headedness, paresthesias, circumoral numbness, and tingling of the extremities. Tetany occurs in severe cases. When anxiety provokes hyperventilation, air rebreathing with a paper bag generally terminates the acute attack.

REFERENCES

Andreoli TE: Disorders of fluid volume, electrolyte, and acid-base balance. In Wyngaarden JB, Smith LH Jr (eds): Cecil Textbook of Medicine, 18th ed. Philadelphia, WB Saunders Co, 1988, pp 528–558.
Ballermann BJ, Brenner BM: Role of atrial peptides in body fluid homeostasis. Circ Res 58:619–630, 1986.
Foster DW, McGarry JD: The metabolic derangements and treatment of diabetic ketoacidosis. N Engl J Med 309:159–169, 1983.
Gabow PA, Kaehny WD, Fennessey PV, et al: Diagnostic importance of an increased serum anion gap. N Engl J Med 303:854–858, 1980.
Kokko JP, Tannen RL (eds): Fluids and Electrolytes. Philadelphia, WB Saunders Co, 1986.
Madias NE: Lactic acidosis. Kidney Int 29:752–774, 1986.
Needleman P, Greenwald JE: Atriopeptin: a cardiac hormone intimately involved in fluid, electrolytic, and blood pressure homeostasis. N Engl J Med 314:828–834, 1986.

28

ARTERIAL HYPERTENSION

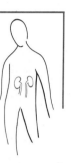

Elevation of the systemic arterial blood pressure represents one of the most common problems in clinical medicine. As many as 60 million Americans are hypertensive. Although the majority of these individuals are asymptomatic, chronic elevation of the systemic arterial blood pressure can lead to significant morbid sequelae, including congestive heart failure, myocardial infarction, cerebrovascular accident, and/or renal insufficiency. Effective therapy is now available for the patient with hypertension. Many of the undesirable complications of this disease can be prevented if hypertension is detected and treated properly.

DEFINITION AND EPIDEMIOLOGY

The dividing line between normal and elevated blood pressure is not absolute, a fact that makes a precise definition of hypertension difficult. Studies indicate that the morbidity and mortality related to an elevation in blood pressure increase in direct proportion to the level of systolic and diastolic blood pressure, beginning at levels well below 140/90. However, a blood pressure in excess of 140/90 is generally considered the point at which a patient can be considered hypertensive, particularly if the elevation is reproduced on at least two occasions. Hypertension is typically classified as mild, moderate, or severe depending on the level of the diastolic blood pressure (Table 28–1). However, isolated systolic hypertension may occur and is defined as a systolic blood pressure greater than or equal to 160 mm Hg associated with a diastolic blood

pressure less than 85 mm Hg. The blood pressure in healthy children and pregnant women is typically lower, so that readings in excess of 120/80 may indicate an abnormal elevation in blood pressure.

In the United States, approximately 15 per cent of the adult white population and 25 per cent of the adult black population can be considered hypertensive. Many factors affect the risk of developing hypertension in an individual patient. The incidence of the disease increases with age. Heredity plays a strong role, with approximately 80 per cent of hypertensive patients displaying a positive family history. Obesity and the dietary intake of sodium are two other variables that increase the risk of hypertension in susceptible individuals. Whereas heredity and age cannot be controlled, factors such as body weight and diet can be modified.

TABLE 28–1. CLASSIFICATION OF HYPERTENSION

RANGE (mm Hg)	CLASSIFICATION
DIASTOLIC	
<85	normal
85–89	high normal
90–104	mild hypertension
105–114	moderate hypertension
>115	severe hypertension
SYSTOLIC (when diastolic <90)	
<140	normal
140–159	borderline systolic hypertension
>160	isolated systolic hypertension

THE PATHOPHYSIOLOGY OF HYPERTENSION

A review of the physiological determinants of normal blood pressure provides a way of introducing the factors that play a role in the development of hypertension. The blood pressure is generated by cardiac contraction, which produces its maximal pressure, the systolic blood pressure, during ejection. This is followed by cardiac relaxation, which results in a fall in blood pressure to its nadir level, the diastolic blood pressure. The mean arterial blood pressure lies between the systolic and diastolic pressure and can be defined as a function of cardiac output and systemic vascular resistance (Fig. 28–1). The mean arterial pressure is tightly regulated within a range that maintains tissue perfusion but minimizes vascular trauma. Multiple factors impact on the control of blood pressure by mechanisms that affect either cardiac output or systemic vascular resistance (Fig. 28–1).

The first of these is the baroreceptor reflex, a virtually instantaneous response that regulates the blood pressure by controlling autonomic discharge from the brain stem. Fluctuations in the mean arterial pressure are detected by specialized receptors in the carotid sinus which relay information rapidly to the brain stem. Adrenergic outflow from the brain stem directly modifies the heart rate, cardiac contractility, and sys-temic vascular resistance to restore the blood pressure toward its prior set point.

The second mechanism involves the renin-angiotensin system. The kidney produces renin, an enzyme that acts on a plasma protein, termed renin substrate, to form angiotensin I, which is subsequently converted, primarily in the lungs, to angiotensin II. Angiotensin II is a potent vasoconstricting hormone that raises systemic vascular resistance. Angiotensin II also stimulates the adrenal gland to synthesize aldosterone, a mineralocorticoid hormone that promotes the reabsorption of sodium and water by the kidney. Stimulation of the renin-angiotensin system, therefore, produces vasoconstriction and renal sodium and water retention. Multiple factors affect the release of renin from the juxtaglomerular cells of the kidney, including alterations in renal perfusion pressure, changes in the sodium content of the distal renal tubule, beta-adrenergic stimuli, and the influence of locally produced prostaglandins.

Third, the extracellular fluid volume affects the systemic arterial blood pressure. The kidney plays an important role in the regulation of extracellular volume at a level that allows for adequate tissue perfusion. In states of extracellular fluid volume depletion, the kidney responds with avid reabsorption of sodium and water from the renal tubules. Conversely, if the blood pressure rises because of an increased plasma volume,

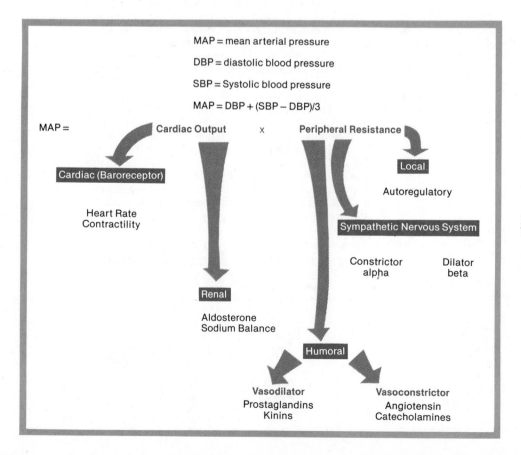

MAP = mean arterial pressure

DBP = diastolic blood pressure

SBP = Systolic blood pressure

MAP = DBP + (SBP − DBP)/3

MAP =   Cardiac Output   x   Peripheral Resistance

Cardiac (Baroreceptor)

Heart Rate
Contractility

Local

Autoregulatory

Sympathetic Nervous System

Constrictor   Dilator
alpha   beta

Renal

Aldosterone
Sodium Balance

Humoral

Vasodilator   Vasoconstrictor
Prostaglandins   Angiotensin
Kinins   Catecholamines

FIGURE 28–1. Determinants of blood pressure.

the kidney undergoes a natriuresis in order to return plasma volume to its baseline.

Other factors including the sympathetic nervous system, vasodilating hormones such as the prostaglandins and kinins, and local autoregulatory forces all impact on systemic vascular resistance and hence on the control of blood pressure.

CLINICAL ASPECTS OF HYPERTENSION

The vast majority of patients with hypertension (90 to 95 per cent) will not have a definable cause for their disease and are given the diagnosis of primary or essential hypertension. Essential hypertension, rather than a discrete entity, represents a heterogeneous syndrome in which multiple factors contribute to the elevated blood pressure through an effect on cardiac output, systemic vascular resistance, and/or sodium balance.

Pathophysiologically, the initial phase of hypertension may be characterized by an increase in cardiac output and/or systemic vascular resistance. Established hypertension, however, is most often maintained by an elevated systemic vascular resistance as cardiac output returns to normal. The kidney likely plays an important role in the maintenance of hypertension by the upward "resetting" of the pressure level at which natriuresis occurs. Furthermore, the enhanced vascular tone in hypertensive patients may be the result of the influence of angiotensin II, sympathetic nervous system discharge, arteriolar hyperplasia, and other factors (Fig. 28–1).

Although essential hypertension is usually detected during middle age, the disease probably begins during the early teenage years. It is typically of insidious onset and asymptomatic for many years. If the hypertensive patient remains undetected or is inadequately treated, morbidity and mortality may be significant. Although elevated blood pressure in itself can lead to vascular injury and end-organ damage, a second major mediator of disease in the hypertensive patient is accelerated atherosclerosis. The most commonly involved target organs are the brain, heart, kidney, and major blood vessels (Table 28–2). The major causes of death in the hypertensive patient relate to these pathological processes, with myocardial infarction and cerebrovascular accident the most common sequelae. These complications can largely be prevented if effective treatment is instituted before the development of irreversible end-organ damage.

The approach to the patient with hypertension begins with an evaluation of the severity of disease as assessed by its effect on target organs. The physical examination should include a careful evaluation of the optic fundus, which provides an assessment of the vascular effects of hypertension. The presence of grade III (hemorrhages and exudates) or grade IV retinopathy (papilledema) indicates severe hypertension. Routine laboratory studies in a newly diagnosed hy-

TABLE 28–2. HYPERTENSIVE COMPLICATIONS

TARGET ORGAN	HYPERTENSIVE	ATHEROSCLEROTIC
Brain/eye	Intracerebral hemorrhage	Thrombotic stroke
	Lacunar infarcts	TIA
	Encephalopathy	
	Fundal hemorrhages, exudates, papilledema	
Heart	Congestive failure	Myocardial infarct
	Ventricular hypertrophy	Angina
Kidney	Nephrosclerosis	Renal artery stenosis
Vessels	Aortic dissection	Diffuse atheromata

pertensive patient should include an electrocardiogram, complete blood count, urinalysis, and blood chemistries such as serum electrolytes, creatinine, glucose, triglycerides, cholesterol, and uric acid.

A subset of patients with hypertension may develop rapidly progressive, aggressive disease that is termed accelerated or malignant hypertension. This disease is characterized by a severe elevation of blood pressure (diastolic values usually in excess of 120 mm Hg and as high as 150 mm Hg) associated with widespread end-organ dysfunction. If untreated, irreversible tissue damage and death is the typical outcome. Diffuse fibrinoid necrosis of arterioles is the common pathological finding. The patient most often appears ill and may have complaints of headache, blurred vision, and dyspnea. The typical retinal findings include papilledema, fundal hemorrhages, and infarctions (cotton wool spots). Encephalopathy and congestive cardiac failure may also occur. Microangiopathic hemolytic anemia is common, and renal function may be significantly impaired.

REMEDIABLE CAUSES OF HYPERTENSION

Only 5 to 10 per cent of patients with hypertension are found to have a secondary cause of their elevated blood pressure (Table 28–3). However, because the management of hypertension in these individuals is significantly different and the disease potentially curable, it is important to consider these conditions. A detailed evaluation designed to exclude all causes of secondary hypertension is not warranted in most patients. However, a more thorough investigation should be pursued in the young patient with severe hypertension, the individual whose blood pressure is poorly controlled on antihypertensive therapy, and the person whose initial screening evaluation is suspicious for the presence of an underlying cause.

A brief description of the major causes of secondary hypertension and the approach to diagnosis are as follows.

Renovascular Hypertension. In this condition one or both renal arteries are affected by a stenotic lesion that causes renal ischemia and subsequent stimulation of the renin-angiotensin system. In the initial phase

TABLE 28–3. SECONDARY CAUSES OF HYPERTENSION

CAUSE	SYMPTOMS/SIGNS	ASSOCIATIONS	CONFIRMATION
Renovascular	Flank bruit, diffuse atherosclerosis	$\downarrow$ K$^+$, $\uparrow$ Creatinine	Arteriogram, $\uparrow$ Renal vein, renin level
Renal disease	Edema	Acute/chronic renal disease	$\uparrow$ Creatinine, $\uparrow$ BUN
Pheochromocytoma	Paroxysmal sweating, palpitations, flushing, headache, weight loss, episodic hypertension, tachycardia, orthostatic hypotension	$\uparrow$ Urine VMA, metanephrines, catecholamines	CT scan, arteriography
Mineralocorticoid excess	Weakness, muscle cramps	Hypokalemia, alkalosis, $\downarrow$ renin	$\uparrow$ Aldosterone level, CT scan
Aortic coarctation	$\uparrow$ BP in arms, $\downarrow$ BP in legs	Rib notching on chest x-ray	Arteriography

of renal artery stenosis, hypertension is mediated by the excessive production of renin, with subsequent vasoconstriction and volume expansion induced by angiotensin II and aldosterone. In this phase, the disease is responsive either to repair of the vascular stenosis or to angiotensin blockade with converting enzyme inhibition. The chronic or late phase of renovascular hypertension is characterized by a poor response to these measures owing to the development of contralateral renal parenchymal disease that sustains the hypertension by mechanisms other than excessive release of renin.

The stenotic renal vascular lesions are of two major varieties. The first, termed fibromuscular dysplasia, is characterized by proliferation of the vascular media and occurs most commonly in young, otherwise healthy women. The second and most common stenotic lesion is an atheromatous plaque that affects the proximal renal artery. Older individuals with widespread atherosclerotic disease are most susceptible. On physical examination, renovascular hypertension is suggested by the presence of a flank or abdominal bruit. Hypokalemic metabolic alkalosis related to chronic stimulation of aldosterone can be observed. Renal dysfunction manifested by an evaluation in serum creatinine may also be present.

The diagnosis of renovascular hypertension usually requires a renal arteriogram to assess the vascular anatomy of the kidney and selective renal vein renin studies to confirm the role of renin excess in the pathogenesis of the hypertension. Unilateral renal artery stenosis is characterized by an elevated venous renin level on the affected side and a suppressed level on the contralateral side. Unfortunately, there are few simple screening tests for renovascular hypertension. The captopril challenge test, however, is emerging as a promising, noninvasive means of assessing for potential renovascular disease. The acute administration of this angiotensin-converting enzyme inhibitor to a patient with hemodynamically significant renal artery stenosis results in an acute rise in the plasma renin activity.

The treatment of renovascular hypertension must be individualized. Surgical revascularization or transluminal angioplasty of the stenotic lesion can be curative in some patients. In others, notably the elderly or those with other complicated medical problems, management with angiotensin-converting enzyme inhibitors and/or other antihypertensive drugs is the better choice.

Parenchymal Renal Disease. Hypertension is commonly associated with a variety of acute or chronic renal diseases. The mechanism is most often the consequence of hypervolemia, although in some patients the renin-angiotensin system mediates the hypertension. Although most chronic renal diseases cannot be reversed, treatment of the associated hypertension may slow the progression of the renal insufficiency and reduce the risk of other morbid complications.

Pheochromocytoma. Hypertension is the hallmark of pheochromocytoma, a rare tumor of chromaffin cells that secretes norepinephrine and/or epinephrine. These tumors are most often located within the adrenal medulla but may arise along the sympathetic ganglia of the abdomen and chest. Patients typically describe symptoms of paroxysmal sweating, flushing, palpitation, and orthostasis in association with intermittent hypertension. However, some patients present with sustained hypertension without these classic findings. The diagnosis is made by detecting elevated excretion of catecholamines or the metabolites vanillylmandelic acid (VMA) and metanephrine in the urine. The tumor can usually be localized by computed tomography of the abdomen or chest. Surgical removal of the tumor is the preferred treatment for pheochromocytoma, but preoperative control of the blood pressure and extracellular fluid volume is critically important.

Mineralocorticoid Excess. Primary aldosteronism is an important cause of mineralocorticoid-mediated hypertension and is most commonly the result of an autonomous, benign adrenal adenoma. Bilateral adrenal hyperplasia or adrenal carcinoma is less frequently observed. Hypertension in these disorders results from volume expansion induced by augmented tubular sodium and water reabsorption by the kidney. The major symptoms in these patients are referable to mineralocorticoid-mediated hypokalemic metabolic alkalosis. The diagnosis is suggested by the detection of elevated levels of aldosterone in the plasma or urine, in association with a low renin level. The hallmark of primary aldosteronism is a lack of aldosterone suppression by maneuvers such as saline volume expansion or converting enzyme inhibition. Anatomic confirmation of the disease requires either computerized scanning of the adrenal gland or selective adrenal venous sampling for aldosterone. Individuals with an adrenal tumor should be considered for surgical removal. Patients who are poor surgical candidates or have bilateral adrenal hyperplasia can often be managed medically with an aldosterone antagonist such as spironolactone in combination with other antihypertensive drugs.

Coarctation of the Aorta. Coarctation of the aorta is a congenital disorder in which the aorta is narrowed, usually just distal to the left subclavian artery. Mechanical impairment of blood flow to the kidneys results in stimulation of the renin-angiotensin axis, which initiates the hypertensive response to aortic coarctation. The hallmark on physical examination is an elevated blood pressure in the arms associated with a lower blood pressure in the legs. The disease is most commonly diagnosed during childhood, and the treatment is surgical repair of the vascular narrowing.

TREATMENT OF HYPERTENSION

The goal of treatment in the hypertensive patient is to reduce the risk of morbid sequelae and death due to cerebrovascular, cardiovascular, and renal disease. Individuals with diastolic blood pressures consistently greater than 95 mm Hg benefit from treatment directed at lowering blood pressure. For individuals with diastolic blood pressures between 90 and 95 mm Hg, the therapeutic approach should be individualized. If other risk factors such as diabetes mellitus or hyperlipidemia are present, treatment should be strongly considered. Antihypertensive therapy should aim to maintain the diastolic blood pressure below 90 mm Hg or at the lowest level consistent with patient tolerance.

Antihypertensive therapy includes nonpharmacological intervention as well as specific drug treatment. The former approach includes such recommendations as dietary sodium restriction, exercise, weight loss, behavior modification, and the limitation of heavy al-

TABLE 28–4. COMMONLY PRESCRIBED ORAL ANTIHYPERTENSIVE DRUGS

CLASSIFICATION	EXAMPLE	MECHANISM	SIDE EFFECTS	PRECAUTIONS/ CONSIDERATIONS
Diuretics	Thiazide, furosemide	Salt/water diuresis	Hypokalemia, hyperuricemia, hyperglycemia	Furosemide is more useful in chronic renal insufficiency
	Spironolactone	Aldosterone antagonist	Hyperkalemia	Should be avoided in renal insufficiency
Beta-adrenergic blockers	Propranolol	↓ Cardiac contractility and heart rate, may ↓ renin release	Bradycardia, fatigue, insomnia	Avoid in patients with obstructive airway disease, congestive heart failure, heart block
Central adrenergic inhibitors	Clonidine, methyldopa	Decreased CNS sympathetic outflow	Drowsiness, dry mouth, fatigue, sexual dysfunction	Rapid clonidine withdrawal may lead to rebound hypertension
Peripheral adrenergic inhibitors	Guanethidine	Vasodilation	Orthostatic hypotension, sexual dysfunction	Use with caution in the elderly
Alpha-1–adrenergic blocker	Prazosin	Vasodilation	"First dose" hypotension, orthostatic hypotension, tachycardia	Tachyphylaxis to drug effect often noted
Combined alpha/beta blocker	Labetalol	↓ Cardiac contractility and heart rate, vasodilation	Dizziness, fatigue, headache	Avoid in patients with obstructive airway disease, congestive heart failure, heart block
Vasodilators	Hydralazine, minoxidil	Vasodilation	Tachycardia, fluid retention	Positive antinuclear antibody, lupus syndrome with hydralazine, hypertrichosis with minoxidil
Calcium channel blockers	Nifedipine	Vasodilation	Tachycardia, fluid retention	Usually combined with beta blockers; useful in patients with hypertension and heart failure
Angiotensin-converting enzyme inhibitor	Captopril	Inhibition of angiotensin II production	Skin rash, neutropenia	May cause worsening of renal function, proteinuria in patients with renal disease

TABLE 28–5. PARENTERAL DRUGS FOR HYPERTENSIVE EMERGENCIES

DRUG	ADVANTAGES	PRECAUTIONS/ CONSIDERATIONS
Vasodilators		
Nitroprusside	Rapid onset, allows effective titration of blood pressure, no sedation	Requires intensive care monitoring with arterial line, thiocyanate toxicity with prolonged use
Diazoxide	Rapid onset	Large boluses may cause severe hypotension, prolonged effect, sodium retention, reflex tachycardia, angina
Hydralazine	IM preparation	Reflex tachycardia, angina
Nitroglycerin	Dilates coronary vessels, rapid onset	Requires intensive care monitoring, may cause flushing and headache
Adrenergic Inhibitors		
Trimethaphan	Rapid onset, allows effective titration of blood pressure	Bowel/bladder atony, useful in hypertensive crisis of aortic dissection
Methyldopa	Gradual fall in blood pressure	Inconsistent effect, sedation
Labetalol	Little reflex tachycardia, prolonged duration	Bronchospasm, bradyarrhythmias; avoid with left ventricular failure

cohol or tobacco consumption. These interventions may be all that is required in the patient with mild hypertension (diastolic blood pressure 90 to 95 mm Hg). Antihypertensive drugs are almost always necessary in the management of most other patients but should be prescribed as an adjunct to the nonpharmacological therapy outlined above.

The majority of individuals with hypertension can be treated effectively in the outpatient setting if the response to antihypertensive therapy is monitored closely and the potential adverse side effects of drug treatment are recognized (Table 28–4). Traditionally, the thiazide diuretics or beta-adrenergic blocking drugs have been the initial choice(s) for the management of hypertensive patients. Other drugs have been added to this regimen to obtain optimal control of the blood pressure. This "stepped care" approach to drug treatment has been superseded in recent years by a more individualized approach to drug therapy which acknowledges the variable efficacy and patient tolerance to antihypertensive agents.

The patient with a mild or moderate elevation in blood pressure is often managed effectively with either a single antihypertensive agent or a combination of two complementary drugs. Although diuretics or beta-adrenergic blockers can be prescribed as initial therapy, the calcium channel blocking drugs and angiotensin-converting enzyme inhibitors are popular choices either as monotherapy or in conjunction with a diuretic for many hypertensive patients. Centrally acting adrenergic inhibitors are also commonly prescribed. The dose of each drug should be increased as needed to achieve the therapeutic goal in blood pressure reduction unless unacceptable side effects occur. In these cases, an alternate drug should be substituted. Individuals with more severe elevations in blood pressure will often require more than two antihypertensive drugs for optimal control. These drug regimens typically include a diuretic, a vasodilator, and an adrenergic inhibitor.

Hypertensive emergencies require a more aggressive approach to treatment. Management in a hospital setting, often in the intensive care unit, is required in order to minimize damage to target organs such as the brain, heart, and kidney. Parenterally administered antihypertensive drugs such as sodium nitroprusside, labetalol, hydralazine, and diazoxide are often indicated for optimal management of these critically ill patients (Table 28–5). In other severely hypertensive individuals without signs of end organ dysfunction, treatment with oral agents such as clonidine or calcium channel blockers may be effective in lowering the blood pressure acutely.

REFERENCES

Detection, evaluation, and treatment of renovascular hypertension. Final Report of the Working Group on Renovascular Hypertension. Arch Intern Med 147:820, 1987.

Ferguson RK, Vlasses PH: Hypertensive emergencies and urgencies. JAMA 255:1607, 1986.

Hypertension prevalence and the status of awareness, treatment, and control in the United States. Final Report of the Subcommittee on Definition and Prevalence of the 1984 Joint National Committee. Hypertension 7:457, 1985.

Joint National Committee on detection, evaluation, and treatment of high blood pressure. The 1988 report of the Joint National Committee. Arch Intern Med 148:1023–1038, 1988.

29

ACUTE RENAL INSUFFICIENCY

Acute or subacute declines in the glomerular filtration rate and/or in tubular function (acute renal insufficiency) can occur in a variety of clinical settings and as a consequence of different types of insults to the kidney (Table 29–1). Decreases in the effective circulating blood volume or in renal blood flow may result in a decline in the glomerular filtration rate with relatively intact tubular function. Such conditions are termed prerenal azotemia. Obstruction to urine flow results in an acute decrease in renal function and the development of obstructive nephropathy. Renal parenchymal inflammatory diseases such as glomerulonephritis and interstitial nephritis can also result in acute changes in kidney function. The term *acute tubular necrosis* (ATN) designates a clinical syndrome in which there is a simultaneous and progressive deterioration of both glomerular and tubular function in the absence of documented glomerular or interstitial nephritis, vascular disease, or obstruction of the collecting system. Although the name acute tubular necrosis is not a valid histological description of this syndrome (see page 213), this terminology is widely used and will be employed in this chapter. Synonyms for acute tubular necrosis include vasomotor nephropathy, toxic nephropathy, and the acute renal failure syndrome. Acute tubular necrosis usually refers to rapid changes in renal function consequent to a severe reduction in the effective circulating extracellular fluid volume and/or the ingestion, administration, or generation of substances that are directly toxic to the renal tubular cells. In the clinical setting, the diagnosis of ATN is often suggested from the history and physical examination of the patient but is, in fact, a diagnosis of exclusion. Said in another way, it is necessary to exclude carefully the other defined renal syndromes before concluding that ATN is present.

CLINICAL PRESENTATION

Renal insufficiency results in signs and symptoms that reflect loss of the regulatory, excretory, and endocrine functions of the kidney. The inability to regulate the volume of body fluid compartments may be expressed as edema, hypertension, or congestive heart failure. The loss of ability to regulate the composition of the body fluids is evidenced by the development of hyperkalemia, metabolic acidosis, and hyperphosphatemia.

The loss of excretory ability of the kidney is expressed by a rise in the plasma concentration of specific substances normally excreted by the kidney. The most widely monitored indices are the concentrations of blood urea nitrogen (BUN) and creatinine in the serum. The rates of rise of the BUN and creatinine reflect the impairment in the filtration function of the kidney and the rates of generation of urea nitrogen and creatinine. Creatinine generation is proportional to muscle mass. Accordingly, a patient with acute renal failure and a large muscle mass may have an increase in the serum concentration of creatinine of several milligrams per deciliter per day. A patient with smaller muscle mass but with the same degree of renal filtration failure may have a slower rate of rise. Urea nitrogen derives from the catabolism of protein. In an average patient with acute renal failure, the BUN rises about 10 to 15 mg/dl/day. In a catabolic patient, blood urea nitrogen may increase by over 40 mg/dl/day. In a patient who is not catabolic and in whom the dietary intake of protein is low, the rate of urea nitrogen generation will be less and the blood level will increase at a slower rate. Thus, while increases in the serum concentration of urea nitrogen and creatinine indicate the presence of renal disease, the absolute blood concentrations obtained and the rate of change are related to both the degree of renal injury and the rate of generation.

DIFFERENTIAL DIAGNOSIS AND DIAGNOSTIC EVALUATION OF THE PATIENT
(Table 29–2 and Fig. 29–1)

History and Physical Examination. The history and physical examination provide useful diagnostic in-

TABLE 29–1. ETIOLOGIES OF ACUTE RENAL INSUFFICIENCY

TYPE	EXAMPLES
Prerenal azotemia	External losses of fluid and electrolytes—vomiting, diarrhea, diuretic administration, burns
	Internal sequestrations of extracellular fluid—peritonitis, pancreatitis
	Decreased effective circulating volume—congestive heart failure, liver disease with ascites
Diseases of the renal arteries or veins	Direct trauma to renal vasculature, dissecting aortic aneurysm
Intrinsic renal disease	
Glomerulonephritis	Postinfectious glomerulonephritis, antibasement membrane antibody disease, collagen vascular diseases
Acute interstitial nephritis	Drug-associated acute interstitial nephritis
Acute tubular necrosis	Vasomotor nephropathy, toxic nephropathy
Intratubular obstruction	Rhabdomyolysis, multiple myeloma, uric acid–induced acute renal failure (tumor lysis syndrome)
Obstruction of collecting system	Bladder outlet obstruction, bilateral ureteral obstruction (rare), ureteral obstruction in a solitary kidney

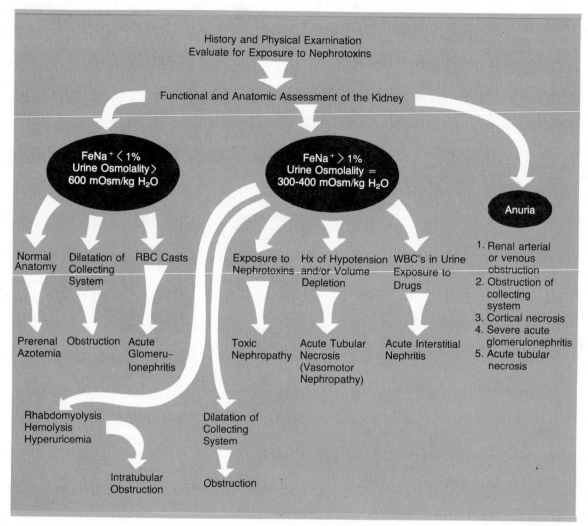

FIGURE 29-1. Diagnostic plan in a patient with acute renal insufficiency.

formation. Careful review of medical records, if available, and medications should be performed. Certain signs and symptoms may provide clues to specific disease entities. For example, the presence of swelling and edema of muscle might indicate rhabdomyolysis; the findings of abdominal or flank pain could be the result of renal infarction, obstruction to urine flow, or acute inflammation of the kidney. The signs and symptoms of specific disease entities are discussed more completely in other chapters. It is important to note that virtually all renal injuries may result in the development of acute renal insufficiency.

Routine and Special Blood Chemistries. A hemogram and a urinalysis should be obtained. The choice of special laboratory tests depends upon the clinical circumstances. If a collagen vascular or immune complex disease is suspected, the serum complement should be measured. Determination of the titer of antinuclear antibodies is indicated in patients suspected to have systemic lupus erythematosus. In patients with a clinical picture consistent with rapidly progressive glomerulonephritis or Goodpasture's syndrome, the serum should be tested for the presence of antiglomerular basement membrane antibodies. Serum and urine protein electrophoresis is indicated in patients in whom the diagnosis of multiple myeloma is suggested.

Determination of Kidney Anatomy and Renal Blood Flow. Sonography provides a noninvasive method of obtaining an estimate of the size of the kid-

TABLE 29-2. DIAGNOSTIC APPROACH TO A PATIENT WITH ACUTE RENAL INSUFFICIENCY

1. History and physical examination and review of medications
2. Routine and special laboratory tests
3. Examination of the urine, measurement of renal tubular function, and determination of the urine flow rate
4. Determination of the anatomy of the kidney and, when indicated, the renal blood flow
5. Other diagnostic tests when indicated

ney, of detecting cysts and masses in or near the kidney, and of determining the presence or absence of dilatation of the collecting system. It is, therefore, an important and safe screening test to rule out obstruction and to differentiate between acute and chronic disease. Large kidneys may indicate inflammatory disease or infiltrative disease of the kidneys. Further delineation of the anatomy of the kidneys may require radiocontrast dyes. In patients with renal insufficiency, the quality of the radiographs obtained with the use of radiocontrast agents may be suboptimal, and the radiocontrast dyes, in and of themselves, may be nephrotoxic.

Radionuclide methods are available to assess renal blood flow and excretory (secretory) function. Blood flow studies can easily discriminate between the presence or absence of renal blood flow and the symmetry of flow to the two kidneys but are less accurate in quantitating the absolute rates of flow. In a patient who presents with anuria or who develops renal failure after abdominal trauma or retroperitoneal surgery, in an elderly individual in whom the etiology of the acute renal insufficiency is obscure, or in a patient with abdominal, flank, or back pain, it is prudent to determine that blood flow to the kidney is intact. Angiography is required if equivocal results are obtained by nuclide scanning, in a patient suspected of acute renal venous disease, or when time does not permit a lengthy evaluation such as in a patient with suspected dissecting aortic aneurysm. Renal blood flow is also clearly decreased in patients with glomerulonephritis or transplant rejection. Assessment of renal blood flow may be of particular value in differentiating between renal transplant ATN and rejection. Renal blood flow as assessed by nuclide scanning is normal or only slightly decreased in a patient with established ATN. Tubular secretory function, however, is impaired. The findings of a normal or nearly normal renal blood flow, but impaired tubular function as assessed by radionuclide scanning, are consistent with the diagnosis of acute renal failure.

Examination of the Urine, Measurement of Renal Tubular Function, and Determination of the Urine Flow Rate (Table 29–3). A careful urinalysis should be performed to determine the presence or absence of red blood cell casts. The presence of red blood cell casts indicates inflammation of the glomerulus. The presence of red blood cells but not red blood cell casts is less diagnostic and may indicate disease in the kidney itself or in the collecting system. White blood cell casts reflect inflammation (but not necessarily infection) of the renal parenchyma. Polymorphonuclear leukocytes may derive from the kidney and/or the collecting system. The presence of lymphocytes and/or eosinophils may suggest the diagnosis of acute interstitial nephritis. The urinalysis of a patient with obstruction to flow in the collecting system is variable. An important diagnostic point is that the presence of azotemia in the face of a normal urinalysis is highly suggestive of obstruction. The presence of red or white blood cells, however, does not rule out the diagnosis of obstruction. The urine of patients with acute tubular necrosis usually contains protein and, on microscopic examination, granular casts. Glucose may be detected in the urine in the absence of hyperglycemia, a finding that reflects tubular damage. In acute tubular necrosis, the urinalysis is almost always abnormal but nondiagnostic.

An important series of diagnostic tests relates to an assessment of renal tubular function. The most widely used and convenient tests are measurements of the concentration of electrolytes and the osmolality of the urine and the calculation of the fractional excretion of sodium. To be of optimal clinical value, such measurements must be obtained prior to the administration of diuretics and should be considered in concert with other assessments of the state of hydration of the individual. The utility of these urinary indices is highest in patients with oliguria and azotemia. The urine indices are not diagnostic in and of themselves. In general, acute tubular necrosis is characterized by defects in tubular absorptive function as expressed by the findings of a urine concentration of sodium of greater than 40 mEq/L on a spot sample, a fractional excretion of sodium of greater than 1 per cent, and a urine osmolality that approaches that of the serum.

Prerenal azotemia is characterized by a decrease in the glomerular filtration rate as manifest by a rise in the BUN and creatinine and by normal tubular function as evidenced by a low urine concentration of sodium, a high urine osmolality, and a fractional excretion of sodium of less than 1 per cent. Patients with acute renal insufficiency secondary to acute glomerulonephritis may also have well-preserved renal tubular function early in the course of their disease, as may patients with the acute onset of partial urinary tract obstruction.

The major value of determining the urine concentration of sodium and the fractional excretion of sodium is in formulating a differential diagnosis in a patient with decreased renal function (Fig. 29–1). Interpretations of these tests, however, must be made in conjunction with other assessments of the patient. While patients with renal tubular disease frequently have isotonic urine and elevated fractional excretions of sodium and patients with prerenal disease manifest sodium avidity, there are clinically important exceptions to these generalizations. Certain types of ATN, such as radiographic dye–induced renal injury, may present with all the clinical characteristics of ATN but with fractional excretions of sodium less than 1 per cent. Conversely, a patient with depletion of the extracellular fluid volume may have a high urine concentration and fractional excretion of sodium if diuretics have been administered, during the generation phase of metabolic alkalosis, and when there was preexisting interstitial renal disease with renal salt wasting. In these latter conditions, the urinary excretion of sodium may not reflect the state of hydration of the patient.

Determination of the urine flow rate is not helpful in formulating a differential diagnosis of the etiology of the acute renal insufficiency but is important in clinical management. Oliguria is considered to be

TABLE 29–3. DIFFERENTIAL DIAGNOSIS OF ACUTE RENAL INSUFFICIENCY

DIAGNOSIS	SERUM BUN:Cr	URINALYSIS	URINE SODIUM (mEq/L)	FeNa (%)	URINE OSMOLALITY (mOsm/kg H$_2$O	COMMENTS
Prerenal azotemia	>20:1	Hyaline casts; may be nearly normal	<20	<1%	>600	Clinical signs of volume depletion. Hx of vomiting, diarrhea, or sweating. Hx of diuretic administration.
Acute arterial or venous disease	<20:1	May present with anuria	—	—	—	Arterial: Hx of abdominal trauma or manipulation of aorta or renal arteries. Venous: Hx of nephrotic syndrome, trauma, or severe dehydration (in children). Renal arteriography or venography may be indicated.
Intrinsic renal disease						
Acute glomerulonephritis	>20:1	RBC's, RBC casts, proteinuria	<20	<1%	>600	Hx of sore throat, pyoderma, or other infections. Renal biopsy may be indicated.
Acute interstitial nephritis	<20:1	WBC's, WBC casts, eosinophiluria	Variable	Variable	Variable	Hx of exposure to drugs that cause interstitial nephritis. Eosinophilia.
Acute tubular necrosis	<20:1	Granular casts, proteinuria, ± RBC's, ± WBC's	>20	>1%	~250–300	Vasomotor nephropathy: Hx of volume depletion or decrease in blood pressure. Toxic nephropathy: Hx of exposure to nephrotoxic drugs or radiocontrast dyes.
Intratubular obstruction	>20:1	Variable	Variable	Variable	Variable	Signs, symptoms, and laboratory findings of rhabdomyolysis or multiple myeloma. Hx of lymphoma or leukemia with hyperuricemia.
Obstruction of collecting system	>20:1	Variable, may be normal	Variable; may be <20	Variable; may be <1%	Variable	Hx of fluctuating urine volume. Sonogram of kidney showing bilateral dilatation of ureters.

present when the urine volume is less than 500 ml/day. Patients with acute tubular necrosis may have oliguria or polyuria. The distinction between these two forms may reflect differences in the etiology and/or the severity of the insult. Acute partial obstruction to urine flow may be associated with a decreased or variable urine output. However, the presence of a normal urine volume does not exclude the diagnosis. Obstruc-

tion of modest duration may result in the loss of concentrating ability by the kidney and, as a consequence, the excretion of an apparently normal volume of urine.

The presence of total anuria provides an important diagnostic clue in the evaluation of a patient with acute renal insufficiency and reduces the differential diagnostic list. Acute arterial or venous catastrophes, total urinary tract obstruction, severe cortical necrosis, severe acute glomerulonephritis, and, occasionally, severe acute tubular necrosis may present with anuria.

Indications for Renal Biopsy and Other Diagnostic Tests. A percutaneous or open renal biopsy may be indicated in patients suspected of having glomerulonephritis or acute interstitial nephritis. The value of a renal biopsy is to confirm the diagnosis and predict outcome prior to use of steroids and other potent immunosuppressive agents and before instituting difficult therapeutic procedures such as plasmapheresis. Other diagnostic tests may be indicated depending upon the clinical circumstances.

PATHOGENESIS AND ANATOMY OF ACUTE TUBULAR NECROSIS

The ATN syndrome is characterized by an acute and usually progressive loss of tubular and glomerular function. The vast majority of patients with ATN have, as their initiating event, either a decrease in renal plasma flow or exposure to a nephrotoxic agent. The vasomotor nephropathy variant of ATN occurs in a patient in whom there is a decrease in blood pressure and/or in the effective circulating volume. The pathophysiological events in the generation of vasomotor nephropathy are not known with certainty. An initial decrease in renal blood flow appears to be a requisite for the development of ATN. However, blood flow returns nearly to normal within 24 to 48 hours after the initial insult. Despite adequate renal blood flow, tubular dysfunction persists and the glomerular filtration rate remains depressed. The factor or factors that sustain the renal functional impairment after the primary insult depend upon the nature of the original insult. Leakage of glomerular ultrafiltrate from the tubular lumen into the renal interstitium across the damaged renal tubular cells, obstruction to flow due to debris or crystals in the lumen of the tubules, loss of high-energy intermediates in renal tubular cells, and a decrease in the glomerular capillary ultrafiltration coefficient (K_f) have all been proposed to play a pathophysiological role in sustaining the clinical picture of ATN.

The toxic nephropathy variant of ATN occurs in clinical circumstances in which the patient has been exposed to a nephrotoxic agent. These agents impair tubular function and result in a secondary decrease in filtration. Many drugs have been implicated in causing toxic nephropathy. Antibiotics, particularly the aminoglycoside antibiotics, and specific cancer chemotherapeutic agents are two classes of drugs commonly associated with ATN. Specific forms of toxic nephropathy are discussed in Chapter 33.

Histologically, the kidney may appear nearly normal. The brush border membranes of the proximal convoluted tubule may be absent, and cellular debris may be observed in the tubule lumina. In patients with rhabdomyolysis and ATN, myoglobin-stained casts may be observed on histological examination of the kidney. Cellular infiltrates are not usually prominent unless there is an associated interstitial nephritis. There is, however, edema of the interstitium. Aminoglycoside antibiotic toxicity is suggested by the presence of lipid whorls in the cytoplasm of the renal tubule cells. It is to be stressed that in the vast majority of patients with ATN, the histological picture is nondiagnostic. Despite the common use of the term acute tubular necrosis, necrosis of the tubules is rarely observed. The glomeruli appear normal by light microscopy. The functional abnormalities of ATN are not expressed in the histology of the kidney.

MANAGEMENT

There are absolute and relative indications for dialysis. Dialytic therapy should be instituted for uremic symptoms such as encephalopathy and pericarditis. Other indications for dialysis include severe fluid overload, hyperkalemia, metabolic acidosis, and life-threatening abnormalities in serum concentrations of electrolytes which cannot be effectively managed by conservative means. In a patient who is asymptomatic and without the above clinical and laboratory findings, a trial of conservative nondialytic management may be attempted. In a patient who is catabolic with increases of BUN of greater than 20 mg/dl/day, it is reasonable to institute dialysis prior to the development of severe clinical symptoms. If instituted, dialysis (hemodialysis or peritoneal dialysis) should be performed as often as is required to obtain the therapeutic goal.

The principles and techniques involved in hemodialysis and peritoneal dialysis are discussed in Chapter 30. The following considerations relate to the use of hemodialysis or peritoneal dialysis in the acute clinical situation. Hemodialysis usually requires the use of heparin to prevent the clotting of blood during its extracorporeal circulation. Hemodialysis is absolutely or relatively contraindicated in patients with acute intracerebral hemorrhage, with active gastrointestinal bleeding, and in the immediate postoperative period. Hemodialysis must also be used with caution in patients with pericarditis and/or pericardial effusions, acute myocardial infarctions, and underlying bleeding disorders. In the above clinical circumstances, peritoneal dialysis may be the preferred type of dialytic therapy. Alternatively, hemodialysis without heparin may be attempted.

The relative inefficiency of peritoneal dialysis may render this form of dialysis suboptimal in the acute treatment of very catabolic patients, in patients with marked hyperkalemia, and in patients with severe metabolic acidosis. Whether or not dialysis is instituted, there are several distinct clinical problems unique to the patient with ATN.

Sodium and Water Balance. The dietary or intravenous administration of sodium and water should be matched to the urinary and nonurinary losses of the patient once a nearly normal state of hydration is achieved. Diuretic administration may be attempted to increase the urine output if the above measures are not effective and the extracellular fluid volume is expanded (see below). If diuretics are unsuccessful in preventing expansion of the extracellular fluid volume, dialysis is required. In patients who require large amounts of intravenously infused fluids, such as patients receiving intravenous alimentation, dialysis may be required on a daily basis. When dialysis is instituted, the removal of sodium and water by dialysis must be considered in the calculation of the net water and sodium balance of the patient.

Potassium Homeostasis. Hyperkalemia is a life-threatening complication of acute renal failure and often necessitates urgent intervention. The cardiac effects of hyperkalemia are the most dangerous and include conduction defects, ventricular tachycardia, and cardiac arrest. Electrocardiographic changes, specifically peaked T waves, prolongation of the PR interval, or widening of the QRS complex, may be observed in hyperkalemic states and are an indication for prompt treatment (Table 29–4). The cardiotoxic effects of severe hyperkalemia can be reduced temporarily by infusions of calcium chloride. Measures such as the administration of glucose and insulin or sodium bicarbonate induced intracellular shifts of potassium. Permanent removal of potassium from the body, however, requires either the administration of resins that bind potassium in the gut or the use of dialytic modalities.

Acid-Base Abnormalities. Most patients with ATN are acidotic. An occasional patient with vomiting or nasogastric suction may develop metabolic alkalosis if the rate of hydrogen ion loss exceeds the rate of production. Acidosis can be treated by administration of bicarbonate or bicarbonate equivalents. Dialysis is required for severe acidosis. Alkalosis can be treated by the oral or intravenous administration of acid or by employing dialysis baths with reduced concentrations of base.

Phosphate Balance. Hyperphosphatemia is treated by limiting the dietary absorption of phosphate by phosphate-binding antacids. If the patient is not eating, hyperphosphatemia can be effectively managed by dialysis.

Diet. A source of protein is required in patients with ATN, since the underlying disease process as well as the presence of renal insufficiency results in increased catabolism and decreased anabolism of protein. However, dietary protein contributes to the generation of urea nitrogen and perhaps other products thought to be involved in the genesis of the "uremic syndrome." In a patient who is not severely catabolic and does not require dialysis, protein intake should be limited to 40 gm/day and should contain a high content of essential amino acids (high biological value protein). Carbohydrates should be administered to provide sufficient calories. If the patient is severely catabolic, as evidenced by a rise in the urea nitrogen concentration of over 20 mg/dl/day, higher intakes of protein are often required to maintain nitrogen balance. Parenteral nutrition that provides amino acids, carbohydrates, and fats is often indicated in the patient with acute renal failure who is unable to meet these demands for nutrients. The added intravenous volume of these solutions, however, may necessitate frequent dialytic intervention for the control of fluid homeostasis, particularly in the oliguric patient. Alternative maneuvers to manage the extra volume include pure ultrafiltration and continuous arteriovenous hemofiltration (CAVH), as outlined in Chapter 30.

Adjustment in Drug Dosing Regimens. Drug-induced renal failure is a common clinical problem. In addition, renal failure is associated with abnormalities in the metabolism of a number of commonly used drugs. The relationship between drugs and renal disease is discussed more fully in Chapter 33. It is critical, however, to carefully review the indications for and the dose of all drugs administered to patients with ATN. Monitoring of blood concentrations of drugs is an important adjunct to effective treatment.

Other. Vitamins are often administered to patients with ATN. Since the water-soluble vitamins and folate are removed by dialysis, they should be provided routinely in patients requiring dialysis. Blood transfusions may be required in some patients with ATN. Because of the potential for overexpansion of the extracellular fluid volume and hyperkalemia consequent to infusion of large amounts of blood to a patient with ATN, elective or semielective blood transfusions are often given during dialysis.

The Use of Diuretics. It has been established that pretreatment of the subject with vigorous hydration, osmotic diuretics, or loop diuretics protects the kidney from some forms of renal injury. Accordingly, patients who will be exposed to potentially injurious stimuli such as radiocontrast dyes, vascular surgery, or nephrotoxic drugs should be maintained with high rates of urine flow and replete extracellular fluid volumes.

TABLE 29–4. TREATMENT OF HYPERKALEMIA

TREATMENT	MECHANISM	INDICATIONS/COMMENTS
Calcium chloride	Opposes cardiotoxic effects of K^+	Severe hyperkalemia with EKG changes; combine with other measures
Glucose/Insulin	Intracellular K^+ shift	Temporary maneuver; repeat doses often necessary; combine with other measures
Na^+ bicarbonate	Intracellular K^+ shift	Temporary maneuver; may cause metabolic alkalosis; combine with other measures
Kayexalate resin	Binds K^+ in the gut in exchange for Na^+	Combine with cathartic, e.g., sorbitol; give P.O. or as enema; slower onset of action
Dialysis	Removal by diffusion	Effective in uncontrolled hyperkalemia; hemodialysis preferred over peritoneal dialysis

The value of diuretics when administered after the injurious insult is controversial. Most studies indicate that diuretics do not alter the severity or the duration of ATN. Loop acting diuretics, however, may convert oliguric ATN into a polyuric form. Some clinicians, therefore, advocate administration of a bolus dose of a loop acting diuretic once the diagnosis is established. If the diuretic fails to induce a diuretic response, it is discontinued. Although the diuretics do not alter the course of ATN, it is generally easier to manage the polyuric than the oliguric form of ATN.

OUTCOME AND PROGNOSIS

The outcome of patients who develop ATN is highly variable and dependent upon the nature of the underlying disease. With the availability of dialysis, death is rarely due to renal failure directly. In modern acute care hospitals, mortality rates may be in excess of 50 per cent, a figure that reflects the advanced age, severity of disease, and number of coexisting illnesses in this patient population. The outcome is considerably more favorable in younger patients with fewer co-existing diseases. As a generalization, patients with antibiotic-induced acute renal failure appear to have a more favorable outcome than those with vasomotor nephropathy. The same generalization applies to patients presenting with nonoliguric as compared to oliguric ATN.

In a patient with established ATN but not exposed to additional insults to the kidney, renal function may recover. The onset of recovery averages 7 to 10 days, although shorter and longer periods of renal dysfunction are not uncommon. In patients who are oliguric, recovery is heralded by an increase in urine output. Generally, in a patient not undergoing dialysis, the urine output doubles every 24 to 48 hours until an output of 3000 to 4000 ml per day is attained. The serum concentration of urea nitrogen and creatinine decreases 48 to 72 hours after the onset of the increase in urine output. The progressive increase in urine output should be monitored carefully. A patient with oliguric ATN who begins to manifest an increase in urine output usually demonstrates complete progression to urine outputs of 3000 ml or more per day. If a patient fails to reach this value or if urine output decreases after an initial increase, the possibility of an additional renal insult should be carefully considered.

REFERENCES

Cooper K, Bennett WM: Nephrotoxicity of common drugs used in clinical practice. Arch Intern Med 147:1213–1218, 1987.

Grantham JJ: Acute renal failure. In Wyngaarden JB, Smith LH Jr (eds): Cecil Textbook of Medicine, 18th ed. Philadelphia, WB Saunders Co, 1988, pp 559–562.

Myers BD, Moran SM: Hemodynamically mediated acute renal failure. N Engl J Med 314:97–105, 1986.

30
CHRONIC RENAL FAILURE

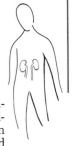

The term chronic renal failure describes the existence of irreversibly advanced and usually progressive renal insufficiency. End-stage renal disease (ESRD) is that stage of chronic renal failure at which renal function is no longer sufficient to sustain life. The incidence of newly diagnosed end-stage renal failure is approximately 50 to 100 new cases per million population. There are approximately 80,000 patients currently maintained on chronic dialysis in the United States.

Specific Etiologies (Table 30–1)

The outcome from any specific form of renal injury and the progression to end-stage renal disease have been reviewed in Chapter 29. The most common etiologies of renal disease in patients being considered for dialysis and transplantation are chronic glomerulo-nephritis, hypertensive nephrosclerosis, chronic interstitial nephritis, polycystic kidney disease, and diabetes mellitus. The inclusion of diabetes mellitus in such a list reflects recent improvement in the care and management of this patient population such that greater numbers of diabetic patients survive the other ravages characteristic of this illness and thus manifest ESRD.

TABLE 30–1. COMMON CAUSES OF END-STAGE RENAL DISEASE

Chronic glomerulonephritis
Hypertensive nephrosclerosis
Chronic interstitial nephritis
Chronic diabetic glomerulosclerosis
Polycystic kidney disease

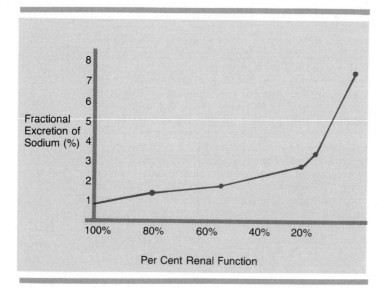

FIGURE 30–1. Changes in the fractional excretion of sodium required to maintain homeostatic balance in a patient ingesting a diet containing 100 mEq of sodium and undergoing progressive loss of renal function.

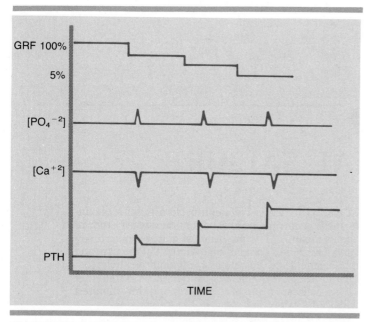

FIGURE 30–2. Schematized representation of the changes in the serum concentrations of calcium (Ca^{+2}), phosphate (PO_4^{-2}), and parathyroid hormone (PTH) in a patient undergoing a stepwise reduction in renal function. The dietary intake of phosphate is constant throughout the time period. The changes in the plasma concentration of calcium and phosphate are not observable clinically owing to the rapid adjustments mediated by PTH. (Adapted from Bricker NS, Slatopolsky E, Reiss E, Avioli LV: Calcium, phosphorus and bone in renal disease and transplantation. Arch Intern Med 123:543–553, 1969.)

ADAPTATION TO NEPHRON LOSS

The kidney has great functional reserve and is able to compensate for progressive loss of functioning nephrons. The homeostatic, the excretory, and, in part, the endocrine functions of the kidney are maintained even when function of the kidney is only 10 per cent of normal. Further degrees of nephron loss usually result in the clinical manifestations of uremia.

The adaptation to nephron loss can be illustrated for a single solute such as sodium (Fig. 30–1). In an individual with a glomerular filtration rate of 100 ml/min and ingesting 100 mEq of sodium per day, the urinary excretion of sodium must be 100 mEq per day in order to maintain body weight and the composition of body fluid compartments constant. In such an individual, 25,000 mEq of sodium are filtered at the glomerulus per day. Since only 100 of the 25,000 mEq of sodium filtered at the glomerulus are excreted, the fractional rate of excretion is 0.4 per cent. If the filtration rate were to be reduced by 50 per cent, the filtered load of sodium would be reduced proportionately. In order to maintain overall balance, 100 mEq of sodium would still have to be excreted. Under these circumstances, the fractional excretion of the filtered load of sodium by the kidney would be increased to 0.8 per cent. In the face of progressive reductions in the rates of filtration, the constancy of the composition and volume of body fluid compartments is maintained by progressive increases in the fractional rates of excretion of filtered sodium such that intake and output are matched. As renal function decreases, however, there is a narrowing of the range of intake which can be tolerated (see Chapter 27). In general, renal adjustments in the rates of excretion are adequate to accommodate normal rates of intake down to rates of filtration of 10 to 20 per cent of normal.

The above example highlights several important points in the adaptation to nephron loss. The nephrons that remain functional in the presence of a decrease in total number of functioning units are not partially damaged units. Rather, they behave in a normal or supernormal manner and respond appropriately to physiologic stimuli. The above defines the concept of the "intact nephron hypothesis." Said in another way, in a kidney that has sustained loss of nephrons, the remaining nephrons display a high degree of organization and respond appropriately to the needs of the organism.

The adaptive changes in nephron function are mediated by stimuli generated outside the kidney and within the kidney itself. The nature of the stimuli is not known for all solutes but has been well studied in the adaptation of calcium and phosphate metabolism to progressive renal disease (Fig. 30–2). In the presence of a constant intake of phosphate and progressive loss of nephrons, the following sequence of events ensues. With each decrease in the glomerular filtration rate, the dietary intake of phosphate results in a transient increase in serum phosphate and, as a consequence, a decrease in the serum concentration of ionized calcium. The decrease in ionized calcium causes release of parathyroid hormone (PTH). PTH, in turn, causes an increase in the urinary excretion of phosphate and a normalization of the serum concentrations of calcium and phosphate. The intact nephrons respond appropriately to PTH. In this example, normal plasma concentrations of calcium and phosphate are maintained, but there is a progressive rise in the concentration of PTH. Thus, the intact nephron hypothesis has been extended to include the "trade-off hypothesis." In this circumstance, normal calcium and phosphate homeostasis is maintained at the expense of development of secondary hyperparathyroidism. The negative aspect of this trade-off is hyperparathyroid-associated disease of bone and dysfunction of other organ systems. The trade-offs for maintenance of balance of other solutes aside from phosphate have not been elucidated clearly, but it is likely that the general thesis applies to multiple regulatory functions of the kidney.

When renal failure is far advanced, the adaptive response of the kidney to changes in the dietary intake of solute is severely compromised and the urinary excretion rates tend to become fixed. This loss of regulatory capacity of the kidney provides an explanation for the findings that in patients with advanced renal failure, alterations in dietary intake can be associated with states of depletion or excess. For example, ingestion of amounts of sodium in excess of the excretory capacity of the kidney results in expansion of the extracellular fluid volume. Conversely, ingestion of amounts of sodium that are less than the fixed rate of urinary excretion results in depletion of the extracellular fluid volume.

FACTORS AFFECTING THE RATE OF LOSS OF NEPHRONS

It has been appreciated for some time that many patients have a slow, steady decline in renal function over a period of months to years (see Fig. 25–1). A number of pathogenetic mechanisms have been implicated in the slow decline in renal function.

Continuing Primary Insult. It is often suggested that the disease initially causing the renal injury is still active and results in progressive damage. Frequently, despite the progressive loss of renal function, it is not possible to identify continued activity of the primary disease or exposure to toxins.

Secondary Renal Insults. In some circumstances, there may be development of secondary insults to the kidney, and these secondary processes could account for the progression of renal insufficiency. Congestive heart failure, hypercalcemia, infection, obstruction to urine flow, exposure to nephrotoxic drugs, or alterations in the extracellular fluid volume may result in further decreases in renal function.

Alterations in Glomerular Hemodynamics, PTH Metabolism, and Systemic Arterial Blood Pressure

ALTERATIONS IN GLOMERULAR HEMODYNAMICS IN RENAL DISEASE. The nephrons that remain functional in the presence of renal injury are, as noted earlier, not partially damaged but rather supernormal. Morphologically and functionally, these nephrons are larger and have higher than normal rates of glomerular plasma flow and filtration. The reason for the increase in the glomerular plasma flow and the rate of filtration is not known with certainty but is related, at least in part, to the dietary intake of protein. Protein or its peptide fragments cause renal vasodilation, an increase in glomerular plasma flow, and an increase in the glomerular hydrostatic pressure. It has been proposed that in renal insufficiency, the superperfusion and hyperfiltration of remaining nephrons, in and of itself, results in glomerulosclerosis and further loss of nephrons. Administration of a low-protein diet containing proteins of high biological value (proteins with a high content of essential amino acids) may lead to a reduction in glomerular blood flow, glomerular hydrostatic pressure, and hyperfiltration and thus slow the progression of the renal disease.

THE ROLE OF PARATHYROID HORMONE. In adapting to a constant intake of phosphate, calcium and phosphate homeostasis are maintained at the expense of development of hyperparathyroidism. PTH, however, has several actions that may be detrimental to the kidney. PTH may contribute to injury of renal cells by facilitating deposition of calcium in the renal parenchyma or by translocating calcium into the cells and the mitochondria. The net effect of PTH would be further loss of nephrons and increasing degrees of hyperparathyroidism.

THE ROLE OF BLOOD PRESSURE. Regardless of the nature of the primary renal insult, the codevelopment of elevation of the blood pressure results in a significant acceleration in the rate of nephron loss. It has been suggested that aggressive and early treatment is indicated for blood pressure elevations, even elevations in the range in which therapy is of questionable value in patients without renal disease.

CLINICAL MANIFESTATIONS OF END-STAGE RENAL DISEASE

The clinical manifestations of ESRD are protean. Clinical signs and symptoms may arise as a direct consequence of organ dysfunction secondary to the "uremic stage" or as an indirect consequence of primary dysfunction of another system. There is not one single compound or pathophysiological event that explains the multiple organ and systems abnormalities in uremia. Urea, monitored as the blood urea nitrogen (BUN) concentration, is not, in and of itself, the "uremic toxin." Much discussion has focused on the possible role of the so-called middle molecules, that is, molecules of molecular weight of 500 to 2000 daltons. These middle molecules are retained in patients with renal disease, but their exact pathophysiological role remains to be defined. It has also been proposed that PTH may be an important factor in the genesis of some of the clinical manifestations of ESRD.

Table 30–2 lists the major clinical manifestations of

TABLE 30–2. MANIFESTATIONS OF END-STAGE RENAL DISEASE

	LIFE-THREATENING	COMMON	UNCOMMON OR VARIABLE FREQUENCY
Blood chemistries	Acidosis, ↑K⁺	↑BUN/creatinine, ↑PO_4^{-2}, ↑alkaline phosphatase, ↑urate, ↑Mg^{+2}	↑Amylase, ↓SGOT
Cardiovascular system	Pulmonary edema, cardiac tamponade	↑Blood pressure, coronary artery disease, arrhythmias, congestive heart failure, pericarditis	Pericarditis ± pericardial effusion
Uremic osteodystrophy		↑Alkaline phosphatase, ↑PTH, ↓1,25 (OH)₂ Vit D	Bone pain, fractures
Nervous system	Encephalopathy	Peripheral neuropathy	
Hematopoietic system		Anemia, ↓platelet function, ↓WBC function, ↓immune responsivity, coagulopathy	
Gastrointestinal system	Gastrointestinal hemorrhage	Gastroenteritis, colitis, hepatitis	Ascites
Skin and conjunctiva		Pruritus	Darkening of skin, conjunctivitis
Endocrine system		Glucose intolerance, ↑blood levels of peptide, hormones, ↓erythropoietin	Gonadal dysfunction, abnormal thyroid function tests
Muscular and articular system			Proximal myopathy, arthritis (pseudogout)
Genitourinary system		Urinary tract infections, cystic degeneration of the kidney, carcinoma of the kidney	
Pulmonary system		Pulmonary congestion, infections	Poor gas exchange, pleural effusions

ESRD and divides them into those that are life-threatening, those that are common but not an immediate threat to existence, and those that occur with variable clinical frequency and expression. This division, however, is arbitrary and in any given patient, one organ system dysfunction may be the major threat to life or rehabilitation. The major causes of death in patients with ESRD are cardiovascular catastrophies and infections. The major morbid complications are the development of uremic bone disease (uremic osteodystrophy) and neuropathy.

Blood Chemistries

Analysis of serum chemistries reveals a variety of abnormalities in patients with ESRD. The BUN and creatinine are increased to a variable degree. Since the blood level attained reflects not only the impairment in filtration function of the kidney but also the rate of generation of these substances, the development of "uremic" symptoms may not correlate directly with blood values. Metabolic acidosis is commonly observed and is usually a hyperchloremic acidosis. In far-advanced renal failure, the acidosis may be associated with an increased anion gap. Hyperkalemia is observed when renal failure is far advanced or in patients with coexisting deficiency or tubular insensitivity to aldosterone. In far-advanced renal failure, the serum concentration of phosphate is increased. Bone-derived alkaline phosphatase increases over time in the ESRD patient and can be used to follow the development of uremic osteodystrophy. Serum concentrations of uric acid and magnesium are often elevated.

Cardiovascular Disease

Cardiovascular disease is one of the most common causes of death in patients with ESRD. The incidence of coronary artery disease in ESRD patients is increased, owing in part to the presence of hypertension, glucose intolerance, and/or abnormalities in lipid metabolism. Renal disease may also result in accelerated atherosclerotic disease and a form of cardiomyopathy. Ingestion of sodium and water in excess of the excretory capacity of the kidney can result in expansion of the extracellular fluid volume. The clinical manifestations of expansion of the extracellular fluid volume include hypertension, congestive heart failure, and peripheral edema.

Involvement of the pericardium is common in ESRD patients. Clinical manifestations may include pericarditis with pain, fever, and a pericardial friction rub or pericardial effusion with or without clinically apparent pericarditis. Pericardial tamponade and constrictive pericarditis are less common manifestations but are more life-threatening. Pericarditis occurs in two distinct clinical situations. In the newly diagnosed uremic patient or in patients who have been inadequately dialyzed, institution of regular dialytic treatment results in resolution of the pericarditis. Pericarditis can also arise in patients who are already established on dialysis and who appear to be well-dialyzed. In this circumstance, increasing the number or duration of dialytic treatments does not hasten the resolution of the pericarditis. Cardiac tamponade requires immediate drainage of the pericardial fluid. Constrictive pericarditis requires surgical intervention.

Uremic Osteodystrophy

The changes in PTH and vitamin D metabolism in patients with chronic renal insufficiency have a profound effect on the activity of osteoblasts and osteoclasts. In general, bone dissolution is accelerated while bone formation is decreased. These changes are relative to one another such that the clinical and laboratory abnormalities may vary widely. Some patients may manifest only laboratory abnormalities, such as a rise in alkaline phosphatase, whereas others may have severe and disabling bone pain and fractures. The development of bone disease in the uremic patient, uremic osteodystrophy, is universal. It is convenient to subdivide the metabolic bone disease of the ESRD patients into three subtypes (Fig. 30–3). Although all are present to a variable degree, one subtype may dominate the clinical picture. Hyperparathyroidism is universal in ESRD; the bone manifestation is the development of osteitis fibrosa cystica. In advanced renal disease, there is a failure to convert vitamin D to its active metabolite, $1,25(OH)_2$ vitamin D, and, as a consequence, rickets or osteomalacia develops. In addition, recent evidence indicates that the accumulation of aluminum metabolites in bone results in a form of vitamin D–resistant rickets. Owing to a variety of factors including sustained acidosis, poor nutrition, and as yet other undefined factors, osteoporosis is common.

Neurological Manifestations

Central nervous system manifestations of ESRD may range from mild changes in mentation to coma, convulsions, and death. The more severe clinical manifestations occur in patients with advanced uremia and are alleviated by the institution of dialysis. In a patient with severe uremic central nervous system manifestations, the initial dialysis treatments should be brief so as to avoid the development of a disequilibrium syndrome, generally manifested by cerebral edema and worsening neurological findings. Usually after a few dialytic treatments, the patient becomes adapted and no longer manifests this dialysis disequilibrium condition. A rare but severe neurological syndrome may occur in patients maintained on dialysis, called "dialysis dementia." This dementing syndrome is also associated with a movement disorder and has a fatal outcome in the majority of patients. Finally, the presence of arteriosclerosis and hypertension makes the ESRD patient vulnerable to the development of cerebrovascular disease.

Involvement of the peripheral nervous system is frequent in advanced renal disease and is manifest by a glove-and-stocking peripheral neuropathy. In some patients, the neuropathy may be quite severe and preclude successful rehabilitation. The institution of dialysis may stabilize the neuropathy, but only rarely is a severe neuropathy reversed. In some patients, the neuropathy may progress despite seemingly adequate dialysis.

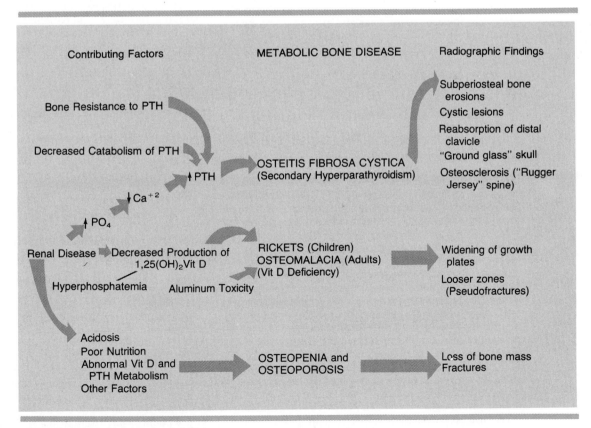

FIGURE 30–3. Uremic osteodystrophy.

The development of ESRD may also result in dysfunction of the autonomic nervous system. Clinical manifestations may include abnormalities in motility of the gastrointestinal tract with the findings of gastroparesis and/or diarrhea, labile blood pressure, and intolerance to dialysis. Dialysis generally does not reverse the overt manifestations of the autonomic neuropathy.

Hematopoietic System

Anemia is a nearly universal finding in patients with advanced renal disease. The etiology of the anemia is multifactorial. Red blood cell production is decreased owing to the lack of erythropoietin production by the kidney, the presence of products retained in uremia which inhibit erythropoiesis, and the fibrosis of the bone marrow. Red blood cell loss may be accelerated by the presence of uremic gastroenteritis and the disordered function of platelets. The anemia may be exacerbated by associated dietary limitations or malabsorption of essential foodstuffs required for red cell production such as folic acid and iron.

Total white blood cell counts are normal to low in ESRD. Some patients manifest poor polymorphonuclear leukocyte chemotaxis. Although not present in all ESRD patients, blunted production of antibodies and/or cellular immune responsivity is present in a significant number of such patients. The nature of the defects in white blood cell function are not known with certainty but appear to include both an inherent defect in the cells themselves and a response to a circulating factor. These defects in white blood cell function, in conjunction with other factors, may provide an explanation for the findings that infections are a common cause of death in ESRD patients.

Platelet counts are normal in patients with advanced renal disease, but qualitative defects in platelet function have been well documented. Abnormalities in activity of clotting factors and in factors mediating the bleeding time have been described in ESRD patients. The abnormalities of hemostasis are not totally reversed by dialysis and may contribute to the frequent findings of gastrointestinal blood loss and subcutaneous hematomas in patients with ESRD. The defects in hemostasis are also important considerations in the evaluation of an ESRD patient who requires surgery.

Gastrointestional Tract

In untreated uremic patients, gastroenteritis and/or colitis is frequently reported. Patients may present with anorexia, nausea, vomiting, or gastrointestinal bleeding. The above symptoms may improve when dialysis is instituted. In addition, there are abnormalities in the motility of the gastrointestinal tract in some patients as well as abnormalities in the absorptive functions of the gut.

Particularly in patients on dialysis, hepatitis is common as a result of exposure to blood and blood products. Transaminase activity in serum, however, may be only minimally elevated in patients with significant liver disease because of suppression in transaminase activity in uremic serum.

Skin and Conjuctiva

Itching and conjunctivitis are common manifestations of end-stage renal disease and appear to represent the clinical sequelae of microcrystallization of calcium. In addition, PTH itself may cause pruritus. As a consequence of poor nutrition and the defects in platelet function, poor skin texture and bruising are common. In long-standing ESRD patients, there is darkening of the skin, perhaps related to retention of substances that stimulate melanin production.

Endocrine Systems

The kidney is the organ that produces erythropoietin and $1,25(OH)_2$ vitamin D, the active metabolite of vitamin D. Renal disease is associated with low or absent levels of both these hormones. The kidney is also the organ of catabolism of several peptide hormones such as insulin, glucagon, PTH, and gonadotropic hormones. Glucose intolerance is common in patients with ESRD, owing, in part, to the abnormal circulating levels of hormones, to alterations in hormone-receptor interactions, and to changes in post–hormone receptor events in given cells. Abnormalities in gonadal function are common in patients with advanced renal insufficiency. Pregnancies and term deliveries are rare in females with ESRD. Menstrual periods also tend to be irregular.

Muscular and Articular System

Generalized malaise, muscle fatigue, weakness, and twitching may be seen in patients with ESRD. A proximal myopathy, perhaps related to hyperparathyroidism, may occur. The fasciculation and twitching of muscles may be related to depolarization of muscle cells secondary to uremia.

Articular symptoms, including overt arthritis, occur in uremic individuals. Although any form of arthritis may occur, pseudogout due to the deposition of calcium pyrophosphate seems to occur with increased frequency in patients with renal disease. Interestingly, despite the presence of hyperuricemia, overt attacks of gout are rare.

Genitourinary System

Urinary tract infection is common in patients with ESRD and may be related to stasis in the collecting system due to low rates of urine flow. In patients maintained on chronic dialysis for a period of time, there is significant incidence of cystic degeneration of the kidney. There is also a significant increase in the incidence of carcinoma of the kidney.

Pulmonary System

Infections of the lung occur more commonly in renal disease patients and may be the consequence of poor clearing of secretions and impaired host defenses. Calcium may be deposited in the lung parenchyma and contribute to poor exchange of gases seen in some uremic individuals. Pulmonary congestion secondary to overexpansion of the extracellular fluid volume and/or congestive heart failure is a common clinical problem. Patients with uremia may also develop pleural effusions not due to other recognizable causes.

TREATMENT OPTIONS

CONSERVATIVE MANAGEMENT

Conservative management of patients with advanced renal disease is feasible in most (but not all) patients even when the glomerular filtration rate is as low as 10 ml/min. Some patients with even lower levels of function can be managed conservatively over short periods of time while awaiting evaluation and preparation for longer-term management.

Regulation of Fluids and Electrolytes

The cardinal pathophysiological abnormality of fluid and electrolyte homeostasis in advanced renal failure is the inability of the kidney to adjust the rates of excretion to widely varying rates of intake. The urinary excretion of *water* and *solutes* tends to be fixed over a narrow range. Thus, when the rate of intake exceeds the rate of output, a state of retention will result. Rates of intake which are less than output will result in states of depletion. Management of such individuals, therefore, requires matching of dietary intake to output. Practically, this involves ingestion of enough sodium and water to maintain the extracellular fluid volume at normal levels. *Potassium* intake usually requires careful monitoring. Once a dietary regimen is instituted, serial measurements of body weights, blood pressure, and blood electrolytes are required to ensure that the patient has achieved the steady-state balance believed to be optimal clinically. Diuretics may be of value in patients unable to restrict their intake of sodium. Oral potassium-binding resins, which allow elimination of potassium by the gut, can be used in patients exhibiting frequent and life-threatening hyperkalemia. *Bicarbonate* or bicarbonate equivalents are used to partially correct systemic acidosis. *Antihypertensive* agents are indicated if hypertension is still evident after control of the fluid and electrolyte status of the patient. In patients who are unable to adjust sodium and water balance by diet, with or without the use of diuretics, and/or those who are persistently hyperkalemic or acidotic, dialysis therapy is usually indicated.

The dietary intake of *phosphate* is intimately involved in the genesis of secondary hyperparathyroidism. It is not feasible to restrict the dietary intake of phosphate severely, since such diets are unpalatable. Aluminum-based antacids bind phosphate in the gastrointestinal tract and prevent its absorption. These antacids can aid in control of the plasma concentration of phosphate and in the correction of the abnormalities in the metabolism of calcium and PTH. If the plasma concentration of phosphate can be controlled, it may be possible to administer calcium and/or analogues of vitamin D to increase calcium absorption in the gut and further suppress the stimulation of PTH release. The net aim of the use of phosphate-binding antacids, calcium, and vitamin D analogues is to restore serum concentrations of calcium and phosphate to values as close to normal as possible.

While the above regimen is widely used, certain cau-

tions need to be considered. Aluminum toxicity may be involved in the development of some types of uremic osteodystrophy and may play a role in the generation of a dementing syndrome reported in dialysis patients. The administration of calcium and/or vitamin D analogues must be carefully monitored so as to avoid elevation of the product of the serum concentration of calcium and phosphate. Deposition of calcium in body tissues may be involved in some of the systemic manifestations of renal failure.

Despite therapeutic maneuvers designed to control the abnormalities in calcium, phosphate, and parathyroid hormone metabolism, progressive hyperparathyroidism may develop. A parathyroidectomy may be indicated in patients with progressive hyperparathyroidism as manifested by overt hypercalcemia, a markedly elevated alkaline phosphatase, bone pain and/or fractures, and radiographic evidence of advanced and progressive changes (Fig. 30–3). If bone disease continues to progress despite optimal medical management and adequate dialysis, renal transplantation may be the preferred treatment option.

Elimination of Waste Products of Metabolism and Drugs

As noted earlier, there is no consensus on the nature of the uremic toxins. Nonetheless, the dietary intake of protein contributes to the genesis of uremic symptoms. While urea is not a toxic product in and of itself, the BUN concentration does correlate both with the dietary intake of protein and with the systemic manifestations of end-stage renal disease. It is generally believed that the BUN reflects the accumulation of other products of protein catabolism, some of which may contribute to clinical symptoms. Restriction of dietary intake of protein can lead to symptomatic improvement in the nausea, vomiting, malaise, and encephalopathy of end-stage renal disease. Such improvements are usually associated with a decrease in the BUN. On the other hand, uremic patients have a decreased protein anabolic rate and an increased rate of protein catabolism. Marked restrictions in protein intake, therefore, can result in protein malnutrition. A patient with end-stage renal disease can usually be maintained in nitrogen balance by restriction of the dietary intake of protein to 40 gm/day. Essential amino acids (high biological value proteins) are indicated to stimulate the reincorporation of urea nitrogen into new protein synthesis and to prevent accumulation of nitrogen metabolites that are not essential. Additional calories need to be provided when protein intake is restricted. The use of a low-protein diet containing proteins of high biological value can lead to symptomatic improvement and prolong the time until a patient must have dialytic therapy or transplantation.

The kidney is a major route of excretion of drugs. Moreover, renal failure is associated with alterations in the binding of drugs by plasma proteins and in the overall metabolism and distribution of drugs within the body. These considerations are reviewed in Chapter 33.

Endocrine and Other Considerations

The relationship between calcium, phosphate, and PTH has already been considered. Glucose intolerance is common in patients with end-stage renal disease. A patient with pre-existing diabetes mellitus may experience marked changes in insulin and carbohydrate requirements as renal function deteriorates. If anorexia limits the intake of carbohydrates, hypoglycemia may ensue if the insulin dose is not adjusted. In addition, some uremic patients have impaired gluconeogenesis. On the other hand, the following factors may result in hyperglycemia. Uremic patients have defects in the tissue uptake and metabolism of glucose and in the number and action of insulin receptors. Carbohydrate intake as a percentage of total calories is increased by the dietary regimen. The plasma concentration of glucagon is also elevated in patients with renal failure. Finally, advanced renal disease limits the urinary excretion of glucose when hyperglycemia is present. In the diabetic patient with advanced renal failure, frequent monitoring of blood sugar concentrations, adjustments in the doses of insulin, and alterations in the diet are required. A variety of abnormalities in thyroid function tests have been described in patients with advanced renal failure. These tests need to be carefully correlated with the clinical assessment of the patient prior to administration of thyroid hormone replacement. Despite laboratory tests that, if considered by themselves, might suggest hypothyroidism, the incidence of hypothyroidism is probably not significantly increased in patients with end-stage renal disease.

Anemia is very common in patients with ESRD, and the average patient on dialysis has hematocrit readings of 20 to 30 ml/dl. Folate is provided to all patients on dialysis since it is removed by dialysis. Iron supplements are given if iron deficiency is documented. Iron should not routinely be provided, since excess iron administration may result in the development of hemochromatosis. Blood transfusions may be indicated in patients who are unable to maintain their red cell mass and are symptomatic from the anemia. Transfusions are also given prior to surgery to improve tolerance to the stress of anesthesia and surgical manipulations. Treatable causes of gastrointestinal bleeding should also be addressed. Administration of androgens may be of value as a stimulus to the production of red blood cells in men. In females, anabolic steroids with low androgenic activity are used to stimulate the bone marrow. Recently, recombinant erythropoietin has been introduced for clinical use in uremic patients. In preliminary studies, recombinant erythropoietin has been demonstrated to increase the hematocrit and the overall well-being of patients with ESRD. However, there have been increases in the serum concentration of potassium and in the frequency of clotting of the dialyzer in patients receiving erythropoietin. Nonetheless, recombinant erythropoietin therapy may prove to be an important adjunct in the treatment of the anemia of ESRD.

Vitamin supplements are indicated in most ESRD patients. Water-soluble vitamins are removed by dialysis, and supplements are clearly indicated in patients on dialysis.

DIALYTIC THERAPY

Principles and Technology of Dialysis

The principles underlying the use of dialysis are those of diffusion and convection (Fig. 30–4). Blood is separated from a dialysis solution by a semipermeable membrane. For hemodialysis, blood is pumped into a dialyzer containing an artificial semipermeable membrane. The dialysis solution bathes the opposite side of the membrane. In peritoneal dialysis, the capillaries of the peritoneal membrane serve as the semipermeable membrane, dialysis solution being instilled into the peritoneal cavity.

The physical separation of blood from the dialysis solution by a semipermeable membrane sets conditions favorable for net transfer of solutes and water from one compartment to the other. If a concentration gradient for a substance can be established, passive diffusion of that substance across the membrane can occur. The rate of transfer depends on the concentration gradient of the substance in question and its permeability across the semipermeable membrane. For example, urea will diffuse from blood into the dialysis bath, which initially contains no urea. In this example, urea removed from the body is associated with a decrease in the blood concentration of urea. Another example is the removal of potassium from plasma by using dialysis baths with concentrations of potassium lower than that of the plasma. By imposing the appropriate gradients, substances can be made to

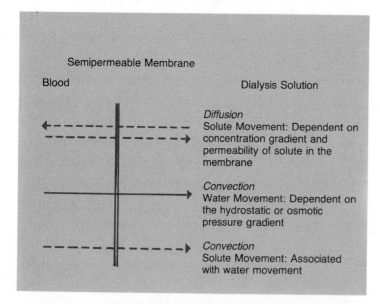

FIGURE 30–4. Representation of the principles of dialysis. Solutes that are permeable in the semipermeable membrane will diffuse along their concentration gradient. Additional solutes may be transferred associated with bulk water flow. Water movement is dependent upon the prevailing hydrostatic and/or osmotic pressure gradient across the semipermeable membrane.

diffuse into or out of the blood. For other substances, such as sodium, it is not advisable to markedly alter the plasma concentration. Net removal of these substances, however, can be accomplished by inducing a flow of water across the membrane. In hemodialysis, water flow is accomplished by imposing a hydrostatic pressure gradient across the membrane. In peritoneal dialysis, water flow is induced by imposing an osmotic gradient across the membrane. In either mode, the membrane behaves as if pierced with large water-filled channels that offer little resistance to flow of solutes dissolved in water. Thus, if the dialysis bath contains sodium in a concentration which approximates that of plasma, this convective pathway will permit net sodium removal from the body without inducing a change in the plasma concentration of sodium.

In some clinical circumstances, there is a requirement for ultrafiltration without dialysis. In patients with volume overload, such as refractory congestive heart failure, the clinical need is to remove extracellular fluid volume rather than to alter the electrolyte composition or remove uremic toxins. To accomplish these ends, two additional "dialytic" procedures have been introduced. The first, called *pure ultrafiltration*, employs standard dialysis techniques and dialyzers. A hydrostatic pressure gradient is imposed across the membrane, but no dialysis solution is introduced on the opposite side of the membrane. Thus, pure ultrafiltrate of blood is obtained. This mode of therapy is very efficient for rapid removal of fluid. The second, called *continuous arteriovenous hemofiltration* (CAVH), utilizes arterial and venous cannulae and a dialysis cartridge containing a membrane that is highly permeable to water. The arteriovenous pressure difference provides the driving force for ultrafiltration. The rate of fluid removal per unit time is less with CAVH than with pure ultrafiltration using hemodialysis techniques, but by virtue of its use on a continuous rather than on an intermittent basis, large amounts of fluid can be removed over longer time intervals. CAVH is indicated for those patients unable to tolerate rapid removal of extracellular fluid. Both pure ultrafiltration and CAVH can be used as primary modes of therapy in patients requiring fluid removal or as additional modes of therapy in patients who also require dialysis. As with conventional hemodialysis, both CAVH and pure ultrafiltration require systemic anticoagulation with heparin to prevent clotting within the dialyzer cartridge.

The vascular access required for chronic hemodialysis is created by forming an arteriovenous fistula by direct anastomosis of native vessels, or by the use of artificial grafts. Blood is pumped into the dialyzer and flows along one side of the artificial membrane. The dialysis solution is pumped in a counterflow direction across the other side of the membrane. The effluent blood is then returned to the patient. Dialysis machines permit regulation of the rate of blood flow, dialysate flow, and hydrostatic pressure gradient across the membrane. The technique of "high flux hemodialysis" utilizes a highly permeable dialysis cartridge and results in more efficient removal of solutes and water than conventional hemodialysis. The technique is attractive to many patients because the length of each dialysis session can be reduced significantly.

Peritoneal dialysis is accomplished by placement of a soft catheter through the abdominal wall into the peritoneal cavity. The external end of the catheter is attached in a closed system to a bag containing dialysis solution. Dialysis solution is instilled into the peritoneal cavity, permitted to dwell for varying periods of time, and then drained from the peritoneal cavity. These fill-dwell-drain cycles may be performed intermittently or continuously. The osmolality of the dialysis solution is adjusted by varying the concentration of glucose. The hypertonic dialysate creates an osmotic gradient for water removal equivalent to the hydrostatic pressure gradient of hemodialysis.

Indications for Dialysis and Adequacy of Dialysis

The major goals of dialysis (hemodialysis or peritoneal dialysis) are to maintain fluid and electrolyte balance and to rid the body of waste products. Dialysis is indicated in patients with severe abnormalities in fluid and electrolyte balance such as fluid overload, volume-dependent hypertension, acidosis, or hyperkalemia; in patients with "uremic" symptoms such as pericarditis or encephalopathy; and in patients whose renal function is 5 per cent or less of normal regardless of symptoms. The adequacy of dialysis has not clearly been defined in quantitative terms. Adequacy, however, may be defined clinically by the well-being of the patient and correction of the regulatory and excretory defects of the kidney. Dialysis is not total renal replacement therapy. The endocrine abnormalities are not corrected by dialysis. Uremic bone disease and neuropathy may persist and accelerate despite seemingly adequate dialysis. Diet and medication must be carefully monitored, as discussed earlier. Owing to the time required for dialysis, the psychological adjustments to the presence of organ failure, and the dependence on machines to sustain life, the impact of end-stage renal disease requiring chronic dialytic therapy on the life style of an individual is significant. Management of dialysis patients, therefore, requires input not only from physicians, but also from individuals in nursing, dietary, social work, and psychology services.

Complications of Dialysis

Clotting and infection of the vascular access are common problems in patients maintained on hemodialysis. In addition, the hemodialysis machine functions as a low-resistance arteriovenous fistula requiring that cardiac output and/or peripheral vascular resistance increase so as to maintain systemic arterial blood pressure. In patients with significant heart disease or autonomic neuropathy (particularly diabetics) or those receiving drugs that inhibit the normal response of the autonomic nervous system, failure to manifest the appropriate cardiovascular response may result in intolerance to hemodialysis. The changes in extracellular fluid volume and in the composition of blood following hemodialysis may also contribute to the patient's intolerance to hemodialysis. Peritonitis is the most common complication of peritoneal dialysis and occurs following the inadvertent introduction of bacteria into the peritoneal space through the peritoneal dialysis catheter. Infections may also occur along the intra-abdominal tract of the catheter. In patients on peritoneal dialysis for extended periods (years), there may be a progressive loss in the efficiency of dialysis.

Factors Involved in the Choice of Type of Dialysis

Chronic hemodialysis can be performed in the home, if the patient has a dialysis partner, or in an outpatient dialysis facility. Chronic peritoneal dialysis is usually a home- rather than a facility-based treatment. The morbidity and mortality of ESRD patients treated with either hemodialysis or peritoneal dialysis are approximately the same. The choice of one modality over the other, therefore, is often predicated on nonmedical considerations, such as the patient's desires to directly participate in his or her care, the home and work situation of the patient, and the proximity of the patient to a kidney treatment center. In certain acute and chronic circumstances, however, one modality may be the preferred treatment option.

1. Cardiovascular instability is more common in patients treated with hemodialysis than in those treated with peritoneal dialysis. Peritoneal dialysis does not require an extracorporeal low-resistance blood circuit. In addition, by virtue of the fact that peritoneal dialysis is a less efficient modality on a per minute basis, the changes in blood chemistries and in the extracellular fluid volume occur more slowly. In a patient who is experiencing instability or intolerance to hemodialysis, peritoneal dialysis may be the preferred treatment option.

2. In the patient with diabetes mellitus, peritoneal dialysis is the preferred choice of dialytic therapy. Peritoneal dialysis avoids the requirement for heparin with the attendant risk of blindness in the diabetic patient with retinopathy. There is a significant increase in the incidence of blindness in diabetic patients treated with chronic hemodialysis. In addition, patients with diabetes mellitus who reach ESRD have a high incidence of associated cardiac disease and autonomic neuropathy and, as a consequence, are less tolerant to hemodialysis.

3. The presence of intra-abdominal adhesions, communications between the pleural and peritoneal spaces, or abdominal wall hernias contraindicates the institution or continuation of peritoneal dialysis. Obesity and abnormalities in serum lipids may be exacerbated by the glucose absorbed from the peritoneal dialysis fluid. The presence or worsening of these conditions is a relative contraindication to peritoneal disease.

Outcomes of Dialysis

Death rates in patients on chronic dialysis averages 10 to 15 per cent per year but are quite variable. In recent years, the age of patients who are maintained on chronic dialysis has increased, as have the number and severity of coexisting illnesses. The major causes of mortality and morbidity are infections and cardiovascular events. Patients can be maintained on dialysis while awaiting renal transplantation, and patients who have undergone unsuccessful attempts at renal transplantation can be returned to chronic dialytic therapy.

TRANSPLANTATION

In suitable individuals, renal transplantation is a valid option for treatment of patients with end-stage renal disease. Although patient survival is approximately equal in patients receiving a renal transplantation and those treated by dialysis, there are significant differences between these forms of replacement therapy. A successful transplant more closely approximates the function of the normal kidney than does dialysis. Dietary restrictions are considerably less, and the patient is no longer obligated to the time required to perform dialysis. The advantages of transplantation are partially offset by the requirement for immunosuppressive drugs with the consequent results of infections and neoplasms and the risks associated with immunological rejection of the transplanted kidney.

The success of a renal transplant is dependent upon a number of factors. Perhaps the most important factor is the immune tolerance of the recipient. In general, the better the match of tissue antigens between donor and recipient, the better the outcome. Organ donation by a living relative, therefore, has a better renal outcome than does donation from a cadaveric source. The inherent immune responsivity of the recipient also determines the tolerance to a transplanted organ. Finally, the ability of drugs to modify the immune response is a factor in the overall success rate of renal transplantation. Tissue typing and measurements of reactivity of the recipient to the donor are determined by clinical laboratory methods. The use of these tests has improved the outcome from transplantation by providing a closer match between donor and recipient and avoiding transplantation in patients with unfavorable immunological parameters. In addition, considerable progress has been made to modulate the immune response of the recipient by the use of immunosuppressive drugs including corticosteroids, azathioprine, cyclophosphamide, and cyclosporine and by the use of other immunomodulating agents such as antilymphocyte globulins, monoclonal antibodies, and pretransplant blood transfusions.

Although the success rate of renal transplantation continues to improve, rejection of the allograft remains a significant concern for all patients with a kidney transplant. Three major patterns of allograft rejection have been identified (Table 30–3). Hyperacute rejection, the least common form, occurs in the immediate perioperative period and is mediated by performed antibodies to the allograft. In these cases, the allograft is rendered nonfunctional and requires immediate removal. Acute rejection of a kidney transplant can occur within the first weeks after engraftment or as a delayed phenomenon months to years after successful transplantation. The rejection process involves cell-mediated immunity and is characterized by infiltration of the renal parenchyma with lymphocytes. A deterioration in renal function, often associated with fever and graft tenderness, is typical in the patient with acute rejection. Rapid intervention with high-dose corticosteroids, antilymphocyte globulin, or monoclonal antibodies is often effective in reversing the acute rejection. Chronic rejection occurs as a slowly progressive immunological injury to the allograft occurring months to years after transplantation and is manifest by microvascular scarring and ischemia. There is no effective treatment that halts the progression of chronic allograft rejection, and loss of the transplant is the eventual outcome.

SUMMARY

End-stage renal disease can result directly from many types of renal injury or as a secondary consequence of processes that are initiated by the original insult. Such factors as hyperfiltration, hyperparathyroidism, and hypertension in the progression of disease may be amenable to therapy. Careful conservative management, therefore, may not only slow the progression of disease but may also relieve some of the clinical consequences of renal disease. Dialysis and transplantation provide renal replacement therapy that can sustain life and allow for medical and social rehabilitation of the patient.

TABLE 30–3. PATTERNS OF RENAL ALLOGRAFT REJECTION

TYPE	TIMING	PATHOPHYSIOLOGY	TREATMENT
Hyperacute	Minutes/hours	Preformed antibodies	Removal of graft
Acute	Days to years, multiple episodes may occur	Cell-mediated	Corticosteroids, antilymphocyte globulin, monoclonal antibodies
Chronic	Usually years	Humoral, vascular injury	None

REFERENCES

Brenner BM, Meyer TW, Hostetter TH. Dietary protein intake and the progressive nature of kidney disease: The role of hemodynamically mediated glomerular injury in the pathogenesis of progressive glomerular sclerosis in aging, renal ablation, and intrinsic renal disease. N Engl J Med 307:652–759, 1982.
Bricker NS: On the pathogenesis of the uremic state: An exposition of the "trade-off hypothesis." N Engl J Med 286:1093–1099, 1972.
Fine LG: The uremic syndrome: Adaptive mechanisms and therapy. Hosp Prac (In Office Edition) 22:63–73, 1987.
Kokko J: Chronic renal failure. In Wyngaarden JB, Smith LH Jr (eds): Cecil Textbook of Medicine. 18th ed. Philadelphia, WB Saunders Co., 1988, pp 563–577.
Slatopolsky E: The interaction of parathyroid hormone and aluminum in renal osteodystrophy. Kidney Int 31:842–854, 1987.

31

RENAL VASCULAR AND GLOMERULAR DISEASES

The renal vasculature includes the renal artery and its major branches, the specialized glomerular capillary bed, and the renal veins. Each of these vascular divisions may contribute to distinct clinical syndromes. *Glomerular disease* rarely causes local symptoms; it is more likely detected by the presence of either edema or hypertension, the cardiovascular complications of the disorder, or the presence of blood or protein in the urine. Deranged glomerular function—either proteinuria consequent to increased glomerular capillary permeability to macromolecules, or a reduced GFR secondary to altered glomerular ultrafiltration dynamics—characterizes these diseases. *Large vessel disease* of the kidney may be associated with flank or abdominal pain and cause alteration of both glomerular and tubular function.

GLOMERULAR DISEASES

CLINICAL PRESENTATION

Proteinuria in excess of 0.5 to 1 gm/24 hr is the hallmark of glomerular disease and indicates an impairment in the ability of the glomerular capillary to retain serum macromolecules (proteins). The second common sign of glomerular disease, red and white blood cells and cellular casts in the urinary sediment, is associated with glomerular inflammation. Regardless of the etiology of the glomerular injury, the clinical presentation and course of glomerular diseases converge on the following general patterns.

Nephrosis is a presentation of glomerular injury characterized predominantly by proteinuria with minimal or no cellular sediment in the urine. Nephrosis is expressed clinically as edema formation, normal to reduced blood pressure, and normal or slowly decreasing rates of glomerular filtration (GFR). The *nephrotic syndrome* is a clinical syndrome in which heavy proteinuria (usually >3 gm/24 hr) leads to a reduction in the serum albumin (usually <3.0 gm/dl) and in which edema formation, the expansion of the interstitial component of the extracellular fluid volume, occurs as a result of renal salt retention in the face of a reduced serum oncotic pressure. Hyperlipidemia and lipiduria are frequent findings in the syndrome.

Nephritis describes a presentation of glomerular injury in which hematuria or a prominent cellular urinary sediment occurs along with moderate to heavy proteinuria. Hypertension and/or heart failure occurs regularly in nephritic glomerulopathies as renal salt retention expands both the intravascular and interstitial components of the extracellular fluid volume. A reduced GFR is usually seen at an early stage in the course of nephritic diseases. Focal glomerulonephritis, which affects portions of some glomeruli, may present only with hematuria and proteinuria; the GFR and systemic hemodynamic functions may be little affected. Diffuse glomerulonephritis, which affects the entirety of most glomeruli, more often presents with clinical signs of ECF volume excess and azotemia in addition to hematuria and proteinuria.

PATHOGENIC MECHANISMS

Mechanisms of Injury

In most primary glomerular diseases, injury is believed to occur through immunological processes. The principal indication of this association is the regular detection by immunofluorescent staining of immune reactants (IgG, IgM, IgA, C3, or C4) within the glomeruli (Fig. 31–1).

Three modes of antigen-antibody interaction have been described for the activation of complement within the glomerulus. *Circulating immune complexes* (CIC) form within the circulation and may be trapped in the glomerular capillary wall during ultrafiltration. *In situ immune complex* formation takes place when circulating free antigen lodges within the glomerulus and antibody subsequently binds to the trapped antigen. Finally, *antirenal antibody* (specifically, anti–glomerular basement membrane antibody) may form, bind to an element of the glomerulus, and activate injury pathways.

Attraction of polymorphonuclear leukocytes (PMN's) appears to be the most direct consequence of immune complex complement activation. However, injury does occur in immune deposit glomerular diseases in which PMN infiltration is minimal or absent. Moreover, in some common human glomerulopathies, immune reactants are absent. Glomerular injury in diseases such as diabetes mellitus and amyloidosis likely proceeds from metabolic derangements. Finally, hemodynamic insults to the glomerular capillary bed may lead to glomerular necrosis, as in the case of severe hypertension, or to sclerosis, as with sustained elevations of glomerular capillary pressure or flow.

Mechanisms of Proteinuria

The serum proteins are excluded from the urine on the basis of both their size and their net negative charge. The latter causes them to be repelled by the fixed negative charge of the glomerular capillary wall. Albumin, with a molecular radius of about 3.6 nm, is almost totally excluded from passage into the urine, but a neutral molecule of equal size would appear in urine at a concentration of approximately 20 per cent that in the blood.

Proteinuria in glomerular disease most likely represents a loss of the functional, negatively charged barrier of the glomerulus rather than a disruption in the structure of the capillary wall. This proteinuria does not represent either a failure by the tubules to reabsorb normally filtered proteins or an increase in the tubular secretion of serum proteins.

Sodium Retention

Renal salt retention, expressed clinically as edema formation and/or volume overload and hypertension, is another common feature of glomerular disease. While a reduction in GFR may account for some of the decreased ability to excrete salt, alterations in glomerular hemodynamics may independently compromise the ability of the kidney to excrete sodium. In this case, a change in postglomerular blood flow and

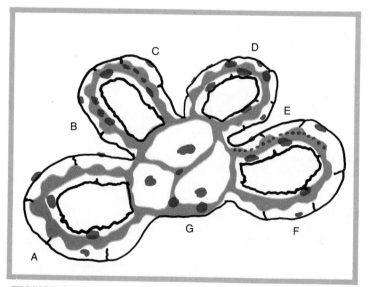

FIGURE 31–1. Patterns of immune deposits in glomeruli. *A,* Normal capillary loop. *B,* Subendothelial deposits. *C,* Intramembranous deposits. *D,* Subepithelial "humps." *E,* Fine, epimembranous deposits. *F,* Linear glomerular basement membrane deposits. *G,* Mesangial deposits.

protein concentration may increase salt and volume absorption in the proximal nephron. Stimulation of the renin-aldosterone axis leading to hormone-dependent renal sodium retention may occur in nephrotic patients who have a reduction in circulating volume attendant to lowered vascular oncotic pressure or in nephritic patients who have gross reductions in renal blood flow.

Reduction in GFR

As noted in Chapter 26, the rate of glomerular filtration may fall as a result of a decrease in capillary hydrostatic pressure or a decrease in the permeability of the capillary wall. Endothelial cell swelling, capillary occlusion or sclerosis, and glomerular scarring all decrease glomerular capillary pressure and blood flow. In other cases, glomerular architecture is little affected. In animals, a reduction in the permeability (K_f) of the glomerular capillary has been found in similar circumstances.

Even when glomerular permeability is reduced, GFR can be maintained near normal by raising the hydrostatic pressure and/or blood flow within the glomerular capillary bed through alteration of glomerular arteriolar tone. In some glomerular disease, a progressive fall in GFR continues long after any evidence for immunological injury can be found. In such cases, these adaptive hemodynamic changes in the glomerulus lead to physical, nonimmunological injury of the glomerular capillaries and result in progressive glomerular sclerosis.

CLASSIFICATION OF GLOMERULAR DISEASES

The classification of glomerulopathies is very confusing because groupings can be made according to the histological pattern of injury, the etiological origin of injury, or the mode of clinical presentation. This section will first divide glomerular diseases by their chief pattern of clinical presentation (nephrosis, nephritis, or mixed) and then order the individual entities by the dominant renal histopathological pattern.

NEPHROTIC GLOMERULOPATHIES

Table 31–1 lists the more common renal lesions which present clinically with nephrotic-range proteinuria. The entries listed in heavy black print present almost solely as the nephrotic syndrome and will be discussed in this section. Each of these histopathological patterns may occur as a primary (idiopathic) renal lesion, in which no contributory disease process has been identified, or secondary to a known disease. Underlined entries may have manifestations other than the nephrotic syndrome and are discussed in subsequent sections.

Minimal Change Nephropathy

This glomerulopathy is the most common cause of childhood nephrotic syndrome, is most prevalent in children aged 2 to 6 years, and displays a 3:1 male

TABLE 31–1. GLOMERULOPATHIES ASSOCIATED WITH THE NEPHROTIC SYNDROME

Minimal Change Nephropathy (Nil Lesion, Lipoid Nephrosis)
  Idiopathic
  Secondary: Hodgkin's lymphoma
Membranous Glomerulopathy (Epimembranous or Perimembranous Nephropathy)
  Idiopathic
  Secondary: Infections—hepatitis B, syphilis
        Neoplasms—carcinoma of lung, stomach, breast
        Drugs—gold, D-penicillamine
        Systemic lupus erythematosus
Focal Glomerular Sclerosis (Focal and Segmental Glomerulosclerosis, Focal Sclerosing Glomerulopathy)
  Idiopathic
  Secondary: Heroin abuse
        Chronic vesicoureteral reflux
Diabetic Glomerulosclerosis (Kimmelstiel-Wilson Glomerulosclerosis)
Amyloidosis
  Idiopathic amyloid
  Secondary amyloid: Multiple myeloma
        Chronic infection—osteomyelitis, tuberculosis
        Familial Mediterranean fever
Essential Cryoglobulinemia
Membranoproliferative Glomerulonephritis
Mesangioproliferative Glomerulonephritis

predominance. Up to 25 per cent of cases of adult nephrotic syndrome may be minimal change. Edema in an otherwise healthy individual is the mode of clinical presentation in over three fourths of cases. Up to one third of childhood cases appear to follow an upper respiratory infection.

Proteinuria greater than 50 mg/kg/day with a serum albumin less than 2.0 gm/dl and a serum cholesterol greater than 300 mg/dl is a typical finding. Lipiduria, seen as lipid droplets or "Maltese crosses" under polarized light, is common, while microscopic hematuria occurs in a distinct minority of patients. Serum complement levels are normal.

Renal insufficiency and azotemia do not occur unless caused by severe vascular volume contraction. Postural hypotension and circulatory collapse may occur in the face of severe reductions of serum oncotic pressure. An increased susceptibility to infection by encapsulated organisms (pneumococcus, *Haemophilus*, *Klebsiella*) is notable when proteinuria is great and may relate to urinary losses of IgG. Thrombosis of renal and peripheral veins, associated with a hypercoaguable state, is not uncommon.

The term minimal change or nil lesion refers to the fact that the glomeruli appear normal on light microscopy (Fig. 31–1A). There is no significant or consistent staining for immune reactants. Electron microscopy reveals nothing more than the "fusion" of epithelial cell foot processes, a nonspecific finding that likely reflects the loss of the anionic charge of the glomerulus and subsequent collapse of the epithelial cell onto the basement membrane. No regular etiological association is known for the disease in children, but some adults with the minimal change lesion are found to have Hodgkin's disease.

The natural course of minimal change nephropathy is that of spontaneous remission, frequently with relapse, but with eventual disappearance of proteinuria. However, because of the exquisite sensitivity of the proteinuria to corticosteroids, almost all patients are treated with these drugs. Steroids are given at an initial dose of about 60 mg/sq m/day of prednisone for 4 weeks, then tapered over 8 to 12 weeks, and discontinued only after the patient has remained free of proteinuria for about 4 weeks.

Of the fewer than 10 per cent who do not respond to the initial course of steroids, some will remit with either prolonged therapy or an increased dose of prednisone. Failure to respond to steroids, or persistent steroid dependency, has been used as an indication for concomitant therapy with an alkylating agent such as cyclophosphamide. However, the considerable risk of this drug, including the danger of gonadal injury or carcinogenesis in children, makes its use highly controversial in the treatment of a disease with a naturally favorable outcome.

About three fourths of individuals will be free of proteinuria, off treatment, at ten years. The mortality rate in children is well below 5 per cent and usually related to vascular complications, occasionally to infections, but not to renal insufficiency. Adults have a response to steroids and an eventual outcome similar to that described for children. Nonresponders to steroids will often be found to have a glomerulopathy other than minimal change, often focal sclerosis.

Membranous Glomerulonephropathy

Membranous glomerulonephropathy (GN) is the most common cause of nephrotic syndrome in adults. It accounts for about 50 per cent of adult cases, has a peak incidence in the fifth decade, and is not common in children. The disease may be detected as asymptomic proteinuria, but as many as 80 per cent of patients present with massive proteinuria and the nephrotic syndrome. While the majority of cases of membranous GN are idiopathic, the membranous lesion may be seen in association with unrelated disorders such as persistent hepatitis B antigenemia, systemic lupus erythematosus (SLE), organic gold exposure, and neoplasia (especially carcinoma).

Proteinuria in excess of 15 to 20 gm/day is not uncommon in membranous GN, and microscopic hematuria occurs in a substantial number of patients. Serum complement levels are normal in the idiopathic disease. A progressive fall in GFR occurs in a majority of patients, and hypertension and azotemia develop late in the disease.

The classic finding on light microscopy is that of uniform basement membrane thickening throughout the glomerulus. Cellular proliferation and infiltration are strikingly absent. IgG and C3 are prominent on immunofluorescent microscopy and show a uniform, finely granular pattern outlining the capillary loops (Fig. 31–1E). Electron microscopy identifies deposits along the epithelial side of the glomerular basement membrane.

While the majority of patients with membranous ne-phropathy present with the nephrotic syndrome, spontaneous complete remission of proteinuria occurs in about 25 per cent of cases and partial remission in a similar number. However, most of the remaining patients will progress to end-stage renal failure by ten years. The fall in GFR is usually gradual, so that sudden drops in renal function may indicate a secondary problem, such as renal vein thrombosis or drug-induced interstitial nephritis. There continues to be controversy regarding the treatment of membranous nephropathy, but some physicians recommend courses of steroids and/or cytotoxic agents as a means of retarding progression to renal failure.

Focal Glomerular Sclerosis (FGS)

Idiopathic FGS is a cause of the nephrotic syndrome in 10 to 20 per cent of children and young adults. The presentation is usually that of edema with heavy proteinuria so that this disorder may be diagnosed as minimal change nephropathy in the absence of a renal biopsy. However, a number of clinical features tend to set focal glomerular sclerosis apart from the more common minimal change lesion. Less than 20 per cent of patients with FGS remit with steroids, compared to a greater than 90 per cent remission rate in minimal change nephropathy. In addition, microhematuria is common in FGS, and hypertension and azotemia are present at the time of diagnosis in a substantial number of patients with FGS. Serum complement levels are normal.

The diagnostic feature of this glomerulopathy on light microscopy is the focal (only some glomeruli involved) and segmental (only parts of each glomerulus affected) finding of hyalin sclerosis in the absence of significant proliferation or necrosis. Because deep, juxtamedullary glomeruli appear to be affected first in FGS, a renal biopsy that samples only superficial glomeruli may be diagnosed as showing minimal change nephropathy. Late in the disease, global sclerosis of individual glomeruli and pronounced interstitial and tubular damage are seen.

Immunofluorescence shows patchy deposits of IgM and C3 confined to areas of the glomeruli identified as sclerosed on light microscopy. The IgM is believed to be trapped nonspecifically in sclerotic glomeruli but not to be causally related to the development of FGS. Likewise, specific immune deposits are absent on electron microscopy.

While remissions do occur, the overall course is one of continuous proteinuria with relentless progression to end-stage renal failure. Persistent nephrotic-range proteinuria has a less favorable prognosis, with at least 50 per cent of these patients having terminal renal failure at ten years. Steroid therapy has been beneficial in producing remission of proteinuria in some, but not all, studies and may slow progression of renal failure in patients whose proteinuria remits. Recurrence of FGS in transplants is common.

Similar pathology has been associated with the nephrotic syndrome in patients who abuse intravenous drugs (heroin nephropathy) and in some, but not all, cases of nephrotic syndrome occurring in patients infected with the HIV virus (AIDS nephropathy). In each of these instances the disease appears much more virulent than in the idiopathic variety. Progression to end-stage renal failure in less than one year is common in these syndromes.

NEPHRITIC GLOMERULOPATHIES

Unlike the glomerular lesions that regularly present as the nephrotic syndrome (edema and heavy proteinuria), other patterns of renal histopathology are associated with nephritic syndromes (hypertension, hematuria, and proteinuria). The common pattern in nephritic glomerular lesions is that of cellular proliferation (mesangial, endothelial, or epithelial cells) and cellular infiltration (polymorphonuclear leukocytes, macrophages). Table 31–2 lists the common histopathological and clinical diseases that present with major manifestations of the nephritic syndrome. Some of these entities are discussed in subsequent sections.

Three general categories of cellular proliferation, each representing one part of the spectrum of clinical nephritis, can be described. *Focal nephritis*, which affects portions of some glomeruli, is most often associated with hematuria and proteinuria but with little or no reduction in GFR. *Diffuse proliferative nephritis* from any etiology, in which nearly all glomeruli show extensive cellular proliferation and/or infiltration, is usually associated with azotemia and hypertension in addition to hematuria and proteinuria. Finally, *glomerulonephritis* with *extensive crescent formation* is almost always associated with progressive deterioration of renal function.

A given case of glomerulonephritis may run its course at any one of the above stages, but crossover from one histological lesion to another is common among most types of GN. The finding of extensive crescent formation on a renal biopsy (≥50 per cent of glomeruli affected) carries an ominous prognosis for reversibility of the renal lesion.

Proliferative Glomerulonephritis

Acute glomerulonephritis (AGN) is the most common nephritic syndrome and can be divided etiologically into post-streptoccocal AGN and nonstreptococcal AGN. In either case, the patient usually presents with oliguria, dependent or facial edema, urine that is grossly bloody or "tea-colored" from hemolyzed RBC's, and a history of a recent or ongoing infectious process. Hypertension is present or develops during the course of the disease in most patients, and the GFR is almost always reduced. Proteinuria is a constant finding but is rarely of sufficient magnitude to produce the nephrotic syndrome. Red blood cell casts are usually present in the urine. Although azotemia is common, the acute renal syndrome with uremia occurs in a minority of patients. Complete recovery of renal function after clearing of the infectious process is the rule, although some patients are left with a partial impairment of GFR and fewer still progress to chronic renal failure.

Acute post-streptococcal GN is most frequent in

TABLE 31–2. GLOMERULOPATHIES ASSOCIATED WITH NEPHRITIC SYNDROMES

Proliferative Glomerulonephritis
  Postinfectious, acute glomerulonephritis
    Streptococcal
    Nonstreptococcal: Staphylococcal, pneumococcal, mumps, varicella, hepatitis B, Ebstein-Barr virus
  Systemic lupus erythematosus
  Anaphylactoid purpura (Schönlein-Henoch purpura)
  Essential cryoglobulinemia
Progressive Crescentic Glomerulonephritis
  Idiopathic rapidly progressive glomerulonephritis
  Anti–glomerular basement membrane disease: Goodpasture's syndrome
Other Glomerulonephritides
  Hemolytic-uremic syndrome
  Hereditary nephritis (Alport's syndrome)
  Vasculitides: Wegener's granulomatosis, periarteritis nodosa

children and young adults and follows group A, beta-hemolytic streptococcal infections of either the pharynx or skin (pyoderma). Signs of nephritis usually appear 10 to 20 days after onset of the infection. The antistreptolysin O (ASO) titer is almost always elevated in streptococcal pharyngitis but is elevated in less than one third of patients with streptococcal pyoderma. Antihyaluronidase titers are usually elevated in the latter patients. Total serum complement activity (CH_{50}) and serum C3 are almost invariably depressed during the acute illness. These return to normal in three to six weeks as the renal disease disappears. About 2 per cent of patients may have minor urinary sediment abnormalities (protein and/or RBC's) for as long as seven to ten years. Progression to chronic renal failure is rare and is usually confined to the older adults who develop acute GN.

Nonstreptococcal, postinfectious GN has been described in association with bacterial endocarditis due to coagulase-positive *Staphylococcus aureus*, with chronically infected atrioventricular shunts due to coagulase-negative *S. epidermidis*, and with pneumococcal pneumonia. Acute viral infections such as hepatitis B, mumps, varicella, infectious mononucleosis, and others have also given rise to acute GN. The pattern of the acute GN is the same as that for post-streptococcal GN, and the prognosis for complete renal recovery is favorable in these diseases. A similar syndrome of acute nephritis may be seen in association with other disease processes, most notably with systemic lupus erythematosus (SLE).

Histologically, these cases are characterized on light microscopy by endothelial and mesangial cell proliferation with leukocyte infiltration. Immunofluorescent staining is usually strongly positive for IgG and C3 and shows a granular pattern of deposition around capillary loops. The classic EM finding in post-streptococcal GN is that of large "humps" of electron-dense deposits in subepithelial spaces (Fig. 31–1D).

Treatment in all of these cases is directed at eradication, where possible, of the infecting organism and management of the consequences of renal injury until recovery occurs. Corticosteroids and immunosuppressive agents are not useful. Edema and hypertension are best managed by salt restriction and diuretic therapy. The azotemia is usually self-limited, but a few patients will require dialysis.

Anaphylactoid purpura, or Henoch-Schönlein purpura, is a chronic recurrent disorder that is most common in young children and is occasionally associated with nephritis. It is characterized by repeated attacks of palpable purpura, chiefly in the lower trunk and legs; episodic bouts of abdominal pain; and transient arthralgias. An acute nephritic picture with hematuria, moderate proteinuria, and a modest reduction in GFR occurs in a number of patients. A few patients develop a rapidly progressive course to renal failure, almost always within the first few years of diagnosis of the purpura. Serum C3 levels are normal, although CH_{50} activity may be mildly depressed.

Light microscopy varies from focal, segmental cellular proliferation to diffuse cellular proliferation with extensive crescent formation; the latter lesion is seen most commonly when renal failure occurs. Immunofluorescent staining for mesangial IgA and C3 is prominent. Importantly, dermal capillaries of affected or unaffected skin stain strongly for IgA and C3 so that a skin biopsy may be useful in diagnosing the etiology of nephritis in such patients.

The basic disease is self-limiting, disappearing after a few months to years. Complete renal healing is seen in over half of patients who develop nephritis, but about 10 per cent progress to renal failure. Steroids ameliorate extrarenal symptoms but do not appear to alter the renal component of the disease. Recurrence has been noted in transplants.

Essential cryoglobulinemia, in which IgG/IgM cryoprecipitates having rheumatoid factor activity occur, may cause an acute nephritic syndrome. Acute renal failure with proteinuria and hematuria occurs along with purpura, fever, and Raynaud's phenomenon. Immunofluorescent microscopy typically shows IgG, IgM, and C3 in granular masses within the mesangium and capillary loops. On EM, large intracapillary "thrombi" of the cryoprecipitate may be seen. Lowering the circulating level of cryoprecipitate with plasmapheresis often induces a clinical remission of the nephritis.

Progressive Crescentic Glomerulonephritis

Rapidly progressive glomerulonephritis (RPGN) describes a nephritic syndrome that is more common after the third decade of life, has a clinical presentation similar to that of acute postinfectious GN, and is characterized by extensive formation of glomerular crescents. The major clinical distinction is that RPGN displays a rapid (<6 month) progression to end-stage renal failure. Serum complement levels are normal, a fact that helps in the early distinction of this syndrome from postinfectious or SLE nephritis.

Two categories of RPGN have been identified, based on the distinctive histopathology and serology of each variety. *Anti–glomerular basement membrane* (anti-GBM) glomerulonephritis occurs in association with circulating anti-GBM antibodies. Goodpasture's syndrome is a form of anti-GBM nephritis in which pulmonary hemorrhage is a major feature of the clinical disease. *Idiopathic* RPGN has a similar renal course but lacks circulating anti-GBM antibody.

Light microscopy of all forms of RPGN is dominated by the appearance of extensive glomerular crescents in greater than 50 per cent of glomeruli. Crescents may be seen in severe forms of other glomerular diseases, including post-streptococcal GN and anaphylactoid purpura.

Anti-GBM disease is identified by continuous, linear staining for IgG and C3 along the basement membranes of glomerular capillaries (Fig. 31–1F). In Goodpasture's syndrome, linear immune staining of pulmonary capillary basement membranes can also be demonstrated. Idiopathic RPGN has variable immune staining that ranges from patchy, segmental staining for C3 and IgM to cases in which no immunofluorescence is seen. Electron microscopy does not regularly show deposits in either form of this disorder, but breaks in the glomerular basement membrane are common.

Treatment in anti-GBM nephritis is directed toward lowering the level of circulating anti-GBM antibody. Plasmapheresis to remove circulating antibody, in combination with corticosteroids and immunosuppressive drugs to reduce antibody production, has been successful in halting progression of disease in some patients. Individuals with an initial serum creatinine greater than 5 mg/dl, or those having crescents in 80 per cent or more of glomeruli on renal biopsy, are not likely to respond to treatment. Anti-GBM disease has recurred in transplanted kidneys. No therapy has been shown to be of consistent benefit in the treatment of idiopathic RPGN.

Other Glomerulonephritides

The *hemolytic-uremic syndrome* (HUS) chiefly affects children under the age of 10 years and almost always follows a nonspecific gastrointestinal or influenzal syndrome. However, an adult form does occur and is seen primarily is women taking oral contraceptives or those in the postpartum period.

The acute phase of HUS is manifest by sudden onset of severe oligoanuria, hematuria, acute gastrointestinal symptoms, and gastrointestinal bleeding. Hypertension and volume overload are common, as are petechiae and ecchymoses. Oligoanuria and azotemia persist for one to two weeks in children, with spontaneous recovery the rule. Acute dialysis during this period has dramatically increased survival. Recurrence of the syndrome in children is well-documented, and these children may have progressive renal disease. The outcome in adults is much less favorable, with the vast majority of survivors requiring chronic dialysis or transplantation.

Another striking feature of this syndrome is microangiopathic hemolytic anemia, evidenced by fragmented circulating RBC's accompanied by thrombocytopenia. The glomeruli may show fibrin thrombi in capillary loops and segmental fibrinoid necrosis on light microscopy. Bilateral renal cortical necrosis occurs in the most severe cases, mostly in adults. A characteristic lesion is seen on EM in which capillary endothelial cells are separated from basement membranes by a space filled with finely granular basement membrane–like material.

Thrombotic thrombocytopenic purpura (TTP), which likely shares certain pathogenic origins with HUS, may also present with signs of nephritis and microangiopathic hemolytic anemia. In TTP, the clinical syndrome is dominated by neurological manifestations and the nephritis is evidenced by modest proteinuria, microhematuria, and modest degrees of azotemia. Glomerular pathology is similar to, but less extensive than, that of HUS.

Hereditary nephritis, or Alport's syndrome, is a chronic GN that seems to follow X-linked inheritance. The clinical manifestations of renal disease are more common and more severe in males. The disease presents in childhood with recurrent bouts of gross hematuria, often with loin or vague abdominal pain. Sensorineural deafness is seen in about half the patients. Proteinuria is usually slight and the nephrotic syndrome is uncommon. Males are especially prone to develop renal failure by age 20 to 30 years. Treatment does not alter the course of the disease, and it is not known to recur in transplanted kidneys.

Light microscopy findings are nonspecific, but an inflammatory interstitial component with foam cells becomes prominent as the disease progresses. There is no consistent immunofluorescent finding in glomeruli, but electron microscopy shows a distinctive lesion. Widespread glomerular basement membrane alterations are evident, with severe GBM attenuation alternating with thick GBM's split by a central lucent zone.

MIXED GLOMERULOPATHIES

Certain glomerular diseases have a mixed clinical presentation (Table 31–3). Either nephrotic or nephritic symptoms may dominate the clinical picture, but signs of both nephrosis and nephritis often occur together. Whatever the initial presentation, these glomerulopathies usually follow a relentless course to end-stage renal failure.

Membranoproliferative Glomerulonephritis (MPGN)

MPGN is a chronic glomerulopathy of unknown etiology which is most common in children and young adults. The majority of patients present with significant manifestations of both nephrosis and nephritis. The presence of glomerular disease is discovered in over one third of patients as a result of finding either hematuria or proteinuria, both of which are present in virtually all patients, on a routine urinalysis. Up to one half of patients present with the nephrotic syndrome and have significant, persistent proteinuria throughout the course of the disease. An acute nephritic picture with hypertension, hematuria, and azotemia is seen in about one third of patients. This pres-

TABLE 31–3. GLOMERULOPATHIES WITH NEPHROTIC AND NEPHRITIC FEATURES

Membranoproliferative Glomerulonephritis (Mesangiocapillary GN, Hypocomplementemic GN)
Idiopathic: Type I
            Type II, dense deposit
Secondary: Chronic infections
            Essential cryoglobulinemia
Mesangioproliferative Glomerulonephritis
Idiopathic: IgA/IgG nephropathy (Berger's disease)
            Non-IgA
Secondary: Systemic lupus erythematosus
            Anaphylactoid purpura

entation, especially in the face of a low serum C3 value, requires differentiation from post-streptococcal GN by ASO titer measurements and from lupus nephritis by measurement of antinuclear antibody (ANA) titers.

On light microscopy the most prominent features are mesangial cell proliferation and apparent thickening of capillary basement membranes. Electron microscopy serves to separate the disease into two varieties. Type I MPGN is characterized by subendothelial deposits and duplication of capillary basement membranes caused by interposition of mesangium within the basement membrane (Fig. 31–1B). Type II, also known as dense deposit disease, displays striking deposits of electron-dense material within the basement membranes of peripheral capillary loops (Fig. 31–1C). The early complement components C1q and C4 are often present in type I but usually absent in type II, while C3 is prominent in both varieties.

Persistent hypocomplementemia in MPGN is often associated with a 7S gamma globulin that is capable of inducing cleavage of C3 in the absence of calcium or properdin. This C3 nephritic factor (C3NeF) is more prevalent in type II MPGN, but its presence does not appear to influence the prognosis of the disease.

Temporary spontaneous remissions are known to occur, but at least half the patients will have end-stage renal failure after ten years, with the rate of progression being somewhat greater in type II MPGN. No therapy has proven successful in arresting the progression to renal failure in either type. The presence either of a persistent nephrotic syndrome or of renal insufficiency at the time of diagnosis is associated with rapid deterioration, but neither the occurrence of gross hematuria nor spontaneous remission of proteinuria affects the outcome. Type II, dense-deposit disease almost invariably recurs in transplanted kidneys, while recurrence of type I is far less common.

Mesangioproliferative Glomerulonephritis

This histopathological pattern is best exemplified by the idiopathic syndrome of IgA nephropathy (Berger's disease). This is a distinctive glomerulopathy found in about half of patients with benign recurrent hematuria, a syndrome predominantly of young adult males. The classic presentation is that of repeated bouts of asymptomatic gross hematuria, which often occur in conjunction with an upper respiratory infection and which are separated by periods when only microscopic hematuria is evident. Proteinuria is usually modest, less than 1 gm/day, but up to 10 per cent of patients develop the nephrotic syndrome. Serum complement levels are normal.

The light microscopy is nondiagnostic, but the most typical finding is that of focal, segmental proliferation within glomeruli. The diagnosis is made by the invariable presence of IgA, accompanied by IgG in about half the cases, seen by immunofluorescence within the mesangium (Fig. 31–1G). Mesangial IgA can also be seen in lupus nephritis and in anaphylactoid purpura. Electron microscopy confirms the presence of deposits within the mesangium.

Originally thought to represent a benign disorder, it is now known that 10 to 20 per cent of patients, especially those with heavy proteinuria, will progress to end-stage renal failure in 10 to 15 years. The course of the disease is not known to be altered by corticosteroids or immunosuppressive agents. Mesangial deposits of IgA, sometimes associated with hematuria, recur regularly in kidneys transplanted into these patients.

RENAL VASCULAR DISEASE

Renovascular disorders can be defined based on the size of the vessel involved (Table 31–4). Thromboembolic occlusion of the renal arteries or veins occurs most frequently in a narrow spectrum of clinical settings and may dramatically affect renal function. Stenosis of one or both renal arteries is the most common cause of curable, secondary hypertension. Nephrosclerosis, the sclerotic narrowing of small, intrarenal vessels, is a frequent complication of long-standing hypertension and is a major factor leading to end-stage renal failure in these patients. In addition, systemic vasculitic diseases frequently involve the smaller intrarenal vessels to produce distinctive renal syndromes (see Chapter 30).

Renal Artery Occlusion

Thrombosis of renal arteries is most often seen in cases of severe abdominal trauma. It is seen less frequently after manipulation of the aorta at surgery or during angiography and can occur in association with aneurysms of the aorta or main renal arteries. Occlusion of renal arteries may also occur as an embolic phenomenon, often in patients with underlying atherosclerotic vascular disease. Clot emboli originate from the heart during atrial fibrillation or after myocardial infarction and may occlude major vessels. Valvular vegetations of bacterial endocarditis sometimes embolize to and obstruct arteries of the kidney. Simultaneous embolization to other organs such as brain, mesentery, skin, and muscle provides clues to the origin and nature of occlusive disease in the kidney.

Renal artery occlusion does not invariably cause renal infarction or symptoms. However, when symptoms occur, they usually reflect tissue ischemia and cell death. Sudden renal infarction may cause severe localized flank pain, nausea and vomiting, and oliguria, but rarely hematuria. A sudden onset or exacerbation of hypertension may occur. A leukocytosis may be seen along with elevations of lactate dehydrogenase (LDH) in serum and urine. Segmental or unilateral renal infarction may be asymptomatic without an evident effect on renal function.

Renal vascular scintiradiography is useful in the initial evaluation of suspected cases of renal infarction. Total lack of renal blood flow in a dynamic study or defects in activity on a static image are highly compatible findings. Renal arteriography may be needed to visualize the extent or location of the occluding embolus/thrombus. Renal artery embolectomy has been successful in restoring blood flow and renal function even if performed two to four days after embolization. However, conservative, nonsurgical management of renal artery occlusion may have a more favorable outcome, especially in patients with unilateral or segmental occlusion.

Atheromatous embolization from aortic plaque usually follows manipulation of an atherosclerotic aorta and affects multiple small vessels. The process presents either as acute oliguric renal failure following a surgical or angiographic procedure of the aorta or as spontaneous progressive renal failure occurring over a period of weeks to months. Asymptomatic atheromatous embolization to segmental arteries appears to occur not infrequently as evidenced by local, healed renal infarcts discovered incidentally at autopsy. Path-

TABLE 31–4. CLASSIFICATION OF RENAL VASCULAR DISEASES

DISORDER	VESSEL AFFECTED	SYNDROME
Renal Artery Occlusion		
Thrombosis	Main or segmental renal arteries	Asymptomatic
Clot/vegetation embolization	Main or segmental renal arteries	Acute renal failure
		Hypertension
Atheromatous embolization	Small or medium renal arteries	Acute renal failure Progressive renal failure
Renal Vein Thrombosis	Main renal vein	Asymptomatic Acute renal failure Pulmonary embolization
Renal Artery Stenosis		
Fibromuscular dysplasia	Main renal artery	Hypertension
Atherosclerotic	Main renal artery	Hypertension Progressive renal failure
Nephrosclerosis		
Benign	Small arteries and arterioles	Slowly progressive renal failure
Malignant	Arterioles and small arteries	Rapidly progressive renal failure with proteinuria

ological examination of the kidney reveals the presence of cholesterol "clefts" surrounded by tissue reaction in small to medium renal arteries. Similar vascular lesions are evident in tissues outside the kidney. There is no treatment for this disorder and the prognosis is very poor, reflecting the severity of the primary atheromatous disease.

Renal Venous Occlusion

Renal vein occlusion is a thrombotic event. The incidence of renal vein thrombosis (RVT) is high in nephrotic glomerulopathies, especially membranous nephropathy, and in certain neoplastic diseases. Renal vein thrombosis may occur in infants who develop severe volume depletion accompanying gastroenteritis or sepsis.

Renal vein thrombosis most often occurs in the absence of direct clinical symptoms. However, two distinct patterns of clinical presentation have been recognized. Acute renal failure is often seen in children or in patients with the nephrotic syndrome who have a reduced, but stable, baseline GFR. The second mode of presentation is that of acute pulmonary embolism and infarction, seen most often in patients with the nephrotic syndrome.

Renal vein thrombosis can sometimes be diagnosed with renal ultrasonography, but renal venography may be required for definitive diagnosis. Prophylactic anticoagulant therapy in patients with nephrotic glomerulopathies, the group at highest risk for RVT, is not of proven value. Acute anticoagulant therapy is indicated in cases of proven or threatened pulmonary embolism; an improvement in renal function may occur.

Renal Artery Stenosis

The consequences of renal artery stenosis (RAS) are two-fold: the development of secondary, renin-dependent hypertension and the progressive loss of renal function from ischemia. Renal artery stenosis probably accounts for no more than 2 to 3 per cent of all cases of hypertension in the general population. However, two distinct clinical circumstances point to the high likelihood of RAS as the etiology of the hypertension. First, the onset of significant hypertension in a young female (<35 years old) is highly likely to be due to fibromuscular dysplasia of the renal arteries. Second, the onset of hypertension in a previously normotensive patient older than 55 years of age is often associated with atherosclerotic renal artery stenosis.

Fibromuscular hyperplasia of the renal artery may involve the intima, media, or adventitia of the vessel. The mid and distal thirds of the renal artery are usually involved, the disease is often bilateral, and the lesion tends to progress with time. Renal arteriography demonstrates a typical beaded appearance of the renal arteries. Percutaneous angioplasty is preferred for opening the stenotic vessels and has a greater than 90 per cent success rate.

Atherosclerotic renal artery stenosis is an extension of atheromatous disease of the aorta. Thus, the renal artery ostium and proximal one third of the renal vessels are most affected. Both renal arteries tend to be involved but often asymmetrically. A number of tests have been devised to predict either improvement of renal function or relief of hypertension following surgical correction of the stenosis. One of the more popular tests, measurement of individual renal vein renin values, depends on the stimulation of renin in the stenosed, ischemic kidney and the suppression of renin in the unaffected kidney. Based on this and similar tests, one can expect improvement in the hypertension in greater than 90 per cent of patients in whom the tests are positive. However, at least one third of patients who have negative test results will have a similarly favorable response to surgery. Therefore, clinical factors such as patient age, operative risk, success of medical therapy, and adequacy of renal function are important considerations in the decision to operate in any single case of renal artery stenosis. Percutaneous dilatation of atherosclerotic stenosis has a good initial success rate, but re-stenosis or vessel closure after one year is relatively high. Treatment of hypertension secondary to RAS with converting enzyme inhibitors (CEI) is highly successful. However, acute renal failure may occur in cases of bilateral RAS treated with these drugs. An abrupt fall in GFR after starting CEI therapy should prompt an investigation for bilateral renal artery stenosis.

Nephrosclerosis

Nephrosclerosis is one of the most common complications of essential hypertension and a significant cause of end-stage renal failure. Two forms of the process can be described based on the severity and duration of the hypertension, the pathology of the vascular lesion in the kidney, and the eventual effect on renal and patient survival.

Benign nephrosclerosis is a misnomer that is used to describe a slow process of intrarenal vascular sclerosis and ischemic change that complicates the course of long-standing essential hypertension. A progressive decrease in kidney size is evident on renal sonography or radiography.

Although all the intrarenal arteries show some signs of sclerotic thickening, the dominant lesion is at the level of the afferent arteriole. Hyaline thickening of the afferent arteriolar wall leads to a homogeneous, eosinophilic appearance of the vessel. The glomeruli have ischemic wrinkling of the basement membranes and become progressively sclerotic while the tubules undergo atrophy and are replaced by fibrotic tissue. These changes occur in the absence of inflammation.

Minimal proteinuria occurs in some patients, but the urinary sediment is usually normal. A slow decline in GFR is generally the only feature of the disorder. End-stage renal failure due to nephrosclerosis is more common in males and blacks, and nephrosclerosis has been estimated to account for 5 to 25 per cent of all cases of end-stage renal failure. Treatment is directed at early control of blood pressure elevations, but even late intervention may slow the progression of renal failure.

Malignant nephrosclerosis is a generalized necrotizing arteritis seen in conjunction with accelerated hypertension. Proteinuria and hematuria occur together with acute decreases in GFR. The diastolic blood pressure is usually, but not necessarily, above 120 mm Hg, and neuroretinal signs of encephalopathy, retinal arteriolar hemorrhage, and papilledema are almost always present. The entire syndrome is most common in black males and most often occurs as an acute exacerbation of essential hypertension.

The kidneys are generally contracted in size and have petechial hemorrhages on the surfaces. Fibrinoid necrosis without inflammation in the renal arterioles and sometimes extending into the glomerular tufts is the characteristic lesion. A second prominent lesion is the "onion skin" endothelial proliferation in small arteries produced by concentric layers of collagen and proliferating endothelial cells. Similar changes are seen in the renal vessels in the adult hemolytic-uremic syndrome and the accelerated hypertension of scleroderma.

Prior to effective antihypertensive therapy, more than three fourths of persons with accelerated hypertension died of renal or cardiac failure within one year. Prompt, effective control of the blood pressure reverses the prognosis, with less than one fourth of the patients suffering a renal or cardiac death in one year. With long-term blood pressure normalization, the vascular lesions heal, demonstrating the contributory role of pressure per se to the pathogenesis of the disorder. The goal of therapy is to rapidly lower the diastolic blood pressure to about 100 mm Hg, with a more gradual lowering to about 80 mm Hg over the course of a few days. The GFR frequently falls further during the early phase of blood pressure control, but improvement of filtration function is to be expected as the vascular lesion heals.

MULTISYSTEM DISEASE WITH RENAL INVOLVEMENT

A number of systemic conditions and diseases are associated with a significant incidence of renal dysfunction. The renal involvement often carries dire consequences for the outcome of the primary disorder. In each of these diseases or processes, vascular and glomerular abnormalities usually dominate the clinical syndromes.

Diabetes Mellitus (DM)

The metabolic and physiological consequences of diabetes mellitus regularly involve the kidney and lead to renal dysfunction. The term *diabetic nephropathy* usually connotes diabetic glomerular injury, but diabetes almost inevitably affects all elements of the kidney simultaneously (Table 31–5). Glomerular proteinuria is the initial clinical manifestation of the diabetic renal lesion in a majority of patients. However, renal disease in some diabetics will present as an interstitial process, typically hypertension and type IV RTA (see Chapter 32).

Diabetic glomerulosclerosis is one of the more significant of the diabetic renal lesions and is the most frequent cause of end-stage renal failure in these patients. Glomerular disease occurs in one third to one half of persons with juvenile-onset, insulin-dependent (type I) diabetes mellitus. The onset of clinically apparent glomerular involvement occurs, in most patients, between 15 and 20 years after the initial diagnosis of DM. Renal disease in DM is first seen as asymptomatic, episodic proteinuria, but progression to fixed, moderate-to-heavy proteinuria occurs rapidly, within one to two years. The time course for development of glomerular disease in type II diabetes, in which significant hypertensive injury may also be present, is not nearly so clear.

Once proteinuria becomes established, a rapid fall in GFR follows, with the course of end-stage renal failure being complete within five years. Although proteinuria is common in type I DM, the incidence of the nephrotic syndrome is low. However, the prevalence of type I DM in the population makes diabetic glomerulopathy a significant cause of adult nephrotic syndrome. The appearance of hypertension usually parallels that of proteinuria. Diabetic retinopathy is an invariant finding in patients with diabetic glomerulopathy; this combination of findings is designated the retinorenal syndrome. The onset of the nephrotic syndrome in an individual having type I DM for less than 10 years, or in the absence of diabetic retinopathy, should alert one to consider a nondiabetic etiology of the renal disease.

The classic glomerular lesion in DM, Kimmelstiel-Wilson nodular glomerulosclerosis, appears as hyalin nodules lying in the center of peripheral capillary loops. This pattern is actually seen in less than 25 per cent of cases of diabetic glomerulopathy. The more typical finding, and that seen most often when heavy proteinuria is present, is that of diffuse glomerular sclerosis associated with arteriosclerosis of *both* afferent and efferent arterioles. Basement membrane thickening and interstitial atrophy may be prominent. Linear immunofluorescent staining for IgG and/or C3 along capillaries appears to represent nonspecific trapping.

Diabetic glomerulopathy seems to result from the metabolic derangements of the diabetic patient. The

TABLE 31–5. CLASSIFICATION OF DIABETIC NEPHROPATHY

DISORDER	CHARACTERISTICS
Diabetic Glomerulosclerosis	
Type I DM	One third to one half of all patients affected
	High correlation with diabetic retinopathy
	Onset with proteinuria after 15-20 yrs diabetes
	End-stage renal failure in 5-6 yrs after onset
	Hypertension common after onset
Type II DM	Incidence and rate of progression uncertain
	Usually occurs in association with hypertension
Diabetic Interstitial Nephropathy	
Types I & II	Mild to moderate reduction in GFR
	Hyporeninemic hypoaldosteronism with type IV RTA
	Papillary necrosis not uncommon

renal lesion may be related to a generalized alteration of basement membranes caused by addition of disaccharide units to the collagen matrix. In glomerular capillaries this may lead to hyperfiltration seen early in type I DM, when the GFR may be 20 to 30 per cent above normal. The biochemical abnormality of the basement membrane, together with altered glomerular capillary hemodynamics, may lead to nonimmune glomerular injury and sclerosis. This superimposed physical injury is like that which follows some cases of immune-mediated glomerular disease.

Control of hypertension may slow the rate of deterioration of renal insufficiency. Results of recent animal studies indicate that intrarenal angiotensin II generation, with its attendant action on the arterioles of the glomerular capillary bed, may be a significant factor in the maladaptive increase in glomerular blood flow and pressure. For this reason, studies are underway to examine the potential protective benefits of treating diabetics with converting enzyme inhibitors early in the course of their disease, thereby preventing or ameliorating the development of glomerular injury. While strict control of hyperglycemia does not affect the course of established renal insufficiency, evidence is now accumulating that such control in newly diagnosed diabetics might prevent early metabolic changes in basement membranes.

Renal insufficiency is a major limit to survival in diabetics under 40 years of age. The life expectancy of diabetics on hemodialysis is somewhat less than that for nondiabetics. Continuous ambulatory peritoneal dialysis (CAPD) offers a better prognosis for many diabetics with renal failure. Death from cardiovascular complications is highly likely for the diabetic on dialysis. The most promising treatment for diabetic renal failure appears to be renal transplantation from a living, related donor. The diabetic lesion does recur in transplanted kidneys but has not been a significant cause of transplant kidney failure.

A significant number of diabetics display a prominent and characteristic interstitial lesion that appears related to ischemic injury. The syndrome of hyporeninemic hypoaldosteronism is a feature of this lesion and is a major cause of type IV RTA (see Chapter 32). These patients typically present with hyperkalemia and hyperchloremic metabolic acidosis with only a modest reduction in GFR. Hypertension is prominent in this syndrome. The clinical features of the interstitial lesion almost inevitably merge into the glomerular syndrome of diabetic glomerulosclerosis as the patient approaches end-stage renal failure.

Two other renal conditions frequently complicate the course of diabetic nephropathy. Papillary necrosis, especially in conjunction with renal infection, is common in diabetics. The sloughing of papillary tissue may cause acute ureteral obstruction with colic, may be associated with hematuria and passage of tissue in the urine, and may be identified as calyceal irregularity seen on IVP. Although bacteriuria is no more prevalent in diabetics than in nondiabetics, the syndrome of acute pyelonephritis is a more frequent outcome of untreated bacteriuria in the diabetic.

TABLE 31–6. RENAL DISEASE IN MULTIPLE MYELOMA

Functional Disorders
    Paraproteinuria—Filtered Bence-Jones protein
    Fanconi syndrome—Secondary amyloidosis
    Vasopressin-resistant polyuria—Secondary amyloidosis or hypercalcemia
Acute Renal Failure
    Prerenal azotemia—Secondary polyuria plus anorexia/emesis of hypercalcemia
    Vasomotor nephropathy—Secondary severe hypercalcemia
    Nephrotoxic ATN—Secondary increased susceptibility to nephrotoxins, intratubular protein precipitation
Chronic Renal Failure
    Myeloma kidney—Intratubular obstruction and interstitial scarring
    Amyloidosis

Multiple Myeloma

This plasma cell dyscrasia, which often presents with bone pain and/or paraproteinuria, is associated with renal dysfunction at some time in about half of all patients (Table 31–6). The etiologies of renal insufficiency in mutiple myeloma include a specific renal lesion known as "myeloma kidney," hypercalcemia, and an increased susceptibility to nephrotoxins.

"Myeloma kidney" refers to a unique renal lesion that is associated with Bence-Jones proteinuria, the excretion of kappa and lambda light chains of immunoglobulins. Renal insufficiency is common with this lesion. Hypercalcemia, commonly greater than 12 to 13 mg/dl, is seen in at least one third of myeloma patients and may cause a vasopressin-resistant hyposthenuria with polyuria. The combination of volume depletion from the polyuria and hypercalcemia may cause reversible renal insufficiency. Finally, patients with multiple myeloma have an increased risk for acute renal failure after exposure to radiocontrast media or aminoglycoside antibiotics. Intravenous saline is indicated prior to exposure to a nephrotoxic agent.

Amyloidosis

Renal involvement is not uncommon in amyloidosis of any etiology. Glomerular, tubular, and vascular deposits of amyloid occur throughout the kidneys. The most common renal presentation is that of asymptomatic proteinuria, often with paraproteinuria (e.g., Bence-Jones proteinuria). Fanconi's syndrome (see Chapter 32), an indicator of concomitant tubular dysfunction, is not uncommon. Hepatosplenomegaly, malabsorption, or peripheral neuropathy may aid in diagnosing the etiology of the glomerulopathy. Enlarged kidneys may be found on intravenous urography (IVP) or renal ultrasonography. On renal biopsy, bland eosinophilic deposits are found in the mesangium or in capillary loops. Special staining by Congo red reveals the green birefringence under polarized light that positively identifies the deposits as amyloid. Amyloid found in a rectal biopsy correlates highly with renal involvement.

Asymptomatic proteinuria may persist for some

years, but the occurrence of the nephrotic syndrome usually heralds a rapid progression of renal failure. Neither steroids nor alkylating agents seem to alter the course, but colchicine may be useful in patients with familial Mediterranean fever.

Sickle Cell Anemia (SS)

Renal damage occurs in almost all patients homozygous for this hereditary disease, but SS is a most unusual cause of renal failure. The primary injury occurs in the renal medulla, where frequent vascular occlusion from erythrocyte sickling in the hypertonic medullary environment causes obliteration of the vasa recta. Hematuria and a reduction in urinary concentrating ability are prominent manifestations of this phenomenon.

Hematuria, usually in the microscopic range, occurs in most SS patients, but dramatic and prolonged bouts of gross hematuria may be seen. Hematuric patients with sickle hemoglobin are most often heterozygotes, owing simply to their greater number. Bed rest, forced hydration, and transfusions are the standards for treating gross hematuria; nephrectomy is rarely indicated.

A decreased concentrating ability is a very common defect in SS but does not usually cause clinically apparent polyuria. Since these patients dilute urine normally, the defect is likely related to a failure to maintain medullary hypertonicity due to the alteration in medullary blood flow. Papillary necrosis commonly follows infarction from occlusion of the vasa recta.

Hepatic Diseases

Renal dysfunction associated with liver disease includes the glomerulopathies seen with hepatitis B, tubular dysfunction seen with primary biliary cirrhosis, and azotemic syndromes seen with cirrhosis of the liver.

Azotemia in decompensated cirrhosis is often associated with an elevated serum bilirubin and ascites. The reduced GFR is most often due to a reduction in effective circulating volume and renal blood flow which occurs in the face of a reduction in serum albumin and oncotic pressure. The *hepatorenal syndrome* is, almost by definition, a terminal event identified by oliguria, a declining GFR, and tremendous renal sodium avidity. The urinary sodium concentration is almost always less than 10 mEq/L, and there is a disproportionately high BUN/creatinine ratio in most cases. The decline in renal function usually follows one of three events in a cirrhotic patient with ascites: sepsis, a vigorous attempt to reduce ascites with diuretics, or a large volume paracentesis. The kidneys appear normal but show intense, segmental vascular spasm on arteriography. It is not known if the functional renal defect is induced by a hepatic toxin.

Ascites and edema in cirrhotic patients represent cosmetic rather than medical problems in most cases. Treatment of these manifestations should include sodium restriction and the sparing use of diuretics in order to reduce the risk of a decline in renal function. Acute expansion of intravascular volume may reverse azotemia in some cirrhotic patients. Dialysis is indicated when there is a reasonable expectation of improved hepatic function.

Disorders of Pregnancy

Three important relations exist between renal disease and the pregnant state: the effect of existing renal disease on the outcome of the pregnancy; the effect of the normal hemodynamic, endocrinological, and immunological changes of pregnancy on pre-existing renal disease; and the occurrence of distinct renal syndromes in association with pregnancy.

Since uremia causes a disruption in normal hormonal cycles, fertility in women is greatly diminished when the BUN is greater than 40 to 50 mg/dl. However, those patients with mild renal insufficiency (BUN <25 mg/dl) have about a 75 per cent chance of completing a normal, full-term pregnancy. Fetal loss is significant at higher levels of azotemia and when hypertension is a prominent part of the renal disease. In the nephrotic syndrome without azotemia, the birth weight of the infant is decreased in the face of significant maternal hypoalbuminemia.

In most cases, pregnancy does not appear to adversely affect the course of pre-existing renal disease. In lupus nephritis (see below) the renal activity of the disease is generally decreased during pregnancy, but a significant number of patients experience an increase in the activity of nephritis post partum. Some patients with severe lupus nephritis experience an exacerbation of nephritis in the first trimester of pregnancy. Increased doses of steroids may prevent this occurrence. Finally, patients with scleroderma will often experience a significant decline in GFR and a rise in blood pressure during pregnancy.

Hypertension in pregnancy requires careful consideration. Blood pressure usually falls in the first weeks of normal pregnancy and returns to pregestational values only near term. Normal pregnancy is characterized by ECF volume expansion, an increased cardiac output, a decreased systemic vascular resistance, and resistance to the vasopressor effects of angiotensin II. Therefore, any absolute elevation of blood pressure or a pattern of rising blood pressure in early pregnancy is abnormal. At least three categories of pregnancy-related hypertension exist.

Toxemia is a syndrome of hypertension, proteinuria, hyperuricemia, and edema that is seen in the third trimester of pregnancy. It occurs predominantly in young primigravidas or in women over the age of 40. The signs may be deceptive, since mild edema is common in normal pregnancies, and the elevated blood pressure and serum uric acid concentrations must be interpreted in light of the values for a normal pregnancy. A blood pressure of 130/80 may be abnormal at 30 weeks' gestation. Likewise, the serum uric acid concentration is often reduced to less than 3 mg/dl in a normal pregnancy, so that a value of 5 to 6 mg/dl is distinctly abnormal.

Treatment of toxemia consists of vigorous control of blood pressure and the delivery of the fetus as soon as it is judged to be viable. Modest azotemia may be seen, but renal failure is rare. Complete normalization of blood pressure and cessation of proteinuria occur post partum. There is no increased risk of developing sustained hypertension after the single occurrence of toxemia in a young woman.

Essential hypertension may be present before pregnancy and may have little effect on the outcome of the pregnancy. Hypertensive patients are more prone to develop toxemia. Only when diastolic blood pressures remain above 100 mm Hg is there significant fetal loss.

A final group of patients consists of those in whom hypertension develops in late (third trimester) pregnancy in successive gestations. These patterns seem to have an increased likelihood of developing sustained hypertension later in life.

Besides toxemia, two other distinct renal syndromes may be seen in association with pregnancy. *Bilateral renal cortical necrosis* is a rare syndrome that almost always follows a dire obstetric complication: abruptio placentae, retained fetal fragments, or septic abortion. The presentation is usually that of a scant output of bloody urine, followed by sudden, virtually complete anuria. Renal failure is always present and evidence of intravascular coagulation is common. Oligoanuria is prolonged in all cases, but a few patients recover sufficient renal function to stop dialysis after weeks to months of treatment.

Postpartum renal failure, or the adult hemolytic-uremic syndrome, is a rare disorder that has an onset from two to three days up to eight to nine weeks post partum. The preceding pregnancy and delivery are usually normal. A microangiopathic hemolytic anemia with prominent fragmentation of red blood cells is evident. The kidneys show marked deposition of fibrin in arterioles and glomeruli. A vascular proliferative lesion identical to that of accelerated hypertension is seen, although patients with post partum renal failure are typically normotensive. About three fourths of patients have permanent renal failure and require dialysis or transplantation.

Systemic Lupus Erythematosus (SLE)

This disease chiefly affects young females and is diagnosed by serological evidence of autoantibodies to cell nuclear components (ANA's) and by clinical evidence of inflammatory processes in multiple organs (skin, joints, brain, and kidney). Five major categories of glomerular histopathology have been described for SLE nephritis (Table 31–7). Virtually all cases of lupus nephritis display a degree of interstitial inflammation uncommon for other glomerulopathies.

In general, the clinical presentation and severity of renal disease in SLE correlates with the underlying histological lesion. About two thirds of patients will have some clinical evidence of renal disease (proteinuria, microhematuria, or azotemia) at the time SLE is diagnosed. Virtually all patients will have some evidence of SLE renal disease if studied by renal biopsy.

Renal disease in SLE may present clinically as either nephrosis or nephritis. The former presentation is more common, with the nephrotic syndrome occur-

TABLE 31–7. RENAL HISTOPATHOLOGY IN SYSTEMIC LUPUS ERYTHEMATOSUS*

CLASS	RENAL SURVIVAL
Type I—Normal Kidneys	~100%
No histological changes	
Type II—Mesangial Glomerulonephritis	~85%
Increased cellularity and immune deposit confined to mesangium	
Type III—Focal Proliferative Glomerulonephritis	~70%
Mesangial changes plus segmental cellular proliferation and necrosis in <50% of glomeruli	
Type IV—Diffuse Proliferative Glomerulonephritis	25–40%
Changes of Type III involving nearly all glomeruli	
Type V—Membranous Glomerulonephritis	~85%
Diffuse, uniform basement membrane thickening due to small subepithelial deposits; normal cellularity	
Type VI—Interstitial Lupus Nephritis	?
Marked interstitial inflammation with minimal or no glomerular changes	

*World Health Organization classification of renal histopathology of SLE. Three additional types may be defined as combinations of these basic categories.

ring in over half of all patients. Even in these patients, however, considerable overlap of clinical manifestations occurs and hematuria, hypertension, and azotemia are frequent findings. A smaller number of patients present with a full-blown nephritic picture with a clinical course resembling that of RPGN. Renal function may deteriorate rapidly over a period of only a few weeks. Serum complement activity, both CH_{50} and C3, are reduced with active renal disease.

As shown in Table 31–7, the glomerular histopathology in SLE is similar to that seen in non-SLE diseases for any given lesion. For instance, type IV, diffuse proliferative lupus glomerulonephritis has similarities to acute, postinfectious GN. Likewise, type V, membranous lupus glomerulopathy, is indistinguishable from idiopathic membranous nephropathy. A separate classification of the histopathology of lupus nephritis is based on the activity (cellular proliferation and infiltration) and chronicity (fibrous crescents and glomerular sclerosis) of the lesions. This scheme has been used successfully to predict responsiveness and prognosis of the renal disease to treatment.

In general, the clinical course and the prognosis of lupus nephritis corresponds to the glomerular lesion. As seen in Table 31–7, the five-year renal survival in untreated patients ranges from greater than 80 per cent in patients with the type V, membranous lesion to about 25 per cent in patients with the type IV, diffuse proliferative lesion.

Corticosteroid therapy is the mainstay of treatment for lupus nephritis. In the absence of advanced renal failure (serum creatinine >6 mg/dl) and extensive glomerular sclerosis, high-dose steroid therapy (prednisone, 40 to 60 mg/day for 6 to 12 months) has had a dramatic effect on survival. The renal survival in diffuse proliferative SLE glomerulopathy with such treatment is up to 80 per cent in five years versus the 25 per cent survival without steroids. The addition of a cytotoxic drug, such as cyclophosphamide, may allow use of a lower dose of prednisone, avoiding complications of high-dose steroid therapy but adding those of a cytotoxic agent. The membranous lesion has been treated with steroids to reduce proteinuria, but the effect of treatment to slow progression to renal failure is unclear.

REFERENCES

Balow JE, et al: Lupus nephritis. Ann Intern Med 106:79–94, 1987.

Couser WG: Glomerular disorders. *In* Wyngaarden JB, Smith LH Jr (eds): Cecil Textbook of Medicine. 18th ed. Philadelphia, WB Saunders Co., 1988, pp 582–602.

Grenfell A, et al: Clinical diabetic nephropathy: Natural history and complications. Clin Endocrinol Metab 15:783–805, 1986.

McCluskey RT: Immunopathogenetic mechanisms in renal disease. Am J Kidney Dis 10:172–180, 1987.

Ponticelli C, et al: Treatment of idiopathic membranous nephropathy. Adv Nephrol 16:195–218, 1987.

Schwartz GL, et al: Renal parenchymal involvement in essential hypertension. Med Clin North Am 71:843–858, 1987.

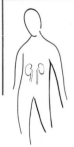

32

TUBULOINTERSTITIAL AND OBSTRUCTIVE DISEASE

Tubulointerstitial diseases are usually asymptomatic until renal damage is far advanced. These disorders characteristically present as abnormalities of urine composition, i.e., failure of urinary concentrating ability, salt wasting, failure of urinary acidification, or failure of complete resorption of organic solutes such as glucose. A decrease in GFR is a late manifestation of these diseases. *Obstruction* of the urinary drainage system usually causes alterations in patterns of urination (oliguria, anuria, nocturia) and may also present with localized pain. Both glomerular and tubular functions are disrupted.

TUBULAR AND INTERSTITIAL DISEASE

CLINICAL PRESENTATION

The clinical manifestations of tubulointerstitial injury reflect the many regulatory functions of the different nephron segments. Tubular disorders may present as alterations in osmotic balance (nephrogenic diabetes insipidus), in acid-base regulation (renal tubular acidosis), in extracellular fluid volume homeostasis (salt-losing nephropathy), and in mineral metabolism (primary phosphaturia). In each case, the function of the segment of the nephron most affected determines the clinical manifestations of the syndrome. Some tubular disorders are purely functional and do not directly affect glomerular filtration. Renal failure, expressed as a reduction in the GFR, occurs only as an indirect effect of altered body homeostasis (see Chapter 26) in these disorders.

Other diseases, in which physical injury to the tubulointerstitial compartment of the kidney occurs, do lead to reductions in GFR. Such disorders include the hereditary cystic diseases of the kidney (polycystic kidney disease) and the chronic interstitial nephritides (lead nephropathy, analgesic nephropathy). The initial presentation of these disorders also reflects the loss of specific tubular functions, and only when far advanced do they display characteristics of a reduction in GFR. Table 32–1 outlines the major tubulointerstitial diseases.

PATHOGENIC MECHANISMS

The great majority of tubulointerstitial disorders occur as a result of one of three general mechanisms: hereditary, toxic injury, or a change in tubule regulation by drugs or hormones. Polycystic kidney disease, familial nephrogenic diabetes insipidus, and Fanconi's syndrome are disorders of hereditary origin. Analgesic nephropathy, lead nephropathy, and some types of renal tubular acidosis are representative of toxic injuries. Pituitary diabetes insipidus (ADH deficiency), adrenal salt wasting (deficient mineralocorticoid), and diuretic administration are examples of the last category (see Chapter 26).

TUBULOINTERSTITIAL DISEASE

Polycystic Kidney Disease (PKD)

This familial disorder is the most significant of a number of renal cystic disorders (Table 32–2). Polycystic kidney disease is inherited as an autosomal dominant trait with high penetrance and has been linked to a gene on chromosome 16. Virtually 100 per cent of persons inheriting the disorder will have cystic changes, but not necessarily renal failure, by age 80 years. The disease will progress to end-stage renal failure in about 25 per cent of individuals by age 50 and in almost 50 per cent by age 70. A separate, infantile form of the disease occurs in association with congenital hepatic fibrosis and causes death from renal failure in the first year of life. Adults may also develop multiple, benign renal cysts that do not cause renal dysfunction or failure.

Clinical manifestations of PKD rarely occur before the age of 20 to 25 years. This accounts for the frequent passage of the genetic trait to offspring by asymptomatic, yet affected, individuals of child-bearing age. Nonspecific, dull lumbar pain is the most frequent initial symptom and usually occurs when the kidneys are sufficiently enlarged to be palpable on examination of the abdomen. Sharp, localized pain may result from cyst rupture or infection or from passage of a renal calculus. Microhematuria without RBC casts is frequently the initial sign of PKD; gross hematuria may also occur.

Hypertension occurs commonly in PKD at early stages of the disease. Polycystic disease may thus be discovered in the course of evaluating hypertension in a young adult. Nocturia due to a urinary concentrating defect is often present at the time of diagnosis, and most patients show impaired salt conservation on a restricted salt intake. Urinary tract infection and pyelonephritis are common complications. Up to one third of patients with polycystic renal disease have multiple, asymptomatic hepatic cysts, and cerebral aneurysms are more prevalent than in unaffected persons.

The diagnosis of polycystic kidney disease is made on the basis of radiographic evidence of multiple cysts distributed throughout the renal parenchyma. The nephrogram phase of intravenous urography (IVP) shows the lucent cysts surrounded by attenuated strands of functional renal tissue. Renal ultrasonography provides a convenient means for demonstrating and following the distribution and size of the cystic lesions. Both studies can be employed to screen younger family members of patients in order to iden-

TABLE 32–1. TUBULOINTERSTITIAL DISORDERS

Structural Disorders
  Cystic Diseases
    Polycystic kidney disease
    Medullary cystic disease
    Medullary sponge kidney
    Simple renal cysts
  Chronic Interstitial Diseases
    Analgesic nephropathy
    Heavy metal nephropathy
    Radiation nephropathy
    Others: nephrosclerosis, diabetic nephropathy
  Renal Tumors
    Benign tumors
    Renal cell carcinoma
Functional Disorders
  Proximal Tubular
    Fanconi syndrome
    Aminocidurias (cystinuria)
    Renal glycosuria
    Vitamin D–resistant rickets (familial hypophosphatemia)
    Proximal (type II) renal tubular acidosis
  Distal Tubular
    Nephrogenic diabetes insipidus
    Bartter's syndrome
    Liddle's syndrome
    Distal (types I and IV) renal tubular acidosis

tify the asymptomatic lesion at a time when genetic counseling may be useful. These tests will identify a significant number of affected persons by ages 10 to 12 years, but a person at risk cannot be judged free of the disease until a negative study is obtained in the age range of 30 to 35 years. The latter fact is especially important in selecting younger family members for donation of a kidney for transplantation to an older, affected sibling or parent. Failure to concentrate the urine above 800 mOsm/kg H_2O after an overnight water fast is highly predictive of PKD in adolescents at risk for the disorder.

Therapy for polycystic kidney disease is directed toward control of hypertension and prevention and early treatment of urinary tract infections. Nephrectomy is occasionally indicated for persistent gross hematuria or for an infected renal cyst. Decompressing cysts by

TABLE 32–2. CYSTIC DISEASES OF THE KIDNEY

DISORDER	DIAGNOSTIC FEATURES	CLINICAL MANIFESTATIONS	OUTCOME
Polycystic			
Infantile	Palpable abdominal masses at birth	Hepatic fibrosis	Death in infancy
Adult	Multiple, bilateral renal cysts on IVP or renal sonography in large kidneys	Hematuria, polyuria, hypertension, abdominal pain	Chronic renal failure (40 to 50 years old)
Medullary Cystic	None	Polyuria, enuresis	Chronic renal failure (15 to 20 years old)
Medullary Sponge	Nephrocalcinosis, radial medullary cysts on IVP	Recurrent renal calculi and urinary infections	Benign
Simple	Single or multiple cysts in normal-sized kidneys	Asymptomatic	Benign

surgical "unroofing" is associated with a high incidence of complications, including complete renal failure, and has no demonstrated therapeutic value. End-stage renal failure is managed by either dialysis or transplantation. Bilateral nephrectomy may be required prior to transplant in patients with inordinately large kidneys or in those with a history of frequent or persistent urinary tract infection.

Cystic Diseases of the Renal Medulla

Medullary cystic disease (nephronophthisis) occurs either as a rare, automosomal recessive disease or as a feature of some cases of retinitis pigmentosa. *Medullary sponge kidney* is a more common, benign disorder that is often detected incidentally on abdominal radiographs.

Medullary cystic disease regularly results in end-stage renal failure during adolescence or early adulthood. Prolonged enuresis in chilhood, due to a urinary concentrating defect, and anemia are early indications of the renal disease. Neither radiography nor renal biopsy has a high rate of success in demonstrating the small medullary cysts.

Medullary sponge kidney is a benign disorder that often presents as a result of passage of a renal calculus. Colicky renal pain, hematuria, or urinary tract infection may herald the disorder, each symptom the result of renal stone formation. Nephrocalcinosis occurs in about half the patients and accounts for identification of asymptomatic patients on routine abdominal radiographs. The diagnosis is made on IVP by the characteristic radial pattern of contrast-filled medullary cysts. Treatment for urinary tract infection and renal calculus formation is indicated. Renal failure does not occur as part of the basic disease.

Chronic Interstitial Nephritis

Distinct causes of chronic interstitial nephritis include analgesic abuse, heavy metal ingestion, and radiation exposure. Diabetes mellitus, multiple myeloma, and essential hypertension, diseases that affect multiple organs, may also cause significant renal interstitial disease. No specific etiology is identifiable for up to one half of all cases of chronic interstitial nephritis. In each case, the disease process may be wholly asymptomatic, with azotemia discovered incidentally on a laboratory screening panel. Hypertension is a regular feature of these disorders and modest proteinuria (<1 to 2 gm/24 hr) is not uncommon. A large number of cases are recognized only when end-stage renal failure occurs and a retrospective diagnosis is made based on a history of toxic exposure.

Analgesic nephropathy follows the ingestion over years of time of combination analgesics, usually aspirin plus either phenacetin or acetaminophen. Use of the single agents alone is not associated with renal injury. The renal medullary lesion may reflect a toxic effect of acetaminophen which is magnified by drug concentration in the medulla. Salicylates, perhaps by blocking production of renal medullary vasodilator prostaglandins, may intensify this concentrating process. Progression of the disease may be halted if analgesic intake is stopped early in the course.

Decreased urinary concentrating ability results from the medullary lesion but frank polyuria is uncommon. Papillary necrosis, visible on renal radiography (IVP) and causing passage of tissue in the urine, is a hallmark of the disease. Treatment consists of withdrawing combination analgesic preparations, rigorously controlling blood pressure, and maintaining surveillance for urinary tract obstruction from sloughed papillary tissue.

Heavy metal nephropathy occurs chiefly with chronic lead ingestion, leaded paints and illicit alochol being prominent sources. The renal disorder is similar to analgesic nephropathy, but coexistence of an anemia disproportionate to the degree of renal insufficiency, prominent peripheral neuropathy, and a high incidence of gouty arthritis are characteristic of lead nephropathy. Interstitial nephritis previously attributed to urate deposition in the kidney (urate nephropathy) is now believed to be lead nephropathy with saturnine gout. Increased urinary lead excretion following EDTA administration is a useful diagnostic test, but EDTA infusion may cause toxic renal failure and is not useful in treating this disorder.

Chronic radiation nephritis may follow some years after local retroperitoneal irradiation. It, too, is associated with progressive, often silent, renal insufficiency; accelerated hypertension is a common complication. There is no treatment for the nephropathy, but strict management of hypertension is important.

Renal Tumors

Most renal tumors appear to originate from the tubulointerstitial components of the kidney. Renal cell carcinoma, for instance, is thought to be of proximal tubular origin. The evaluation of a patient for any renal mass may proceed according to the scheme given in Figure 32–1. This plan attempts to differentiate benign cystic lesions from solid masses and to identify malignant characteristics in solid renal masses.

Benign tumors of the kidney include cortical adenomas and angiomyolipomas (hamartomas). The former are more common in older males and frequently harbor nests of malignant cells. Therefore, adenomas are usually diagnosed after surgical evaluation of a solid renal mass. Angiomyolipomas are highly vascular fatty tumors that mimic renal cell carcinomas in both presentation and angiographic appearance. Significantly, over half of these tumors are seen in patients with tuberous sclerosis. Surgical exploration may be necessary for differentiating angiomyolipoma from renal cell carcinoma in patients without tuberous sclerosis, especially if CT scan results are equivocal.

Renal cell carcinoma, or hypernephroma, is the most frequent malignant renal neoplasm in adults and accounts for about 2 per cent of cancer deaths in both sexes. The term hypernephroma originated from the gross appearance of most of these tumors which, because of their high lipid content, resemble adrenal tissue.

The classic clinical presentation of renal cell car-

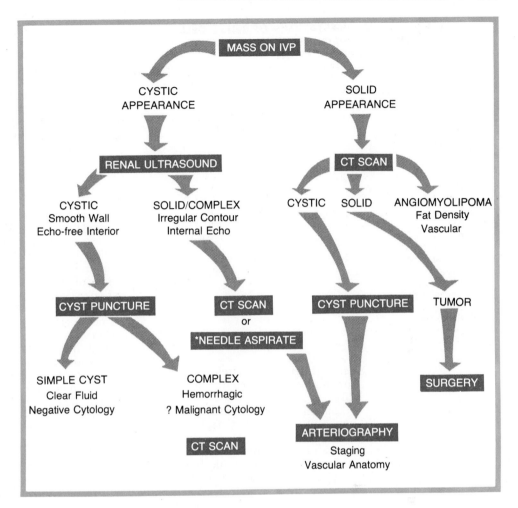

FIGURE 32–1. Scheme for work-up of renal mass.

cinoma, a triad of hematuria, flank pain, and palpable flank mass, is seen in only about 10 per cent of patients (Table 32–3). However, any one of these features is present in well over half of all patients as an initial manifestation of the tumor.

Renal cell carcinoma is notable for the large number of systemic, extrarenal manifestations of the tumor. Fever is seen in about one fifth of cases, and an elevated erythrocyte sedimentation rate (ESR) is seen in half the patients. Anemia is seen in about one third of patients, but polycythemia is a striking finding in some cases. Reversible hepatic dysfunction has been described, as has peripheral neuropathy. Ectopic hormone syndromes associated with renal cell carcinoma include hypercalcemia from osteoclast-stimulating factors and Cushing's syndrome from tumor production of an ACTH-like factor. Hypercalcemia in renal cell carcinoma is frequently associated with bone metastasis of the tumor.

The tumors usually have three cell types: clear cells, granular cells, and spindle cells; the latter cell type and extensive nuclear anaplasia carry a poor prognosis. The tumors are highly vascular, supplied by vessels with thin, amuscular walls. Extension of the tumor into normal renal veins and even into the vena cava is not uncommon. Metastatic spread is chiefly via vascular routes, and the lungs, bone, and liver are most frequently sites of metastasis. The tumors often undergo cystic, internal degeneration, thus mimicking benign renal cysts. Calcification within a renal mass, the result of internal necrosis, is a significant radiographic indicator of malignancy.

As shown in Figure 32–1, needle aspiration of a sonographically cystic lesion is useful in confirming the diagnosis of a simple renal mass. Sonographically solid masses should not undergo needle puncture owing to the risk of rupturing a degenerating carcinoma. Computed tomography (CT) is the preferred means of examining solid renal masses. Renal arteriography may be important when the CT results are indeterminate or for delineation of tumor vascular supply. Renal cell carcinomas are highly vascular tumors; avascular masses may sometimes be carcinomas (<5 per cent of renal cell tumors) or may represent abscesses. The abnormal vessels of renal cell carcinomas constrict poorly in response to epinephrine, a finding of signif-

TABLE 32–3. MANIFESTATIONS OF RENAL CELL CARCINOMA: APPROXIMATE INCIDENCE AT PRESENTATION

MANIFESTATION	PER CENT OF TOTAL
Local	
Hematuria	60
Abdominal mass	45
Pain	40
"Classic triad"—hematuria/mass/pain	10
Systemic	
Common	
Weight loss	30
Anemia	20
Fever	10
Uncommon	<5 (each)
Erythrocytosis	
Leukemoid reaction	
Varicocele	
Hepatopathy	
Hypercalcemia	
Cushing's syndrome	
Galactorrhea	

icance during renal arteriography. Careful needle aspiration for culture may be performed if renal abscess is judged to be likely.

Treatment of renal cell carcinoma requires surgical excision of the tumor, usually by radical nephrectomy. A small, localized tumor may be removed by heminephrectomy, or even ex vivo dissection when preservation of renal functional mass is critical. The tumors respond poorly to radiation and chemotherapy. Vena caval angiography may be valuable preoperatively to ascertain the presence of venous tumor thrombus. Survival is related to cellular morphology, local extension, and distant metastases and ranges from about 10 to 50 per cent ten-year survival based on these factors.

DISORDERS OF TUBULAR FUNCTION

The Fanconi Syndrome

This disorder represents a generalized failure of specialized proximal tubular reabsorption. The Fanconi syndrome is identified by concomitant aminoaciduria, glycosuria, phosphaturia, uricosuria, and bicarbonaturia. The tubulopathy itself does not lead to renal failure, but the condition in which Fanconi's syndrome occurs may cause renal insufficiency.

The Fanconi syndrome is commonly seen as a part of some hereditary disorders, is rarely seen as a single hereditary defect, and may occur as an acquired defect in association with an underlying disease or drug. The most common cause of the syndrome in children is the hereditary disease cystinosis, a disorder characterized by the cellular accumulation of cystine in various organs, including the kidney. Wilson's disease, characterized by excess body copper accumulation, is also a cause of hereditary Fanconi syndrome. The tubu-

lopathy may be acquired as a feature of such diseases as multiple myeloma, amyloidosis, and Sjögren's syndrome.

Aminoaciduria

Abnormal excretion of amino acids may occur as a single defect in proximal tubular reabsorptive function. The aminoacidurias are grouped according to the class of amino acids affected, i.e., basic, neutral, or acidic, and reflect a specific defect in the cellular transport system for each group. The most significant of these many disorders is cystinuria, which is actually a failure of reabsorption of the dibasic amino acids lysine, ornithine, arginine, and cystine. Cystine is singled out because of its very low solubility over the urinary pH range of 4.5 to 7.0. Renal stone formation is the most prominent feature of cystinuria, and renal failure due to repeated bouts of urinary tract obstruction and/or urinary tract infection is a common outcome of untreated cystinuria. No cellular accumulation of cystine occurs, reflecting the defect in tubular amino acid transport in cystinuria compared with the defect in cellular processing of the amino acid in cystinosis.

Flat, hexagonal cystine crystals are seen on urinalysis, and a definitive diagnosis is made by the demonstration of the isolated appearance of the four dibasic amino acids in the urine. Urinary cystine excretion of more than 400 mg/gm creatinine is characteristic. The most effective treatment is forced water intake to keep urine cystine concentrations below saturation levels.

Renal Glycosuria

The persistent urinary excretion of glucose at normal blood glucose levels, and therefore, normal filtered loads of glucose, is a benign disorder. The specific proximal tubular defect is inherited by either autosomal dominant or autosomal recessive genetics. Renal glycosuria is not associated with the risk of developing diabetes mellitus and requires no treatment.

Vitamin D–Resistant Rickets

Also called familial hypophosphatemia, this X-linked hereditary disorder is characterized by hypophosphatemia (usually <2.5 mg/dl), inappropriate phosphaturia (phosphate/creatinine clearance ratio >0.25), rachitic bone disease, and normal serum calcium and PTH levels. The primary defect is unknown, but a decrease in intestinal calcium and phosphate absorption accompanies the renal phosphate "leak." Vigorous treatment with both high-dose vitamin D (20,000 to 50,000 IU/day) and oral phosphate is required to heal the rachitic bone lesions.

Nephrogenic Diabetes Insipidus (NDI)

Nephrogenic DI is a specific defect in the response of the collecting tubule to ADH. ADH release in response to osmotic or volume stimulation and circulating levels of ADH are normal, yet the urine is persistently hypotonic to plasma. Aside from this specific concentrating defect, renal function is normal. Nephrogenic DI may occur either as a rare, X-linked hereditary disorder or as an acquired defect secondary to lithium or demeclocycline therapy.

Hereditary nephrogenic DI presents in infancy as repeated bouts of fever and altered mental status, the consequences of hypertonic volume depletion and encephalopathy. In later life, persistent polyuria and incessant thirst dominate the clinical picture. Urinary tract dilation may result from the massive volumes of urine excreted daily, 15 to 20 liters in adults. Permanent neurological damage may result from repeated bouts of hypertonic encephalopathy.

The diagnosis is made by family history, a failure to concentrate the urine after 12 to 18 hours dehydration, and a failure to raise urine osmolality above that of plasma in response to exogenous ADH. Treatment consists of assurance of ready access to and intake of water, plus a thiazide diuretic along with salt restriction. This regimen modestly reduces ECF volume, leading to increased isotonic fluid absorption in the proximal nephron. In turn, a lesser volume of hypotonic fluid is generated in the loop of Henle and delivered to the ADH-unresponsive collecting duct for excretion in the final urine.

Acquired NDI is generally incomplete and is expressed as a dramatic reduction in maximal urinary concentration. The defect almost always disappears with cessation of the demeclocycline or lithium.

Bartter's Syndrome. This rare disorder affects mostly females, who present with stunted growth plus symptoms of polyuria and recurrent muscular weakness. The biochemical profile is that of hypochloremic metabolic alkalosis, profound hypokalemia (1.5 to 2.5 mEq/L), hyperreninemia, and hyperaldosteronism. Despite high renin values the patients are normotensive and are insensitive to the pressor effect of angiotensin II (A II). Urinary excretion of potassium and chloride remains high despite the hypochloremic, hypokalemic state. Chronic vomiting and excess use of diuretics produce the same clinical manifestations and must be excluded before entertaining the diagnosis of Bartter's syndrome. Juxtaglomerular apparatus hyperplasia is the distinguishing renal lesion.

The renal manifestations of Bartter's syndrome are associated with excessive renal prostaglandin E_2 (PGE_2) activity and excretion. PGE_2 has been shown to stimulate renin secretion, to block vasoconstriction produced by A II, and to inhibit salt absorption in the thick ascending limb of Henle. Treatment of these patients with cyclo-oxygenase inhibitors (aspirin, indomethacin) reduces urinary PGE_2 excretion, restores vascular sensitivity to exogenous A II, and reduces urinary chloride losses. The lack of total correction of hypokalemia by these drugs has led to the notion that Bartter's syndrome is due to a primary defect in the tubular handling of chloride or of potassium, and that the increased PGE_2 production is secondary to hypokalemia.

Renal Tubular Acidosis

The term renal tubular acidosis describes a group of disorders whose individual features reflect the site and mechanisms of failure in tubular hydrogen ion transport (Fig. 32–2). Type I, or classic distal RTA, represents an inability of the collecting duct to maintain a gradient of free hydrogen ion between the blood and the urine. This failure may be due to increased backleak of hydrogen ion from the tubular lumen to blood or to a failure in the hydrogen secretory mechanism. Type I RTA is expressed as an inability to lower urine pH (the free hydrogen ion concentration) in the face of an acid challenge. Type II, or proximal RTA, involves an impairment in the rate of hydrogen ion secretion and, therefore, bicarbonate reabsorption in the proximal tubule. Proximal RTA is expressed as bicarbonaturia that persists until the serum bicarbonate concentration and the filtered load of bicarbonate fall to levels that match the reduced proximal tubular absorptive capacity. Finally, the designation type IV RTA is used to describe a defect in mineralocorticoid-dependent hydrogen ion secretion in the distal nephron. Type IV RTA usually accompanies some form of renal interstitial disease (as in lead or diabetic nephropathies) and results either from diminished aldosterone secretion or from a failure of collecting duct response to aldosterone.

Distal RTA (type I) may occur sporadically as an isolated disorder, or may be secondary to a systemic disease or toxin. Prominent causes of distal RTA include primary and secondary hypergammaglobulinemia, nephrocalcinosis, amyloidosis, sickle cell disease, and amphotericin B administration.

Children often present with lethargy, anorexia, stunted growth, and bone disease. Adults often present with bone pain, pathological fractures, or renal stones. These problems appear to result from bone buffering of hydrogen ion over an extended period, leading to bone calcium loss and hypercalciuria. Disordered calcium metabolism is expressed as rickets in children and osteomalacia, nephrocalcinosis, and nephrolithiasis in adults. The distinguishing laboratory features include hyperchloremic metabolic acidosis with hypokalemia and a urinary pH that is consistently above pH 6.0 to 6.5

An inability to lower pH below 5.3 in the face of spontaneous acidosis or an acid load (given as oral NH_4Cl) is diagnostic. After administration of a single dose of the loop diuretic furosemide, normal individuals and those with type I, gradient-limited RTA increase urinary acid secretion concomitant with the increased delivery of Na^+ to the distal nephron.

Treatment of distal RTA is accomplished by oral alkali replacement, either as sodium bicarbonate or Shohl's solution, at the rate of 1 to 3 mEq/kg/day. The 60 to 70 mEq of bicarbonate required to treat type I RTA corresponds to the normal contribution of the distal nephron to H^+ excretion. Correction of acidosis by this means leads to cessation of hypercalciuria and renal stone formation and correction of hypokalemia. However, normal growth and bone development in children may require administration of several hundred milliequivalents of bicarbonate daily.

Proximal RTA (type II) occurs rarely as an isolated lesion and is most often seen as a part of the Fanconi

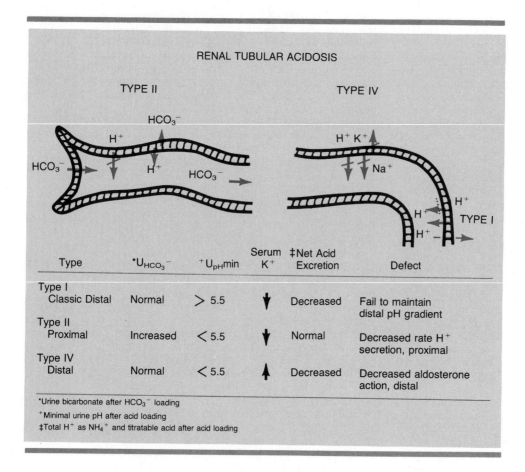

FIGURE 32–2. Differentiation of varieties of renal tubular acidosis.

RENAL TUBULAR ACIDOSIS

Type	$^*U_{HCO_3}^-$	$^+U_{pH}$min	Serum K^+	$\ddagger$Net Acid Excretion	Defect
Type I Classic Distal	Normal	> 5.5	↓	Decreased	Fail to maintain distal pH gradient
Type II Proximal	Increased	< 5.5	↓	Normal	Decreased rate H^+ secretion, proximal
Type IV Distal	Normal	< 5.5	↑	Decreased	Decreased aldosterone action, distal

*Urine bicarbonate after HCO_3^- loading
$^+$Minimal urine pH after acid loading
$\ddagger$Total H^+ as NH_4^+ and titratable acid after acid loading

syndrome. Proximal RTA is a self-limiting process in that normal acidification of urine, measured both as a maximum reduction in urine pH and as a normal excretion of ammonia and titratable acid, is possible when the serum bicarbonate level reaches a reduced, steady-state value. This value is usually 14 to 18 mEq/L and represents the maximal resorptive capacity of the proximal tubule in the disorder. At this moderate level of extracellular buffer reduction, daily H^+ excretion is complete and long-term buffer deficits do not develop as in distal RTA.

Clinical signs and symptoms are few in proximal RTA and relate to growth retardation. Hyperchloremic metabolic acidosis and hypokalemia, the result of increased delivery of sodium bicarbonate to the distal nephron, are evident, but hypercalciuria, nephrocalcinosis, and nephrolithiasis are absent. The urine pH can reach values of 4.5 to 5.0 as long as the serum bicarbonate level is below the proximal tubular resorptive threshold. The diagnosis is confirmed by the infusion of bicarbonate and observation of an increase in urine pH plus bicarbonaturia at subnormal levels of serum bicarbonate.

The treatment of proximal RTA with alkali replacement is virtually impossible because any elevation of the serum bicarbonate above the absorptive capacity of the proximal tubule results in quantitative urinary excretion of the added bicarbonate. Modest salt depletion, thereby increasing general proximal tubular absorption, will aid in raising the serum bicarbonate concentration.

Type IV RTA results from a diminished mineralocorticoid effect in the distal nephron and is expressed as a decrease in the secretory rates of potassium and hydrogen. There are two forms of the disorder. Aldosterone levels may be reduced, either from primary adrenal disease, in which case renin levels are elevated, or from renal interstitial disease, in which case renin levels may be reduced. Alternatively, adequate levels of aldosterone may be present but the distal nephron is unresponsive to its effect. This type of the disorder may be caused either by disease of the distal nephron, by the aldosterone-blocking diuretic spironolactone, or by the potassium-sparing diuretics triamterene and amiloride.

Since both potassium and hydrogen secretion are blunted, hyperkalemia accompanies the hyperchloremic metabolic acidosis of type IV RTA. This is in contrast to the hypokalemia seen in types I and II. Hyperkalemia decreases the renal generation and excretion of the major urinary buffer ammonium, so that total acid excretion is reduced although the urine pH may be appropriately acidic. A mild degree of renal insufficiency is present in many of these patients.

Relative salt wasting, that is, an inability to reduce urinary sodium excretion during salt restriction, is not uncommon. Basal and stimulated renin plus aldosterone levels should be measured in these patients.

Mineralocorticoid replacement, as fludrocortisone, is effective therapy in patients with an absolute reduction in aldosterone. Because increased sodium delivery to the distal nephron augments potassium and hydrogen secretion even in the absence of aldosterone, a high-salt diet plus a loop diuretic (furosemide) will increase both potassium and hydrogen excretion in all these patients. Reduction of the serum potassium alone increases urinary ammonium excretion and net urinary acid excretion and restores the hydrogen balance in some of these patients.

DISEASES OF THE URINARY CONDUITS

There are three disease processes that primarily affect the urinary drainage system: obstruction, infection, and urinary tract stone formation. These processes are closely interactive and often share a cause-effect relationship.

Urinary Tract Obstruction

Obstruction to urine flow may occur at any point from the renal pelvis to the urethral meatus. The causes of obstruction are manifold but may be classified into a few general groups as given in Table 32–4. The age and sex of the patient obviously influence the likelihood of a given pairing of etiology and site.

The obstruction may occur suddenly, as with a lodged calculus, and be associated with flank and radiating groin pain, or it may occur slowly, as with compression by cervical carcinoma, and be associated with no symptoms until uremia from renal failure appears. So long as urine formation proceeds, the urinary tract proximal to the obstruction dilates (hydronephrosis). However, long-standing obstruction causes tubular and interstitial atrophy, eventual glomerular sclerosis, and cessation of urine formation. Urinary tract dilation may no longer be evident at this time.

A change in urinary habits is often the presenting sign of urinary tract obstruction. Complete urinary tract obstruction is the most common cause of true anuria. However, polyuria, especially nocturia, is not uncommon in partial obstruction and may occur as a consequence of defective urinary concentration. Overflow incontinence is a common occurrence in lower tract obstruction. Prolonged enuresis in childhood is a common symptom of congenital obstructive disorders.

Unilateral ureteral obstruction usually causes no detectable change in urinary flow nor in total renal function, and the asymptomatic loss of one kidney in this manner is not rare. Azotemia or renal failure occurs only if the drainage of both kidneys is significantly compromised. While red and/or white blood cells are frequently found in the urinalysis of patients with obstruction, the combination of a normal urinalysis and acute azotemia correlates highly with the presence of urinary tract obstruction.

Renal sonography is the preferred means of diagnosing urinary tract obstruction and depends on identification of hydronephrosis. Dilation of the urinary tract may not be evident within the first 24 hours of obstruction, in which case an IVP, showing a prolonged nephrogram phase with delayed filling, can provide valuable diagnostic information. A 24-hour or 48-hour film may show contrast media concentrated either in dilated calyces or in the renal pelvis. Retrograde examination of the ureters is rarely required to make the diagnosis but may be necessary to define the anatomy of the obstruction before surgical intervention.

Long-term partial obstruction is associated with functional defects in urinary acidification and urinary concentration. Total obstruction eventually leads to tubular atrophy and glomerular sclerosis, grossly dilated and distorted calyces, and profound cortical thinning. Recovery of renal function after relief of obstruction is adversely affected by the presence of superimposed urinary tract infection or by a lengthy duration of obstruction. Total urinary tract obstruction is a significant cause of end-stage renal failure.

Management of urinary tract obstruction is directed toward identification of the site and cause of obstruction and relief of the obstruction, usually through surgical intervention. Elimination of obstruction is at times associated with a postobstructive diuresis, due partially to a solute diuresis from salt and urea retained during obstruction and partially to the renal concentrating defect. In some cases, definitive relief of obstruction is not possible and urinary diversion may be required. This may be as simple as an indwelling urethral catheter or more complex, such as an ileal conduit. In all cases, control of urinary tract infection is of paramount concern. Urinary tract infection in an obstructed kidney constitutes a urological emergency and requires prompt relief of the obstruction.

Multiple myeloma, rhabdomyolysis, and acute uric acid nephropathy cause renal failure by mechanisms

TABLE 32–4. CAUSES OF URINARY TRACT OBSTRUCTION

Congenital Urinary Tract Malformation
  Meatal stenosis
  Ureterocele
  Posterior urethral valves
Intraluminal Obstruction
  Calculi
  Blood clots
  Sloughed papillary tissue
Extrinsic Compression
  Pelvic tumors
  Prostatic hypertrophy
  Retroperitoneal fibrosis
Acquired Anomalies
  Urethral strictures
  Neurogenic bladder
  Intratubular precipitates

that include intrarenal tubular obstruction. In acute uric acid nephropathy, uric acid crystals precipitate within the collecting ducts and renal pelvis. Acute, dramatic hyperuricemia plus hyperkalemia and hyperphosphatemia occur as part of a tumor lysis syndrome. These products issue from massive cell death that follows chemotherapy for exquisitely sensitive tumors, often lymphomas. The poorly soluble uric acid "sludge" may be flushed from the kidney and renal pelvis by a forced alkaline diuresis if renal function is not severely compromised. Dialysis is indicated to reduce the uric acid load and/or life-threatening levels of hyperkalemia.

URINARY TRACT INFECTION

Bacterial infection of the urinary tract is one of the more common infectious processes and is dealt with in Chapter 94. Infection of the renal parenchyma, pyelonephritis, is much less common than infection of the lower urinary tract. A large fraction of cases of end-stage renal failure have been attributed to chronic pyelonephritis based on postmortem findings of renal interstitial inflammation and scarring. It is probable that the majority of these cases represent forms of the noninfectious interstitial renal diseases discussed earlier. However, pyelonephritis may contribute significantly to permanent renal damage in patients with urinary tract obstruction, polycystic kidney disease, and renal calculi.

UROLITHIASIS

Renal stone formation and its significant morbidity are common, affecting up to 50 per cent of the general population at least once during a lifetime. Calcium, usually calcium oxalate or phosphate, is the most common constituent of renal calculi and is present in some form in almost 90 per cent of all renal stones (Table 32–5). Uric acid, cystine, and magnesium are the other major stone constituents. Up to three fourths of all stones, composed predominantly of calcium oxalate, occur in the syndrome of idiopathic urolithiasis. About 5 per cent of calcium stone formation is attributable to hyperparathyroidism. Some degree of uric acid lithiasis is contributory to about one fifth of all renal calculi.

Urinary stone formation depends on a number of factors. The saturation of urine with a mineral is governed by the amount excreted and the volume of urine in which it is contained. Urine is frequently supersaturated with respect to calcium. Crystallization from solution requires a nidus, or "seed," upon which to grow, and crystal precipitation may be inhibited by certain compounds.

Idiopathic urolithiasis, in which no underlying metabolic or infectious etiology is evident, accounts for the majority of cases of renal stone formation. Hypercalciuria, defined as the excretion of greater than 4 mg calcium/kg/24 hr, without hypercalcemia, occurs in about 80 per cent of these cases. At least two subtypes of hypercalciuria appear to exist: in "renal" hypercalciuria, a deficiency in renal calcium reabsorption appears to drive increased intestinal calcium absorption, whereas in "absorptive" hypercalciuria, there is a primary increase in intestinal calcium absorption necessitating an increase in urinary calcium excretion. In both circumstances, serum calcium, phosphate, and PTH levels are normal. Stone formation in idiopathic hypercalciuria depends heavily on the constant supersaturation of urine with calcium.

The cause of stone formation in patients with normal levels of urinary calcium excretion is less certain. However, hyperuricosuria has been observed in a large number of patients with idiopathic urolithiasis and may coexist with hypercalciuria in up to 20 per cent of patients. The uric acid may serve as the nidus for further calcium oxalate deposition.

Secondary hypercalciuria, in which the serum calcium concentration may be elevated, occurs in only 5 to 7 per cent of recurrent stone formers. Hyperparathyroidism, distal RTA, sarcoidosis, and hypervitaminosis D account for a large number of these cases.

Chronic urinary tract infection with urea-splitting organisms (i.e., *Proteus* species) is associated with struvite (triple phosphate) stones containing ammonium, magnesium, and calcium. These frequently form as "staghorn" calculi, outlining the renal calyces. A vicious dependency develops in which urinary tract in-

TABLE 32–5. CHARACTERISTICS OF RENAL CALCULI

CHEMICAL COMPOSITION	PER CENT ALL STONES	URINARY MANIFESTATION	RADIOGRAPHIC APPEARANCE
Calcium oxalate/phosphate	75%	Hypercalciuria (40–75%) Hyperuricosuria (30–50%) Hyperoxaluria (<5%) Hypocitraturia ($\cong$50%) None ($\cong$5%)	Opaque, round, multiple calculi
Magnesium–ammonium phosphate + (calcium phosphate·carbonate)	20%	Infection with urease(+) organism	Opaque, staghorn calculus
Uric acid	5%	Hyperuricosuria	Radiolucent
Cystine	1–2%	Hypercystinuria	Opaque, staghorn ± round calculi

fection cannot be cleared owing to the presence of the foreign body (calculus) and stone formation continues as long as the urine is infected.

Passage of a renal stone is often the initial manifestation of renal stone disease and presents as ureteral colic, sharp unilateral flank pain that radiates to the groin. Hematuria is characteristically present in the urinalysis, and crystalluria may be obvious. A plain abdominal radiograph will demonstrate the densely opaque calcium stones and the faintly opaque, sulfur-containing cystine stones. Only pure uric acid stones are radiolucent. An excretory urogram (IVP) may be required to demonstrate small stones or the site along the urinary tract at which a stone has lodged.

The work-up for renal calculus is indicated in Table 32–6. Serial plain abdominal radiographs identify changes in stone size and number, serum calcium determinations identify hypercalcemic disorders associated with stone formation, and urine cultures identify etiological (urea-splitting) and complicating bacterial involvement. Hypercalciuria and hyperuricosuria are identified by appropriate 24-hour urine collections. Any stone passed in the urine should be subjected to analysis to determine its mineral composition.

Treatment for an obstructing stone may be as simple as the promotion of a *brisk* diuresis to enhance spontaneous passage of a stone. Removal of stones by surgical intervention may be required, especially when renal compromise secondary to obstruction is evident. The introduction of extracorporeal shockwave lithotripsy has provided a safe and effective means of removing existing renal calculi in most patients. The major effort of medical management is directed toward reducing the likelihood of stone growth and recurrent formation.

In all cases, prevention of urolithiasis includes forced hydration with water to produce a dilute urine. This suffices to prevent recurrence in some individuals, especially in hot climates. If hypercalcemia is present, parathyroidectomy for hyperparathyroidism or specific therapy for the elevation in serum calcium is indicated. In cases of idiopathic hypercalciuria, dra-

TABLE 32–6. PATIENT EVALUATION IN UROLITHIASIS

INITIAL	SECONDARY
Blood: Serum calcium	Serum PTH
Serum uric acid	Serum 1,25(OH)$_2$
Serum phosphate	vitamin D$_3$
Alkaline phosphatase	
Urine: Urinalysis for crystalluria	24-hour urine calcium
Urinalysis for pyuria	24-hour urine uric acid
	Urine culture
Radiography: Plain film (KUB)	Serial KUB's
IVP	

matic reductions in urinary calcium excretion and stone formation can be achieved with thiazide diuretics and salt-restricted diet. Thiazide therapy should reduce the 24-hour urinary calcium excretion by almost half. If hyperuricosuria coexists, the addition of allopurinol to reduce the uric acid load is advantageous. Successful treatment of struvite stones may require specific, long-term antibiotic therapy in combination with surgical lithotomy.

REFERENCES

Ettinger B, et al: Randomized trial of allopurinol in the prevention of calcium oxalate calculi. N Engl J Med 315:1386–1389, 1986.

Gardner KD: Cystic kidneys. Kidney Int 33:610–621, 1988.

Kurtzman NA: Renal tubular acidosis: A constellation of syndromes. Hosp Pract 22:131–144, 1987.

McKinney TD: Tubulointerstitial diseases and toxic nephropathies. *In* Wyngaarden JB, Smith LH Jr (eds): Cecil Textbook of Medicine. 18th ed. Philadelphia, WB Saunders Co, 1988, pp 602–614.

Rector FC Jr: Obstructive nephropathy. *In* Wyngaarden JB, Smith LH Jr (eds): Cecil Textbook of Medicine. 18th ed. Philadelphia, WB Saunders Co, 1988, pp 614–617.

Ritchie AN, et al: The natural history and clinical features of renal cell carcinoma. Semin Nephrol 7:131–139, 1987.

Ritz E, et al: Lead nephropathy. Contrib Nephrol 55:185–191, 1987.

33
RENAL PHARMACOLOGY

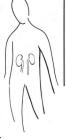

Renal pharmacology encompasses a range of important topics in clinical nephrology including the pharmacokinetics of drugs in patients with impaired renal function as well as the spectrum of drug-induced renal injury. The principles of extracorporeal removal of specific drugs or toxins from the body are also included in a discussion of renal pharmacology.

RENAL EXCRETION OF DRUGS

A number of drugs and drug metabolites are eliminated from the body by renal excretion. Excretion of drugs by the kidney may involve glomerular filtration, tubular secretion, and/or tubular reabsorption de-

TABLE 33–1. DRUGS WHOSE RENAL EXCRETION IS AFFECTED BY URINE pH

Augmented Excretion in Acidic Urine (Weak Bases)
Amphetamines
Chloroquine
Diazepam
Meperidine
Morphine
Quinidine
Trimethoprim

Augmented Excretion in Alkaline Urine (Weak Acids)
Acetazolamide
Cephaloridine
Diazoxide
Furosemide/ethacrynic acid
Hydrochlorothiazide
Methotrexate
Penicillin
Phenobarbital
Acetylsalicylic acid
Sulfonamides

pending upon the agent in question. Filtration of a drug through the glomerulus depends on the chemical characteristics of the drug as well as the degrees of binding of the drug to plasma proteins. Drugs that are highly bound to plasma proteins are poorly filtered, while those that are bound less avidly or not at all can gain access to the tubular fluid via glomerular filtration. Drugs that are organic anions or cations can be secreted from the peritubular capillary blood into the tubular lumen by specific transport mechanisms in renal tubular cells. Some drugs that gain access to the tubular fluid by filtration and/or secretion may be reabsorbed back into the systemic circulation by mediated or passive tubular transport mechanisms. The net rate of excretion of drugs that undergo this form of bidirectional transport across renal tubules depends on the relative activites of the secretory and absorptive processes. The rate of excretion of an organic anionic or cationic drug whose pK is the range of the pH normally attainable in the tubular fluid can be affected

significantly by a change in the pH of the urine. This effect of "nonionic diffusion" describes the difference in permeability of a drug across the renal tubule when the drug is in its ionized versus un-ionized form. Alkalinization of the urine will increase significantly the excretion of organic acids such as aspirin and phenobarbital by trapping the drug in tubular fluid in its ionized form. Conversely, acidification of the urine will increase the renal excretion of organic bases such as amphetamine (Table 33–1).

PHARMACOKINETICS OF DRUGS IN RENAL INSUFFICIENCY

A decrease in the glomerular filtration rate and/or a loss of secretory and absorptive transport functions of the kidney occurs in patients with renal insufficiency. These changes in renal function may have a major effect on the elimination of drugs that are excreted by the kidney. In addition, advanced renal failure is characterized by the retention of endogenous organic compounds in the blood which may compete with certain drugs for specific renal transport systems involved with excretion.

Renal insufficiency may affect the metabolism of drugs not only by decreasing the rates of excretion in the urine, but also by a number of nonrenal mechanisms. Renal disease is associated with alterations in the binding of drugs by plasma proteins and, as a consequence, may affect the bioavailability of some drugs. A common example occurs in patients with renal failure who are taking Dilantin (phenytoin). An increase in the free concentration of the drug in plasma can be observed because of reduced binding of Dilantin to plasma proteins in the uremic state. In addition, renal insufficiency may be associated with a change in the volume of distribution of certain drugs or with the rate of absorption of drugs from the gastrointestinal tract. The secondary consequences of renal failure may also alter the metabolic pathways of drugs in other organs.

ALTERATIONS IN DRUG DOSES IN PATIENTS WITH RENAL FAILURE

A number of commonly prescribed drugs require alterations in either the amount or the timing of administration in patients with renal dysfunction. In patients who are dialysis-dependent, the problem is compounded further by the effects of drug removal during hemodialysis or peritoneal dialysis. Drugs listed in Table 33–2 require no alteration in dose in the patient with renal insufficiency. The metabolism of these agents is predominantly by nonrenal routes and is not altered significantly by the presence of renal failure or the "uremic" environment. Table 33–3 lists drugs that should be avoided, if possible in patients with renal failure because of adverse drug-related side-effects. Table 33–4 provides a partial listing of drugs whose

TABLE 33–2. DRUGS REQUIRING LITTLE OR NO ALTERATION IN DOSE IN PATIENTS WITH RENAL FAILURE

ANTIBIOTICS	OTHERS
Cloxacillin	Codeine
Nafcillin	Morphine
Clindamycin	Propoxyphene
Erythromycin	Benzodiazepines
Rifampin	Lidocaine
Isoniazid	Quinidine
Chloramphenicol	Propranolol
Amphotericin B	Hydralazine
	Clonidine
	Prazosin
	Phenytoin
	Theophylline

metabolism is altered significantly in the patient with renal disease. These agents can be used with caution if the proper adjustments in dose are made.

One of two methods can be used to adjust drug dosing regimens in patients with renal disease who are receiving drugs that are excreted by the kidney. The dosing interval can be held constant and the dose of medication reduced, or the medication dose can be held constant and the dosing interval lengthened. Various nomograms are available which provide guidelines regarding drug dosage adjustments in patients with varying degrees of renal dysfunction. Exclusive reliance on a nomogram alone can result in drug concentrations that are below therapeutic range or in the toxic range. Whenever possible, blood levels should be monitored as a guide to therapy.

DRUG-ASSOCIATED RENAL INJURY

Nephrotoxicity associated with the administration of various pharmaceutical agents is a common clinical problem. The precise classification of drug-related renal dysfunction is arbitrary, and a single drug may be associated with more than one mechanism of injury. The classification shown in Table 33–5 indicates a primary separation into those drugs that are associated with an acute change in kidney function and a clinical picture of either the "acute renal failure" syndrome or isolated defects in tubular function, and those that can lead to chronic renal failure. The acute category is further subdivided into drugs that directly affect kidney function ("toxic nephropathy") and those that result in renal dysfunction by secondary processes. Although the toxic nephropathy variant of the acute renal failure syndrome is usually taken to imply drug-associated injury to the renal tubules, the term has been extended in recent years to include drugs that cause immunological injury to the kidney (glomerulonephritis and acute tubulointerstitial nephritis) and those that affect the regulation of renal blood flow. The more common forms of toxic nephropathies are discussed separately.

ACUTE DRUG-RELATED RENAL DYSFUNCTION

Direct (Toxic Nephropathy)

Immunological Drug-Induced Renal Disease. Drugs such as penicillins, sulfonamides, phenytoin, and allopurinol are associated with the development of hypersensitivity vasculitis, a systemic disorder characterized by the deposition of immune complexes in the small blood vessels of the kidney and the skin. The renal histopathology is typically that of a proliferative glomerulonephritis. The renal prognosis of this disease is favorable when the offending agent is discontinued.

Isolated glomerular injury is associated with drugs such as gold salts, penicillamine, and captopril. The

TABLE 33–3. DRUGS THAT SHOULD BE AVOIDED IN PATIENTS WITH RENAL FAILURE

ANTIBIOTICS	OTHERS
Tetracycline	Aspirin
Nitrofurantoin	Oral hypoglycemics
Nalidixic acid	Lithium carbonate
	Acetazolamide
	Spironolactone
	Triamterene

TABLE 33–4. DRUGS REQUIRING SIGNIFICANT DOSE ADJUSTMENT IN PATIENTS WITH RENAL FAILURE

ANTIBIOTICS	OTHER
Aminoglycosides	Digoxin
Cephalosporins	Procainamide
Carbenicillin/ticarcillin	Cimetidine
Penicillin G	
Sulfonamides	
Vancomycin	

TABLE 33–5. DRUG-INDUCED NEPHROTOXICITY

Acute Renal Dysfunction
  Indirect Injury
    Prerenal azotemia
      nonsteroidal anti-inflammatory agents
      vasodilators
    Postrenal azotemia
      methysergide
      practolol
      sulfonamides
  Direct Injury: Immunological Mechanism
    Hypersensitivity vasculitis
      penicillins
      sulfonamides
      allopurinol
    Glomerulonephritis
      gold
      penicillamine
      nonsteroidal anti-inflammatory agents
    Tubulointerstitial nephritis
      penicillins—particularly methicillin
      sulfonamides
      cephalosporins
      rifampin
      cimetidine
      phenytoin
      nonsteroidal anti-inflammatory agents
  Direct Injury: Nonimmunological Mechanism
    Tubular damage
      Aminoglycosides
      cis-platinum
    Renal tubular acidosis
      amphotericin B
      lithium carbonate
      nonsteroidal anti-inflammatory agents
    Nephrogenic diabetes insipidus
      lithium carbonate
      demeclocycline
      methoxyflurane
Chronic Renal Disease
  Chronic Interstitial Nephritis
    phenacetin-aspirin combination
    lithium carbonate
    nitrosoureas

histologic lesion is that of membranous glomerulopathy. The clinical manifestations of heavy proteinuria and hematuria as well as the histologic abnormalities frequently resolve when the drugs are stopped.

The interstitium of the kidney may be affected by immunologically mediated inflammatory reactions in response to the ingestion of certain drugs. Agents such as the penicillin derivatives, particularly methicillin, are associated with the development of acute allergic interstitial nephritis. Allopurinol, cimetidine, phenytoin, rifampin, and sulfonamides, and the nonsteroidal anti-inflammatory drugs (NSAIDs) may result in a similar syndrome. An interstitial inflammatory response characterized by infiltration of white blood cells is typical of the acute allergic interstitial nephritis syndromes. The patient may have fever, rash, and eosinophilia in addition to renal dysfunction. Many patients with this drug-related syndrome may manifest only the renal functional impairment. The prognosis is generally good, with renal function returning when there is no longer exposure to the offending agent. A short course of corticosteroids may be indicated in certain patients to hasten the recovery phase.

Direct Tubular Toxicity. Certain classes of drugs are capable of causing direct damage to renal tubular cells. The clinical presentation is that of the acute renal failure syndrome as reviewed in Chapter 29. The aminoglycoside antibiotics and the cancer chemotherapeutic agent cisplatin are common causes of this form of drug-related renal injury.

In addition to the morphological and functional disturbances associated with the development of acute renal insufficiency, a number of drugs may produce specific defects in renal tubular function. In these conditions, the glomerular filtration rate may or may not be affected. Derangements in proximal tubular function occur after exposure to heavy metals and outdated tetracycline. The manifestations may include renal tubular acidosis, aminoaciduria, phosphaturia, uricosuria, and glycosuria. Impairment in the ability to concentrate the urine may be seen in patients taking lithium carbonate, demethylchlortetracycline, or amphotericin B. Diabetes insipidus is the clinical expression of this defect. Drugs such as vincristine, cyclophosphamide, and chlorpropamide may be associated with impaired ability to excrete a dilute urine, a defect that may result in hyponatremia. Hyperkalemia and distal renal tubular acidosis may be seen in patients receiving amphotericin B, beta-adrenergic blocking agents, and nonsteroidal anti-inflammatory drugs.

Indirect Renal Injury

Drugs that affect the systemic vascular resistance, the blood pressure, and/or the extracellular fluid volume may cause a decrease in renal blood flow and in glomerular filtration rate. These hemodynamic changes can result in the development of prerenal azotemia, particularly in individuals whose autoregulation of renal blood flow is impaired and in those receiving other drugs that inhibit the autoregulatory response of the kidney. Nonsteroidal anti-inflammatory drugs, as well as vasodilator drugs, may cause this type of renal injury.

Although less common, a postrenal or obstructive pattern of renal injury can occur as a manifestation of drug administration. Retroperitoneal fibrosis and obstructive nephropathy have been reported following the long-term administration of methysergide. Intratubular precipitation of crystals derived from drugs such as the sulfonamides may result in acute renal dysfunction. Although an important cause of acute renal dysfunction when the sulfa drugs were initially introduced, this drug-related renal effect is now infrequent, as the newer sulfonamides are more soluble. Acute renal failure may develop from the intratubular precipitation of uric acid in patients receiving cancer chemotherapy. Renal dysfunction due to precipitation of oxalic acid crystals within the renal tubules has been observed in patients ingesting ethylene glycol and in a rare patient exposed to the anesthetic agent methoxyflurane.

CHRONIC RENAL FAILURE DUE TO DRUGS OR TOXINS

Chronic renal failure related to the long-term ingestion of analgesics, particularly drug combinations containing aspirin and phenacetin, has been recognized as a frequent cause of end-stage renal disease in some areas of the world, notably Australia, Britain, and Scandinavia. The typical patient has ingested analgesic drugs in kilogram amounts over a period of years. Often there is a history of chronic pain such as headache or backache. Peptic ulcer disease and iron deficiency anemia may also be present. When these findings are associated with renal insufficiency, the possibility of analgesic nephropathy should be considered. An accurate drug history, however, may be difficult to obtain owing to the personalities of these patients and the fact that these agents are often not considered medications. The pathogenesis of analgesic nephropathy is uncertain but is likely related to a chronic decrease in renal papillary blood flow induced by aspirin which allows for the accumulation of toxic metabolites of phenacetin in the interstitium and papillae of the kidney. The clinical presentation is that of progressive renal insufficiency and hypertension. Papillary necrosis can occur. The histological abnormalities include interstitial fibrosis and atrophy of renal tubules. It has been suggested that the deterioration in renal function may be slowed or reversed when the drugs are stopped. Since there are no specific characteristics of this disease entity, a strong clinical suspicion and a careful drug history are mandatory.

IMPORTANT NEPHROTOXINS

Nonsteroidal Anti-inflammatory Drugs (NSAIDs). Renal toxicity related to NSAIDs has emerged as a very common form of drug-induced nephrotoxicity. NSAIDs are potent inhibitors of prostaglandin synthesis, a property that contributes to their nephrotoxic potential in certain high-risk patients. Several distinct patterns of nephrotoxicity have been associated with these agents (Table 33–6). The most frequent pattern of injury related to NSAIDs is a prerenal azotemia. In settings where renal blood flow is highly dependent on the activity of vasodilating prostaglandins, the administration of NSAIDs may precipitate the development of acute renal failure. Susceptible individuals include those with congestive heart failure, cirrhosis, chronic renal disease, and volume depletion. A hyperchloremic metabolic acidosis, often associated with hyperkalemia, has also been recognized as an effect of the NSAIDs, particularly in individuals with pre-existing chronic interstitial renal disease. Hyporeninemic hypoaldosteronism occurs in these individuals in states of renal prostaglandin inhibition. Hyponatremia is occasionally identified in patients taking NSAIDs and is the result of an impairment in the ability of the kidney to generate a maximally dilute urine when renal prostaglandin production is inhibited. Finally, NSAIDs have been associated with the development of an acute interstitial nephritis, often associated with renal insufficiency. Heavy proteinuria or frank nephrotic syndrome may accompany the interstitial lesion. The glomerular lesion is typically that of minimal change glomerulopathy. Discontinuation of the offending agent usually results in a resolution of this disorder.

Aminoglycoside Antibiotics. Although there are differences in the nephrotoxic potential of the various aminoglycosides, all agents of this type can cause renal injury. The aminoglycosides are excreted unchanged in the urine and are transported across both the luminal and antiluminal borders of the cells of the proximal tubule. The drug accumulates in these cells in concentrations up to one hundred times the serum concentration. The cationic properties of the aminoglycosides allow them to bind to tubular membrane acidic phospholipids and to induce disruptions in a number of membrane and subcellular functions of the proximal tubule. The nephrotoxicity of the aminoglycosides is related to the cumulative dose of the drug administered. The potential for developing nephrotoxicity from exposure to these antibiotics is increased in patients who have underlying renal disease, vascular instability, depletion of the extracellular fluid volume, concurrent exposure to other potentially nephrotoxic agents, and hypokalemia. Prevention of aminoglycoside nephrotoxicity depends upon the recognition of high-risk patients, the use of drug dosing nomograms to estimate an appropriate daily dose of drug, the measurement of serum levels of the drug, and frequent monitoring of renal function tests. If a decline in renal function develops during administration of these agents, the drug should be discontinued if possible. Although the renal dysfunction induced by aminoglycoside antibiotics is usually mild and reversible, when combined with other nephrotoxic insults, acute renal failure requiring dialytic support may develop.

Cancer Chemotherapeutic Agents. A number of drugs used in the treatment of patients with cancer can be associated with the development of renal injury and/or specific defects in the function of the kidney. *Cis*-diamminedichloroplatinum (cisplatin) is a potent nephrotoxin. The pattern of injury observed with this agent resembles that seen with other heavy metals such as lead, arsenic, and mercury. Vigorous intravenous hydration prior to administration of the drug and the use of mannitol may reduce the risk of renal injury. However, if significant renal dysfunction occurs with cisplatin, the injury is often irreversible.

Radiographic Contrast Agents. Although not strictly drugs, radiographic contrast materials are increasingly recognized as a cause of an acute decline in renal function. These agents are iodinated organic compounds that are excreted by glomerular filtration. The nephrotoxic potential of these agents is multifactorial. Intense renal vasoconstriction, tubular precipitation of proteinaceous debris, and direct tubular toxicity have all been described to occur in radiographic contrast–mediated acute renal failure. Although the nephrotoxicity of these agents can manifest unexpectedly, clinical evidence of renal dysfunction is most commonly observed in high-risk settings. Individuals with pre-existing renal disease, diabetes mellitus, multiple myeloma, or dehydration are considered at greatest risk. The acute renal dysfunction induced by radiographic contrast agents is typically mild and the prognosis for recovery of renal function is good. In some patients, particularly those at high risk, radiographic contrast–induced renal dysfunction may evolve into an oliguric acute renal failure syndrome requiring temporary dialytic support. Thus, identification of susceptible patients is important, as are maneuvers such as hydration and the establishment of brisk urine flow rates prior to the administration of these agents.

TABLE 33–6. THE SPECTRUM OF RENAL TOXICITY ASSOCIATED WITH NONSTEROIDAL ANTI-INFLAMMATORY DRUGS (NSAIDs)

TYPE	PATHO-PHYSIOLOGY	FEATURES	ASSOCIATED CONDITIONS
Acute renal failure	↓ Renal blood flow	Prerenal azotemia, sodium retention	Congestive heart failure, cirrhosis, volume depletion, renal insufficiency
Hyperchloremic metabolic acidosis	↓ Renin/aldosterone production	$\uparrow K^+$, $\uparrow Cl^-$, $\downarrow CO_2$	Interstitial renal disease
Acute interstitial nephritis	Lymphocytic infiltration of renal interstitium	Acute renal failure, +/− heavy proteinuria	Unknown

TABLE 33–7. INDICATIONS FOR HEMODIALYSIS AND HEMOPERFUSION IN TOXIC OVERDOSES

1. Hypotension, hypoventilation, or hypothermia in a severe intoxication with a drug removable by hemodialysis or hemoperfusion (see below).
2. Prolonged coma, particularly in patients with pulmonary disease.
3. Significant hepatic or renal disease which impairs drug metabolism or excretion.
4. Presence of a drug or metabolite directly toxic to tissue (e.g., methanol, ethylene glycol).
5. Presence of a potentially fatal blood level of a drug or toxin.

HEMODIALYSIS	HEMOPERFUSION
Aspirin	Digoxin
Lithium carbonate	Glutethimide
Phenytoin	Ethchlorvynol
Aminoglycosides	Benzodiazepines
Ethanol	Meprobamate
Methanol	Methaqualone
Ethylene glycol	Phenobarbital
	Theophylline

HEMODIALYSIS AND HEMOPERFUSION IN THE TREATMENT OF DRUG OVERDOSES

The vast majority of drug intoxications can be managed by routine supportive measures. The excretion of drugs that are eliminated from the body by the kidney can be augmented by increasing the urine flow rate and expanding the extracellular fluid volume. Altering the pH of the urine may increase the renal excretion of certain anionic or cationic drugs (see Table 33–1). In selected patients with life-threatening drug overdoses, the use of extracorporeal methods to remove drugs is a valuable procedure.

Hemodialysis/Hemoperfusion for Drug Removal. Hemodialysis is most efficacious in the removal of small molecular weight drugs or toxins that are water-soluble and not highly protein-bound. Hemodialysis may also be a useful adjunctive measure for correction of severe metabolic acidosis associated with the ingestion of aspirin, methanol, or ethylene glycol. Hemoperfusion is a technique that removes drugs by a process of adsorption onto an activated charcoal column or other resin material (e.g., Amberlite). Hemoperfusion is most beneficial in the removal of lipid-soluble or highly protein-bound drugs (Table 33–7). Peritoneal dialysis is rarely used in the management of drug overdoses owing to its low efficiency (see Chapter 30).

Complications and Indications. The use of extracorporeal techniques to remove drugs and toxins is not without risk, particularly in the patient who is hemodynamically unstable. Both hemodialysis and hemoperfusion require systemic heparinization and insertion of vascular catheters. Hypotension may complicate hemoperfusion, as the extracorporeal volume of blood is about 500 ml. Thrombocytopenia associated with adherance of platelets to the resin column has also been described. The removal of highly lipid-soluble drugs such as glutethimide and ethchlorvynol may require sequential hemofiltration treatments because of the slow rate of equilibration of these drugs between body fat stores and the extracellular space. The use of extracorporeal modalities in the management of drug intoxications should be considered only when there are clear indications as outlined in Table 33–7.

REFERENCES

Blye E, Lorch J, Cortell S: Extracorporeal therapy in the treatment of intoxication. Am J Kidney Dis 4:321, 1984.

Cooper K, Bennett WM: Nephrotoxicity of common drugs used in clinical practice. Arch Intern Med 147:1213, 1987.

Hart D, Lifschitz MD: Renal physiology of the prostaglandins and the effects of non-steroidal antiinflammatory agents on the kidney. Am J Nephrol 7:408, 1987.

Reed WE, Sabatini S: The use of drugs in renal failure. Semin Nephrol 6:259, 1986.

Ries F, Klastersky J: Nephrotoxicity induced by cancer chemotherapy with special emphasis on cisplatin toxicity. Am J Kidney Dis 8:368, 1986.

SECTION IV

GASTROINTESTINAL DISEASE

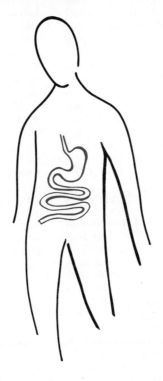

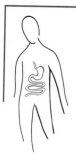

34

THE COMMON CLINICAL MANIFESTATIONS OF GASTROINTESTINAL DISEASE

A.   ABDOMINAL PAIN

Pain, a subjective sensation that generally heralds tissue damage, is the most frequent symptom of gastrointestinal disease and the one that usually brings the patient to the physician. Specific patterns of pain are often helpful in suggesting or establishing a correct diagnosis and may be the most sensitive and specific sign of abdominal disease. For example, the diagnosis of acute appendicitis is established on clinical findings alone; a characteristic, localized, right lower quadrant pain and tenderness occur at a time when the most sophisticated imaging studies, such as computed tomography, may be normal. This section will review the etiology, characteristics, and patterns of abdominal pain, concluding with a discussion of the approach to the patient with acute abdominal pain and a brief overview of the irritable bowel syndrome.

ORIGIN OF ABDOMINAL PAIN

Pain-sensitive neurons from visceral organs and the peritoneum travel in sympathetic pathways to spinal sensory neurons. The afferent endings are located in the smooth muscles of hollow organs, in organ capsules, in the peritoneum, and in intra-abdominal blood vessels. Abdominal organs are insensitive to stimuli such as cutting, tearing, and burning. Generally only three processes produce pain in the alimentary tract: (1) stretching or tension in the wall of a hollow organ or the capsule of a solid organ as a result of forceful muscular contraction, muscle spasms, distention, or traction; (2) inflammation with associated release of substances, such as bradykinin, prostaglandins, histamine, and serotonin, that stimulate or sensitize nerve endings; (3) ischemia, which releases noxious tissue metabolites. Spinal sensory neurons also receive input from peripheral nonpain neurons, thus establishing the basis for referred pain to extra-abdominal sites.

CHARACTERISTICS OF ABDOMINAL PAIN

The location, timing, quality, and progression of abdominal pain are important diagnostic clues. Abdominal pain usually takes one or a combination of three patterns: (1) Visceral pain is usually dull, poorly localized due to the multisegmental bilateral innervation of abdominal organs, and often midline in location. It originates in an abdominal viscus and may have a crampy or gnawing quality. (2) Parietal (somatic) pain is intense and often well-localized and lateralized. The pain is due to stimulation, usually inflammatory in nature, of the parietal peritoneum. (3) Referred pain is localized superficial or deep pain perceived in areas remote from the diseased viscus and innervated by the same spinal segment. The pain is sometimes associated with hyperesthesia.

Although visceral pain is usually poorly localized, certain useful generalizations can be made. Pain from the esophagus is usually substernal, may be discretely localized, and, if severe, may penetrate to the middle of the back or the left arm. Pain from the stomach, duodenum, and pancreas is epigastric, often with radiation to the back. Liver, gallbladder, and bile duct pain may be epigastric but is usually located in the right upper quadrant. Gallbladder or biliary pain may be referred to the tip of the scapula. Pain from a subphrenic abscess or hepatic abscess may be referred to the shoulder tip. Jejunal and ileal pain is often periumbilical, although terminal ileal pain may be felt in the right lower quadrant. Colonic pain is poorly localized but is usually felt in the lower abdomen or hypogastric area, as is pain from the pelvic organs. Finally, rectal pain may be felt over the sacrum. Unusual but diagnostically important patterns of abdominal pain include angina-like left upper quadrant discomfort from the transverse colon, and left back/hip pain resembling L4 root disease or ovarian disease but emanating from the transverse or the descending colon. Posterior appendiceal rupture sometimes produces similar pain in the right lumbar-gluteal area.

The quality and progression of pain may also be helpful. The pain of esophageal reflux (heartburn) is usually burning in nature, whereas the characteristic pain of peptic ulcer disease gnaws or burns and often subsides following ingestion of food or antacids. Pain due to bowel obstruction is described as recurrent, severe, and cramping (colic), often interposed with short periods of little or no pain. Furthermore, patients with bowel colic pain are often restless. In contrast, the term biliary colic is a misnomer, as the pain associated with cystic duct obstruction is usually steady rather than intermittent in nature. Pain due to inflammation, particularly of the parietal peritoneum, transmits a

TABLE 34–1. PAIN PATTERNS OF ABDOMINAL DISEASE

LOCATION	DISEASES	PAIN QUALITY/ CHARACTERISTICS	PAIN REFERRAL	PAIN PROGRESSION	ASSOCIATED FINDINGS
Acute Onset Pain Epigastric	Perforated duodenal ulcer	Severe; may have history of chronic ulcer pain	Back	Rapidly progresses over the entire abdomen	Abdominal guarding Free air in peritoneal cavity on x-ray
	Acute cholecystitis	Colicky or steady	Tip of scapula	Pain intensity steadily increases over hours Pain localizes to right upper quadrant	Fever Localized tenderness Gallstones visible on ultrasound examination; ^{99m}Tc-HIDA scan fails to visualize gallbladder
	Acute pancreatitis	Steady Boring	Back	Peritoneal signs may appear later in severe cases	Nausea and vomiting Epigastric tenderness
Periumbilical	Small bowel obstruction	Cramping	Back	—	Hyperactive bowel sounds Nausea and vomiting Dilated bowel loops with air-fluid levels on x-ray Abdominal distention
	Appendicitis	Cramping Steady	Back or groin in some cases	Pain localizes to right lower quadrant	Localized tenderness on abdominal and rectal examination Occult blood in feces
	Intestinal infarction	Severe aching May be diffuse	—	Progresses to peritonitis	Decreased or absent bowel sounds Initial examination may be unimpressive Lactic acidosis, shock
Lower quadrants	Dissecting aortic aneurysm	Sudden, severe Boring, tearing May be periumbilical	Flank Inguinal regions	—	Shock Abdominal bruit Abdominal mass
	Diverticulitis	Steady Aching Often left lower quadrant	Back	—	Palpable inflammatory mass Constipation Fever, leukocytosis
	Colon obstruction	Crampy	Back	—	Vomiting Constipation (sometimes diarrhea) Abdominal distention Hyperactive bowel sounds
Chronic Pain Substernal	Reflux esophagitis	Burning Often after meals or at night	Left arm	Into upper chest	Bitter or sour fluid in the mouth
Epigastric	Duodenal ulcer	Gnawing, burning Often between meals and at night	Occasionally to the back	—	Relief with food or antacids
	Nonulcer dyspepsia	Same as duodenal ulcer Bloating	—	—	Occasional relief with food or antacids
	Gastric ulcer	Gnawing Worsened by food	Occasionally to the back	—	Some relief by antacids
Periumbilical	Intestinal angina	Colicky Aching May be diffuse, lower quadrants Occurs after meals	—	Pain remits in 1-2 hours	Weight loss
	Inflammatory bowel disease	Cramping Aching May be in lower quadrants	—	—	Diarrhea Blood and pus in stools Urgency, tenesmus
Lower quadrants	Irritable bowel syndrome	Cramping Steady Often intermittent	—	—	Alternating constipation and diarrhea Bloating, "gassy" sensation

steady quality, felt locally, if the peritoneum is irritated focally by an underlying diseased organ such as an inflamed appendix or gallbladder, or diffusely if material such as gastric juice, intestinal contents, blood, or pus has leaked into the peritoneal cavity. Peritoneal irritation is accompanied by tenderness, by guarding (voluntary tensing) and rigidity (involuntary spasm) of the overlying abdominal muscles, and by rebound tenderness. Such patients usually lie still to minimize the discomfort. Pain due to intestinal ischemia is usually severe, poorly localized, and steady, often with little abdominal tenderness in the early stages. The pain related to dissection of an abdominal aortic aneurysm occurs suddenly and is severe and often described as "tearing."

Some types of abdominal pain change characteristically with time. For example, sudden severe pain that subsequently becomes generalized concomitant with the appearance of signs of peritoneal irritation suggests that a hollow viscus has perforated to cause generalized peritonitis. In contrast, the pain of acute appendicitis or cholecystitis may begin as a poorly localized midline pain that later moves directly over the inflamed organ as localized peritoneal inflammation develops.

The characteristic pain patterns of those abdominal diseases for which pain is an important clinical clue are summarized in Table 34–1.

NAUSEA AND VOMITING

Nausea and vomiting are often associated with abdominal pain, and their presence may provide clues to the underlying diagnosis. Vomiting most commonly occurs with obstruction and distention of the stomach or intestine (pyloric stenosis, small bowel obstruction), motility disorders (diabetic gastroparesis), or irritation and inflammation of the peritoneum. In these disorders, vagal afferents are thought to stimulate the medullary chemoreceptor trigger zones, which in turn induce vomiting. Drugs and gastric mucosal irritants may also induce vomiting via this pathway. Other disorders associated with vomiting include increased intracranial pressure, psychogenic vomiting, hypersecretion of gastric acid (Zollinger-Ellison syndrome), and the early morning vomiting of alcoholics, pregnant women, and uremics.

APPROACH TO THE PATIENT WITH ACUTE ABDOMINAL PAIN

The evaluation and care of patients with acute abdominal pain ("acute abdomen") provide one of the great challenges in clinical medicine because of the potentially lethal nature of many of the causes and the frequent need for prompt surgical or medical intervention. Although one can enlarge the differential diagnosis, the most common causes are acute appendicitis, cholecystitis or pancreatitis, bowel obstruction, perforated viscus, intestinal infarction, strangulated viscus, acute diverticulitis, ruptured ectopic pregnancy, and ruptured aortic aneurysm. During the evaluation of these patients, it is essential to remember that pulmonary (pneumonia), pelvic, renal (renal stone), hematologic (sickle cell crisis), hepatic (acute hepatitis), and metabolic (acute porphyria) disorders can cause acute abdominal pain.

The history of patients with acute abdominal pain should focus on the onset, nature, and radiation of pain, and the presence of associated symptoms such as fever, nausea, vomiting, constipation, and diarrhea. Crucial facts also can come from the patient's medical history. For example, prior surgery or peptic ulcer disease might suggest possible bowel obstruction (adhesions) or perforation (ulcer). The physical examination includes observation of the patient for restlessness (more common with intestinal colic) or immobility (more common with diffuse peritonitis), as well as examination for the typical signs of peritonitis, bowel obstruction, shock, and cardiovascular collapse (due to hypovolemia from acute peritonitis, bowel obstruction, or hemorrhage). The chest examination must rule out pulmonary causes of abdominal pain such as pneumonia or hepatic congestion due to congestive heart failure. The abdominal examination particularly addresses the following: (1) the nature of bowel sounds, (2) the presence of localized or diffuse severe tenderness, (3) the presence of masses or incarcerated hernias, and (4) the presence of fluid in the abdomen. Evidence for peritoneal tenderness and abdominal guarding is best sought with gentle palpation and light percussion. Vigorous palpation and maneuvers to elicit rebound are extremely painful and usually unnecessary. Adequate rectal and pelvic examinations are essential and provide important clues to genitourinary, colonic, and appendiceal disease.

Useful laboratory tests include a hematocrit, white blood count and differential, urinalysis, and examination of the stool for blood or pus. Tests for serum amylase, bilirubin, and transaminases and inspection for gross lipid are usually rapidly available and may be helpful. The diagnosis of acute pancreatitis is one of exclusion because an elevated serum amylase can accompany other causes of abdominal pain, including bowel ischemia, biliary tract disease, perforated ulcer, and ruptured ectopic pregnancy.

Helpful radiographic procedures include plain films of the abdomen in a supine and upright position (to evaluate intestinal gas patterns and search for free intra-abdominal air), as well as a chest radiograph. Certain other tests such as barium or Gastrografin studies of the small bowel or colon, CT imaging, ^{99m}Tc-HIDA scans, ultrasound, and endoscopic procedures are useful in selected patients.

Adequate pain relief should be provided to all patients even while awaiting a definitive diagnosis. Ultimate management depends upon the underlying disease process. Because many disorders causing abdominal pain require prompt surgical intervention, surgical consultation should be obtained early. Few pathognomonic signs or symptoms exist for many of the processes under consideration, and an early diagnostic laparotomy may sometimes be necessary.

IRRITABLE BOWEL SYNDROME

The term irritable bowel syndrome (IBS) refers to a common symptom complex, including abdominal pain and altered bowel habits, usually constipation or alternating diarrhea and constipation, for which no organic cause can be demonstrated. IBS is extremely common, constituting up to 50 per cent of referrals to gastroenterologists in the United States. Symptoms usually begin during adolescence or young adulthood, last for many years, and affect women more than men. Although the etiology and pathogenesis of IBS are not well-understood, the syndrome probably is derived from a variety of disorders. For example, patients with lactase deficiency were previously thought to have IBS. Current concepts of the pathogenesis of IBS focus on two major factors: (1) abnormal colonic motility, including high-amplitude segmental contractions, particularly after stimulation by meals, emotion, mechanical distention, or pharmacological agents; and (2) increased inherent sensitivity to physiological levels of discomfort produced by normal amounts of intestinal gas or intraluminal sigmoid pressures.

Abdominal pain, the most frequent symptom of IBS, varies widely in pattern and degree, ranging from dull, aching discomfort in the lower quadrants to sharp, knifelike hypogastric pain. Pain is often related to meals, possibly reflecting an exaggeration of the normal food-stimulated increase in colonic motility, and may be relieved by passing flatus or stool. The pain rarely occurs at night. Some disturbance of bowel habit is always present in the form of constipation, diarrhea, or a combination of the two. Stools are often described as marble- or pellet-like and may be accompanied by mucus. Bleeding does not occur except perhaps from accompanying hemorrhoids; IBS is never an explanation for occult fecal blood. Certain personality characteristics, such as rigidity, meticulousness, and obsessive-compulsiveness, as well as emotional lability, lethargy, and headaches have been associated with IBS.

Evaluation includes a history, physical examination, stool analysis, screening laboratory tests, proctosigmoidoscopy, and barium enema to eliminate the possibility of underlying organic disease.

Most importantly, treatment should include education regarding the benign nature of the condition and the pathophysiological nature of the symptoms, as well as sympathetic reassurance and continued support by the physician. Psychological counseling or treatment of psychoneuroses may be helpful in selected patients. Drug treatment has little place, and narcotic analgesics must be avoided. Bulk agents such as Metamucil and increased dietary fiber are useful adjuncts in the therapy of constipation. Anticholinergic spasmolytics sometimes may relieve pain. Special diets (aside from increased dietary fiber) offer little or no help, unless it is evident that specific foods repeatedly cause symptoms.

Complications of IBS include potential drug abuse, sigmoid hypertrophy, and the formation of diverticula.

REFERENCES

Connell AM: Motility and its disturbances. Clin Gastroenterol 11:3, 1982.
Schuster MM: Irritable bowel syndrome. *In* Sleisenger MH, Fordtran JS (eds): Gastrointestinal Disease. 4th ed. Philadelphia, WB Saunders Co, 1989, pp 1402–1418.
Silen W (ed): Cope's Early Diagnosis of the Acute Abdomen. 16th ed. Oxford, Oxford University Press, 1983.
Wyngaarden JB, Smith LH Jr (eds): Cecil Textbook of Medicine. 18th ed. Philadelphia, WB Saunders Co, 1988, pp 656–662, 722–723.

B. GASTROINTESTINAL HEMORRHAGE

DEFINITION

Bleeding from the gastrointestinal (GI) tract is an important and common clinical problem. Blood loss may be massive and acute or occult and chronic from a large variety of pathological lesions. A few common lesions, however, account for most GI bleeding episodes. In approximately 80 per cent of patients acute GI bleeding stops spontaneously, but bleeding may recur, often during hospitalization, or persist to constitute a life-threatening emergency.

The goals of management in the patient with GI hemorrhage, in order of priority, are to (1) correct hypovolemia, (2) arrest hemorrhage by the least invasive means, and (3) prevent recurrent hemorrhage. The latter two goals are more rationally attained by accurate identification of the site and pathological nature of the bleeding lesion. However, prompt and adequate hemodynamic resuscitation of the patient takes priority over all diagnostic procedures.

PRESENTATION OF GI HEMORRHAGE

Blood loss from the GI tract may be either (1) *acute*, implying sudden or massive bleeding, often with accompanying signs of hypovolemia, or (2) *chronic*, in which case blood loss is usually occult.

Acute bleeding may present in several ways:

Hematemesis. Vomiting of bright red blood or blood altered by contact with gastric acid (which displays a "coffee-grounds" appearance) is called hematemesis. This extremely valuable clinical clue limits the field of search for a bleeding site considerably, since it denotes bleeding proximal to the ligament of Treitz.

Melena. Melena, the passage of black, tarry stools, usually implies blood loss greater than 500 ml originating anywhere between the oropharynx and the right hemicolon. Melena occurs most often, however, from upper GI bleeding lesions and may be their only manifestation.

Hematochezia. Passage of bright red or maroon-colored stool, termed hematochezia, generally results from a lesion in the GI tract distal to the ligament of Treitz. Rarely, however, it may also result from rapid, massive GI bleeding proximal to this point.

Chronic gastrointestinal blood loss may present as an incidentally discovered positive test for fecal occult blood or with the manifestations of iron-deficiency anemia: fatigue, dyspnea, syncope, and, not infrequently, angina in older patients with underlying ischemic heart disease. A history of intermittent melena may often be elicited, although confirmation of GI blood loss will usually require a positive guaiac test (e.g., Hemoccult test) for occult blood in the stool. Occasionally, a bleeding lesion in a patient may result in both chronic and acute blood loss, which may present either simultaneously or separated in time.

TABLE 34–2. CAUSES OF GI BLEEDING

UPPER GI	UPPER OR LOWER GI	LOWER GI
Duodenal ulcer	Neoplasms	Hemorrhoids
Gastric ulcer	Arterial-enteric fistulas	Anal fissure
Anastomotic ulcer	Vascular anomalies	Diverticulosis
Esophagitis	Angiodysplasia	Ischemic bowel disease
Gastritis	Arteriovenous	Inflammatory bowel
Mallory-Weiss tear	malformations	disease
Esophageal varices	Hematologic disease	Meckel's diverticulum
Hematobilia	Elastic tissue diseases	Solitary colonic ulcer
	Pseudoxanthoma	Intussusception
	elasticum	
	Ehlers-Danlos	
	syndrome	
	Vasculitis syndrome	

ETIOLOGY OF GASTROINTESTINAL BLEEDING

Many lesions in the GI tract may bleed (Table 34–2), although comparatively few account for the vast majority of encountered cases. Bleeding is defined as upper or lower according to its origin above or below the ligament of Treitz.

Upper GI Bleeding

Upper GI bleeding is attributable to peptic ulceration, erosive gastritis, or esophagogastric varices in approximately 90 per cent of cases.

Peptic Ulcer. Bleeding may occur from duodenal, gastric, and post-surgical anastomotic ulcers. A typical history of ulcer pain or dyspepsia may be absent, with bleeding being the first manifestation of peptic ulcer disease.

Gastritis. Erosive gastritis may result from ingestion of alcohol or anti-inflammatory drugs, such as aspirin or indomethacin. Gastric erosions also frequently develop as so-called stress gastritis in hospitalized patients with major trauma, severe systemic illness, extensive burns, or head injury. Since the risk of bleeding from erosive gastritis is high (about 20 per cent) with a high mortality rate in such severely ill hospitalized patients, preventive measures aimed mainly at raising gastric pH above 4 are usually instituted through the hourly administration of antacids or through the intravenous administration of H_2-receptor blocking agents. Although clearly successful in preventing bleeding, these measures do not affect mortality in these critically ill patients.

Esophagogastric Varices. Bleeding occurs most frequently from varices in the esophagus and is characteristically abrupt and massive. Varices arise mainly as a result of portal hypertension secondary to cirrhosis. Alcoholic cirrhosis is by far the most common cause of variceal bleeding in the United States, although any cause of portal hypertension (e.g., portal venous thrombosis, schistosomiasis) may lead to variceal hemorrhage. Three factors complicate the course of GI bleeding in *patients with cirrhosis.* (1) Although varices are usually suspected as the cause of bleeding, other causes (e.g., gastritis, ulcers) actually account for up to 50 per cent of bleeding lesions in these patients. These other causes of bleeding must invariably be considered in the diagnostic work-up of the cirrhotic patient. (2) Sustained portal hypertension leads to recurrent bleeding in 70 per cent of patients with cirrhosis. Thus portal decompression by means of a surgically created portosystemic shunt is the only absolutely effective means for preventing recurrence of bleeding. This in turn carries a high morbidity and appreciable mortality, especially when performed as an emergency procedure. (3) Cirrhosis often leads to the development of encephalopathy, which may manifest or exacerbate during bleeding, as well as to the development of coagulation defects, which contribute to continued bleeding. Because of these three factors,

GI bleeding in patients with cirrhosis often poses difficult therapeutic problems.

Other Lesions. The Mallory-Weiss syndrome, which refers to hemorrhagic laceration of the mucosa of the esophagogastric junction produced by vomiting, is characterized by a history of retching and nonbloody vomiting followed by hematemesis. Several other lesions of the upper GI tract, including esophagitis, carcinoma, and other tumors of the stomach, generally cause chronic blood loss but may also produce massive bleeding. Arterial-enteric fistulae may occur as a result of the use of synthetic bypass grafts for aortic aneurysms and must be suspected in any patient who has had such a bypass and presents with GI bleeding.

Lower GI Bleeding

Lesions of the anorectum and colon are by far the most common causes of lower GI bleeding.

Non-neoplastic Anorectal Lesions. Small amounts of bright red blood on the stool and toilet tissue usually arise from hemorrhoids, anal fissures, and fistulae. Proctitis from a variety of infectious causes is seen most frequently in male homosexuals and may give rise to hematochezia.

Neoplastic Lesions of the Colon and Rectum. Carcinoma of the colon and colonic polyps usually present with chronic blood loss but may produce brisk bleeding as well.

Ulcerative, Bacterial, and Ischemic Colitis. Bleeding may accompany diarrhea in ulcerative colitis as well as in infectious diarrhea due to *Entamoeba histolytica*, *Shigella*, and *Campylobacter*. In these cases, diarrhea is usually prominent, with mucus and leukocytes in the stool along with constitutional symptoms (e.g., malaise, fever). Ischemic colitis may cause bloody diarrhea in the elderly.

Colonic Diverticula. The sigmoid colon is the most common site in which large numbers of colonic diverticula occur. Those that bleed, however, are most frequently located in the ascending colon and constitute the most common cause of massive lower GI bleeding. Diverticulitis, in contrast to diverticulosis, is an uncommon source of blood loss.

Angiodysplastic Lesions. Relatively small, acquired submucosal arteriovenous malformations called angiodysplastic lesions are a common source of bleeding from the cecum and right colon in the elderly. Angiodysplastic lesions, which may also occur in the upper GI tract, are often difficult to diagnose either endoscopically or radiographically because they are flat, are located in the submucosa, and may be completely obscured by even minor bleeding. These lesions appear to develop with aging and may be responsible for a substantial proportion of bleeding previously ascribed to right-sided diverticula. There seems to be an increased association of these lesions with calcific aortic stenosis.

Small Intestinal Lesions. Small intestinal lesions rarely cause GI hemorrhage. Meckel's diverticulum is present in the distal ileum of 2 per cent of the population and is the most common discrete lesion of the lower small bowel to bleed acutely.

Bleeding Diatheses

Blood dyscrasias (leukemia, thrombocytopenia), disorders of coagulation (hemophilia, disseminated intravascular coagulation), vascular malformations (Osler-Weber-Rendu disease), vasculitides (Henoch-Schönlein purpura), and connective tissue disorders (pseudoxanthoma elasticum) may all produce GI blood loss originating from upper or lower sites.

THE APPROACH TO THE PATIENT WITH GASTROINTESTINAL HEMORRHAGE

Steps in the approach to the patient who presents with GI bleeding are considered in this section in order of priority (Table 34–3), i.e., (1) initial assessment, (2)

TABLE 34–3. DIAGNOSTIC APPROACH TO THE PATIENT WITH GASTROINTESTINAL HEMORRHAGE

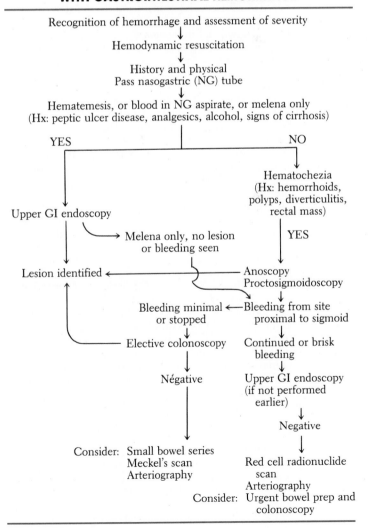

resuscitation, (3) diagnosis, and (4) treatment. The management of GI bleeding must be individualized according to the nature and extent of bleeding. Thus in cases of massive, continuous bleeding, for example, more urgent diagnostic and therapeutic intervention may be called for, as transfusions may fail to keep pace with the rapid rate of blood loss.

Initial Assessment

If it is established or suspected that a patient has bled acutely from the gastrointestinal tract, pulse and blood pressure are noted and large-bore intravenous lines inserted for the initial infusion of saline or other plasma expanders prior to any further inquiry or examination. Blood is sent for typing and cross-matching, a complete blood count, prothrombin time, and platelet count. The latter two help to rule out a bleeding diathesis, which commonly accompanies bleeding in patients with cirrhosis, and establish a baseline for assessment of coagulation disturbances that may supervene with massive transfusion. Blood sent for electrolytes, BUN, creatinine, and liver function tests at this stage will aid in evaluating renal function, which may become compromised as a result of hypovolemic shock, as well as the presence of liver disease, which would alert the physician to a variceal source of hemorrhage.

Vital signs are the most reliable means for assessing the degree of volume loss. An orthostatic fall in blood pressure of greater than 10 mm Hg usually signifies a 20 per cent or greater loss of blood volume. Hypotension is usually accompanied by tachycardia, but heart rate alone is unreliable. When blood loss approaches 40 per cent of blood volume, signs of shock are usually present with pallor, cool extremities, pronounced tachycardia, and hypotension. A small amount of hematemesis or melena is misleading in that it may represent only a small proportion of the blood lost into the gastointestinal tract, while even small losses may seriously compromise an elderly patient or a patient with pre-existing anemia or dehydration. The hematocrit is initially unreliable for evaluating acute blood loss, because a fall in hematocrit following acute blood loss requires equilibration of the contracted intravascular space with the extravascular space, which takes several hours. Thus, soon after even substantial bleeding, the hematocrit may be normal. An initially low hematocrit may suggest pre-existing chronic blood loss, and this may be confirmed by the presence of microcytic red cell indices.

Resuscitation

Unless bleeding is mild or chronic, patients are placed in an intensive care unit. Although initial management is usually conducted by internists, surgical consultation at this stage is mandatory, as surgical intervention may be urgently required, and the decision to intervene surgically is greatly facilitated by the patient's being jointly followed by both medical and surgical teams. Resuscitation is directed toward maintaining the intravascular volume and providing adequate tissue oxygenation. Nasal oxygen may be used, particularly in the elderly or in patients with cardiac or pulmonary disease. Vital signs, urine output, and, in some cases, central venous or pulmonary wedge pressure are monitored.

Crystalloid solutions are given via large-bore intravenous lines to begin volume replacement. Actively bleeding patients are given whole blood or packed red cells and fresh-frozen plasma to replace volume losses. However, if the patient is hemodynamically stable as a result of plasma volume restoration from the extravascular space and intravenous administration of crystalloids, packed cells alone may be given.

Blood is given according to the volume lost, the presence of continued bleeding, pre-existing anemia, and the ability of the patient to withstand blood loss. Thus, severe active bleeding may require whole blood administration under pressure via several intravenous lines. On the other hand, an otherwise healthy young person who is hemodynamically stable and who has stopped bleeding from a duodenal ulcer may tolerate a hematocrit of 25 per cent quite well and may be treated with oral iron. In general, evidence of hypotension, diminished tissue perfusion, or continued bleeding is an indication for transfusion.

Diagnosis

The first step in the diagnosis of the cause of gastrointestinal bleeding is to differentiate between upper and lower bleeding. The patient's *history* may be of considerable value in this differentiation. Hematemesis, for example, suggests bleeding proximal to the ligament of Treitz, and recent ingestion of anti-inflammatory drugs or alcohol suggests gastritis. A typical history of peptic ulcer pain may be helpful, as will a prior or family history of GI bleeding. Recent retching followed by hematemesis points to the possibility of Mallory-Weiss syndrome. A change in bowel habits may suggest colonic cancer, and acute abdominal pain with bleeding may indicate ischemic colitis. The history may also reveal the presence of an aortic bypass graft.

Physical examination may reveal stigmata of chronic liver disease, suggesting a variceal source of bleeding, whereas enlargement of lymph nodes or an abdominal mass may reflect an intra-abdominal malignancy. Examination of the skin may show the telangiectasia characteristic of Osler-Weber-Rendu disease. Rectal examination will help to rule out a mass.

A simple and expedient diagnostic procedure is the passage of a nasogastric tube. A clear aspirate rules out active bleeding proximal to the pylorus. Active bleeding from a duodenal ulcer may be missed but is ruled out if clear bile is aspirated. If bleeding from an upper GI source is intermittent, the aspirate may be negative. An elevated BUN also suggests upper, as opposed to lower, GI bleeding, because blood constitutes a "high-protein diet."

Further *diagnostic procedures* are selected according to the clinical suspicion of upper versus lower GI bleeding and the rate of blood loss. In acute bleeding, barium studies are generally inappropriate, and if very rapid bleeding is present, particularly if the source is colonic, endoscopic examination may fail to visualize the site of bleeding. Under such conditions, angiography is often the procedure of first choice and may be preceded by a radiolabeled red-cell scan to localize further the region of blood loss. If bleeding is moderate, angiography often fails to show extravasation of contrast at the site of bleeding, and endoscopic procedures are preferred.

In most cases of suspected upper GI bleeding, upper GI endoscopy will provide a rapid, safe, definitive means for diagnosis of the site of blood loss. If bleeding has stopped, a double-contrast barium upper GI series will detect most malignancies and peptic ulcers, although gastritis is often missed. Endoscopy, a more specific and sensitive diagnostic tool, has occasional therapeutic advantages as well as the advantage of allowing biopsy of lesions suspicious of malignancy. Thus endoscopy is preferred by many physicians for upper GI hemorrhage even in the patient who has stopped bleeding.

Bleeding from the lower GI tract is first evaluated by anoscopy and proctosigmoidoscopy, which will detect lesions in the rectosigmoid region, including hemorrhoids, polyps, carcinoma, and inflammatory bowel disease. More proximal colonic lesions may be detected by colonoscopy after colonic cleansing, but if bleeding is brisk, colonoscopy may prove futile and recourse to angiography may be necessary. If bleeding has stopped, double-contrast barium enema studies may be considered, but they are often inconclusive and make colonoscopy and angiography difficult to perform in the event of early recurrent bleeding. Colonoscopy is thus often performed even after lower GI bleeding has stopped. If evaluation of presumed lower GI bleeding is unrewarding, an upper GI source should always be excluded. Small bowel lesions below the ligament of Treitz are difficult to detect, but may be seen with a small bowel barium series.

For patients with chronic GI blood loss, the initial search for a responsible lesion is undertaken with barium studies followed, as indicated, by endoscopic evaluation and biopsy of lesions suspicious of malignancy. Angiography is occasionally employed, particularly to search for vascular lesions of the bowel.

In spite of the use of sophisticated diagnostic techniques, the site of bleeding is not established in many patients with GI bleeding. Sometimes this reflects a subtle or inaccessible lesion, at other times a multitude of lesions without identification of the one responsible for the bleeding. This does not necessarily compromise the patient, although repeated hospitalization for bleeding from an undiagnosed site is the lot of an unfortunate few and represents a difficult challenge to the physician.

Treatment

Approximately 80 per cent of patients presenting with gastrointestinal hemorrhage will stop bleeding spontaneously. In such cases, management is directed toward prevention of further bleeding by either medical or surgical treatment. Thus, following bleeding from a duodenal ulcer, treatment with antacids, sucralfate, or an H_2-receptor blocker is often initiated. Conservative management is usually undertaken in cases of gastritis, Mallory-Weiss tears, angiodysplasia, or diverticulosis in which bleeding ceases spontaneously. On the other hand, malignant lesions and polyps are resected either surgically or endoscopically when possible. If bleeding does not cease or recurs, further management will depend upon the site and nature of the lesion as well as upon the assessed ability of the patient to withstand surgery. For example, most cases of peptic ulcer that fail to cease bleeding will require urgent surgery.

Several nonsurgical techniques for arresting gastrointestinal hemorrhage have been widely used, although their role is far from clear. These include radiological procedures such as intra-arterial infusion of vasopressin, a powerful vasoconstrictor, and selective embolization of bleeding arterial foci. Endoscopic electrocoagulation and laser photocoagulation are also becoming increasingly used, particularly for elderly, poor-risk patients with angiodysplastic lesions.

Variceal hemorrhage requires special consideration. Most patients with variceal bleeding are poor operative candidates and run a high risk of rebleeding. Additional precautions and supportive measures are required in these patients, as bleeding may precipitate hepatic encephalopathy while renal function may deteriorate rapidly (see Chapter 44). Cleansing of blood from the bowel using enemas as well as administration of lactulose helps to lessen the risk of encephalopathy. Volume should be replaced using blood or blood products, with care taken to avoid overtransfusion, which can worsen variceal bleeding. Since these patients often retain sodium and water avidly, infusion of large volumes of saline should be avoided as far as possible, as this will invariably aggravate ascites. Initial measures to arrest hemorrhage nonoperatively include intravenous infusion of vasopressin (which is as effective as, but safer than, intra-arterial administration) and clotting factor replacement, usually in the form of fresh frozen plasma and platelets. Balloon tamponade is resorted to when bleeding fails to cease, but it is often only a temporary measure. Currently, continued bleeding is usually treated by endoscopic injection of the varices with sclerosant solutions (sclerotherapy), which is successful in arresting bleeding in up to 90 per cent of cases. Emergency decompression of the portal system by means of portosystemic shunt surgery is, at times, the only means for arresting acute variceal hemorrhage. Prevention of recurrent bleeding from varices may be achieved through either repeated endoscopic sclerotherapy or elective portosystemic shunt surgery. Both options carry distinct advantages and disadvantages (Chapter 45).

REFERENCES

Cello, JP, Crass RA, Grendell, JH, Trunkey, DD: Management of the patient with hemorrhaging esophageal varices. JAMA 256:1480, 1986.

Peterson WL: Gastrointestinal hemorrhage. *In* Wyngaarden JB, Smith LH Jr (eds): Cecil Textbook of Medicine. 18th ed. Philadelphia, WB Saunders Co, 1988, pp 796–800.

Steer ML, Silen W: Diagnostic procedures in gastrointestinal hemorrhage. N Engl J Med 309:646, 1983.

C. MALABSORPTION

The gastrointestinal tract has as its main purpose the digestion and absorption of nutrients, either macronutrients required predominantly for energy or micronutrients, for example, trace elements and vitamins. Only 1 μg of vitamin B_{12} needs to be absorbed daily in a highly specific and complex process in the terminal ileum. Conversely, the gastrointestinal tract may be called upon to digest, solubilize, transport, and resynthesize 80 gm of fat daily. Beyond the net absorption of dietary components, the gut has a large daily internal circulation of water, electrolytes, and bile salts that are secreted in gastric juice, pancreatic juice, bile, and intestinal secretions and then reabsorbed in the small intestine and colon for reutilization. The gastrointestinal tract must first prepare for subsequent absorption of the crude mixtures of nutrients and non-nutrients ingested as "food." These preparatory processes of *digestion* consist of (a) the controlled release into the intestine of food that has been fragmented to small particle size by the grinding action of the stomach; (b) the release of appropriate amounts of enzymes, cofactors, buffers (bicarbonate), detergents (bile salts), and water into the lumen under hormonal control to allow digestion of food to an isotonic mixture of simple components; and (c) further digestion of disaccharides and oligopeptides by brush border–bound enzymes. All of these steps must precede actual absorption.

Absorption of nutrients occurs from an enormous surface area supplied by the intestinal villi and microvilli during an average transit time of approximately 1½ to 2 hours between the stomach and the ileocecal valve. (Colonic absorption consists largely of salvage of fluid and electrolytes only.) The absorption of a given substance may occur diffusely throughout the intestine or be localized to specific sites (e.g., vitamin B_{12} and bile salts in the terminal ileum). In view of the complexities of the above coordinated chemical and physiological processes, it is not surprising that a large number of disorders can result in maldigestion or malabsorption, either with considerable specificity or more globally. The purpose of this section is to present a general classification of the disorders of maldigestion and malabsorption, based on current knowledge of pathophysiology, together with a rational approach to their differential diagnosis.

NORMAL ABSORPTION

Malabsorption can be understood only in the context of normal absorption. Only the absorption of the three major classes of caloric nutrients will be described here. The intestinal absorption of water and electrolytes is described in Section D of this chapter, since this analogous form of "malabsorption" largely results in diarrhea. The important specific mechanisms for the absorption of iron (ferrous and heme forms), calcium (under the control of vitamin D), and vitamin B_{12} are described elsewhere.

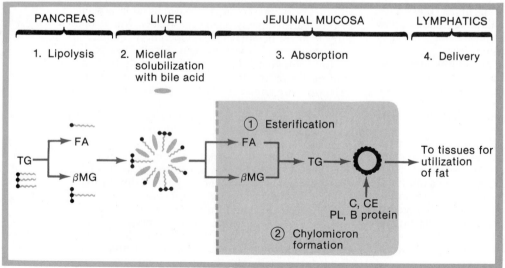

FIGURE 34–1. Schematic of intestinal absorption, showing the participation of pancreas, liver, and intestinal mucosal cells in fat absorption. TG = triglycerides; FA = fatty acids; βMG = beta-monoglyceride; C = cholesterol; CE = cholesterol esters; PL = phospholipids. (From Wilson FA, Dietschy JM: Gastroenterology 61:911, 1971. Copyright 1971, The Williams & Wilkins Company, Baltimore.)

Digestion and Absorption of Fat (Fig. 34–1).
Most dietary fat is in the form of triglycerides of long-chain fatty acids (e.g., saturated—palmitic and stearic; unsaturated—oleic and linoleic). Fat from the stomach enters the duodenum as an oil-liquid emulsion; long-chain fatty acids and oligopeptides in the duodenum stimulate the flow of bile (via cholecystokinin [CCK]) and pancreatic juice (via secretin and CCK) (see Fig. 34–1). Pancreatic lipase, bound to the lipid surface by colipase in the presence of the detergent action of amphophilic bile salts, releases two free fatty acids from each molecule, leaving a 2-monoglyceride. These products of lipolysis are incorporated into complex mixed micelles with bile salts, which enhance their solubility and allow them to traverse the unstirred water layer that overlies the surface of the epithelial cells. The fatty acids and 2-monoglycerides then diffuse from the micelles into the cell cytosol, where they are largely resynthesized into triglycerides and packaged into chylomicrons and very low density lipoproteins (VLDL) for transport via lymphatics. The bile salts remain in the intestinal lumen for reutilization and are finally reabsorbed from the terminal ileum. The process of fat absorption is normally highly efficient; approximately 95 per cent of ingested neutral fat is absorbed. Fat-soluble vitamins are probably "carried along" in this same general process.

Digestion and Absorption of Proteins. The digestion and absorption of proteins are simpler than those for fat, which may explain why malabsorption of fat figures more prominently in most malabsorptive syndromes. Hydrolysis of proteins begins in the stomach with pepsin but continues more completely in the upper small intestine catalyzed by pancreatic trypsin, chymotrypsin, and carboxypeptidase. The products of hydrolysis are free amino acids, dipeptides, and oligopeptides, the latter of which may undergo further hydrolysis by dipeptidases or oligopeptidases in the brush border of microvilli on the surface of the enterocytes. Many amino acids are absorbed as dipeptides, which are subsequently hydrolyzed to the free amino acids in the mucosal cells. There are several specific transport systems for amino acids: (a) the dibasic amino acid system, which is often abnormal in cystinuria; (b) the neutral amino acid system, which is abnormal in Hartnup disease; (c) the imino acid–glycine system; and (d) the dicarboxylic acid system. Amino acids are absorbed by active cotransport with sodium, predominantly in the jejunum.

Digestion and Absorption of Carbohydrates. Ingested carbohydrates consist largely of starch (a complex hexose polysaccharide) and the disaccharides sucrose and lactose. Salivary and pancreatic amylases hydrolyze starch intraluminally to oligosaccharides and disaccharides. In contrast to dipeptides, disaccharides cannot be absorbed. The final stages of digestion are catalyzed by specific enzymes in the microvillous surface—limit dextrinase, sucrase, lactase, and maltase. The released glucose and galactose are absorbed by active transport in association with sodium; fructose absorption is by facilitated diffusion.

CLASSIFICATION OF THE MALABSORPTION SYNDROMES (Table 34–4)

A very large number of disorders can produce or be associated with intestinal malabsorption, varying from specific genetic defects to acquired diffuse mucosal diseases. It will not be possible to discuss all of these entities in this section, which is devoted to a general understanding of malabsorption, but they are described in detail in the articles to which reference is made at the end of this section. In general it is useful to think of malabsorption as resulting from abnormalities in one or more of the normal processes of digestion and absorption described earlier.

Inadequate Digestion. Ingested food must be broken down to its proper components for absorption through intraluminal or surface enzymatic processes.

TABLE 34–4. CLASSIFICATION OF THE MALABSORPTION SYNDROMES

Inadequate Digestion
  Pancreatic exocrine deficiency
    primary—e.g., chronic pancreatitis, cystic fibrosis, carcinoma of the pancreas
    secondary—gastrinoma with acid inactivation of pancreatic lipase
  Intraluminal bile salt deficiency
    liver disease—especially biliary cirrhosis
    disease or bypass of the terminal ileum—impaired recycling mechanism
    bacterial overgrowth syndrome—increased deconjugation of bile salts
  Specific abnormalities—disaccharidase deficiencies

Inadequate Absorption
  Inadequate absorptive surface—e.g., short bowel syndrome, bypass fistulas, extensive Crohn's disease
  Specific mucosal cell defects
    genetic—abetalipoproteinemia, Hartnup disease, cystinuria, monosaccharide absorptive defects
    acquired—hypovitaminosis D
  Diffuse disease of the small intestine
    immunologic or allergic injury—celiac disease (gluten-sensitive enteropathy), ? eosinophilic enteritis, ? Crohn's disease
    infections and infestations—Whipple's disease, giardiasis, tropical sprue, bacterial overgrowth syndrome
    infiltrative disorders—lymphoma, mastocytosis, amyloidosis
    fibrosis—systemic sclerosis, radiation enteritis

Lymphatic Obstruction
  Lymphangiectasia
  Whipple's disease
  Lymphoma

Multiple Mechanisms
  Postgastrectomy steatorrhea
  Bacterial overgrowth syndrome
  Disease or bypass of the distal ileum
  Scleroderma, lymphoma, Whipple's disease
  Diabetes mellitus

Drug-induced Malabsorption
  Neomycin, cholestyramine, antacids, ethanol, chronic ingestion of laxatives, biguanides

Hyperabsorptive "Malabsorption"
  Hemochromatosis, hypervitaminosis D
  Enteric hyperoxaluria

The exocrine secretion of the pancreas, described in Chapter 40, is of particular importance in the supply of lipase, colipase, and certain proteases, especially trypsin. One of the cardinal manifestations of chronic pancreatitis, either acquired or secondary to cystic fibrosis, is malabsorption. Even in the presence of normal pancreatic secretion of lipase, however, a gastrinoma (the Zollinger-Ellison syndrome) may stimulate enough gastric acid to lower the duodenal pH sufficiently to impair the activity of lipase and produce fat malabsorption.

The pancreatic component of fat digestion must be supplemented with a sufficient concentration of intraluminal bile salts for normal lipolysis and micelle formation. Inadequacy of bile salts can result from (a) decreased synthesis by the liver, although this is rarely severe enough to result in major malabsorption; (b) prolonged cholestasis (see Chapter 47) especially in biliary cirrhosis; (c) deconjugation of the bile salts within the intestine by bacterial action in the bacterial overgrowth syndrome; or (d) interference in the ileal reabsorption of bile salts for recycling, either due to the use of cholestyramine or more commonly in the presence of ileal disease or an ileal bypass. In these circumstances, the liver is not able to synthesize enough bile salts de novo to maintain critical intraluminal levels so that maldigestion and malabsorption of fat and fat-soluble substances (e.g., vitamins A, D, E, and K) occur.

In addition to these more global disorders of digestion associated with deficiencies of pancreatic enzymes or bile salts, more selective defects in digestion can occur. For example, deficiency of lactase, an intestinal brush border enzyme that normally hydrolyzes lactose to glucose and galactose, impairs the absorption of this disaccharide and may result in milk intolerance with symptoms of flatulence, distention, and diarrhea. Lactase deficiency may be inherited (lactase deficiency is common in certain ethnic groups such as blacks and Orientals) or may occur secondary to other causes of diffuse mucosal injury (e.g., celiac disease).

Inadequate Absorption. The components of food may not be adequately absorbed even after they have been normally digested. This may result from an insufficient available absorptive surface even though that remaining is normal. The simplest example is that of the postsurgical short bowel syndrome, which may follow surgery for mesenteric infarction or bypass surgery for morbid obesity or Crohn's disease.

Conversely, the absorptive surface may be normal in area but defective in function. This type of defect can be within the mucosal cell and then is usually highly specific and genetic in origin. Examples are selective absorptive defects for certain amino acids in cystinuria and Hartnup disease and for fat in abetalipoproteinemia, due to defective intracellular synthesis of apolipoproteins. Selective defects can also be acquired, such as the reduced absorption of calcium when there is insufficient synthesis of 1,25-dihydroxycholecalciferol.

More frequently malabsorption, especially that of fat, is found in conditions in which there is a diffuse disease process involving the small intestinal mucosa and/or submucosa. Several causes of such diffuse injury are recognized, although the mechanisms involved are often obscure:

IMMUNOLOGIC OR ALLERGIC INJURY. It is thought that gluten-sensitive enteropathy (to be discussed subsequently) falls in this category, as well as possibly some forms of the rare disorder eosinophilic enteritis.

INFECTIONS AND INFESTATIONS. Whipple's disease is a systemic disorder, the presumed bacterial etiology of which has not been clearly defined. In this disorder marked by malabsorption, the intestinal submucosa is packed with macrophages containing PAS-staining granules. Patients may also have fever, arthralgias, lymphadenopathy, pigmentation changes, and neurological manifestations. Whipple's disease is rare, but the diagnosis is important, since it usually responds to prolonged antibiotic therapy. Infestation with *Giardia lamblia* may be sufficient to cause malabsorption, although flatulence, nausea, and diarrhea are more common symptoms. In addition to causing deconjugation of bile salts, bacterial overgrowth may also produce diffuse mucosal injury.

INFILTRATIVE DISORDERS. The mucosa and/or submucosa may be diffusely infiltrated in a number of disorders sufficient to impair its absorptive function. Examples include primary lymphoma of the bowel, particularly important as a cause of malabsorption in certain parts of the world such as the Near East, and such rare disorders as systemic mastocytosis and amyloidosis.

FIBROSIS. The intestinal wall may become thickened and fibrotic in such disorders as systemic sclerosis and radiation injury. The causes of impaired absorption may be complex in these entities, however, and may result in part from abnormal motility and bacterial overgrowth.

LYMPHATIC OBSTRUCTION. After their absorption, long-chain fatty acids are largely resynthesized as triglycerides and secreted into the lymphatics as chylomicrons or as very low density lipoproteins (VLDL). Diffuse obstructive lesions of the mesenteric lymphatics can therefore impair fat absorption. This is not infrequently a second cause of malabsorption in diffuse intestinal lymphoma and may also occur in Whipple's disease and in the rare congenital disorder lymphangiectasia. The latter entity more commonly presents as protein-losing enteropathy with secondary hypoalbuminemia.

Multiple Mechanisms. In view of the complexity of the digestive and absorptive processes, it is not surprising that a number of disorders may impair two or more steps. For example after subtotal gastrectomy with a gastroenterostomy (Billroth II procedure) a modest degree of malabsorption is very common. This may result from rapid gastric emptying and rapid intestinal transit, poor mixing of the pancreatic and biliary secretions from the blind duodenal loop with intestinal contents, decreased stimulus for pancreatic

TABLE 34–5. SOME DRUG-INDUCED ABSORPTIVE DEFECTS

DRUG	SUBSTANCE MALABSORBED
Ethanol	Folates, vitamin B_{12}
Antacids	Phosphate
Phenytoin	Folates
Neomycin	Fatty acids, vitamin B_{12}
Cholestyramine	Bile acids, thyroxine
Tetracycline	Iron

and biliary secretion due to decreased release of secretin and cholecystokinin, and bacterial overgrowth due to stasis in the afferent blind loop. As noted, bacterial overgrowth itself not only deconjugates bile salts but may cause diffuse injury to the intestinal epithelium. In diabetes mellitus there may be an associated exocrine deficiency of the pancreas and/or a motility disorder of the small intestine presumed to be due to diabetic neuropathy of the autonomic nervous system. This may be associated with bacterial overgrowth due to stasis.

Drug-induced Malabsorption. A number of drugs have been shown to cause malabsorption of specific dietary elements, some of which are listed in Table 34–5.

Hyperabsorptive "Malabsorption." Although we are accustomed to think of malabsorption as too little absorption, it can also represent too much absorption. In hemochromatosis, for example, there is inherited continued excessive absorption of iron. In hypervitaminosis D there is excessive absorption of calcium. Enteric hyperoxaluria is an acquired abnormality characterized by excessive absorption of dietary oxalate, largely in the colon, and results in a tendency to form calcium oxalate kidney stones.

CLINICAL MANIFESTATIONS OF MALABSORPTION

There are a large number of diseases associated with malabsorption, only some of which are listed in Table 34–4. In many of these diseases the major clinical manifestations may not be related directly to malabsorption. In others the defects are highly specific, such as pernicious anemia with selective malabsorption of vitamin B_{12} or osteomalacia or rickets with poor absorption of calcium. In this brief discussion we shall be concerned only with the symptoms and signs associated with the more general forms of malabsorption, especially those forms including malabsorption of fat.

Early Manifestations. The early manifestations of malabsorption may be subtle and easily missed. There is usually a change in bowel habits with somewhat more bulky and sometimes oily stools that are difficult to flush (they are sticky and tend to float because of increased gas content). This may be associated with some weight loss, fatigue, depression, and a sense of bloating. Nocturia may be noted, thought to be caused by nocturnal reabsorption of excessive intestinal fluid. It is important to consider the diagnosis at this early stage in order to define the cause of malabsorption and to institute appropriate treatment.

Late Manifestations. The major late manifestations of the malabsorption syndrome are summarized in Table 34–6. By and large they represent the results of specific deficiencies secondary to malabsorption. Typically these patients are wasted with poor muscle mass but have distended abdomens with hyperactive bowel sounds. They tend to be hypotensive and often have increased pigmentation of the skin. Abdominal

TABLE 34–6. CORRELATION OF DATA IN MALDIGESTION AND MALABSORPTION*

CLINICAL FEATURES	LABORATORY FINDINGS	PATHOPHYSIOLOGY
Wasting, edema	↓ Serum albumin	↑ Albumin loss (gut), ↓ protein ingestion, ↓ protein absorption
Weight loss, oily bulky stools	↑ Stool fat excretion, ↓ serum carotene	↓ Ingestion and absorption fat, CHO, protein
Paresthesias, tetany	↓ Serum Ca^{++}, ↑ alkaline phosphatase, ↓ mineralization bones (x-ray), ↓ serum Mg^{++}	↓ Absorption Ca^{++}, vitamin D, Mg^{++}
Ecchymoses, petechiae, hematuria	↑ Prothrombin time	↓ Absorption vitamin K
Anemia	Macrocytosis, ↓ serum vitamin B_{12}, ↓ absorption vitamin B_{12} and/or folic acid, microcytosis, hypochromia, ↓ serum iron, no iron in marrow	↓ Absorption vitamin B_{12} and/or folic acid, ↓ absorption iron
Glossitis	↓ Serum vitamin B_{12}, folic acid	↓ Absorption B vitamins
Abdominal distention, borborygmi, flatulence, watery stools	↓ Xylose absorption, ↓ disaccharidases in intestinal biopsy, fluid levels, small intestine (x-ray)	↓ Hydrolysis disaccharides and ↓ absorption, monosaccharides and amino acids

* From Gray GM: Maldigestion and malabsorption: Clinical manifestations and specific diagnosis. *In* Sleisenger MH, Fordtran JS (eds): Gastrointestinal Disease. 3rd ed. Philadelphia, WB Saunders Co, 1983, p 230.

pain is uncommon except in the presence of certain specific disorders, e.g., chronic pancreatitis or primary intestinal lymphoma. At this time the clinical diagnosis is easy to make. The determination of the specific cause of the malabsorption may be more difficult.

CLINICAL TESTS OF DIGESTION AND ABSORPTION

A large number of tests of varying degrees of complexity and specificity are potentially useful in the study of patients suspected of having abnormalities of digestion and/or absorption. Some of the most useful of these tests will be described briefly.

Fecal Fat Analysis. As a screening measure a qualitative test for stool fat using a Sudan III stained smear is useful in the detection of steatorrhea. The standard, however, is to measure quantitatively the amount of fat in a three-day stool specimen after the patient has ingested a diet containing 80 to 100 gm of fat daily. Normal fat excretion in these circumstances is less than 6 gm/24 hr (usually < 2.5 gm). Values higher than this reliably indicate fat malabsorption (steatorrhea) but do not indicate the pathogenesis of the abnormality.

Tests of Pancreatic Exocrine Function. Some of these tests are described in Chapter 40 (see Table 40–1). The bentiromide test determines the split of an orally administered synthetic peptide by pancreatic chymotrypsin. An excretion in 6 hr of less than 50 per cent of a 500-mg dose of bentiromide, as urinary arylamines, is virtually diagnostic of pancreatic exocrine insufficiency. Pancreatic disease may also be suspected from the diffuse calcification on a plain film of the abdomen and from elevation of serum trypsin-like immunoactivity. Occasionally a secretin test may be required.

Xylose Absorption-Excretion Test. The absorption of D-xylose, a poorly metabolized 5-carbon sugar, reflects the integrity of carbohydrate absorption by the proximal small intestine. Since no enzymatic digestion or solubilization is required prior to absorption, the rate of absorption is unaffected by pancreatic or hepatic (biliary) disease and is a more selective test of mucosal integrity. Usually 25 gm of D-xylose is given orally to a well-hydrated subject, and the amount of the sugar excreted in the subsequent five-hour urine is measured. Normal values exceed 4.5 gm/5 hr, but this figure may be reduced by age, decreased renal function, excessive body fluid (ascites, edema), or intestinal bacterial overgrowth. In the latter case the test should return to normal with the use of antibiotics. As a variation the plasma xylose can be measured one hour after xylose is ingested and should exceed 30 mg/dl.

Radiographic Studies. Radiographic studies of the stomach and small intestine in malabsorption are usually nonspecific, with thickening of the mucosal folds, modest dilatation of the intestinal lumen, and occasionally clumping and segmentation of the barium in a so-called moulage pattern. Rarely the study may be diagnostic with the demonstration of a stricture, a fistula, or a "blind-loop" (e.g., a small bowel diverticulum).

Small-intestinal (Jejunal) Biopsy. Peroral biopsy of the small intestinal mucosa is frequently indicated in the investigation of malabsorption. Table 34–7 summarizes the conditions in which the biopsy is likely to be diagnostic and those in which it is often abnormal but in a nonspecific way.

Vitamin B_{12} Absorption (the Schilling Test). Vitamin B_{12} (cobalamin) is selectively absorbed in association with intrinsic factor in the distal ileum. An abnormality in its absorption usually represents one or more of four abnormalities: (a) disease of the distal ileum (e.g., Crohn's disease), (b) deficiency of intrinsic factor, (c) deficient pancreatic exocrine function (pancreatic trypsin is necessary to release cobalamin from a binding "R-protein" of gastric juice so that it is free to combine with intrinsic factor), and (d) increased utilization of cobalamin during transit (e.g., bacterial overgrowth). In the usual form of the test, radioactive vitamin B_{12} is given orally either alone, with intrinsic factor, or after therapy with a broad-spectrum antibiotic in suspected bacterial overgrowth, and its urinary excretion is measured over 24 hours. A flushing dose of 1.0 mg vitamin B_{12} is given simultaneously to prevent its hepatic storage and to enhance excretion. Normally more than 7 per cent of the orally administered radioactive vitamin B_{12} will be recovered in the urine. The pattern of abnormalities found in the sequential Schilling test may suggest (a) all three stages abnormal—intrinsic intestinal disease or pancreatic exocrine insufficiency; (b) stage 1 abnormal, stage 2 normal—intrinsic factor deficiency (pernicious anemia); (c) stages 1 and 2 abnormal, stage 3 normal—bacterial overgrowth.

Other Breath Tests. Several breath tests that assess abnormal rates of intraluminal bacterial metabolism of specific compounds have been developed. In the ^{14}C-xylose breath test the amount of $^{14}CO_2$ expired is measured at 30 and 60 minutes after giving the radioactive sugar orally (1 gm, 5 to 10 μCi). In the presence of bacterial overgrowth in the small intestine the sugar is catabolized by gram-negative aerobes, which

TABLE 34–7. UTILITY OF SMALL BOWEL BIOPSY SPECIMENS IN MALABSORPTION

Often diagnostic

Whipple's disease	Giardiasis
Amyloidosis	Abetalipoproteinemia
Eosinophilic enteritis	Agammaglobulinemia
Lymphangiectasia	Mastocytosis
Primary intestinal lymphoma	

Abnormal but not diagnostic

Celiac sprue	Bacterial overgrowth
Systemic sclerosis	syndrome
Radiation enteritis	Tropical sprue
	Crohn's disease

leads to an increased release of $^{14}CO_2$, especially at 30 minutes. In an analogous fashion, intraluminal bacterial metabolism of sugars (usually lactulose is given as a test substance) releases free hydrogen, which can be measured in expired air. This test can also be used to assess specific disorders of carbohydrate digestion and absorption, such as lactase deficiency, in which expired H_2 is measured after the ingestion of 50 gm of lactose.

Miscellaneous Tests. There are many other important although nonspecific tests that may reflect malabsorption, such as body weight, serum albumin, the prothrombin time (absorption of the fat-soluble vitamin K), and serum levels of cholesterol, carotene, folic acid, calcium, and magnesium. All of these tests measure only the results of malabsorption and are, in general, of little help in its differential diagnosis.

APPROACH TO THE PATIENT WITH SUSPECTED MALDIGESTION AND/OR MALABSORPTION

In view of the large number of tests that are available to study patients suspected of having malabsorption, a logical sequence in their use is indicated in order to arrive at a diagnosis most expeditiously (Fig. 34–2). In general the diagnosis of malabsorption of fat is best established by a quantitative 72-hour fecal fat analysis. Since this may be difficult to obtain, steatorrhea can also be established with a qualitative stool fat examination and a measurement of serum carotene. If the stool fat is normal, the patient may still have a selective abnormality for the absorption of carbohydrates, especially if symptoms are largely those of watery diarrhea, cramps, and excessive flatus. The most frequent cause of abnormal carbohydrate absorption is that of lactase deficiency (acquired or congenital). Specific tests for carbohydrate malabsorption include oral tolerance tests with the suspected carbohydrate associated with measurement of H_2 in expired air or the level of the sugar in the blood, checking also to see if the symptoms are reproduced. Typically the feces have a low pH (<6) and there is a significant fecal osmotic gap due to the high concentration of fecal short chain fatty acids produced by colonic bacteria from unabsorbed carbohydrates.

If malabsorption for fat is demonstrated (>6 gm/24 hr in the stool or abnormal qualitative stool fat and decreased serum carotene), a next logical step would be a xylose absorption-excretion test. A normal xylose test makes a diffuse mucosal abnormality highly unlikely and suggests an abnormality in digestion, such as pancreatic deficiency or deficiency of bile salts. Specific tests for pancreatic insufficiency can then be carried out as noted (Fig. 34–2). If the urinary xylose excretion test is abnormal, a breath test should be carried out to check for the presence of bacterial overgrowth (^{14}C-xylose to $^{14}CO_2$; or lactulose to H_2). A radiographic study may demonstrate either diffuse or segmental disease, including fistulas, blind loops, or other areas of stasis conducive to overgrowth. If no bacterial overgrowth is indicated because of normal breath tests, a diffuse mucosal abnormality should be suspected. At this point a small bowel radiograph and a peroral jejunal biopsy should be performed. The approach to the patient suspected of having bacterial overgrowth is described later in this section.

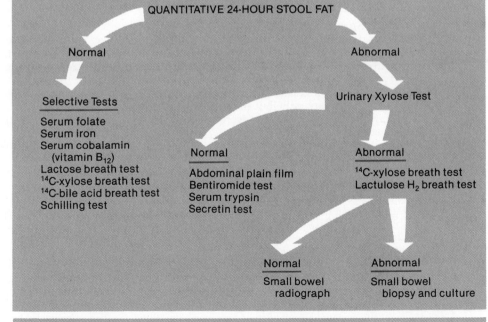

FIGURE 34–2. Approach to the patient with suspected maldigestion or malabsorption. (From Toskes PP: Malabsorption. *In* Wyngaarden JB, Smith LH Jr [eds]: Cecil Textbook of Medicine. 18th. ed. Philadelphia, WB Saunders Co, 1988, p 740.)

This sequence of tests is usually sufficient to establish the cause of malabsorption, although other tests, such as the response to a gluten-free diet for celiac disease or the study of pancreatic exocrine function, may also be indicated.

TREATMENT OF MALABSORPTION

The treatment of malabsorption is too diverse to be summarized in general terms and depends in considerable measure on the stage at which the defect occurs as well as its direct causation. Treatment may include cimetidine or ranitidine for a gastrinoma; the daily use of pancreatic enzyme preparations; antibiotics for the bacterial overgrowth syndrome or Whipple's disease; the use of a gluten-free diet for celiac disease; the use of medium chain fatty acids, which are more readily absorbed; surgical repair of biliary obstruction, blind loops, or fistulas; or the chemotherapy of lymphoma. It may also require replacement therapy with fat-soluble vitamins and other specific nutrients. Rarely total parenteral nutrition may be indicated (e.g., for the short bowel syndrome).

DISORDERS ASSOCIATED WITH MALABSORPTION

A very large number of disorders may result in intestinal malabsorption of varying degrees of severity. Some but not all of these have been listed in Table 34–4 as examples of the potential causes of the syndrome. This section will discuss only two of these entities, celiac sprue and the bacterial overgrowth syndrome. Other specific disorders are discussed elsewhere in this book or are discussed in detail in the appended references.

Celiac Sprue (Gluten-sensitive Enteropathy, Nontropical Sprue). Celiac sprue is a chronic, seemingly familial disorder associated with a life-long sensitivity to dietary gluten, a protein found in wheat and wheat products. When this protein (or certain peptides derived from it) is ingested, a diffuse mucosal injury results that is characteristic but nonspecific. The villi are shortened and blunted with decreased absorptive surface area, the crypts are hyperplastic, and the lamina propria is usually heavily infiltrated with lymphocytes.

PATHOGENESIS. The pathogenesis of the injury has not been established, although the best evidence suggests an immunological mechanism. Patients with celiac sprue have a high prevalence of certain histocompatibility types (HLA-B8 and Dw3), suggesting a linkage on chromosome 6 and strengthening the possibility of an immunological origin. On careful examination as many as 10 per cent of first-degree relatives of patients with celiac sprue may have the disorder. A second hypothesis postulates that an incomplete hydrolysis of peptides derived from gluten leads to the accumulation of toxic intermediates that directly injure the mucosal cell and that the immunological phenomena are secondary to this direct cell injury. Whatever the cause, it is known that the lesion is locally produced, disappears when gluten is withdrawn, and recurs within a few days when gluten is reintroduced. The pathogenesis of the resulting malabsorption is largely that of a diffuse mucosal abnormality. It has also been suggested that the abnormal mucosa has a reduced ability to secrete secretin and cholecystokinin-pancreozymin and therefore that pancreatic and biliary functions are secondarily impaired.

SYMPTOMS AND SIGNS. The symptoms and signs of celiac sprue are largely those that have been described for malabsorption in general. Symptoms tend to be more severe in childhood, diminishing after adolescence. Once again it must be emphasized that the gastrointestinal symptoms may be very mild and the patient may present with other manifestations such as anemia (iron or folate deficiency), a bleeding diathesis (vitamin K deficiency), or metabolic bone disease (vitamin D or calcium deficiency).

DIAGNOSIS. Patients with sprue usually exhibit fat malabsorption, an abnormal xylose test, and an abnormal pattern of dilated intestinal loops with thickened mucosal folds and flocculation of barium on radiographic examination. The Schilling test is usually normal but may be abnormal if the disorder extends to the ileum. Peroral biopsy shows the characteristic but not pathognomonic lesion. Finally, and most importantly, there is a clinical and histological response to a gluten-free diet.

TREATMENT AND PROGNOSIS. Treatment is by lifelong adherence to a gluten-free diet. Corn flour and rice products can safely be substituted for wheat, barley, and oats. A clinical response usually begins within a few weeks and the patient may continue to improve over a number of months. Reversion to a regular diet usually leads to a rapid return of symptoms. The long-term prognosis is excellent, although patients with celiac sprue appear to have a higher incidence of non-Hodgkin's lymphoma in later life.

Bacterial Overgrowth Syndrome. The small intestine usually harbors very few microorganisms ($<10^4$ colonies per ml). This comparatively sterile sanctuary is thought to result from the combined effects of gastric acidity, the rapid sweeping action of normal intestinal motility, and the secretion into the intestine of immunoglobulins. When bacteria are present in increased numbers in the small intestine, malabsorption is a frequent consequence. Loss of the normal sweeping function of the gut due to motility disorders or to "blind loops" (e.g., spontaneous or surgically created diverticula) and decreased gastric acid secretion (especially in the elderly) are the most common causes of upper intestinal bacterial overgrowth.

PATHOGENESIS. As noted previously, the malabsorption associated with bacterial overgrowth may result from three mechanisms: (a) deconjugation of bile salts, leading to impaired micelle formation; (b) a patchy injury to mucosal cells thought to be due to direct injury by bacteria or bacterial products; and (c) direct utilization of nutrients by bacteria, best established for vitamin B_{12}.

CONDITIONS ASSOCIATED WITH BACTERIAL OVERGROWTH. A large number of disorders may be associated with bacterial overgrowth. In addition to such gross structural derangements as blind loops, fistulas, or strictures, this syndrome may be found in the impaired intestinal motility of systemic sclerosis, amyloidosis, diabetes mellitus, and chronic pseudo-obstruction. It may also occur in hypogammaglobulinemia and in pancreatic insufficiency. Damage to the ileocecal valve, including surgical resection of the ileocecal area, may also introduce colonic organisms into the small intestine.

DIAGNOSIS. The initial approach to a patient with malabsorption of any cause has been described above and in Figure 34–2. If bacterial overgrowth is suspected based on the finding of an abnormal xylose test in the presence of a normal jejunal biopsy, with or without radiographic abnormalities, this can be best confirmed by an abnormal ^{14}C-xylose breath test (or a lactulose H_2 test) as described above. Other approaches that can be used include: (a) a positive three-stage Schilling test, (b) direct culture of jejunal fluid (usually $>10^7$ organisms/ml with a mixed culture of anaerobes for significant bacterial overgrowth), or (c) a 10- to 14-day therapeutic trial using a broad-spectrum antibiotic.

TREATMENT. The treatment depends upon the anatomical and functional cause of the impaired sweeping function of the intestine. Sometimes surgery is indicated. More often patients will require chronic or intermittent antibiotic therapy for both aerobic and anaerobic organisms on an indefinite basis. The most frequently used agents are tetracycline, metronidazole, and trimethoprim-sulfamethoxazole. A cephalosporin in combination with metronidazole may be required; in some forms of malabsorption, parenteral nutrition may be required. This form of therapy will not be described in this introductory textbook.

REFERENCES

Wright TL, Heyworth MF: Maldigestion and malabsorption. *In* Sleisenger MH, Fordtran JS (eds): Gastrointestinal Disease. 4th ed. Philadelphia, WB Saunders Co, 1989, pp 263–282.

Toskes PP: Malabsorption. *In* Wyngaarden JB, Smith LH Jr (eds): Cecil Textbook of Medicine. 18th ed. Philadelphia, WB Saunders Co, 1988, pp 732–745.

Toskes PP, Donaldson RM Jr: The blind loop syndrome. *In* Sleisenger MH, Fordtran JS (eds): Gastrointestinal Disease. 4th ed. Philadelphia, WB Saunders Co, 1989, p 1289–1297.

Trier JS: Celiac sprue. *In* Sleisenger MH, Fordtran JS (eds): Gastrointestinal Disease. 4th ed. Philadelphia, WB Saunders Co, 1989, pp 1134–1152.

D. DIARRHEA

DEFINITION

Diarrhea is best defined as an increase in stool liquidity and weight (>200 gm/day) that may be associated with increased stool frequency, urgency, perianal discomfort, and/or fecal incontinence. This chapter will discuss normal water and solute handling by the intestine, the pathophysiology of diarrhea, and the evaluation of diarrhea. Other specific clinical entities that lead to diarrhea are discussed in Section C of this chapter and in Chapter 38. Infectious causes of diarrhea are discussed in Chapter 92.

NORMAL INTESTINAL PHYSIOLOGY

The intestine normally receives 8 to 10 liters of fluid per day, 1500 to 2000 ml from injested food and liquids and the rest from salivary, gastric, pancreatic, biliary, and small intestinal secretions. The small bowel absorbs all but about 1 liter of this fluid, and the colon absorbs 90 per cent of the remaining fluid, resulting in a fecal fluid output of 100 to 150 ml per day.

The mechanisms responsible for solute and fluid absorption differ in different regions of the gut. All obey the general principle, however, that solutes (salts and other substances) are absorbed by specific mechanisms, while water follows passively according to osmotic gradients. The principal cellular mechanisms responsible for small intestinal solute transport, several of which are shown in Figure 34–3, appear to be sodium-coupled processes; i.e., they use the energy of the sodium gradient (established by the sodium pump) to drive entry or exit of a wide range of compounds, including protons, chloride, glucose, amino acids, and bile acids across cell membranes. Bicarbonate secretion, driven by sodium/hydrogen exchange, accounts for the relatively alkaline nature of ileal and colonic contents. Thus, jejunal and ileal fluid typically contains Na^+, 140 mM; K^+, 6.0 mM; Cl^-, 100 mM; and HCO_3^-, 30 mM.

Colonic solute transport is limited to electrolytes and occurs through slightly different mechanisms. Sodium absorption, which occurs via a specific sodium channel, generates an electrical potential across the

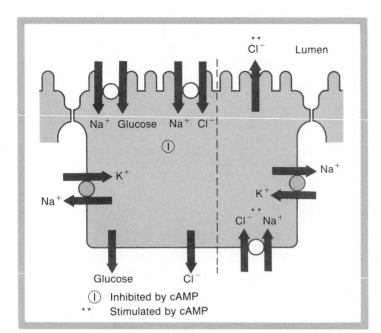

FIGURE 34–3. Schematic representation of electrolyte and glucose transport mechanisms in the small intestine. Absorptive mechanisms (shown on the left) and secretory mechanisms (shown on the right) are driven by Na$^+$, K$^+$-ATPase (shown in closed circles). Cyclic AMP produces a secretory diarrhea by both inhibiting absorption and stimulating secretion of sodium and chloride. Coupled absorption of sodium and glucose is unaffected, and this is the basis for current oral rehydration formulas.

colon wall, which in turn drives both chloride absorption and potassium secretion, leading to the typically high potassium concentration of colonic contents. In addition, organic acids, produced by colonic bacteria from nonabsorbed carbohydrate or fat, react with bicarbonate to produce organic anions and CO_2. Thus, colonic fluid typically contains Na$^+$, 40 mM; K$^+$, 90 mM; Cl$^-$, 15 mM; HCO$_3$$^-$, 30 mM; and organic anions, 85 mM.

Both small bowel and colon also secrete electrolytes and water. In the small bowel, secretion probably originates in crypt cells and may be due to sodium-coupled entry of anions (Cl$^-$) across the serosal cell membrane, followed by secretion of chloride across the luminal cell membrane. Sodium and water are thought to follow chloride passively according to electrical and osmotic gradients (Fig. 34–3). Colonic chloride secretion may occur via a similar mechanism in which chloride uptake across the serosal membrane is coupled to both sodium and potassium entry.

Although intestinal water movement is passive, it is not inconsequential. Since water absorption is linked to solute absorption, the presence of poorly absorbed, osmotically active solutes such as Mg^{+2}, SO$_4$$^{-2}$, and PO$_4$$^{-3}$ in the gut lumen will impair water absorption or cause water secretion.

CLASSIFICATION AND PATHOPHYSIOLOGY

Diarrhea may result if one or more of the following occur: (1) decreased normal absorption of solute and water; (2) increased secretion of electrolytes; (3) presence of poorly absorbed, osmotically active solutes in the gut lumen; (4) abnormal intestinal motility; and (5) inflammation with exudation of mucus, blood, or pus (Table 34–8).

Secretory Diarrhea. Secretory diarrhea, usually due to abnormalities in both absorption and secretion of electrolytes, is a common cause of watery diarrhea (Table 34–9). For many of the disorders listed here, the ultimate cause of intestinal secretion is an increase in cellular cyclic adenosine monophosphate (cAMP) levels. As shown in Figure 34–3, cAMP has two effects: it inhibits neutral NaCl absorption and stimulates chloride secretion without altering other solute transport mechanisms. For example, cholera, the archetypal secretory diarrhea, is due solely to the action of a small, heat-labile toxin that binds to intestinal mucosal cells and specifically stimulates the enzyme adenylate cyclase to produce cAMP. Since other sodium-coupled transport mechanisms function normally, hydration can be maintained by oral administration of sodium-glucose solutions.

Other causes of secretory diarrhea exist but remain poorly understood. Ion secretion in some cases may be due to increases in intracellular calcium or other cyclic nucleotides (cGMP). Small bowel disorders that produce villous atrophy ("flat gut"), such as celiac disease, are often associated with electrolyte secretion, probably due to unopposed secretion from the remaining crypt cells. Finally, disorders that cause malabsorption (see Section C of this chapter) and osmotic diarrhea (see below) may also be associated with secretory diarrhea. Nonabsorbed bile acids and fatty acids may stimulate ion secretion by colonic mucosal cells.

Secretory diarrhea usually presents as copious watery diarrhea that persists during a two-day fast. Because the diarrheal fluid is composed of electrolytes and water, fecal osmolality can be entirely accounted for by the usual cations and anions (Na$^+$, K$^+$, Cl$^-$, HCO$_3$$^-$, and organic anions) and there is little or no fecal solute gap [solute gap = fecal or plasma osmolality − 2(Na$^+$ + K$^+$). The factor of 2 is to account for the anions in stool.]

Osmotic Diarrhea. Osmotic diarrhea is due to the accumulation of poorly absorbed solutes in the gut lumen. This may occur by (1) ingestion of poorly absorbed solutes such as lactulose, Mg^{+2}, SO$_4$$^{-2}$, or PO$_4$$^{-3}$; (2) generalized malabsorption; or (3) failure to absorb a specific dietary component such as lactose. Examples of osmotic diarrhea are listed in Table 34–10.

Osmotic diarrhea typically stops when the patient fasts (or stops ingesting the responsible solute). Because osmotic diarrhea is due to the presence of poorly absorbed, unmeasured solutes, fecal fluid exhibits a large solute gap (>50 mOsm·L^{-1}). In this case, the

TABLE 34–8. CLASSIFICATION OF DIARRHEA*

TYPE	MECHANISM	EXAMPLES	CHARACTERISTICS
1. Secretory	Increased secretion and/or decreased absorption of Na$^+$ and Cl$^-$	Cholera VIP-secreting tumor Bile salt enteropathy Fatty acid–induced diarrhea	Large volume, watery diarrhea No blood or pus No solute gap Little or no response to fasting
2. Osmotic	Nonabsorbable molecules in gut lumen	Lactose intolerance (lactase deficiency) Generalized malabsorption (particularly carbohydrates) Mg^{2+}-containing laxatives	Watery stool, no blood or pus Improves with fasting Stool may contain fat globules or meat fibers and may have an increased solute gap
3. Inflammatory	Destruction of mucosa Impaired absorption Outpouring of blood, mucus	Ulcerative colitis Shigellosis Amebiasis	Small frequent stools with blood and pus Fever
4. Decreased absorptive surface	Impaired reabsorption of electrolytes	Bowel resection Enteric fistula	Variable
5. Motility disorder	Increased motility with decreased time for absorption of electrolytes and/or nutrients Decreased motility with bacterial overgrowth	Hyperthyroidism Irritable bowel syndrome Scleroderma Diabetic diarrhea	Variable Malabsorption

* Diarrhea is, in many instances, due to a combination of mechanisms. The diarrhea of generalized malabsorption, for example, is attributable to osmotic and secretory diarrhea as well as to decreased absorptive surface.

measured stool electrolytes [2(Na$^+$ + K$^+$)] usually do not account for all of fecal fluid osmolality. However, in the case of ingestion of anions such as SO$_4^{-2}$ or PO$_4^{-3}$, the fecal solute gap will be low (normal) and specific measurement of stool SO$_4^{-2}$ and PO$_4^{-3}$ must be performed. In individuals with carbohydrate malabsorption, stool pH is acidic owing to products of fermentation, and reducing substances are readily measured in the stool.

Abnormal Intestinal Motility. At least three types of motility disorders may result in diarrhea: (1) reduced peristalsis leading to bacterial overgrowth (see Section C of this chapter); (2) increased small bowel motility leading to decreased contact time between small bowel mucosa and intestinal contents and thus delivery of increased volume to the colon; and (3) increased colonic emptying with decreased contact time and increased stool liquidity. Diarrhea due mainly or in part to motility disorders includes that associated with irritable bowel syndrome, postvagotomy and postgastrectomy syndromes, diabetic neuropathy, scleroderma, and thyrotoxicosis.

EVALUATION OF DIARRHEA

The evaluation of diarrhea requires attention to the history and physical examination and careful selection and interpretation of laboratory tests.

History and Physical Examination

The patient's description (or better yet, the physician's observation) of the diarrheal stool is often informative. Large, voluminous stools suggest a source from the small bowel or proximal colon, whereas small stools associated with frequent urges to defecate sug-

TABLE 34–9. SOME CAUSES OF SECRETORY DIARRHEA

Agents that activate the adenylate cyclase–cAMP system
Cholera toxin
Escherichia coli heat-labile toxin
Vasoactive intestinal polypeptide (VIP)
Prostaglandins
Salmonella enterotoxin
? Dihydroxy bile acids and fatty acids
Agents that probably do not activate the adenylate cyclase–cAMP system
Escherichia coli heat-stable toxin
Serotonin
Enterotoxins of *Clostridium perfringens, Pseudomonas aeruginosa, Klebsiella pneumoniae,* and *Shigella dysenteriae*
Calcitonin
Castor oil, phenolphthalein
Villus atrophy (e.g., celiac sprue)

TABLE 34–10. SOME CAUSES OF OSMOTIC DIARRHEA

Disaccharidase deficiencies
Glucose-galactose or fructose malabsorption
Lactulose, mannitol, sorbitol ("chewing gum diarrhea") ingestion
Magnesium ingestion (antacids, laxatives)
Sulfate, phosphate ingestion (laxatives)
Sodium citrate ingestion
Steatorrhea (pancreatic insufficiency)
Generalized malabsorption
    Small bowel mucosal disease (celiac disease)
    Bacterial overgrowth (bile acid deconjugation, villous atrophy)

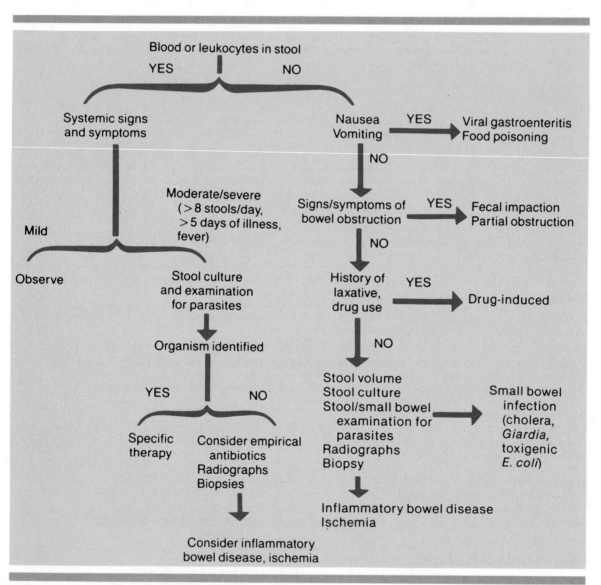

FIGURE 34–4. Evaluation of acute diarrhea.

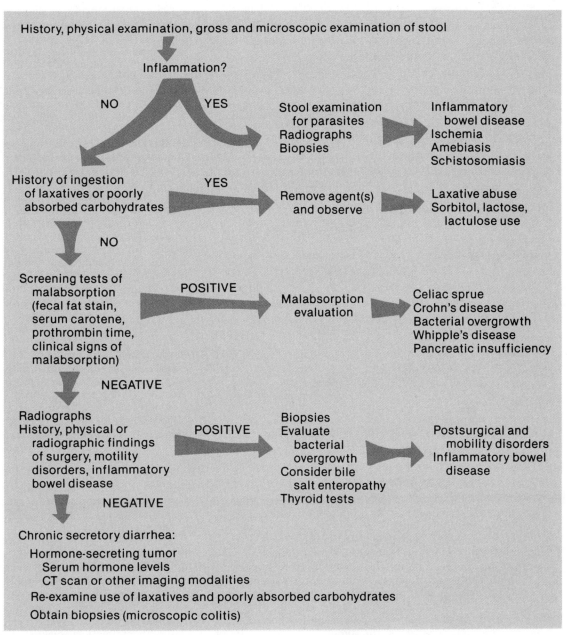

FIGURE 34–5. Evaluation of chronic diarrhea.

TABLE 34–11. TESTS THAT MAY BE USEFUL IN THE WORK-UP OF DIARRHEA*

Stool
Consistency
Frequency/24 hr
Volume/24 hr
WBC's by Wright's stain
Blood
Sudan stain for fat
Quantitative fat/24 hr
NaOH for phenolphthalein and other laxatives
Cultures for enteric pathogens
Ova and parasites
Clostridium difficile toxin
Osmolality
Na, K, Cl
pH
Reducing substances
Mg, SO$_4$, PO$_4$
Proctoscopy
Mucosal appearance
Biopsy
Blood
Electrolytes
Immunoglobulins, albumin
T$_3$, T$_4$
Ameba serology
Folate, vitamin B$_{12}$
Ca, Mg, PO$_4$
Erythrocyte sedimentation rate
Eosinophil count
Special Assays
Vasoactive intestinal polypeptide (VIP)
Calcitonin
Gastrin
Prostaglandins
Other

Gastric Analysis
X-ray Studies
Upper GI, small bowel, barium enema
Abdominal and pelvic sonogram, CT scan
Abdominal angiogram
Small Bowel Studies
Aspirate (O and P, colony count, cultures)
Biopsy
Mucosal disaccharidase assay
D-Xylose absorption test
Schilling test with intrinsic factor
^{14}C–bile acid absorption
Carbohydrate breath tests
Exocrine Pancreatic Function
Upper Endoscopy
Colonoscopy
Urine
5-Hydroxyindoleacetic acid (5-HIAA)
Metanephrines, vanillylmandelic acid (VMA)
NaOH (for phenolphthalein)
Heavy metals, drug screen
Room Search for Drugs
Intestinal Perfusion Studies
Therapeutic Trials

* From Krejs GJ, Fordtran JS: Diarrhea. *In* Sleisenger MH, Fordtran JS (eds): Gastrointestinal Disease. 3rd ed. Philadelphia, WB Saunders Co, 1983.

gest disease in the left colon or rectum. Blood suggests mucosal inflammation, whereas frothy stools and flatus suggest carbohydrate malabsorption. Greasy, foul-smelling stools with visible oil or fat indicate severe steatorrhea. A thorough drug history is also important, as antibiotics, antacids, antihypertensive agents, thyroxine, digitalis, propranolol, quinidine, colchicine, lactulose, ethanol, and laxatives may be associated with diarrhea. Other pertinent information includes the time course of the present illness (acute or chronic), previous surgery, systemic complaints, recent travel, family history, and sexual orientation (male homosexuals have a high incidence of intestinal infections). For example, acute diarrhea is usually due to infectious agents or toxins (food poisoning) whereas chronic diarrhea is not.

The physical examination may provide clues to the diagnosis of diarrhea, including signs of weight loss and malabsorption, systemic signs of inflammation such as fever or arthritis, adenopathy (lymphoma), neuropathy (diabetic diarrhea), or flushing (malignant carcinoid syndrome).

Laboratory tests

Although the cause of diarrhea may be apparent from information obtained through the history and physical examination, selected laboratory tests are often needed to establish or confirm a diagnosis. Table 34–11 lists a number of tests that may be useful in evaluating diarrhea, although for most patients only a few of these will be necessary. In selecting appropriate tests, it is useful to group patients into two categories: (1) Those with acute diarrhea, generally due to infection, drugs, food poisoning, or fecal impaction. Inflammatory bowel disease and bowel ischemia are less frequent causes of acute diarrhea. Traveler's diarrhea, a specific subset of this group, occurs within two weeks of travel to a tropical or developing area and runs a self-limited course of one to ten days. (2) Those with chronic diarrhea, which in turn may be divided into (a) secretory diarrhea, generally due to drugs, hormones, bile acids, or fatty acids; (b) osmotic diarrhea, generally due to drugs, laxatives, or malabsorption; (c) inflammatory diarrhea due to inflammatory bowel disease (ulcerative colitis, Crohn's disease), ischemic colitis, or parasitic infection; (d) motility disorders such as irritable bowel syndrome, scleroderma, and diabetic autonomic neuropathy; (e) disorders of impaired absorptive surface such as post-surgical diarrhea. General algorithms for evaluation of acute and chronic diarrhea are shown in Figures 34–4 and 34–5.

Tests that should be performed on all patients include examination of the stool for consistency, fecal leukocytes (Wright's stain), and blood. In patients with acute diarrhea, fecal leukocytes suggest either infection with invasive organisms such as *Shigella, Escherichia coli, Entamoeba histolytica*, gonococci, or *Campylobacter*, or antibiotic-associated colitis. In patients with chronic diarrhea, pus suggests colitis such as ulcerative colitis, Crohn's disease, or ischemic colitis. Pus is not seen in toxin-induced secretory diarrhea, malabsorption, laxative abuse, or giardiasis. Fecal blood generally indicates inflammation and has the same significance as pus.

The physician selects further tests depending upon the clinical picture. Patients with moderate to severe or prolonged acute diarrhea, in whom an infectious cause is likely, should have stools examined for ova and parasites and appropriately cultured for bacterial pathogens. Proctosigmoidoscopy is generally of little help in acute diarrhea except to visualize pseudomembranes in antibiotic-associated diarrhea. Blood cultures and a white blood cell and differential count may be useful in individuals with signs of systemic infection, whereas serological tests for amebiasis are helpful as they are usually positive in the presence of tissue invasion.

In evaluating chronic diarrhea, the initial selection of tests is designed to answer the following questions: (1) Is inflammation present? If so, proceed with imaging studies of the bowel (enteroclysis, barium enema, endoscopic procedures) and obtain tissue biopsies. (2) Is malabsorption present? Evaluate stool fat and D-xylose absorption. (3) Are structural, mucosal, or motility abnormalities present? Evaluate appearance with radiographic or endoscopic procedures and biopsies if appropriate. The answers to these questions will determine selection of more specific and specialized tests listed in Table 34–11. Certain of these tests deserve brief discussion.

Stool examination and culture should always precede enemas or radiographic studies, as fluid or barium may interfere with demonstration of pathogens. Similarly, proctosigmoidoscopy, which rapidly allows examination and biopsy of the distal colon, should be performed without enemas or other preparation, as these may distort or obscure evidence of disease. Mucosal smears may be obtained at sigmoidoscopy for culture and examined for pus. Rectal biopsies may be performed to detect amyloidosis, Whipple's disease, inflammation, or schistosomiasis.

Quantitative fecal fat determination (see Section C of this chapter) is one of the most sensitive tests for steatorrhea and, if elevated, the differential diagnosis of malabsorption should be pursued. Test results must be interpreted in light of dietary fat intake, which is usually standardized at 100 gm/day for the entire three days of the collection. Other tests for malabsorption are discussed in Section C of this chapter.

Hormone assays (vasoactive intestinal polypeptide, prostaglandins, calcitonin, gastrin, and others) are likely to be helpful only in the rare subgroup of patients with chronic, severe (>1 liter/day) secretory diarrhea in whom laxative abuse and intrinsic gastrointestinal tract disease have been ruled out.

Therapeutic trials may also be indicated in certain cases as diagnostic tests, including pancreatic enzymes (for pancreatic exocrine insufficiency), antibiotics (for bacterial overgrowth), metronidazole (for giardiasis), cholestyramine (for bile acid malabsorption), and various diets (lactose-free).

Therapy

Optimal therapy is to cure the underlying disorder. However, if this is not possible, certain drugs may ameliorate the disease (prednisone in inflammatory bowel disease) or treat the diarrhea (cholestyramine to bind bile acids). Specific antisecretory drugs are not yet available; however, supportive and symptomatic therapy is often required. Fluid and electrolyte replacement is an important aspect of therapy for diarrhea, particularly in infants and elderly individuals. Oral sodium-glucose solutions or intravenous fluids may be required. Opiates (codeine, diphenoxylate, or loperamide) reduce urgency, frequency, and stool volume in a wide range of diarrheal illnesses, probably via decreased gut motility and increased contact time. Opiates should not be used in patients with severe ulcerative colitis and impending toxic megacolon, and they may actually prolong illness in patients with infectious diarrhea (shigellosis). However, they are extremely useful agents in patients with chronic, disabling diarrhea.

Antibiotics are generally not necessary for acute or traveler's diarrhea, as these are self-limited processes and antibiotics may not shorten the duration of the illness. The new oral broad-spectrum fluoroquinolone antibiotics may, however, prove useful for empirical treatment of virtually all types of bacterial diarrhea. Use of antibiotics and antiparasitic agents is discussed in Chapter 83.

SPECIFIC CLINICAL DISORDERS

Infectious causes of diarrhea, the "gay bowel syndrome," sexually transmitted diarrheal diseases, and food poisoning are discussed in Chapters 92 and 96 to 99. The evaluation and differential diagnosis of malabsorption are covered in Section C of this chapter and inflammatory bowel disease in Chapter 38.

REFERENCES

Fedorak RN, Field M: Antidiarrheal therapy. Digest Dis Sci 32: 195, 1987.

Field M, Fordtran JS, Schultz SG (eds): Secretory Diarrhea. Bethesda, MD, American Physiological Society, 1980.

Fine KD, Krejs GJ, Fordtran JS: Diarrhea. In Sleisenger MH, Fordtran JS (eds): Gastrointestinal Disease. 4th ed. Philadelphia, WB Saunders Co, 1989, pp 290–316.

Krejs GJ: Diarrhea. In Wyngaarden JB, Smith LH Jr (eds): Cecil Textbook of Medicine. 18th ed. Philadelphia, WB Saunders Co, 1988, pp 725–732.

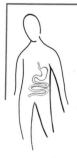

35

RADIOGRAPHIC AND ENDOSCOPIC PROCEDURES IN GASTROENTEROLOGY

Over the past years a wide variety of techniques have been introduced in radiology for the detection of disease in the gastrointestinal tract. There has been a concomitant explosion of new endoscopic techniques designed to address many of the same diagnostic (and therapeutic) problems. Indeed, often the most difficult task for the physician is selecting the most appropriate procedure(s) to use in each clinical setting. This chapter will review briefly the various radiographic and endoscopic procedures currently available and their optimal use.

RADIOGRAPHIC PROCEDURES

Table 35–1 summarizes the radiographic procedures in general use.

Plain Radiographs and Barium Contrast Studies

Plain radiographs of the abdomen in the supine and upright or lateral decubitus positions are simple to obtain and relatively inexpensive. They provide information of value in select circumstances. They are highly sensitive for clinical entities that involve abnormal gas patterns such as bowel obstruction, perforation of a hollow organ (free intraperitoneal air), pneumotosis intestinalis, and infections with gas-forming organisms (emphysematous cholecystitis) and are usually the first test obtained when these entities are considered. Plain films are also useful in detecting intra-abdominal calcifications such as gallbladder or renal stones or pancreatic calcifications in chronic alcoholic pancreatitis.

Contrast studies using barium sulfate (or occasionally the water-soluble iodinated contrast agent Gastrografin) provide more information about the anatomy of the tubular gastrointestinal tract. Single-contrast studies are performed using a bolus of contrast material and generally detect mass lesions but frequently miss small or mucosal lesions. Double-contrast studies, in which barium is administered first followed by a radiolucent substance such as air to produce a thin layer of barium coating the mucosa, are better able to detect all types of lesions, including those confined to the mucosa.

Single- and double-contrast barium swallows detect esophageal strictures and masses, and double-contrast studies may detect lesions of the mucosa such as ulcerations or varices. Endoscopy, which may miss submucosal mass lesions, is much more sensitive for mucosal lesions. Use of fluoroscopy during a barium swallow, particularly when combined with cine or video recordings, allows evaluation of esophageal motility disorders.

The standard single- or double-contrast examination of the upper gastrointestinal tract (upper GI series) is widely used to detect gastric mass lesions, gastric ulcers, and duodenal ulcers. Major changes in gastric motility can be evaluated using fluoroscopy, and markedly reduced motility may provide the first clue to a submucosal gastric cancer, a disease often difficult to detect by endoscopy. Most gastric ulcers (benign and malignant) are visualized radiographically; however, it is not possible to identify correctly all malignant ulcers on the basis of their radiographic appearance, so that biopsy is generally recommended. Double-contrast upper GI examinations may detect mucosal disorders such as erosive gastritis, Mallory-Weiss tears, stress ulcers, and anastomotic ulcers; however, endoscopy is more sensitive for such lesions. Overall, in the initial evaluation of common clinical problems such as dysphagia and epigastric pain, the upper GI series remains a primary diagnostic imaging test.

Satisfactory radiographic examination of the small bowel is more difficult to achieve owing to pooling and dilution of barium during passage through the small bowel and to obscuring of bowel segments by overlapping loops. The standard small bowel series, in which barium is introduced orally, can evaluate the caliber of the small bowel and provide some information regarding bowel mucosa, thickness of folds, and fluid transit time, particularly in the proximal bowel. Mass lesions, obstructions, and fistulas are usually detected. An improved view of the entire small bowel can be obtained by performing a small bowel enema (enteroclysis) in which barium, followed by radiolucent methylcellulose solution, is delivered directly into the jejunum via an orogastric tube. Imaging of the terminal ileum is improved by a per oral pneumocolon, in which air is introduced (per rectum) after opacification of the terminal ileum by barium (introduced orally). Specific radiographic evaluation of the small intestine is generally utilized when evaluating malabsorption, inflammatory bowel disease, or bowel obstruction. Endoscopic techniques to visualize the small bowel beyond the C-loop of the duodenum are not available.

TABLE 35–1. RADIOGRAPHIC AND ENDOSCOPIC PROCEDURES

PROCEDURE	ADVANTAGES	DISADVANTAGES	COST*
Plain film of the abdomen	Identifies gas (intramural, intraperitoneal, as well as luminal) and calcifications	Few specific features	$106–143
Barium swallow	Shows mass lesions and motility disorders well	Misses many superficial mucosal lesions	$215
Double-contrast barium examination of the upper gastrointestinal tract ("UGI series")	Delineates ulcers and tumors well	Misses some superficial mucosal lesions Misclassifies 9–17% of malignant gastric ulcers	$296
Small bowel series	Simple to perform Evaluates transit time, caliber, and proximal mucosa and often shows mass lesions	May miss distal or subtle lesions	$212
Enteroclysis (small bowel enema)	Improved definition of mucosa and bowel wall of entire small bowel	Requires per oral intubation	$400
Double-contrast barium enema ("pneumocolon")	Shows polyps, tumors, fistulas, diverticula, and other structural changes (e.g., inflammatory bowel disease) well	Uncomfortable for some patients Impossible in those with lax anal sphincter May miss superficial mucosal and rectal lesions Misses angiodysplastic lesions	$335
Oral cholecystography	Outlines most gallstones May delineate tumors or polyps	Will not visualize gallbladder in jaundiced patients and often fails to visualize the inflamed gallbladder	$168
Percutaneous transhepatic cholangiography	Excellent definition of intrahepatic bile ducts Option for therapeutic intervention	Extrahepatic bile ducts may not be well visualized Nondilated ducts may be missed	$575
Angiography	Demonstration of acutely bleeding lesions Definition of vascularity of mass lesions	Invasive Large contrast load Bleeding lesions visualized only if blood loss exceeds 0.5 ml/min Expensive	~$2000
Ultrasound	No radiation exposure Real-time examination Best for fluid-filled lesions, gallstones, and bile ducts	Gas obscures examination Bowel poorly visualized	$241 •
Computed tomography	Excellent anatomical definition Visualizes bowel wall thickness, mesentery, retroperitoneum, aorta well Density changes may indicate nature of diffuse parenchymal disease	Expensive Radiation exposure Bowel sometimes not well visualized Possible reactions to iodinated intravenous contrast media	$834
MRI of the abdomen	Excellent anatomical definition Identifies patency of vessels Sensitive detection of hepatic tumors No radiation	Expensive Patient must be cooperative No contrast agents available Operator-dependent	$809
Liver-spleen scan	Demonstrates mass lesions (>1–2 cm in size) Increased bone marrow uptake suggests portal hypertension	Limited anatomical definition	$393
^{99m}Tc-HIDA liver scan	Best test for cystic duct obstruction	Will not visualize if bilirubin >6 mg/dl Poor anatomical definition	$400
^{99m}Tc-RBC scan	Approximate localization of intermittently bleeding lesion	Poor anatomical definition	$565
Esophagogastroduodenoscopy	Direct visualization of upper gastrointestinal tract Identifies virtually all mucosal lesions Permits biopsy, electrocautery	Expensive Invasive May miss motility and compressive lesions	$916
Flexible sigmoidoscopy (to 25 cm)	Direct visualization of rectum, sigmoid, and distal descending colon Permits biopsy and polypectomy Useful for monitoring of inflammatory bowel disease	Invasive Misses lesions in more proximal colon	$211
Colonoscopy	Direct visualization of large bowel Permits biopsy and polypectomy, electrocautery, and laser treatment of bleeding	Expensive Invasive Higher rate of complications than barium enema	$1076
Endoscopic retrograde cholangiopancreatography	Only method for visualizing pancreatic ducts; permits biopsy of ampullary lesions and sphincterotomy for common duct stones	Requires considerable skill Expensive	$1551

* Costs are those charged at the University of California, San Francisco, in 1988.

Single- and double- (pneumocolon) contrast (or "air-contrast") radiographs of the colon have long been the standard for identifying lesions in the colon. With the use of pneumocolon, radiographic detection of even subtle lesions such as polyps and early inflammatory bowel disease is excellent, although generally colonoscopy detects more lesions and allows a more thorough examination of the rectum. Therefore, the choice of double-contrast barium enema or colonoscopy to evaluate patients with occult fecal blood, suspected inflammatory bowel disease, a tumor, diarrhea, or obstruction often depends upon the need for tissue for histological examination and the availability, cost, and comfort of the procedure.

The studies discussed thus far are usually performed using barium sulfate as the contrast agent. Water-soluble iodinated compounds, which produce images of lesser quality and are more expensive, are generally used only when a perforation is suspected (as barium is toxic when it escapes into body cavities) or when a colonic obstruction is suspected (barium caught above a colonic obstruction will dehydrate and possibly worsen the obstruction, whereas the water-soluble agents will not).

Ultrasound and Computed Tomography

Ultrasound (US) and computed tomography (CT) markedly extend the diagnostic capacity of the ra-diologist far beyond that which was possible with barium studies alone. Indeed, organs such as the pancreas, which were previously radiologically invisible, are now readily imaged. The information provided by US and CT is complementary to that provided by barium studies: US and CT are most useful in examining the solid abdominal organs (liver, spleen, pancreas, kidney, retroperitoneal lymph nodes) and gallbladder, whereas barium studies excel in depicting the lumen of the tubular gastrointestinal tract. Table 35–2 outlines the relative merits of US and CT.

Ultrasound, which employs high-frequency sound waves rather than x-rays, allows the examination of solid and fluid-filled structures noninvasively. Air or gas obscures the ultrasound beam; thus, structures under gas-filled loops of bowel cannot be visualized. US requires great skill on the part of the operator; however, real-time images allow examination of dynamic as well as static processes. Images, like those of CT, are displayed in cross-section. US has the ability (1) to detect abdominal masses as small as 2 cm in diameter, particularly in the right and left upper quadrants and pelvis; (2) to differentiate fluid-filled cysts from solid masses; (3) to identify gallstones rapidly and more efficiently than is possible with oral cholecystography or CT; (4) to identify dilated bile ducts; and (5) to detect ascites and some vascular abnormalities such as abdominal aortic aneurysms.

Computed tomography uses multiple x-ray beams and detectors in conjunction with computer analysis to identify and display small differences in tissue density. Anatomical definition is more precise with CT than with US and imaging quality is not affected by bowel gas, but the equipment is expensive. Current scanners obtain high-quality images quickly (2 to 3 seconds). CT is primarily used for the detection of mass lesions (tumors, cysts, abscesses), although it also detects dilated bile ducts, pancreatic inflammation, and some gallstones. Newer scanners also can detect changes in intestinal wall thickness (such as in ischemia, Crohn's disease, or appendicitis) and mesenteric abnormalities. Some diffuse hepatic parenchymal lesions that alter liver density, such as fatty liver or hemochromatosis, can also be identified by CT. Finally, CT is better than US in detecting retroperitoneal lesions and parenchymal processes such as ruptures or hematomas of the liver, spleen, and kidney, aortoenteric fistulas, and retroperitoneal adenopathy.

Both US and CT also offer the option of performing guided thin needle aspiration of lesions virtually anywhere in the abdomen to obtain cells or fluid for cytological examination and culture.

Radionuclide Imaging

Improvements in radiopharmaceuticals and imaging devices have resulted in new techniques that are of value in selected circumstances. The traditional liver-spleen scan, using ^{99m}Tc-sulfur colloid that undergoes phagocytosis by reticuloendothelial cells, has largely been supplanted by US or CT but is still useful in the evaluation of benign hepatic neoplasms

TABLE 35–2. COMPARISON OF ULTRASOUND AND COMPUTED TOMOGRAPHY

	ULTRASOUND	COMPUTED TOMOGRAPHY
Organs best visualized	Kidney Gallbladder Liver and bile ducts Pancreas Spleen Blood vessels	Liver and dilated bile ducts Retroperitoneal lymph nodes Mesentery Gallbladder Aorta Spleen Pancreas Kidney Pelvic organs

Lesions best visualized	Fluid-filled masses/
	  cysts
	Gallstones
	Dilated bile ducts
	Aortic aneurysms
	Pancreatic tumor
	Ascites
		Tumors/cysts/abscesses
		Lymphadenopathy
		Mass lesions
		Abdominal aortic aneurysm
		Trauma or parenchymal
		  hematoma of liver, spleen,
		  and kidney
		Fatty liver
		Hepatic iron overload
		  (hemochromatosis)

Advantages	Real-time examination
	Noninvasive
	Guided needle
	  aspiration
		Less dependent upon a
		  skilled operator
		Guided needle aspiration

Disadvantages	Skilled operator
	  necessary
	Gas obscures deeper
	  organs
		Absence of fat makes
		  examination more difficult

(see Chapter 46) and, when combined with a lung scan, subphrenic abscesses. Newer agents, such as ^{99m}Tc-HIDA, which are taken up by hepatic parenchymal cells and excreted in bile, outline the shape of the liver and are useful in the evaluation of acute cholecystitis (see Chapter 47) or of biliary atresia in infants. In general, they are not useful in other biliary tract disorders, as anatomical definition is poor. The affinity of ^{99m}Tc-pertechnetate for gastric mucosa makes this agent useful for the detection of Meckel's diverticula, 85 per cent of which contain ectopic gastric mucosa. Radiolabeled foods are used to measure gastric emptying of solids and liquids. Indium-111–labeled leukocytes injected intravenously may be useful in localizing abseses. Finally, ^{99}Tc-sulfur colloid and ^{99m}Tc-labeled red blood cells have been used in some centers to detect the site of bleeding in patients with gastrointestinal hemorrhage.

Visceral Angiography

Specially trained radiologists are now able to introduce catheters into virtually any artery or vein and, by injecting contrast agents, to visualize the vasculature of most organs. Because angiography is an invasive procedure with a small but significant morbidity, it is generally reserved for the detection of vascular tumors (e.g., hepatoma, angioma, angiosarcoma) and acutely bleeding lesions of the gastrointestinal tract, particularly of the colon or small bowel, that cannot be visualized endoscopically. Angiography also offers the option to treat bleeding by intra-arterial infusion of vasopressin or occlusion of bleeding vessels.

Magnetic Resonance Imaging (MRI)

Cross-sectional images of the body can also be obtained without x-ray by the use of a magnetic field and radiofrequency radiation combined with computer analysis. Current detectors, available in only a few centers, detect protons and thus display organs by their chemical composition rather than x-ray density. MRI may offer better resolution than CT and also offers the opportunity to follow in situ chemical reactions. MRI is particularly sensitive to intrahepatic tumors, hepatic fat, and hepatic iron. MRI visualizes patent blood vessels extraordinarily well and may be the most useful procedure for assessing patency of shunts, grafts, and veins. The equipment is even more expensive than that used for CT, however, and the final role of MRI in clinical medicine is not yet established.

Visualization of the Biliary Tree

Oral cholecystography (OCG), the time-honored method for imaging the gallbladder, involves the oral administration of an iodinated compound, which is concentrated in the gallbladder, followed 12 hours later by a radiograph of the gallbladder. The technique identifies most gallstones in patients with a functioning gallbladder. However, in many patients with chronic cholecystitis, and in all patients with a serum bilirubin greater than 2 mg/dl, the gallbladder will not opacify. US is more sensitive (> 98 per cent verus 90 per cent) in detecting gallstones and has replaced the OCG in most centers.

Bile ducts and disorders involving them are well seen only when contrast material is used to fill them. Contrast may be injected into the biliary tree from the upstream side via a thin (23-gauge) needle introduced percutaneously into the hepatic parenchyma (percutaneous transhepatic cholangiogram, PTC) or from below via a small catheter placed endoscopically into the papilla of Vater (endoscopic retrograde cholangiopancreatography, ERCP, see page 280). Table 35–3 compares these two procedures, both of which pro-

---

TABLE 35–3. COMPARISON OF PERCUTANEOUS TRANSHEPATIC CHOLANGIOGRAPHY AND ENDOSCOPIC RETROGRADE CHOLANGIOPANCREATOGRAPHY

	PERCUTANEOUS TRANSHEPATIC CHOLANGIOGRAPHY	ENDOSCOPIC RETROGRADE CHOLANGIOPANCREATOGRAPHY
Lesions best visualized	Intrahepatic ductal lesions Multiple lesions in a single duct system Several punctures may be made to examine ducts in all lobes	Extrahepatic ductal lesions Pancreatic duct Ampulla of Vater
Therapeutic implications	Temporary external drainage of bile Placement of stents through bile duct obstructions Balloon dilatation of biliary stricture	Sphincterotomy for removal of common duct stones Placement of stents Balloon dilatation of strictures Biopsy of ampullary lesions

Success rate
  dilated ducts
  non-dilated ducts
	100%
	60–80%
		80–90%
		80–90%

Disadvantages	Experienced operator required May miss additional lesions in left lobe	Experienced operator required May not visualize ducts proximal to a lesion
Complications	Bleeding Biliary infection/sepsis Hemobilia	Pancreatitis Biliary infection/sepsis Bile duct perforation

vide an excellent view of the biliary tree, although PTC is generally preferred for intrahepatic bile duct lesions and ERCP for extrahepatic duct lesions.

ENDOSCOPIC PROCEDURES

Endoscopic examination of the gastrointestinal (GI) tract was first achieved using rigid, multi lensed instruments that were difficult to use, permitted limited visualization, and were often traumatic to the patient. The development of fiberoptic instruments has revolutionized gastrointestinal endoscopy and hence the management of many gastrointestinal disorders. Currently, a wide range of instruments is available, some tailor-made for specialized applications. The modern fiberoptic endoscope provides a true extension of the eyes and hands of the physician. These instruments combine wide-angle visualization of the GI tract with flexibility and ability to control the movement of the tip of the scope up to 360 degrees, as well as good patient tolerance.

Most endoscopes include multipurpose channels for passage of air and water, as well as for aspirating fluid out of the GI tract. They also permit the passage of a number of instruments, including cytology brushes, biopsy forceps, injection needles, electrocautery snares, wire baskets, and laser probes.

As discussed earlier, endoscopy has certain distinct advantages over barium contrast radiological examination of the GI tract: (1) It has greater sensitivity for mucosal lesions often missed by barium studies. (2) Endoscopy allows greater diagnostic specificity in certain situations. For example, in a patient with gastrointestinal hemorrhage, a lesion identified by barium contrast radiology will not necessarily be responsible for the bleeding. This uncertainty is eliminated by the direct visualization of actively bleeding lesions permitted by endoscopy. (3) Endoscopy permits biopsy or cytology of lesions at the time of visualization. (4) Endoscopy combines therapeutic capabilities with direct visualization of the gastrointestinal tract, e.g., enabling injection of bleeding esophageal varices at the time of diagnosis. Endoscopy carries the two disadvantages of higher cost (see Table 35–1), and higher patient morbidity and mortality, although the latter is extremely small for nontherapeutic endoscopy (0.0004 per cent). Endoscopy is also often inferior to radiology in identifying submucosal or compressive lesions of the gastrointestinal tract as well as disorders of esophageal motility.

Whether endoscopic or radiological examination should be undertaken as a first procedure depends upon the clinical problem (e.g., acute bleeding versus abdominal pain), the range of likely diagnoses, the possible need for therapeutic intervention, locally available skill, and cost factors, as well as the fact that radiological and endoscopic techniques are often complementary to one another in obtaining a diagnosis.

Endoscopic examination is generally performed under sedation with parenteral sedation, with topical anesthetic spray applied to the pharynx for upper endoscopy

Esophagogastroduodenoscopy

Visualization of the GI tract up to the duodenum is also referred to as upper GI endoscopy or panendoscopy. Major indications are diagnosis of suspected upper GI hemorrhage and upper GI malignancy. Endoscopy is the diagnostic procedure of first choice in virtually all instances of upper GI hemorrhage (see Chapter 34B); even when bleeding is brisk, responsible lesions are readily visualized by experienced endoscopists. Endoscopic biopsy and cytology yield a diagnostic accuracy for upper GI cancer of close to 100 per cent, although accuracy is less in submucosal and/ or infiltrative lesions. Other indications include investigation of some cases of acid-peptic disease, abdominal pain, esophageal symptoms, removal of foreign bodies, and injection of varices.

Endoscopic "Retrograde" Cholangiopancreatography (ERCP)

Cannulation of the ampulla of Vater is carried out using a special side-viewing endoscope. This is technically the most difficult endoscopic examination to perform. Once cannulation is achieved, selective intubation of the pancreatic and common bile ducts is undertaken followed by injection of a radiographic contrast medium. Radiographs are taken of the contrast-outlined ducts. Indications for ERCP include the diagnosis of pancreatic cancer, investigation of obstructive jaundice, placement of biliary stents, and performance of endoscopic sphincterotomy. In obstructive jaundice, ERCP is preferred to percutaneous cholangiography if duct dilatation is absent, if there is associated pancreatic or duodenal pathology, or if a coagulation defect is present. Detailed comparison of ERCP with percutaneous cholangiography is given in Table 35–3.

Endoscopic sphincterotomy entails an electrocautery incision into the duodenal papilla and is used to release retained common duct gallstones in patients who have already undergone cholecystectomy (and who would otherwise require a second operation) and in those patients considered poor surgical risks. The morbidity rate from sphincterotomy is 4 to 8 per cent, and the mortality rate is 0.4 per cent.

Sigmoidoscopy and Colonoscopy

Both rigid and flexible fiberoptic sigmoidoscopes are employed in clinical practice. Rigid sigmoidoscopy is a rapid, inexpensive procedure, but it is less well tolerated by the patient and permits less extensive examination of the rectosigmoid area. Sigmoidoscopy (especially flexible sigmoidoscopy) is commonly used to evaluate the cause of bloody diarrhea and to look for neoplastic disease of the rectosigmoid area. When the rectosigmoid area is involved, sigmoidoscopic biopsy will often suffice in making the diagnosis of inflammatory bowel disease without the need for colonoscopy. Colonoscopy enables visualization of the entire colon to the level of the cecum. Indications for colonoscopy include investigation of suspected colonic neoplastic disease, evaluation of lower GI bleeding, surveillance for the development of malignancy in ulcerative colitis and polyposis syndromes, and diagnosis and evaluation of the extent of inflammatory bowel disease. Complications, including bleeding or perforation, may occur in 0.5 per cent of patients.

Removal of colonic polyps for bleeding or to exclude malignancy is an important therapeutic application of colonoscopy. Colonoscopy plays only a modest role in patients with active lower gastrointestinal bleeding, as considerable blood within the relatively narrow confines of the colon tends to obscure vision (see Chapter 34B). Angiography or ^{99m}Tc-RBC scanning may be preferable in this situation.

Laparoscopy

Laparoscopy is a procedure occasionally used in gastroenterology. Its major value is in permitting biopsy under direct vision of suspected metastatic tumor nodules on the hepatic or peritoneal surface.

REFERENCES

Federle MP, Goldbert HI: Conventional radiography of the alimentary tract. *In* Sleisenger MH, Fordtran JS (eds): Gastrointestinal Disease: Pathophysiology, Diagnosis and Management. 3rd ed. Philadelphia, WB Saunders Co, 1983, pp 1634–1667.

Mueller PR, Harbin WP, Ferrucci JT, et al: Fine needle transhepatic cholangiography: Reflections after 450 cases. AJR 136:85, 1981.

Sleisenger MH, Fordtran JS (eds): Gastrointestinal Disease: Pathophysiology, Diagnosis and Management. 4th ed. Philadelphia, WB Saunders Co, 1989.

Vennes JA: Gastrointestinal endoscopy. *In* Wyngaarden JB, Smith LH Jr (eds): Cecil Textbook of Medicine. 18th ed. Philadelphia, WB Saunders Co, 1988, pp 668–674.

Wall SW: Diagnostic imaging procedures in gastroenterology. *In* Wyngaarden JB, Smith LH Jr (eds): Cecil Textbook of Medicine. 18th ed. Philadelphia, WB Saunders Co, 1988, pp 662–668.

36

DISEASES OF THE ESOPHAGUS

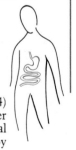

Although the esophagus appears to be a simple organ, esophageal disease is common and ranges from trivial complaints of heartburn to major clinical problems of aspiration, obstruction, and hemorrhage. This chapter will briefly outline normal esophageal function and describe a group of unique symptoms characteristic of most esophageal disorders. The major benign categories of esophageal disorders, gastroesophageal reflux disease, and motility disorders will be discussed with a brief review of other common esophageal diseases. Malignant disease of the esophagus will be discussed in Chapter 39.

NORMAL ESOPHAGEAL PHYSIOLOGY

The esophagus serves a single function: conveying solids and liquids from the mouth to the stomach while preventing aspiration and movement of gastric contents in the opposite direction (gastroesophageal reflux). Swallowing is a complex and well-coordinated motor activity that includes (1) movement of a food bolus into the pharynx concomitant with protection of the airway, (2) relaxation of the upper esophageal sphincter, (3) initiation and distal propagation of peristaltic contractions by the esophageal muscle, and (4) relaxation of the lower esophageal sphincter. After passage of the food bolus, the lower esophageal sphincter re-establishes a tonic contraction, thereby preventing regurgitation of gastric contents.

CLINICAL SYMPTOMS OF ESOPHAGEAL DISEASE

Dysphagia, the sensation that a food bolus arrests ("sticks") during swallowing, indicates esophageal disease, and the patient can often indicate the exact site. Dysphagia may be due to motility disorders or to narrowing of the esophageal lumen by benign or malignant disease (Table 36–1). A motility disorder is more likely if dysphagia occurs with both liquids and solids, or if the patient can force the bolus down by altering posture, performing a Valsalva maneuver, or repeated swallowing.

Heartburn (pyrosis), a common esophageal symptom, is a burning pain that radiates up behind the sternum. It is due to reflux of gastric contents into the esophagus. It is usually relieved by antacids, is precipitated by bending over or lying down, and may be accompanied by regurgitation of sour- or bitter-tasting

TABLE 36–1. ETIOLOGY OF DYSPHAGIA

TYPE	EXAMPLE
Esophageal motility disorder	Achalasia
	Aperistalsis (scleroderma)
	Diffuse esophageal spasm
Luminal narrowing	Inflammatory disease (reflux, *Candida* infection)
	Malignant tumor (squamous cell or adenocarcinoma)
	Benign stricture (reflux, lye ingestion)
	Esophageal web

material. Nocturnal reflux and regurgitation may present as recurrent aspiration pneumonia, wheezing, or hoarseness.

Odynophagia, or pain on swallowing, is usually associated with esophageal obstruction or mucosal disease such as reflux esophagitis, radiation-induced damage, or infection by viral or fungal agents.

Severe substernal chest pain that is often indistinguishable from angina pectoris may result from abnormal esophageal motor function, such as diffuse esophageal spasm.

GASTROESOPHAGEAL REFLUX DISEASE

Definition. Gastroesophageal reflux disease (GERD) refers to a spectrum of clinical manifestations due to reflux of stomach and duodenal contents into the esophagus. (See Chapter 37 for a general discussion of acid-peptic disease.)

Etiology and Pathogenesis. The esophagus is normally protected from prolonged exposure to acid, pepsin, bile acids, and pancreatic enzymes by three mechanisms: (1) the antireflux barrier provided by tonic contraction of the lower esophageal sphincter, (2) rapid clearance of refluxed material via peristalsis, and (3) alkalinization of acidic material by swallowed saliva. Patients with symptomatic GERD usually exhibit

TABLE 36–2. TREATMENT OF GASTROESOPHAGEAL REFLUX DISEASE

Simple Measures
1. Elevation of the head of the bed
2. Avoidance of food or liquids before bedtime
3. Liquid antacid (aluminum hydroxide–magnesium hydroxide), 30 ml one hour and three hours after meals and at bedtime
4. Avoidance of cigarettes, alcohol
5. Weight loss

Measures for Resistant Cases
1. H_2-receptor blockers (cimetidine 300 mg four times a day or ranitidine 150 mg twice a day)
2. Bethanechol (urecholine) 10 or 15 mg four times a day
3. Alginic acid-antacid (Gaviscon) 15 ml four times a day
4. Antireflux surgery (Nissen fundoplication, Hill repair, Belsey repair)

one or more of the following: decreased or absent tone in the lower esophageal sphincter, inappropriate relaxation of the lower esophageal sphincter unassociated with swallowing, and decreased acid clearance due to impaired peristalsis. Other factors such as abnormal saliva and reflux of bile salts and pancreatic enzymes may be implicated in some patients.

Clinical Manifestations. Heartburn, ranging in degree from mild to severe, is the most common symptom of GERD and is often associated with regurgitation of acidic (bitter-tasting) material. Aspiration pneumonia, nocturnal wheezing, and hoarseness may be seen in patients with frequent regurgitation, occasionally in the absence of heartburn. Dysphagia, bleeding from esophageal erosions, and stricture formation also occur. Smoking, alcohol or caffeine intake, and pregnancy, all of which decrease lower esophageal sphincter tone, may precipitate or exacerbate GERD.

Diagnosis. The diagnosis of GERD is best made based on the history and clinical manifestations. Objective tests are useful to quantify the extent and severity of disease and to address three questions: (1) Does reflux exist? (2) Is acid reflux responsible for the patient's symptoms? (3) Has reflux led to esophageal damage? Reflux may be demonstrated during a barium swallow or by a radionuclide scintiscan after placement of ^{99}Tc-sulfur colloid in the stomach. Esophageal manometry is useful to demonstrate abnormal peristalsis and lower esophageal sphincter tone but will not show reflux. More sensitive tests for the presence of acid reflux include monitoring esophageal pH with a luminal pH probe for periods of 30 minutes to 24 hours either after instillation of HCl in the stomach (Tuttle test) or under near-physiological conditions. The presence of reflux does not necessarily mean that reflux is responsible for the patient's symptoms. If chest pain is not typical of heartburn, the Bernstein test may be performed to determine whether acid, but not saline, dripped into the esophagus via a nasogastric tube reproduces the patient's symptoms. Finally, symptoms due to acid reflux do not always correlate with the extent of damage to the esophageal mucosa. Severe esophageal damage, such as a stricture or deep ulcer, can be assessed by barium swallow. However, endoscopy with biopsy is the most sensitive test for reflux-induced mucosal damage. Endoscopic changes range from very shallow linear erosions to confluent ulceration to complete mucosal denudation. Microscopically, basal cell hyperplasia, polymorphonuclear cell infiltration, or frank ulceration can be seen. A few patients will exhibit Barrett's epithelium, the presence of columnar epithelium in the esophagus, which is produced by severe chronic reflux and is associated with an increased risk of malignant transformation.

Treatment and Prognosis. Medical management of GERD is successful in all but the most severe cases, and, as outlined in Table 36–2, consists of maneuvers designed to decrease reflux and administration of antacids or H_2-receptor blockers to decrease acid secretion. Chronic therapy may be necessary in patients with severe reflux. Surgical management, which is reserved for those few patients with objective evidence of reflux who fail to respond to an adequate trial of medical management, attempts to restore lower esophageal sphincter function by wrapping the lower esophagus with a cuff of gastric fundal muscle. These procedures are often successful but cannot be performed in patients with aperistalsis (e.g., scleroderma), who may have severe GERD.

Complications. GERD complications include esophageal (peptic) stricture, esophageal ulcer, Barrett's esophagus, pulmonary aspiration, and upper gastrointestinal hemorrhage.

MOTOR DISORDERS OF THE ESOPHAGUS

Definition and Pathogenesis. Motility disorders may arise from disease of smooth muscle (scleroderma) or of the intrinsic nervous system (achalasia, Chagas' disease). In achalasia, degeneration of the ganglion cells in Auerbach's plexus leads to increased tone and impaired relaxation of the lower esophageal sphincter, which is often associated with absent peristalsis. The etiology of other motility disorders, such as diffuse esophageal spasm, is uncertain.

Clinical Manifestations. The three most common motility disorders are achalasia, scleroderma, and diffuse esophageal spasm, each of which exhibits a unique pattern of symptoms (Table 36–3).

Diagnosis. The clinical history is often characteristic, and a cine esophagogram (Fig. 36–1) combined with esophageal manometric studies (Table 36–3) will confirm the diagnosis in most cases. An infiltrating carcinoma of the gastric cardia can mimic achalasia; thus, biopsies of the lower esophagus are an important part of the evaluation of these patients.

Treatment and Prognosis. Achalasia often responds to brisk dilatation of the lower esophageal sphincter with a pneumatic bag, a procedure thought

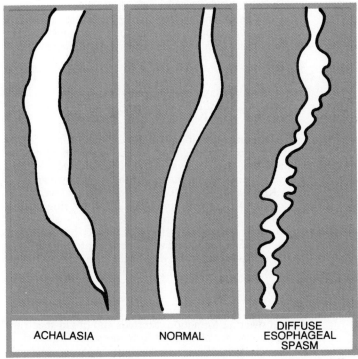

FIGURE 36–1. Radiological appearance of achalasia (*left*) and diffuse esophageal spasm (*right*). In achalasia the esophageal body is dilated and terminates in a narrowed segment or "bird beak." The appearance of numerous simultaneous contractions is typical of diffuse esophageal spasm. (Courtesy of Drs. FE Templeton and CA Rohrmann. From Pope CE II: *In* Sleisenger MH, Fordtran JS [eds]: Gastrointestinal Disease. 3rd ed. Philadelphia, WB Saunders Co, 1983.)

to rupture some of the sphincter muscle fibers. Surgical myotomy (Heller procedure) may be beneficial for those few who do not respond to pneumatic dilatation. Therapy for scleroderma includes chronic treatment of GERD with H₂ blockers or antacids (see Table 36–2). Patients with diffuse esophageal spasm

TABLE 36–3. ESOPHAGEAL MOTOR DISORDERS

	ACHALASIA	SCLERODERMA	DIFFUSE ESOPHAGEAL SPASM
Symptoms	Dysphagia Bolus often passes with time or various maneuvers	Gastroesophageal reflux disease Dysphagia	Substernal chest pain (angina-like) Dysphagia with pain
X-ray appearance	Dilated, fluid-filled esophagus Distal "bird beak" stricture	Aperistaltic esophagus Free reflux Peptic stricture	Simultaneous noncoordinated contractions
Manometric findings			
Lower esophageal sphincter	High resting pressure No or incomplete relaxation with swallow	Low resting pressure	Normal pressure
Body	Low-amplitude, simultaneous contractions after swallow	Low-amplitude peristaltic contractions or no peristalsis	Some peristalsis Diffuse and simultaneous nonperistaltic contractions, often of high amplitude

may respond to nitroglycerin, anticholinergic agents, or calcium-channel blocking drugs, although results are often disappointing. Occasionally, good long-term results have been obtained from a longitudinal myotomy.

OTHER ESOPHAGEAL DISORDERS

Tumors. Carcinoma of the esophagus is discussed in Chapter 39. Benign neoplasms (leiomyoma, lipoma, papilloma, and fibrovascular polyps) are very rare and usually are asymptomatic or present as dysphagia.

Rings and Webs. Congenital rings and webs may occur in the proximal or distal (Schatzki's ring) esophagus. The Plummer-Vinson syndrome consists of an upper esophageal web, dysphagia, and iron-deficiency anemia. Most rings and webs are asymptomatic or may present as intermittent dysphagia for a bolus of meat. They can be disrupted mechanically with peroral dilators.

Esophageal Injury. Caustic ingestion causes severe esophageal injury leading to necrosis and eventual stricture formation. Steroids and broad-spectrum antibiotics are often used to treat caustic injuries, although their efficacy is uncertain. Strictures often respond to peroral dilatation.

Trauma. Vomiting may lead to mucosal (Mallory-Weiss) or full-thickness (Boerhaave's syndrome) tears of the lower esophagus. Mallory-Weiss tears usually occur just below the gastroesophageal junction. They often present with hemorrhage and will heal spontaneously. Esophageal rupture often occurs just above the gastroesophageal junction into the mediastinum and requires immediate diagnosis and surgical repair.

Infection. Esophageal infection with *Candida* or *Herpesvirus* can occur, particularly in the immunosuppressed host, often with severe mucosal inflammation and ulceration. Severe odynophagia is a common symptom and dysphagia may occur. Diagnosis is best made by endoscopic visualization and biopsy.

REFERENCES

Pope CE II: Diseases of the esophagus. *In* Wyngaarden JB, Smith LH Jr (eds): Cecil Textbook of Medicine. 18th ed. Philadelphia, WB Saunders Co, 1988, pp 679–689.
Pope CE II: The esophagus. *In* Sleisenger MH, Fordtran JS (eds): Gastrointestinal Disease. 4th ed. Philadelphia, WB Saunders Co, 1989, pp 541–547.
Spechler SJ, Goyal RK: Barrett's esophagus. N Engl J Med 315:362, 1986.
Vantrappen G, Janssens J, Hellemans J, et al: Achalasia, diffuse esophageal spasm and related motility disorders. Gastroenterology 76:450, 1979.
Ward PH (moderator): Complications of gastroesophageal reflux. West J Med 149:58, 1988.

37

ACID-PEPTIC DISEASES

The normal stomach can secrete H$^+$ up to one million times its concentration in extracellular fluid in association with potent proteolytic enzymes. It is not surprising, therefore, that gastric juice is fully capable of injuring the host as well as digesting components of the diet. Acid-peptic disease, which refers nonspecifically to disorders associated with such injury, includes peptic ulcer of the duodenum and stomach (and rarely of the jejunum or of a Meckel's diverticulum), some forms of gastritis, and reflux esophagitis. The latter entity has been discussed in Chapter 36.

NORMAL GASTRIC PHYSIOLOGY

The stomach serves as a reservoir in which ingested food is churned and fragmented into small particles prior to its timed release into the duodenum. Beyond these important mechanical functions, the stomach also initiates the processes of digestion by the secretion of HCl and pepsinogen, which in the presence of HCl is rapidly converted to proteolytic pepsin. Acid-peptic disease occurs when there is an imbalance between the processes of secretion and the normal processes of defense against chemical self-injury.

Normal Secretion. HCl is secreted by the parietal cells and pepsinogen primarily by the chief cells, both found in the gastric mucosa, predominantly in the body and fundus of the stomach. These two agents are secreted in parallel; no condition is known in which there is selective secretion of either HCl or pepsinogen. Three endogenous chemicals stimulate the secretion of acid: gastrin, histamine, and acetylcholine (Fig. 37–1). Acetylcholine is released locally from vagal (cholinergic) nerve terminals in the stomach, stimulated by stretch reflexes within the stomach or by the cephalic phase of gastric secretion. Gastrin is released from "G cells" in the antrum of the stomach and in the duodenum, stimulated largely by the products of protein digestion and by alkalinization. It circulates as a hormone before acting on the parietal cell. Histamine is found in mastlike cells in the gastric wall in close proximity to the chief cells. The role and control of local histamine release are unknown, but histamine and its structural analogues are powerful gastric secretagogues when administered systemically, and the use of H_2-receptor antagonists markedly inhibits HCl (and pepsinogen) secretion by the stomach. There is also evidence of a nongastrin gut-derived secretagogue stimulated by the products of protein digestion, but its structure has not been defined. The interaction of these various agents at the final common parietal cell pathway for acid secretion is unclear. In brief, gastric secretion seems to result largely from the cephalic phase (via the vagus), the gastric phase (stretch stimulation of the vagus; protein and alkalinization stimulation of gastrin release), and the intestinal phase (further release of gastrin and of the nongastrin secretagogue). Secretion of pepsinogen is largely under vagal control (i.e., acetylcholine) and to a lesser extent by the other described mechanisms as well.

Basal secretion of acid averages about 1.0 to 2.0 mEq/hr in men but less in women. The normal range, however, varies widely from 0 to 10.5 mEq/hr for men and from 0 to 5.6 mEq/hr for women. When maximally stimulated with a secretagogue—usually betazole (a histamine analogue) or pentagastrin—the secretory rate may rise as high as 50 mEq/hr for men and 30 mEq/hr for women. The ratio of basal to maximal acid output (MAO) is sometimes determined in the study

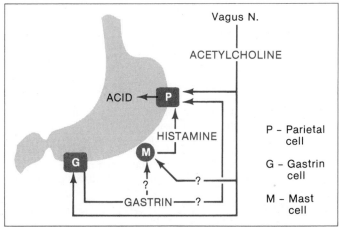

FIGURE 37–1. The parietal cell with three receptors, histamine, gastrin, and acetylcholine. All act to stimulate a potassium-hydrogen ATPase (the hydrogen pump at the luminal side of the cell). However, the characteristics of each compound differ enough to suggest that each acts at a different receptor. Histamine causes increases in intracellular adenyl cyclase and cyclic AMP, which in turn activate or increase the amount of the potassium-hydrogen ATPase. Cholinergic drugs and gastrin cause influx of Ca^{++}, which in turn activates the potassium-hydrogen ATPase. (From Richardson CT: Peptic ulcer: Pathogenesis. *In* Wyngaarden JB, Smith LH Jr [eds]: Cecil Textbook of Medicine. 18th ed. Philadelphia, WB Saunders Co, 1988, p 693.)

of patients with suspected abnormal secretory drives.

Normal Defense. The stomach and the duodenum have developed several defense mechanisms to protect the mucosa from the acid-pepsin mix of gastric juice (Fig. 37–2). A thin coating of mucus is con-

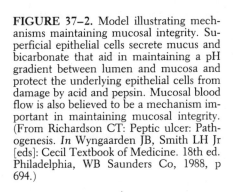

FIGURE 37–2. Model illustrating mechanisms maintaining mucosal integrity. Superficial epithelial cells secrete mucus and bicarbonate that aid in maintaining a pH gradient between lumen and mucosa and protect the underlying epithelial cells from damage by acid and pepsin. Mucosal blood flow is also believed to be a mechanism important in maintaining mucosal integrity. (From Richardson CT: Peptic ulcer: Pathogenesis. *In* Wyngaarden JB, Smith LH Jr [eds]: Cecil Textbook of Medicine. 18th ed. Philadelphia, WB Saunders Co, 1988, p 694.)

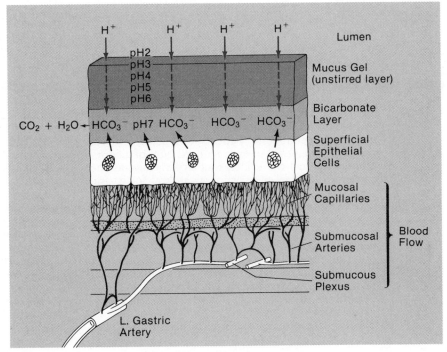

tinuously formed and spreads out protectively over the mucosal cells. This diminishes the exposure of these cells to luminal gastric juice. The surface apical cells secrete bicarbonate within and under the mucin layer, which serves to neutralize the H^+ that diffuses back from the lumen. The epithelial cells are constantly being shed and renewed so that damaged cells are promptly replaced. Epithelial cells also migrate to cover denuded areas and in this way contribute to epithelial restitution. Prostaglandins may play a role in stimulating all of these repair mechanisms, including an increase in mucosal blood flow. The average individual can secrete more than 100 mmol of HCl daily throughout life without significant mucosal injury.

PEPTIC ULCER DISEASE OF THE STOMACH AND DUODENUM

For convenience peptic ulcer of the stomach and duodenum will be discussed together, although there are a number of differences that will warrant comment.

Incidence. Peptic ulcers are very common causes of morbidity but rarely cause death of the patient. As many as one fourth of men and one sixth of women develop a peptic ulcer sometime during life, as judged by typical scars at autopsy, but far fewer (5 to 10 per cent) develop symptomatic ulcers during life. Furthermore, the incidence of duodenal ulcer seems to be declining in the United States. Duodenal ulcers are more frequent than gastric ulcers; men have a higher incidence of duodenal ulcers but the same incidence of gastric ulcers when compared to women.

Pathogenesis. Peptic ulcers are presumed to represent some breakdown in the balance of acid-pepsin secretion and the mucosal defense mechanisms (Fig. 37–2). The mechanisms involved may be multifactorial for a given individual and certainly are so in different patients with peptic ulcers. Patients with duodenal ulcer tend as a group to have increased basal and maximal acid output rates of HCl secretion, but to have normal acid output and gastrin release after eating. The higher basal acid output in patients with duodenal ulcer may result from higher basal serum gastrin concentrations. Patients with gastric ulcers usually have normal or even reduced rates of acid secretion. Overall the evidence of hyperacidity as the cause of duodenal ulcer is marginal, and for gastric ulcer it is nonexistent.

Genetic factors seem to be important in some patients with peptic ulcer. There is an increased incidence in first-degree relatives of patients with duodenal ulcers and a positive association with high levels of serum pepsinogen I, which appears to be inherited as a dominant trait and may reflect total chief cell mass. There are weaker associations with blood group O and with HLA-B5. Familial gastrinomas will be discussed later.

There is a strong association of peptic ulcer with cigarette smoking, possibly due to diminished bicarbonate secretion by the pancreas as a cause for duodenal ulcers and to diminished pyloric sphincter tone with reflux of duodenal juice for gastric ulcers. Furthermore, peptic ulcer has been reported to be increased in uremia, chronic obstructive pulmonary disease, alcoholic cirrhosis, hyperparathyroidism (hypercalcemia), mastocytosis (histamine), cluster headaches (Horton's cephalgia), and polycythemia vera. The use of nonsteroidal anti-inflammatory agents definitely increases the incidence of superficial gastric mucosal erosions and gastric ulcers, but the possible role of these agents, and of glucocorticoids, in the pathogenesis of duodenal ulcers is more controversial. Reflux of bile and pancreatic juice from the duodenum through an incompetent pyloric sphincter has been postulated to play a role in some cases of gastric ulcer. The possible role of psychological factors is unclear, but emotional distress may increase gastric secretion.

Campylobacter pylori infections of the gastric mucosa have recently been detected by antral biopsies in patients with duodenal or gastric ulcers (in approximately 90 per cent and 70 per cent of such patients, respectively). This infection can also be detected indirectly by the release of $^{14}CO_2$ from orally administered ^{14}C-urea, because of the action of bacterial urease. Approximately 20 per cent of normal subjects harbor *C. pylori* in gastric biopsies. Further study is necessary to define whether this organism has a role in the pathogenesis or natural history of peptic ulcer disease.

Clinical Manifestations. The cardinal manifestation of peptic ulcer is *epigastric pain* that is relieved by the ingestion of food or antacids. The pain, frequently described as burning or gnawing, most typically occurs one to three hours after eating. This is related to gastric emptying, when the continuing secretion of gastric acid is unbuffered and presumably produces pain by direct irritation of nerve endings in the ulcer or, as some think, by inducing spasm. The pain tends to occur in clusters, perhaps over several weeks, with subsequent periods of remission of varying duration. The pain of peptic ulcer may be atypical in location, in character, and in its relationship to meals. It may also be absent despite the presence of an active peptic ulcer demonstrated radiographically or endoscopically.

In addition to pain, patients with peptic ulcer tend to have a variety of symptoms that can be best summarized as *"dyspepsia"*—bloating, nausea, anorexia, excessive eructations, and epigastric discomfort. Not infrequently patients present with one of the complications of peptic ulcer.

In the absence of complications, the physical examination is rarely of help in the diagnosis of peptic ulcer disease. Most frequently there is a moderate amount of epigastric tenderness. The physical examination may give evidence of one of the diseases associated with ulcer diathesis, as noted above.

Complications. Complications are not infrequent

in peptic ulcer disease. It has been estimated that as many as one third of patients in whom the diagnosis is made in life will have one or sometimes more than one of these complications during the course of illness. These complications are also the main indications for surgery for peptic ulcer disease, to be discussed subsequently.

BLEEDING.   Bleeding from peptic ulcer disease, the most common cause of upper gastrointestinal bleeding, occurs in about 10 to 15 per cent of patients. It may be the first manifestation of the disease and carries an overall mortality rate of about 7 per cent. Death from peptic ulcer bleeding is more likely to occur in older patients (above age 60), in those with other illnesses, with gastric ulcers, or with severe and recurrent bleeding (>3 units of blood required per day), and when there is an exposed bleeding vessel in the ulcer visualized endoscopically. The approach to the patient with upper gastrointestinal bleeding is described in Chapter 34B. In approximately 85 per cent of patients, bleeding from peptic ulcer disease will stop under medical therapy; about 15 per cent of patients require emergency surgery. This usually consists of ligation of a bleeding vessel for duodenal ulcer together with a truncal vagotomy and pyloroplasty. Distal gastrectomy is usually indicated for emergency surgery for gastric ulcer in the distal stomach and biopsy, ligation of bleeding vessels, and distal gastrectomy for more proximal ulcers. Patients who have bled once from a peptic ulcer have an increased chance of bleeding again (30 to 50 per cent chance).

PERFORATION.   A peptic ulcer may erode through the entire wall of the duodenum or stomach. Sometimes this leads to penetration of an adjacent organ such as the pancreas, with resulting pancreatitis and intractable pain. More frequently, especially with anterior duodenal ulcers and lesser curvature gastric ulcers, there is free perforation into the peritoneal cavity. This complication occurs in 5 to 10 per cent of patients with duodenal ulcers and 2 to 5 per cent with gastric ulcers. Not infrequently there is associated hemorrhage. Rarely perforation is the first symptom of a peptic ulcer; more frequently the patient has a long history of more typical symptoms. The presentation is typically that of an acute abdomen with the sudden onset of severe abdominal pain, peritoneal signs (abdominal muscle rigidity, rebound tenderness), and hypotension with tachycardia. Free air in the abdominal cavity can usually be demonstrated by an upright radiograph. In most patients with free perforation, emergency surgery is indicated to repair the site and to wash out the peritoneal cavity. Depending upon the state of the patient, more definitive surgery (proximal gastric vagotomy and antrectomy, for example) may be carried out at the same operation. In some poor-risk patients the perforation is allowed to seal spontaneously while the patient is maintained on nasogastric suction, fluids, and antibiotics.

OBSTRUCTION.   The gastric outlet may become obstructed by the inflammation, spasm, and fibrosis induced by an ulcer. This complication is most frequent in ulcers involving the pyloric channel. The symptoms are usually those of early satiety, nausea, vomiting after eating, epigastric pain, and fullness. On physical examination the patient may present with a succussion splash and signs of dehydration. Laboratory studies may show metabolic alkalosis and hypokalemia. Most patients with this complication, which occurs in about 5 per cent of patients diagnosed as having peptic ulcer, have had long-standing clinical illness. It is very unusual for this complication to be the initial presentation. Obstruction can be readily demonstrated by a positive saline load test (>400 ml of gastric juice recovered 30 minutes after instilling 750 ml of saline by nasogastric tube into an empty stomach). This test may not be necessary if there is 200 ml of gastric juice in the stomach after an overnight fast. The obstruction can be directly demonstrated by endoscopy or indirectly by an upper GI series. An attempt should be made to treat all patients with gastric outlet obstruction initially by medical means—nasogastric tube drainage, repair of fluid and electrolyte deficits, cimetidine or ranitidine (to reduce HCl loss by the drainage), and parenteral nutrition. At least half of patients so treated, presumably those in whom spasm and edema are of particular importance, will respond to this therapy over several days and can be spared surgical therapy.

INTRACTABLE PAIN.   The pain of a peptic ulcer is rarely intractable if the patient is compliant with a treatment regimen. When present it may represent penetration posteriorly or into an adjacent viscus.

Diagnosis.   The diagnosis of a peptic ulcer can be established only by the demonstration of the ulcer by direct inspection endoscopically (the most sensitive and specific method) or indirectly by radiographic studies (an upper GI series). An upper GI series is usually the first screening study because it is less expensive than endoscopy. If no ulcer is found radiographically, however, and the suspicion of peptic ulcer is still high, endoscopic examination is indicated, since as many as one fifth of such ulcers may be missed by an upper GI series. If a gastric ulcer is found radiographically, it is imperative to demonstrate that it is benign rather than malignant. A number of findings make a malignant ulcer more or less likely (age of the patient, location and size of the ulcer, the topography of the mucosal folds around the ulcer), but this can be established with acceptable clinical accuracy only by inspection and multiple biopsies of the lesion. Some physicians supplement this approach by cytological examinations.

When the presence of a typical peptic ulcer has been established radiographically or endoscopically, other studies are rarely indicated, since the pathogenesis of these lesions is still obscure in most cases. In only a few clinical situations is the measurement of serum gastrin or of the basal and peak acid outputs of the stomach indicated (Table 37–1), primarily for the suspicion of a gastrinoma (to be discussed subsequently).

In addition to the occasional need to rule out a gastrinoma, after the presence of a peptic ulcer has been

TABLE 37–1. CLINICAL SITUATIONS IN WHICH MEASUREMENT OF SERUM GASTRIN LEVELS IS INDICATED

Family history of peptic ulcer
Ulcer associated with hypercalcemia or other manifestations of multiple endocrine neoplasia type I
Multiple ulcers
Peptic ulceration of postbulbar duodenum or jejunum
Peptic ulceration associated with diarrhea*
Chronic unexplained diarrhea*
Enlarged gastric folds on upper GI x-ray
Before surgery for "intractable" ulcer
Recurrent ulcer after ulcer surgery

* Not due to antacid ingestion. (Adapted from Schiller LR: Peptic ulcer: Epidemiology, clinical manifestations, and diagnosis. In Wyngaarden JB, Smith LH Jr [eds]: Cecil Textbook of Medicine. 18th ed. Philadelphia, WB Saunders Co, 1988, p 698.)

demonstrated, the nonspecific symptoms of peptic ulcer must be differentiated from those of functional dyspepsia, gastric cancer, biliary tract disease, pancreatitis, and a wide variety of other abdominal disorders.

Treatment. Most patients with peptic ulcer can be treated successfully by medical methods. Surgery is usually required only for the complications of the disease noted above: bleeding, perforation, gastric outlet obstruction, and rarely intractable pain. In addition to the specific measures to be described, all patients with peptic ulcer disease should be advised to discontinue cigarette smoking, to drink alcohol only in moderation, and to discontinue the use of nonsteroidal antiinflammatory agents. Although diet was once considered to be of great importance in the treatment of peptic ulcer, there is no good evidence that changes in diet influence the rate of healing. Patients are best advised simply to avoid foods that in their personal experience lead to dyspeptic symptoms and to limit eating between meals and at bedtime, since eating during that time further enhances gastric secretion.

Medical management of peptic ulcer is in general directed either toward reducing the concentration of gastric acid or toward reducing mucosal damage from acid-pepsin exposure.

REDUCTION OF GASTRIC ACID. A number of agents can reduce substantially the rate of secretion of acid by acting at various sites in the normal or hyperstimulated parietal cell (Fig. 37–3). Of these agents only the H$_2$-receptor antagonists are being currently used as primary therapy in the United States. Cimetidine (in a usual dose of 800 mg at night or 400 mg twice daily), ranitidine (300 mg at night or 150 mg twice daily), and famotidine (40 mg at bedtime) are all highly effective in blocking the secretion of HCl. Cimetidine in its usual doses may cause confusion in some older patients, especially in the presence of renal insufficiency, and with long-term treatment sometimes has an antiandrogenic effect characterized by gynecomastia and impotence. It may also inhibit the metabolism of certain other drugs by the liver as an important example of drug interaction. Ranitidine is thought to be less likely to cause mental symptoms in susceptible patients, is not antiandrogenic, and inhibits the metabolism of other drugs less markedly. The substituted benzimidazoles (omeprazole as a prototype) show considerable promise but have not as yet come into general use.

The concentration of gastric acid can be reduced not only by inhibiting its secretion but also by neutralizing it intraluminally with antacids. The antacids more frequently used contain magnesium and/or aluminum hydroxide as their main ingredient. Calcium-containing antacids are no longer in favor because of the effect of ionized calcium in stimulating the secretion of gastrin, and sodium-containing antacids are generally too brief in their effectiveness and often add too much sodium to the diet with the danger of edema, hypertension, or metabolic alkalosis. The aluminum- and magnesium-containing antacids have comparatively few side effects (constipation for Al, diarrhea for Mg, the potential for phosphate depletion due to its enteric trapping), but they are often inconvenient to the patient. About 7 to 10 ml of the liquid antacid, or 2 tablets 7 times per day (equivalent to approximately 200 mmol of buffer per day) is a reasonable general regimen.

IMPROVEMENT OF MUCOSAL DEFENSE. Mucosal defense is a general concept that covers many aspects of susceptibility that cannot be readily measured, as can the secretion and concentration of HCl. Only one drug is widely used currently in the United States for this purpose, sucralfate. This agent, an aluminum hydroxide salt of sucrose that has been modified by sulfation, is unabsorbed following its usual dose of 1 gm four times daily. Its mechanism of action is unclear, but it is thought to adhere to and protect the surface of the ulcer as an artificial mucin and may also locally stimulate prostaglandin synthesis. Exogenous prostaglandins may also be useful in this mechanism of treatment in the future.

The five main first-line agents—cimetidine, raniti-

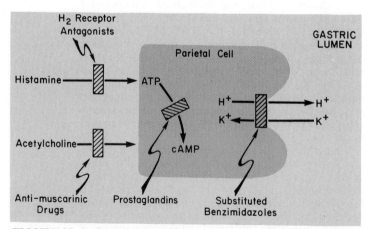

FIGURE 37–3. Sites of action of drugs employed to inhibit acid secretion. (From Peterson WL: Peptic ulcer: Medical therapy. In Wyngaarden JB, Smith LH Jr [eds]: Cecil Textbook of Medicine. 18th ed. Philadelphia, WB Saunders Co, 1988, p 700.)

dine, famotidine, antacids, and sucralfate—have been roughly equally effective in bringing about the healing of peptic ulcer, and all tend to be more effective with duodenal than with gastric ulcer. It has been shown that ranitidine given as a single 300-mg dose at bedtime is as effective as the other less convenient regimens. Treatment for four to six weeks will be associated with healing in approximately 90 per cent of patients. Treatment is then discontinued unless symptoms recur.

If this initial approach to treatment of a duodenal ulcer is not successful, care should be taken to ensure that the patient is compliant and that an unhealed ulcer is actually present endoscopically. Other doses or combinations of the above agents can then be tried. True intractability, or the development of a complication, may then indicate the need for surgery.

A gastric ulcer requires special consideration because of the danger of carcinoma (about 4 per cent of gastric ulcers) and should be carefully followed until healing. If healing does not occur on one of the above regimens by eight weeks, it is advisable to carry out endoscopy again with further biopsies and cytological studies. If they prove negative, a trial of another eight weeks on a different regimen may be indicated prior to the consideration of elective surgery.

The indications for long-term maintenance therapy are not certain. In many patients with primary healing and without complications, treatment can be discontinued. In those who are considered at high risk for recurrence or who have had complications of peptic ulcer disease, long-term therapy is indicated (Fig. 37–4).

SURGICAL MANAGEMENT.   Surgery for peptic ulcer is indicated usually for complications of the disease and when medical management has failed. The surgical procedures most frequently employed are shown in Figure 37–5. In various combinations they are devised to decrease acid secretion by reducing the cephalic phase of gastric secretion (vagotomy) or the gastric phase of gastric secretion (antrectomy to remove a major source of gastrin). Various drainage procedures are then employed to maintain gastric emptying in the postvagotomy state. Increasingly proximal ("superselective") vagotomy rather than truncal vagotomy is being employed to reduce acid secretion more selectively without the adverse effects on gastric motility and emptying. In patients with intractable benign gastric ulcers, vagotomy may not be required, since acid production is usually normal or low. Antrectomy or subtotal gastrectomy may be the treatment of choice.

Complications of Treatment.   Although surgical treatment of peptic ulcer is usually successful in relieving symptoms and preventing recurrence and carries a low mortality rate, there are infrequent complications that may be distressing to the patient:

THE DUMPING SYNDROME.   With disruption of the normal storage function of the stomach, for which the pylorus is the gatekeeper, ingested food may be prematurely dumped in excessive amounts into the small intestine, leading to nausea, vomiting, weakness, abdominal pain, and diarrhea. These symptoms occur

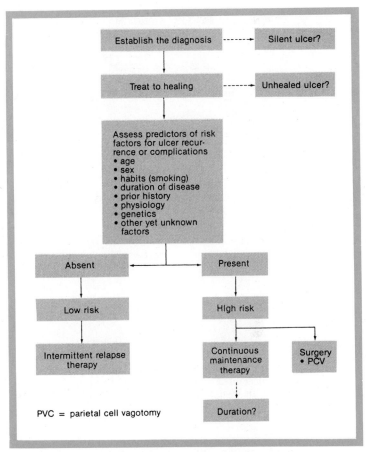

FIGURE 37–4. Algorithm for the treatment of the patient with peptic ulcer disease. (From Van Deventer GM: Approaches to the long-term treatment of duodenal ulcer disease. Am J Med 77(5B):15, 1984.)

soon after eating. More rarely there are late symptoms (one to three hours after eating), which probably result from reactive hypoglycemia from excessive rapidity of carbohydrate absorption followed by an overshoot of insulin release.

WEIGHT LOSS.   Many patients lose weight after partial gastric resection procedures. In part this is due to early satiety, but sometimes there is an associated malabsorption syndrome of complex pathogenesis (see Chapter 34C).

POSTVAGOTOMY DIARRHEA.   Many patients have diarrhea after truncal vagotomy for reasons that are unclear. The diarrhea may be related to the associated pyloroplasty. In a very few these symptoms may be persistent and incapacitating.

AFFERENT LOOP SYNDROME.   When the afferent

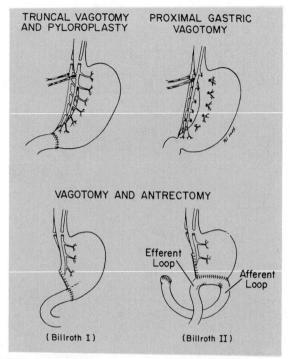

FIGURE 37–5. Model illustrating surgical procedures for peptic ulcer disease. (From Thirlby RC: Peptic ulcer: Surgical therapy. *In* Wyngaarden JB, Smith LH Jr [eds]: Cecil Textbook of Medicine. 18th ed. Philadelphia, WB Saunders Co, 1988, p 703.)

loop formed in a Billroth II procedure (Fig. 37–5) becomes partially occluded, pancreatic and biliary secretions accumulate and cause distention and pain. This is typically followed by opening up of the obstruction to release these secretions into the gastric remnant where they commonly cause vomiting. This complication may require reconstructive surgery. In patients with Billroth II anastomoses, bacteria may proliferate in the afferent loop. This may cause malabsorption of fat and vitamin B_{12}, as described more fully in Chapter 34C.

ANEMIA. Anemia is common after reconstructive surgery for peptic ulcer and is often complex in pathogenesis—iron deficiency, vitamin B_{12} deficiency, and/or folate deficiency.

THE ZOLLINGER-ELLISON SYNDROME

The Zollinger-Ellison syndrome, caused by a functioning islet cell tumor that secretes gastrin, accounts for well under 1 per cent of clinically diagnosed peptic ulcers. The possibility of this rare entity should be considered in several circumstances: (1) ulcers in unusual locations such as the second or third portions of the duodenum or the jejunum, (2) unusually severe peptic ulcer disease that is refractory to treatment or that is recurrent after surgery, (3) ulcer disease accompanied

by diarrhea and sometimes malabsorption (see Chapter 34), and (4) a strong family history of ulcer disease, especially if there is evidence of other endocrine tumors.

Pathogenesis. Single or often multiple gastrinomas in the pancreas, or more rarely in other abdominal but extrapancreatic sites, secrete excessive amounts of gastrin. This hormone drives acid secretion by the parietal cells as well as having a trophic effect in increasing their number (as much as three to five times). Although these tumors are slow-growing, most are histologically and biologically malignant with early metastases regionally and to the liver. In approximately one fourth of patients the gastrinoma is associated with other endocrine adenomas, most commonly in the pattern known as the multiple endocrine neoplasia type I syndrome (MEN I), in which adenomas or hyperplasia may involve the islet cells, the parathyroid glands, the thyroid, and the pituitary.

Clinical Manifestations. The clinical manifestations are usually those of severe peptic ulcer disease as noted above. Rarely diarrhea may precede peptic ulcer formation or be a more prominent part of the symptomatology.

Diagnosis. The diagnosis of the Zollinger-Ellison syndrome is not usually difficult if it is considered. In general it depends on the demonstration of an elevation of serum gastrin in the presence of increased basal secretion of gastric acid. Intravenous secretin (1 unit/kg) produces a marked increase in serum gastrin levels in most patients with gastrinoma, but not in patients with ordinary duodenal ulcers.

Treatment. An attempt should be made to find and remove a resectable tumor, although this can be done in only about one quarter of patients. If not successful, patients should be treated with very high doses of an H_2-receptor antagonist or a substituted benzimidazole (e.g., omeprozole). Total gastrectomy may still be required for the rare patient who does not respond to medical therapy.

GASTRITIS

Gastritis does not represent, strictly speaking, an acid-peptic group of diseases, but it will be discussed here for convenience, since it does reflect a breakdown in the interaction of injurious agents and mucosal defense mechanisms. Gastritis can be acute or chronic, specific or nonspecific.

Acute Gastritis. In acute gastritis there is infiltration of the lamina propria by inflammatory cells, often accompanied by superficial erosions that may be diffuse or localized. The mechanism of the mucosal injury is often unclear. Certain drugs, especially aspirin, nonsteroidal anti-inflammatory agents, and ethanol, are thought to disrupt the mucosal barrier to back-diffusion of acid and thereby to initiate chemical injury. "Stress ulcers" represent acute erosive injury to the stomach in many severe surgical or medical conditions with complicating bleeding. Stress ulcers are thought to result from ischemia, but again back-diffusion of acid may be the common final pathway of injury. Gastritis can sometimes be attributed to specific events such as irradiation, ingestion of alkali, or rarely bacterial infection (phlegmonous gastritis). Following surgery, reflux of bile salts and/or pancreatic enzymes may produce acute gastritis.

Most cases of acute gastritis are probably mild and escape diagnosis. The diagnosis is established by endoscopic examination. When present, symptoms are usually those of dyspepsia, epigastric pain, nausea, and vomiting. The most important complication of acute gastritis is that of bleeding from the superficial erosions. This usually responds to conservative management and omission of the precipitating agent if known (aspirin, alcohol). Antacids and/or cimetidine or ranitidine are often used as well but have not been shown to affect healing. The overall prognosis of acute, erosive gastritis is excellent, with rapid healing of the lesions within days.

Chronic Gastritis. Chronic gastritis has been classified by the histological severity of the process (superficial, atrophic, or gastric atrophy) and by the anatomical location in the stomach where it is most manifest (type A—fundus and body of the stomach; type B—antrum). In most patients no pathogenesis can be firmly established, although chronic use of the same drugs implicated in acute gastritis and chronic exposure to bile salts and pancreatic enzymes are postulated to be of importance in some patients. In type A atrophic gastritis there are usually circulating antibodies against parietal cells whether or not pernicious anemia is present; in some patients with type B atrophic gastritis antibodies against gastrin-producing cells have been reported.

There are no definite clinical manifestations of idiopathic chronic gastritis. Patients with type A gastritis may have pernicious anemia alone or linked with one or more other autoimmune diseases. Chronic gastritis may be associated with a higher incidence of benign gastric ulcer and gastric cancer. No specific treatment is indicated for idiopathic chronic gastritis.

REFERENCES

Wolfe MM, Soll AH: The physiology of gastric acid secretion. N Engl J Med 319:1707, 1988.

Richardson CT, Schiller LR, Peterson WL, Thirlby RC, Feldman M: Peptic ulcer. *In* Wyngaarden JB, Smith LH Jr (eds): Cecil Textbook of Medicine. 18th ed. Philadelphia, WB Saunders Co, 1988, pp 692–709.

Soll AH, Isenberg JI: Peptic ulcer diseases. *In* Sleisenger MH, Fordtran JS (eds): Gastrointestinal Disease. 3rd ed. Philadelphia, WB Saunders Co, 1983, p 625.

Talley NJ, Phillips SF: Non-ulcer dyspepsia: potential causes and pathophysiology. Ann Intern Med 108:865, 1988.

Weinstein WM: Gastritis. *In* Sleisenger MH, Fordtran JS (eds): Gastrointestinal Disease. 4th ed. Philadelphia, WB Saunders Co, 1989, pp 792–813.

38

INFLAMMATORY BOWEL DISEASE

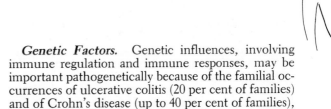

Definition

Inflammatory bowel disease (IBD) refers to both idiopathic ulcerative colitis and Crohn's disease, important chronic medical disorders of unknown etiology. For convenience, ulcerative colitis (UC) and Crohn's disease will be discussed together as IBD in order to emphasize their similarities and to point out their differences. In general IBD is more common in whites than in nonwhites, is equal in men and women, and is more common in Ashkenazic Jews than in Sephardic Jews. The incidence of UC is now approximately equal to that of Crohn's disease in many medical centers worldwide. Symptoms characteristically begin in early adult life (15 to 30 years) but may begin at any age. A comparison of the pathological and clinical features of UC and Crohn's disease is given in Table 38–1.

Etiology and Pathogenesis

The cause of IBD is not known; therefore speculations abound:

Genetic Factors. Genetic influences, involving immune regulation and immune responses, may be important pathogenetically because of the familial occurrences of ulcerative colitis (20 per cent of families) and of Crohn's disease (up to 40 per cent of families), the high concordance rates of IBD in monozygotic twins, and the familial clustering of sclerosing cholangitis and ulcerative colitis.

Infectious Origin. Despite many studies, no agent has been consistently isolated.

Immunological Origin. The extraintestinal manifestations (see below), the reported presence of antibodies to colonic epithelial cells and of cytotoxic T cells, and the clinical and histological responses to immunosuppressive agents have suggested an immunological basis for intestinal injury. Current interest is directed to a possible defect in immunoregulatory activity in the intestinal epithelium (e.g., abnormally increased T helper cell or diminished T suppressor cell response to antigen).

TABLE 38–1. COMPARISON OF THE PATHOLOGICAL AND CLINICAL FEATURES OF ULCERATIVE COLITIS AND CROHN'S DISEASE

FEATURE	ULCERATIVE COLITIS	CROHN'S DISEASE
Pathology		
Discontinuous involvement	0	+ +
Transmural inflammation	0/+ *	+ + +
Deep fissures and fistulas	0	+ +
Confluent linear ulcers	0	+ +
Crypt abscesses	+ + +	+
Focal granulomas	0	+ +
Clinical		
Rectal bleeding	+ + +	+
Malaise, fever	+	+ + +
Abdominal pain	+	+ + +
Abdominal mass	0	+ +
Fistulas	0	+ + +
Endoscopic		
Diffuse, continuous involvement	+ + +	0/+
Friable mucosa	+ + +	0/+
Rectal involvement	+ + +	+
Cobblestoning	0	+ + +
Linear ulcers	0	+ +

* In toxic megacolon.

Psychological Origin. Few believe that emotional factors are etiologic, but they may exacerbate symptoms and impair the ability to cope with the chronicity and debility of IBD.

In brief, environmental factors (infectious?, noninfectious antigens or toxins?) may trigger a sequence of events in which altered immunological responses and/or genetic responses become critical in the pathogenesis of IBD. With increasing technological development in parts of Asia, for example, the incidence of IBD is increasing.

Pathology

The pathology is of particular importance in IBD. It is the basis for the clinical manifestations described below and also for the distinction that is made between UC and Crohn's disease.

Ulcerative Colitis. The acute lesion is a *diffuse* (without skip areas), *superficial* (mucosal and submucosal) inflammation that almost always involves the rectum (>95 per cent) and may extend from the rectum throughout the colon. With pancolitis the terminal ileum may be slightly involved (a "backwash ileitis"), but UC is essentially a colonic disease. Infiltrated with neutrophils, the epithelium is typically diffusely inflamed, granular, and friable and may show small superficial ulcerations or occasionally deep linear ulcers. Multiple microabscesses may develop in and around the crypts. When severely inflamed, the colon may become markedly distended (diameter >6 cm) with attenuation of its walls, a condition known as "toxic megacolon." This is associated with an immediate danger of perforation. In chronic UC hyperplasia of the muscularis mucosae secondary to the continuous processes of injury and repair may produce a smooth, foreshortened colon with loss of normal haustral markings (the lead-pipe colon radiographically). Heaped-up, rounded patches of granulation tissue develop as outcroppings between areas of ulcerative injury; they are called postinflammatory pseudopolyps, since they are not neoplastic. Ultimately with long-standing disease the epithelial cells may show dysplastic changes that are considered to be harbingers of malignancy. Unless carcinoma occurs UC rarely produces a stricture or a fistula.

Crohn's Disease. In Crohn's disease, also termed regional enteritis, the inflammation is *transmural* (involving all layers of the bowel and the serosal surface), may be *discontinuous* (with skip areas of normal bowel between), and involves the rectum in fewer than 50 per cent of cases. In contrast to UC, Crohn's disease may involve any area of the GI tract (mouth, esophagus, stomach, duodenum); approximately one third is colonic; one third is ileal; and one third is ileocolonic. Rarely the more proximal small bowel, the stomach, or even the mouth may be involved. With transmural and even mesenteric involvement, inflamed loops of bowel may become adherent to each other or to other organs, producing palpable masses, fistulas, or obstruction. The mucosa may appear grossly normal or exhibit a cobblestone appearance. Deep linear ulcers may be present, most characteristically in the long axis of the bowel. The infiltrate in the thickened, stiffened walls contains not only neutrophils but also lymphocytes and macrophages, with granuloma formation in about 50 per cent of cases. As noted, fistula formation, including perirectal disease, is common, but dysplasia of epithelial cells is not noted. Fibrosis and intestinal stenosis result from excess collagen production.

Clinical Manifestations

The clinical manifestations of IBD can be conveniently considered as those relating directly to the bowel disease and the systemic response to it and those that are extraintestinal and of more obscure origin.

Intestinal Manifestations. The cardinal manifestations of acute *UC* are diarrhea, rectal bleeding, fever, weight loss, and abdominal pain. The disease can be mild with only a gradual slight increase in the number of stools and can be limited anatomically to the rectum (ulcerative proctitis). Conversely in a minority of patients (10 to 15 per cent) it begins explosively, so that the patient is acutely ill and requires immediate hospitalization to prevent complications of toxic megacolon such as shock, hypokalemia, and colonic perforation. Depending upon the severity of the diarrhea and the extent of ulceration and inflammation, the patient may exhibit electrolyte abnormalities (particularly hypokalemia), anemia, leukocytosis, fever, and all of the symptoms and signs of toxicity—e.g., weakness, anorexia, tachycardia, and hypotension. The abdomen may be distended and diffusely tender, but generally no masses are felt. Most treated patients with UC have remissions of their symptoms that may last for months or even years, followed by recurrent acute exacerbations.

In *Crohn's disease* the onset of symptoms is often more subtle than in UC, and the type of presentation is influenced by the anatomical site of the major lesion. If the ileum is primarily involved, the symptoms may suggest low-grade intestinal obstruction with post-cibal colicky pain, modest diarrhea, and sometimes the presence of a right lower quadrant palpable mass. Gross rectal bleeding is rare in all forms of Crohn's disease, although occult blood loss is common. The onset of Crohn's ileitis may simulate acute appendicitis in a young person. With colonic involvement diarrhea may be more prominent as well as perirectal disease, comprising fissures, fistulas, and perirectal abscesses. Colonic Crohn's disease is also associated with a higher incidence of the extraintestinal manifestations described below. "Toxic megacolon" may occur in Crohn's disease but less often than in UC. Free perforation of the bowel as opposed to fistula formation is uncommon. In brief, consistent with their respective pathological lesions, Crohn's disease is more likely to produce fistulas or strictures and less likely to produce hemorrhage or perforation than is UC. Aphthous ulcers of the buccal mucosa are not infrequent.

Extraintestinal Manifestations. Similar extraintestinal manifestations may occur with UC and with Crohn's disease of the colon (Table 38–2). These will be considered together and discussed briefly. *Nutritional deficiencies*, occurring secondary to anorexia, fever, diarrhea, blood loss, and malabsorption, may result in growth retardation or severe weight loss.

IBD may be associated with two forms of *arthritis*, sometimes termed enteropathic arthritis: (a) nondeforming acute inflammatory arthritis of unknown cause affecting large joints more frequently, and (b) sacroiliitis and ankylosing spondylitis, which occur in those patients who also have HLA-B27. The former tends to parallel the colonic disease, but it may precede the onset of IBD by months or years. The process is characteristically a mono- or oligoarticular, asymmetric synovitis affecting the knees or ankles. Sacroiliitis and ankylosing spondylitis generally persist, even after colectomy for UC. The clinical and radiographic findings in the HLA-B27 associated arthritis of IBD are similar to those observed in the idiopathic process. *Hepatobiliary abnormalities* are diverse in nature and severity. Many patients have fatty liver and mild pericholangitis, often manifested chemically only by an elevated serum alkaline phosphatase. Rarely sclerosing cholangitis involving both intrahepatic and extrahepatic ducts may develop, presenting the full picture of obstructive jaundice and leading to cirrhosis. Sclerosing cholangitis is much more often associated with UC than with Crohn's disease. There is an increased incidence of cholelithiasis, especially with Crohn's disease of the ileum, thought to be secondary to deficient ileal reabsorption of bile salts. Primary carcinoma of the bile ducts is rare but is increased in incidence. *Ocular manifestations* of IBD include episcleritis, iritis, and uveitis. *Erythema nodosum* may occur in about 5 per cent of patients, especially in women, and a peculiar indolent necrotic skin lesion termed *pyoderma gangrenosum* may be found in about 1 to 2 per cent, especially with active UC. *Renal lesions* may include (a) kidney stone diathesis, especially calcium oxalate stones due to absorptive hyperoxaluria in Crohn's disease, (b) obstructive uropathy or fistulas to the urinary tract in Crohn's disease, (c) kaliopenic nephropathy, or, very rarely, (d) amyloidosis. An increased tendency to develop *thrombophlebitis* has also been noted. Osteoporosis and osteomalacia may complicate the course of IBD (see Chapters 77 and 78).

These extraintestinal manifestations may rarely precede overt bowel symptoms or may be the most important source of disability. Most of them tend to remit with improvement of colitis or following colectomy except for sclerosing cholangitis, cirrhosis, and sacroiliitis/spondylitis.

Diagnosis

The diagnostic challenge is to determine whether a patient who presents with diarrhea, abdominal pain, rectal bleeding, fever, or any of the other manifestations listed above has IBD or not and, if so, whether the disease represents UC or Crohn's disease. The list of disorders that must be considered varies with the clinical presentation and may be a long one: acute bacillary dysentery, amebiasis, pseudomembranous colitis, ischemic colitis, colonic neoplasms, angiodysplasia, "microscopic colitis," and "collagenous colitis." Laboratory studies are generally not helpful in the diagnosis of IBD except to exclude other possi-

TABLE 38–2. EXTRAINTESTINAL MANIFESTATIONS OF INFLAMMATORY BOWEL DISEASE*

1. Nutritional abnormalities
   weight loss, hypoalbuminemia, vitamin deficiencies, deficiencies of calcium, zinc, magnesium, phosphate
2. Hematologic abnormalities
   anemia (Fe loss, folate deficiency), leukocytosis, thrombocytosis
3. Skin manifestations
   pyoderma gangrenosum, erythema nodosum
4. Arthritis
   ankylosing spondylitis and sacroiliitis (B27-associated), peripheral large joint involvement
5. Hepatic and biliary abnormalities
   fatty liver, pericholangitis, sclerosing cholangitis, gallstones, carcinoma of the bile ducts
6. Renal abnormalities
   kidney stone diathesis (calcium oxalate, uric acid), obstructive uropathy, fistulas to urinary tract
7. Eye abnormalities
   iritis, conjunctivitis, episcleritis
8. Miscellaneous
   fever, increased thrombophlebitis, osteoporosis, osteomalacia

* Modified from Rosenberg IH: Crohn's disease. *In* Wyngaarden JB, Smith LH Jr (eds): Cecil Textbook of Medicine. 18th ed. Philadelphia, WB Saunders Co, 1988, p 745.

bilities. The diagnosis rests on (1) direct visualization of the colonic mucosa by sigmoidoscopy or colonoscopy, with biopsy of an abnormal area if indicated; (2) a radiological study of the colon, and of the ileum if indicated, preferably using an air-contrast barium enema technique; (3) exclusion of other possibilities by appropriate bacterial cultures for *Campylobacter*, *Yersinia*, *Chlamydia*, and other organisms; measurement of the toxin of *Clostridium difficile*, or the search for trophozoites of *Entamoeba histolytica*, for example.

The characteristic endoscopic findings in acute UC are those described under "Pathology" above: a friable, granular, diffuse uniform lesion of the mucosa that may exhibit superficial ulcerations or that bleeds easily when rubbed with a cotton swab. With more chronic disease, deeper ulcers and pseudopolyps may be found. In Crohn's disease the mucosa is often involved focally and may even appear normal except for a "cobblestone appearance" due to distortions caused by submucosal inflammation and linear ulcerations. When present, ulcers may be shallow and superficial or deep and longitudinal.

Radiographic studies are of particular importance in the diagnosis of IBD and in demonstrating the extent of its involvement. An air-contrast barium enema usually demonstrates the diffuse lesions of UC and may show the presence of pseudopolyps (Fig. 38–1). The study may be normal in early disease, however, and is less sensitive than direct visualization of the mucosa by endoscopy. Late in the disease a smooth "lead-pipe" foreshortened colon with loss of haustral markings may be noted. Radiographic studies of Crohn's colitis most typically show skip areas, rectal sparing, longitudinal ulcers, and asymmetrical, segmental narrowing of the bowel. Fistulas may be present. In the small bowel, especially the terminal ileum, there is usually loss of the normal mucosal pattern and reduction in the size of the lumen to produce the characteristic "string sign."

Although the classic differences between UC and Crohn's disease of the colon as described above usually allow this distinction to be made, these two entities are sometimes difficult to distinguish at the time that IBD is diagnosed.

Treatment and Prognosis

The treatment of UC and Crohn's disease is similar in that both disorders require chronic, nonspecific therapeutic programs employing many of the same agents. In addition, the general treatment of the patient's nutrition, psychological problems, anemia, and other systemic disabilities may be similar. Therapy and prognosis differ enough, however, to warrant separate brief discussions.

Ulcerative Colitis. No single drug is curative, and a comprehensive therapeutic approach usually is required. Sulfasalazine, various antibacterial compounds (e. g., tetracycline, metronidazole), steroids, and symptom-controlling medication (e. g., mild antispasmodics, sedatives) remain drugs of choice. Immune suppressants, such as 6-mercaptopurine, azathioprine, and cyclosporine, continue to be used cautiously and in very special circumstances.

Mild to moderate acute colitis may respond to supportive measures supplemented by sulfasalazine (3 to

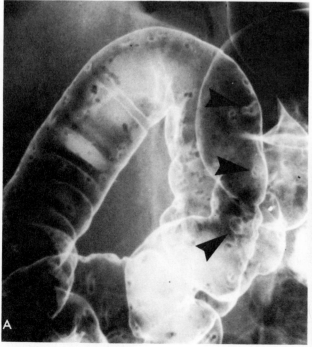

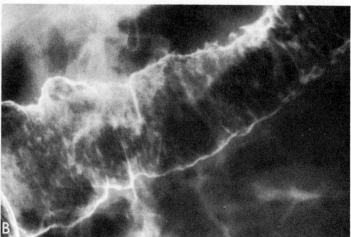

FIGURE 38–1. Double-contrast barium enema in a patient with ulcerative colitis demonstrating (A) pseudopolyps and (B) multiple, irregular serrations in the transverse colon representing mucosal ulcerations. (From Sleisenger MH, Fordtran JS [eds]: Gastrointestinal Disease. 3rd ed. Philadelphia. WB Saunders Co, 1983, pp 1134–1135.)

4 gm daily) alone. Sulfasalazine is split by bacterial action in the colon to yield sulfapyridine and 5-aminosalicylate (5-ASA), the latter considered to be the active agent through its local inhibition of prostaglandin and leukotriene synthesis. Newer preparations of 5-ASA alone are becoming available with mechanisms for colonic release. These may be particularly useful for patients who are sensitive to the sulfapyridine moiety of sulfasalazine. If this regimen is insufficient, it can be supplemented by corticosteroid therapy, given either as oral prednisone 20 to 40 mg daily or, especially for left-sided colonic involvement, as hydrocortisone (100 mg) administered as a bedtime enema. When the acute exacerbation is over, the use of sulfasalazine (2 gm daily) should be continued indefinitely to maintain control of the disease and to prevent recurrence.

Acute, severe UC merges into the entity of toxic megacolon, described below. This represents a medical emergency requiring immediate hospitalization, close attention to replacement of blood and electrolytes, systemic corticosteroids in large doses, coverage by broad-spectrum antibiotics, and surgical consultation. Emergency colectomy may be required for failure of toxic megacolon to improve clinically and radiographically in 36 to 48 hours, for excessive hemorrhage, or for perforation. The medical regimens for the individual patient must be determined within this spectrum for intensity and for duration.

Surgical treatment for UC is usually that of total colectomy with a permanent ileostomy and is ultimately required in approximately 20 to 25 per cent of patients. The operation is "curative" in that UC as a disease is confined to the colon. The indications for elective as opposed to emergency colectomy described above are generally the following: (a) Failure of medical management. This can be either during the first acute episode or after some years of treatment during which therapy is insufficiently effective in suppressing the disease or suppression requires unacceptably large amounts of corticosteroids. (b) Concern about the presence or future development of carcinoma. This may arise because of the detection of dysplastic, presumably premalignant changes in the epithelium or of gross changes on radiographic or endoscopic examination that are suspicious for carcinoma. Of course colectomy may also be indicated for demonstrated carcinoma complicating UC.

Few patients (<1 per cent) die during an acute attack of UC. Most patients (>90 per cent) respond to therapy or have spontaneous remissions, but unfortunately most have recurrence of the disease months or even years later. Most patients with UC have a reasonably normal life span. Death from UC usually results either from an acute complication (perforation, hemorrhage, sepsis, shock) or from the late development of carcinoma of the colon.

Crohn's Disease. The medical treatment of Crohn's disease is similar to that for UC, with sulfasalazine and corticosteroids being the main agents used beyond general supportive and dietary measures.

Crohn's disease is seldom acute, in contrast to UC, although it may present acutely as intestinal obstruction, for example. The response to treatment tends to be less striking than that of UC, and remissions are not as complete. Sulfasalazine is not effective in preventing exacerbations of Crohn's disease, as documented in long-term trials. Some success has been noted with Crohn's disease by putting the bowel to rest with use of parenteral hyperalimentation, which may also be helpful in preparing patients for surgery.

Surgical treatment of Crohn's disease is not curative and is always undertaken with reluctance, since the disease tends to recur proximal to the site of excision and the patients are especially prone to forming postoperative adhesions. Surgery is most frequently required for obstruction, fistula formation, or abscesses (especially perirectal disease). The key principle is to remove as little of the bowel as possible.

The prognosis for Crohn's disease is generally less favorable than for UC, since it responds less well to medical management and cannot generally be cured by surgery. As is the case with UC, most patients with Crohn's disease live a normal life span. Death from Crohn's disease is usually from sepsis rather than from hemorrhage or carcinoma of the colon.

Complications

The complications associated with IBD have been largely discussed as part of the clinical or extraintestinal manifestations of these diseases. In addition to the more specific and acute complications such as hemorrhage or perforation, one must be concerned about some of the long-term nonspecific problems such as retardation of growth in children, malnutrition, weakness, lassitude, recurrent pain, and depression. These are complications of many chronic debilitating diseases. Two other complications, alluded to previously and found mostly but not exclusively with UC, will be further described in brief.

Toxic Dilatation of the Colon (Toxic Megacolon). This complication, which represents perhaps the extreme range of acute UC, describes the presence of a markedly distended atonic colon with attenuation of its wall thickness, usually associated with signs of systemic toxicity—hypotension, tachycardia, fever, and leukocytosis. Diarrhea may be diminished rather than enhanced, because of loss of colonic motor function. Hypokalemia and hypoalbuminemia are common. Toxic megacolon may occur spontaneously, or be induced by injudicious use of drugs (anticholinergics, opiates), by preparation for a barium enema examination, by colonoscopic manipulation in the severely ill patient, or by hypokalemia. The diagnosis is usually made with a plain film of the abdomen showing a colonic diameter greater than 6 cm, usually seen in the transverse colon. There is an immediate and continuing danger of perforation until the dilatation is reversed. The treatment of this medical emergency has been described above.

Carcinoma of the Colon. A general discussion of carcinoma of the colon is found in Chapter 39. There is increased risk of neoplasia in IBD, particularly in chronic UC. The incidence of carcinoma in UC relates to two variables: (a) the presence of extensive mucosal disease, i.e., pancolitis, and (b) the duration of active colitis. The incidence begins to rise after 10 years of active disease. Carcinoma complicating UC has the following characteristics as compared to that occurring spontaneously: (a) it is distributed more evenly in the colon, (b) it is more likely to occur in multiple sites, (c) it is usually discovered at a more advanced stage and has a worse prognosis, and (d) it is more difficult to diagnose because its associated symptoms are mimicked by those of the underlying disease. Because of this it is imperative to institute long-term follow-up protocols in patients with chronic pancolitis, using colonoscopy and biopsies of suspicious lesions and of the colonic mucosa in general. The latter may show the development of dysplastic changes, thought to be premalignant, and therefore suggest the advisability of preventive colectomy.

ISCHEMIC COLITIS

In older patients inflammatory bowel disease may be simulated by ischemic injury to the colon. This ischemic injury, which may be acute or chronic, usually occurs as a complication of severe atherosclerosis. More rarely it results from vascular injury secondary to surgery or a dissecting aneurysm, from a low cardiac output state, from vasculitis, or from a hypercoagulable state. The ischemia is more likely to occur in "watershed areas" between the distributions of two major vessels (splenic flexure, rectosigmoid area) and is usually secondary to hypoperfusion rather than to complete obstruction. The rectum is almost always spared because of its collateral blood supplies. The clinical picture may be acute or chronic, with all gradations between.

Acute ischemic colitis is usually manifested by the sudden onset of localized abdominal pain, tenderness, and rectal bleeding, which is sometimes associated with fever, hypotension, tachycardia, and peritoneal signs. Sigmoidoscopy or colonoscopy may show no abnormalities but more frequently shows multiple ulcers or bulging areas of submucosal hemorrhage. Barium enema examination is hazardous during the acute phase, but when carried out later most characteristically shows areas of narrowing and the changes in the bowel outline called "thumbprinting" caused by mucosal hemorrhage and edema. Acute ischemic colitis may initially be difficult to distinguish from IBD or diverticulitis. Most acute ischemic episodes resolve over the subsequent several weeks with general supportive measures. Angiography is rarely indicated, and surgery is reserved for patients with clear evidence of perforation and/or infarction. The patient who recovers from an acute episode may remain well subsequently or may enter a more chronic phase of the illness.

Subacute or chronic ischemic colitis may lead to longer periods of vague abdominal pain and diarrhea

with or without significant bleeding, fear of eating, and substantial weight loss. This may closely simulate IBD in older people clinically as well as endoscopically. Over a period of time fibrosis may follow ischemic injury, leading to areas of narrowing of the colon. If such strictures lead to obstruction, surgery may be required. Rarely are attempts at revascularization indicated.

DIVERTICULITIS

Diverticula, serosa-covered saccules that include mucosa, extend from the lumen through the colonic muscular layer and are very common in later life in Western societies. These small herniations occur usually through areas of the colonic wall weakened by penetration of an arteriole. The incidence of diverticula is thought to be enhanced by any factor that chronically increases intraluminal pressure, particularly by refined diets of low fiber content that yield stools of small bulk. Most diverticula are found in the sigmoid area and are asymptomatic. They become important because of two complications: bleeding and infection. Vessels in or around a diverticulum may bleed briskly in older people, and diverticular bleeding must be differentiated from bleeding from other causes, especially from angiodysplasia or carcinoma. The differential diagnosis of gastrointestinal bleeding is discussed in Chapter 34B.

Diverticulitis refers specifically to infection in or more likely around diverticula (micro- or macroperforations of the diverticulum), thought to result usually from obstruction by fecoliths or inspissated feces with impairment of the blood supply and drainage. This walled-off, localized infection, caused by intestinal organisms, may produce a microabscess that heals spontaneously, may perforate to cause localized or more rarely generalized peritonitis, or may extend to cause larger abscesses that may be local or that may rarely penetrate other adjacent organs. Acute diverticulitis is said to simulate "left-sided appendicitis" with left lower quadrant pain (often exacerbated during defecation), tenderness, fever, leukocytosis, and sometimes a palpable inflammatory mass. Bleeding during the acute illness, if present at all, is usually microscopic. Rectal examination may reveal a tender mass; sigmoidoscopy characteristically shows extrinsic narrowing of the colonic lumen and inflamed mucosa. Barium enema, which is hazardous during the acute phase, generally confirms the presence of an inflammatory mass and often shows leakage of barium beyond the lumen of a diverticulum. The acute illness is treated by withholding solid food and by the use of broad-spectrum antibiotics. Surgical treatment may be required acutely for perforation, fistula formation, or a large abscess and electively for recurrent attacks of diverticulitis, especially when these result in fibrosis and obstruction. Many physicians recommend high-fiber diets to promote regular daily bowel movements and to reduce colonic intraluminal pressures in an attempt to prevent the progression of diverticulosis and the recurrence of diverticulitis.

REFERENCES

Cello JP, Schneiderman DJ: Ulcerative colitis. *In* Sleisenger MH, Fordtran JS (eds): Gastrointestinal Disease. 4th ed. Philadelphia, WB Saunders Co, 1989, pp 1435–1477.

Danzi, JT: Extraintestinal manifestations of idiopathic inflammatory bowel disease. Arch Intern Med 148:297, 1988.

Donaldson RM Jr: Crohn's disease. *In* Sleisenger MH, Fordtran JS (eds): Gastrointestinal Disease. 4th ed. Philadelphia, WB Saunders Co, 1989, p 1327.

Grendell JH, Ockner RK: Vascular diseases of the bowel. *In* Sleisenger MH, Fordtran JS (eds): Gastrointestinal Disease. 4th ed. Philadelphia, WB Saunders Co, 1989, p 1903.

Kirsner JB, Shorter RG: Inflammatory Bowel Disease. 3rd ed. Philadelphia, Lea and Febiger, 1988.

Rosenberg IH, Levin B: Inflammatory bowel disease. *In* Wyngaarden JB, Smith LH Jr (eds): Cecil Textbook of Medicine. 18th ed. Philadelphia, WB Saunders Co, 1988, p 745.

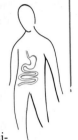

39

NEOPLASMS OF THE GASTROINTESTINAL TRACT

Neoplasms of the gastrointestinal tract are among the most common and important malignant tumors. Only the most important tumors will be discussed in this chapter. Tumors of the pancreas and of the liver are described in the chapters devoted to those organs.

CARCINOMA OF THE ESOPHAGUS

Tumors of the esophagus are usually malignant squamous cell carcinomas; less than 10 per cent are benign (most frequently leiomyomas). Adenocarcinomas account for about 5 per cent; all other malignant lesions are exceedingly rare.

Incidence

The incidence of esophageal carcinoma in white men is about 5 per 100,000, about three times that in white women. It is about four times higher in blacks and more than 30 times higher in certain other parts of the world (North China, Caspian Sea area).

Etiology and Pathogenesis

The cause of carcinoma of the esophagus is not known, but there are certain important associations. The incidence varies widely geographically, as noted above, but the presumed environmental factors have not been established with certainty. The incidence of esophageal carcinoma is increased in those who smoke or drink alcohol to excess and in those who have or have had squamous cell tumors of the head and neck. Injury due to lye ingestion, irradiation, or long-term stasis (usually achalasia) increases the incidence. Adenocarcinoma is strongly associated with columnar (Barrett's) epithelium, a complication of long-term gastric reflux. A rare inherited disorder with thickened skin in the palms and soles (tylosis) and gluten-sensitive enteropathy are both associated through unknown mechanisms with an increased incidence of esophageal carcinoma.

Clinical Manifestations

Dysphagia is the most frequent and important symptom of esophageal carcinoma (see Chapter 36). This symptom usually begins with difficulty in swallowing solids and then progresses steadily over six to nine months to involve liquids as well. *Anorexia* and *weight loss* commonly occur simultaneously. Regurgitation and aspiration may lead to coughing after swallowing fluids or to recurrent episodes of bronchopneumonia.

Substernal pain usually follows dysphagia and most frequently reflects extension of the tumor into mediastinal structures. These tumors rarely bleed briskly (about 5 per cent) but may result in slow, steady blood loss. With extension of the tumor the recurrent laryngeal nerve may be involved, resulting in hoarseness. Nail clubbing may occur, and very rarely paraneoplastic endocrine abnormalities (hypercalcemia, Cushing's syndrome) have been described.

Complications

A number of the clinical manifestations are in effect complications of the disease, such as pain, aspiration pneumonia, and bleeding. Esophagotracheal or esophagobronchial fistulas may occur, resulting in more frequent episodes of pulmonary infection. Metastases are most frequently to regional nodes, the liver, and the lung.

Diagnosis

Dysphagia occurring in anyone over the age of 40 must be assumed to be secondary to carcinoma of the esophagus until proved otherwise. The diagnosis depends on biopsy of a suspicious lesion or on cytological examination. An esophagogram, preferably a double-contrast study, is usually the first step in the evaluation of a patient suspected of having an esophageal carcinoma. If a suspicious area is noted, fiberoptic esophagoscopy is then carried out in order to obtain a number of biopsy specimens from deep within the abnormal area, sometimes supplemented by brush cytology specimens. The distinction between a tumor and a benign stricture can be very difficult to make on radiographic grounds alone, so that esophagoscopy should be carried out in most cases.

CT of the chest is very useful in delineating the extent of the tumor and its mediastinal spread, as part of staging. Ultrasound or CT scans of the liver are indicated as well as part of staging if the diagnosis has been established.

Treatment and Prognosis

Unfortunately esophageal tumors spread and metastasize early; not more than 25 per cent are surgically resectable at the time of diagnosis. The results of surgery, which is usually carried out only for carcinomas of the lower two thirds of the esophagus, are highly unsatisfactory for cure. There is an operative hospital mortality of about 10 to 15 per cent, and only about 5 per cent survive for five years. On the other hand, resection with reanastomosis often gives considerable palliation from dysphagia, pain, and aspiration. Tumors of the upper middle third of the esophagus are most frequently treated for palliation by irradiation using about 6000 rads. Symptomatic relief can often be obtained by dilating a malignant stricture, by placing a plastic prosthetic tube across the site of obstruction, or by coagulation of the tumor using a laser or heat.

CARCINOMA OF THE STOMACH

Most tumors of the stomach are adenocarcinomas. Only about 5 per cent are primary lymphomas of the stomach, and other malignant lesions (e.g., leiomyosarcoma) are rarer still. Since the clinical characteristics and diagnostic measures are similar for all malignant tumors of the stomach, this chapter will focus on adenocarcinoma. Benign tumors (e.g., leiomyomas and adenomas) are rarely the cause of symptoms, most often being found incidentally.

Incidence

The incidence of gastric carcinoma in the United States (now about 20,000 cases annually) has declined dramatically for unknown reasons during the past 30 to 40 years from being the single most common malignant disease to its current rank of approximately seventh. Similar but lesser declines have occurred in Western European and in other Anglo-Saxon countries, but the incidence remains very high in some parts of the world, especially in Japan, certain parts of

South America, and Eastern Europe. When population groups emigrate from areas of high incidence to those of low incidence, they tend to attain over several generations the usual rates found in their new environment. An interesting inverse relationship has been noted between the incidence of carcinoma of the stomach and carcinoma of the colon in population groups.

Etiology and Pathogenesis

Because of the marked geographical differences in the incidence of gastric carcinoma cited above, together with the change in incidence in migrant populations, it is assumed that there are important environmental factors in the etiology of this disease, but none has been clearly demonstrated. Some association patterns can be described however (Table 39–1). Gastric cancer is more common in men than women, blacks than whites, those with a positive family history, those with blood group A, and those of a lower socioeconomic status. Diet is thought to be an important determinant of risk, possibly relating to high nitrate and salt content. Nitrates can be reduced to nitrites by bacterial action (perhaps more readily in achlorhydric stomachs, since more bacteria are present), which in turn can react with a number of amines to form nitroso compounds. The latter have been demonstrated to be gastric carcinogens in animals. Gastric cancer seems to have a positive association with a diet high in salted fish and meat and pickled vegetables and a negative association with ascorbic acid and fresh vegetables. It is increased in patients with atrophic gastritis (with or without pernicious anemia) and with large (>2 cm) gastric polyps, and after partial gastrectomy for peptic ulcer disease. None of these factors can be clearly related to the decreasing incidence of gastric cancer in the United States cited above.

Pathology

Adenocarcinomas of the stomach derive from mucous cells, not from parietal or chief cells. Subtypes have been described related to differentiation and characteristics of growth and spread: the *intestinal type* (resembling colonic carcinoma) has a better prognosis than the *diffuse type*; the *expanding type* (cells maintaining a close relationship) has a better prognosis than the *infiltrative type*. The tumors are most frequently found in the distal third of the stomach and may be exophytic (with or without a stalk), diffusely infiltrative throughout the stomach (sometimes termed linitis plastica), or ulcerated.

Clinical Manifestations (Table 39–1)

Gastric carcinoma usually presents with nonspecific symptoms and signs. *Epigastric pain* is highly variable. In about one quarter of patients it may resemble the pain of peptic ulcer. More frequently it is a dull epigastric discomfort that may be exacerbated rather than relieved by food and may be associated with *nausea* and *early satiety*. Almost all patients have *anorexia* and *weight loss*. *Vomiting* may be prominent, especially with distal tumors leading to pyloric obstruction. Tumors arising in the cardia may infiltrate into the gastroesophageal junction and cause *dysphagia*. The tumors commonly bleed, producing iron deficiency anemia and more rarely hematemesis with corresponding symptoms of weakness, fatigue, and shortness of breath. More rarely the patient may present when symptoms and signs relating to metastases, direct extension, or paraneoplastic syndromes are prominent. These include, for example, obstructive jaundice, malignant ascites, a gastrocolic fistula, Trousseau's syndrome (thrombophlebitis), dermatomyositis, and acanthosis nigricans.

Physical examination may reveal an epigastric mass, evidence of one or more of the complications noted above, or other evidence of metastasis, such as a left supraclavicular Virchow's node, a Blumer's shelf (a mass in the perirectal pouch), or Krukenberg tumors (metastases to the ovaries) on pelvic examination.

Diagnosis

The first diagnostic study in a patient with the symptoms noted above is usually a radiographic examination of the stomach, preferably using a double-contrast technique and multiple projections for adequate demonstration of mucosal detail. The radiographic appearance of the tumor may vary considerably, from an ulcerated or nonulcerated exophytic mass to simply a thickened, nondistensible gastric wall. There are certain characteristics that suggest malignancy in an ulcer—an irregular ulcer base, an ulcer within a mass, the type of convergent folds—but the true differentiation can be made only by biopsy.

Endoscopic examination with multiple biopsies of a suspicious area is now the standard means of diagnosing carcinoma of the stomach. This should be supplemented with brush cytology obtained at the time of endoscopy, since cytology will sometimes (about 15 per cent) be positive even when the biopsy specimens do not reveal carcinoma. No other laboratory studies are diagnostic.

Treatment and Prognosis

Surgery offers the only chance for cure of gastric cancer, but it is a rare chance. After the diagnosis is established, staging must be carried out to determine insofar as possible if there is distant spread or local spread (beyond the wall of the stomach but confined to adjacent nodes) or whether the tumor seems to be confined to the stomach. This staging is usually carried out by biopsy of suspected nodes, liver function tests, and scans, ultrasonography, and increasingly by CT of the abdomen. Occasionally laparoscopy and biopsy are indicated. If distant spread is found, surgery should be confined to palliative procedures, usually for obstruction. If the tumor is localized, subtotal gastrectomy is usually carried out for tumors of the distal or middle third and total gastrectomy for the proximal third. In either case extensive resection of regional lymphatics is indicated. Less than 10 per cent of patients with gastric carcinoma survive for 5 years.

TABLE 39–1. ADENOCARCINOMA OF THE STOMACH

ASSOCIATED WITH	CLINICAL MANIFESTATIONS
Environment—geographical differences	Anorexia, early satiety, weight loss
Diet—? nitrosamines	Dysphagia, vomiting, weakness
Blood group A	Epigastric distress to severe, boring pain
Atrophic gastritis	Anemia, occult blood in stools
Adenomatous polyps (>2 cm)	Epigastric mass, signs of metastases
Subtotal resection for benign ulcer disease	Rare—Virchow's node, Blumer's shelf, Trousseau's syndrome, acanthosis nigricans

Irradiation of gastric carcinoma is generally unsatisfactory and has been palliative at best. A number of chemotherapeutic programs have been tried with very modest effects, if any, on survival.

CARCINOMA OF THE COLON

Adenocarcinoma is the most important malignant disease of the large bowel and will be considered to include rectal cancer as well for purposes of discussion. Other tumors of the large bowel, other than polyps (to be discussed subsequently), are much rarer and will not be considered here.

Incidence

Carcinoma of the large bowel is the third most common cancer in the United States (after carcinoma of the lung and breast) and is second in frequency in both men and women. Approximately 145,000 new cases are diagnosed annually, accounting for about 15 per cent of all malignant tumors in both men and women. The incidence is much higher in North America, Western Europe, Australia, and New Zealand than in Japan, South America, or Africa. Population groups that emigrate tend to acquire the risk characteristic of their new environment.

Etiology and Pathogenesis

The cause of colonic cancer is not known, but there are certain interesting associations. The geographical differences in incidence noted above, together with shifts in incidence in migrant groups, strongly suggest environmental factors. Particular attention has been directed to diet, since the incidence seems to be greater in those whose diet is low in fiber but high in animal fat and protein, perhaps particularly that derived from beef. It is thought that the type of colonic flora associated with such a diet may produce carcinogens that are in contact with colonic mucosa for longer periods of time due to the prolonged colonic transit times of low-fiber diets. These speculations,

TABLE 39–2. RISK FACTORS FOR CARCINOMA OF THE COLON

Increasing age
Inflammatory bowel disease
Personal history of colonic cancer or adenoma
Family history of colon cancer
Familial polyposis syndromes (adenomatous polyps)
History of breast or female genital cancer
Peutz-Jeghers syndrome (hamartomas)
Acromegaly

and those concerning the possible protective effect of dietary selenium, ascorbic acid, and alpha-tocopherol, await confirmation.

In addition to these possible environmental factors within populations, a number of risk factors are known for the individual (Table 39–2). The risk of colorectal carcinoma begins to increase around age 40 and roughly doubles for each succeeding decade. A number of conditions associated with increased mucosal cell turnover may lead to increased risk, e.g., inflammatory bowel disease, especially ulcerative colitis (see Chapter 38), and certain familial polyposis syndromes (to be discussed subsequently). A history of previous cancer or adenoma of the colon, a history of colon cancer in a first-degree relative, and the "family cancer

syndrome" (multifocal cancers in other organs, especially the female sex organs, as well as the colon) carry increased risk for carcinoma of the colon as well. There is increasing evidence that activation of an oncogene may be of key importance in the origin of colorectal tumors.

Pathology

Adenocarcinomas of the colon vary considerably in histological appearance (scirrhous, papillary, medullary, or colloid), but the prognosis relates to the degree of invasion of the wall or spread at the time of discovery rather than the pathological description. The distribution of tumors in the colon (Fig. 39–1) is predominantly left-sided, with fully 50 per cent being within reach of a sigmoidoscope, although there seems to be an increasing tendency for tumors to be found more proximally in the colon.

Clinical Manifestations

The early symptoms of carcinoma of the colon are often mild and nonspecific, especially with tumors in the area of the cecum or ascending colon where obstruction is rare and where blood that is lost is well mixed with feces and therefore less apparent. *A change in bowel habits*, especially with left-sided lesions, may be the first symptoms. This can be diarrhea, constipation, alternation of diarrhea and constipation, a change in the caliber of the stool, or tenesmus. *Pain* with left-sided tumors usually results from partial obstruction, but pain with right-sided tumors may represent invasion of the colonic wall or adjacent structures. *Hematochezia* is common, as is constant occult bleeding, leading to iron deficiency *anemia* with its associated symptoms of weakness, fatigability, and shortness of breath. The generalized symptoms of many malignancies—weight loss, anorexia, and malaise—are usually present late in the illness. Rarely patients may present with peritonitis due to tumor invasion and perforation of the colonic wall or with complications from metastases such as jaundice or ascites.

Diagnosis

Carcinoma of the bowel must be suspected in any patient over age 40 who presents with change of bowel habits or in the caliber of stools, ill-defined abdominal pain, hematochezia, or iron deficiency anemia. Bright red blood on the stools should not be attributed to hemorrhoids or diverticulosis until malignancy has been carefully excluded. If the patient has any of the special risk factors listed in Table 39–2, the threshold for suspicion is further lowered. Even in the absence of such symptoms or findings, careful testing of stools for occult blood (using the Hemoccult test, for example) may pick up early malignant lesions.

Diagnostic studies usually start with a careful digital rectal examination followed by proctoscopy or sigmoidoscopy, since radiographic studies are often not satisfactory for the rectum or lower sigmoid. If no lesion is found, a double-contrast barium enema is performed after careful bowel cleansing. If a suspicious lesion is noted, or indeed even if the study is normal

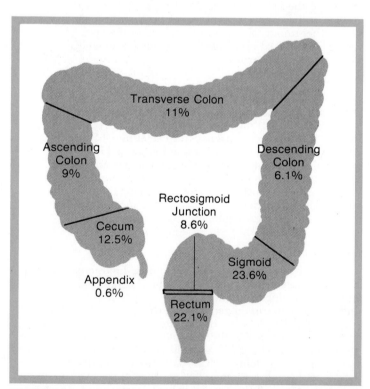

FIGURE 39–1. Distribution of large bowel cancer by anatomical segment according to the third national cancer survey (segment unspecified). (From Shottenfeld D, Fraumeni J Jr [eds]: Cancer Epidemiology and Prevention. Philadelphia, WB Saunders Co, 1982, pp 703–727.)

and the suspicion is high, colonoscopy is performed with multiple biopsies and brush cytological preparations from abnormal sites. These combined studies are successful in the detection of the vast majority of carcinomas of the colon. Measurement of carcinoembryonic antigen (CEA) is not useful in diagnosis but may be of value in following a patient after resection of a tumor, as a rise in CEA may then herald recurrence.

The differential diagnosis includes a large number of diseases associated with any of the above symptoms, particularly diverticulitis, ischemic colitis, angiodysplasia, inflammatory bowel disease, and benign polyps.

Treatment and Prognosis

The only effective treatment is surgical removal of the tumor and the adjacent colon and mesentery. Hemicolectomy is usually performed for right-sided and left-sided tumors; anterior resection with anastomosis to the rectal stump for sigmoid or upper rectal tumors; and a combined abdominal-perineal resection with a permanent colostomy for lesions within 5 cm of the anal verge. Surgery may also be indicated for palliation even in the presence of obvious metastatic disease when there is obstruction, perforation, or hemorrhage. Radiation therapy is used most frequently for pelvic recurrences or painful metastases, particularly in bone and sometimes in liver. Chemotherapy, usually with 5-fluorouracil, has been used in the treatment of hepatic metastases, but with only modest success.

The results of the surgical treatment of early carcinoma of the large bowel are excellent, with 80 to 90 per cent 10-year survival for mucosal lesions, 60 to 80 per cent with bowel wall invasion, and as high as 50 to 60 per cent even when regional nodes are involved. Postoperatively each patient must be followed closely for recurrence using colonoscopy, radiographic procedures, and measurements of CEA in a regular schedule over many years.

Screening and Prevention

The process of colonic carcinogenesis probably evolves over years. Neoplastic polyps and early localized carcinomas can be resected readily with excellent long-term results. There is therefore considerable interest in screening certain populations for colonic polyps and carcinomas using annual testing for occult fecal blood and periodic (every three to five years) proctosigmoidoscopy beginning at age 40 to 50. The finding of occult blood in the stool should be followed up rigorously with radiological or endoscopic examination of the entire colon. There is still some debate about the cost effectiveness of this approach in the general population. Quite clearly, however, individuals known to be at high risk for developing carcinoma of the colon (familial polyposis syndrome, prior colonic polyp or cancer, long-standing ulcerative colitis) should be screened, but may require other methods such as colonoscopy.

POLYPS OF THE GASTROINTESTINAL TRACT

A polyp, a mass of tissue that arises from the surface and extends into the lumen of the gastrointestinal tract, usually represents an overgrowth of epithelial cells. Polyps can be single or multiple, sporadic or familial, pedunculated (on a stalk) or sessile (flat based), neoplastic or non-neoplastic, as well as benign or malignant. They can also occur virtually anywhere in the gastrointestinal tract. The polyps of greatest importance, however, are those found in the colon, so these will receive primary attention. A simplified classification of colonic polyps is given in Table 39–3. Only the neoplastic polyps and those benign polyps associated with the familial polyposis syndromes will be discussed here.

Incidence

Colonic adenomatous polyps, usually less than 1 cm in diameter, are very common and are found with increased frequency with age. After the age of 65, for example, two thirds of individuals will have at least one polyp. Patients with one demonstrated polyp have a considerably enhanced chance of having another coincident one or of developing an additional polyp subsequently.

Etiology and Pathogenesis

Nothing is known directly about the cause of colonic polyps other than the role of inheritance in the familial polyposis syndromes to be noted later. There is considerable evidence, albeit most of it indirect, that most if not all carcinomas of the colon derive from previously benign polyps, most commonly after at least 10 to 15 years. If this is so, one would expect that the risk factors that have been defined for colonic carcinoma (Table 39–2) might also prove to pertain to benign polyps as well. Clearly only a very small percentage of benign polyps progress to malignancy, although the definite existence of this potential usually makes it advisable to remove any demonstrated colonic adenomatous polyp.

Clinical Manifestations

As might be expected from lesions that vary so widely in size, shape, number, and location, the as-

TABLE 39–3. POLYPS OF THE COLON

Neoplastic Polyps
  Benign adenomatous polyps (tubular, mixed, or villous)
    random occurrence
    familial—familial polyposis of the colon, Gardner syndrome (Fig. 39–2), Turcot's syndrome, cancer family syndrome
  Malignant polyps—carcinomatous changes, in situ or invasive
Non-neoplastic Polyps
  Inflammatory "pseudopolyps"
  Peutz-Jeghers syndrome—hamartomas
  Mucosal polyps with normal epithelium
  Juvenile polyps

sociated clinical manifestations are diverse. In fact most polyps cause no symptoms and are found incidentally at autopsy or on radiographic or colonoscopic studies done for other purposes. The most frequent abnormalities are those of *bleeding* (hematochezia, anemia) or more rarely *abdominal pain*, if the polyp is large enough to obstruct the bowel partially. With large polyps patients may note a *change in bowel habits* with diarrhea or constipation. Very rarely large villous adenomas may produce *watery diarrhea* containing enough potassium to produce significant hypokalemia.

Diagnosis

The diagnosis of a colonic polyp is readily made with use of a double-contrast barium enema, or even more effectively by colonoscopy. The nature of the polyp is usually documented by excisional biopsy.

Treatment

Although only a few polyps in the colon undergo malignant transformation, a polyp that has been discovered should usually be removed. Fortunately this can now be readily accomplished in most patients with polyps by colonoscopic polypectomy. Large sessile polyps may require surgery, especially if the suspicion

of malignancy is high. Patients who have required polypectomy should be closely followed (colonoscopy or double-contrast barium enema every two to three years) in order to detect the development of new polyps.

THE FAMILIAL POLYPOSIS SYNDROMES

The familial polyposis syndromes are rare, dominantly transmitted disorders in which multiple polyps are found within the gastrointestinal tract (Table 39–3). Some of the best delineated syndromes will be described briefly here.

Familial Polyposis of the Colon

In this rare genetic disorder (1 in 8000 births) multiple adenomatous polyps develop gradually during childhood such that they characteristically carpet the entire colon. An association with activation of certain human oncogenes has been reported. More than 1000 grossly visible polyps may form with many other nascent polyps demonstrable microscopically. Very rarely the ileum may be involved as well. The symptoms are those of bleeding and diarrhea, but the main clinical

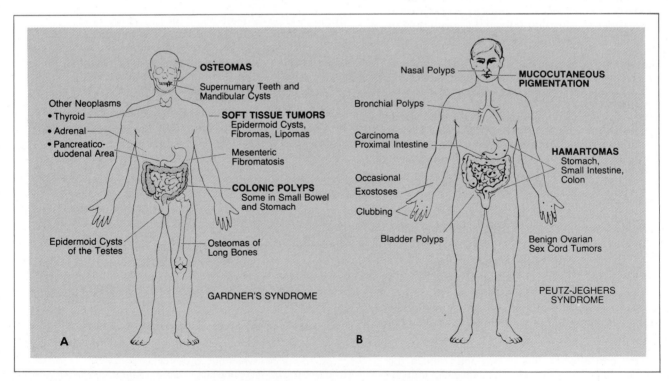

FIGURE 39–2. *A*, Schematic representation of Gardner's syndrome. The triad of colonic polyposis, bone tumors, and soft tissue tumors (heavy print) are the primary features; other features are indicated in lighter print. *B*, Schematic presentation of the Peutz-Jeghers syndrome. Mucocutaneous pigmentation and benign gastrointestinal polyposis (heavy print) are the primary features of this syndrome. Lighter print shows the secondary features. (From Boland CR, Kim YS: *In* Sleisenger MH, Fordtran JS [eds]: Gastrointestinal Disease. 3rd ed. Philadelphia, WB Saunders Co, 1983.)

consequence is that of the virtual 100 per cent occurrence of carcinoma of the colon by age 40. When the diagnosis of familial polyposis is made, therefore, elective complete colectomy is required (usually after full growth has been attained). Because of its dominant transmission, other members of the family must be carefully surveyed.

Gardner's Syndrome

This rare entity resembles familial polyposis of the colon with certain other associated features, especially osteomas and benign soft-tissue tumors (see Fig. 39–2 for illustration of the complete syndrome). The stomach and small bowel (especially the duodenum) may also be involved. Because of the malignant potential of the colonic polyps, total colectomy is indicated.

Peutz-Jeghers Syndrome

In this familial disorder the polyps are more generally distributed throughout the gastrointestinal tract and are associated with characteristic mucocutaneous pigmentation, especially in the buccal mucosa, the lips, the soles of the feet, and the dorsum of the hands (Fig. 39–2). The polyps are hamartomas rather than adenomas and therefore have a much lower incidence of neoplastic transformation, although this complication may occur, especially in the small intestine. Surgery is usually indicated only for complications from the polyps—bleeding, pain, or obstruction.

REFERENCES

Boland CR, Itzkowitz SH, Kim YS: Colonic polyps and the gastrointestinal polyposis syndromes. *In* Sleisenger MH, Fordtran JS (eds): Gastrointestinal Disease. 4th ed. Philadelphia, WB Saunders Co, 1989, pp 1483–1518.
Boyce HW Jr: Tumors (of the esophagus). *In* Sleisenger MH, Fordtran JS (eds): Gastrointestinal Disease. 4th ed. Philadelphia, WB Saunders Co, 1989, pp 619–631.
Davis GR: Neoplasms of the stomach. *In* Sleisenger MH, Fordtran JS (eds): Gastrointestinal Disease. 4th ed. Philadelphia, WB Saunders Co, 1989, pp 745–771.
Vogelstein B, Fearon ER, Hamilton SR, et al: Genetic alterations during colorectal-tumor development. N Engl J Med 319:525, 1988.
Winawer SJ: Neoplasms of the large and small intestine. *In* Wyngaarden JB, Smith LH Jr (eds): Cecil Textbook of Medicine. 18th ed. Philadelphia, WB Saunders Co, 1988, p 766.
Winawer SJ: Neoplasms of the stomach. *In* Wyngaarden JB, Smith LH Jr (eds): Cecil Textbook of Medicine. 18th ed. Philadelphia, WB Saunders Co, 1988, p 709.
Bresalier RS, Kim YS: Malignant neoplasms of the large and small intestine. *In* Sleisenger MH, Fordtran JS (eds): Gastrointestinal Disease. 4th ed. Philadelphia, WB Saunders Co, 1989, pp 1519–1560.

40

THE PANCREAS

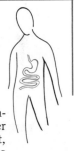

NORMAL STRUCTURE AND FUNCTION

The pancreas is a relatively small (70 to 110 gm) but versatile organ containing two specific and seemingly independent components: (a) *the endocrine pancreas* and (b) *the exocrine pancreas*. The endocrine pancreas consists of the islets of Langerhans, packets of endocrine cells peppered randomly throughout the pancreas that secrete insulin, glucagon, and other polypeptide hormones. The endocrine pancreas will be discussed in other chapters and will not be considered further here. The cells of the exocrine pancreas cluster into acini that are further grouped in lobules. Acinar cells are drained by ductules that converge into ducts of increasing size, terminating in the duct of Wirsung, which drains through the sphincter of Oddi and the papilla of Vater into the second portion of the duodenum. The head of the pancreas lies within the curvature of the duodenum, and the body and tail extend for about 12 to 15 cm retroperitoneally toward the hilum of the spleen (Fig. 40–1). The head of the pancreas is in close anatomical relationship with a number of vital structures, including the common bile duct, the inferior vena cava, the aorta and the origin of the superior mesenteric artery, the splenic artery and vein, and the right adrenal gland and kidney.

The normal pancreas secretes a large volume (up to 1500 ml per day) of a distinctive fluid.

Electrolyte Composition. Acinar cells secrete fluid that resembles extracellular fluid: ductular cells progressively add a bicarbonate-rich liquid so that the relative amount of bicarbonate increases and may reach as high as 120 mEq/L. Pancreatic bicarbonate is an important factor in neutralizing gastric acid in the duodenal bulb.

Protein Content. Pancreatic fluid is protein-rich, more than 90 per cent of which represents enzymes or proenzymes secreted by acinar cells: (1) active form—lipase, amylase, and ribonuclease, and (2) inactive form—proteases and phospholipase. The inactive proenzymes are activated in cascade fashion in

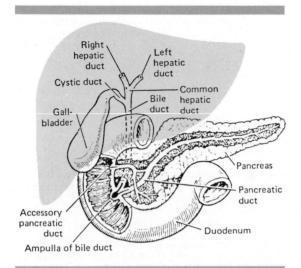

FIGURE 40–1. Connections of the ducts of the gallbladder, liver, and pancreas. (Reproduced, with permission, from Bell GH, Emslie-Smith D, Paterson CR: Textbook of Physiology and Biochemistry. 9th ed. Edinburgh, Churchill Livingstone, 1976.)

the gut: enterokinase converts trypsinogen to trypsin; trypsin then activates all of the other proenzymes. Other proteins in pancreatic juice are colipase, which binds to and enhances lipase activity, and trypsin inhibitors.

Control of Secretion. The small basal secretion of the exocrine pancreas is stimulated by a variety of factors, the relative importance of which is unknown. Most pancreatic secretion occurs postprandially in response to one or more of three stimuli: (1) *Hormones.* Two hormones seem most important and potentiate each other: secretin, which stimulates ductular cells to increase water and bicarbonate; cholecystokinin

(CCK), which stimulates acinar cells to secrete enzymes and proenzymes. (2) *Cephalic stimulation.* Vagal, cholinergic pathways stimulate an increase in enzyme-rich fluid. (3) *Enteropancreatic cholinergic reflex pathways.* The role of pancreatic fluid in digestion is further considered in the chapter on Malabsorption (Chapter 34C).

Studies of Pancreatic Structure and Function

The pancreas until recently was frustratingly difficult to study in the presence of suspected disease. It can now be successfully imaged noninvasively by ultrasonography and computed tomography (CT) (Fig. 40–2) and invasively by endoscopic retrograde cholangiopancreatography (ERCP). Biopsy by fine needle with ultrasound or CT guidance and selective angiography are also useful in selected cases, and imaging by nuclear magnetic resonance (MRI) is proving to be increasingly useful.

Acute injury to the pancreatic acini is reflected by leakage of the enzyme amylase into blood, which can be measured as an increase in serum amylase or more rarely as urinary amylase. Normal serum amylase (25 to 125 U/L) largely originates in salivary glands (about two thirds). In addition to the pancreatic isozyme of amylase, lipase and trypsinogen are also released into the plasma during pancreatic injury. Pancreatic secretion is estimated, by aspiration of duodenal contents through a tube following stimulation with secretin, secretin-CCK, or a test meal, as summarized in Table 40–1. The bentiromide test, which measures the intraintestinal hydrolyses of a synthetic peptide by pancreatic chymotrypsin, is described in Chapter 34C on malabsorption. Such quantitative studies of secretion are occasionally needed to determine the presence or absence of pancreatic exocrine insufficiency.

TABLE 40–1. RANGE OF NORMAL RESPONSES TO SECRETORY TESTS OF THE PANCREAS

Secretin test*
   Volume (ml/80 min): 117–392
   HCO_3^- concentration (mEq/L): 88–137
   HCO_3^- output (mEq/80 min): 16–33
   Amylase output (units/80 min): 439–1921
Secretin + CCK*
   Volume (ml/80 min): 111–503
   HCO_3^- concentration (mEq/L): 88–144
   HCO_3^- output (mEq/80 min): 10–86
   Amylase output (units/80 min): 441–4038
Lundh Test
   Mean tryptic activity (IU/L): 61
Bentiromide test
   Excretion of arylamine in urine >57% in 6 hours of that administered in the test dose of the synthetic peptide

* Modified from Dreiling DA, Janowitz HD, Perrier CV: Pancreatic Inflammatory Disease. A Physiologic Approach. New York, Hoeber Medical Division, Harper & Row, Publishers, 1964.

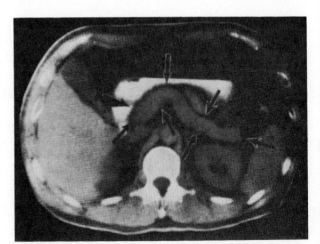

FIGURE 40–2. Normal pancreas demonstrated by computed tomography. (Courtesy of Dr. Eugene P. DiMagno, Mayo Medical School, Rochester, Minnesota.) (Reprinted from Grendell JH: The pancreas. *In* Smith LH Jr, Thier SO [eds]: Pathophysiology: The Biological Principles of Disease. 2nd ed. Philadelphia, WB Saunders Co, 1985, p 1225.)

ACUTE PANCREATITIS

Definition. Acute pancreatitis is an acute, inflammatory disorder of the pancreas associated with edema, swelling, and various amounts of autodigestion, necrosis, and hemorrhage. It is usually defined clinically by a symptom complex with an associated elevation of serum amylase. It is useful to consider acute pancreatitis as a single clinical entity, although it may be of diverse etiologies, may vary greatly in severity, and may shade into chronic relapsing pancreatitis and chronic pancreatitis (to be considered subsequently).

Etiology and Pathogenesis. The disorders most commonly associated with acute pancreatitis in the United States are listed in Table 40–2. Of these, alcoholism and biliary tract disease are the most important. The pathogenesis of acute pancreatitis is thought to be autodigestion due to inappropriate intrapancreatic activation of proteases (Fig. 40–3). Just why this occurs usually is unknown, although it is speculated that alcohol produces obstructive inspissated proteinaceous plugs in pancreatic ducts and that gallstones, passing through the sphincter of Oddi,

TABLE 40–2. RISK FACTORS IN ACUTE PANCREATITIS

Alcohol abuse
Gallstones
Abdominal trauma (including surgery)
Infections: mumps, coxsackie, hepatitis, other viruses
Hypertriglyceridemia
Hypercalcemia
Drugs: steroids, diuretics, isoniazid, immunosuppressives, sulfonamide
Cancer of the pancreas
Pancreas divisum (?)
Hereditary: (familial) pancreatitis
Posterior penetration of a duodenal ulcer
Endoscopic retrograde cholangiopancreatography (ERCP)
Very rare—ischemic vascular disease, systemic lupus erythematosus

Modified from Brooks FP: Diseases of the Exocrine Pancreas. Philadelphia, WB Saunders Co, 1980, p 8.

cause intermittent obstruction. Simply ligating the pancreatic duct does not usually cause acute pancreatitis, however, so that other unexplained factors are probably involved. Knowledge of the association of acute pancreatitis with the conditions listed in Table 40–2 is important for two reasons: (a) it suggests the possibility in a given patient, and (b) preventing re-

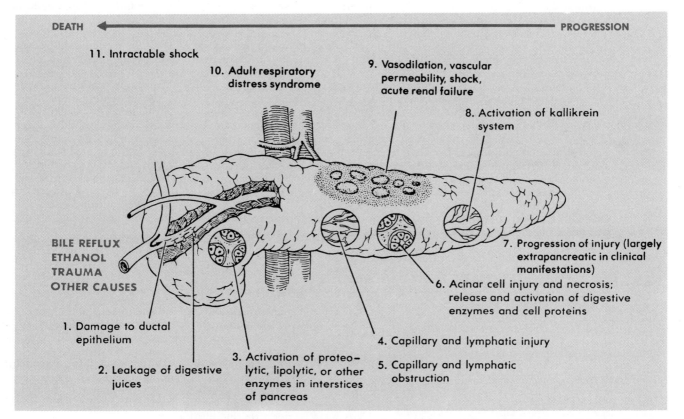

FIGURE 40–3. The pathophysiology of acute pancreatitis is not fully understood, but, as the schematic above implies, a cascade of events seems likely, beginning with the release of toxic substances into the parenchyma and ending with shock and death. Damage to the ductal epithelium or acinar cell injury may result from bile reflux, increased intraductal pressure, alcohol, or trauma. (Modified from Grendell JH: The pancreas. *In* Smith LH Jr, Thier SO [eds]: Pathophysiology: The Biological Principles of Disease. 2nd ed. Philadelphia, WB Saunders Co, 1985, p 1228.)

TABLE 40–3. SOME CONDITIONS OTHER THAN ACUTE PANCREATITIS THAT MAY BE ASSOCIATED WITH HYPERAMYLASEMIA

Macroamylasemia	Peptic ulcer
Diabetic ketoacidosis	Mesenteric infarction
Renal insufficiency	Parotitis, mumps
Burn injury	Opiate administration
Postoperative state	Cholecystitis

current pancreatitis often depends on reversal of these associated abnormalities.

Clinical Manifestations. The most important symptom of acute pancreatitis is abdominal *pain*, which is characteristically steady, severe, and epigastric in location with later radiation to the back and partially relieved by leaning forward. The pain is highly variable, however, and may be relatively mild or diffuse. The abdomen is usually tender, without signs of peritoneal irritation, and nausea and vomiting are absent. Severe cases distend the abdomen with ileus and produce high fever, confusion, tachycardia, and, sometimes, impending shock. Rarer features are (1) discoloration in the flanks (Grey-Turner's sign) or around the umbilicus (Cullen's sign) in hemorrhagic pancreatitis, (2) subcutaneous fat necrosis presenting as tender, red subcutaneous nodules, (3) ascites, (4) atelectasis and/or left-sided pleural effusion, (5) adult respiratory distress syndrome, (6) jaundice, and (7) an epigastric mass representing a pseudocyst.

Diagnosis. The diagnosis of acute pancreatitis must be entertained in any patient with the acute onset of severe, noncolicky epigastric pain, especially in the presence of one of the known associated disorders (Table 40–2). The differential diagnosis usually includes biliary colic, a perforated viscus (especially a duodenal ulcer), acute cholecystitis, abdominal vasculitis, acute bowel infarction, renal colic, and a number of other causes of "the acute abdomen."

Most patients with clinically defined acute pancreatitis have an enlarged pancreas as defined by ultrasonography and/or CT, but the diagnosis cannot be made without concomitant evidence of acinar cell injury as reflected in an elevation of serum amylase. Conversely, other causes of an elevated serum amylase must be considered also (Table 40–3). After the onset of symptoms serum amylase rises early (2 to 12 hours) and usually remains elevated for three to five days. Some believe that in the face of an elevated serum amylase, an associated increased renal clearance of amylase (amylase clearance >4 per cent of that of creatinine) is a useful indication of the presence of pancreatitis, but the test is not diagnostic. It is of greater use in indicating the presence of macroamylasemia.

Other laboratory abnormalities may include hyperglycemia, hypocalcemia, an increase in serum lipase, and leukocytosis.

Treatment and Prognosis. The treatment of acute pancreatitis is largely supportive: (1) careful monitoring and volume replacement for fluids lost retroperitoneally; (2) relief of pain, preferably using meperidine; (3) nasogastric suction—this traditional approach to "putting the pancreas at rest," however, will not affect outcome in mild to moderate cases; (4) treatment of complications as they arise—calcium for hypocalcemia, insulin for excessive hyperglycemia, etc. Other measures that have been advocated, including administration of cimetidine, aprotinin, and glucagon, appear to be without benefit.

About 90 per cent of patients recover, usually within one to two weeks. About 10 per cent die despite therapy, most frequently from the adult respiratory distress syndrome or from shock.

Complications. The complications most frequently seen in the course of acute pancreatitis are listed in Table 40–4. A phlegmon is a solid mass of inflamed pancreas, which usually subsides spontaneously. A pseudocyst is a liquefied collection of necrotic debris surrounded by a rim of pancreatic tissue and/or other tissue. Small pseudocysts may disappear, but large ones may persist to cause pain or bleeding, erode into adjacent tissues, or become infected, requiring surgical drainage. Pancreatic or peripancreatic abscess can be a serious complication and an occasional cause of death.

TABLE 40–4. COMPLICATIONS OF ACUTE PANCREATITIS

Pancreatic—phlegmon, pseudocyst, abscess, ascites, hemorrhage
Contiguous organs—portal venous thrombosis, bowel necrosis, intraperitoneal bleeding, obstruction of common duct
Systemic
  Cardiovascular—hypotension, nonspecific ST-T changes, pericardial effusion
  Pulmonary—pleural effusion, shock lung, atelectasis
  Renal—acute renal failure
  Gastrointestinal—gastritis
  Hematologic—disseminated intravascular coagulation
  Metabolic—hypocalcemia, hyperglycemia
  Fat necrosis—subcutaneous, bone
  Central nervous system—psychosis

Reprinted from Levitt MD: Pancreatitis. *In* Wyngaarden JB, Smith LH Jr (eds): Cecil Textbook of Medicine. 18th ed. Philadelphia, WB Saunders Co, 1988, p 778.

CHRONIC PANCREATITIS

Definition. Chronic pancreatitis and chronic relapsing pancreatitis can be considered together, since both represent a slowly progressive destruction of pancreatic acini, varying amounts of inflammation, fibrosis, and dilatation and distortion of the pancreatic ducts. In chronic relapsing pancreatitis there are associated episodes of acute inflammation. The end result is that of varying degrees of pancreatic destruction and exocrine insufficiency.

Etiology and Pathogenesis. By and large the same conditions listed in Table 40–2 as being associated with acute pancreatitis may also lead to chronic pancreatitis. Biliary tract disease, however, is rarely associated with chronic pancreatitis. In the United States the

TABLE 40–5. SYMPTOMS AND SIGNS OF CHRONIC PANCREATITIS

Abdominal pain	Jaundice
Weight loss	Palpable pseudocyst
Diabetes mellitus	Pancreatic ascites
Steatorrhea	Gastrointestinal bleeding

major associated conditions are alcoholism in adults and cystic fibrosis in children; in the developing countries the most common cause seems to be protein-calorie malnutrition. The cause is unknown in many cases. Injury is presumed to be secondary to auto-digestion, as in acute pancreatitis (Fig. 40–3), but this has not been established. Alcohol seems to lead to duct obstruction due to protein plugs.

Clinical Manifestations. The most important symptoms and signs of chronic pancreatitis are summarized in Table 40–5. In general, severe, intractable abdominal *pain* is the cardinal symptom, although pain may be mild or even absent in a minority of patients or episodic with relapsing pancreatitis. The pain may persist for some years before other manifestations such as pancreatic calcification, diabetes, and malabsorption appear. The pain may go through to the back, be partially relieved by sitting up and leaning forward, be exacerbated by eating or drinking alcohol, or exhibit none of these features. Patients usually lose weight because of anorexia and/or an associated malabsorption (steatorrhea and azotorrhea). Encasement of the common bile duct in fibrous tissue may produce obstructive jaundice. The islets of Langerhans often become sufficiently destroyed to produce diabetes mellitus. Gastrointestinal bleeding may rarely result from thrombosis of the splenic vein, leading to gastric varices, or more commonly from gastritis, resulting from the associated excessive use of ethanol or aspirin (in an attempt to relieve pain). Rarely, an abdominal mass representing a pseudocyst may be palpated.

Diagnosis. The diagnosis of chronic pancreatitis as a cause of pain is usually easy in the presence of the classic triad of pancreatic calcification, pancreatic exocrine deficiency (malabsorption), and diabetes mellitus, especially if any of the known risk factors are present. However, only a minority of patients present with this complete clinical picture. The differential diagnosis usually includes abdominal malignancy, especially carcinoma of the pancreas or of the stomach or colon. Biliary tract disease, peptic ulcer disease, mesenteric vascular disease, and functional abdominal complaints may occasionally simulate the pain of chronic pancreatitis.

Measurement of serum amylase is of no help in the diagnosis of chronic pancreatitis, since it is usually elevated only during acute exacerbations of chronic, relapsing pancreatitis. Three structural features may be of help: (1) the demonstration of pancreatic calcification by a plain abdominal radiograph or, with greater sensitivity, by CT; (2) the demonstration of dilated, distorted ducts, best shown by ERCP; (3) the demonstration of pseudocysts by ultrasonography and/or CT.

Malabsorption can be demonstrated by fecal analysis for fat, and its pancreatic origin can be deduced by the tests described in Chapter 34C. In chronic pancreatitis pancreatic stimulation tests characteristically show reductions in pancreatic juice volume, bicarbonate content, amylase output, and tryptic activity.

Treatment and Prognosis. The treatment of chronic pancreatitis is directed toward (1) prevention of further injury, (2) relief of pain, and (3) replacement of lost exocrine function. Prevention of further injury usually depends upon attempting to reverse one or more of the factors listed in Table 40–2, especially alcoholism. The replacement of lost exocrine function is described in Chapter 34C on Malabsorption. The treatment of pain is usually the most difficult and important challenge. There are three general approaches:

ANALGESICS. Attempts should be made to begin with nonaddictive analgesics before resorting to narcotics. The severity and duration of the pain may require narcotics with the attending dangers of addiction.

"PUTTING THE PANCREAS AT REST." The ingestion of large amounts of pancreatic enzymes may reduce pain, presumably by diminishing stimuli to its exocrine secretion. Avoiding large meals and alcohol also may help.

SURGICAL THERAPY. Surgery to relieve a ductal obstruction or drainage of a pseudocyst may be effective in selected cases of intractable pain, although the results are often unsatisfactory. Resection of the pancreas is occasionally performed.

Fortunately, the pain of chronic pancreatitis tends to diminish over time, presumably because of the destruction of most of the residual functioning exocrine cells. Patients seldom die of uncomplicated chronic pancreatitis.

Complications. The complications that may be associated with chronic pancreatitis are listed in Table 40–6. An increased incidence of carcinoma of the pancreas probably occurs only in rare forms of hereditary pancreatitis.

CARCINOMA OF THE PANCREAS

Definition. Carcinoma of the pancreas is an almost universally fatal malignancy, over 90 per cent representing an adenocarcinoma arising from ductal

TABLE 40–6. COMPLICATIONS OF CHRONIC PANCREATITIS

Pseudocyst formation	Peptic ulcer
Pancreatic abscess	Drug addiction
Obstruction of the common bile duct	Exocrine insufficiency
Diabetes mellitus	Carcinoma (rare)

cells. Much rarer are islet cell tumors (not discussed here), epidermoid tumors, or adenocarcinomas arising from acinar cells. Carcinoma of the pancreas seems to be increasing in incidence and is now the fourth most common malignant tumor (after tumors of the lung, colon, and breast), accounting for about 5 per cent of deaths from cancer.

Etiology and Pathogenesis. The cause of carcinoma of the pancreas is not known. Epidemiological studies have suggested the following risk factors: advancing age, smoking, diabetes mellitus, some forms of chronic pancreatitis, and certain dietary habits (increased consumption of animal fat and protein). A reported association with excessive consumption of coffee is unconfirmed.

Clinical Manifestations. The clinical manifestations tend to be nonspecific and are often insidious in onset, so that the malignancy reaches an advanced stage by the time diagnosis is made. The cardinal manifestations are *epigastric pain* and *weight loss*. The pain is usually persistent, dull, and noncolicky and may radiate to the back but can be individually variable. Anorexia, nausea, and vomiting occur frequently, sometimes in association with a strange aversion to meat. Emotional disturbances (anxiety, depression) have been described as occurring more frequently and earlier than in other malignancies. Obstructive jaundice results commonly from carcinoma of the head of the pancreas, sometimes in association with a large, palpable gallbladder. A number of other abnormalities can accompany the illness: migratory thrombophlebitis (Trousseau's sign), acute pancreatitis, diabetes mellitus, paraneoplastic endocrine syndromes (Cushing's syndrome, hypercalcemia), upper gastrointestinal bleeding (direct invasion of stomach or duodenum, involvement of the splenic vein with production of varices), or an abdominal mass. Rarely, with adenocarcinoma of acinar cells, fat necrosis may produce painful nodules subcutaneously or bone pain from intramedullary involvement.

Diagnosis. Carcinoma of the pancreas must be considered in older patients with unexplained abdominal pain, excessive weight loss, the sudden onset of diabetes mellitus without obesity or appropriate family history, acute pancreatitis without a known risk factor (Table 40–2), or obstructive jaundice. Laboratory studies, including the serum tumor markers carcinoembryonic antigen (CEA), α-fetoprotein (AFP), and galactosyltransferase isoenzyme II (GT-II), rarely help because of their nonspecificity.

The diagnosis is made most frequently by a combination of imaging and fine needle biopsy. Figure 40–4 provides an algorithm for using these modalities. The diagnostic sensitivity for carcinoma of the pancreas by these techniques is ultrasonography 70 to 90 per cent, CT approximately 80 per cent, and ERCP 75 to 85 per cent. Selective arteriography rarely may be required.

Treatment and Prognosis. The treatment of pancreatic carcinoma is inadequate and disappointing. Only about 10 to 20 per cent of tumors are resectable

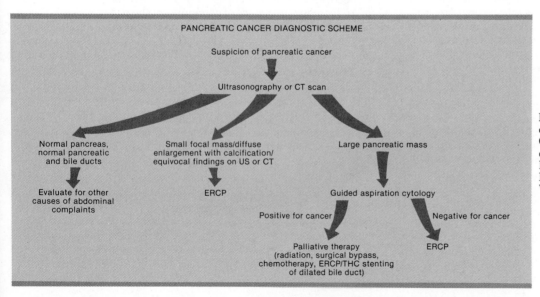

FIGURE 40–4. Pancreatic cancer diagnosis. (Reprinted from Cello JP: Carcinoma of the pancreas. *In* Wyngaarden JB, Smith LH Jr [eds]: Cecil Textbook of Medicine. 18th ed. Philadelphia, WB Saunders Co, 1988, p 783.)

at the time of diagnosis, and surgical treatment of even this group produces no demonstrated increase in five-year survival. Surgery is often confined to palliative decompression of the biliary system to relieve obstructive jaundice or severe pruritus or cholangitis. This can now be effected in many patients by percutaneous transhepatic stenting of the common bile duct with internal or external drainage. Stents may be placed also during ERCP. Supravoltage radiation or multidrug chemotherapeutic programs may somewhat palliate symptoms but do not prolong survival. Approximately 10 per cent of patients survive diagnosis by one year and only 1 to 2 per cent by five years.

Complications. The complications of pancreatic carcinoma have largely been listed as part of the clinical manifestations. In addition, there may be extensive local invasion of vital structures and metastases, especially to the liver.

REFERENCES

Cello JP: Carcinoma of the pancreas. *In* Sleisenger MH, Fordtran JS (eds): Gastrointestinal Disease. 4th ed. Philadelphia, WB Saunders Co, 1989, pp 1872–1884.

Cello JP: Carcinoma of the pancreas. *In* Wyngaarden JM, Smith LH Jr (eds): Cecil Textbook of Medicine. 18th ed. Philadelphia, WB Saunders Co, 1988, p 781.

Grendell JH, Cello JP: Chronic pancreatitis. *In* Sleisenger MH, Fordtran JS (eds): Gastrointestinal Disease. 4th ed. Philadelphia, WB Saunders Co, 1989, pp 1842–1872.

Levitt MD: Pancreatitis. *In* Wyngaarden JB, Smith LH Jr (eds): In Cecil Textbook of Medicine. 18th ed. Philadelphia, WB Saunders Co, 1988, p 774.

Soergel KH: Acute pancreatitis. *In* Sleisenger MH, Fordtran JS (eds): Gastrointestinal Disease. 4th ed. Philadelphia, WB Saunders Co, 1989, pp 1814–1842.

Van Dyke JA, Stanley RJ, Berland LL: Pancreatic imaging. Ann Intern Med 102:212, 1985.

SECTION

V

DISEASES OF THE LIVER AND BILIARY SYSTEM

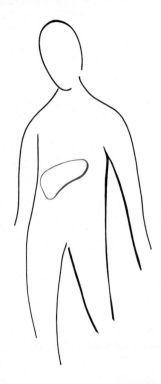

41

LABORATORY TESTS IN LIVERDISEASE

TABLE 41–1. CLINICAL MANIFESTATIONS OF LIVER DISEASE

SIGN/SYMPTOM	PATHOGENESIS	LIVER DISEASE
Constitutional		
Fatigue, anorexia, malaise, weight loss	Liver failure	Severe acute or chronic hepatitis Cirrhosis
Fever	Hepatic inflammation or infection	Liver abscess Alcoholic hepatitis Viral hepatitis
Fetor hepaticus	Sulfur compounds, produced by intestinal bacteria, not cleared by the liver	Acute or chronic liver failure
Cutaneous		
Spider telangiectasias, palmar erythema	Altered estrogen and androgen metabolism with altered vascular physiology	Cirrhosis
Jaundice	Diminished bilirubin excretion	Biliary obstruction Severe liver disease
Pruritus	Uncertain	Biliary obstruction
Xanthomas and xanthelasma	Increased serum cholesterol	Biliary obstruction/cholestasis
Endocrine		
Gynecomastia, testicular atrophy, diminished libido	Altered estrogen and androgen metabolism	Cirrhosis
Hypoglycemia	Decreased glycogen stores and gluconeogenesis	Acute liver failure Alcohol binge with fasting
Gastrointestinal		
Right upper quadrant abdominal pain	Liver swelling, infection	Acute hepatitis Hepatocellular carcinoma Liver congestion (heart failure) Acute cholecystitis Liver abscess
Abdominal swelling	Ascites	Cirrhosis, portal hypertension
Gastrointestinal bleeding	Esophageal varices	Portal hypertension
Hematological		
Decreased red cells, white cells, and/or platelets	Hypersplenism	Cirrhosis, portal hypertension
Ecchymoses	Decreased synthesis of clotting factors	Liver failure
Neurological		
Altered sleep pattern, subtle behavioral changes, somnolence, confusion, ataxia, asterixis, obtundation	Hepatic encephalopathy	Liver failure, portosystemic shunting of blood

The liver, the largest organ in the body, plays a central role in many essential physiological processes, including glucose homeostasis, plasma protein synthesis, lipid and lipoprotein synthesis, bile acid synthesis and secretion, and vitamin storage (B_{12}, A, D, E, and K), as well as biotransformation, detoxification, and excretion of a vast array of endogenous and exogenous compounds. The clinical manifestations of liver disease are, likewise, varied and may be quite subtle. Clues to the existence, severity, and etiology of liver disease may be obtained from a careful history and physical examination or by routine laboratory screening tests. Clinical clues to the presence of liver disease will be briefly mentioned here and are discussed more fully in other chapters. This chapter will focus on the use of laboratory tests in the evaluation of liver disease.

CLINICAL APPROACH TO LIVER DISEASE

Table 41–1 outlines useful clinical clues to the presence of liver disease that may be elicited from the history and physical examination. Other important information to be obtained includes a history of jaundice or liver disease in family members, recent travel, exposure to individuals or animals with liver or parasitic disease, sexual promiscuity, use of intravenous drugs, and exposure to alcohol, toxins, or drugs.

LABORATORY TESTS OF LIVER FUNCTION AND DISEASE

Unlike tests used to assess function of other organ systems (e.g., arterial blood gas, creatinine clearance), "liver function" tests often do not measure liver function, nor do they accurately reflect etiology or severity of a disease process. Nevertheless, if their limitations are understood, they can be very useful. In general, the tests currently available can be divided into two categories: (1) tests of hepatic function or capacity, and (2) screening tests that suggest the presence and/or type of liver disease. Specific diagnostic tests such as serological tests for hepatitis B infection are covered in other chapters.

TESTS OF HEPATIC FUNCTION

Although the liver performs a great variety of presumably testable functions, it has proved difficult to devise a test that is simple, cheap, reproducible, and noninvasive and that accurately reflects hepatic capacity for all functions. Instead, currently available tests of liver function are indirect, static measurements of serum levels of compounds that are synthesized, metabolized, and/or excreted by the liver. The liver has a large reserve capacity, and therefore "function" tests may remain relatively normal until liver dysfunction is severe. Table 41–2 outlines the most widely available and useful liver function tests. The serum albumin level and prothrombin time both reflect the hepatic capacity for protein synthesis. The prothrombin time responds rapidly to altered hepatic function because the serum half-lives of Factors II and VII are short (hours). In contrast, the serum half-life of albumin is 14 to 20 days, and serum levels fall only with prolonged liver dysfunction.

Serum bile acid levels, particularly when measured two hours after a meal, have proved to be the most sensitive test of liver disease, and this is due to the high efficiency with which the liver normally extracts bile acids from portal blood. Small changes in hepatic blood flow, portosystemic shunting, or liver function all result in a substantial elevation of serum bile acid levels, while terminal ileal dysfunction (e.g., Crohn's disease) leads to fecal loss of bile acids and decreased serum levels. Although exquisitely sensitive, bile acid levels are nonspecific and fail to reflect accurately overall liver function.

The ^{14}C-aminopyrine breath test was originally developed as a test of liver function. It measures the rate at which the liver metabolizes ^{14}C-labeled aminopyrine to $^{14}CO_2$, which is collected and measured in exhaled breath. This test is performed only in some academic centers.

SCREENING TESTS OF HEPATOBILIARY DISEASE

Screening tests of hepatobiliary disease (Table 41–2) are conveniently divided into two categories: (1) tests of biliary obstruction, and (2) tests of hepatocellular damage, based on the mechanisms responsible for the abnormal test. However, none of the tests is specific for either category, and it is the pattern and magnitude of abnormalities that often provide diagnostic clues to the type of liver disease present.

The *serum bilirubin* level is the result of bilirubin production, bilirubin conjugation, and excretion of bilirubin into bile. Bilirubin's bright orange color made it the first, and the most striking, of liver test indicators. However, the differential diagnosis for hyperbilirubinemia (see Chapter 42) requires consideration of an extensive list of disorders, including hematological disorders, congenital abnormalities of bilirubin metabolism, and a wide array of liver diseases. Serum bilirubin determination is nonspecific and only moderately sensitive as a test of liver function. Elevation of serum bilirubin, however, should prompt a search for the cause, including potentially treatable biliary obstruction. Serum bilirubin levels may not return promptly to normal after relief of biliary obstruction

TABLE 41–2. CLINICAL TESTS OF HEPATIC FUNCTION

	PROPERTY EXAMINED	SIGNIFICANCE OF ABNORMAL RESULTS
Tests of Hepatic Function (Normal values)		
Serum albumin (30–50 gm/L)	Protein synthetic capacity (over days to weeks)	Decreased synthetic capacity; Protein malnutrition; Increased protein loss (nephrotic syndrome, protein-losing enteropathy); Increased extracellular fluid volume
Prothrombin time (10.5–13 sec)	Protein synthetic capacity (hours to days)	Decreased synthetic capacity (especially Factors II and VII); Vitamin K deficiency; Consumptive coagulopathy
Serum bilirubin (0.2–1.0 mg/dl)	Extraction from blood and excretion into bile	Hemolysis; Impaired hepatic function; Cholestasis (intrahepatic); Bile duct obstruction
Serum bile acids (fasting: 0.7–5.6 μM)	Extraction from blood and excretion into bile	Diffuse liver disease; Cholestasis; Terminal ileal disease; Portosystemic shunting of blood
^{14}C-aminopyrine breath test (5–19.5% of dose excreted at 2 hours)	Drug-metabolizing capacity	Decreased metabolic capacity (diffuse liver disease); Severe portosystemic shunting of blood
Screening Tests of Hepatobiliary Disease		
Tests of Biliary Obstruction		
Serum bilirubin (0.2–1.0 mg/dl)	Extraction of bilirubin from blood, conjugation and excretion into bile	Hemolysis; Diffuse liver disease; Cholestasis; Extrahepatic bile duct obstruction; Congenital disorders of bilirubin metabolism
Serum alkaline phosphatase (also 5'-nucleotidase and gamma glutamyl transpeptidase) (56–176 U/L)	Increased enzyme synthesis and release	Bile duct obstruction; Cholestasis; Infiltrative liver disease (neoplasms, granulomas); Bone destruction/remodeling; Pregnancy
Tests of Hepatocellular Damage		
Aspartate aminotransferase (AST; SGOT) (10–30 U/L)	Release of intracellular enzyme	Hepatocellular necrosis; Cardiac or skeletal muscle necrosis
Alanine aminotransferase (ALT; SGPT) (5–30 U/L)	Release of intracellular enzyme	Same as AST; however, more specific for liver cell damage

TABLE 41–3. CHARACTERISTIC PATTERNS OF LIVER FUNCTION TESTS

DISORDER	BILIRUBIN	ALKALINE PHOSPHATASE	PROTHROMBIN TIME	AST	ALT
Gilbert's syndrome	↑	nl	nl	nl	nl
Bile duct obstruction (pancreatic carcinoma)	↑↑↑	↑↑↑	↑-↑↑	↑	↑
Acute viral or toxic hepatitis	↑-↑↑↑	↑-↑↑	nl-↑↑↑	↑↑↑	↑↑↑
Cirrhosis	nl-↑	nl-↑	nl-↑↑	nl-↑	nl-↑

nl = normal

or improvement in liver disease, because some bilirubin binds covalently to albumin and is removed from the circulation only as albumin is catabolized (half-life 14 to 20 days).

Serum alkaline phosphatase activity reflects a group of isoenzymes derived from liver, bone, intestine, and placenta. Serum levels are elevated in association with cholestasis, partial or complete bile duct obstruction, and bone regeneration, and also with neoplastic, infiltrative, and granulomatous liver diseases. An isolated elevated alkaline phosphatase level may be the only clue to partial obstruction of the common bile duct, to obstruction of ducts in a single lobe or segment of liver, or to neoplastic or granulomatous disease. Alkaline phosphatase is located on the plasma membrane of hepatocytes. In cholestasis, accompanied by increased serum and tissue levels of bile acids, bits of hepatocyte membrane containing alkaline phosphatase are solubilized into the blood stream. Increased hepatic bile acid levels also stimulate synthesis of alkaline phosphatase, contributing to the elevation of serum levels. 5'-Nucleotidase and gamma glutamyl transpeptidase, other hepatocyte plasma membrane enzymes, are similarly released into the circulation during bile duct obstruction or cholestasis.

Aspartate (AST) and alanine (ALT) aminotransferases are intracellular amino-transferring enzymes present in large quantities in liver cells. Following injury or death of liver cells, they are released into the circulation. In general, the serum transaminases are sensitive (albeit nonspecific) tests of liver damage, and the height of the serum transaminase activity reflects the severity of hepatic necrosis, but there are important exceptions. Both enzymes require pyridoxal 5-phosphate as a cofactor, and the relatively low serum transaminase values seen in patients with severe alcoholic hepatitis (often <300 U/L) may reflect deficiency of this cofactor. Although transaminase levels are increased in a wide array of liver diseases, high levels (>15 times the upper limit of normal) are rare in bile duct obstruction and almost always indicate acute hepatocellular necrosis (e.g., viral or toxic hepatitis).

Liver function tests usually do not indicate the nature of the underlying liver disease; however, the *pattern* of liver test abnormalities may provide insight in this regard. Table 41–3 outlines the most common patterns of liver test abnormalities.

LIVER BIOPSY

Biopsy and histological examination of liver tissue are of value in the differential diagnosis of diffuse or localized parenchymal diseases (e.g., cirrhosis, hepatitis, hemochromatosis) or hepatomegaly. Liver biopsy is safe (serious complications <0.5 per cent); however, it is contraindicated in uncooperative patients and those with coagulation abnormalities or thrombocytopenia.

REFERENCES

Kaplowitz N, Eberle D, Yamada T: Biochemical tests for liver disease. *In* Zakim D, Boyer T (eds): Hepatology: A Textbook of Liver Disease. Philadelphia, WB Saunders Co, 1982, pp 583–611.

Ockner RK: Laboratory tests in liver disease. *In* Wyngaarden JB, Smith LH Jr (eds): Cecil Textbook of Medicine. 18th ed. Philadelphia, WB Saunders Co, 1988, pp 814–817.

42

JAUNDICE

DEFINITION

The term jaundice or icterus describes the yellow pigmentation of skin, sclerae, and mucous membranes produced by increased serum bilirubin (hyperbilirubinemia). Jaundice, the most colorful and often the earliest sign of a variety of liver and biliary diseases, is a starting point for evaluating many of these disorders. Serum bilirubin normally ranges from 0.5 to 1.0 mg/dl. Jaundice usually becomes clinically evident at levels exceeding 2.5 mg/dl and is most readily detected in the sclerae.

BILIRUBIN METABOLISM

About 4 mg/kg of bilirubin is produced each day, mainly (80 to 85 per cent) derived from the catabolism of the hemoglobin heme group of senescent red blood cells. The heme ring is cleaved in the reticuloendothelial system to form biliverdin, which in turn is oxidized to bilirubin, a water-insoluble tetrapyrrole. A smaller proportion of bilirubin (15 to 20 per cent) is derived from the destruction of maturing erythroid cells in the bone marrow (ineffective erythropoiesis) and from the heme groups of predominantly hepatic hemoproteins such as cytochrome P-450 and cytochrome c (Fig. 42–1).

Bilirubin liberated into the plasma is transported to the liver bound tightly but reversibly to albumin. Three phases of hepatic bilirubin metabolism are recognized: (1) uptake, (2) conjugation, and (3) excretion into the bile, the last step being overall rate-limiting. Uptake is reversible and follows dissociation of bili-

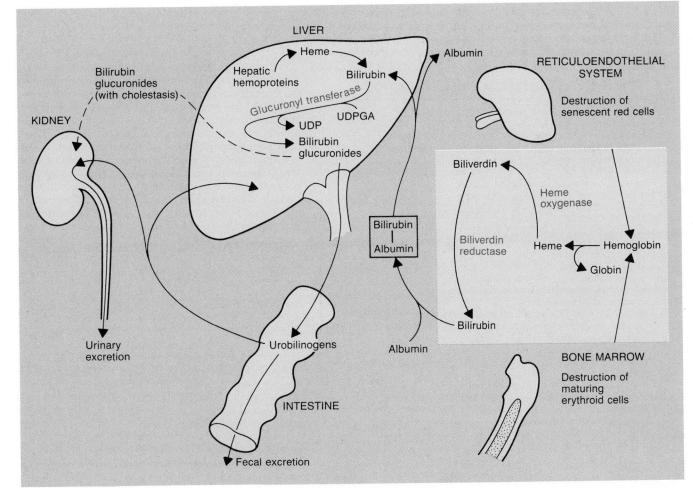

FIGURE 42–1. The pathway of bilirubin formation, metabolism, and excretion.

rubin from albumin. Unconjugated bilirubin is insoluble in water and is virtually incapable of being excreted in bile. This apolar molecule, however, dissolves in lipid-rich environments and readily traverses the blood-brain barrier and placenta.

Bilirubin is rendered water-soluble and hence capable of being excreted in the aqueous bile by its conjugation with a sugar, glucuronic acid. Mono- and diglucuronides of bilirubin are formed in the hepatic endoplasmic reticulum catalyzed by the enzyme UDP-glucuronyl transferase. If the biliary excretion of conjugated bilirubin is impaired, the pigment from hepatocytes regurgitates into plasma. Conjugated bilirubin is both water-soluble and less tightly bound to albumin than unconjugated pigment, so that it is readily filtered by the glomerulus and appears in the urine when its plasma levels are increased (Fig. 42–1). Unconjugated bilirubin is not excreted in urine. With sustained conjugated hyperbilirubinemia (e.g., obstructive jaundice), a proportion of the conjugated bilirubin becomes covalently bound to albumin and is therefore unavailable for renal or biliary excretion.

Conjugated bilirubin excreted in the bile is not reabsorbed by the intestine but is converted by bacterial action in the gut to colorless tetrapyrroles termed urobilinogens. Up to 20 per cent of urobilinogen is reabsorbed and undergoes an enterohepatic circulation, a proportion being excreted in the urine. Thus, both impaired hepatocellular excretion and marked overproduction of bilirubin lead to increased appearance of urobilinogen in the urine.

LABORATORY TESTS FOR BILIRUBIN

The van den Bergh reaction is the most commonly used test for bilirubin in biological fluids. When carried out in an aqueous medium, the test shows a colored reaction only with water-soluble bilirubin derivatives (called the *direct* van den Bergh fraction). The addition of methanol enables a colored reaction to take place with water-insoluble bilirubin (called the *indirect* van den Bergh fraction). Direct and indirect van den Bergh fractions provide clinically useful estimations of conjugated and unconjugated bilirubin, respectively. However, the correlation between actual levels of conjugated bilirubin and levels estimated by the direct-reacting fraction is poor. Normal plasma actually contains more than 95 per cent unconjugated bilirubin.

Qualitative estimation of bilirubin in urine is carried out with Ictotest tablets or dipsticks, which are positive in cases of conjugated hyperbilirubinemia.

CLINICAL CLASSIFICATION OF JAUNDICE

A logical first step in the study of a jaundiced patient is to determine whether there is an unconjugated or a conjugated hyperbilirubinemia. This question is usually easily resolved by testing the urine for bilirubin. If positive, conjugated hyperbilirubinemia is present, and this is confirmed by finding greater than 50 per cent conjugated bilirubin on serum testing.

Classification of jaundice according to this distinction is shown in Table 42–1. Mechanisms contributing to predominantly unconjugated hyperbilirubinemia include (1) overproduction, (2) decreased hepatic uptake, and (3) decreased conjugation. Conjugated hyperbilirubinemia implies either (1) a defect in hepatocellular secretion of bilirubin or (2) mechanical obstruction to the major extrahepatic bile ducts. Occasionally jaundice may result from a single abnormality in the complex pathway from bilirubin production to its biliary excretion, e.g., from hemolysis and from rare conditions, such as Crigler-Najjar syndrome (decreased or absent conjugation) and Dubin-Johnson syndrome (defective hepatocellular excretion of bilirubin). More frequently there are multiple rather than isolated causes of jaundice. For example, the jaundice occurring in patients with hepatocellular disease (i.e., hepatitis, cirrhosis) may result from a combination of diminished red cell survival and impairment of all three stages of hepatocellular bilirubin transport and metabolism.

Unconjugated Hyperbilirubinemia

Overproduction. Hemolysis from a variety of causes may lead to bilirubin production sufficient to exceed the clearing capacity of the liver with subse-

TABLE 42–1. CLASSIFICATION OF JAUNDICE

Predominantly Unconjugated Hyperbilirubinemia
Overproduction
  Hemolysis (spherocytosis, autoimmune, etc.)
  Ineffective erythropoiesis (e.g., megaloblastic anemias)
Decreased hepatic uptake
  Gilbert's syndrome
  Drugs (e.g., radiographic contrast agents)
  Sepsis
Decreased conjugation
  Gilbert's syndrome
  Crigler-Najjar syndrome types I and II
  Neonatal jaundice
  Hepatocellular disease
  Sepsis
  Drug inhibition (e.g., chloramphenicol)
Predominantly Conjugated Hyperbilirubinemia
Impaired hepatic excretion
  Familial disorders (Dubin-Johnson syndrome, Rotor syndrome, benign recurrent cholestasis, cholestasis of pregnancy)
  Hepatocellular disease
  Drug-induced cholestasis
  Primary biliary cirrhosis
  Sepsis
  Postoperative
Extrahepatic ("mechanical") biliary obstruction
  Gallstones
  Tumors of head of pancreas
  Tumors of bile ducts
  Tumors of ampulla of Vater
  Biliary strictures (post-cholecystectomy, primary sclerosing cholangitis)
  Congenital disorders (biliary atresia, Caroli's syndrome)

quent development of jaundice. This *hemolytic jaundice* is characteristically mild; serum bilirubin levels rarely exceed 5 mg/dl. Ineffective erythropoiesis, which may be substantially increased in megaloblastic anemias, may also lead to mild jaundice.

Impaired Hepatic Uptake. Impaired uptake is very rarely encountered as an isolated cause for clinical jaundice, but may play a role in the mild jaundice following administration of radiographic contrast media (competition for bilirubin uptake) and in Gilbert's syndrome (see below).

Impaired Conjugation. A genetically determined decrease or absence of UDP-glucuronyltransferase is encountered in the Crigler-Najjar syndrome, whereas mild, acquired defects in the enzyme may be produced by drugs (e.g., chloramphenicol).

Neonatal Jaundice. All steps of hepatic bilirubin metabolism are incompletely developed in the neonatal period, while increased production is also present. The major defect is in conjugation, however, leading to unconjugated hyperbilirubinemia between the second and fifth days of life. When increased production of bilirubin occurs in the neonatal period, usually as a result of hemolytic disease secondary to blood-group incompatibility, severe unconjugated hyperbilirubinemia may occur, carrying the risk of neurological damage (kernicterus).

Gilbert's Syndrome. This very common disorder affects up to 7 per cent of the population, with a marked male predominance. It commonly manifests during the second or third decade of life as a mild unconjugated hyperbilirubinemia, exacerbated by fasting, and noted clinically or as an incidental laboratory finding. The mechanism appears to involve increased production, diminished uptake, and defective conjugation of bilirubin to varying proportions in different individuals. Nonspecific gastrointestinal symptoms and fatigue are commonly associated, but this condition is entirely benign. The diagnosis is strongly suggested by unconjugated hyperbilirubinemia with normal hepatic enzymes and the absence of overt hemolysis. Liver biopsy is always normal and is rarely, if ever, indicated to confirm the diagnosis.

Conjugated Hyperbilirubinemia

Determining the cause of unconjugated hyperbilirubinemia rarely poses difficulty. Usually, the major difficulty in evaluating jaundice is encountered in differentiating an intrahepatic defect in excretion from that of obstruction in a patient with predominantly conjugated hyperbilirubinemia. This clinical situation is often described as *cholestatic jaundice*, and the approach to its differential diagnosis is discussed in detail below.

Cholestasis implies that bile formation or flow is impaired. Typically, a patient with cholestatic jaundice has predominantly conjugated hyperbilirubinemia and an elevated alkaline phosphatase, usually to at least three to four times normal. When prolonged, cholestasis may lead to hypercholesterolemia, malabsorption of fat and fat-soluble vitamins, and reten-

tion of bile salts, which may lead to pruritus. Biochemical evidence of liver cell damage (elevated transaminases, prolonged prothrombin time uncorrected by administration of vitamin K) may be minimal or marked, depending upon the cause of the cholestasis. All of the features of cholestasis may be present in some patients *without jaundice*.

Impaired Hepatic Excretion. This pathogenetic category of jaundice, also called intrahepatic cholestasis, is applied to all disorders in the transport of conjugated bilirubin from the hepatocyte to the radiologically visible intrahepatic bile ducts. Thus it includes a wide range of conditions from drug-induced cholestasis (impaired canalicular transport) to primary biliary cirrhosis (destruction of the small intrahepatic bile ductules). The following are some important causes of intrahepatic cholestasis.

DRUG-INDUCED CHOLESTASIS. Typical cholestatic jaundice may be produced by phenothiazines, oral contraceptives, and methyltestosterone. Eosinophilia may accompany drug-induced jaundice.

SEPSIS. Systemic sepsis, mainly due to gram-negative organisms, may produce a predominantly conjugated hyperbilirubinemia, usually accompanied by mildly elevated serum alkaline phosphatase levels.

POSTOPERATIVE JAUNDICE. This increasingly recognized syndrome has an incidence of 15 per cent following heart surgery and 1 per cent following elective abdominal surgery. Occurring one to ten days postoperatively, and multifactorial in origin, the elevated

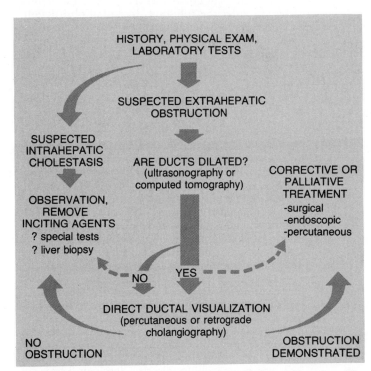

FIGURE 42–2. Approach to the patient with cholestatic jaundice. The algorithm demonstrates the systematic consideration of the available diagnostic options.

bilirubin is predominantly of the conjugated variety with increased alkaline phosphatase and minimally abnormal transaminases.

HEPATOCELLULAR DISEASE. Hepatocellular disease (i.e., hepatitis and cirrhosis) from a variety of causes (see Chapters 43 and 45) may result in a typical cholestatic jaundice. Evidence of hepatocellular damage and dysfunction is usually prominent and includes marked elevation of transaminases, prolonged prothrombin time, hypoalbuminemia, and clinical features of hepatic dysfunction (see Chapter 44). In hepatocellular disease all three steps of hepatic bilirubin metabolism are impaired. Excretion, the rate-limiting step, is usually the most profoundly disturbed, leading to a predominantly conjugated hyperbilirubinemia. Jaundice may be profound in acute hepatitis (see Chapter 43) without prognostic implications. In contrast, in chronic liver disease, jaundice usually implies severe decompensation of hepatic function with a poor prognosis.

Extrahepatic Biliary Obstruction. Complete or partial obstruction of the extrahepatic bile ducts may result from a variety of causes, including impaction of gallstones, carcinoma of the head of the pancreas, tumors of the bile ducts, bile duct strictures, and chronic pancreatitis with bile duct compression. In complete obstruction, conjugated hyperbilirubinemia is prominent and usually plateaus at 30 to 40 mg/dl in the absence of renal failure, hepatocellular damage, or infection within the bile ducts, all of which may develop during the course of mechanical obstruction. Stools may become clay colored as a result of the failure of bile to enter the intestine. In partial obstruction, jaundice may be mild or even absent, becoming prominent when infection of the ducts complicates the obstruction.

APPROACH TO THE DIAGNOSIS OF JAUNDICE

A careful history and physical examination are of paramount importance in obtaining clues to the nature and cause of jaundice. A history of darkened urine invariably implies conjugated hyperbilirubinemia, while pale stools and pruritus suggest a cholestatic process. An inquiry about use of drugs or alcohol, exposure to jaundiced persons (drug or viral hepatitis), recurrent abdominal pain and nausea (gallstones), epigastric pain radiating into the back accompanied by weight loss and a distended gallbladder (carcinoma of the head of the pancreas), and pre-existing liver disease will often go far in delineating the probable cause for the jaundice. Routine laboratory tests are helpful in that serum transaminases are usually less than 5- to 10-fold elevated in patients with bile duct obstruction, while alkaline phosphatase levels are usually greater than two to three times normal. Conversely, a greater than 10- to 15-fold elevation of serum transaminases indicates hepatocellular disease. Serological tests for hepatitis may be helpful (see Chapter 43), whereas autoantibodies, if strongly positive, may be of diagnostic value, e.g., the antimitochondrial antibody in primary biliary cirrhosis.

Clinical evaluation and routine laboratory tests serve to identify the cause of jaundice in up to 85 per cent of cases. More sophisticated diagnostic procedures are often needed, however, to determine the cause, especially whether the cholestatic jaundice in a given patient is intrahepatic or due to extrahepatic obstruction.

A diagnostic approach to this question is illustrated in Figure 42–2. If extrahepatic obstruction is suspected, it is necessary to determine first by noninvasive means whether or not the major bile ducts are dilated. In jaundiced patients, dilatation of the ducts is usual when a mechanical obstruction is present but is absent in cases of intrahepatic cholestasis. Either ultrasound or CT scanning may be used to determine the caliber of bile ducts, the former generally preferred because of lesser cost and absence of radiation. Additional definitive clues, such as the presence of stones in the common duct or gallbladder, may be obtained as well. However, both imaging techniques may give rise to false-positive and false-negative results in a small number of patients. Thus, in a patient with cholestatic jaundice, the absence of dilated ducts on ultrasound should not dissuade the clinician from proceeding to cholangiography if the suspicion of extrahepatic obstruction based on clinical evaluation is high. If dilated ducts are found on noninvasive imaging, direct cholangiography provides the most reliable approach to nonoperative diagnosis of cholestatic jaundice. This may be accomplished by either percutaneous puncture of the intrahepatic biliary tree with a thin needle (percutaneous transhepatic cholangiography) or by means of endoscopic retrograde cholangiography. The percutaneous route is simpler technically, has a success rate of close to 100 per cent in the presence of dilated ducts, and is less expensive. The endoscopic route, although more demanding both technically and in terms of time and cost, is of value in demonstrating duct pathology when the bile ducts are not dilated (in which case the percutaneous route may often fail) or when associated pancreatic disease is suspected. It may also permit direct biopsy of lesions at the ampulla of Vater and sphincterotomy and stone extraction in appropriate instances.

Liver biopsy may be indicated when an intrahepatic cause for cholestasis is strongly suspected on clinical grounds or when extrahepatic obstruction is ruled out by definitive cholangiography. Liver histology itself is often a poor guide to whether cholestasis is intra- or extrahepatic. The decision to perform a biopsy thus will rest on the certainty with which extrahepatic obstruction has been excluded in a patient with cholestasis and on the clinical course of the disease. Thus, for example, in a patient with cholestatic jaundice in whom recent ingestion of chlorpromazine is documented and in whom the jaundice is beginning to resolve following cessation of the drug, the best course may be to observe without further investigation.

REFERENCES

Ockner RK: Approaches to the diagnosis of jaundice. *In* Wyngaarden JB, Smith LH Jr (eds): Cecil Textbook of Medicine. 18th ed. Philadelphia, WB Saunders Co, 1988, pp 817–818.

Scharschmidt BF: Bilirubin metabolism and hyperbilirubinemia. *In* Wyngaarden JB, Smith LH Jr (eds): Cecil Textbook of Medicine. 18th ed. Philadelphia, WB Saunders Co, 1988, pp 811–814.

43

ACUTE AND CHRONIC HEPATITIS

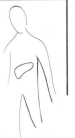

DEFINITION

The term hepatitis is applied to a broad category of clinicopathological conditions that result from the damage produced by viral, toxic, pharmacological, or immune-mediated attack upon the liver. The common pathological features of hepatitis are hepatocellular necrosis, which may be focal or extensive, and inflammatory cell infiltration of the liver, which may predominate in the portal areas or extend out into the parenchyma. Clinically, the liver may be enlarged and tender with or without jaundice, and laboratory evidence of hepatocellular damage is invariably found in the form of elevated transaminase levels. Independent of its cause, the clinical course of hepatitis may range from mild or inapparent to a dramatic illness with evidence of severe hepatocellular dysfunction, marked jaundice, impairment of coagulation, and disturbance of neurological function. Hepatitis is further divided into acute and chronic types on the basis of clinical and pathological criteria.

Acute hepatitis implies a condition lasting less than six months, culminating either in complete resolution of the liver damage with return to normal liver function and structure or in rapid progression of the acute injury toward extensive necrosis and a fatal outcome.

Chronic hepatitis is defined as a sustained inflammatory process in the liver lasting longer than six months.

Differentiation of acute from chronic hepatitis on histological criteria alone may be impossible. Extension of inflammatory cells beyond the limits of the portal tracts surrounding isolated nests of hepatocytes (piecemeal necrosis) and connection of portal and/or central areas of the hepatic lobules by swaths of inflammation, necrosis, and collapse of architecture (bridging necrosis) are seen in liver biopsies taken from patients with severe forms of chronic hepatitis. These features may also be seen, however, in uncomplicated acute hepatitis that will ultimately undergo complete resolution. A purely histological diagnosis of chronic hepatitis usually requires evidence of progression toward cirrhosis such as significant fibrous scarring and disruption of the hepatic lobular architecture.

ACUTE HEPATITIS

Agents causing acute hepatic injury are listed in Table 43–1. The mechanisms whereby these agents produce hepatic damage include direct toxin-induced necrosis (e.g., acetaminophen, *Amanita phalloides* toxin) and host immune-mediated damage, which probably plays an important, but not well understood, role in viral hepatitis. In the case of frank hepatotoxins such as *Amanita* poisoning, massive hepatic necrosis is the dominant process, and the clinical course is more aptly described as fulminant hepatic failure (see Chapter 44) rather than acute hepatitis. Such a course is less common, but well recognized, with all the causative agents listed in Table 43–1.

Acute Viral Hepatitis

Etiology. Viral hepatitis is caused by four main viruses: hepatitis viruses A, B, and D and the so-called non-A, non-B agents, of which there appear to be at least two (Table 43–2). Cytomegalovirus and Epstein-Barr virus occasionally cause hepatitis. Hepatitis D

TABLE 43–1. CAUSES OF ACUTE HEPATITIS

Viral Hepatitis
  Hepatitis A virus
  Hepatitis B virus
  Hepatitis non-A, non-B viruses
  Hepatitis D virus ("delta agent")
  Epstein-Barr virus
  Cytomegalovirus
Alcohol
Toxins
  Amanita phalloides mushroom poisoning
  Carbon tetrachloride
Drugs
  Acetaminophen
  Isoniazid
  Halothane
  Chlorpromazine
  Erythromycin
Other
  Wilson's disease

TABLE 43–2. CHARACTERISTICS OF COMMON CAUSATIVE AGENTS OF ACUTE VIRAL HEPATITIS

	HEPATITIS A	HEPATITIS B	HEPATITIS D	HEPATITIS NON-A, NON-B (TWO OR MORE AGENTS)
Causative agent	27-nm RNA virus	42-nm DNA virus; core and surface components	36-nm hybrid particle with HBsAg coat	Apparent similarities to hepatitis B virus
Transmission	Fecal-oral; water-, food-borne	Parenteral inoculation or equivalent; direct contact	Similar to HBV	Same as for B; epidemic form similar to HAV
Incubation period	2–6 weeks	4 weeks–6 months	Similar to HBV	2–20 weeks
Period of infectivity	2–3 weeks in late incubation and early clinical phase	During HBsAg positivity (occasionally only with anti-HBc positivity)	During HDV RNA or anti-HDV positivity	Unknown
Massive hepatic necrosis	Rare	Uncommon	Yes	Uncommon
Carrier state	No	Yes	Yes	Yes (? for epidemic form)
Chronic hepatitis	No	Yes	Yes	Yes (not for epidemic form)
Prophylaxis	Hygiene; immune serum globulin	Hygiene; hepatitis B immune globulin; vaccine	Hygiene, HBV vaccine	Hygiene; ? immune serum globulin; avoid commercial blood

virus, an incomplete RNA virus, causes hepatitis either simultaneously with the B virus or in individuals already chronically infected with the B virus. Of these agents, the B virus has been most extensively characterized, whereas least is known regarding the non-A, non-B agents. The complete B virus (Dane particle) consists of several antigenically distinct components (Fig. 43–1), including a surface coat (hepatitis B surface antigen, HBsAg) and a core of circular DNA, DNA polymerase, hepatitis B core antigen (HBcAg), and hepatitis e antigen (HBeAg). HBsAg may exist in serum either as part of the Dane particle or as free particles and rods. Surface antigen as well as HBcAg and HBeAg each elicit distinct antibody responses from the host, which are of value in serological diagnosis and characterization of the state of B virus replication in the liver.

Transmission. Hepatitis A virus (HAV) is excreted in the feces during the incubation period (Fig. 43–2) and is transmitted by the fecal-oral route. It is thus implicated in most instances of water-borne and food-transmitted infection and in epidemics of viral hepatitis. The hepatitis B virus is present in virtually all body fluids and excreta of carriers and is transmitted mainly by parenteral routes. Thus, transmission occurs most commonly via blood and blood products, contaminated needles, and intimate personal contact. Persons at high risk of infection with the B virus therefore include sexual partners of acutely as well as chronically infected individuals, with male homosexuals being at particularly high risk; health professionals, particularly surgeons, dentists, and workers in clinical laboratories and dialysis units; intravenous drug abusers; and infants of infected mothers ("vertical transmission"). Patients with increased exposure to blood or blood products and/or with impaired im-

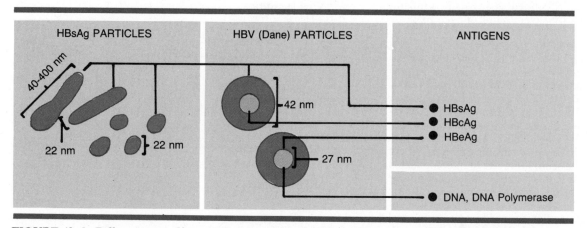

FIGURE 43–1. Different types of hepatitis B virus particles in plasma. The locations of the various antigenic components are indicated.

munity (e.g., dialysis patients, patients with leukemia or Down's syndrome) are also highly susceptible to B virus infection.

Non-A, non-B hepatitis, similar to hepatitis B, is largely a parenterally transmitted disease. Since no diagnostic marker exists for this group of viruses as yet, non-A, non-B hepatitis is currently the main cause of post-transfusion hepatitis. An epidemic, water-borne form of non-A, non-B hepatitis has also been associated with outbreaks, mainly in Asia.

Clinical and Laboratory Manifestations. Acute viral hepatitis typically begins with a prodromal phase lasting several days and characterized by constitutional and gastrointestinal symptoms including malaise, fatigue, anorexia, nausea, vomiting, myalgia, and headache. A mild fever may be present. Symptoms suggestive of "flu" may be prominent; arthritis and urticaria, attributed to immune complex deposition, may be present, particularly in hepatitis B. Smokers often describe an aversion to cigarettes. Jaundice soon appears with bilirubinuria and a loss of stool color, often accompanied by an improvement in the patient's sense of well-being. Jaundice may be absent (anicteric hepatitis); in such cases—probably the majority of cases of acute viral hepatitis—medical attention is often not sought. The liver is usually tender and enlarged; splenomegaly is found in about one fifth of patients.

Transaminases (ALT and AST) are released from the acutely damaged hepatocytes and serum transaminase levels rise, often to levels exceeding 20-fold normal. Bilirubinuria and an elevated serum bilirubin are usually found, with mild elevations in serum alkaline phosphatase levels. The white cell count is normal or slightly depressed.

The icteric phase of acute viral hepatitis may last from days to weeks, followed by gradual resolution of symptoms and laboratory tests.

Complications

POSTHEPATITIS SYNDROMES. In some patients, prolonged fatigue and malaise may persist for months after return of liver function tests to normal. Reassurance is all that is required, and normal activity is encouraged. Isolated elevation of unconjugated serum bilirubin may persist (an expression of Gilbert's syndrome; see Chapter 42) and requires no treatment.

CHOLESTATIC HEPATITIS. In some patients, a prolonged, although ultimately self-limited, period of cholestatic jaundice may supervene with marked conjugated hyperbilirubinemia, elevation of alkaline phosphatase, and pruritus. Investigation may be required to differentiate this condition from mechanical obstruction of the biliary tree (see Chapter 47).

FULMINANT HEPATITIS. Massive hepatic necrosis occurs in less than 1 per cent of patients with acute viral hepatitis, leading to a devastating and often fatal condition called fulminant hepatic failure. This is discussed in detail in Chapter 44.

CHRONIC HEPATITIS. This may develop following acute hepatitis B, D, or non-A, non-B. Hepatitis A never progresses to chronicity. Persistence of transaminase elevation beyond six months suggests evo-

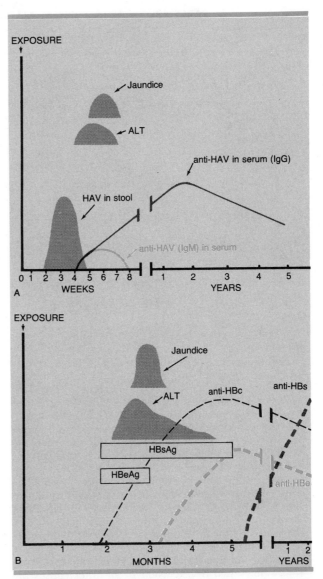

FIGURE 43–2. Sequence of clinical and laboratory findings in (A) a patient with hepatitis A and (B) a patient with hepatitis B.

lution to chronic hepatitis, although a slowly resolving acute hepatitis may occasionally lead to abnormal liver function tests well beyond six months with eventual complete resolution. Chronic hepatitis is considered in detail later in this chapter. Hepatitis B virus infection without evidence of any liver damage may persist, resulting in asymptomatic or "healthy" hepatitis B carriers. In Asia and Africa, many such carriers appear to have acquired the virus from infected mothers during infancy.

RARE COMPLICATIONS. Rarely, acute viral hepatitis may be followed by aplastic anemia, while cryoglobulinemia, glomerulonephritis, and vasculitis may complicate the course of hepatitis B. Pancreatitis with elevation of serum amylase may also occur.

TABLE 43–3. SEROLOGICAL MARKERS OF VIRAL HEPATITIS

AGENT	MARKER	DEFINITION	SIGNIFICANCE
Hepatitis A virus (HAV)	Anti-HAV IgM type IgG type	Antibody to HAV	Current or recent infection or convalescence Current or previous infection; confers immunity
Hepatitis B virus (HBV)	HBsAg HBeAg	HBV surface antigen e antigen; a component of the HBV core	Positive in most cases of acute or chronic infection Transiently positive in acute hepatitis B May persist in chronic infection Reflects presence of viral replication and whole Dane particles in serum Reflects high infectivity
	Anti-HBe	Antibody to e antigen	Transiently positive in convalescence May be persistently present in chronic cases Reflects low infectivity
	Anti-HBc (IgM or IgG)	Antibody to HBV core antigen	Positive in all acute and chronic cases Reliable marker of infection, past or current IgM anti-HBc reflects active viral replication Not protective
	Anti-HBs	Antibody to HBV surface antigen	Positive in late convalescence in most acute cases Confers immunity
Hepatitis D virus (HDV)	Anti-HDV (IgM or IgG)	Antibody to HDV antigen	Acute or chronic infection; not protective

Serodiagnosis. The ability to detect the presence of viral components in hepatitis B and antibodies to components of hepatitis A, B, and D agent has enabled considerable progress to be made in the study of the epidemiology of viral hepatitis. These so-called viral markers can be diagnostic of the cause of acute viral hepatitis (Table 43–3). An etiological diagnosis is of great importance in planning preventive and public health measures pertinent to the close contacts of infected patients and in evaluating the prognosis. The time course of appearance of these markers in acute hepatitis A and B is shown in Figure 43–2. Epstein-Barr virus and cytomegalovirus hepatitis may also be diagnosed by the appearance of specific antibodies of the IgM class. No reliable markers have as yet been described for non-A, non-B hepatitis, which is currently diagnosed by exclusion of all other causes of hepatitis. In acute hepatitis B, HBsAg and HBeAg are present in serum. Both are usually cleared within a period of three months, but HBsAg may persist in some uncomplicated cases for six months to one year. Clearance of HBsAg is followed after a variable "window" period by emergence of anti-HBs, which confers long-term immunity. Anti-HBc and anti-HBe appear in the acute phase of the illness, but neither provides immunity. During the serological window period, anti-HBc may be the only evidence of hepatitis B infection, and IgM anti-HBc, a marker of active viral replication, is suggestive of recent infection. Hepatitis D infection superimposed on B virus infection may be detected by specific antibody to this agent.

Management. There is no specific treatment for acute viral hepatitis. Management is largely supportive, including rest in proportion to the severity of symptoms, maintenance of hydration, and adequate dietary intake. Most patients show a preference for a low-fat, high-carbohydrate diet. Vitamin supplementation is of no proven value, although vitamin K administration may be indicated if prolonged cholestasis occurs. Activity is restricted to limit fatigue. Alcohol should be avoided until liver enzymes return to normal. Measures to combat nausea can include small doses of metoclopramide and hydroxyzine. Hospitalization is indicated in patients with severe nausea and vomiting, or with evidence of deteriorating liver function such as hepatic encephalopathy (Chapter 44) or prolongation of the prothrombin time. In general, hepatitis A may be regarded as noninfectious after two to three weeks, whereas hepatitis B is potentially infectious to intimate contacts throughout its course, although the risk is very small once HBsAg has cleared.

Prevention. Both feces and blood from patients with hepatitis A contain virus during the prodromal and early icteric phases of the disease. Raw shellfish concentrate the virus from sewage pollution and may serve as vectors of the disease. General hygienic measures should include handwashing by contacts and careful handling, disposal, and sterilization of excreta and contaminated clothing and utensils. Close contacts of patients with hepatitis A should receive immune serum globulin (ISG) as soon as possible. Travelers to endemic areas where sanitation facilities are poor may be protected by prior administration of ISG.

Hepatitis B is rarely transmitted by the fecal-oral route, but it is still prudent to avoid contact with the excreta of patients. Far more important is the meticulous disposal of contaminated needles and other blood-contaminated utensils.

ISG is of very limited value in preventing hepatitis B. However, administration of immune serum globulin enriched in anti-HBs (hyperimmune globulin, hepatitis B immune globulin, HBIG) may afford protection after a needlestick exposure or mucosal exposure (e.g., during pipetting of infectious serum in a clinical laboratory or following eye splash) and is also recommended for sexual contacts of patients with acute hepatitis B. It also appears to be protective to neonates born to mothers who are acutely or chronically infected. The usefulness of HBIG in household contacts is less well-established.

An important advance in the field of hepatitis B prevention has been the development of a safe, highly effective vaccine. Available vaccines include the original one manufactured from triple-inactivated HBsAg obtained from the serum of chronic carriers of the B virus, as well as a recombinant vaccine. The vaccine is given in three doses over six months and confers immunity in close to 100 per cent of recipients for a period of at least five years. Vaccination is currently recommended for high-risk groups and individuals, including health professionals, dialysis patients, hemophiliacs, residents and staff of custodial care institutions, and sexually active homosexual males. It appears also to be of value in combination with HBIG after acute exposure to the virus, e.g., accidental needlestick and particularly in infants born to HBsAg-positive mothers.

Alcoholic Fatty Liver and Hepatitis

Alcohol abuse is the most common cause of liver disease in the Western world. Three major pathological lesions resulting from alcohol abuse are (1) fatty liver, (2) alcoholic hepatitis, and (3) cirrhosis. The first two lesions are potentially reversible, may sometimes be confused clinically with viral hepatitis, and are described in this chapter. Alcoholic cirrhosis is discussed in Chapter 45.

Mechanism of Injury. Alcohol appears to produce liver damage by several mechanisms that are still incompletely understood. Fatty liver may be related to increased NADPH generated during alcohol metabolism, which promotes fatty acid synthesis and triglyceride formation. Since alcohol also impairs the release of triglyceride in the form of lipoproteins, fat accumulates in hepatocytes. Acetaldehyde produced from oxidation of alcohol may be directly hepatotoxic and is implicated in the production of the more severe hepatic lesions seen in alcoholics. Immune-mediated hepatic damage may also play a role in producing the lesion of alcoholic hepatitis.

Individuals vary considerably in their ability to withstand the effects of alcohol on the liver. Nevertheless, consumption by men in excess of 40 gm of ethanol per day carries a substantial risk of the development of alcoholic liver disease, while women appear to have a lower threshold of injury. Malnutrition may potentiate the toxic effects of alcohol on the liver, and genetic factors may contribute to individual susceptibility.

Clinical and Pathological Features. Alcoholic *fatty liver* may present as an incidentally discovered tender hepatomegaly. Some patients will consult a physician because of right upper quadrant pain. Jaundice is very rare. Transaminases are usually mildly elevated (less than five times normal). Liver biopsy shows diffuse or centrilobular fat occupying most of the hepatocyte.

Alcoholic hepatitis, a much more severe and prognostically ominous lesion, is characterized by the histological triad of (1) alcoholic hyalin, an eosinophilic aggregate usually seen near or around the cell nuclei; (2) infiltration of the liver by polymorphonuclear leukocytes; and (3) a network of intralobular connective tissue surrounding hepatocytes and central veins. Patients with this histological lesion may be asymptomatic or extremely ill with hepatic failure. Anorexia, nausea, vomiting, weight loss, and abdominal pain are common presenting symptoms. Hepatomegaly is present in 80 per cent of patients with alcoholic hepatitis, and splenomegaly is often present. Fever is common, but bacterial infection should always be excluded, since patients with alcoholic liver disease are prone to develop pneumonia as well as infection of the urinary tract and peritoneal cavity. Jaundice is commonly present and may be pronounced with cholestatic features (Chapter 42). Cutaneous signs of chronic liver disease may be found, including spider angiomata, palmar erythema, and gynecomastia. Parotid enlargement, testicular atrophy, and loss of body hair may be prominent (see Chapter 45). Ascites and encephalopathy may be present and indicate severe disease. The white cell count may be strikingly elevated, whereas transaminases are only modestly raised, an important differentiating feature from other forms of acute hepatitis. The AST/ALT ratio frequently exceeds 1, in contrast to viral hepatitis in which the transaminases are usually increased in parallel. A prolonged prothrombin time, hypoalbuminemia, and hyperglobulinemia may be found.

Diagnosis. A history of excessive, prolonged alcohol intake is often difficult to elicit from patients with alcoholic liver disease, whereas others suspected of imbibing to excess are often found to have liver disease from causes other than alcohol. Liver biopsy is extremely helpful in establishing the diagnosis.

Complications and Prognosis. Alcoholic fatty liver will revert to complete histological normality with cessation of alcohol intake. Alcoholic hepatitis can also revert to normal but more commonly either progresses to cirrhosis, which may already be present at the time of initial presentation, or runs a rapid course to hepatic failure and death. Not infrequently its course is complicated by the development of encephalopathy, ascites, and deteriorating renal function with increasing BUN and creatinine levels (hepatorenal syndrome) or gastrointestinal bleeding from varices.

Treatment. Treatment of acute alcoholic hepatitis is supportive. Attempts should be made to treat the underlying alcoholism, although this is often unrewarding. A high-calorie diet is instituted and may require administration by nasogastric tube in severely anorectic patients. Protein should be included, but

TABLE 43–4. CLASSIFICATION OF DRUG-INDUCED LIVER DISEASE

CATEGORY	EXAMPLES
Predictable hepatotoxins with zonal necrosis	Acetaminophen
	Carbon tetrachloride
Nonspecific hepatitis	Aspirin
	Oxacillin
Viral hepatitis-like reactions	Halothane
	Isoniazid
	Phenytoin
Cholestasis	
Noninflammatory	Estrogens
	17α-substituted steroids
Inflammatory	Chlorpromazine
	Antithyroid agents
Fatty liver	
Large droplet	Ethanol
	Corticosteroids
Small droplet	Phenylbutazone
	Allopurinol
Chronic hepatitis	Methyldopa
	Nitrofurantoin
Tumors	Estrogens
	Vinyl chloride
Vascular lesions	6-Thioguanine
	Anabolic steroids
Fibrosis	Methotrexate
Granulomas	Allopurinol
	Sulfonamides

may need to be restricted in patients with encephalopathy (see Chapter 45). The use of corticosteroids is of no proven benefit.

Drug- and Toxin-Induced Hepatitis

A broad spectrum of hepatic pathology may result from a variety of therapeutic drugs and nontherapeutic toxins (Table 43–4). The pathophysiological mechanisms whereby this wide variety of hepatic lesions is produced are complex. At one end of the spectrum is a predictable, dose-dependent, direct toxic effect upon hepatocytes leading to frank hepatocellular necrosis. This is typified by the effects of acetaminophen and carbon tetrachloride, both of which will produce centrilobular hepatocellular necrosis in virtually all individuals in whom a sufficient quantity is ingested. Other reactions are generally not predictable and usually occur for unknown reasons in susceptible individuals (idiosyncratic drug reaction). In some instances, genetically determined differences in pathways of hepatic drug metabolism may result in metabolites with greater toxic potential. Examples include viral hepatitis–like reactions (halothane, isoniazid), cholestatic hepatitis (chlorpromazine), granulomatous hepatitis (allopurinol), chronic hepatitis (methyldopa), and pure cholestasis without inflammatory cell infiltration or hepatocellular necrosis (estrogens, androgens). Immune-mediated hepatic damage may contribute in some, possibly resulting from the drug or its metabolites acting as a hapten on the surface of hepatocytes.

A few important examples of drug-induced hepatitis are discussed here.

Acetaminophen. Acetaminophen is converted by the hepatic cytochrome P-450 drug-metabolizing system to a potentially toxic metabolite that is subsequently rendered harmless through conjugation with glutathione. When massive doses are taken (in excess of 10 to 15 gm), the formation of excess toxic metabolites depletes the available glutathione and produces necrosis. Acetaminophen overdose, commonly taken in a suicide attempt, leads to nausea and vomiting within a few hours. These symptoms subside and are followed in 24 to 48 hours by clinical and laboratory evidence of hepatocellular necrosis (raised transaminases) and hepatic dysfunction (prolonged prothrombin time, hepatic encephalopathy). Extensive liver necrosis may lead to fulminant hepatic failure and death. Severe liver damage may be predicted on the basis of blood levels of the drug from 4 to 12 hours after ingestion. Early treatment of patients at high risk with N-acetylcysteine (within 16 hours of the ingestion), which is thought to promote hepatic glutathione synthesis, may be life-saving.

Isoniazid (INH). INH as a single-drug prophylaxis against tuberculosis commonly produces subclinical hepatic injury (20 per cent incidence) as evidenced by raised serum transaminase levels. This appears to be transient and self-limiting in most cases. There is, however, a 1 per cent incidence of overt hepatitis with clinical and pathological features of viral hepatitis, which progresses to massive, fatal hepatic necrosis in one tenth of affected patients. The incidence of severe hepatic damage increases with age, such that significant elevation of transaminases in persons over the age of 35 is an indication for discontinuing the drug.

Halothane. The commonly used anesthetic agent halothane rarely causes a viral hepatitis–like reaction in susceptible individuals within a few days of exposure. Complete recovery is the rule, but massive hepatic necrosis may occur, usually following repeated exposure.

Chlorpromazine. Chlorpromazine produces a cholestatic reaction, often weeks to months after the drug is begun. Fever, anorexia, and a rash may accompany jaundice and pruritus. Eosinophilia is common. Erythromycin may produce a similar picture, but right upper quadrant pain, mimicking acute cholecystitis, is often prominent.

CHRONIC HEPATITIS

An inflammatory process within the liver that fails to resolve after six months is called chronic hepatitis.

Etiology. Many of the causes of acute hepatitis can ultimately lead to chronic hepatitis (Table 43–5). A notable exception is hepatitis A virus. Hepatitis B virus is a common cause of chronic hepatitis worldwide, and it is thought that superimposition of hepatitis D virus infection may produce a more severe outcome. Several drugs may produce a chronic hepatitis, the best recognized being methyldopa. In contrast to acute hepatitis, an etiological agent is frequently difficult to identify in cases of chronic hepatitis. The pathogenesis of these idiopathic forms of chronic hepatitis is probably autoimmune in some cases, whereas others are likely to have a viral origin.

Pathology and Clinical and Laboratory Manifestations

CHRONIC PERSISTENT HEPATITIS. Chronic persistent hepatitis is defined as a chronic inflammatory process confined to the portal areas without involvement of the periportal region. This is the most common form of chronic hepatitis, particularly following hepatitis B. The prognosis is generally excellent, with nonprogression or resolution being the rule. Patients with this lesion may be asymptomatic or complain of fatigue and/or right upper quadrant pain. Laboratory abnormalities are usually confined to mildly raised transaminase levels.

CHRONIC LOBULAR HEPATITIS. Chronic lobular hepatitis, an uncommon form of chronic hepatitis, consists of scattered necrosis throughout the hepatic lobule similar to a late-resolving acute viral hepatitis. Most cases are of viral etiology; progression is uncommon.

CHRONIC ACTIVE HEPATITIS. Chronic active hepatitis, the most serious form of chronic hepatitis, may progress to cirrhosis and liver failure. Histologically, the portal areas are expanded with lymphocytes and plasma cells, with spillover into the adjacent lobule (periportal hepatitis, piecemeal necrosis). Bridging necrosis, collapse, and fibrosis, as well as the features of cirrhosis (see Chapter 45), may be present. Twenty per cent of cases are caused by chronic hepatitis B infection; others may follow non-A, non-B hepatitis. Drugs (Table 43–5) may cause an identical picture. Some cases show associated features that suggest autoimmunity ("lupoid hepatitis").

The clinical course ranges from asymptomatic disease to a severe illness with constitutional symptoms, cutaneous signs of chronic liver disease, jaundice, and hepatosplenomegaly. The variety of chronic active hepatitis called *lupoid hepatitis* predominates in young females and is often accompanied by prominent extrahepatic manifestations, including amenorrhea, skin rashes, acne, vasculitis, thyroiditis, and Sjögren's syndrome. In chronic active hepatitis, transaminase levels are elevated over a wide range and are characteristically accompanied by polyclonal hypergammaglobulinemia. Laboratory evidence of liver failure may be present (hyperbilirubinemia, prolonged prothrombin time, hypoalbuminemia). Antibodies to smooth muscle and antinuclear antibodies may be found, particularly in lupoid hepatitis. Wilson's disease may present clinically and histologically as a chronic active hepatitis and should be excluded in patients under the age of 35 (Chapter 45).

Liver biopsy is of great value in making the diagnosis of chronic active hepatitis, in differentiating it from milder forms of chronic hepatitis, and in assessing the progression of the disease to cirrhosis. Liver biopsy is

TABLE 43–5. CAUSES OF CHRONIC HEPATITIS

Viral Infections
  Hepatitis B virus
  Hepatitis B virus with superimposed hepatitis D virus
  Hepatitis non-A, non-B pathogens
Drugs and Toxins
  Methyldopa
  Amiodarone
  Isoniazid
Idiopathic
  Idiopathic with prominent autoimmune features (lupoid hepatitis)
  Idiopathic with minimal or no autoimmune features
Metabolic Liver Disease
  Wilson's disease
  Alpha$_1$-antitrypsin deficiency

considered prerequisite to any attempt to treat the disease with immunosuppressive agents.

Treatment. In certain, selected cases of chronic active hepatitis, corticosteroid therapy may lead to dramatic improvement in clinical, laboratory, and histological features of the disease as well as to reduced mortality. Azathioprine is also used, but mainly for its steroid-sparing effect. Patients likely to benefit from corticosteroids are those with severe symptoms, a fivefold or greater elevation in transaminases, and marked necroinflammatory activity on liver biopsy. In patients with HBsAg-positive chronic active hepatitis, immunosuppression will enhance viral replication, and corticosteroids are of no benefit in the course of the liver disease. Patients with drug-induced chronic hepatitis or Wilson's disease also will not respond to corticosteroids. Non-A, non-B chronic hepatitis is often mild and may undergo spontaneous improvement; patients with non-A, non-B hepatitis are therefore not usually considered candidates for immunosuppressive therapy.

Patients successfully managed with corticosteroids frequently relapse on discontinuation of the drug and may require its reinstitution. Liver transplantation is described in Chapter 44.

REFERENCES

Alter H (ed): Hepatitis. Semin Liver Dis, 6:1, 1986.
Centers for Disease Control: Update on hepatitis B prevention. Ann Intern Med 107:353, 1987.
Ockner RK: Acute viral hepatitis. *In* Wyngaarden JB, Smith LH Jr (eds): Cecil Textbook of Medicine. 18th ed. Philadelphia, WB Saunders Co, 1988, pp 818–826.
Ockner RK: Toxic and drug-induced liver disease. *In* Wyngaarden JB, Smith LH Jr (eds): Cecil Textbook of Medicine. 18th ed. Philadelphia, WB Saunders Co, 1988, pp 826–830.
Ockner RK: Chronic hepatitis. *In* Wyngaarden JB, and Smith LH Jr (eds): Cecil Textbook of Medicine. 18th ed. Philadelphia, WB Saunders Co, 1988, pp 830–833.
Zakim D, Boyer TD, Montgomery CM, Kanas N: Alcoholic liver disease. *In* Zakim D, Boyer TD (eds): Hepatology: A Textbook of Liver Disease. Philadelphia, WB Saunders Co, 1982, pp 739–789.

44

FULMINANT HEPATIC FAILURE

Fulminant hepatic failure is defined as hepatic failure with Stage III or IV encephalopathy (deep somnolence or coma) which develops in less than eight weeks in a patient *without pre-existing liver disease*. It results from severe widespread hepatic necrosis, commonly due to acute viral infection with B, A, D, or non-A, non-B viruses. It may also result from fatty liver of pregnancy, ischemic necrosis, or exposure to hepatotoxins such as acetaminophen, isoniazid, halothane, valproic acid, tetracycline, mushroom toxins (e.g., those of *Amanita phalloides*), or carbon tetrachloride. Reye's syndrome, a disease predominantly of children that is characterized by microvesicular fatty infiltration and little hepatocellular necrosis, often resembles fulminant hepatic failure.

Diagnosis

The diagnosis rests on the combination of hepatic encephalopathy, acute liver disease (elevated serum bilirubin, transaminases), and liver failure, the last-named usually indicated by hypoprothrombinemia.

Treatment

Treatment of fulminant hepatic failure remains supportive, as the underlying etiology of liver failure is rarely treatable (see Hepatic Transplantation, below). However, most processes that result in widespread liver cell necrosis and fulminant hepatic failure are transient events, and liver cell regeneration with recovery of liver function often occurs if patients do not succumb to the complications of liver failure in the interim. Meticulous supportive treatment in an intensive care unit setting has been shown to improve survival. Patients with fulminant hepatic failure should be cared for in centers with experience with this disease. Numerous complications (Table 44–1) attend fulminant hepatic failure, and careful identification and treatment of each are essential.

Hepatic encephalopathy, the sine qua non of fulminant hepatic failure, is often the first and most dramatic sign of liver failure. The pathogenesis of hepatic encephalopathy, discussed in Chapter 45, remains unclear; however, most clinical observations suggest a role for protein- and gut-derived toxins that are normally taken up and detoxified by the liver. Abnormal neurotransmitters synthesized from excess aromatic amino acids may also play a role in hepatic encephalopathy. Hepatic encephalopathy that accompanies fulminant hepatic failure differs from that associated with chronic liver disease in two important aspects: (1) It is rarely due to a reversible precipitating factor (see Table 45–6) and often responds to therapy only when liver function improves. (2) It is frequently associated with two other, potentially treatable, causes of coma—hypoglycemia and cerebral edema. Therapy for hepatic encephalopathy follows the principles outlined in Chapter 45. Because these patients are severely ill, all protein intake is stopped, intravenous glucose (1000

TABLE 44–1. MANAGEMENT OF FULMINANT HEPATIC FAILURE

COMPLICATION	PATHOGENESIS	MANAGEMENT
Hepatic encephalopathy	Liver failure	Stop protein, cleanse gut, administer lactulose or neomycin

Hypoglycemia	Decreased gluconeogenesis	Monitor blood sugar
		  10% glucose IV infusion
		  50% glucose IV if needed

Hemorrhage	Decreased synthesis of clotting factors	Vitamin K
	Stress ulcers	Prophylactic oral antacids or IV cimetidine to maintain alkaline gastric pH
	Disseminated intravascular coagulopathy	Fresh frozen plasma if serious bleeding occurs
Hyponatremia	Impaired free water clearance	Monitor blood electrolytes and fluid balance Water restriction
Hypokalemia	—	Potassium supplementation
Respiratory alkalosis	Hyperventilation	No therapy required usually
Metabolic acidosis	Lactic acidosis	IV bicarbonate if necessary
Cerebral edema	—	Consider intracranial pressure monitoring and treatment with IV mannitol
Azotemia	Hypovolemia	Identify and correct hypovolemia
	Hepatorenal syndrome	Dialysis is usually not necessary
	Acute tubular necrosis	
Infection	Impaired synthesis of complement	Prevent aspiration and catheter-related infection
Hypotension, hypoxia, pulmonary edema	Reduced systemic vascular resistance Pulmonary right-to-left shunts	Employ standard measures as needed

to 1500 calories per day) is administered, and lactulose is administered orally, per nasogastric tube, or by enema to cleanse the colon.

Hypoglycemia is a common complication of liver failure. All patients should receive 10 per cent glucose IV infusions with frequent monitoring of blood glucose levels. Other metabolic abnormalities commonly occur, including *hyponatremia, hypokalemia, respiratory alkalosis,* and *metabolic acidosis.* Thus frequent monitoring of blood electrolytes and pH is indicated.

Gastrointestinal hemorrhage may occur from stress ulcers, particularly in the face of impaired synthesis of clotting factors. All patients should receive vitamin K and prophylactic oral antacids or IV cimetidine to maintain gastric pH above 5. Fresh frozen plasma should be used only if clinically significant bleeding occurs.

Renal insufficiency is common in patients with liver failure (see Chapter 29). It is essential that hypovolemia be excluded as a cause of azotemia, by measuring central venous pressure if necessary. Survival of patients with either hepatorenal syndrome or acute tubular necrosis does not appear to be improved by dialysis.

Cerebral edema, the pathogenesis of which is unknown, is a particularly common complication of fulminant hepatic failure in children and young adults. It may result in intracranial herniation and generally portends a fatal outcome. Corticosteroid therapy is not useful; however, improved survival has been reported with intracranial pressure monitoring and IV administration of mannitol in selected patients.

Many other forms of therapy for fulminant hepatic failure have been tried, including corticosteroid administration, exchange transfusion, plasmapheresis, hemodialysis, charcoal hemoperfusion, and extracorporeal perfusion through a human cadaver or pig liver. None has been shown to offer any advantage over conventional supportive therapy, however.

Hepatic Transplantation

Hepatic transplantation (see Chapter 45) has been attempted in a few patients with fulminant hepatic failure with encouraging results. Because of the need for urgent transplantation, potential candidates should be transferred to transplant centers before they develop significant complications (such as coma, cerebral edema, hemorrhage, or infection).

Prognosis

Short-term prognosis is very poor, with the average reported survival being about 20 per cent. Long-term prognosis for those who survive is excellent. Follow-up studies have shown normal liver function and histology in virtually all surviving patients, regardless of the cause of the fulminant hepatic failure.

REFERENCES

Jones EA, Schafer DF: Fulminant hepatic failure. *In* Zakim D, Boyer TD (eds): Hepatology: A Textbook of Liver Disease. Philadelphia, WB Saunders Co, 1982, pp 415–445.

Scharschmidt BF: Acute and chronic hepatic failure with encephalopathy. *In* Wyngaarden JB, Smith LH Jr (eds): Cecil Textbook of Medicine. 18th ed. Philadelphia, WB Saunders Co, 1988, pp 852–856.

45

CIRRHOSIS OF THE LIVER AND ITS COMPLICATIONS

DEFINITION

Cirrhosis is the irreversible end result of fibrous scarring and hepatocellular regeneration that constitute the major responses of the liver to a variety of long-standing inflammatory, toxic, metabolic, and congestive insults. In cirrhosis, the normal hepatic lobular architecture is replaced by interconnecting bands of fibrous tissue surrounding nodules derived from foci of regenerating hepatocytes.

Regenerative nodules may be small (<3 mm, micronodular cirrhosis), a typical feature of alcoholic cirrhosis, or large (>3 mm, macronodular cirrhosis). The latter, also termed postnecrotic cirrhosis, is more commonly seen as a sequel to chronic active hepatitis. The pathology of cirrhosis determines its natural history and clinical manifestations. Thus, fibrous scarring and disruption of the hepatic architecture distort the vascular bed, leading to portal hypertension and intrahepatic shunting. Normal hepatocyte function is dis-

TABLE 45–1. CAUSES OF CIRRHOSIS

Alcohol
Hepatitis viruses (B and non-A, non-B)
Drugs
    Methyldopa
    Methotrexate
    Amiodarone
Autoimmune chronic active hepatitis
Biliary cirrhosis
    Primary biliary cirrhosis
    Secondary biliary cirrhosis
      bile duct strictures
      sclerosing cholangitis
      biliary atresia
      tumors of the bile ducts
      cystic fibrosis
Chronic hepatic congestion
    Budd-Chiari syndrome
    Chronic right-heart failure
    Constrictive pericarditis
Genetically determined metabolic diseases
    Hemochromatosis
    Wilson's disease
    Alpha$_1$-antitrypsin deficiency
    Galactosemia
Cryptogenic

turbed by the resulting inadequacy of blood flow and ongoing direct toxic, inflammatory, and/or metabolic damage to the hepatocytes.

TABLE 45–2. CLINICAL AND LABORATORY FEATURES OF CIRRHOSIS

CLINICAL	LABORATORY
Size and Consistency of the Liver	
Hepatomegaly, or small shrunken liver	
Firm to hard consistency	
Hepatocellular Dysfunction	
Jaundice	Hyperbilirubinemia
Spider angiomata	
Palmar erythema	
Gynecomastia	
Loss of body hair	
Testicular atrophy	
Dupuytren's contracture	
Muscle wasting, edema	Hypoalbuminemia, low BUN
Bruising	Prolonged prothrombin time
Signs of hepatic encephalopathy	
Fetor hepaticus	
Portal Hypertension	
Splenomegaly	Thrombocytopenia, leukopenia
Ascites	
Caput medusa	
Variceal bleeding	
Signs of Specific Diseases	
CREST syndrome	Antimitochondrial antibody (primary biliary cirrhosis)
Kayser-Fleischer rings	Low ceruloplasmin (Wilson's disease)

ETIOLOGY

Most of the conditions that may lead to cirrhosis (Table 45–1) are rarely encountered. Alcohol abuse is by far the most common cause of cirrhosis in the Western world, whereas hepatitis B is a major cause in the Third World. Cryptogenic cirrhosis is a diagnosis of exclusion, but many cases are likely to be an end result of chronic non-A, non-B infection. Causes of hepatic fibrosis alone (e.g., schistosomiasis, which leads to fibrosis of portal venous radicles and portal hypertension) are not classified as causes of cirrhosis, because the hepatic lobular pattern is well preserved and hepatocellular dysfunction (e.g., disordered protein synthesis) is usually lacking.

CLINICAL AND LABORATORY FEATURES

The presence of cirrhosis may remain undetected until autopsy. Individuals with cirrhosis who experience no symptoms and show little clinical evidence of hepatocellular dysfunction are often said to have *well-compensated* cirrhosis. As evidence of complications develops, particularly signs implying disturbed hepatocellular function, the clinical condition is referred to as *decompensated* cirrhosis. If the disease process leading to cirrhosis primarily affects the hepatocytes, e.g., excessive alcohol intake (parenchymal liver disease), evidence of failing hepatocellular function may be prominent in the clinical presentation. If the biliary system is primarily affected, as occurs in primary or secondary biliary cirrhosis, the clinical features of cholestasis predominate and hepatic failure is a late event.

It is convenient to divide the main clinical and laboratory features of cirrhosis into four categories (Table 45–2):

1. *Size and consistency of the liver.*
2. *Features attributable to hepatocellular dysfunction.* These result from both intrinsically "sick" hepatocytes and the shunting of portal blood away from hepatocytes with consequent failure to extract toxins and metabolites.
3. *Features attributable to portal hypertension.*
4. *Extrahepatic features related to specific diseases causing cirrhosis.*

Liver size depends upon the underlying pathological process. In end-stage liver disease due to hepatitis B virus infection, the liver is often small, scarred, and shrunken. In alcoholic cirrhosis, fat infiltration may lead to marked enlargement of the liver. Impaired hepatic detoxification of estrogens, as well as disturbed hypothalamic-pituitary function, produces several cutaneous signs (often called "stigmata" of cirrhosis, e.g., spider angiomata, palmar erythema). Marked jaundice in the absence of complete bile duct obstruction is often a grave prognostic sign implying advanced hepatocellular dysfunction. Impaired hepatocellular protein synthesis leads to hypoalbuminemia and hypoprothrombinemia.

SPECIFIC CAUSES OF CIRRHOSIS

Alcohol. Alcoholic cirrhosis may coexist with alcoholic hepatitis. Features of hepatocellular dysfunction are thus often marked and may improve with abstinence. Micronodular cirrhosis is the rule but is not specific for alcoholic cirrhosis. Evidence of malnutrition and vitamin deficiency is frequently found, particularly in the severely alcoholic patient. Anemia of mixed etiology is common, often with macrocytic indices.

Chronic Active Hepatitis. Chronic active hepatitis from any cause may progress to cirrhosis. The liver is typically small with a macronodular pattern. Evidence of continued inflammatory activity is often present, including moderate elevation of transaminase levels and hypergammaglobulinemia. HBsAg is usually persistently positive in cirrhosis due to hepatitis B virus infection.

Primary Biliary Cirrhosis. Almost exclusively a disease affecting women, primary biliary cirrhosis manifests mainly between the ages of 30 and 65 and results from a progressive, probably immune-mediated destruction of the intralobular bile ductules. Cholestatic features predominate with high serum levels of alkaline phosphatase and cholesterol. Pruritus is a major early symptom, followed later in the course of the disease by xanthomas, hyperpigmentation, and bone pain due to osteoporosis or osteomalacia. Commonly associated conditions include Sjögren's syndrome, scleroderma, and the CREST syndrome (calcinosis, Raynaud's syndrome, esophageal dysfunction, sclerodactyly, telangiectasia). Antimitochondrial antibodies are present in high titer, and serum IgM levels are elevated. Liver biopsy may show characteristic destructive lesions of the bile ductules and is of value in confirming the diagnosis. Jaundice is a prominent feature late in the course of the disease.

Hemochromatosis. See Chapter 63.

Wilson's Disease. See Chapter 63.

MAJOR COMPLICATIONS OF CIRRHOSIS

The major sequelae of cirrhosis are:

1. Portal hypertension, with its attendant complications of (a) variceal hemorrhage, and (b) splenomegaly and hypersplenism.
2. Liver failure.
3. Ascites, which may be further complicated by spontaneous bacterial peritonitis.
4. The hepatorenal syndrome.
5. Portosystemic (hepatic) encephalopathy.
6. Hepatocellular carcinoma.

The pathophysiological interrelationships among these complications are shown diagrammatically in Figure 45–1.

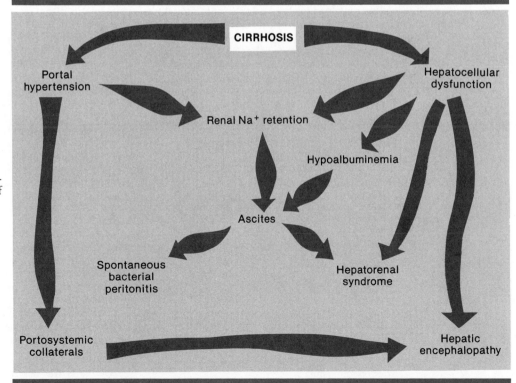

FIGURE 45–1. Interrelationships among the complications of cirrhosis.

Portal Hypertension

The normal liver offers little resistance to portal venous blood flow (about 1 L/min), and portal pressure is normally less than 5 mm Hg above inferior vena caval pressure. The distortion of hepatic architecture in cirrhosis leads to a marked increase in resistance to portal venous flow, which in turn leads to an increase in portal venous pressure.

Although cirrhosis is the most important cause of portal hypertension, any process leading to increased resistance to portal blood flow into (presinusoidal) or through the liver (sinusoidal) or to hepatic venous outflow from the liver (postsinusoidal) will result in portal hypertension (Table 45–3). Since the pressure within any vascular system is proportional to both resistance and blood flow, a marked increase in blood flow will also result in portal hypertension, although such situations are rare.

Portal hypertension leads to the formation of venous collaterals between the portal and systemic circulations. Collaterals may form at several sites, the most important clinically being those connecting the portal to the azygos vein, which form dilated, tortuous veins (varices) in the submucosa of the gastric fundus and esophagus.

Variceal Hemorrhage. Hemorrhage occurs most frequently from varices in the esophagus and is a common and serious complication of portal hypertension, with a mortality rate of 30 to 60 per cent. Large varices bleed most commonly, and bleeding occurs when high tension in the walls of these vessels leads to rupture. Bleeding may present as hematemesis, hematochezia, melena, or any combination of these (see Chapter 34B). Bleeding may lead to shock, stop spontaneously, or recur. Impaired hepatic synthesis of coagulation factors (hepatocellular dysfunction) and thrombocytopenia (hypersplenism) may further complicate the management of variceal bleeding. The management of variceal bleeding has been discussed in Chapter 34B, and here we will emphasize a few important details.

VASOPRESSIN. When given by intravenous infusion, this posterior pituitary hormone causes constriction of splanchnic arterioles and a reduction in portal flow and pressure. Bleeding may be controlled by this measure but recurs in about 50 per cent of patients. The use of vasopressin does not reduce mortality.

BALLOON TAMPONADE. Compression of the varices by inserting a tube with inflatable gastric and esophageal balloons (Sengstaken-Blakemore tube) is an effective, although often temporary, measure. Complications such as aspiration and esophageal rupture may occur, and rebleeding occurs in up to 60 per cent of patients after the tube is removed.

ENDOSCOPIC INJECTION SCLEROTHERAPY. During endoscopy, varices may be injected with sclerosing solutions to arrest acute bleeding. Repeated courses of injection can lead to variceal obliteration, and this approach has been used to prevent recurrent bleeding. However, bleeding frequently recurs prior to complete variceal obliteration, and esophageal strictures are a common complication.

PORTOSYSTEMIC SHUNT SURGERY. Portal decompression may be achieved by a variety of operative procedures aimed at creating a large connection between the high-pressure portal and low-pressure systemic venous systems. Nonselective shunts (e.g., portacaval anastomoses) decompress the entire portal system. Selective shunts (e.g., the distal splenorenal shunt) decompress the varices only. Survival is not improved by shunt surgery, and hepatic encephalopathy is a major complication. Shunt surgery is usually performed electively to prevent recurrent bleeding in patients with good preservation of liver function. Emergency shunt surgery carries a 50 per cent mortality and is rarely undertaken.

OTHER THERAPEUTIC MEASURES. Long-term treatment with beta-blocking drugs, mainly propranolol, reduces portal pressure and variceal blood flow. Beta-blockers have shown promise in the prevention of variceal bleeding, but this form of treatment is still regarded as experimental.

Splenomegaly. Portal hypertension leads to *congestive splenomegaly*, which is often, but not always, clinically apparent. Thrombocytopenia and, less commonly, leukopenia occur as a result of sequestration of platelets and leukocytes in the enlarged spleen (hypersplenism). Diminished numbers of these formed elements is usually of little clinical significance.

Liver Failure

The cirrhotic liver is often impaired in the synthesis of proteins by hepatocytes (hypoalbuminemia, impaired synthesis of coagulation factors) and in normal hepatic detoxification processes. The latter accounts for the development of signs such as spider angiomata and contributes to the development of hepatic encephalopathy, as well as to poorly understood hemodynamic and hormonal disorders that foster the development of ascites and the hepatorenal syndrome.

Ascites

Ascites is the accumulation of excess fluid in the peritoneal cavity. Although cirrhosis is the most com-

TABLE 45–3. CAUSES OF PORTAL HYPERTENSION

I. Increased resistance to flow
   Presinusoidal
      Portal or splenic vein occlusion (thrombosis, tumor)
      Schistosomiasis
      Congenital hepatic fibrosis
      Sarcoidosis
   Sinusoidal
      Cirrhosis (all causes)
      Alcoholic hepatitis
   Postsinusoidal
      Veno-occlusive disease
      Budd-Chiari syndrome
      Constrictive pericarditis
II. Increased portal blood flow
   Splenomegaly not due to liver disease
   Arterioportal fistula

mon cause of ascites, it may result from numerous other causes (Table 45–4). Ascites due to cirrhosis is commonly a transudate (protein concentration <3 gm/dl), whereas inflammatory and neoplastic causes usually lead to formation of an exudate (protein >3 gm/dl). Ascites becomes clinically detectable when more than 500 ml has accumulated. Shifting dullness to percussion is the most sensitive clinical sign of ascites but ultrasound more readily detects small fluid volumes.

Ascites in cirrhosis is the result of several pathogenetic factors: (a) portal hypertension with increased hepatic and splanchnic lymph production and transudation, (b) impaired renal sodium and water excretion secondary to hyperaldosteronism, increased levels of antidiuretic hormone, and other less well-understood factors, and (c) hypoalbuminemia.

Treatment of ascites consists initially of bed rest with restriction of sodium intake. Restricted fluid intake may be necessary if hyponatremia is present. These measures are commonly inadequate, and administration of spironolactone, an aldosterone antagonist, supplemented with a loop diuretic (e.g., furosemide) is often effective. Diuresis should be promoted cautiously, as aggressive diuretic therapy may result in hypokalemia and a depleted plasma volume, leading to hepatic encephalopathy and impaired renal function. A few patients may be extremely refractory to medical measures and may benefit from a surgically implanted plastic shunt between the peritoneal cavity and the superior vena cava (LeVeen shunt). Patients with massive ascites may benefit from abdominal paracentesis of 1 to 2 liters of ascitic fluid, but repeated paracentesis is a poor form of long-term therapy.

Two important complications occur in patients with cirrhotic ascites: spontaneous bacterial peritonitis and the hepatorenal syndrome.

Spontaneous Bacterial Peritonitis. Infection of ascitic fluid usually with coliform bacteria may occur in patients with cirrhosis. Fever, abdominal pain, and tenderness may be present or the infection may be clinically silent. Hepatic encephalopathy may be precipitated. The diagnosis is strongly suspected if the ascitic fluid white cell count is greater than 500/cu mm with greater than 50 per cent polymorphonuclear leukocytes, and is confirmed by Gram's stain and culture. Vigorous antibiotic treatment is indicated, but mortality from this complication is high.

Hepatorenal Syndrome. Serious liver disease from any cause may be complicated by a form of functional renal failure termed the hepatorenal syndrome. It almost invariably occurs in the presence of severe ascites. Typically, the kidneys are histologically normal, with the capacity of regaining normal function in the event of recovery of liver function. The renal dysfunction is characterized by a declining glomerular filtration rate (GFR), oliguria, low urine sodium (<10 mEq/L), and azotemia, often with a disproportionately high BUN/creatinine ratio. The decline in renal function often follows one of three events in a cirrhotic patient with ascites: sepsis, a vigorous attempt to re-

TABLE 45–4. CAUSES OF ASCITES

Exudative Ascites
  Tuberculous peritonitis
  Pancreatitis
  Ruptured viscus (including bile peritonitis)
  Tumors (most commonly metastatic to liver and peritoneal lining)
Transudative Ascites
  Cirrhosis
  Chronic hepatic congestion
    Budd-Chiari syndrome
    Constrictive pericarditis
    Right-heart failure
  Nephrotic syndrome
  Myxedema
  Meigs' syndrome
Chylous Ascites
  Thoracic duct or abdominal lymphatic trauma
  Mediastinal tumors

Differential diagnosis of ascites: ovarian cyst, pancreatic cyst, mesenteric cyst, urinary tract rupture

duce ascites with diuretics, or a large-volume paracentesis.

The hepatorenal syndrome is usually progressive and fatal. It should be diagnosed only after plasma volume depletion (a common cause of reversible, prerenal azotemia in patients with cirrhosis, particularly with diuretic use) and other forms of acute renal injury have been ruled out.

Hepatic Encephalopathy

Hepatic encephalopathy (also called hepatic coma or portosystemic encephalopathy) is a complex neuropsychiatric syndrome that may complicate advanced liver disease and/or extensive portosystemic collateral formation (shunting). Two major forms of hepatic encephalopathy are recognized:

Acute hepatic encephalopathy usually occurs in the setting of fulminant hepatic failure. Cerebral edema plays a more important role in this setting: coma is common and mortality is very high (see Chapter 44).

Chronic hepatic encephalopathy usually occurs with chronic liver disease, commonly manifests as subtle disturbances of neurological function, and is often reversible.

The pathogenesis of hepatic encephalopathy is thought to involve the inadequate hepatic removal of predominantly nitrogenous compounds or other toxins ingested or formed in the gastrointestinal tract. Inadequate hepatic removal results from impaired hepatocyte function as well as the extensive shunting of splanchnic blood directly into the systemic circulation via portosystemic collaterals. Nitrogenous and other absorbed compounds are thought to gain access to the central nervous system, leading to disturbances in neuronal function. Ammonia, derived from both amino acid deamination and bacterial hydrolysis of nitrogenous compounds in the gut, has been strongly implicated in the pathogenesis of hepatic encepha-

TABLE 45–5. STAGES OF HEPATIC ENCEPHALOPATHY

STAGE	CLINICAL MANIFESTATIONS
I	apathy restlessness reversal of sleep rhythm slowed intellect impaired computational ability impaired handwriting
II	lethargy drowsiness disorientation asterixis
III	stupor (arousable) hyperactive reflexes, extensor plantar responses
IV	coma (response to painful stimuli only)

Stage 0 encephalopathy is used to describe subclinical impairment of intellectual function.

lopathy, but its blood levels correlate poorly with the presence or degree of encephalopathy. Other proposed neurotoxins include gamma-aminobutyric acid, mercaptans, and short-chain fatty acids. Mercaptans are also thought to produce the characteristic breath odor (fetor hepaticus) of patients with chronic liver failure. Another hypothesis suggests that an imbalance between plasma branched-chain and aromatic amino acids, a common consequence of severe liver disease, leads to decreased synthesis of normal neurotransmitters and to increased formation of "false neurotransmitters" from aromatic amino acids in the central nervous system.

The clinical features of hepatic encephalopathy include disturbances of higher neurological function (intellectual and personality disorders, dementia, inability to copy simple diagrams [i.e., constructional apraxia], disturbance of consciousness), disturbances of neuromuscular function (asterixis, hyperreflexia, myoclonus), and rarely, a Parkinson-like syndrome and progressive paraplegia. As with other metabolic encephalopathies (which may show many of the signs of hepatic encephalopathy), asymmetrical neurological findings are unusual but can occur, and brain stem reflexes (e.g., pupillary light, oculovestibular, and oculocephalic responses) are preserved until very late. Hepatic encephalopathy is usually divided into stages according to its severity (Table 45–5). Subtle disorders of psychomotor function may exist in many patients with cirrhosis in whom conventional neurological examination is normal. Such subclinical encephalopathy (termed stage 0 encephalopathy) is of importance in that it may impair work performance.

The differential diagnosis of hepatic encephalopathy includes hypoglycemia, subdural hematoma, meningitis, and sedative drug overdosage, all of which are common in patients, particularly alcoholics, with liver disease.

Treatment   Treatment of hepatic encephalopathy is based on four simple principles:

IDENTIFICATION AND TREATMENT OF PRECIPITATING FACTORS.   Table 45–6 lists several important factors that may precipitate or severely aggravate hepatic encephalopathy in patients with severe liver disease. Gastrointestinal bleeding and increased protein intake may provide increased substrate for the bacterial or metabolic formation of nitrogenous compounds that induce encephalopathy. In patients prone to develop hepatic encephalopathy there is a markedly increased sensitivity to central nervous system–depressant drugs, and their use should be avoided in these patients.

REDUCTION AND ELIMINATION OF SUBSTRATE FOR THE GENERATION OF NITROGENOUS COMPOUNDS.   (a) **Dietary protein restriction.** Patients in coma should receive no protein, whereas those with mild encephalopathy may benefit from restriction of protein intake to 40 to 60 gm/day. Vegetable protein diets also appear to be less encephalopathogenic. (b) **Bowel cleansing.** This is important mainly in patients with encephalopathy precipitated by gastrointestinal bleeding or constipation and is achieved by administration of enemas.

REDUCTION OF COLONIC BACTERIA.   Neomycin administered orally reduces the number of bacteria that are responsible for production of ammonia and other nitrogenous compounds.

PREVENTION OF AMMONIA DIFFUSION FROM THE BOWEL.   This is achieved by administration of lactulose, a nonabsorbable disaccharide, which, when fermented to organic acids by colonic bacteria, leads to a lower stool pH. This lowered pH traps ammonia in the colon as nondiffusible NH_4^- ions, but other mechanisms such as inhibition of bacterial ammonia production may also be important.

Hepatocellular Carcinoma

Hepatocellular carcinoma and its relationship to cirrhosis are discussed in Chapter 46.

TABLE 45–6. HEPATIC ENCEPHALOPATHY: PRECIPITATING FACTORS

Gastrointestinal bleeding
Increased dietary protein
Constipation
Infection
CNS-depressant drugs (benzodiazepines, opiates)
Deterioration in hepatic function
Hypokalemia ⎫
Azotemia ⎬ most often induced by diuretics
Alkalosis ⎪
Hypovolemia ⎭

HEPATIC TRANSPLANTATION

Liver transplantation is a highly successful procedure in patients with progressive, advanced, and otherwise untreatable liver disease. Advances in surgical techniques and supportive care, the use of cyclosporine for immunosuppression, and careful selection of patients have all contributed to the recent encouraging results of liver transplantation. Seventy to 80 per cent of patients undergoing liver transplantation will survive at least three years, usually with good quality of life. The types of liver disease for which transplantation now is most commonly performed include nonalcoholic cirrhosis (e.g., primary biliary cirrhosis, chronic active hepatitis) and sclerosing cholangitis in adults and biliary atresia and metabolic disorders (e.g., alpha$_1$-antitrypsin deficiency) in children. Encouraging results have also been obtained in patients with fulminant hepatic failure (see Chapter 44). Transplantation for malignant hepatobiliary disease and hepatitis B virus–related disease has been less successful owing to recurrent disease in the transplanted liver.

The timing of liver transplantation presents a particular challenge because no technology for artificial support, analogous to hemodialysis, is yet available. The survival of ambulatory patients undergoing liver transplantation electively is greater than that of those who are critically ill at the time of the operation. Thus, transplantation is usually considered when deterioration in liver function (e.g., increasing jaundice, encephalopathy, ascites, or variceal bleeding) or declining quality of life becomes evident.

REFERENCES

Ascher NL: Liver transplantation—the first 25 years. West J Med 149:316, 1988.

Boyer TD: Cirrhosis of the liver. In Wyngaarden JB, Smith LH Jr (eds): Cecil Textbook of Medicine. 18th ed. Philadelphia, WB Saunders Co, 1988, pp 842–847.

Boyer TD: Major sequelae of cirrhosis. In Wyngaarden JB, Smith LH Jr (eds): Cecil Textbook of Medicine. 18th ed. Philadelphia, WB Saunders Co, 1988, pp 847–852.

Rocco V, Ware AJ: Cirrhotic ascites; pathophysiology, diagnosis, and management. Ann Intern Med 105:573, 1986.

Scharschmidt BF: Acute and chronic hepatic failure and hepatic transplantation. In Wyngaarden JB, Smith LH Jr (eds): Cecil Textbook of Medicine. 18th ed. Philadelphia, WB Saunders Co, 1988, pp 852–856.

Sherlock S: Chronic portal systemic encephalopathy: Update 1987. Gut 28:1043, 1987.

46

HEPATIC NEOPLASMS AND GRANULOMATOUS AND VASCULAR LIVER DISEASE

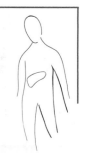

HEPATIC NEOPLASMS

Hepatic neoplasms can be divided into three groups: (1) benign neoplasms, (2) primary malignant neoplasms, and (3) metastatic malignant neoplasms. The last-named category, that of metastatic tumors, constitutes the bulk of hepatic neoplasms in this country. This chapter will briefly review all three categories of hepatic neoplasms and will conclude with a brief discussion of the diagnostic approach to these lesions.

Benign Neoplasms

The group of benign neoplastic lesions includes hepatocellular adenoma, focal nodular hyperplasia, hemangioma, bile duct adenoma, and other rare tumors of mesenchymal origin (e.g., fibromas, lipomas, leiomyomas). Hemangiomas, the most common hepatic neoplasm, are often readily identified by CT or MRI imaging. No further evaluation is necessary unless lesions are large and symptomatic. Hepatocellular adenomas occur almost exclusively in women, and there is strong circumstantial evidence to implicate estrogens, especially oral contraceptives, in their development and growth. Adenomas consist of a monotonous array of normal hepatocytes without bile ducts, portal tracts, or Kupffer cells. Although they are not regarded as premalignant lesions, they have a predilection for hemorrhage, tumor infarct, and rupture. Patients usually have signs and symptoms of an abdominal mass or hemorrhage (pain, fever, circulatory collapse). When circulatory collapse occurs, usually emergency surgery with resection of the adenoma is required.

Adenomas usually appear as cold spots on ^{99m}Tc-sulfur colloid scans and as vascular lesions on angiography. Management of asymptomatic lesions is controversial, although elective surgical excision is usually performed. A trial period of observation may be warranted if oral contraceptives can be discontinued, and some adenomas have been noted to regress under this regimen.

Hepatocellular Carcinoma

Hepatocellular carcinoma is rare in the United States (accounting for less than 2.5 per cent of all malignancies). In other areas of the world, including sub-Sahara Africa, China, Japan, and Southeast Asia, it is one of the most frequent malignancies and is an important cause of mortality, particularly in middle-aged males. Hepatocellular carcinoma usually arises in a cirrhotic liver and is closely associated with chronic hepatitis B virus infection, particularly in those parts of the world, enumerated above, in which infants acquire persistent infection with hepatitis B virus at birth from chronically infected mothers. The advent and widespread use of vaccination to prevent infection with hepatitis B virus are expected to reduce markedly the incidence of this disease, the only disease for which effective immunization against a malignancy is currently available. The risk of hepatocellular càrcinoma is low in cirrhosis associated with primary biliary cirrhosis and Wilson's disease, intermediate in cirrhosis due to alcohol, and high in hemochromatosis. Other risk factors for development of hepatocellular carcinoma, as well as its clinical manifestations, are listed in Table 46–1. Diagnosis of small, potentially treatable lesions, even in high-risk areas, is difficult, as the efficacy of screening for elevated α-fetoprotein levels has been equivocal. Most patients present with widespread, often multifocal disease, and the median survival from the time of diagnosis is less than six months. Hepatic resection can be attempted in patients with small, solitary lesions if the remaining liver is not cirrhotic. Chemotherapy, radiation therapy, and hepatic transplantation have yielded disappointing results.

Other primary hepatocellular malignancies include cholangiocarcinoma, angiosarcoma (related to exposure to vinyl choride, arsenic, or Thorotrast), hepatoblastoma, and cystadenocarcinoma.

Tumor Metastases to the Liver

Metastases constitute the bulk of hepatic malignancies and most commonly derive from tumors of the stomach, pancreas, colon, lung, oropharynx, and bladder and from melanoma. The liver is also a frequent site of involvement by Hodgkin's disease, non-Hodgkin's lymphoma, and malignant histiocytosis.

Diagnostic Approach to Hepatic Neoplasms

Most patients with hepatic neoplasms have right upper quadrant abdominal pain or an abdominal mass. Hemorrhage, systemic manifestations, and biliary obstruction (from strategically located tumors) may also occur. Visualization of discrete focal lesions and histological examination of tissue are generally required for diagnosis. Thus evaluation employs one or more imaging procedures followed by percutaneous, laparoscopic, or surgical biopsy of one or more lesions. Radionuclide scanning is a reasonable first step in the work-up, although imaging by computed tomography or ultrasound may be more sensitive in detecting small lesions and offers the advantage of performing guided percutaneous biopsy or aspiration cytology. MRI may be particularly helpful in this regard. Localization of lesions is generally followed by biopsy; however, additional factors must be considered. Percutaneous biopsies of vascular lesions such as hemangiomas, angiosarcomas, and perhaps hepatocellular adenomas are potentially dangerous, whereas cells obtained by aspiration cytology frequently fail to differentiate hepatocellular adenoma, hepatocellular carcinoma, and normal hepatic tissue. Thus, the choice of procedures will depend on the diagnostic and therapeutic options under consideration.

GRANULOMATOUS LIVER DISEASE

Hepatic granulomas are common, being found in 2 to 10 per cent of all liver biopsies, often in association with an elevated serum alkaline phosphatase level. However, they are rarely a specific finding and have been reported in association with a wide variety of infections, systemic illnesses, hepatobiliary disorders, drugs, and toxins, some of which are listed in Table 46–2. Although granulomas are a nonspecific finding, occasionally specific features are seen, such as acid-fast bacilli in tuberculosis, ova in schistosomiasis, larvae in toxocariasis, and birefringent granules in starch, talc, or silicone granulomas. The differential diagnosis of hepatic granulomas is one of the most extensive in medicine, and the work-up requires meticulous atten-

TABLE 46–1. HEPATOCELLULAR CARCINOMA

Incidence	**Unusual Manifestations**
From 1–7 per 100,000 to >100 per 100,000 in high-risk areas	Bloody ascites
	Tumor emboli (lung)
Sex	Jaundice
4:1 to 8:1 male preponderance	Hepatic or portal vein obstruction
Associations	Metabolic effects:
Chronic hepatitis B infection	erythrocytosis
Hemochromatosis (with cirrhosis)	hypercalcemia
Cirrhosis (alcoholic, cryptogenic)	hypercholesterolemia
Aflatoxin ingestion	hypoglycemia
Thorotrast	gynecomastia
Alpha₁-antitrypsin deficiency	feminization
Androgen administration	acquired porphyria
Common Clinical Presentations	**Clinical/Laboratory Findings**
Abdominal pain	Hepatic bruit or friction rub
Abdominal mass	Serum α-fetoprotein level >400 ng/ml
Weight loss	
Deterioration of liver function	

tion to details of the history, physical examination, and laboratory tests. Indeed, in 20 per cent or more of patients, no cause for granulomas is found despite extensive investigation. A subset of these patients have a syndrome consisting of fever, hepatomegaly, and hepatic granulomas which responds to administration of corticosteroids, described as "granulomatous hepatitis." These patients may possibly have a variant of sarcoidosis.

Liver biopsy (and culture, particularly of acid-fast bacteria) is of considerable value in the diagnosis of sarcoidosis, miliary tuberculosis, and histoplasmosis, as virtually all patients with these disorders will have hepatic granulomas. Characteristic granulomas are seen in many patients with primary biliary cirrhosis, and granulomas may be the first clue to Hodgkin's disease.

VASCULAR DISEASE OF THE LIVER

Portal vein thrombosis, hepatic vein thrombosis (Budd-Chiari syndrome), and veno-occlusive disease are uncommon disorders of hepatic vasculature; affected patients usually present with portal hypertension with or without associated liver dysfunction.

Portal vein thrombosis may develop after abdominal trauma, umbilical vein infection, sepsis, or pancreatitis or in association with cirrhosis or hypercoagulable states; in most cases, however, and particularly in children, the cause is unknown. The disease produces the manifestations of portal hypertension (see Chapter 45); however, liver histology is usually normal. The diagnosis is established by angiography. Surgical management is difficult owing to the absence of suitable patent vessels for portal-systemic shunting.

The *Budd-Chiari syndrome* is associated with abdominal trauma, use of oral contraceptives, polycythemia vera, paroxysmal nocturnal hemoglobinuria, other hypercoagulable states, and congenital webs of the vena cava. Illness may be acute or chronic with abdominal pain, hepatomegaly, ascites, and portal hypertension as prominent features. The diagnosis is usually suspected when centrilobular necrosis is seen on liver biopsy and is established angiographically by inability to catheterize the hepatic veins. Although elevation of serum bilirubin and transaminases is often mild, liver function is often poor and mortality rates of 40 to 90 per cent are reported. Anticoagulants have not proven useful; however, side-to-side portacaval shunts, performed to relieve hepatic congestion, may improve survival.

Veno-occlusive disease, or nonthrombotic occlusion of hepatic venules, is a small-vessel variant of the Budd-Chiari syndrome. Veno-occlusive disease develops in humans and animals exposed to native medicinal teas containing pyrrolozidine alkaloids from *Senecio* and *Crotalia* genera of plants. Cases have also been reported in association with the use of certain chemotherapeutic agents and with bone marrow

TABLE 46–2. DISEASES ASSOCIATED WITH HEPATIC GRANULOMAS

Infections	Hepatobiliary Disorders
Bacterial, spirochetal	Primary biliary cirrhosis
Tuberculosis and atypical	Granulomatous hepatitis
mycobacterial infections	Jejunoileal bypass
Tularemia	**Systemic Disorders**
Brucellosis	Sarcoidosis
Leprosy	Wegener's granulomatosis
Syphilis	Inflammatory bowel disease
Whipple's disease	Hodgkin's disease
Listeriosis	Lymphoma
Viral	**Drugs/Toxins**
Infectious mononucleosis	Beryllium
Cytomegalovirus infections	Parenteral foreign material
Rickettsial	(starch, talc, silicone, etc.)
Q fever	Phenylbutazone
Fungal	Alpha methyldopa
Coccidioidomycosis	Procainamide
Histoplasmosis	Allopurinol
Cryptococcal infections	Phenytoin
Actinomycosis	Nitrofurantoin
Aspergillosis	Hydralazine
Nocardiosis	
Parasitic	
Schistosomiasis	
Clonorchiasis	
Toxocariasis	
Ascariasis	
Toxoplasmosis	
Amebiasis	

transplantation. The occluded venules can be seen on liver biopsy, and a distinctive abnormal vascular pattern may be seen when contrast is injected into the hepatic vein. Patients with alcoholic liver disease also frequently exhibit some degree of hepatic venule sclerosis or occlusion. No specific treatment is available. Some patients appear to recover spontaneously, whereas others require therapy for the complications of portal hypertension.

LIVER ABSCESS

Pyogenic and amebic liver abscesses are important mass lesions of the liver. Unlike hepatic neoplasms, abscesses often present as a relatively acute febrile illness associated with pain in the right upper quadrant of the abdomen. Lesions can be localized by radionuclide scan, ultrasound, or computed tomography. The clinical presentation, diagnosis, and treatment of these lesions are discussed in Chapter 91.

REFERENCES

Di Bisceglie AM, Rustgi VK, Hoofnagle JH, et al: Hepatocellular carcinoma. Ann Intern Med 108:390, 1988.
Kew MC: Hepatic tumors. Semin Liver Dis 4:89, 1984.
Margolis S, Homcy C: Systemic manifestations of hepatoma. Medicine 51:381, 1972.

Scharschmidt BF: Hepatic tumors. *In* Wyngaarden JB, Smith LH Jr (eds): Cecil Textbook of Medicine. 18th ed. Philadelphia, WB Saunders Co, 1988, pp 856–859.
Scharschmidt BF: Parasitic, bacterial, fungal, and granulomatous liver disease. *In* Wyngaarden JB, Smith LH Jr

(eds): Cecil Textbook of Medicine. 18th ed. Philadelphia, WB Saunders Co, 1988, pp 834–838.
Zakim D, Boyer T (eds): Hepatology: A Textbook of Liver Disease. Philadelphia, WB Saunders Co, 1982, pp 464–498, 723–738.

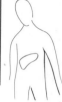

47

DISORDERS OF THE GALLBLADDER AND BILIARY TRACT

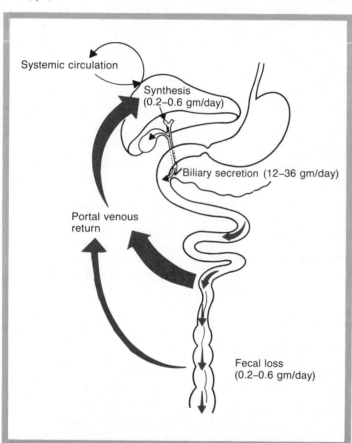

FIGURE 47–1. The enterohepatic circulation of bile salts in humans. The liver secretes 12 to 36 gm of bile salts per day in bile. Ninety five per cent of these bile salts are reabsorbed, with specific bile salt transporters in the terminal ileum accounting for much of the uptake. Bile salts recycle to the liver via portal blood where they are efficiently extracted by hepatocytes and resecreted into bile. The liver also synthesizes sufficient bile salts to equal daily fecal losses (0.2 to 0.6 gm/day). Because of efficient uptake of bile salts by both intestine and liver, delivery of 12 to 36 gm of bile salts to the intestine daily is achieved by recycling a small pool (3 gm) of bile salts 4 to 12 times per day. (Modified from Carey MC: The enterohepatic circulation. *In* Arias IM, Popper H, Schacter D, et al (eds): The Liver: Biology and Pathobiology. New York, Raven Press, 1982.)

The liver produces 500 to 1500 ml of bile per day. The major physiological role of the biliary tract and gallbladder is to concentrate this material and to conduct it silently and efficiently, in well-timed aliquots, to the intestine. In the intestine, biliary bile acids participate in normal fat digestion while cholesterol and a wide variety of other endogenous and exogenous compounds carried in bile are excreted in the feces. Normally unobtrusive, the gallbladder and biliary tree are the source of considerable pain and disability when they become infected or obstructed. This chapter will briefly outline the normal physiology of the biliary system and then focus on the pathophysiology and clinical consequences of gallstones, the most important biliary tract disorder, closing with a brief discussion of neoplasms and other causes of bile duct obstruction. The reader is referred to Chapter 42 for a detailed discussion of the diagnostic approach to jaundice and biliary obstruction and to Chapter 35 for a review of the various imaging techniques used to study the biliary tract.

NORMAL BILIARY PHYSIOLOGY

Bile, a complex fluid secreted by hepatocytes, passes via the intrahepatic bile ducts into the common bile duct. Tonic contraction of the sphincter of Oddi during fasting diverts about half of hepatic bile into the gallbladder where it is stored and concentrated. Cholecystokinin, released after food ingestion, causes contraction of the gallbladder and relaxation of the sphincter of Oddi, allowing delivery of a nicely timed bolus of bile, rich in bile acids, into the intestine. Bile acids, detergent molecules possessing both fat-soluble and water-soluble moieties, convey phospholipids and cholesterol from the liver to the intestine, where the latter undergoes fecal excretion. In the intestinal lumen, bile acids solubilize dietary fat and promote its digestion and absorption. Bile acids are, for the most part, efficiently reabsorbed by the small intestinal mucosa, particularly in the terminal ileum, and are recycled to the liver for re-excretion, a process termed enterohepatic circulation (Fig. 47–1).

PATHOPHYSIOLOGY OF GALLSTONE FORMATION (CHOLELITHIASIS)

Gallstones, the most common cause of biliary tract disease in the United States, occur in 20 to 35 per cent of people by the age of 75 and are of two types: 75 per cent consist primarily of cholesterol, whereas 25 per cent, termed pigment stones, are composed of calcium bilirubinate and other calcium salts. Cholesterol, which is insoluble in water, normally is carried in bile solubilized by bile acids and phospholipids. However, in many individuals, not all of whom will develop gallstones, bile contains more cholesterol than can be maintained in stable solution (Fig. 47–2); i.e., it is supersaturated with cholesterol. In the supersaturated bile of many, but not all, such individuals, microscopic cholesterol crystals form. The interplay of nucleation (mucus, stasis) and "antinucleating" (apo-lipoprotein A-I) factors may determine whether cholesterol gallstones form in supersaturated bile. Gradual deposition of additional layers of cholesterol leads to the appearance of macroscopic cholesterol gallstones. The gallbladder is key to gallstone formation; it constitutes an area of bile stasis in which slow crystal growth can occur and it also may provide mucus or other material to act as a nidus to initiate cholesterol crystal formation. Many of the recognized predisposing factors for cholelithiasis can be understood in terms of the pathophysiological scheme just outlined: (1) biliary cholesterol saturation is increased by estrogens, multiparity, oral contraceptives, obesity, and terminal ileal disease (which decreases the bile acid pool); (2) bile stasis is increased by bile duct strictures, parenteral hyperalimentation, fasting, and choledochal cysts.

The pathophysiology of pigment stones is less well understood; however, increased production of bilirubin (hemolytic states), cirrhosis, and bacterial deconjugation of bilirubin to a less soluble form are all associated with pigment stone formation.

CLINICAL MANIFESTATIONS OF GALLSTONES

Most individuals with gallstones are asymptomatic. Duct obstruction is the underlying cause of all manifestations of gallstone disease. Obstruction of the cystic duct distends the gallbladder and produces biliary pain, while superimposed infection or inflammation leads to acute cholecystitis. Obstruction of the common duct may produce pain, jaundice, infection (cholangitis), pancreatitis, and/or hepatic damage and biliary cirrhosis. The natural history of gallstone disease is outlined in Figure 47–3.

Asymptomatic Gallstones. Approximately 60 to 80 per cent of patients with gallstones in the United

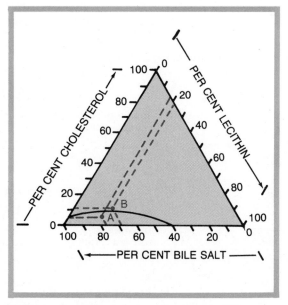

FIGURE 47–2. Phase diagram for plotting different mixtures of bile salt, lecithin, and cholesterol. The curved line represents the boundary of the micellar zone for aqueous solutions containing 4 to 10 per cent solids. Any mixture, such as A, falling within this area contains all its cholesterol in solution. Any mixture, such as B, falling outside this area has excess cholesterol as a precipitate or supersaturated solution. The points A and B actually depict the average composition of gallbladder bile obtained from normal persons and patients with cholesterol gallstones, respectively.

States are asymptomatic, and over a 20-year period it appears that only about 18 per cent of these individuals will develop biliary pain and only 3 per cent will require a cholecystectomy. Asymptomatic patients should be followed expectantly, with prophylactic cholecystectomy considered in three high-risk groups: (1) diabetics, who have a greater mortality (10 to 15 per cent) from acute cholecystitis; (2) persons with a calcified gallbladder, which is often associated with carcinoma of the gallbladder; and (3) persons with sickle cell anemia, in whom hepatic crises may be difficult to differentiate from acute cholecystitis. Attempts to dissolve cholesterol gallstones by orally administered chenodeoxycholic acid or ursodeoxycholic acid have been successful in some patients; however, a policy of expectant management followed by cholecystectomy is probably more cost-effective. Alternative methods under development to eliminate gallstones include (a) dissolution of cholesterol stones by instillation of methyl-tert-butyl ether into the gallbladder and (b) fragmentation of stones by extracorporeal shock-wave lithotripsy.

Chronic Cholecystitis and Biliary Pain. The term chronic cholecystitis has been used to denote nonacute symptoms due to the presence of gallstones. A better term is biliary (pain), as there is only a loose correlation between the presence of symptoms and pathologic findings such as inflammation in the gall-

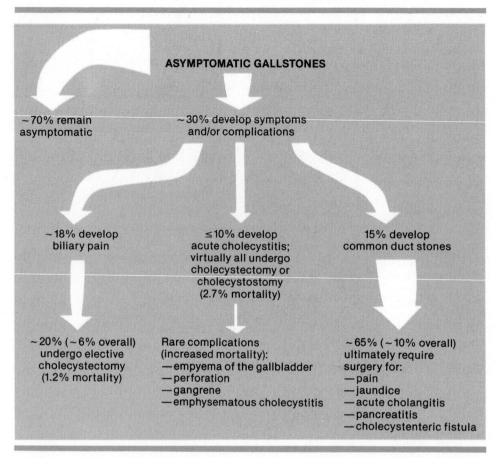

ASYMPTOMATIC GALLSTONES

~70% remain asymptomatic

~30% develop symptoms and/or complications

~18% develop biliary pain

≤10% develop acute cholecystitis; virtually all undergo cholecystectomy or cholecystostomy (2.7% mortality)

15% develop common duct stones

~20% (~6% overall) undergo elective cholecystectomy (1.2% mortality)

Rare complications (increased mortality):
—empyema of the gallbladder
—perforation
—gangrene
—emphysematous cholecystitis

~65% (~10% overall) ultimately require surgery for:
—pain
—jaundice
—acute cholangitis
—pancreatitis
—cholecystenteric fistula

FIGURE 47–3. Natural history of asymptomatic gallstones. The clinical syndromes associated with gallstones are shown here, and the numbers represent the approximate percentage of adults who develop one or more of these symptoms or complications over a 15- to 20-year period. Over this period, approximately 30 per cent of individuals with gallstones will undergo surgery. (The risk of developing complications of gallstones varies considerably among series. The figures shown here represent those derived from more recent studies.)

bladder wall. Gallbladders from symptomatic patients may be grossly normal with mild histological inflammation or may exhibit shrinking, scarring, and thickening, often as a result of previous attacks of acute cholecystitis. Symptoms arise from contraction of the gallbladder during transient obstruction of the cystic duct by gallstones. Biliary pain usually is a steady, cramplike pain in the epigastrium or right upper quadrant which comes on quickly, reaches a plateau of intensity over a few minutes, and begins to subside gradually over 30 minutes to several hours. Referred pain may be felt at the tip of the scapula or right shoulder. Nausea and vomiting may accompany biliary pain, whereas fever, leukocytosis, and a palpable mass (signs of acute cholecystitis) do not. Attacks occur at variable intervals (days to years). Other symptoms such as dyspepsia, fatty food intolerance, flatulence, heartburn, and belching may occur in patients with gallstones; however, they are nonspecific and frequently occur in individuals with normal gallbladders. Gallstones can be best demonstrated by ultrasound (which demonstrates gallstones in more than 95 per cent of patients). Alternatively, one can use oral cholecystography (which demonstrates stones in two thirds of patients; the gallbladder is not visualized in one third of patients, a finding taken to indicate gallbladder disease). Cholecystectomy, which carries a mortality of less than 0.5 per cent, is the treatment of choice for recurrent biliary pain, and may be accompanied by examination of the common duct for concomitant choledocholithiasis. Surgery relieves symptoms of biliary pain in virtually all patients and will prevent development of future complications such as acute cholecystitis, choledocholithiasis, and cholangitis. Alternative approaches to eliminating gallstones, including dissolution and fragmentation, are less commonly employed.

Acute Cholecystitis. Acute cholecystitis refers to

acute right subcostal pain and tenderness due to obstruction of the cystic duct and subsequent distention, inflammation, and secondary infection of the gallbladder. Acalculous cholecystitis, accounting for 5 per cent of cases, is associated with prolonged fasting, e.g., trauma, surgery, or parenteral hyperalimentation, and gallbladder bile that is viscous or "sludgelike." Acute cholecystitis usually begins with epigastric or right upper quadrant pain that gradually increases in severity and usually localizes to the area of the gallbladder. Unlike biliary pain, the pain of acute cholecystitis does not subside spontaneously. Anorexia, nausea, vomiting, fever, and right subcostal tenderness are commonly present, as is Murphy's sign (increased subhepatic tenderness and inspiratory arrest during a deep breath). In approximately one third of patients, a tender, enlarged gallbladder may be felt. Mild jaundice occurs in about 20 per cent of patients as a result of concomitant common duct stones or bile duct edema. Complications of acute cholecystitis include emphysematous cholecystitis (bacterial gas present in gallbladder lumen and tissues), empyema of the gallbladder, gangrene, and perforation. Approximately 10 per cent of patients will present with or develop one of these complications and require emergency surgery. The onset of severe fever, shaking chills, increased leukocytosis, increased abdominal pain or tenderness, or persistent severe symptoms, alone or in combination, indicates progression of disease and suggests development of one of these complications.

Radionuclide scanning following intravenous administration of ^{99m}Tc-DISIDA is the most accurate test with which to confirm the clinical impression of acute cholecystitis (cystic duct obstruction). If the gallbladder fills with the isotope, acute cholecystitis is unlikely, whereas if the bile duct is visualized but the gallbladder is not, the clinical diagnosis is strongly supported. An ultrasound examination that shows the presence of gallstones (or sludge in acalculous cholecystitis) along with localized tenderness over the gallbladder also provides strong supportive evidence for acute cholecystitis. Oral cholecystograms are of no value in this clinical setting, as they are unreliable in the acutely ill patient.

Most patients with acute cholecystitis will improve over one to seven days with conventional expectant management, which includes nasogastric suction, intravenous fluids, and judicious pain medication. Because of the high risk of recurrent acute cholecystitis, it is recommended that most patients undergo elective cholecystectomy within four to eight weeks of an acute episode.

An alternative course of management, outlined in Figure 47–4, is to perform early (acute) cholecystectomy. This approach is less costly and involves no increase in morbidity or mortality. Emergency surgery is performed on those patients with advanced disease and complications, usually associated with infection and sepsis. Cholecystostomy (either operative or percutaneous), rather than cholecystectomy, may be a useful technique in patients in whom there is a high

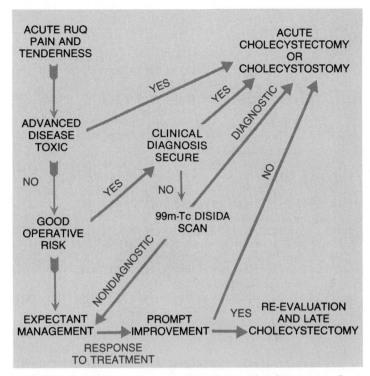

FIGURE 47–4. Scheme for managing patients with right upper quadrant pain and tenderness who are thought to have acute cholecystitis. This scheme is based on a policy of early operation for appropriate patients, and use of cholecystostomy (operative or percutaneous) for patients who are poor operative risks.

operative risk. Patients who are good operative risks and in whom the diagnosis is certain are scheduled for prompt cholecystectomy within 24 to 48 hours. Antibiotics are used in patients with suppurative complications. Expectant management is reserved for those with uncomplicated disease who are not good operative candidates or those in whom the diagnosis is not clear.

The mortality of acute cholecystitis of 5 to 10 per cent is almost entirely confined to patients over 60 years of age with serious associated diseases and to those with suppurative complications. Complications of acute cholecystitis include infectious complications already listed and gallstone ileus (intestinal obstruction due to a gallstone that has eroded through the gallbladder and duodenal walls into the intestinal lumen).

Choledocholithiasis and Acute Cholangitis. In the United States, most gallstones in the common duct come from the gallbladder; this occurs in up to 15 per cent of persons with cholelithiasis. Less commonly, stones may form de novo in the biliary tree. Ductal stones may be asymptomatic (30 to 40 per cent) or may produce biliary colic, jaundice, cholangitis, pancreatitis, or a combination of these. Secondary hepatic effects include biliary cirrhosis and hepatic abscesses.

Intermittent cholangitis, consisting of biliary pain, jaundice, and fever plus chills (Charcot's triad), is the most common manifestation of choledocholithiasis. Biliary infection may be mild or it may be severe, with suppurative cholangitis, sepsis, and shock. Diagnosis is based on a compatible clinical picture and radiological or endoscopic evidence of ductal stones. Treatment includes hospitalization, treatment of infection, and removal of stones. The latter may be accomplished surgically in patients with an intact gallbladder by cholecystectomy and choledochotomy. In individuals with a previous cholecystectomy or those who are poor surgical candidates, endoscopic sphincterotomy, which opens the sphincter of Oddi and allows passage of gallstones up to 1 cm in size, is the preferred approach.

The severest form of cholangitis, suppurative cholangitis, rapidly results in life-threatening sepsis. Initially, the patients may have only mild signs of biliary obstruction, yet they require rapid evaluation and treatment, including intravenous fluids and antibiotics and emergency procedures (surgical, endoscopic, or percutaneous) to drain the biliary tree. The high mortality of 50 per cent for this disease reflects the age of the patients generally affected, the speed with which sepsis develops, and the frequent failure to identify the biliary tree as the source of sepsis.

Other Disorders of the Biliary Tree. A number of other processes, all of which may present as biliary obstruction, jaundice, or infection, may involve the biliary tree. The approach to evaluating these entities is outlined in Chapter 35.

Benign biliary strictures usually result from surgical injury and may cause symptoms days to years later. Early diagnosis is important, as strictures that partially obstruct and are clinically asymptomatic may cause secondary biliary cirrhosis. Biliary stricture should be suspected in anyone with a history of right upper quadrant surgery and a persistently elevated serum alkaline phosphatase level. A similar type of benign stricture is seen in alcoholics in whom the intrapancreatic portion of the common bile duct is compressed by pancreatic fibrosis. Surgical repair or bypass of these lesions is successful in 75 per cent of patients. Balloon catheter dilatation may be useful in selected individuals.

Sclerosing cholangitis is an idiopathic condition of nonmalignant, nonbacterial chronic inflammatory narrowing of the intra- and extrahepatic bile ducts. It most commonly occurs in males, often in association with ulcerative colitis. Patients usually present with pruritus or jaundice, and percutaneous transhepatic cholangiography or endoscopic retrograde cholangiopancreatography shows characteristic changes ("beading") of the bile ducts. Therapy is supportive.

Structural abnormalities such as choledochal cysts, Caroli's disease (saccular intrahepatic bile duct dilation), and duodenal diverticuli may also cause bile duct obstruction, often with secondary choledocholithiasis. Hemobilia and intermittent bile duct obstruction by blood clots are caused by hepatic injury, neoplasms, or hepatic artery aneurysms.

Biliary neoplasms are rare, but include carcinoma of the gallbladder, scirrhous or papillary adenocarcinoma of the bile ducts, and carcinoma of the ampulla of Vater. The latter two neoplasms usually present as unremitting painless jaundice, although necrosis and sloughing of tumor may cause intermittent obstruction and the appearance of occult fecal blood. The term "Klatskin tumor" specifically refers to an adenocarcinoma located at the bifurcation of the common hepatic duct. Carcinoma of the gallbladder often presents as advanced disseminated disease, although symptoms also may resemble those of acute or chronic cholecystitis or bile duct obstruction. Resection of most of these tumors is difficult or impossible and prognosis is poor. For patients with unresectable tumor the goal is palliation, and for those with severe symptoms due to obstruction, percutaneous or endoscopic stenting of the biliary tree may be helpful. Stents should *not* be used in patients with benign disease because complications due to biliary infection and plugging of the stent invariably occur; rather, definitive surgical repair or bypass is preferred.

Motility disorders of the biliary tree have not been well recognized in the past. With the use of newer endoscopic techniques for measuring biliary pressures and motility, it has become apparent that a small group of patients with biliary-type pain have symptoms due to hypertension, dysmotility, and/or stenosis of the sphincter of Oddi, and in this select group, surgical or endoscopic sphincterotomy is of value.

REFERENCES

Gracie WA, Ransohoff DF: The natural history of silent gallstones. The innocent gallstone is not a myth. N Engl J Med 307:798, 1982.

Malet PF, Soloway RD: Diseases of the gallbladder and bile ducts. *In* Wyngaarden JB, Smith LH Jr (eds): Cecil Textbook of Medicine. 18th ed. Philadelphia, WB Saunders Co, 1988, pp 859–872.

Sleisenger MH, Fordtran JS (eds): Gastrointestinal Disease: Pathophysiology, Diagnosis and Management. 4th ed. Philadelphia, WB Saunders Co, 1989.

Thistle JL, Cleary, PA, Lachin, JM, et al: The natural history of cholelithiasis: The national cooperative gallstone study. Ann Intern Med 101:171, 1984.

Wiesner RH, LaRusso NF: Clinicopathological features of the syndrome of primary sclerosing cholangitis. Gastroenterology 79:200, 1980.

Zakim D, Boyer T (eds): Hepatology: A Textbook of Liver Disease. 2nd ed. Philadelphia, WB Saunders Co, 1989.

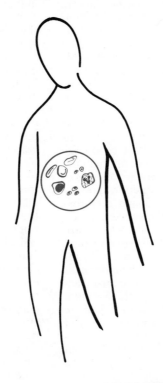

48

HEMATOPOIESIS

Bone marrow in the adult occupies the vertebrae, sternum, ribs, pelvic bones, and, to a lesser extent, the long bones and skull, and comprises about 1 kg of tissue. In the child, hematopoiesis is more prominent in the long bones and skull, whereas in adulthood fatty tissue replaces the hematopoietic marrow in these peripheral areas. In addition, liver and spleen, primary sites of hematopoiesis in the fetus, may regain hematopoietic acitivity in certain adult diseases, including severe anemias, skeletal marrow failure, myelofibrosis, and hematologic malignancies such as leukemia.

Normal bone marrow consists of about 50 per cent hematopoietic cells and 50 per cent fat, with the hematopoietic cells being arranged in cords around sinusoids; blood vessels are abundant. The space occupied by fat increases during adulthood, although hematopoietic tissue can replace it under appropriate conditions at any age. The hematopoietic cells include a small pluripotential stem cell compartment, consisting of small cells resembling lymphocytes, a large compartment of proliferating cells of committed lineage (the ratio of myeloid:erythroid precursors is normally 3 to 5:1), and a large compartment of postmitotic maturing cells of both myeloid and erythroid lineage. Smaller numbers of megakaryocytes, which differentiate into platelets, plasma cells (which produce immunoglobulins), reticulum cells, and lymphocytes are also present. It requires about one week for a stem cell to differentiate into mature daughter cells of either erythroid or myeloid type; the marrow additionally contains about one week's worth of mature leukocytes and erythrocytes. The circulating half-life of polymorphonuclear leukocytes is about 6 hours, of platelets 8 to 10 days, and of erythrocytes 120 days; thus, the granulocyte pool is released much faster than the erythrocyte pool, which is renewed at a rate of 0.8 per cent per day. Because the ratio in the peripheral blood of granulocytes:erythrocytes:platelets is about 1:1000:100, approximately equal numbers of these three cell types are released from the bone marrow each day.

Erythropoiesis is under the control of the hormone erythropoietin, released from the kidney under the stimulus of tissue hypoxia. A glycoprotein of molecular weight 46,000, erythropoietin may also be produced in the liver. It stimulates primitive pluripotential or stem cells into erythropoietic differentiation, acting mainly on the CFU-E (colony forming unit-erythroid) to promote differentiation into proerythroblasts. The earliest recognizable red cell precursor, the *erythroblast*, eventually gives rise to eight or more mature erythrocytes. The erythroblast is a large cell with abundant endoplasmic reticulum, which decreases in size as it matures, incorporates transferrin-bound iron via specific membrane receptors, and begins to form hemoglobin. In more mature stages the developing erythroblasts, the basophilic, then polychromato-

philic, then orthochromic *normoblasts*, lose the capacity to divide. Their nuclei become pyknotic and are finally extruded prior to release of the erythrocytes from the bone marrow. Newly released erythrocytes, or *reticulocytes*, have active mitochondrial function and retain the capacity to form hemoglobin; about 25 per cent of hemoglobin is synthesized after these cells leave the bone marrow, but the mature erythrocyte in the circulation lacks the capacity for protein synthesis and is anucleate. Its energy is supplied by glycolysis.

The earliest recognizable granulocyte precursor is the *myeloblast*, although developmentally committed stem cells, CFU-C, can be identified in tissue culture. Colony stimulating factors (CSF) produced by monocytes and lymphocytes in response to stimuli such as bacterial endotoxin stimulate mitosis in granulocyte precursors. Prostaglandin E_2 inhibits granulocyte production. *Promyelocytes*, the next stage of myeloblast differentiation, are the largest marrow cells except for megakaryocytes. They contain primary lysosomal granules and give rise to neutrophilic, eosinophilic, or basophilic *myelocytes*, which display the specific granules that identify each myeloid subtype. Myelocytes form the most abundant type of myeloid cell in the marrow and represent the last proliferating cell pool; their descendants, *metamyelocytes*, *bands*, and *neutrophils* (or eosinophils or basophils) are incapable of cell division but show increasing functional activity concomitant with maturation of membrane functions: chemotaxis, phagocytosis, bactericidal action. After extrusion from the bone marrow, granulocytes occupy two geographic pools in free equilibrium: a marginated pool of cells adhering to blood vessel walls and a circulating pool of roughly equal size. Once in the peripheral blood, granulocytes, like erythrocytes, do not normally re-enter the bone marrow. They follow a "one-way traffic" pattern, spending a relatively short time in the peripheral blood (average, 6 hours) and exiting into the tissues.

The *megakaryocyte*, the only giant, multinucleated cell in the hematopoietic lineage, also derives from the primitive stem cell, and undergoes endomitosis, reaching DNA contents of 32 to 64 n. Specific surface markers characteristic of mature platelets appear at very early stages in megakaryocyte differentiation and persist through maturation. Megakaryocytes tend to stay near marrow sinusoids, where they mature, developing internal membranes that mark off platelet fields. Each megakaryocyte eventually breaks up, releasing some 5000 *platelets* at the edge of a marrow sinusoid into the blood. Some megakaryocytes circulate and may release their platelets in the lung. Although platelets are anucleate fragments of megakaryocytes, they possess a highly organized structure and glycogen energy stores (and some mitochondria) and circulate for 7 to 10 days.

Marrow lymphocytes are mainly of B cell origin, arising also in spleen and lymph nodes. Primitive T cell precursors arise in the marrow, travel to the thymus, where they undergo further differentiation, and thence to spleen, lymph nodes, or marrow as fully functional mature T cells. Lymphocytes are generally much longer-lived than other marrow cells and may survive for years.

Bone marrow functions include hematopoiesis, the differentiation of antibody-producing plasma cells, and the monitoring of hematopoietic cell quality. Normal bone marrow has an 8- to 10-fold capacity to increase blood cell production in response to humoral signals, which include erythropoietin, colony-stimulating factors, and prostaglandins. Normal bone marrow function depends upon intact marrow architecture, the availability of key nutrients including iron, folic acid, and vitamin B_{12}, and regulatory hormones.

Two types of injury can induce marrow failure: damage that affects the capacity for stem cells to undergo differentiation (e.g., in aplastic anemia) and damage that alters the marrow microenvironment (e.g., invasion of marrow by infection or tumor).

REFERENCES

Golde DW, Takaku F (eds): Hematopoietic Stem Cells. New York, Marcel Dekker, Inc, 1984.
Seiff CA: Hematopoietic growth factors. J Clin Invest 79:1549–1557, 1987.

49

ANEMIA

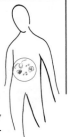

Definition

Anemia represents a decrease in red cell mass or hemoglobin content of blood below physiological need as set by tissue oxygen demand. The conventional limits for normal range of hemoglobin represent the values obtained for 95 per cent of a normal, healthy population, assuming a normal distribution of individuals (Table 49–1). In physiological terms, different ranges exist for men and women, for infants and growing children, and for different metabolic states. Anemia is an expression of many pathological conditions and is not itself a disease state but a clinical sign of such disorders. Therefore, analysis of any anemia should follow a tripartite logical pathway: (1) seek mechanisms by which the anemia occurs, e.g., bleeding, lack of red cell production, or excessive red cell destruction; (2) identify associated diseases that cause anemia; (3) evaluate morphologically the peripheral blood smear (Fig. 49–1).

Determinants of the normal range for hemoglobin, hematocrit, and red cell count include age, sex, and ambient altitude. Newborn infants have high values, which soon decline with rapid growth in infancy. Prepubertal boys and girls have similar values. At puberty, male sex hormones produce a rise in erythropoiesis so that adult males have hemoglobin levels approximately 2 to 4 gm/dl higher and hematocrits 5 to 7 per cent higher than adult females. The healthy elderly normally suffer no decline in hemoglobin or hematocrit values; however, because of increased incidence of chronic diseases, elderly populations may show slight decreases in these values. Populations living at altitudes over 4000 feet above sea level show increased hematocrits, which appear to represent physiological adaptation to the desaturation resulting from diminished atmospheric oxygen tension.

Clinical Assessment of Anemia

Signs and symptoms of anemia vary with the rapidity of onset and with underlying disease of the cardiovascular system (Table 49–2). Thus, rapid blood loss, especially if plasma volume decreases rapidly, or brisk hemolysis may result in cardiovascular compensatory reactions, including tachycardia, postural hypotension, vasoconstriction in skin and extremities, dyspnea on exertion, and faintness. Slowly developing anemias, such as those resulting from nutritional deficiency, permit gradual expansion of the plasma volume so that increased cardiac output gradually compensates. The subject may remain asymptomatic, noting only slight exertional dyspnea or, in the case of pre-existing coronary artery disease, increased angina. Pallor of skin and mucous membranes, jaundice, cheilosis (fissuring of the angles of the mouth), a beefy red, smooth tongue, and koilonychia (spoon-shaped nails) are signs that accompany more advanced anemias of different types. The level of anemia at which

TABLE 49–1. NORMAL VALUES FOR HEMOGRAM IN ADULTS

	MALE	FEMALE
Hemoglobin (gm/dl)	13.5–17.5	11.5–15.5
Hematocrit (%)	40–52	36–48
Red cell count (× 10^{12}/L)	4.5–6.5	3.9–5.6
Mean cell hemoglobin (MCH) (pg)	27–34	
Mean cell volume (MCV) (fl)	80–95	
Mean cell hemoglobin concentration (MCHC) (gm/dl)	30–35	
White blood cell count (× 10^9/L)	4–11	
Platelet count (× 10^9/L)	150–450	
Reticulocyte count (%)	0.5–1.5	

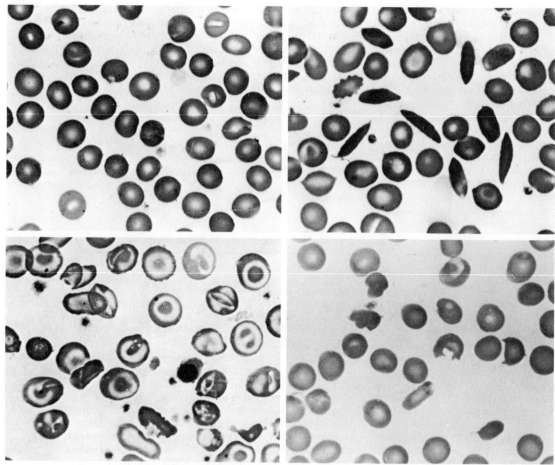

FIGURE 49–1. Photomicrographs of peripheral blood smears. *Upper left*, Spherocytes, round dense cells lacking a central pallor, in a patient with hereditary spherocytes. *Upper right*, Sickle cells, typical of sickle cell anemia. *Lower left*, Target cells, typical of thalassemia. *Lower right*, Schistocytes, typical of microangiopathic hemolytic anemia.

TABLE 49–2. CLINICAL CLUES IN EVALUATION OF ANEMIA

History
1. Family history: anemia, splenomegaly, jaundice, splenectomy
2. Rejection as blood donor
3. Exercise intolerance, syncope, easy fatigue
4. Pallor, jaundice
5. Blood loss or bleeding tendency
6. Malnutrition, malabsorption, alcoholism
7. Chronic disease
8. Transfusion or iron therapy
9. Multiple pregnancy, menorrhagia

Physical Examination
1. Skin and mucous membranes: pallor, jaundice, purpura, smooth or beefy tongue, cheilosis, koilonychia, telangiectasia
2. Adenopathy
3. Hepatomegaly or splenomegaly
4. Tachycardia, cardiomegaly, murmurs
5. Bone tenderness
6. Neuropathy
7. Stool exam (for blood)

signs of cardiovascular decompensation occur varies considerably with underlying disease, age, level of activity, and the individual's stoicism. For example, in the sedentary elderly person, a change in mentation can be an important clue to anemia, whereas decreased activity can mask exercise intolerance.

Evaluation of the anemic patient is best served by a systematic evaluation of the clinical and laboratory findings together (Fig. 49–2). First, is the patient truly anemic? Increased plasma volume, fluid overload, or congestive heart failure may produce a dilutional anemia that disappears when fluid balance is restored. Second, is the anemia acquired or inherited? Family history is important, especially in hemolytic anemias, and a positive family history of jaundice, splenomegaly, or gallstones may suggest such a condition. Hemoglobinopathies are frequent in Mediterranean, African, and Far Eastern populations, making ethnic background pertinent. For the immediate problem, a lifelong history versus recent onset is a key differential point. Third, is there evidence for blood loss? The most common reason for anemia is iron loss and iron deficiency. While in growing children and pregnant women iron deficiency may result from dietary lack, the overwhelming cause of iron deficiency in adults is loss of blood from the gastrointestinal or genitourinary tract. Fourth, is there evidence for nutritional deficiency or malabsorption? In the urban Westerner, folic acid deficiency is a common form of malnutrition, seen especially in the elderly living alone and in alcoholics. Fifth, is there evidence for hemolysis? Inherited hemolytic anemias are common in certain populations, whereas acquired hemolytic anemia is rare, occurring mainly in settings of autoimmune disease and drug ingestion. Sixth, is there evidence for toxic exposure or drug ingestion that could cause bone marrow depression and anemia? Finally, does the patient have a chronic inflammatory disease, renal insufficiency, or cancer, each of which is associated with secondary mild anemias, the "anemia of chronic disease"?

Laboratory Evaluation of Anemia

Laboratory evaluation of anemia starts with the hemogram, that is, the complete blood count (hemoglobin, hematocrit, white blood cell count, differ-

ential, platelet count, and red cell indices) plus the peripheral blood smear. In addition, initial evaluation should include a reticulocyte count, examination of the stool for occult blood, and urinalysis. Automated cell counters directly determine the number and size (volume) of blood cells and measure hemoglobin chemically; the hematocrit is then derived from these values. This complete examination can be carried out on capillary blood from a fingerstick. Automated differential counters are available that report the white cell differential in absolute numbers based on scanning of large populations of leukocytes either on fixed smears or in cell suspensions. Nevertheless, the visual differential performed on stained smears remains an important method and permits evaluation of the morphology of individual leukocytes and of erythrocytes and platelets. Direct examination of the morphology of a stained peripheral blood smear is particularly important in evaluating abnormal cells, as in leukemia. An advantage of automated cell counting is the ability to use the standard deviation of the variable being measured, e.g., red cell volume, to provide information on population heterogeneity, an important factor in certain disease states.

The *red cell indices* give information about the av-

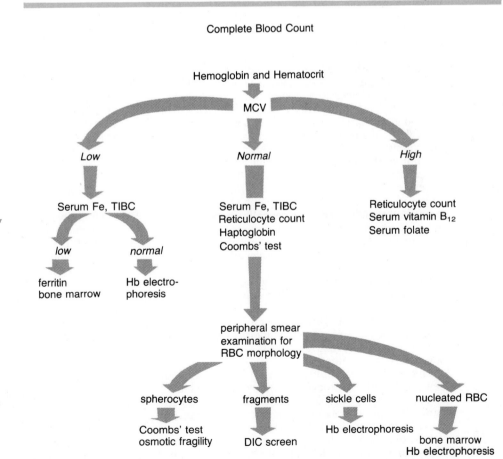

FIGURE 49–2. Laboratory screening for anemia.

erage red cell volume (MCV, mean corpuscular volume) and red cell hemoglobin content (MCH, mean corpuscular hemoglobin) or concentration (MCHC, mean corpuscular hemoglobin concentration). The MCV is the most useful, since it permits separation of microcytic anemia (MCV <80 cu μm) from normocytic (MCV 80 to 100 cu μm) and macrocytic anemias (MCV >100 cu μm). These morphologic categories correlate well with several common types of anemia. *Microcytosis* most commonly occurs in iron deficiency, thalassemia trait, and chronic renal insufficiency, whereas normocytosis accompanies acute blood loss. *Macrocytosis* is characteristic of nutritional anemias, including folic acid deficiency and vitamin B_{12} deficiency. Mild macrocytosis (MCV 100 to 110 cu μm) may also be associated with hemolytic anemias with a raised reticulocyte count and with the refractory anemias found in myelodysplastic syndromes. The MCH is generally low in thalassemia trait, thalassemia, and iron deficiency; the MCHC may be high in spherocytic hemolytic anemias.

Inspection of the peripheral blood smear gives information about individual blood cells not readily obtained from the average values reported by the automated blood counters (Fig. 49–1). The appearance and heterogeneity of red cells can be of diagnostic importance. For example, the microcytes of iron deficiency are relatively homogeneous, whereas in thalassemia major much more diversity in red cell size and shape occurs. In general, the further red cells diverge from the ideal shape (biconcave disc) and size (8 μm diameter), the shorter their lifespan in the circulation. The appearance of sickle cells, cells with inclusion bodies, e.g., Howell-Jolly bodies (nuclear remnants) or basophilic stippling (RNA remnants), parasitized cells (e.g., malaria), microspherocytes, and schistocytes (e.g., microangiopathic anemias, disseminated intravascular coagulation) is rapidly appreciated by inspection of the peripheral blood smear. Similarly, the appearance of individual leukocytes discloses blasts, hypersegmented polymorphonuclear cells, atypical lymphocytes, toxic granulation, and other morphologic abnormalities of disease generally inaccessible to machine recording. Platelet clumping versus true thrombocytopenia and the appearance of very large or small platelets also adds clinically relevant information to the numerical counts.

Evaluation of the leukocyte and platelet counts is an integral part of investigating anemia, since low counts may signify marrow failure or replacement, and high counts may be associated with leukemia or infection. Suspicion of pancytopenia or of marrow invasion with a pathological process should lead to a bone marrow examination.

The *reticulocyte count* measures the per cent of newly released erythrocytes in the circulating blood; these are larger than mature red blood cells and contain traces of endoplasmic reticulum, signifying the continuing capacity for hemoglobin synthesis. After one to two days in the circulation, these methylene blue–stained traces of RNA disappear. Since the normal red cell lifespan is 120 days, the normal reticulocyte count is approximately 1 per cent. Anemia increases the apparent reticulocyte count by decreasing the denominator by which the reticulocyte percentage is calculated (reticulocytes/1000 RBC); hence reticulocyte counts should be corrected to a "normal" hematocrit of 45 (corrected reticulocyte count = retic count × patient's hematocrit/45). Further corrections may be needed during severe anemias when reticulocytes circulate for longer than 24 hours. An elevated reticulocyte count (corrected) signifies increased erythropoietic activity, which may represent a normal response to bleeding, replacement of an appropriate hematinic such as iron, folate, or vitamin B_{12}, or a response to hemolysis. A very low reticulocyte count or absence of reticulocytes occurs after transfusion or in aplastic states.

Blood loss from the gastrointestinal tract is such a common cause of anemia that any initial evaluation of anemia should include testing one to three stool specimens for occult blood. Because bleeding is often intermittent, it is best to obtain several stool specimens on different days. While blood loss into the urine is less common, it is nevertheless desirable to examine the urine for the presence of red cells or blood as well.

ANEMIAS REPRESENTING BONE MARROW FAILURE

Primary disorders of bone marrow function are rare causes of anemia except as a result of drug or toxin action. These disorders include aplastic anemia, pure red cell aplasia, marrow replacement with fibrotic tissue or tumor (myelophthisis and myelodysplastic syndromes), and certain anemias secondary to cancer.

Aplastic anemia is characterized by a peripheral pancytopenia and markedly decreased hematopoietic activity in the bone marrow without a change in normal marrow architecture or replacement with other cell types. The disorder is considered to be severe when the corrected reticulocyte count is less than 1 per cent, platelets are less than 20,000 per cu mm, neutrophil count is less than 500 per cu mm, and marrow cellularity is less than 25 per cent of marrow space. Aplastic anemias, or the tendency toward their development, may be inherited (e.g., Fanconi's anemia) or may develop after a viral infection or as a reaction to a drug. Some drugs, such as cytostatic agents used in cancer chemotherapy, regularly cause marrow hypoplasia as part of their cytotoxic action; such aplasia is dose-dependent and usually reversible. The effect of cycle-specific agents such as cytosine arabinoside and methotrexate on more rapidly dividing mature stem cells tends to spare the earlier, pluripotent stem cells, so that marrow recovery occurs after the drug is stopped. Other drugs induce idiosyncratic marrow hypoplasia or aplasia that is unrelated to drug dose and tends to be less reversible. Chloramphenicol, which also induces a dose-related suppression of erythropoiesis, and phenylbutazone are examples of drugs that produce idiosyncratic marrow aplasia in one of every 24,000 to 40,000 exposed individuals. An inherited stem cell sensitivity or defect is postulated in such cases because of the findings in family and twin studies. A variety of environmental toxins, including solvents such as benzene and insecticides, also can cause a long-lasting marrow aplasia. Radiation exposure of bone marrow also can produce aplastic anemia. Viral infections, particularly hepatitis, Epstein-Barr virus infection, and parvovirus, can result in severe aplasia. An increased incidence of acute leukemia is observed in patients who have had aplastic anemia, and preleukemia may present as marrow hypoplasia.

Pure red cell aplasia, producing a severe anemia with absent reticulocytes, but normal leukocyte and platelet counts, is characterized by selective absence of erythroid precursors in the bone marrow. It is associated with immunological deficiency states, including thymoma.

Two mechanisms have been postulated for aplastic anemia: immunological suppression of hematopoiesis and damage to marrow stem cells. Suppressor T cells as well as immunoglobulins that inhibit erythropoietin or block differentiation of hematopoietic stem cells in vitro have been demonstrated in some cases. Immunosuppressive therapy has led to remission in certain of these cases, especially in pure red cell aplasia. In other cases, no inhibitory immunological mechanisms can be demonstrated, and patients respond to bone marrow transplantation, which presumably repopulates the marrow by new stem cells. Early transplantation of normal, HLA-matched bone marrow, before the patient becomes alloimmunized to blood cells given as supportive therapy, is the treatment of choice in young patients, especially if the patient has an HLA-compatible donor. For patients in whom transplantation is not possible, androgens have been used in addition to supportive transfusion therapy. Recent studies indicate that treatment with a course of antithymocyte globulin is effective in 40 to 50 per cent of cases. Availability of commercially prepared antithymocyte globulin now makes this treatment a feasible early step in the approach to aplastic anemia, especially in the patient who does not have a bone marrow donor.

Marrow invasion by infection (e.g., tuberculosis), tumor, or fibrosis can produce hypoplastic anemias characterized by a normocytic red cell, low reticulocyte count, and the presence of nucleated red blood cells on the peripheral smear: *myelophthisic anemia*. Cancer also can produce a hypoplastic, normocytic anemia without direct marrow invasion. Such anemias involve a subnormal response to erythropoietin and represent one type of the anemia of chronic disease.

HYPOCHROMIC ANEMIAS

Inadequate or defective hemoglobin synthesis results in poorly hemoglobinized erythrocytes in the peripheral blood, a decreased hemoglobin level, and frequently a small erythrocyte volume (microcytosis). Any lesion in the pathway of heme or of globin synthesis can produce a hypochromic anemia (Table 49–3). By far, the most common cause of hypochromic anemia throughout the world is iron deficiency resulting from blood loss (at any age) or inadequate di-

TABLE 49–3. EVALUATION OF HYPOCHROMIC ANEMIA

A. Iron lack or inability to utilize iron in heme production
   1. Iron deficiency
     a. Blood loss
     b. Dietary lack during high demand (childhood, pregnancy)
     c. Poor absorption of food iron (postgastrectomy, small bowel disease, pica)
   2. Poor iron mobilization from body stores
     a. Chronic inflammatory disease
     b. Malignancy
   3. Sideroblastic anemia; failure of iron incorporation into protoporphyrin
   4. Lead poisoning (similar to No. 3)
B. Defective globin synthesis
   1. Alpha-thalassemia
   2. Beta-thalassemia

etary iron (mainly in children and pregnant women). Other important causes of hypochromic anemia include poor iron utilization, as in the anemia of chronic disease, defective heme or porphyrin synthesis, as in the porphyrias or lead poisoning, or impaired globin synthesis, as in the thalassemic syndromes (see below). In the thalassemias, abnormal globin synthesis results in a secondary impairment of heme production and leads to a hemolytic state; this problem will be discussed in the section on hemolytic anemias.

The characteristic findings in iron deficiency anemia reflect exhaustion of body iron stores: absent marrow iron, low plasma iron and ferritin concentrations, a low transferrin saturation (<15 per cent) and high iron binding capacity, and hypochromic, microcytic erythrocytes on the peripheral smear. The reticulocyte count is reduced.

Normal Iron Metabolism

Iron is the most abundant metal in the human body, yet is a trace metal totalling only 3 to 4 gm. Two thirds of total body iron exists as hemoglobin iron in circulating erythrocytes, about one quarter remains in iron stores, and small amounts are found in myoglobin, enzymes, and the plasma. Body iron is tightly regulated and conserved; the daily absorption from the diet averages 1 to 2 mg, and iron balance is maintained by efficient reutilization of hemoglobin iron from red cells removed from circulation by the reticuloendothelial system or enzyme iron except for a small amount lost from the body in sweat, shed skin, and intestinal mucosal cells. Elemental iron is extremely toxic and insoluble, and iron within the body is almost entirely bound to protein carriers. The distribution of iron in body compartments is shown in Table 49–4.

Food iron is absorbed in the ferrous form, after being released from foodstuffs by gastric acid. Heme iron is absorbed directly as hemin (Fe^{+++} heme). The duodenum is the optimal locus of absorption, with less occurring further down the small intestine. An active process transports ferrous iron across the intestinal mucosal cell, governed by the iron content of the cells, with local storage as ferritin if the content is high. The average Western diet contains 10 to 30 mg of iron per day, of which only 5 to 10 per cent is absorbed. In iron

TABLE 49–4. IRON DISTRIBUTION AND TURNOVER

	AMOUNT OF IRON IN AVERAGE ADULT			
	Male (gm)	Female (gm)	Per Cent of Total	DAILY TURNOVER
Hemoglobin	2.4	1.7	65	20 mg
Ferritin and hemosiderin	1.0	0.3	35	
Myoglobin	0.15	0.12	3.5	
Heme enzymes	0.02	0.015	0.5	
Transferrin-iron	0.004	0.003	0.1	
Total daily requirement	0.001	0.002*		

* Menstruating and pregnant women require two to three times the daily Fe requirement of adult men because of increased blood loss and the iron requirement of the fetus. One ml of blood contains approximately 0.5 mg iron.

deficiency states absorption increases to 20 to 30 per cent. Many common foodstuffs and other materials that contain iron-binding substances interfere with iron absorption. These include phytates in cereals and vegetables, casein in milk, clay, and the drug tetracycline. Clay-eating or starch-eating (pica) by children or young women, many of whom are already iron-deficient, can produce severe iron deficiency.

Absorbed iron is transported from the intestine to storage in the bone marrow complexed to the plasma protein transferrin, each molecule of which binds two iron molecules. Transferrin-bound iron (Fe^{+++}, reoxidized by ceruloplasmin) is delivered to reticuloendothelial macrophages for storage as ferritin and to developing erythroblasts, where it is released intracellularly for incorporation into protoporphyrin. Since 25 mg of iron are needed daily for new red cell production, and only 1 to 2 mg are absorbed from the diet, most of the iron being utilized for erythropoiesis is recycled, derived from effete red cells destroyed by the reticuloendothelial system. The transferrin concentration in plasma (measured as the iron-binding capacity) varies widely diurnally, is decreased in inflammatory diseases or infection, and is increased in iron deficiency.

Iron is delivered to developing erythrocytes by the binding of transferrin to a specific cellular receptor. This step is followed by micropinocytotic internalization of the iron-transferrin complex within acidic vacuoles where the iron is released, and from which the apotransferrin-receptor complex is recycled to the cell surface and the apotransferrin liberated. The iron then enters the mitochondria and is enzymatically incorporated into protoporphyrin to form heme; the heme is bound by globin in the cytoplasm to produce hemoglobin. The level of free heme regulates the uptake of iron by normoblasts and reticulocytes.

Iron is stored as ferritin or hemosiderin. Ferritin consists of a spherical protein shell of apoferritin units surrounding a central core of ferric phosphate; up to 4000 iron molecules may be present per molecule of ferritin. Aggregates of ferritin can be detected in bone marrow smears as ferricyanide-positive granules, having a bright blue-green color. Ferritin circulates at concentrations that generally reflect body iron stores, with a normal range of 12 to 325 ng/ml (mean 125 ng/

ml for men, 55 ng/ml for women). In iron deficiency the serum ferritin is less than 10 ng/ml and in iron overload the level may be several thousand ng/ml. Infection tends to reduce the serum ferritin level; liver disease or hepatitis raises the level. *Hemosiderin* is an insoluble, partially dehydrated derivative of ferritin; iron contained in hemosiderin is less accessible for erythropoiesis than is iron in ferritin, which is readily available. Fixed tissue macrophages also serve as a store of ferritin and hemosiderin, derived from phagocytized aged red blood cells. Such iron is rapidly made available after hemorrhage but is poorly available for hemoglobin production during infection, inflammation, and malignancy.

Iron Deficiency

Iron deficiency anemia is a sign of underlying disease, not a disease in itself. The major cause for iron deficiency in adults is blood loss, whereas in growing children and pregnant women dietary iron lack is more common. Malabsorption also can lead to iron deficiency, for example following partial gastrectomy or in adult celiac disease. Rarer associations include esophageal webs (Plummer-Vinson syndrome) and clay or starch pica.

The usual Western diet provides sufficient iron to cover normal losses of adult men, but for menstruating women (who require twice as much iron daily as adult men) dietary iron intake may not be adequate. Women with repeated pregnancies are also at risk of iron lack, since each fetus requires about 400 mg of iron. Gastric acid facilitates iron absorption, since acid is needed to reduce ferric iron in food to the absorbable ferrous form; gastrectomy not only removes the source of acid but by increasing transit time in the intestine may impair duodenal absorption (this is why delayed release forms of iron are less efficacious).

Gastrointestinal bleeding is the most common cause of iron deficiency in men, and the second after gynecologic bleeding in women. In less developed countries, hookworm infestation is the leading cause of iron deficiency. Both benign and malignant gastrointestinal lesions may produce iron deficiency, and investigation for possible colon cancer is imperative in adults over the age of 40. Peptic ulcer disease, hiatal hernia, bleeding due to aspirin ingestion, diverticulitis, and chronic hemorrhoidal bleeding are other frequent causes of gastrointestinal blood loss. Hematuria may also produce iron deficiency. Frequent blood donations may deplete iron stores even in males and lead to latent iron deficiency.

Clinical Manifestations. Clinical manifestations may be subtle, if the iron deficiency is gradual in onset. The most common symptoms include fatigue, exercise intolerance, irritability, and dizziness, i.e., symptoms common to any type of anemia. In severe iron deficiency there may be koilonychia, pallor, and cheilosis. Splenomegaly has been reported in about 10 per cent but not in American adults.

Laboratory Findings. Laboratory findings range from a normocytic anemia in mild cases to microcytic, hypochromic anemia in severe cases. The blood smear shows an increased central pale area in red blood cells, and increased anisocytosis and poikilocytosis. If bleeding is chronic or active, the platelet count may be increased. The serum iron is depressed early in iron deficiency and the transferrin level or total iron-binding capacity is increased to more than 350 μg/dl, with a transferrin saturation of less than 15 per cent. The plasma ferritin concentration is low, below 10 ng/ml. Free erythrocyte protoporphyrin is elevated. The reticulocyte count is usually normal. The bone marrow characteristically reveals erythroid hyperplasia, with small, poorly hemoglobinized normoblasts. Iron stores are absent.

The sequence of changes in laboratory variables follows a definite pattern as iron deficiency develops. First, iron stores are depleted and serum ferritin falls. The iron-binding capacity increases, plasma iron concentration falls, and transferrin desaturation follows. The hemoglobin decreases. Red cell morphology initially remains normochromic and normocytic while the total red cell count falls. Eventually, microcytic, hypochromic red cells appear (Table 49–5).

Diagnostic Evaluation. As iron deficiency represents a manifestation of underlying disease, the cause must be sought. The iron deficiency is easily documented by laboratory tests indicating reduced serum iron, increased transferrin level (or alternatively, a low serum ferritin), and absence of iron stores in the bone marrow. Urinalysis and stool examinations are part of the initial evaluation. In the older patient especially, investigation for a source for gastrointestinal blood loss requires serial examinations of stool for blood, plus, if indicated, appropriate radiographs and endoscopy. Women should have a careful gynecologic history recorded and a pelvic examination.

Therapy. The goals include treating the cause for the iron loss, correcting the anemia, and replenishing body iron stores. Simple iron salts, ferrous sulfate or ferrous gluconate, are effective treatments. Slow-release preparations or enteric-coated tablets are not recommended because they may bypass upper duodenal absorption, thereby reducing absorption. All iron salts are irritating to the gastrointestinal tract in a dose-dependent manner and may cause diarrhea, constipation, or epigastric distress. Accordingly, iron salts are best given in divided doses, gradually increasing to a full dose of 200 mg of elemental iron (about three tablets of ferrous sulfate, 325 mg) daily. This dose provides an optimal response. Iron is best absorbed when the stomach is empty, but gastric irritation may be more common. Absorption after meals is sufficient, and the decrease in GI symptoms is offset by better patient compliance. Ascorbic acid taken with the iron enhances absorption by 20 to 30 per cent but adds to expense. Because of the limited extent of iron absorption even in the iron-deficient patient, it is important to continue therapy for 6 to 12 months, by which time anemia will be corrected and iron stores replenished. Patients should be instructed to continue taking their iron tablets for the full period of time.

Subjective improvement in fatigue or lassitude may occur within a few days, well before a detectable hematologic response, which takes about two weeks. A mild reticulocytosis can be observed, followed by a slow rise in hemoglobin of about 1 gm per two weeks. "Unresponsiveness" to iron therapy is most commonly a sign of poor compliance or continued blood loss. Intercurrent disease, malabsorption, or an ineffective preparation (e.g., sustained-release products) may also impair response.

Parenteral iron therapy should be reserved for patients who cannot tolerate oral iron, have malabsorp-

TABLE 49–5. STAGES IN DEVELOPMENT OF IRON DEFICIENCY ANEMIA

HEMOGLOBIN (gm/dl)	PERIPHERAL SMEAR*	SERUM Fe (μg/dl)	BONE MARROW	SERUM FERRITIN (ng/ml)
13+ (normal)	nc/nc	50–150	Fe 2+	40–340 (male) 14–150 (female)
10–12	nc/nc	↓	Fe absent, erythroid hyperplasia	<12
8–10	hypo/nc	↓↓	Fe absent, erythroid hyperplasia	<12
<8	hypo/micro	↓↓	Fe absent, erythroid hyperplasia	<12

* nc/nc = normochromic, normocytic; hypo/nc = hypochromic, normocytic; hypo/micro = hypochromic, microcytic.

tion, fail to comply, or have a rapid and chronic blood loss. An example of the latter condition is hereditary hemorrhagic telangiectasia (Osler-Weber-Rendu), which in some cases demonstrates a frequency or rate of bleeding exceeding the capacity for oral iron absorption. Iron-dextran complex (Imferon) contains 50 mg iron/ml and is the preparation of choice. It can be administered intramuscularly or intravenously. Because of occasional hypersensitivity to the dextran moiety, a test dose of 0.5 ml should be given first and the patient observed for anaphylactic reactions. The replacement total dose is calculated from the patient's hemoglobin level:

$$\text{mg Imferon needed} = [15 - \text{Hgb(gm/dl)}] \times \text{body weight (kg)} \times 3.$$

The amount is administered in divided doses, 2.5 ml injected into each buttock daily in a Z-track manner, to provide about 250 mg iron daily, or is given intravenously as a single infusion at a rate of up to 1 ml/min.

MEGALOBLASTIC ANEMIAS

Definition. Megaloblastic anemias are anemias in which DNA synthesis is impaired, leading to delayed division of all rapidly proliferating cells—skin, gastrointestinal tract, mucosae, hematopoietic cells—and cellular gigantism. Since all hematopoietic cell lines proliferate rapidly, megaloblastic anemias usually manifest not only macrocytic anemia but also pancytopenia. Ineffective hematopoiesis results from intramedullary loss of a large proportion of developing cells, related to the asynchrony of DNA synthesis, hence producing a hemolytic state.

Causes. The major causes of megaloblastic anemias are folic acid or vitamin B_{12} deficiency, which may be related to nutritional deficiency, disease of the stomach or small bowel, pregnancy, alcoholism, or cancer chemotherapy. Rarer inherited defects in DNA synthesis also occur.

Pathophysiology. Pathophysiology of the megaloblastic anemias relates to the interlocking roles of folic acid and vitamin B_{12} in DNA synthesis. Folic acid (in the reduced 5,10-methylene tetrahydrofolate form) is the carrier for one-carbon fragments that are donated to desoxyuridine to form desoxythymidine, the characteristic pyrimidine in DNA. This methylation of desoxyuridine is essential for thymidine synthesis, and subsequent regeneration of 5,10-methylene tetrahydrofolate is necessary for continued delivery of methyl groups to desoxyuridine. Vitamin B_{12} is the cofactor of the reaction that regenerates tetrahydrofolate from 5-methyl tetrahydrofolate, a major form of folate in the body that is unable to donate its methyl group to desoxyuridine. The 5-methyl group is transferred to homocysteine to form methionine in a methyltransferase-catalyzed reaction in which vitamin B_{12} acts as intermediate methyl acceptor. In addition, vitamin B_{12} is the coenzyme in the conversion of methylmalonyl CoA to succinyl CoA, a reaction necessary

for myelin metabolism in the nervous system. Thus, deficiency of vitamin B_{12} leads to neurologic changes as well as megaloblastic anemia, whereas folate deficiency leads only to megaloblastic anemia. In folate deficiency, the inadequate generation of thymidylate leads to increased incorporation of uridylate into developing hematopoietic cell DNA. The incorporated uridylate is then enzymatically excised, leading to fragmentation of the DNA, blocking of DNA synthesis at a normal rate, and impaired cell proliferation. RNA and protein synthesis, however, can proceed normally.

The ineffective hematopoiesis that results from the impaired DNA synthesis in vitamin B_{12} or folate deficiency leads to megaloblastosis, the production of giant leukocytic forms and large platelets, and is characterized by early intramedullary death of these abnormal cells and shortened lifespan of circulating blood cells. A hemolytic state involving both intramedullary and extramedullary hemolysis results, accompanied by leukopenia and thrombocytopenia.

Clinical and Laboratory Manifestations. Signs and symptoms of megaloblastic anemia are identical for folic acid and vitamin B_{12} deficiency, whereas effects of these vitamin deficiencies on tissues other than hematopoietic tissue may vary. Thus, a profound and slowly developing macrocytic anemia is observed, with large, oval, well-hemoglobinized red cells, considerable anisocytosis, and frequent nuclear remnants. The reticulocyte count is very low. There is leukopenia with hypersegmentation of polymorphonuclear leukocyte nuclei and thrombocytopenia. The platelets are large. The bilirubin is elevated. The bone marrow is markedly hypercellular with megaloblasts showing "nuclear-cytoplasmic dissociation," that is, normal maturation of the cytoplasm in the face of nuclear immaturity, a finely dispersed chromatin pattern, and large nuclear size. Nuclear condensation is delayed in erythroid cells. The myeloid series also shows megaloblastosis, with giant band forms and hypersegmented polymorphonuclear leukocytes. The number of mitotic figures is increased. Megakaryocytes are large and decreased in number and show decreased budding. The iron stores in the marrow are typically increased (because of the intramedullary hemolysis). Epithelial cells of mucosal surfaces such as the mouth, intestinal tract, stomach, and vagina also show gigantism. The gastric and intestinal mucosae tend to atrophy, leading to further malabsorption of folate.

In vitamin B_{12} deficiency neurologic changes may occur, although their presence correlates poorly with the development of the hematologic abnormalities: some patients develop severe neurologic manifestations with only mild anemia, and vice versa. Morphologically, the neurologic abnormality initially produces demyelination, first of the large fibers in peripheral nerves, later of the dorsal and lateral columns of the spinal cord, and sometimes in the cerebrum. Irreversible nerve cell damage is a late complication. Earliest symptoms typically include distal paresthesias in the extremities, with a glove-stocking peripheral neuropathy, and impairment of position and vibration sense in combination with increased deep tendon reflexes. Later a typical spastic ataxia, motor weakness, and paraparesis may occur. Mental changes may also occur with "megaloblastic madness," i.e., dementia in severe cases. Autoimmune phenomena are common with vitiligo, early graying of hair, autoantibody formation, and emergence of other autoimmune diseases.

Vitamin Requirements, Absorption, Metabolism, and Action

FOLIC ACID. Folic acid (pteroylglutamic acid) is derived from leafy plants, liver, or yeast and exists as a family of compounds consisting of a pteroyl ring, para-aminobenzoic acid, and one or more glutamates in a gamma glutamyl linkage (Table 49–6). Food folate comprises polyglutamates, whereas medicinal folate is pteroylmonoglutamic acid. The daily requirement for folate is 50 to 200 μg; the body stores of folate (in the liver) of 5 to 20 mg suffice only for weeks to three or four months. Folate requirements are increased during growth, pregnancy, and hemolytic anemias.

Food polyglutamates must be cleaved to the monoglutamate form in the intestinal tract by folate conjugases in the intestinal mucosa before efficient uptake by an active transport mechanism. Absorption takes place mainly in the upper portion of the small intestine. Certain drugs, such as Dilantin and oral contraceptives, or intrinsic small bowel disease can impair absorption by interfering with conjugase action. Folate is heat labile and is destroyed by prolonged heating or cooking. Absorbed folate is mainly converted to 5-methyl THF, the main transport and storage form. The rate of folate absorption is dependent upon tissue stores and on the integrity of the intestinal mucosa. Accordingly, diseases of the small intestine such as sprue and celiac disease can impair folate absorption.

Because of the relatively low body stores of folic acid, dietary deficiency is a common cause of folate-related megaloblastic anemia. Thus, a diet devoid of fresh vegetables or limited mainly to alcohol frequently leads to folate deficiency. In the elderly, "tea and toast" diets frequently result in folate deficiency. In alcoholism, several factors combine to produce fo-late deficiency: poor diet, a toxic effect of alcohol on the intestinal mucosa, and interference by alcohol with folate utilization in the bone marrow. Increased demands for folate occur during pregnancy, lactation, and rapid growth in childhood. Folate requirements also rise in any chronic hemolytic anemia such as sickle cell anemia, immune hemolytic anemia, or thalassemia, in patients on hemodialysis, and in psoriasis or exfoliative dermatitis. Pregnancy increases the folate requirement 5- to 10-fold. Malabsorption syndromes are commonly accompanied by folic acid deficiency, as food polyglutamates are poorly absorbed by abnormal intestinal mucosa (monoglutamate folic acid is normally absorbed) especially if villous atrophy is present. As a result, celiac disease and nontropical and tropical sprue may result in folate deficiency. Bacterial overgrowth, as in the blind loop syndrome, more commonly causes vitamin B_{12} deficiency. Folate deficiency may lead to low serum B_{12}, whereas in B_{12} deficiency serum folate may be high because of underutilization, although red cell folate may be low.

Folic acid is reduced by the enzyme dihydrofolate reductase to forms capable of carrying one carbon fragments. Once fully reduced by dihydrofolate reductase, folate as tetrahydrofolate again can transport the appropriate 5,10-methylene group needed in thymidylate synthesis. Inhibitors of dihydrofolate reductase therefore inhibit DNA synthesis: the first antimetabolite successfully used in leukemia chemotherapy, aminopterin, is an inhibitor of dihydrofolate reductase. Antimalarial drugs such as pyrimethamine also are dihydrofolate reductase inhibitors. Therefore, megaloblastic changes are observed in patients receiving pyrimethamine for malaria, trimethoprim (present in the drug Bactrim) for bacterial infections, or methotrexate. The toxicity induced by such drugs may be counteracted by administration of folinic acid, which bypasses the need for dihydrofolate reductase by supplying the fully reduced folate.

VITAMIN B_{12}. Vitamin B_{12} is synthesized in nature only by microorganisms and is obtained by eating animal foods (Table 49–6). This vitamin consists of a group of cobalamins, which contain a porphyrin-like corrin ring similar in structure to heme but with a cen-

TABLE 49–6. COMPARISON OF FOLIC ACID AND VITAMIN B_{12}

	FOLIC ACID	VITAMIN B_{12}
Source	Leafy vegetables, yeast, liver	Animal products
Dietary intake	500–1000 μg	7–30 μg
Effect of cooking	Destroyed	Unchanged
Minimal daily need	100–200 μg	1–2 μg
Body stores	10–12 mg (four months)	2–3 mg (2–4 years)
Absorption	Active transport, upper small bowel	Carrier-mediated (intrinsic factor), terminal ileum
Physiological forms	Reduced polyglutamates	Methylcobalamin, adenosylcobalamin
Serum level	3–15 ng/ml	200–900 pg/ml
Function	Transfer 1-carbon fragments in thymidine synthesis	Regenerate reduced folate from 5-CH_3 THF; succinyl CoA formation in CNS

tral cobalt molecule linked to a nucleoside instead of iron. The normal diet contains a large excess of B_{12} (5 to 30 μg) over the daily requirement of 1 μg; only the strictest vegetarian diet is B_{12}-deficient. The chief body storage site for vitamin B_{12} is the liver, where 3 to 5 mg are normally present, representing stores sufficient for several years. The much greater body storage of B_{12} compared to folic acid means that in malnutrition or after GI surgery, vitamin B_{12} deficiency develops much more slowly than does folate deficiency. In the stomach, food vitamin B_{12} is released by pepsin from protein complexes at acid pH and binds with intrinsic factor, a glycoprotein produced by the parietal cells. Other binding proteins, R-factors, present in saliva and gastric juice, also bind vitamin B_{12}. These complexes stabilize the vitamin during intestinal transit. In the small intestine, pancreatic proteases and an alkaline pH further convert B_{12} bound to R proteins to intrinsic factor–B_{12} complexes. In the distal small ileum, specific mucosal receptors permit attachment of intrinsic factor–B_{12} complexes necessary for absorption of the vitamin (without the intrinsic factor) across the gut wall. R protein–B_{12} complexes are not absorbed. Plasma B_{12} is complexed to several types of transcobalamins or transport proteins. Only TC II transports B_{12} to hematopoietic and other proliferating cells; TC I (from leukocytes) and TC III bind the vitamin avidly and may be important in preventing its loss. The normal plasma level of vitamin B_{12} ranges between 175 and 725 pg/ml. Most of this represents B_{12} bound to TC I. In myeloproliferative diseases, in which granulocyte production is high, serum levels of either TC I or TC III and B_{12} are greatly increased.

An enterohepatic circulation of vitamin B_{12}, ensuring recycling of the vitamin, contributes to the low daily requirement. After partial gastrectomy, which may result in loss of intrinsic factor production, this recycling mechanism is interrupted and the requirement increases to 5 to 10 μg/day. The result is that clinical B_{12} deficiency arises earlier after gastric surgery than after dietary depletion. B_{12} deficiency is inevitable after total gastrectomy; after partial gastrectomy, owing to the large amount of intrinsic factor normally produced in the gastric antrum, the development of B_{12} deficiency is variable in time of onset and in rate of occurrence, depending upon the extent of surgery.

Different forms of vitamin B_{12} mediate different chemical reactions. Methylcobalamin, which acquires methyl groups from folate, is the form that acts as a coenzyme for the methyltransferase that converts homocysteine to methionine and is key for the regeneration of biologically active folate. Adenosylcobalamin is the form that is involved in the isomerization of methylmalonyl CoA to succinyl CoA. Medicinal vitamin B_{12} is cyanocobalamin; the binding of cyanate to the B_{12} molecule may represent a natural detoxification mechanism.

Diagnosis. Diagnosis of megaloblastic anemia is usually made from the blood smear and MCV and is confirmed by the finding of a megaloblastic bone marrow and low plasma level of folic acid, vitamin B_{12}, or both (Fig. 49–3). Plasma folic acid falls to low levels (less than 3 ng/ml) quickly, within days to weeks of dietary deprivation, whereas red cell folate better reflects total body stores. Vitamin B_{12} levels fall only when body stores are depleted. Both vitamins were formerly measured by bioassays employing vitamin-requiring microorganisms, which thus assessed biological activity of vitamin; recent development of sensitive radioimmunoassays involving a vitamin B binder has sometimes led to falsely high values for plasma B_{12} because certain assays also measure biologically inactive analogues of B_{12} that bind to R proteins. Assays

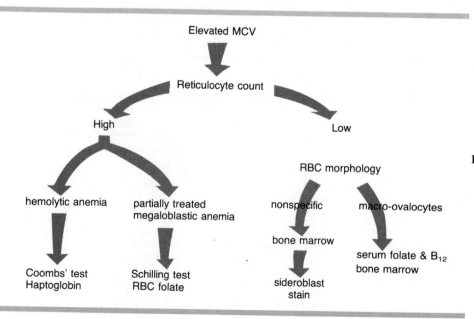

FIGURE 49–3. Evaluation of macrocytosis.

using intrinsic factor only as the binding protein give true values for plasma B_{12}; the action of the analogues is unknown.

Once a folic acid or vitamin B_{12} deficiency state is verified, the underlying cause must be sought. For folic acid, an accurate dietary history plus an evaluation for possible malabsorption usually uncovers a cause. Vitamin B_{12} deficiency is most commonly seen as a result of pernicious anemia, prior partial gastrectomy, or small bowel disease. Pernicious anemia involves an atrophic gastritis that leads to deficient intrinsic factor secretion, hence vitamin B_{12} malabsorption. The disease is accompanied by numerous autoimmune phenomena (unknown whether primary or secondary), including frequent occurrence of anti–parietal cell and anti–intrinsic factor antibodies. The latter impair the absorption of B_{12}-intrinsic factor complexes in the ileum. Finding anti–intrinsic factor antibodies in the serum is considered diagnostic for pernicious anemia, whereas the presence of anti–parietal cell antibodies is a more common, nonspecific phenomenon found in association with gastric disease in older persons. Impaired absorption of oral vitamin B_{12} occurs in several types of B_{12} deficiency and serves as the basis of the Schilling test, which can be used to distinguish between pernicious anemia, small intestinal bacterial overgrowth, and other malabsorption syndromes. In this test a trace amount (1 μg) of radiolabelled B_{12} is administered by mouth, and a large dose of unlabelled B_{12} (1000 μg) is injected intravenously to saturate body stores. The patient's urine is then collected for 48 hours and the amount of excreted labelled B_{12}, representing what was absorbed from the oral dose, is measured. Normally more than 7 per cent of the oral dose is excreted in 48 hours. If the excretion is less than 5 per cent, vitamin B_{12} malabsorption is present. If pernicious anemia is suspected, the test is repeated giving intrinsic factor by mouth together with the radiolabelled B_{12}. If urinary excretion of the radiolabelled B_{12} rises into the normal range, pernicious anemia is confirmed. Villous atrophy caused by the B_{12} deficiency occurs in untreated patients and may prevent normal absorption of B_{12} in the presence of intrinsic factor if the test is carried out before therapy or early after therapy has been started. Repeating part 2 of the Schilling test after one month of replacement therapy, when the gut mucosa has regenerated, gives more accurate results. If small intestinal bacterial overgrowth is suspected as the cause of the B_{12} deficiency, administration of a course of antibiotics before repeating the test will normalize B_{12} absorption and excretion. A special advantage of the Schilling test is that it can be carried out after treatment has begun, because it measures absorption of vitamin independent of therapy.

A therapeutic trial can also be undertaken to determine whether a megaloblastic anemia is due to vitamin B_{12} deficiency. Administration of 1 to 5 μg of vitamin B_{12} intramuscularly daily will lead to a reticulocytosis within three to four days, peaking within ten days. Continuation of the therapy will correct the anemia within a month. Administration of 200 μg of folic acid daily to a patient on a folate-deficient diet will lead to a reticulocytosis in folic acid deficiency but not in vitamin B_{12} deficiency; larger doses of folate will induce a reticulocyte response in the vitamin B_{12}–deficient patient, but will not fully correct the megaloblastic anemia and may lead to worsening or induction of the neurologic abnormalities.

The response to specific therapy of megaloblastic anemia is prompt and follows a predictable pattern. Symptoms improve within 48 hours and the bone marrow red cell morphology reverts to normal in 24 to 48 hours. Serum potassium may fall within 48 hours, representing a return of potassium to intracellular sites. Reticulocytosis is observed within three to four days and may rise to over 25 per cent; leukopenia and thrombocytopenia regress within ten days. Hypersegmented polys and giant bands (in the marrow) disappear within about a week. The elevated bilirubin and LDH, indicating the ineffective erythropoiesis, disappear within one to three weeks. Anemia is corrected within one to two months (if iron stores are adequate). Neurologic improvement in corrected vitamin B_{12} deficiency occurs more slowly and may take 6 to 12 months; long-standing neurologic defects, especially long tract dysfunction, may be irreversible.

Less Common Causes of Megaloblastic Anemia. About 5 per cent of megaloblastic anemias are due to inherited disorders of pyrimidine metabolism such as orotic aciduria, absence of ileal receptors for the intrinsic factor–B_{12} complex (Immerslund's syndrome) or to dyspoietic anemias that may represent preleukemia or may be familial. Megaloblastic anemia may also be induced by antimetabolite therapy that interferes with DNA synthesis, as in cancer chemotherapy.

HEMOLYTIC ANEMIAS

Definition. Hemolytic anemias result from an increased rate of red cell destruction. Because the bone marrow can increase red cell production eight-fold, the rate of red cell destruction may increase considerably without causing anemia (compensated hemolytic state). Normally, red cells survive 120 days in the circulation, gradually losing enzyme activities and becoming denser and less deformable. In hemolytic anemias, the red cell survival ranges from only slightly shortened to a few hours. Hemolytic anemias result from abnormalities of the red cell membrane, enzymes, or hemoglobin, from antibody interactions with the red cell membrane, from toxins or microbial products, or from heat or mechanical trauma. In a hemolytic anemia the red cell morphology may be normal or abnormal, reticulocytes are usually increased, nucleated red cells may be present in the peripheral blood, the bilirubin and LDH increased, urine urobilinogen raised, and red cell survival short. In chronic hemolytic anemias splenomegaly or hepatomegaly may be present, gallstones are common, jaundice and pallor may be present, and the bone marrow shows erythroid hyperplasia.

Hemolysis may be intravascular or extravascular, i.e., takes place in the reticuloendothelial system

TABLE 49–7. MECHANISMS OF HEMOLYSIS

Type of Red Cell Defect
1. Intrinsic (usually inherited)
   a. Membrane (e.g., hereditary spherocytosis)
   b. Enzyme (e.g., glucose 6-phosphate dehydrogenase deficiency)
   c. Hemoglobinopathy (e.g., sickle cell disease, Hb C disease)
   d. Globin synthesis (e.g., thalassemia)
   In all of the above, the red cell defect leads to membrane or cellular rigidity, splenic sequestration, short RBC lifespan.
2. Extrinsic (usually acquired)
   a. Antibody-induced (e.g., Coombs' positive hemolytic anemia)
      1. warm antibody
      2. cold antibody
   b. Drug-induced (e.g., penicillin)
   c. Toxin-mediated (e.g., burns, sepsis)
   d. Red cell fragmentation, mechanical hemolysis (e.g., after heart valve surgery)
   In all of the above, induced changes in red cell membrane lead to splenic removal, and in some, intravascular hemolysis with hemoglobinemia and hemoglobinuria may occur.

Laboratory Features of Hemolysis
1. Increased red cell breakdown
   a. Increased serum bilirubin (unconjugated)
   b. Increased urine urobilinogen
   c. Decreased serum haptoglobin
2. Increased red cell production
   a. Reticulocytosis and polychromasia
   b. Erythroid hyperplasia in bone marrow
   c. Increased requirement for folic acid (low serum folate)
3. Red cell damage
   a. Morphology: fragments, microspherocytes, spherocytes
   b. Increased osmotic fragility
   c. Short red cell survival
   d. Intraerythrocytic inclusions

(Table 49–7). *Intravascular hemolysis* is relatively rare and occurs with acute transfusion reactions, prosthetic heart valve dysfunction, paroxysmal cold or paroxysmal nocturnal hemoglobinuria (PNH), cold agglutinin disease, heat stroke, and clostridial infections. Hemoglobin is released from injured red cells into the plasma, where it is rapidly bound to haptoglobin, hemopexin, or albumin. Haptoglobin-hemoglobin or hemopexin-hemoglobin complexes are promptly cleared from the circulation by the liver, lowering the plasma levels of these proteins. Methemalbumin (the complex of heme with albumin) circulates for some days. If the binding capacity of these proteins is exceeded, hemoglobinuria occurs. Acute hemoglobinuria is not toxic to the kidney, but the accumulation of red cell stroma in renal vessels can lead to acute renal failure. Chronic hemoglobinuria leads to iron deficiency due to the sloughing of renal tubular cells loaded with hemosiderin derived from reabsorbed heme iron. In acute intravascular hemolysis, serum haptoglobin is very low and lactate dehydrogenase (LDH), an enzyme abundant in red cells, is elevated.

Extravascular hemolysis occurs commonly and represents early removal of red cells sequestered by the fixed phagocytes of the spleen and liver. Only a small amount of the hemoglobin removed reaches the plasma, and the heme iron is recycled for further red cell production, so that serum iron levels tend to be high during active hemolysis. Haptoglobin levels also tend to be reduced, but hemoglobinemia is not present. The level of serum lactic dehydrogenase (LDH), representing LDH released from destroyed red cells, is elevated. The level of unconjugated (indirect) bilirubin reflects the net effect of the briskness of hemolysis and the ability of the liver to process bilirubin.

Differential Diagnosis. Differential diagnosis of hemolytic anemias requires evaluation of whether the process is congenital or acquired, is due to abnormality of the red cell or to an abnormality in the plasma or circulatory system (including red cell antibodies, mechanical trauma, infection, etc.), or reflects other underlying disease, and whether it is acute or chronic. An important differentiating point is whether antibodies against red cell antigens are present on the red cell surface (direct Coombs' test) or in the plasma (indirect Coombs' test). Hence, an accurate family history and knowledge of the patient's prior history of jaundice, anemia, splenomegaly, or gallstones are of great importance. Physical findings depend upon the rate and chronicity of hemolysis, and range from scleral icterus and pallor in mild cases to splenomegaly and bony changes in severe chronic hemolysis.

Hemolysis due to intracorpuscular abnormalities may be caused by intrinsic defects in the red cell membrane, hemoglobin (or hemoglobin production), or enzymes. The most common membrane defect is hereditary spherocytosis, which has an incidence of 1:5000 in northern Europeans and less in other population groups. The peripheral blood smear shows a uniform population of spherocytes lacking central pallor. The mean cellular hemoglobin concentration (MCHC) is increased. The osmotic fragility of the red cells is increased, and red cell survival is short. Splenomegaly is usually present, bilirubin gallstones commonly develop, and intermittent jaundice is frequent, particularly in conjunction with stress states such as infection or pregnancy. Aplastic crises may occur during infection, as with parvovirus, due to bone marrow suppression in the face of a short red cell survival. The pathogenesis of the hemolysis is sequestration of the poorly deformable spherocytes, which require extra expenditure of ATP to maintain membrane flexibility. The underlying molecular defect is not fully understood, although abnormalities of the red cell cytoskeletal protein, spectrin, appear to be responsible. In addition, permeability to sodium ion is excessive, requiring increased ATP-dependent cation pump activity to prevent water accumulation by the red cells. Treatment of hereditary spherocytosis includes folic acid administration and splenectomy, which improves red cell survival without altering the red cell defects. Other membrane abnormalities resulting in hemolytic anemia include hereditary elliptocytosis and hereditary stomatocytosis.

The most common red cell enzyme defect worldwide is *glucose 6-phosphate dehydrogenase (G6PD) deficiency*, which affects over 100 million individuals. Other abnormalities in the Embden-Meyerhof enzyme pathway also lead to hemolytic states, but these are extremely rare (pyruvate kinase and hexokinase deficiencies, the next most common, have been reported in a few hundred cases). Normal red cells depend upon aerobic glycolysis to metabolize 90 per cent of glucose in producing ATP and 2,3-diphosphoglycerate. ATP is necessary to preserve membrane flexibility and to support membrane cation pumps, whereas 2,3-DPG influences the binding of oxygen to hemoglobin so as to facilitate oxygen unloading in tissues. Ten per cent of glucose is metabolized via the hexose monophosphate shunt, which generates NADPH, the major reducing compound produced by the red cell. NADPH is required for regeneration of reduced glutathione, which prevents hemoglobin denaturation, preserves the integrity of red cell membrane sulfhydryl groups, and detoxifies hydrogen peroxide and oxygen radicals in and on the red cell. Since G6PD is the initial enzyme in the hexose monophosphate shunt pathway, functionally abnormal enzyme or a low level of G6PD leads to increased red cell oxidative damage, particularly during periods of oxidant stress. G6PD deficiency is a sex-linked trait that is clinically expressed in male heterozygotes. Over 100 inherited variants of G6PD are recognized; young red cells have higher levels of the enzyme in general than do older cells. The common A− variety seen in the black population is less severe than the Mediterranean type, as red cell enzyme levels are about 15 per cent of normal in blacks but less than 5 per cent in the latter group. G6PD deficiency leads to hemolysis in the setting of hepatitis, severe infections, fava bean ingestion, or ingestion of oxidant drugs. Black males with G6PD deficiency and falciparum malaria develop severe intravascular hemolysis (blackwater fever) when treated with antimalarial drugs such as primaquine. G6PD deficiency in persons of Greek or Mediterranean lineage is associated with favism, or hemolysis after ingestion of the fava bean. Acquired G6PD deficiency has been observed in bacterial overgrowth of the bowel and in uremia.

ACQUIRED HEMOLYTIC DISORDERS

Red cell lifespan can become shortened in the course of infectious, malignant, cardiovascular, or immunological diseases. In most of these, hemolysis results from an extracorporeal abnormality such as altered hemodynamics, antibody against red cell antigens, or exposure to toxins. Rarely, the red cells themselves may undergo membrane changes that lead to hemolysis (e.g., in paroxysmal nocturnal hemoglobinuria). For convenience, acquired hemolytic anemias are divided into two categories: Coombs' positive (antibody-mediated) and Coombs' negative hemolytic anemia.

Antibody-mediated hemolytic anemias

These represent a wide variety of conditions in which antibodies directed against red cell antigens (or neoantigens) coat the red cells and are directly or indirectly responsible for hemolysis. Antibodies that arise after transfusion or sensitization to foreign red cells, as during pregnancy, are called *alloantibodies*. Antibodies that arise without sensitization, representing abnormalities in the subject's own immune regulation, are called *autoantibodies*. The presence of antibody on the red cell surface can alter the behavior of the red cells, making them less deformable and more susceptible to phagocytosis by macrophages in the spleen or liver. Macrophages ingest antibody- or complement-coated portions of the red cell membrane, via Fc or complement receptors. Red cells that have lost part of their plasma membrane reseal but assume a more spherical shape (spherocytosis) associated with decreased pliability in the circulation and a shortened lifespan.

Autoimmune hemolytic anemias (AIHA) are characterized by antibodies directed against the patient's own red cell antigens (Table 49–8). In contrast to alloantibodies resulting from transfusion of imperfectly matched red cells, autoantibodies can arise spontaneously, in response to drugs acting as haptens, or in 40 per cent of cases as manifestations of systemic disease. Diseases of disordered immunity such as collagen vascular diseases, chronic inflammatory bowel disease, chronic lymphocytic leukemia, or lymphomas manifest an increased incidence of autoimmune hemolytic anemia. Autoantibodies increase in frequency with age, but only a small proportion of red cell autoantibodies actually cause hemolytic anemia. Whether or not hemolysis occurs depends on the density of red cell coating by antibody, the capacity of the antibody to fix complement on the red cell membrane, the thermal amplitude of the antibody, and the tendency for antibody-coated red cells to be phagocytized by splenic macrophages. AIHA fall into two groups, the warm antibody and the cold antibody autoimmune hemolytic anemias.

Warm antibody hemolytic anemias are mediated by IgG antibodies that attach to red cells at body temperature and that may fix complement (Table 49–8). Clinically important antibodies tend to be of the IgG_1 and IgG_3 subclasses. The AIHA may be associated with collagen vascular disease, lymphoma, chronic lymphocytic leukemia, ovarian teratoma, or ulcerative colitis. Almost half of cases with AIHA are idiopathic, although the hemolytic anemia may be the harbinger of a later-appearing systemic disease; such cases may have a very variable course. The clinical picture relates to the rate of hemolysis; thus, the spectrum varies from a mild asymptomatic jaundice with splenomegaly, when the rate of hemolysis is mild and bone marrow production of red cells can compensate for shortened red cell lifespan, to severe anemia with cardiovascular symptoms, when the rate of hemolysis is rapid. A positive Coombs' (antiglobulin) test using an antiglobulin antiserum detects the coating of the red cell membrane by the autoantibody (Fig. 49–4); if the amount of autoantibody is high, free antibody in the plasma (positive indirect Coombs') is also detected. Complement coating on the red cell, usually the biologically inactive cleavage products of the third component of

TABLE 49–8. AUTOIMMUNE HEMOLYTIC ANEMIAS

	Ab COATING ON RBC	OPTIMUM TEMPERATURE FOR DETECTING Ab
Warm Type		
Idiopathic	IgG or IgG + C	37°C
Secondary	Rarely, IgA or IgM	
Systemic lupus erythematosus		
Other "autoimmune disease"		
Lymphoma		
Chronic lymphocytic leukemia		
Drug induced		
Cold Type	IgM (in cold only) anti-I or anti-i	4°C
Idiopathic	C3b or C3d	4° or 37°C
Secondary		
Infections		
Mycoplasma pneumoniae		
Infectious mononucleosis		
Lymphoma (diffuse histiocytic lymphoma)		
Paroxysmal cold hemoglobinuria	IgG (anti-P)	4°C—antibody binding 37°C—complement-mediated lysis

complement, C3b or C3d, may be detected by specific anticomplement antisera or by broad-spectrum Coombs' antisera that incorporate anticomplement as well as antiglobulin antibodies for screening. AIHA may be accompanied by immune thrombocytopenia (Evan's syndrome). As in other hemolytic anemias, the reticulocyte count is elevated, the serum haptoglobin is low, and spherocytes of varied sizes are present on the peripheral blood smear. The bilirubin may be elevated; usually it is mostly conjugated, but if the total bilirubin exceeds 4 mg/dl, the unconjugated fraction may be increased.

Therapy is directed toward decreasing the rate of

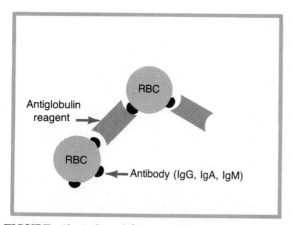

FIGURE 49–4. Coombs' or antiglobulin test. In the Coombs' test, an antibody directed against human immunoglubulin is used to detect the presence of antibody on the surface of the red cells by agglutination. Complement coating on the red cells (C3) can similarly be detected by an anticomplement Coombs' reagent. Broad-spectrum Coombs' reagents can be prepared which detect either immunoglobulin or complement or both; these are used for screening.

hemolysis. The first approach is oral corticosteroids, using 1 to 2 mg/kg/day of prednisolone (or equivalent) and tapering after the hematocrit returns to normal. Steroid therapy diminishes the binding of antibody to fixed macrophages and thereby limits the rate of red cell destruction. Steroids have a slower and less marked effect on inhibition of autoantibody production. Splenectomy is helpful in steroid-dependent or unresponsive cases. Splenectomy also removes an important source of antibody production. Immunosuppressive drugs such as azathioprine or cyclophosphamide are reserved for refractory cases. Transfusion is avoided if possible, as the transfused red cells are usually destroyed as quickly as the patient's own cells. Folic acid supplementation is often necessary because the rapid rate of red cell turnover depletes body stores of this vitamin.

Cold antibody autoimmune hemolytic anemia has a complex etiology. While many naturally occurring antibodies react with red cells in the cold, certain IgM autoantibodies with wide thermal amplitude may mediate autoimmune hemolysis (Table 49–8). The term thermal amplitude describes the temperature range over which these antibodies attach to red cells. Cold agglutinins causing hemolytic anemia are those with a wide thermal amplitude; that is, the capacity to bind to red cells occurs over a broad range from 4°C to a few degrees below body temperature, i.e., at temperatures that may occur in the nose, ears, or extremities during cold exposure. Polyclonal cold-reacting, IgM autoantibodies may arise transiently during infectious mononucleosis, cytomegalovirus infection, mycoplasma pneumonia, or protozoal infections and can cause significant hemolysis. Such polyclonal cold-reacting antibodies tend to be present transiently for days or weeks and resolve spontaneously following convalescence from the infection. In addition, "idiopathic cold agglutinin syndrome," characterized by monoclonal IgM antibodies, may precede the development of lymphoma or Waldenström's macroglobulinemia or may continue for years in the absence of malignant transformation. Unlike the polyclonal IgM cold antibodies, which appear briefly after infections, the monoclonal cold antibodies can persist for years. They show specificity for the I-i antigen system, glycoprotein precursors of ABO antigens. These IgM antibodies bind directly to red cells in the cold, fixing complement to the red cell surface; at warmer temperatures the antibodies dissociate from the red cells, leaving only activated complement bound to the red cell membrane. The C3b fixed on the red cell surface leads to removal of the coated red cells by macrophages in the spleen; in addition, bound C3 is converted to inactive C3d on the red cell membrane, which interferes with further binding or activation of C3 and limits the rate of hemolysis.

In addition to chronic hemolytic anemia, the patient with cold agglutinin disease may suffer from painful, blue fingers and toes on exposure to cold (acrocyanosis). The mainstay of therapy is to minimize cold exposure. In the rare case of severe hemolysis, plasmapheresis (using warmed equipment) or chemotherapy may be necessary.

Paroxysmal cold hemoglobinuria is a rare form of cold-reactive hemolysis in which a polyclonal IgG directed against the red cell P antigen system binds to red cells in the cold and fixes complement, so that when rewarming occurs, the complement cascade is activated and brisk intravascular hemolysis follows. This condition is found uncommonly in syphilis or after viral infections. The hemolysis is self-limited so that protection from cold is the most important therapy.

Drug-induced immune hemolytic anemia is a relatively common disorder that can result from three different mechanisms of hemolysis (Fig. 49–5). (1) *Hapten type*. Haptenic drugs bind to red cell membranes, forming neoantigens to which antibodies develop; a Coombs' positive hemolytic process follows with mainly extravascular destruction of red cells. The drug must be present for hemolysis to occur. Penicillins and cephalosporins are the chief offenders. (2) *Innocent bystander type*. Drugs that bind to plasma proteins elicit antibodies that form circulating immune complexes and activate complement. Red cells as "innocent bystanders" become coated with complement and may undergo intravascular or extravascular hemolysis depending on the rates of activation and inactivation of complement. Red cells show only complement coating. This represents the hemolytic mechanism for most drugs that produce immune hemolysis, including sulfonamides, phenothiazines, quinine, and isoniazid. (3) *Alpha methyldopa type*. Upon chronic use of alpha methyldopa, 15 per cent of patients develop a positive direct Coombs' test, with IgG present on the red cells; only 1 in 10 has hemolysis. The autoantibodies show Rh specificity, suggesting that the drug may somehow modify this red cell antigen system. The positive Coombs' test may persist for months after cessation of the drug. Levodopa and mefenamic acid (an anti-in-

flammatory drug) may also produce this type of autoimmune phenomenon.

Hypersplenism represents excessive sequestration of blood cells, particularly red cells, by an enlarged or abnormally functioning spleen. While senescent red cells are normally removed by trapping in the tortuous, poorly oxygenated sinusoids of the spleen, an enlarged spleen can randomly remove nonsenescent red cells. Pancytopenia, rather than anemia, may result from hypersplenism, but it appears that platelets and leukocytes are merely sequestered in enlarged spleens rather than being excessively destroyed. Hypersplenism is characterized by the picture of "empty blood and full marrow," which distinguishes this condition from the pancytopenias of marrow failure. It may occur in chronic hemolytic anemias of any cause, chronic infections, chronic leukemias and myeloproliferative diseases, lipid storage diseases, lymphomas, and rheumatoid arthritis (Felty's syndrome).

Paroxysmal nocturnal hemoglobinuria (PNH) is an acquired hemolytic disorder associated with increased susceptibility of a red cell subpopulation to complement-mediated damage. It is extremely rare, is considered a stem cell defect, and may be associated with eventual bone marrow aplasia and leukemia. Not only red cells but also granulocytes and platelets are sensitive to the lytic effects of complement and bind increased amounts of C3b compared to normal cells. PNH red cells fail to facilitate inactivation of comple-

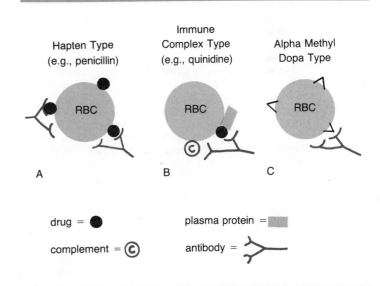

FIGURE 49–5. Mechanisms of drug-induced hemolysis. *A*, The drug binds to the red cell membrane as a hapten. Antibodies to the drug-membrane complex can lyse the red cells, but only in the presence of bound drug. *B*, The drug binds to a plasma protein or antibody, and the complex attaches to the red cell membrane. Antibodies produce binding of complement, and lysis follows. *C*, There appears to be a change in the red cell membrane after long-term treatment with the drug, often with Rh specificity. Antibodies develop which bind to the altered membrane, producing a positive Coombs' test and, rarely, hemolysis.

ment by the plasma C3b inactivator, which may account for their susceptibility to lysis. Clinical manifestations include pancytopenia, intravascular hemolysis, back pain, a tendency to venous thrombosis, and iron deficiency secondary to recurrent hemoglobinuria from intravascular hemolysis. Bone marrow may be hypocellular; the Coombs' test is negative. Hemolysis can be demonstrated by placing the patient's red cells in acidified serum (which permits activation of the alternative complement pathway) or in hypotonic medium (sugar-water test). Other markers associated with PNH include a low leukocyte alkaline phosphatase and a low red cell acetylcholinesterase.

Chemical, Toxic, and Parasitic Causes of Hemolytic Anemia

Either inorganic or complex organic toxins, including snake venoms and heavy metals, can cause hemolytic anemia. Arsenic and copper cause hemolysis by binding red cell membrane sulfhydryl groups; copper-induced hemolysis is seen in Wilson's disease and in hemodialyzed patients. Chloramine, generated in urban water supplies purified with chlorine, and alum may cause hemolysis in hemodialysis patients dialyzed against tap water. The lipophilic antifungal drug amphotericin can cause hemolysis, and snake venoms are directly lytic to red cells because of their content of lysolecithinases. Patients with advanced cirrhotic liver disease often develop spur cell anemia, a hemolytic disorder in which red cell membranes absorb excessive cholesterol present in abnormal circulating low density lipoproteins that contain an excess of cholesterol compared to phospholipid. Acanthocytes with irregular "spurs" are typically found in the peripheral blood.

Malaria commonly causes hemolytic anemia. Parasitized red cells become metabolically depleted, change membrane permeability and deformability characteristics, and may develop neoantigens that produce a positive antiglobulin test. The parasitized red cells also are prone to adhere to the vascular endothelium, which may contribute to local thrombosis. Babesiosis and bartonellosis also cause hemolytic anemia via red cell parasitism.

Hemolysis Resulting from Red Cell Trauma

Red cells exposed to excessive mechanical stress intravascularly or during extracorporeal circulation can undergo *fragmentation hemolysis*. Abnormal shear forces arise during passage of red cells through prosthetic heart valves, damaged natural valves, or vascular shunts. Chronic intravascular hemolysis due to abnormally functioning heart valves or valve prosthesis is relatively uncommon today, when ball valves are less frequently used. Its occurrence usually signals the existence of valve malfunction. Because of higher shear stresses associated with systemic pressures, malfunctioning aortic valves most often cause this type of intravascular hemolysis, but similar syndromes have occurred with mitral valve pathology. In both acute and chronic intravascular hemolysis, the blood smear shows red cell fragments (schistocytes), microspherocytes, and increased polychromasia (indicating reticulocytosis). The plasma haptoglobin is depressed, and the bilirubin and LDH may be elevated. If the process is chronic, hemosiderinuria and consequent iron deficiency may occur, because the hemolysis is intravascular and iron is lost in the urine. Iron therapy is needed to counteract the urinary losses and to correct the anemia. A similar process may occur acutely during extracorporeal circulation as in cardiopulmonary bypass. Red cell fragmentation also occurs after severe burns covering large areas of body surface, or in heat exhaustion. Intravascular hemolysis, without fragmentation of red cells, develops occasionally after prolonged marching or marathon running (march hemoglobinuria).

Microangiopathic hemolytic anemias result when normal red cells are fragmented while traversing intravascular fibrin strands in microvessels partially occluded by thrombi. Acute causes of microangiopathic hemolytic anemia include disseminated intravascular coagulation (DIC), thrombotic thrombocytopenic purpura, hemolytic-uremic syndrome, malignant hypertension, rejection of renal grafts, and mitomycin C toxicity. Certain vascular malformations such as giant hemangiomas (Kasabach-Merritt syndrome), in which sluggish blood flow through abnormally formed vessels triggers localized DIC, produce microangiopathic hemolytic anemia. In each of these settings, localized shearing of red cells within microthrombi results in intravascular hemolysis, usually accompanied by thrombocytopenia because of the concomitant intravascular clotting. In contrast, the schistocytic (fragmentation) hemolytic anemias related to large vessel pathology generally are not accompanied by thrombocytopenia.

Trousseau's syndrome represents chronic DIC in the setting of visceral cancer, with typical schistocytes and thrombocytopenia on the peripheral smear. Coagulation factor levels may be normal or decreased, depending upon the rate of consumption of clotting factors.

HEMOGLOBINOPATHIES

Hemoglobin, the major protein in the red cell, binds oxygen reversibly and is responsible for the capacity of red cells to transport oxygen to the tissues. Hemoglobin is present as a 5 mM solution in red cells. Each hemoglobin molecule consists of two identical alpha globin chains and two nonalpha chains, which in the adult comprise mainly beta globin, with a small amount of delta globin; in the fetus the main nonalpha polypeptide is gamma globin. Two genes on chromosome 16 code for the alpha chains, whereas the genes for the nonalpha globins are clustered on chromosome 11.

Each polypeptide subunit of hemoglobin holds a single heme group in a hydrophobic pocket. The iron of the heme is bound to the porphyrin ring and is also bound to a histidine residue to the globin chain; its hydrophobic environment protects the Fe^{++} from being oxidized even in the presence of oxygen. Oxygen is bound to each heme group via the central iron atom. The structure of the tetrameric hemoglobin molecule changes with the binding of oxygen so that the interactions of the globin chains alter the sequential release of oxygen from the four heme groups, thereby producing the sigmoidal shape of the oxygen dissociation curve. These interactions facilitate the uptake of oxygen in the lungs and its unloading at the tissues, with the steepest part of the curve lying within the ambient oxygen tensions of these two locations. Normal synthesis of alpha and beta chains is balanced, with little excess of either type produced within red cells. Excess globin chains are unstable and tend to precipitate at the red cell membrane (forming Heinz bodies), shortening red cell lifespan.

During transport of red cells from arterial oxygen tension (P_{O_2} 100 mm Hg) to tissue oxygen tension (P_{O_2} 40 mm Hg), the saturation of hemoglobin oxygen decreases from 100 to 75 per cent, although the capacity for O_2 delivery is much greater. Oxygen unloading is facilitated by the binding to hemoglobin of the molecule 2,3-diphosphoglyceric acid (2,3-DPG), an intermediate product of glycolysis; acidic pH and the binding of CO_2 also assist in the release of oxygen from hemoglobin, as do configurational changes in the hemoglobin molecule itself during oxygen release. Changes in the structure of the globin polypeptide chains, or in the heme itself, can affect the oxygen affinity of hemoglobin.

Mutations in the DNA sequences controlling globin synthesis either can produce structurally abnormal hemoglobins (hemoglobinopathies) or can decrease the rate of hemoglobin synthesis (thalassemias) (Table 49–9). The term *hemoglobinopathy* connotes structurally abnormal hemoglobins with altered function, whereas *thalassemia* refers to mutations resulting in decreased synthesis of one globin type. Since the alpha globin chain contains 241 amino acids and the beta chain 246, and single amino acid substitutions resulting from single mutations produce abnormally functioning molecules, a very large number of mutant forms are possible. Only mutations of certain types, however, lead to functional alterations in hemoglobin resulting in abnormal oxygen carriage or anemia. Examples of these functionally important mutations include surface substitutions that alter hemoglobin solubility (e.g., Hb S), substitutions in internal nonpolar residues resulting in hemoglobin instability (e.g., Hb Koln), substitution for the histidine that binds iron, permitting oxidation of heme iron (e.g., Hb M), or substitution at the alpha-beta contact points, which alters heme-heme interactions and changes oxygen affinity (Hb Kansas or Chesapeake). Mutations causing thalassemic syndromes include deletions, removal of stop codons, and frameshift mutations leading to nonsense sequences; these all tend to alter globin synthesis and to decrease the rate of normal globin production, a process that secondarily regulates heme synthesis and leads to hemolytic anemias. In addition, mutations affecting the normal sequence of expression of the beta cluster genes may result in hereditary persistence of Hb F synthesis after birth.

TABLE 49–9. CLINICAL SYNDROMES RELATED TO ABNORMAL HEMOGLOBINS

TYPE OF DEFECT	CLINICAL FEATURES
A. Decreased hemoglobin solubility	
1. Crystalline hemoglobin Hb S, C, D, E	Hemolytic anemia with microvascular occlusion
2. Unstable hemoglobin	Hemolytic anemia
B. Abnormal oxygen transport	
1. Increased O_2 affinity	Polycythemia
2. Decreased O_2 affinity	Normochromic "anemia"
C. Heme oxidation (Hb M)	Cyanosis Methemoglobinemia

Anemias Resulting From Abnormalities in Hemoglobin Structure or Function (Fig. 49–6)

Sickle Cell Anemia. By far the most important disease resulting from a mutation to an abnormally functioning hemoglobin is sickle cell disease, in which a single base change in the DNA results in a substitution of valine for glutamic acid at the sixth position in the beta globin chain. The ensuing insolubility of Hb S under deoxygenated conditions results in polymerization of Hb S molecules within the red cells, leading to distortion of shape, membrane changes, cellular dehydration, and decreased deformability. Microvascular occlusion results from the altered behavior of sickled red cells and produces progressive microinfarction of vital organs, painful bony crises, splenic autoinfarction, and renal damage. Patients have a shortened lifespan. The Hb S gene is present

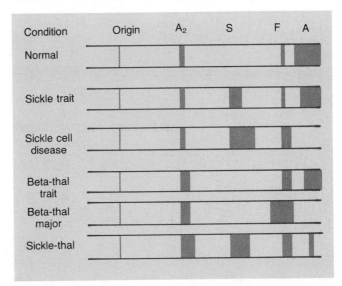

FIGURE 49–6. Common patterns of hemoglobin electrophoresis. Note that in sickle cell anemia, 95 per cent of Hb is S; in sickle trait, 40 per cent is S and 60 per cent is A, but in sickle-thal, 60 to 70 per cent of Hb is A. In beta-thal trait, either Hb A_2 or F (or both) is elevated, whereas in beta-thal major, Hb A is absent and Hb F makes up most of the hemoglobin.

in 10 per cent of American blacks and up to 25 per cent of the population in Western Africa. In the heterozygote (Hb S trait, Hb SA), protection against falciparum malaria is associated with the hemoglobinopathy. The heterozygote state usually has 60 per cent Hb A and 40 per cent Hb S; both types of globins are present in the same cell, but not in the same molecule. The homozygous state (Hb SS, sickle cell disease) has over 90 per cent Hb S, with small amounts of Hb F or Hb A_2. The concurrent presence of thalassemia trait or persistence of Hb F tends to ameliorate the clinical course of SS disease, in the first case by decreasing the rate of synthesis of the β^S chain in relation to other globins, and in the second case by introducing a nonaggregating hemoglobin that interferes with Hb S polymerization (Table 49–10).

Clinical manifestations of SS disease begin in infancy, when Hb F levels begin to fall. Major symptoms and signs include painful crises, swelling of the extremities and spleen (in infants and children), bony and pulmonary infarctions, and cerebrovascular accidents. Any organ may be affected. Intrahepatic sickling can produce marked hepatic swelling, dysfunction, and hyperbilirubinemia; intrarenal sickling can cause renal papillary necrosis and hematuria, with loss of renal concentrating ability (usually by age five); intracutaneous sickling produces necrotic skin ulceration, usually of the ankles and feet; retinal sickling can produce neovascularization and retinal detachment; bony sickling can produce aseptic necrosis and predispose to osteomyelitis. Growth is disturbed, with typical elongated limbs and asthenic habitus. Chronic hemolysis results in a markedly increased incidence of cholelithiasis with multiple bilirubin stones and cholecystitis, a tendency to folic acid deficiency, impaired immunity partially due to loss of spleen tissue and partly related to poor IgM production, and an increased tendency to infections. Cardiomyopathy is common, as is delayed puberty.

Typical laboratory findings in sickle cell anemia include Hb ranging from 6 to 8 gm/dl, hematocrit 18 to 24 per cent, and a normal MCV. WBC and platelets are normal to increased. The reticulocyte count is chronically elevated, often to more than 20 per cent, and nucleated red blood cells are frequently present. Sickle-shaped, holly-leaf–shaped, or otherwise distorted red cells appear in variable numbers on the peripheral smear and in large numbers in deoxygenated wet preparations (see Fig. 49–6). Hemoglobin electrophoresis shows 90 to 95 per cent Hb S. The serum bilirubin is elevated, with mainly direct-reacting bilirubin; the haptoglobin level is low; and the serum LDH level is elevated. Screening for Hb S is most simply performed with a "sickle cell prep" by mixing the patient's blood with sodium metabisulfite, which deoxygenates the red cells and induces sickling observable with a microscope; commerical tests that demonstrate the insolubility of Hb S (Sickledex) are easier to perform for mass screening, as they do not require a microscope. Hemoglobin electrophoresis after positive screening tests is needed to delineate the specific hemoglobinopathy (Table 49–10).

Other sickle cell syndromes representing concomitant SS-thalassemia trait or a mixed hemoglobinopathy (SC, SD) usually have milder clinical courses than does sickle cell anemia (SS). They produce a less severe anemia and may present with splenomegaly rather than an absent spleen. Patients with Hb SC disease, however, can have severe morbidity in pregnancy and a higher rate of ocular complications than patients with SS disease; Hb C, also a β^6 substitution, also results in intracellular hemoglobin polymerization, but anemia and vaso-occlusive manifestations are milder in homozygous Hb C disease than in SS disease. In sickle–beta thalassemia trait, the red cells show microcytosis and hypochromia, the percentage of Hb S is less than 80 per cent, with increased Hb F in a heterogeneous distribution, and some Hb A may be present. If hereditary persistence of Hb F is present, the Hb F distribution among the red cells is homogeneous rather than variable, as it is in beta thalassemia trait.

Management of sickle cell anemia is largely symptomatic and supportive. Painful crises are treated with oxygen administration, intravenous and oral fluids, correction of acidosis, analgesics, and attention to precipitating causes such as dehydration, fever, and infection. Sickle cell crisis itself does not cause fever,

TABLE 49–10. COMPARISON OF SICKLE CELL SYNDROMES

GENOTYPE	CLINICAL CONDITION	Hb A	Hb S	Hb A_2	Hb F	Hb C	OTHER FINDINGS
SA	Sickle cell trait	55–60	40–45	2–3	—	—	Asymptomatic
SS	Sickle cell anemia	0	85–95	2–3	5–15	—	Clinically severe anemia Hb F heterogeneous in distribution
S-β^0thal	Sickle cell–beta thalassemia	0	70–80	3–5	10–20	—	Moderately severe anemia Splenomegaly in 50% Smear: hypo, micro
S-β^+thal	Sickle cell–beta thalassemia	10–20	60–75	3–5	10–20	—	Hb F distributed heterogeneously
SC	Hb SC disease	0	45–50	—	—	45–50	Moderately severe anemia Splenomegaly; target cells
S-HPFH	Sickle—hereditary persistence of Hb F	0	70–80	1–2	20–30	—	Asymptomatic; Hb F is uniformly distributed

but infection or tissue infarction does. Because of the increased risk of infection, pneumococcal vaccine should be administered to all sickle cell patients. Transfusion is not useful in treatment of acute sickle cell crises, but chronic transfusion programs (exchange transfusions are preferred to avoid iron overload) have been tried in patients at high risk of recurrent cerebral infarction. Transfusion prior to surgery appears to help prevent initiation of intraoperative and postoperative crises and perhaps to improve healing. Special attention to good oxygenation during surgery and avoidance of hypothermia are imperative to avoid intraoperative sickling and tissue infarction. Transfusions are also given during the later stages of pregnancy in women with SS disease to counteract placental dysfunction and placental infarction caused by sickling.

Recently, therapies designed to enhance production of Hb F in patients with SS disease have entered clinical trial; these include administration of the drugs 5-azacytidine and hydroxyurea, which may derepress the gene for Hb F or initiate differentiation of more primitive stem cells in which this gene is active. Since the presence of Hb F in SS red cells tends to decrease the intracellular polymerization and precipitation of Hb S, leading to less sickling and improved red cell survival, induction of Hb F production is highly desirable. However, because these drugs are cytotoxic (and 5-azacytidine is potentially carcinogenic), such therapy may depress bone marrow function and have adverse long-term effects. The use of these drugs is considered experimental at present.

Genetic counselling of heterozygotes for Hb S has not been very successful in decreasing reproductive activity of persons at risk of having children with SS disease. Prenatal diagnosis is now possible using restriction enzyme techniques applied to amniocentesis samples, taking advantage of several restriction fragment polymorphisms.

Unstable Hemoglobins. Unstable hemoglobins represent a varied group of disorders, usually autosomal dominant mutants, in which either heme association with globin is defective or the forces holding the globin tetramer together are altered. The result is intracellular precipitation of the denatured hemoglobin as Heinz bodies that bind to the red cell membrane. Such cells are either "pitted" of these inclusions by splenic or hepatic macrophages, resulting in shortened red cell lifespan, or are totally removed in the reticuloendothelial system. Exposure of red cells containing unstable hemoglobin to oxidant stress exacerbates the hemolysis and may cause acute jaundice.

Hemoglobins of Altered Oxygen Affinity. The parital pressure of oxygen at which hemoglobin is half-saturated with oxygen (P_{50}) provides a useful guide to measurement of functional oxygen affinity. The normal P_{50} is about 25 mm Hg. Although more than 80 mutations producing altered oxygen affinity have been found, only a few are of clinical consequence. When hemoglobin is fully oxygenated, it normally assumes the R, or relaxed state, which manifests a high affinity for oxygen; when it is deoxygenated, it is in the T, or tense state, having a low oxygen affinity. Mutations that affect hydrogen bonding or hydrophobic interactions at the $\alpha_1\beta_2$ interface change the R-T balance and alter oxygen affinity. Hemoglobins of high oxygen affinity are clinically associated with erythrocytosis, sometimes with thrombotic tendencies; hemoglobins of low oxygen affinity are associated with apparent anemias, which actually represent a functional marrow response to the increased tissue oxygen delivery. The latter may be accompanied by an asymptomatic cyanosis.

Methemoglobinemia. Methemoglobinemia represents the oxidation of heme iron, which prevents its capacity to transport oxygen, and may result from enzyme deficiency (e.g., NADH-methemoglobin reductase), abnormal hemoglobins with substitutions in the heme pocket (M hemoglobinopathies), or exposure to oxidant drugs. The clinical manifestation is cyanosis without hypoxemia. The blood is brownish and does not turn red upon shaking with air. The reducing agents methylene blue and ascorbic acid can improve the cyanosis in patients with methemoglobinemia due to enzyme deficiency or oxidant drug exposure, but not in patients with M hemoglobinopathies. The drugs that induce methemoglobinemia in normal individuals include nitrites (especially toxic to infants), primaquine, dapsone, aniline dyes, and sulfanilamide.

Thalassemias

As mentioned above, hemolytic anemia in the thalassemias results from mutations that affect globin synthesis (Table 49–11). The hemoglobin that is produced is less than normal in amount but is structurally normal. A decreased synthetic rate of one type of globin chain results in ineffective erythropoiesis, with markedly enhanced intramedullary loss of developing red cells. Several mechanisms are involved: a primary decrease in globin synthesis; the accumulation and precipitation of the other type of globin chain, which is produced in relative excess; and secondarily depressed heme synthesis. The red cells are hypochromic and markedly microcytic and have a shortened circulating lifespan. Because of the complexity of hemoglobin synthesis, thalassemic states can vary clinically from "silent" carrier (heterozygotes for alpha thalassemia) to severely anemic thalassemia major (homozygotes for beta thalassemia) to death in utero from hydrops fetalis (homozygotes for alpha thalassemia). The incidence of beta thalassemia is greatest in persons of Mediterranean and African origin and that of alpha thalassemia in persons of Far Eastern origin; the trait is present in 3 to 5 per cent of such populations. In the United States as many as 20 per cent of blacks and persons of Mediterranean origin carry thalassemia trait.

Beta thalassemia syndromes include thalassemia trait (heterozygous β thalassemia), thalassemia intermedia, and thalassemia major (Cooley's anemia). The genetic alterations that produce these syndromes are many. Mutations of the β-globin gene that depress synthesis of β-globin include the following: deletions, nonsense mutation, or frame shifts that prevent any

TABLE 49–11. COMPARISON OF THE THALASSEMIA SYNDROMES

GENETIC ABNORMALITY	PER CENT Hb A	PER CENT Hb A$_2$	PER CENT Hb F	OTHER	CLINICAL SYNDROME
Normal β β	90–98	2–3	2–3		None
Beta Thalassemias					
Thalassemia major					
β thal^0 β thal^0	0	2–5	95	—	Severe anemia, abnormal growth, iron overload, needs transfusion
β thal$^+$ β thal$^+$	very low	2–5	20–80	—	
Thalassemia intermedia (varied genetic globin abnormalities)		overlaps with Thalassemia major			Severe hypo/micro anemia with Hb 7–9 gm/dl, hepatosplenomegaly, bone changes, iron overload, less need for transfusion
Thalassemia minor					
β β thal^0 or β β thal$^+$	90–95	5–7	2–10		Hypo/micro blood smear, mild to no anemia
Alpha Thalassemias					
Homozygous α-thalassemia − − / − −	—	—	—	Hb H (β$_4$) Hb Barts (γ$_4$)	Hydrops fetalis, stillborn
Hemoglobin H disease − − / − α	60–70	2–5	2–5	Hb H 30–40	Hypo/micro anemia, Hb 7–10 gm/dl, Heinz bodies
α-thalassemia trait − α / − α α α / − −	90–98	2–3	2–3		Hypo/micro smear, no anemia
Silent carrier − α / α α	90–98	2–3	2–3		Normal

mRNA production (β°), and mutations affecting promoter or splice sites, which permit reduced levels of mRNA and hence some hemoglobin synthesis (β$^+$). The clinical features of thalassemia trait are a mild anemia that is markedly microcytic in relation to the hemoglobin level and is sometimes accompanied by splenomegaly. The MCV is frequently in the 60's, with a hemoglobin level of 10 to 12 gm/dl and marked anisocytosis on the peripheral smear. Serum iron and transferrin levels are normal. Hemoglobin electrophoresis (see Fig. 49–5) reveals elevation of Hb A$_2$ to 3 to 5 per cent, and Hb F to 2 to 3 per cent. Morbidity is not associated with thalassemia trait, and iron therapy should not be given.

In contrast to this asymptomatic picture, the homozygous *thalassemia major* is a lethal, severe hemolytic anemia characterized by growth abnormalities, dysfunction of almost all organ systems, and iron overload. Because both β genes are abnormal, very little to no β chain synthesis occurs, and the excess of insoluble α-globin chains in the red cells leads to intracellular precipitation that affects both erythropoiesis and red cell lifespan. The resulting ineffective erythropoiesis causes extreme expansion of marrow space into long bones, skull, and facial bones, as well as the development of extramedullary hematopoiesis in liver, spleen, and around the spinal vertebrae. Growth abnormalities and cortical bone fragility ensue, with an increased rate of fractures. Growth retardation and delay of puberty are universal. The peripheral smear shows severe microcytosis and anisocytosis, many nucleated red blood cells, and hypochromia. The hemoglobin level in the untransfused patient is 3 to 6 gm/dl. Hemoglobin A is very low to absent, and the major hemoglobin is Hb F, with a variably increased amount of Hb A$_2$. Early death by age two to three years was common before transfusion therapy was instituted. With regular transfusion, the hemoglobin level can be maintained at 8 to 10 gm/dl and many of the growth and bony abnormalities decreased.

An absolute increase in iron absorption, plus severe iron overload from transfusion therapy, has led to a different set of complications, that of tissue fibrosis from iron deposition. This abnormality results in cardiomyopathy, diabetes mellitus, and adrenal, parathyroid, and thyroid hypofunction. Affected children also show increased susceptibility to infection and functional hyposplenism; splenectomy is usually performed in late childhood to lessen the transfusion requirements and adds to the risk of sepsis. Iron chelation therapy with subcutaneous desferrioxamine, now begun in early childhood, appears to decrease the devastating consequences of iron overload if chronically maintained; use of carefully phenotyped frozen blood can decrease alloimmunization and prevent transfusion refractoriness. With the most modern of these supportive therapies, the lifespan of patients with thalassemia major has been extended from early childhood to the 20's. Newer approaches, still highly experimental, include bone marrow transfusion and agents that increase Hb F production, such as 5-azacytidine and hydroxyurea (see above). Prenatal diagnosis by restriction enzyme polymorphism techniques is currently more useful in alpha than in beta thalassemia, but direct measurement of depressed β-globin synthesis in fetal blood can be made.

Thalassemia intermedia is genetically variable and frequently appears to represent double heterozygosity for two different thalassemic mutations. Affected persons can maintain an untransfused Hb level of 8 to 10 gm/dl. They have more normal growth and sexual maturation, suffer fewer clinical complications than patients with thalassemia major, and frequently live into midadulthood. Iron overload, however, may occur, as can the tendency to infections, bony fragility, and organ dysfunction, but with a slower time course.

Alpha thalassemia syndromes depend upon the combination of mutations in the four α-gene loci. In order of increasing severity they are α-thal$_2$ trait, α-thal$_1$ trait, hemoglobin H disease, and hydrops fetalis. The first condition is asymptomatic without anemia, except that the MCV and MCH are decreased, while the second condition results in a mild microcytic anemia. Hb H disease presents a mild, variable degree of hemolytic anemia characterized by red cell inclusions, which result from precipitation of the unstable β$_4$ hemoglobin. Hydrops fetalis, the absence of all α-globin production, consistently leads to death in utero or to stillbirth. The amount of Hb Bart's (γ$_4$) present in the blood of an infant with alpha thalassemia corresponds directly to the number of thalassemic α-gene loci. The occurrence of alpha thalassemia trait together with another hemoglobinopathy such as Hb SS tends to ameliorate the latter disease, probably by decreasing the intracellular concentration of the abnormal hemoglobin. There is a high incidence of α-thalassemia trait in American blacks, and this factor ameliorates the clinical severity of sickle cell disease in this population. Silent carrier states for both alpha and beta thalassemia genes are common and can be detected only by family studies.

REFERENCES

Jandl JH: Blood: Textbook of Hematology. Boston, MA, Little, Brown & Co, 1987, pp 153–406.

Orkin SH: Disorders of Hemoglobin Synthesis: The Thalassemias. *In* Stamatogamapoulos G, Nienhuis P, Leder P, Majerus P (eds): Molecular Basis of Blood Diseases. Philadelphia, WB Saunders Co, 1986, pp 106–126.

50

THERAPY WITH BLOOD PRODUCTS

Human blood is an invaluable resource in the supportive therapy of patients with hemorrhage, severe anemias, and coagulation deficits, and yet a dangerous substance if improperly used. Modern blood banking has been made possible by the science of immunohematology and by the development of special methods for the maintenance and preservation of blood ex vivo. Each unit of 450 ml of blood is mixed with 63 ml of an anticoagulant solution containing citrate to prevent clotting, as well as glucose, phosphate, and adenine to prolong red cell viability. The shelf life is 35 days. Transfusion of whole blood is rarely necessary: it is physiologically and economically more reasonable to separate each unit of fresh blood into components that can be used to treat as many as five different recipients (Table 50–1). These components include red blood cells, platelets, and granulocytes; plasma and its protein constituents including albumin, Factor VIII:antihemophilic factor (AHF), other coagulation factors, and gamma globulin.

Red blood cells can be transfused as packed red cells (most of plasma removed); leukocyte-poor (buffy coat–poor) red cells, from which about 80 per cent of the leukocytes have been removed; or frozen red cells (from which about 90 per cent of leukocytes have been removed). Each unit of red cells transfused should raise the hematocrit by 3 to 5 per cent. Platelets are separated from red cells by differential centrifugation and are administered as concentrates of 4 to 10 units suspended in a small volume of plasma. Platelet transfusion is indicated as therapy for severely thrombocytopenic patients who are bleeding, or as prophylaxis for patients with aplastic anemia or with leukemia during myelosuppressive chemotherapy. A rise in platelet count can be expected for one to three days following transfusion, unless the patient has fever, which shortens the survival of transfused platelets, or immune thrombocytopenia, which destroys transfused platelets as fast as autologous ones. Patients who require repeated platelet transfusion may become allosensitized and refractory to random donor platelets and require HLA-matched platelets. Granulocytes can be separated from whole blood by leukapheresis and administered to neutropenic patients or given as buffy coat

TABLE 50–1. BLOOD COMPONENT THERAPY

COMPONENT	INDICATION FOR USE
Whole blood	Rarely needed except in massive hemorrhage
Packed red cells	Standard unit for transfusion
Frozen red cells	Useful in multitransfused patient to decrease, sensitization to HLA and leukocyte antigens
Fresh frozen plasma	Replaces coagulation factors
Plasma protein fraction	Plasma expansion (hepatitis-free)
Cryoprecipitate	Replaces Factor VIII and fibrinogen
Platelet concentrates	Raise platelet count in nonimmune thrombocytopenia
Granulocyte concentrates	May be of *transient* use in infected, granulocytopenic patient; rarely used
Lyophilized Factor VIII concentrate	Treatment of choice in hemophilia A
Lyophilized prothrombin complex concentrate	Treatment of choice in hemophilia B; emergency correction of oral anticoagulant effect
"FEIBA"	Bypasses acquired inhibitors to clotting factors

preparations; both preparations contain considerable lymphocyte and platelet admixture. Because the effect of granulocyte transfusions is transitory (the half-life is about 6 hours), such therapy is usually reserved for treating life-threatening neutropenia. Fresh frozen plasma supplies several of the labile coagulation factors. Fibrinogen and Factor VIII:AHF can be concentrated in cryoprecipitate prepared from individual units of plasma. At the present time the only approved form of fibrinogen for replacement therapy is cryoprecipitate.

BLOOD COMPATIBILITY TESTING

Over 300 different antigenic determinants have been identified on human red blood cells, the most important being the ABO system (Table 50–2). Almost all human red cells belong to one of the four major blood groups—A, B, AB, or O. Subjects of one type, for example A, carry in their plasma natural IgM antibodies to the B antigen. Serum from type AB individuals contains no such natural antibodies, whereas serum from type O carries both anti-A and anti-B. These antibodies are easily demonstrable in saline solution. The ABO types are inherited as autosomal co-

dominant traits. ABO compatibility is essential for blood transfusion. Acquired antibodies against ABO antigens, produced by alloimmunization following transfusion, pregnancy, or exposure to heterologous antigens, usually microbial, are IgG in type.

A second important blood antigen group is Rh, which consists of at least three linked loci—Cc, D, and Ee. IgG antibodies can develop to the Rh antigens after sensitization by prior transfusion or pregnancy. These antibodies are more difficult to detect than the natural ABO isoagglutinins and usually require testing in the presence of protein-containing medium rather than saline. The most clinically important locus in the Rh system is D; the absence of D is called Rh negative. Transfusion of Rh+ (D+) blood to a sensitized Rh− person can provoke acute hemolysis. An Rh+ fetus carried by a sensitized Rh− mother can develop erythroblastosis fetalis. In the past, maternal sensitization in such cases occurred at the time of delivery of the first child. This problem has been prevented in about 80 per cent of potential cases by treating Rh− mothers immediately after delivery, amniocentesis, or abortion with Rh immune globulin (RhoGAM) to prevent Rh immunization of the mother. In Rh− mothers who incur transplacental hemorrhage during pregnancy (diagnosed by the appearance of Rh alloantibody in maternal blood), Rh immune globulin should be administered during the pregnancy. Intrauterine transfusion of the fetus can also be carried out in those Rh− mothers who become sensitized.

Antibodies to Kell, Duffy, and Kidd antigens occur after sensitization by allogeneic red cells and may cause hemolytic transfusion reactions. Antibodies to many other antigens, such as the MN system, Lewis, P, or Ii, occur commonly but generally are inactive at body temperature and do not usually cause clinical problems (Table 50–3).

Compatibility testing for red cell transfusion consists of several sequential steps. First, the potential recipient's own red cells are typed. Then an antibody screen is performed, i.e., testing the potential recipient's serum against a panel of red cells selected to include the most frequent antigens that cause clinical reactions. Third, cross-matching is carried out, that is, testing the recipient's serum with samples of the red cells from units intended for transfusion. Under emergency circumstances, packed type O red cells can be given to a recipient of any ABO type. Rh+ cells can, in an emergency, be transfused to an Rh− recipient if the latter's serum contains no anti-D; the likelihood of sensitizing the recipient is 70 per cent. In the pres-

TABLE 50–2. ABO BLOOD GROUP SYSTEM

PHENOTYPE	GENOTYPES	ANTIGENS	NATURAL ANTIBODIES	FREQUENCY*
O	OO	O	anti-A, anti-B	45%
A	AA or AO	A	anti-B	40%
B	BB or BO	B	anti-A	9%
AB	AB	AB	none	3%

ence of sudden hemorrhage, plasma expanders such as albumin can be used until cross-matched blood becomes available.

HAZARDS OF BLOOD TRANSFUSION

The hazards of administering blood products include transfusion reactions, circulatory overload, transmission of disease, iron overload, coagulation disturbances, and graft-versus-host disease (Table 50–4).

Transfusion reactions include acute hemolytic reactions, anaphylaxis, and febrile reactions. Most commonly, acute hemolytic reactions result from errors made by the persons who label blood samples intended for typing and cross-matching or from administering to one patient a unit of blood intended for another. Most such errors are made on the hospital floor or clinic. Less commonly, such reactions may result from errors made in the blood bank procedures. Hemolytic reactions may also occur when blood has been properly typed and cross-matched by standard techniques but unusual alloimmunization has escaped detection.

Since acute hemolytic reactions may lead to anaphylaxis and renal failure or death, rapid and orderly response to such catastrophes is essential. The blood transfusion must first be discontinued, a tube of blood drawn from the patient for inspection and for evaluation at the blood bank, and intravenous fluids immediately started. Urine output and vital signs must be monitored, and diuretics or mannitol administered in an effort to maintain a brisk urine flow. A hematocrit tube should be immediately centrifuged and the plasma inspected for the presence of hemoglobin; pink plasma confirms an intravascular hemolytic transfusion reaction. Hemoglobinuria also should be sought but may be delayed in time of appearance. If oliguria or anuria occurs, dialysis is warranted. In all cases, fluid and electrolyte balance requires careful monitoring, especially to guard against hyperkalemia.

Hemolytic transfusion reactions may be immediate or delayed. ABO incompatibility can activate the complement cascade and therefore produce acute reactions with intravascular hemolysis. Rh or Kell antibodies do not activate complement at a rapid rate and tend not to produce acute hemolysis. Instead, they cause shortened red cell lifespan and produce extra-

TABLE 50–3. MAIN BLOOD GROUP SYSTEMS

NAME	FREQUENCY OF ANTIBODIES	CAUSE OF HEMOLYTIC REACTIONS
ABO	Very common	Yes
Rhesus	Common	Yes
Kell	Occasional	Yes
Duffy	Occasional	Yes
Kidd	Occasional	Yes
Lutheran	Rare	Yes
Lewis	Rare	No
P	Rare	Rare
MNS	Rare	No
Ii	Rare	Yes

vascular hemolysis. Acute hemolytic transfusion reactions usually present with the sudden onset of back pain, hypotension, sweating, fever, and chills. Patients receiving incompatible blood while under anesthesia fail to exhibit such reactions, and postoperative oliguria, hemoglobinuria, or renal failure may be the first sign that a prior hemolytic transfusion reaction has occurred. Delayed hemolysis is common in the repeatedly transfused patient owing to anamnestic increases in antibody after prior sensitization, and takes place 5 to 10 days after the transfusion. Such delayed transfusion reactions produce a rapid fall in hematocrit accompanied by jaundice or a rise in bilirubin. A previously negative alloantibody screen often becomes positive at this time.

Febrile reactions or urticaria are much more common than hemolytic transfusion reactions. They usually represent alloimmunization to leukocyte antigens, which may be acquired during pregnancy (20 per cent of women) or prior multiple transfusion (70 to 90 per cent of multitransfused recipients). They range in severity from simple fever, to urticaria plus fever and chills, to vomiting and hypotension. These symptoms can usually be prevented by administering leukocyte-poor blood or by pretreatment of the patient with chlorpheniramine and hydrocortisone. Both drug pretreatment and the administration of leukocyte-poor blood may be needed. If these measures do not suffice, then frozen-thawed, washed red cells should be sub-

TABLE 50–4. EVALUATION OF TRANSFUSION REACTIONS

TYPE OF REACTION	CLINICAL SIGNS	MANAGEMENT OF PROBLEM
Major hemolytic (incompatibility)	Shock, back pain, flushing, fever, intravascular hemolysis	1. Stop transfusion. Return blood to blood bank with fresh sample of patient's blood. 2. Hydrate IV; support BP, maintain high urine flow. 3. Check for hemoglobinemia and hemoglobinuria.
Febrile	Fever, urticaria (usually due to sensitization to WBC antibodies)	Pretreat with hydrocortisone, Benadryl, or both Use buffy coat–poor RBC
Allergic	Fever, urticaria, anaphylactoid reaction (often due to sensitivity to donor plasma proteins)	Benadryl, hydrocortisone Use washed RBC or frozen RBC

stituted. Anaphylactoid reactions (3 to 5 per cent of transfusion recipients develop urticaria) may also be caused by recipient antibody to IgA, especially in transfusion recipients who are IgA-deficient. IgA-deficient patients should receive washed red cells and should avoid plasma-containing preparations.

Transmission of disease by transfused blood components rarely involves bacterial infection, because modern blood banking practices utilize closed blood collecting systems that guard effectively against bacterial contamination. Hepatitis transmission, however, remains a serious hazard of blood transfusion, despite the reduction in transmission of hepatitis B. Thanks to the development of sensitive methods of detecting HB Ag positivity, hepatitis B now represents only 10 per cent of all post-transfusion hepatitis. Non-A, non-B hepatitis and delta agent account for the balance of cases. Up to 4 per cent of patients receiving blood products will develop hepatitis, the highest risk being in recipients of commercial coagulation factor concentrates. Patients receiving red cells, platelets, or plasma also incur considerable risk. Transfusion can also transmit cytomegalovirus infection, particularly to patients undergoing organ grafts who have activated lymphocytes in which this virus multiplies. Malaria and babesiosis can also be transmitted by transfusion, but syphilis is now rare.

Acquired immune deficiency syndrome (AIDS) develops in a small percentage of persons receiving transfusion of red cells, platelets, or commercial coagulation factor concentrates. By the end of 1987, about 2000 persons with no risk factors other than transfusion had developed AIDS out of some 60,000 total reported cases of AIDS. The risk overall is low, calculated at 1 in 10^6 transfusions. Hemophiliacs who receive coagulation factor concentrates are at highest risk. Several cases of AIDS have been reported in infants following neonatal exchange transfusion. Elimination of high-risk individuals from blood donor pools will reduce this risk further, as will more sensitive screening for anti-HTLV III antibodies in prospective blood donors.

Circulatory overload, especially with whole blood transfusion, may occur in patients with cardiopulmonary dysfunction or congestive heart failure and can be avoided by using packed red cells or other concentrated components. In patients with congestive heart failure who need red cells, exchange transfusion consisting of removal of a unit of the patient's own blood before administering one to two units of packed red cells may avoid circulatory overload.

Problems Associated with Massive Transfusions

A bleeding tendency may occur in patients receiving multiple units of blood over a short time period. This is due in part to dilutional thrombocytopenia, since blood stored longer than 24 hours contains few viable platelets. Conditions requiring massive transfusion support are often accompanied by disseminated intravascular coagulation, adding the problems of consumption of platelets and coagulation factors. In such cases, it may be necessary to replace platelets, coagulation factors (using fresh frozen plasma), or fibrinogen (as cryoprecipitate) in addition to red cells. In addition, administration of large amounts of citrated blood may temporarily depress the serum calcium level and require calcium supplementation.

Graft-versus-host disease, representing engraftment of donor lymphocytes in the recipient, can be observed after transfusion of blood products to immunocompromised recipients, such as patients with congenital T cell defects or those being prepared for bone marrow transplantation. Irradiation of the blood products prior to transfusion prevents this complication.

Bone marrow transplantation is discussed in Chapter 52.

REFERENCES

Mollison PL: Blood Transfusion in Clinical Medicine. 7th ed. New York, Blackwell Scientific Publications, 1987.

51

LEUKOCYTE DISORDERS

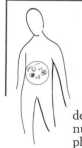

The main function of leukocytes is to maintain host defenses against disease, especially infection. Mononuclear phagocytes (monocytes and tissue macrophages) and granulocytes accomplish this by ingestion and killing of microorganisms and by digestion of tissue debris. Lymphocytes participate in the activation and effector functions of the immune system, and macrophage/monocytes play essential roles in the responses of lymphocytes.

Quantitative disorders of granulocytes are more common than functional disorders; the latter are frequently incompatible with normal lifespan and are mainly confined to children, although some acquired disorders of granulocyte function occur in the setting of hematologic diseases or drug therapy. Acquired leukopenia, especially neutropenia and its extreme form, agranulocytosis, is the most common quantitative disorder of clinical significance.

NEUTROPHIL STRUCTURE AND FUNCTION

Polymorphonuclear leukocytes make up the largest percentage of circulating leukocytes (50 to 70 per cent). They are nondividing, terminally differentiated cells that are motile, phagocytize a variety of microorganisms and inert particles, and release enzymes from cytoplasmic granules both into phagocytic vacuoles, and, under many circumstances, into the extracellular milieu. The three phases of microbial attack by neutrophils include chemotaxis, the directed movement along a concentration gradient of attractant substance toward a target organism; phagocytosis, the engulfment of the microbe in a membrane-lined phagocytic vacuole; and microbial killing, a chemical attack on the ingested microorganisms via the release of granule contents into the phagocytic vacuoles (bactericidal proteins, myeloperoxidase, cathepsins) plus the formation of oxygen free radicals such as superoxide and hydroxyl ion. In the presence of halides, such as Cl^-, toxic substances are generated that kill the ingested microbes.

Chemotaxis involves the margination of circulating neutrophils along the endothelial lining of vessels, usually in postcapillary venules, their penetration through the vascular wall via intercellular junctions, and their directed migration toward the extravascular source of the infection. The migration of the neutrophils takes place along a chemical gradient of an attracting substance, which may be n-methylated bacterial peptides, complement fragments (C5a), or leukotriene B_4. Leukocyte proteases are responsible for the production of complement-derived chemotaxins, whereas lipoxygenases mediate production of arachidonic acid–derived leukotrienes and hydroxyacids. These latter substances also have chemotactic and leukocyte-activating functions. Chemotactic substances binding to tissue sites may also serve to localize neutrophil accumulation.

Recognition of microorganisms or other particulate substances is required for subsequent ingestion by phagocytes. Opsonins, or proteins that coat microorganisms and promote their avid uptake by neutrophils, include the complement fragment C3b, the large plasma protein fibronectin, and immunoglobulins. These substances adhere to the surface of microorganisms and promote binding to the C3b and Fc receptors on the neutrophil plasma membrane. *Phagocytosis,* the localized invagination of the leukocyte surface membrane to form a vacuole or vesicle, follows, with internalization and then fusion of the phagocytic vacuoles with intracellular enzyme-containing granules.

Microbicidal activity of neutrophils combines two interacting functions: degranulation and activation of the respiratory burst. Neutrophils possess a double set of cytoplasmic granules. The primary or azurophilic granules contain lysozyme, acid hydrolases, neutral proteases including cathepsin G and elastase, myeloperoxidase, and basic proteins. Specific granules contain lysozyme, transcobalamin III, apolactoferrin, collagenase, and the C5-cleaving protease. Azurophilic granules fuse mainly with the phagocytic vesicles, pouring their contents into the acidic interior of the vesicles. Specific granules fuse both with phagocytic vesicles and with the plasma membrane, so that their contents are also released outside the neutrophil. These enzymes aid in the digestion of the bacterial cell wall, dissolve connective tissue, degrade cellular debris, or bind specific substances useful to bacterial metabolism such as iron.

The same stimuli that activate phagocytosis and granule release also initiate the respiratory burst by activating a plasma membrane–bound oxidase that catalyzes one-electron reduction of oxygen to superoxide (O_2^-) in the presence of the electron acceptor NADPH. Interaction of O_2^- with H_2O yields hydroxyl radical $OH\cdot$, which is directly bactericidal. In addition, H_2O_2 and Cl^- in the presence of myeloperoxidase form the microbicidal hypochlorite ion OCl^-. These reactions are essential for the killing of catalase-positive microorganisms.

Granulocytes have a short lifespan in the circulation (half-life about 6 hours) and undergo one-way traffic from the bone marrow through the blood into the tissues, where they may live for a few days. In the blood, about 50 per cent of granulocytes normally are marginated along vascular endothelium, remaining in dynamic equilibrium with the circulating neutrophil pool. Epinephrine, stress, or certain steroids shift more granulocytes to the circulating pool.

MONOCYTE STRUCTURE AND FUNCTION

Monocytes represent a second type of circulating and fixed (tissue macrophage) phagocyte of even greater functional versatility than neutrophils. They comprise a much smaller fraction of the leukocytes, about 10 per cent, and are longer-lived. Monocytes contain granules that are not clearly divided into subtypes. The circulating monocytes display slower chemotaxis than do neutrophils and appear later at sites of inflammation. Their major phagocytic role relates to the killing of intracellular microorganisms, both bacterial and parasitic. When monocytes are exposed to lipopolysaccharide or gamma interferon, they become "activated" and display increased motility, metabolic activity, size, and microbicidal potency. The three basic functions of mononuclear phagocytes are secretion, ingestion, and interaction with lymphocytes. Monocytes synthesize more than 50 different protein mediators and enzymes, release interleukins that affect lymphocyte function and cause fever, present antigen to T cells for immune responses, and have very active arachidonic acid metabolism resulting in production of prostaglandins (PGE_2, which regulates bone marrow and immunologic cell proliferation), leukotrienes, and thromboxane. In addition to complement and immunoglobulins, fibronectin also serves as an opsonin for mononuclear phagocytes. The process of pinocytosis permits macrophages to ingest and pro-

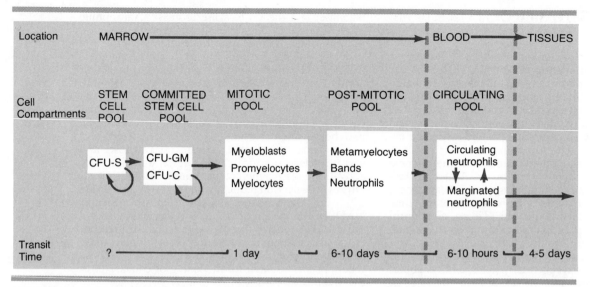

FIGURE 51–1. Neutrophil granulocyte maturation and kinetics.

TABLE 51–1. ACQUIRED ABNORMALITIES OF NEUTROPHIL FUNCTION

1. **Adhesiveness**
   Increased: Bacteremia, hemodialysis (early)
   Decreased: Corticosteroids, epinephrine (demargination), aspirin, alcohol
2. **Chemotaxis**
   Increased: Bacterial infection
   Decreased: Diabetes mellitus, uremia, cirrhosis
   Severe burns
   Hodgkin's disease, leprosy, sarcoid
   Neonates
   Myeloproliferative syndromes
3. **Phagocytosis**
   Decreased: Diabetes mellitus, acute infections
   Myeloproliferative syndromes
   Leukemia

TABLE 51–2. CAUSES OF NEUTROPENIA

Benign familial
Drug-induced
  Anti-inflammatory drugs
  Antibacterial drugs (chloramphenicol, cotrimoxazole)
  Anticonvulsants
  Antithyroid drugs
  Phenothiazines
Cyclical
Disease-related
  Viral infection
  Bacterial sepsis
  Anaphylaxis
  Autoimmune
  Felty's syndrome
  Systemic lupus erythematosus
  Bone marrow failure
  Hypersplenism
  Vitamin B_{12} and folic acid deficiency
  Leukemia

cess large volumes of fluid, including plasma. Activated monocytes are also tumoricidal.

A series of reciprocal interactions between monocytes and lymphocytes is necessary for normal immune function. Monocytes and macrophages activate T cells by presenting antigen; special subpopulations of monocytes subserve this function, especially dendritic and Langerhans (skin) cells. Dendritic cells are a recently identified minor population of monocytic cells with long surface processes that appear to be the antigen-presenting cells of the blood, whereas Langerhans cells have a similar function in the skin. Lymphokines secreted by activated T cells cause accumulation and activation of monocytes. One such lymphokine, interleukin 2, is the T cell growth factor that permits expansion of T cell populations in immune responses. In addition, macrophages stimulate proliferation and differentiation of B lymphocytes via secretion of interleukin 1. Prostaglandin E_2 secreted by monocytes and macrophages, in contrast, downregulates lymphocytic responses.

NEUTROPENIA

The normal white blood cell count varies between 5,000 and 10,000/μl, with 50 to 70 per cent neutrophils. The normal lower limit for neutrophil concentration is approximately 2000/μl for Caucasians and 1500/μl for blacks, the difference resulting from different sizes of marginated pools. Normal bone marrow contains a postmitotic compartment of mature neutrophils sufficient for 7 to 10 days, although under stress, neutrophil transit time in the marrow from early differentiation to the appearance of mature forms in the blood can be as short as five days (Fig. 51–1).

Neutropenia can result from depressed production of leukocytes, increased peripheral destruction, increased pooling in the spleen, or an increased rate of loss into tissues (Tables 51–1 and 51-2). The most common cause of neutropenia is marrow depression caused by drugs or radiation. Idiosyncratic drug reactions, that is, reactions rarely caused by a given drug, may result in sudden marrow suppression (e.g., chlorpromazine) or neutrophil destruction (e.g., amidopyrine); removal of the drug usually results in recovery. The latter situation often involves an antineutrophil antibody or an innocent bystander mechanism, in which drug-antibody complexes attach to the neutrophil surface (cephalosporins).

In *agranulocytosis*, the bone marrow appears normocellular except for the absence of granulocyte precursors; profound neutropenia is present in the blood, and sore throat and fever are common symptoms. Drugs commonly causing this syndrome include antithyroid drugs, phenylbutazone, chlorpromazine, and sulfonamides.

Neutropenia also is frequent in collagen vascular diseases such as systemic lupus erythematosus, and accompanies hypersplenism, as in Felty's syndrome. It is also seen in vitamin B_{12} or folic acid deficiency, acute leukemia, and viral infections including infectious mononucleosis and viral hepatitis, and it is common in alcoholism. Many types of congenital neutropenias and benign familial neutropenias have been described. A rare form is *cyclic neutropenia*, which is familial or sporadic and is characterized by periodic falls in the neutrophil count to near zero; granulocyte precursors are absent from the marrow at such times. Marrow production spontaneously resumes to restore granulocyte counts to normal levels; then the entire cycle repeats. A defective stem cell is postulated and other blood cells may also cycle, but less dramatically. Fever and sepsis may occur during the granulocyte nadirs. A temporary neutropenia or "pseudoneutropenia" can be found early in hemodialysis, when complement activation on the dialyzer membrane induces neutrophil aggregation and temporary sequestration in the lungs.

Evaluation of neutropenia involves a search for underlying disease, examination of the bone marrow, testing for antibodies directed against leukocytes, and elimination of drugs. An absolute neutrophil count of less than 1000/μl is considered life-threatening. Meticulous oral and anal hygiene, stool softener therapy, and immediate evaluation of fever or any sign of infection are required throughout the duration of neu-

TABLE 51–3. CAUSES OF NEUTROPHIL LEUKOCYTOSIS

Bacterial infections (pyogenic)
Inflammation; tissue necrosis
Acute hemolysis or hemorrhage
Corticosteroid therapy
Lithium therapy
Myeloproliferative disease
Metastatic cancer
Familial

tropenia. Rapid initiation of broad-spectrum antibiotics for fever or infection is needed, with attention to the danger of superinfection. Transfusion of neutrophil concentrates has not proved to be of benefit in recent controlled trials, probably because of a combination of dysfunction of neutrophils that occurs during preparation of the cells for transfusion and the rapid half-life of neutrophils following their infusion.

NEUTROPHIL LEUKOCYTOSIS

Neutrophil leukocytosis, or a persistent increase in circulating neutrophil levels above 7500/μl, is frequently observed in bacterial infection, inflammatory diseases, and hemorrhage and in association with malignancy or myeloproliferative disease (Table 51–3). There are also familial leukocytoses, which are benign. Transient leukocytosis can be induced by stress or severe exercise. A leukemoid reaction can usually be distinguished from the high white cell count of myeloproliferative disease or leukemia by the maturity of the leukocytes, an orderly "left shift" or appearance of band forms and a few metamyelocytes, and an elevated leukocyte alkaline phosphatase.

REFERENCES

Gallin JI, Fauci AS (eds): Advances in Host Defense Mechanisms. Vol 1. Phagocytic Cells. New York, Raven Press, 1982.

Jandl JH: Granulocytes. *In* Blood: Textbook of Hematology. Boston, MA, Little, Brown & Co, 1987, pp 441–471.

Williams WJ, Beutler E, Erslev AJ, Lichtman MA (eds): Hematology. 3rd ed. New York, McGraw-Hill Book Co, 1983.

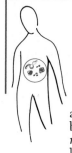

52

HEMATOLOGIC MALIGNANCIES

The hematologic malignancies include diseases that arise in bone marrow and lymph nodes. The primary bone marrow disorders are the *leukemias*, the *"immunoproliferative diseases"* such as multiple myeloma, and the *myeloproliferative syndromes* such as polycythemia vera and myelofibrosis with myeloid metaplasia. Evidence suggests that all of these diseases arise from single cell mutations that develop into malignant clones having a growth advantage over normal cells in the marrow. The evidence has arisen from different avenues. In chronic lymphocytic leukemia, for example, the malignant lymphocytes all express an identical surface immunoglobulin, and in multiple myeloma the malignant plasma cells express the identical cytoplasmic and secreted immunoglobulin. In chronic myelogenous leukemia, all the cells of the myeloid series as well as the erythroid precursors, the megakaryocytes, and the B lymphocytes bear the same marker chromosome, the Philadelphia chromosome. Further evidence for the clonal nature of the hematologic malignancies has come from the study of females who are heterozygous for the X-linked enzyme, glucose-6-phosphate dehydrogenase (G6PD). Because only one X chromosome is active in any single cell (inactivation of a maternal or paternal X chromosome occurring at random), half of all the somatic cells of a female heterozygote carry the gene for one G6PD type (e.g., $G6PD^A$) and the other half carry the gene for the other type (e.g., $G6PD^B$). Figure 52–1 demonstrates a study of G6PD expression in the cells of

A woman with polycythemia vera has two X chromosomes in each cell of her body; by mere chance, one bears the gene for isoenzyme $G6PD^A$ and the other for isoenzyme $G6PD^B$.

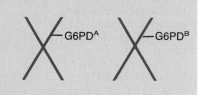

Because of X-chromosome inactivation, each cell expresses only one isoenzyme. For example, 50 per cent of fibroblasts express $G6PD^A$ and 50 per cent express $G6PD^B$.

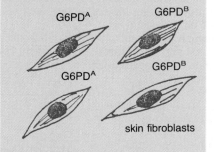

skin fibroblasts

FIGURE 52–1. Polycythemia vera represents a clonal expansion of an abnormal pluripotent stem cell: Analysis using G6PD expression as a marker of clonality.

In contrast to other cell types, all the granulocytes, erythrocytes, platelets, and B lymphocytes express only one G6PD isoenzyme. The finding indicates that the hematopoietic cells of polycythemia vera arise from a single stem cell.

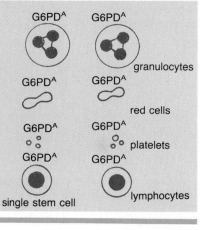

single stem cell

such a woman who developed polycythemia vera. Whereas the skin fibroblasts express either one or the other G6PD isoenzyme, the malignant cells express only one isoenzyme. This finding indicates that the malignant cells arise from a single cell that has expanded into a malignant clone.

THE MYELOPROLIFERATIVE DISORDERS

Four diseases are commonly grouped together as the myeloproliferative disorders: polycythemia vera, myelofibrosis with myeloid metaplasia, essential thrombocythemia, and chronic myelogenous leukemia. All represent clinical conditions that result from uncontrolled expansion of all bone marrow elements. The increased production of erythroid, myeloid, and megakaryocytic lines results from a malignant transformation of a pluripotent stem cell. The increased marrow fibrosis often present in these diseases represents a reaction of normal fibroblasts to growth stimuli provided by the neoplastic cells. Present evidence suggests that the fibroblast growth factor is produced by the bone marrow megakaryocytes that are increased in the myeloproliferative disorders. Chronic myelogenous leukemia will be discussed separately.

The myeloproliferative disorder *polycythemia vera* is a neoplastic disease of a bone marrow stem cell which affects primarily the erythroid line. Hyperplasia of all bone marrow elements is characteristic, but the increase in erythroid precursors with an elevated red cell mass is the most prominent feature. The increased red blood cell production is autonomous; that is, there is no secondary stimulus such as hypoxia or elevated erythropoietin levels driving red cell production. The typical clinical presentation is that of a patient with an elevated hematocrit. The physician must approach all

TABLE 52–1. EVALUATION OF THE PATIENT WITH AN ELEVATED HEMATOCRIT

1. History
     Family history? Social history (e.g. smoking)?
2. Physical examination
     Splenomegaly? Cardiac or pulmonary disease?
3. Chromium 51 red blood cell mass

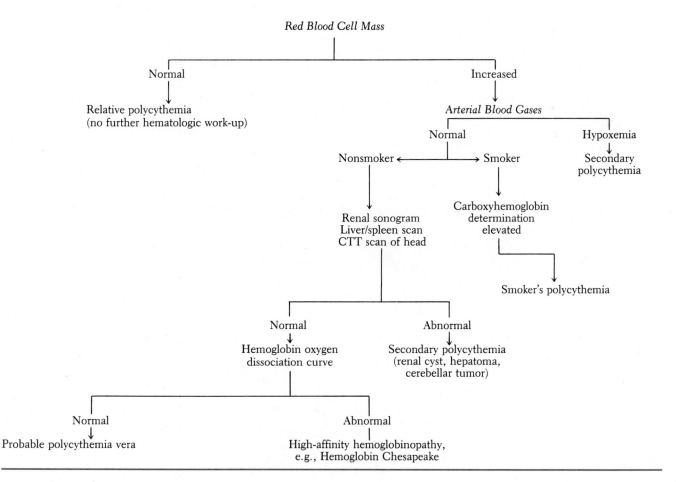

patients with elevated hematocrits in a systematic way (Table 52–1) to decide first whether the high hematocrit actually represents an increased red cell mass and, if so, whether the increased red cell mass is secondary to a stimulus external to the bone marrow or whether it represents true polycythemia, polycythemia vera.

A hematocrit above 54 per cent for men or 50 per cent for women should lead the physician to question whether the patient has polycythemia. The hematocrit or per cent packed red cell volume reflects the ratio of red cells to plasma. Thus, the hematocrit may be elevated either if there is truly an excess of red cells or if there is decreased plasma volume, as in dehydration. The best available direct measurement of red cell mass is the ^{51}Cr-labelled red cell mass. This test will distinguish between absolute polycythemia, in which the red cell mass is truly expanded, and "relative" polycythemia, in which the red cell mass is normal but the plasma volume is contracted (Fig. 52–2).

Relative polycythemia (also called spurious, stress, or Gaisbock's polycythemia) is a chronic condition that typically affects obese, hypertensive, tense men who present with hematocrit values between 55 and 60 per cent. The red cell mass is normal; the plasma volume is contracted for unknown reasons. The pathophysiology of relative polycythemia is not well understood. Because the red cell mass is normal, aggressive phlebotomy is not indicated.

As noted, an elevated red cell mass (men > 36 ml/kg; women > 32 ml/kg) defines *absolute polycythemia*.

Absolute polycythemia may be primary, as in the autonomous increase in red cell production that occurs in polycythemia vera, or it may be secondary to a physiological mechanism driving red cell production to a higher than normal level. The most common cause for secondary polycythemia is decreased tissue oxygen delivery, usually due to decreased arterial oxygen saturation, as, for example, in chronic obstructive pulmonary disease. In this setting, the tissue hypoxia causes an increase in renal erythropoietin production. The erythropoietin in turn stimulates the bone marrow erythroid precursors and increases the number of red cells produced in order to increase tissue oxygen delivery. The increase in red cell mass may be beneficial to the hypoxic tissue; however, the associated increase in total blood viscosity and the marked increase in total blood volume may be clinically detrimental. For example, patients with cyanotic congenital heart disease with a hematocrit of 75 per cent require repeated phlebotomy to decrease the total blood volume and whole blood viscosity. The consequences of the marked hyperviscosity that accompanies a hematocrit greater than 60 per cent include decreased cerebral blood flow, decreased cardiac output, and a tendency to thrombosis.

The approach to the patient with absolute polycythemia should follow a logical pathway to determine whether the patient has secondary or primary polycythemia, polycythemia vera. The history and physical examination may provide the answer. A wheezing, cyanotic, barrel-chested man with severe chronic obstructive pulmonary disease can be distinguished quickly from the plethoric patient with splenomegaly who most likely has typical polycythemia vera. Simple laboratory data will complete the analysis in the majority of patients. White blood count and platelet count are elevated in most patients with polycythemia vera; they are normal in most patients with secondary polycythemia. A low arterial oxygen saturation will indicate that the polycythemia is a compensatory mechanism for hypoxemia. Thus, the history, physical examination, and screening laboratory data should distinguish between primary and secondary polycythemia. Sometimes, however, the cause of the secondary polycythemia may not be obvious and requires further testing for rare causes; these include abnormal hemoglobins with increased oxygen affinity, erythropoietin-secreting renal cysts, cerebellar hemangioblastoma, and hepatocellular carcinoma (Table 52–1).

In polycythemia vera, normal control of bone marrow cell production is lost. Although the erythroid line is primarily affected, resulting in an elevated red cell mass, increased granulocyte and platelet production are frequently found as well. Polycythemia vera shares some clinical features with the other myeloproliferative disorders: myelofibrosis with myeloid metaplasia, essential thrombocythemia, and chronic myelogenous leukemia. In all these diseases, there is abnormal (although variable) expansion of all the bone marrow elements: the myeloid precursors, the megakaryocytes, the erythroid precursors, and the fibroblasts of the bone marrow.

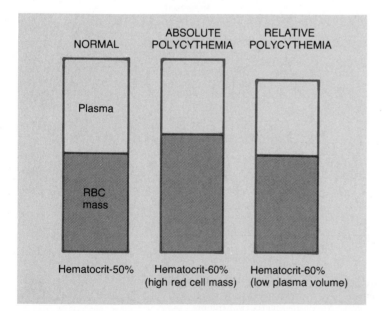

FIGURE 52–2. The relative volume of plasma to red cell mass in normal and polycythemic patients. In a normal man, the red cell mass represents approximately 50 per cent of the total blood volume and the hematocrit is 50 per cent. In a patient with absolute polycythemia, the plasma volume is normal and the red cell mass is elevated, resulting in a hematocrit of 60 per cent. In relative polycythemia, the plasma volume is contracted and the red cell mass is normal; this results in an elevated hematocrit.

32171

The cause of polycythemia vera is not known. The disorder occurs sporadically in both sexes, with a mean age of presentation of about 60 years. Some affected patients are asymptomatic, while others can suffer symptoms due to hypervolemia, hyperviscosity, or platelet dysfunction.

The combination of intravascular hyperviscosity due to a high red cell mass and a high platelet count with functionally abnormal platelets puts patients with polycythemia vera at high risk for stroke, myocardial infarction, and venous thromboembolism.

The metabolic consequences of increased cell turnover also can cause symptoms such as gout or itching (Table 52–2).

The diagnosis of polycythemia vera may be readily apparent or may require extensive laboratory testing to exclude secondary polycythemia (see Table 52–1). Clinical criteria diagnostically useful for the disease are outlined in Table 52–3. If a full evaluation does not convince the physician that a patient has polycythemia vera, two other laboratory tests may be helpful when available: a serum erythropoietin level (which should be zero in polycythemia vera) and an assay of bone marrow erythroid colony growth (which should demonstrate growth of erythroid colonies independent of added erythropoietin in polycythemia vera).

Polycythemia vera, appropriately treated, is compatible with many years of active life. The treatment involves two steps: lowering the hematocrit by phlebotomy and, if necessary, decreasing bone marrow red cell and platelet production by chemotherapy or radioactive phosphorus. Initially, phlebotomy serves to lower the hematocrit, which optimally should be brought to 45 per cent or less. With repeated phlebotomies, bone marrow iron stores (which may be low at the time of diagnosis in polycythemia vera) are further depleted, and red cell production is retarded. In response to repeated phlebotomy, however, platelet production may be increased by as yet incompletely understood mechanisms. If the platelets increase to more than $10^6/\mu l$, the risk of thrombosis or hemorrhage increases. Accordingly, treatment with chemotherapy or radioactive phosphorus may be indicated in this setting. Use of antiplatelet drugs such as aspirin has not proved beneficial in preventing thrombosis in patients with polycythemia vera and may promote hemorrhage. In patients over age 50 the risk of thrombosis is high enough, however, to warrant myelosuppressive therapy with hydroxyurea to control platelet counts.

With appropriate therapy, the median survival for patients with polycythemia vera is at least 10 years. Thrombosis is a major cause of death. Acute leukemia occurs in a small percentage. This tendency to malignant transformation is increased if the patient receives an alkylating agent or radioactive phosphorus for treatment. The current choice of chemotherapy in polycythemia vera is the antimetabolite hydroxyurea, which so far has not been associated with an increased incidence of acute leukemia. Late in the course of polycythemia vera, the "spent" phase may occur. This is marked by increasing bone marrow fibrosis with de-

TABLE 52–2. CLINICAL MANIFESTATIONS OF POLYCYTHEMIA VERA

Hyperviscosity and/or **hypervolemia** may lead to:
1. Decreased cerebral blood flow with:
   a. Tinnitus
   b. Lightheadedness
   c. Stroke (rarely)
2. Congestive heart failure
3. Thrombosis

Platelet dysfunction may lead to:
1. Thrombosis due to:
   a. Thrombocytosis
   b. Intrinsically abnormal platelets (e.g., prolonged bleeding time, absent aggregation to epinephrine, abnormal prostaglandin metabolism, increased Fc receptor expression)
2. Hemorrhage:
   a. Upper gastrointestinal bleeding may occur.
   b. Aspirin aggravates bleeding tendency.
3. Microvascular thrombosis may produce painful toes and fingers.

Increased cell turnover can lead to:
1. Gout (due to hyperuricemia)
2. Itching (due to increased histamine production from basophils)

creased red cell production and, commonly, the development of anemia and marked splenomegaly. At this stage of the disease, the patient's clinical picture resembles that of myelofibrosis with myeloid metaplasia.

Myelofibrosis with myeloid metaplasia (MMM) (agnogenic myeloid metaplasia) is a myeloproliferative disorder in which, as in the other myeloproliferative disorders, there is expansion of all bone marrow elements due to malignant transformation of a pluripotent stem cell. Bone marrow fibrosis is a reaction to this event and may progress to cause almost complete obliteration of normal marrow space. Extramedullary hematopoiesis in the liver and spleen is a cardinal feature of the disease. The extramedullary hematopoiesis due either to reactivation of a fetal site of hematopoiesis or to new migration of bone marrow stem cells may produce marked hepatosplenomegaly.

The clinical presentation of MMM may be subtle,

TABLE 52–3. CRITERIA FOR THE DIAGNOSIS OF POLYCYTHEMIA VERA

A1—Elevated red cell mass
    Male: >36 ml/kg
    Female: >32 ml/kg
A2—Normal arterial O_2 saturation (>92%)
A3—Splenomegaly

B1–Thrombocytosis: Platelet count >400,000/μl
B2—Leukocytosis: White cell count >12,000/μl
B3—Elevated leukocyte alkaline phosphatase (LAP): >100
B4—Elevated serum B_{12}: >900 pg/ml (due to elevated transcobalamin)

Diagnosis requires:
A1 + A2 + A3
or
A1 + A2 and any two from B category

(Polycythemia Vera Study Group, 1975)

TABLE 52–4. DIFFERENTIAL DIAGNOSIS OF AN ELEVATED WHITE BLOOD COUNT

	MYELOFIBROSIS WITH MYELOID METAPLASIA	CHRONIC MYELOGENOUS LEUKEMIA	LEUKEMOID REACTION
WBC	Usually <100,000/μl with early myeloid forms	May be >100,000/μl with early myeloid forms	Rarely >100,000/μl; promyelocytes or blasts are rare.
RBC morphology	Nucleated RBC and teardrop cells	Occasional nucleated RBC	Usually normal
Leukocyte alkaline phosphatase (LAP score)	Normal or high	Low (<20)	High
Bone marrow	Usually "dry tap" with fibrosis	Panhypercellular	Myeloid hyperplasia
Philadelphia chromosome	Absent	Present (about 90% of cases)	Absent

consisting of no more than nucleated red blood cells detected in a peripheral blood smear. Such cells are a hallmark of extramedullary hematopoiesis. Anemia with teardrop forms and nucleated red cells on peripheral smear, leukocytosis with a shift to the left, and splenomegaly provide additional suggestive features. The diagnosis is strengthened by bone marrow aspiration (usually a "dry tap") and confirmed by biopsy showing fibrosis. The differential diagnosis of MMM includes a leukemoid reaction or chronic myelogenous leukemia as outlined in Table 52–4.

The course of MMM is one of slowly progressive splenomegaly, hepatomegaly, and anemia with thrombocytopenia. The spleen may become so massive that the patient can barely eat or sit comfortably. Portal hypertension due to increased splenic blood flow may become a major clinical problem late in the course of the disease. Unfortunately no treatment alters the natural history of MMM. Supportive care includes treatment with folic acid and iron supplementation when indicated, but most patients eventually require transfusion to counteract anemia. Androgens may decrease the transfusion requirement, at least temporarily. Splenectomy is used cautiously for those selected patients in whom the enlarged organ produces unbearable pressure symptoms, pain, or poor nutrition. The procedure carries a substantial morbidity and mortality. Furthermore, following splenectomy, the liver may enlarge rapidly. Patients may live five or even ten years after the diagnosis of MMM is made, but most suffer serious morbidity during this time.

Essential thrombocythemia is a myeloproliferative

disorder characterized by platelet counts consistently elevated over 1 million/μl. The differential diagnosis between essential thrombocythemia and benign reactive thrombocytosis is outlined in Table 52–5. The major presenting symptom of this disease is hemorrhage, although thrombotic events also may occur. Many patients, particularly young ones, remain totally asymptomatic. The optimum therapy is not known. Because the natural history may include a long lifespan, aggressive therapy with alkylating agents usually is not indicated. Occasionally, a patient will present with very painful or even gangrenous fingers and toes due to microvascular thrombosis. Such patients respond well to antiplatelet drugs (e.g., aspirin) and/or to decreasing the platelet count with a cytotoxic drug such as hydroxyurea. Acute management with plateletpheresis is rarely indicated.

THE LEUKEMIAS

Leukemia is a condition in which the bone marrow is replaced by a malignant clone of lymphocytic or granulocytic cells. The course of the disease may be chronic or explosive; if left untreated, all leukemias are fatal. Lymphomas, by contrast, are tumors arising from cells of the lymphatic system. The bone marrow may be involved by lymphoma cells, but this is rarely the primary site of a lymphoma.

Chronic Leukemias

Chronic myelogenous leukemia (CML) is often classified as a myeloproliferative disease as well as a leu-

TABLE 52–5. DIFFERENTIAL DIAGNOSIS OF AN ELEVATED PLATELET COUNT

	ESSENTIAL THROMBOCYTHEMIA	BENIGN REACTIVE THROMBOCYTOSIS
Platelet number	>1 $\times$ 10^6/μl; may have bizarre morphology	Usually >4 $\times$ 10^5–1 $\times$ 10^6/μl; may have large platelets
Platelet function	Prolonged bleeding time may be present; absent aggregation response to epinephrine	Normal
Spleen	Usually palpable	Normal
Course	Platelets remain elevated without treatment	Platelets return to normal after inciting event is past (e.g., splenectomy, GI bleeding, infection)
Complications	Hemorrhagic events more common than thrombosis	Rare

kemia, since it shares the major feature of the myeloproliferative diseases: uncontrolled expansion of all marrow elements. All marrow cell lines in CML express a marker chromosome, the Philadelphia chromosome, pointing to a mutation in a pluripotent stem cell as the initiating event. The Philadelphia chromosome represents a reciprocal translocation of part of the long arm of chromosome 22 to chromosome 9. Recent work suggests an association of the Philadelphia chromosome with activation of cellular oncogenes (see Chapter 55).

Although CML is usually a disease of adults, it sometimes affects children as well. The average age at onset is between 40 and 50 years. The disorder is not familial, and most patients have no history of excess exposure to carcinogenic chemicals or increased radioactivity. Nonetheless, the incidence of CML did increase markedly seven years after the atomic bomb explosion in Japan in 1945.

The typical patient with CML presents with few symptoms, and the disease may be discovered on routine blood count. Leukocytosis with early myeloid precursors in the peripheral blood and splenomegaly are almost always present at the time of diagnosis. Thrombocytosis is also common. Table 52–4 outlines the differential diagnosis between CML, MMM, and a leukemoid reaction. Initially, affected patients are managed easily with periodic oral chemotherapy (alkylating agents or hydroxyurea) to normalize the blood count and reduce splenomegaly. This chronic phase of CML lasts three to five years. Subsequently, the course of the disease accelerates. The white count and spleen size become more difficult to control. Anemia and, eventually, thrombocytopenia develop, and fever and increasing weakness may appear. Eventually, white cell maturation ceases, so that the peripheral blood contains increasing numbers of promyelocytes and myeloblasts. This is termed the "blast phase," and it heralds death within three to six months.

The events that transform CML from the chronic to the blast phase are not understood. Hyperdiploidy or other chromosome abnormalities in addition to the Philadelphia chromosome often develop. In approximately 20 per cent of blast crises, the blast cells bear markers of lymphoid cell origin such as the enzyme terminal deoxynucleotidyl transferase (Tdt). This finding is important in therapeutic management, since drugs that are effective in lymphoid malignancies (e.g., vincristine and prednisone) may be useful in a lymphoid type (Tdt-positive) of blast crisis. Overall, however, the treatment of blast crisis is unsatisfactory, and any remissions are short.

Preliminary reports that the use of recombinant human alpha interferon in the chronic phase of CML may induce hematologic remission and suppress the Philadelphia chromosome point to new therapeutic strategies in this disease. At present, allogeneic bone marrow transplantation in highly selected patients with CML offers the only chance of producing long-term disease-free survival (and possibly cure).

Chronic lymphocytic leukemia (CLL) was described by Dr. William Dameshek as an "accumulative disease of immunologically incompetent lymphocytes," a concise definition that describes the majority of patients. CLL is a disease of older persons, and fewer than 10 per cent of cases are patients under 50 years old. Men develop CLL twice as often as women and, as in all forms of leukemia, the disorder is more common in whites than blacks.

The diagnosis of CLL is based on an absolute and sustained lymphocytosis in the peripheral blood of no less than 15,000 cells/μl. The bone marrow is hypercellular, and more than 40 per cent of the cells are lymphocytes. The lymphocytes in the peripheral blood and marrow are of the small, well-differentiated type. Slowly enlarging lymph nodes and gradual enlargement of the liver and spleen due to the accumulation of neoplastic lymphocytes may occur early or late in the course of the disease. The immunological incompetence of the expanding lymphocyte population expresses itself in hypogammaglobulinemia with predisposition to infections and in the emergence of such autoimmune phenomena as the production of antibodies against host red blood cells, causing Coombs' positive hemolytic anemia. Table 52–6 outlines the immune disorders in CLL.

Lymphocytes in chronic lymphocytic leukemia usually consist of a clonal proliferation of B lymphocytes (Fig. 52–3). The malignant cells all display immunoglobulin molecules on their plasma membranes bearing the same idiotype and the same single light chain type. The most common surface immunoglobulins represented are IgM and IgD. The finding of two heavy chain classes does not preclude the concept of monoclonality, as the IgD and IgM have the same idiotype specificity and presumably reflect an early, frozen stage of differentiation of normal B lymphocytes. CLL lymphocytes also express the Ia antigen, the receptor for C3, and the receptor for the Fc portion of immunoglobulin.

About 1 per cent of patients with CLL demonstrate predominantly T lymphocytes in their peripheral blood. These lymphocytes form rosettes with sheep red blood cells and do not bear surface immunoglobulin. The T cell form of CLL appears to carry a poorer prognosis than the B cell type. Skin involvement is

TABLE 52–6. IMMUNE DISORDERS IN CLL

Autoantibody Production
  Autoimmune hemolytic anemia
    Coombs' test positive in 20 to 30% of patients with CLL
    Hemolysis rare
    Usually responds to corticosteroids
  Autoimmune thrombocytopenic purpura
    Thrombocytopenia may also be due to bone marrow replacement by CLL or to splenic sequestration.
    Usually responds to corticosteroids
Disorder of Immunoglobulin Synthesis
  Monoclonal gammopathy
    Monoclonal spike present in 10% of patients with CLL—IgG or IgM.
    Usually not of clinical importance
  Hypogammaglobulinemia
    Present in majority of cases, particularly stages III and IV
    Results in increased susceptibility to bacterial infection

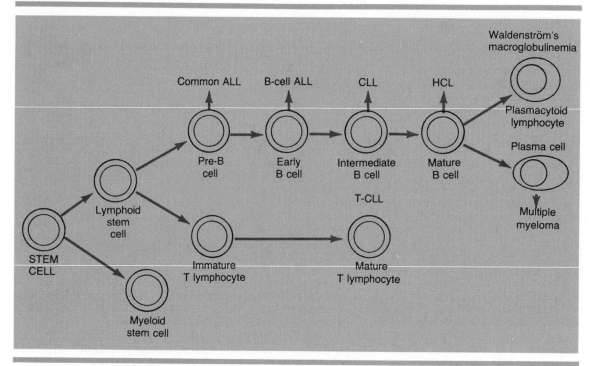

FIGURE 52–3. Lymphocyte development and the stages at which maturation arrest will result in various immunological subtypes of lymphoid leukemia or in an "immunoproliferative" malignancy. B cell = bursa or bone-marrow derived lymphocyte; T cell = thymus-derived lymphocyte; ALL = acute lymphoblastic leukemia; CLL = chronic lymphocytic leukemia; HCL = hairy cell leukemia. (Adapted from Markowitz MJ, Mouradian J, Moore A: Acute and chronic lymphocytic leukemia. *In* Molander DW (ed): Disease of the Lymphatic System. New York, Springer-Verlag, 1984.)

seen frequently in these patients, and standard forms of therapy for CLL are less effective.

The etiology of CLL is unknown. Despite occasional familial clusterings of CLL, no firm genetic basis for the disease has been found, nor does exposure to radiation or other potentially mutagenic agents such as alkylating agents appear to predispose. Chromosome abnormalities (particularly involving chromosomes 12 and 14) have been described in about half of patients with CLL. To date, no convincing data support a viral etiology.

A major contribution to understanding the natural history of CLL is the clinical staging system devised by Rai et al, which identifies prognosis according to the state of illness at the time of first diagnosis (Table 52–7). The stages of the disease reflect the concept of the "accumulative" nature of CLL. Stage 0 is lymphocytosis alone. Stages I and II reflect the development of increasing tumor mass (nodes, liver, or spleen), while the anemia and thrombocytopenia of stages III and IV indicate bone marrow replacement interfering with normal hematopoiesis, and splenomegaly causing decreased red blood cell and platelet survival. Most patients are in stage 0, I, or II at the time of diagnosis.

Figure 52–4 plots the median duration of survival from the time of diagnosis of 125 patients studied by Rai et al. As can be seen, although the median survival was 71 months, the duration depended considerably on the clinical stage. Although palliative treatment exists, there is no cure for CLL. Treatment is generally withheld in the asymptomatic stage. When symptoms such as enlarging lymph nodes, splenomegaly, progressive anemia, and/or thrombocytopenia occur, alkylating agents (e.g., chlorambucil) and prednisone prove beneficial. Radiotherapy to the spleen or to areas of bulky adenopathy may be useful.

Unlike CML, there is no predictable blast phase in CLL. However, the disease sometimes can transform into a clinically more malignant lymphocytic neoplasm called diffuse histiocytic lymphoma ("Richter's syndrome"). Prolymphocytic leukemia, a more ag-

TABLE 52–7. CRITERIA FOR CLINICAL STAGING OF CLL (RAI)

Stage 0:	Lymphocytosis alone >15,000/μl in peripheral blood >40% marrow lymphocytosis
Stage I:	Lymphocytosis and enlarged nodes
Stage II:	Lymphocytosis and splenomegaly, hepatomegaly, or both
Stage III:	Lymphocytosis and anemia: hemoglobin <11 gm/dl
Stage IV:	Lymphocytosis and thrombocytopenia: platelets <100,000/μl

gressive form of CLL, may also arise in a patient with CLL.

Hairy cell leukemia (HCL) (also called leukemic reticuloendotheliosis) is a neoplastic disorder characterized by "hairy cells" in the peripheral smear and bone marrow. Hairy cells look like lymphocytes with fine cytoplasmic projections. Unlike typical B cells, they are capable of phagocytosis. The cells stain positive for tartrate-resistant acid phosphatase (TRAP).

HCL is more common in men than women and usually presents as a slowly developing pancytopenia with splenomegaly. Splenectomy may be useful if the spleen enlarges painfully or severe cytopenia develops. Chemotherapy has not helped most patients with hairy cell leukemia. Most patients with HCL, however, will respond to alpha interferon with improvement in blood counts. Additionally, recent studies with an investigational agent, 2'-deoxycoformycin, have shown that a complete hematologic remission is possible in some patients with HCL. The median survival for patients with hairy cell leukemia is three to five years; some patients live many years after diagnosis with little treatment.

Acute Leukemias

In acute leukemias immature hematopoietic cells proliferate without differentiation into normal mature blood cells. The proliferating cells, whether myeloblasts or lymphoblasts, do not allow the normal production of erythrocytes, granulocytes, and platelets to take place. This leads to the major clinical complications of the disease: anemia, susceptibility to infection, and bleeding.

In most cases of acute leukemia, one finds no recognizable predisposing condition or event. In a few circumstances, however, an association with a possible leukemogenic agent(s) has been identified. Known agents associated with the development of acute leukemia include radiation, viruses, genetic predisposition, and chemicals (Table 52–8). How these agents interact with normal marrow stem cells so as to produce a malignant clone that lacks the ability to differentiate is not known.

Acute leukemias are divided into two broad categories: *acute lymphoblastic leukemia* (ALL) and *acute myeloblastic leukemia* (AML). ALL is primarily a disease of children, AML primarily of adults. Approximately 20 per cent of adult leukemias, however, are of the lymphoblastic type. Because the natural history and the treatment of these two types of leukemia differ, it is important to distinguish between them. The major distinction lies in bone marrow morphology; histochemical stains and surface and cytoplasmic markers are also useful (Table 52–9). Chromosome changes in acute leukemia reveal some correlation with cell type. For example, the chromosome rearrangement t(15;17) is found in acute promyelocytic leukemia. There is a subgroup of patients with atypical ALL whose cells demonstrate the Philadelphia chromosome.

Because of heterogeneity within the two broad categories of acute leukemia, a French, American, and

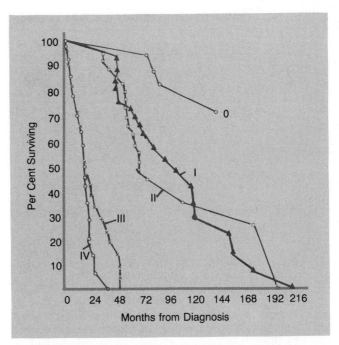

FIGURE 52–4. Chronic lymphocytic leukemia: Median survival from time of diagnosis of 125 patients staged by the Rai criteria. (Adapted from Rai KR, Sawitsky A, Cronkite EP, et al: Clinical staging of chronic lymphocytic leukemia. Blood 46:219, 1975.)

British (FAB) group developed a subdividing classification that has proved useful in studying the course and therapy of the acute leukemias (Table 52–10). Among the myeloblastic leukemias the morphologic subtypes possess relatively distinctive clinical correlation. For example, acute promyelocytic leukemia (M_3) is associated with disseminated intravascular coagulation (DIC); the prominent cytoplasmic granules in the promyelocytes release enzymes that stimulate the coagulation cascade and promote intravascular coagulation. Acute monocytic leukemia (M_5) is associated with skin and gum infiltration with leukemic cells. Among lymphoblastic leukemias, the L_1 subtype is found predominantly in children and the L_2 subtype

TABLE 52–8. EXAMPLES OF AGENTS ASSOCIATED WITH THE DEVELOPMENT OF ACUTE LEUKEMIA

AGENT	EXAMPLE
Ionizing radiation	Incidence of leukemia increased in persons exposed to atomic bombings in Japan, 1945.
Viruses	A T cell leukemia that clusters in Southern Japan and Caribbean is associated with a human type C retrovirus (HTLV).
Genetic predisposition	An identical twin of a young child with acute leukemia has a 20% chance of developing the disease.
Chemicals	Alkylating agents: Chlorambucil, a treatment for polycythemia vera, leads to increased development of acute leukemia.

TABLE 52–9. LABORATORY AIDS TO DISTINGUISH BETWEEN AML AND ALL

	AML	ALL
1. Morphology of leukemic blasts	Granules in cytoplasm; Auer rods* may be present	Agranular, basophilic cytoplasm
	Multiple nucleoli	Regular, folded nucleus with one prominent nucleolus
	FAB (see Table 52–10) subclassification, M_1–M_7	FAB subclassification, L_1–L_3
2. Histochemistry	Myeloperoxidase positive	Myeloperoxidase negative; PAS positive
3. Cytoplasmic markers	—	Terminal deoxynucleotidyl transferase (TDT) positive
4. Surface markers (% of cases)	—	B cell markers (5%)
		T cell markers (15–20%)
		CALLA† (50–65% cases)

* Auer rods are a linear coalescence of cytoplasmic granules that stain pink with Wright's stain.
† CALLA = Common acute lymphoblastic leukemia antigen.

is found primarily in adults. The L_3 subtype is uncommon and carries a poor prognosis.

The diagnosis of acute leukemia is rarely difficult. The patient is usually acutely ill and presents with symptoms that indicate abnormal bone marrow function: infection due to granulocytopenia, bleeding due to thrombocytopenia, and/or anemia due to lack of erythroid maturation. Bone pain due to the expanded leukemic marrow may be present. In ALL, lymphadenopathy and splenomegaly are common. The total white blood count usually is elevated, sometimes above 100,000/µl, but can be normal or even low (<3000/µl). The blood smear is almost always abnormal, showing predominantly blast cells with only a few normal mature leukocytes present. The hemoglobin and platelet count are almost always depressed. The blood uric acid is usually elevated due to the increased white cell turnover; clinical gout is rare but renal damage due to the hyperuricemia may occur. A bone marrow aspirate and biopsy make the diagnosis. The marrow is almost always hypercellular or "packed" with sheets of monotonous undifferentiated cells that replace the normal marrow elements.

The diagnosis of acute leukemia represents a medical emergency. The initial hours or days after diagnosis should be spent stabilizing the patient and pre-

TABLE 52–10. FRENCH-AMERICAN-BRITISH (FAB) CLASSIFICATION OF ACUTE LEUKEMIA

Acute Myelocytic Leukemia
M_1—Acute myelocytic leukemia without differentiation
M_2—Acute myelocytic leukemia with differentiation (predominantly myeloblasts and promyelocytes)
M_3—Acute promyelocytic leukemia
M_4—Acute myelomonocytic leukemia
M_5—Acute monocytic leukemia
M_6—Erythroleukemia
M_7—Megakaryocytic leukemia
Acute Lymphocytic Leukemia
L_1—Predominantly "small" cells (twice the size of normal lymphocyte), homogeneous population
L_2—Larger than L_1, more heterogeneous population
L_3—"Burkitt-like" large cells, vacuolated abundant cytoplasm

paring him for treatment. If the white blood count is greater than 100,000/µl, the patient is at high risk for cerebral hemorrhage caused by leukostasis, that is, obstruction of and damage to blood vessels plugged with rigid blasts. In this setting, immediate steps should be taken to reduce the white count by initiating chemotherapy, if possible, or performing leukapheresis. Allopurinol, a xanthine oxidase inhibitor, is given concurrently to decrease the uric acid formation that results when treatment begins to destroy leukocytes. Antibiotics may be needed to treat infections, which can be life-threatening when patients have few or no mature granulocytes. Transfusion with red cells to maintain adequate blood hemoglobin levels and/or platelets to prevent hemorrhage is usually required. Acute leukemia is one of the most dreaded diagnoses that a patient can receive. The initial management must include enough time spent with the patient and his family to reassure them and to explain the treatment and support programs.

The specific treatment of acute leukemia consists primarily of chemotherapy; radiotherapy sometimes may be used as an adjunct. The total leukemic cell burden is estimated to be from 10^{11} to 10^{12} cells at clinical presentation. Chemotherapeutic drugs follow first-order kinetics. This means that the drugs kill a constant percentage of cells (e.g., 99 per cent) with each administration. A clinically complete remission with disappearance of all detectable leukemia in the blood and bone marrow may mean a reduction in tumor burden from 10^{12} to 10^9 cells. A similar amount of treatment is needed to reduce the number of cells from 10^9 to 10^7. Thus, the eradication of the last leukemia cell by chemotherapy becomes almost an impossible task.

Chemotherapeutic drugs are administered with the goal of stopping cells from proliferating. The drugs are targeted against different phases of the cell cycle, with specific programs designed to follow the kinetics of the cell cycle. An example of a treatment program for acute lymphoblastic leukemia is outlined in Table 52–11. Similar programs are used to treat AML, cytosine arabinoside and daunorubicin being the agents of choice.

TABLE 52–11. A TYPICAL PROGRAM FOR TREATMENT OF ACUTE LYMPHOBLASTIC LEUKEMIA

PHASE	PURPOSE	TREATMENT
Induction of complete remission	To eradicate all detectable leukemia cells	Vincristine, prednisone, daunorubicin, L-asparaginase
Central nervous system prophylaxis	To treat a potential "sanctuary" of leukemia	Intrathecal methotrexate (? cranial radiotherapy)
Intensification or consolidation during remission	To decrease further the leukemic burden	Chemotherapy similar to induction
Maintenance of remission	Continual suppression of the leukemic clone	Methotrexate, 6-mercaptopurine, vincristine, and prednisone

Cure of acute leukemia with rigorous chemotherapy programs and meticulous supportive care is sometimes possible, although the encouraging results achieved in children with ALL (i.e., over 60 per cent alive in complete remission and probably cured at five years) have not been reproduced in adults. About 30 per cent of adults with ALL may obtain a long-term remission. The percentage is considerably smaller in AML, with only 10 to 20 per cent surviving five years in remission, although 60 to 70 per cent of patients achieve a first remission averaging one year in duration.

Bone marrow transplantation from a related HLA-matched donor is being investigated as a treatment for patients with acute leukemia. Patients under age 30 who achieve an initial complete remission with chemotherapy can be considered possible candidates for this experimental procedure if they have a suitable donor. The complications of bone marrow transplantation are substantial, however, and include acute and/or chronic graft-versus-host disease, interstitial pneumonias, and the infections and hemorrhagic complications expected during an initial period of bone marrow aplasia. Late recurrence of the leukemia is still a major concern and is believed to represent inadequate eradication of the leukemic clone by the initial cytotoxic treatment. Since in one case, however, post-transplant recurrence in a male patient involved a female's donor cells, it appears possible that the recipient passed a transmittable agent to the new cell line.

Other innovative approaches to the cure of acute leukemias include the use of monoclonal antibodies directed to leukemia-associated cell surface antigen. The technology of this approach is progressing rapidly and may be incorporated into future treatment programs in which autologous bone marrow transplantation during remission may become more widely utilized in combination with purging of leukemia residual cells by monoclonal antibody treatment.

MYELODYSPLASTIC SYNDROMES

In contrast to the explosive nature of acute leukemia, the myelodysplastic syndromes are characterized by the slow development of an anemia refractory to standard therapy. Affected patients are usually elderly; however, in recent years an increasing number of younger patients have developed myelodysplastic syndromes following prior treatment with radiotherapy, combination chemotherapy, or both, for another neoplasm such as Hodgkin's disease or ovarian carcinoma. Typically, the patient presents with the insidious onset of increasing fatigability and decreasing exercise tolerance; often the patient ascribes the symptoms to "growing old." Physical examination may reveal pallor, and laboratory examination shows an anemia that may be profound. The anemia is typically macrocytic, with an MCV of 100 to 110 μ^3; the peripheral smear may show a dimorphic erythrocyte population, and the patients may also have leukopenia with or without thrombocytopenia. The bone marrow is hypercellular, with increased iron stores and morphologically abnormal erythroid precursors (dyserythropoiesis) as well

TABLE 52–12. CLASSIFICATION OF THE MYELODYSPLASTIC SYNDROMES

DIAGNOSIS (RELATIVE INCIDENCE)	PATIENT CHARACTERISTICS	PERIPHERAL BLOOD	BONE MARROW
Refractory anemia (56%)	Elderly patient; anemia	May have abnormal red cell morphology	<5% blasts
Refractory anemia with ringed sideroblasts (21%)	Elderly; anemia	May have dimorphic picture (microcytic/hypochromic and macrocytic)	Hypercellular; iron stain shows iron in a ring around red cell nuclei.
Refractory anemia with excess blasts (10%)	May have pancytopenia	<5% blasts	5–20% blasts
Chronic myelomonocytic leukemia (11%)	Similar to above	Absolute monocytosis <5% blasts	5–20% blasts
Refractory anemia in transformation (1%)	Any age; symptoms of brief duration	>5% blasts	20–30% blasts

TABLE 52–13. COMMON CAUSES OF LYMPHADENOPATHY

Infection
  Bacterial: Localized infection with regional adenopathy (e.g., streptococcal pharyngitis, foot ulcer with inguinal adenopathy)
  Viral: Infectious mononucleosis, cytomegalovirus, cat scratch fever
  Parasite: Toxoplasmosis
  Spirochete: Syphilis
  Mycobacterial: Tuberculosis, *Mycobacterium avium* (in immunosuppressed patients)
  Fungal: Actinomycosis, cryptococcosis (in immunosuppressed patients)
Drug Reaction
  Serum sickness
  Phenytoin (may cause "pseudolymphoma")
Malignancy
  ·Solid tumors—metastatic patterns:
    Cervical adenopathy: head and neck cancer
    Supraclavicular adenopathy: gastrointestinal tumors
    Axillary adenopathy: breast cancer
    Inguinal adenopathy: carcinoma of the anus
  Lymphoma
Miscellaneous
  Sarcoidosis
  Generalized lymphadenopathy in homosexual men (AIDS-related complex)

as an increased percentage of early myeloid cells. This syndrome has been called "refractory anemia" or "preleukemia" in the past. Because the initial presentation and the course are variable, the condition is now referred to as the myelodysplastic syndrome and further defined according to a classification proposed by the FAB co-operative group mentioned above. Table 52–12 outlines the major clinical features and relative incidence of the five types of myelodysplastic syndromes. For refractory anemia (with or without ringed sideroblasts), the median survival time is approximately three to four years. The other three categories (refractory anemia with excess blasts, chronic myelomonocytic leukemia, and refractory anemia in transformation) carry a survival of one to two years or less. The risk of developing acute leukemia increases with the number of blasts in the bone marrow at presentation; thus, about 20 to 30 per cent of patients with refractory anemia (type 1 or 2) develop acute leukemia, but over 60 per cent of patients with refractory anemia with excess blasts in transformation will develop acute leukemia.

Treatment of the myelodysplastic syndrome is primarily directed toward improving the anemia. Blood transfusions are a mainstay of treatment. A few patients with refractory anemia with ringed sideroblasts respond to large doses of vitamin B_6. Chemotherapy has been used when increased numbers of blasts appear in the bone marrow. The role for chemotherapy, either in conventional doses or in low doses, is still being studied.

THE LYMPHOMAS

The lymphomas are a group of malignant neoplasms that arise in lymph nodes or extranodal lymphoid tissue. They are a heterogeneous group of malignancies from both a pathological and a clinical viewpoint. The two major subgroups are Hodgkins' disease and the non-Hodgkin's lymphoma. In both these subgroups, the most common clinical presentation is that of a patient who notices an enlarged lymph node. Before the physician considers a biopsy of the enlarged node, he must obtain a thorough history and perform a physical examination and selected laboratory tests to evaluate possible causes of the swollen lymph node. Cervical lymphadenopathy most commonly is associated with infections such as streptococcal pharyngitis, infectious mononucleosis, and toxoplasmosis. Axillary lymphadenopathy, particularly if it is unilateral, should direct the physician to perform a careful breast examination for possible cancer. Inguinal adenopathy may reflect skin infections of the legs or infection of the genitalia or anus such as syphilis. Scrofula, or tuberculous lymphadenitis, may present as asymptomatic isolated lymphadenopathy. Table 52–13 outlines various common causes of lymphadenopathy. If the cause of the enlarged lymph node(s) is not obvious after consideration of the above, the physician should consider lymph node biopsy for diagnosis.

Hodgkin's Disease.   This is primarily a disease of young adults but also appears in children and the elderly. The patient usually presents with asymptomatic lymphadenopathy; for example, on a routine pre-employment chest x-ray the radiologist finds mediastinal lymphadenopathy. Some patients with Hodgkins' disease have symptoms of fever, night sweats, or loss of weight; the factor or factors responsible for the production of these symptoms are not known.

Hodgkin's disease is classified by pathological subtype, by clinical stage, and by the presence or absence of symptoms. The four pathological subtypes are nodular sclerosis, lymphocyte predominance, mixed cellularity, and lymphocyte depletion (Table 52–14). In all four subtypes the finding of Reed-Sternberg cells assures the pathologist that the diagnosis of Hodgkin's disease is correct. The typical Reed-Sternberg cell is a large cell with two prominent nuclei. Each nucleus contains a prominent nucleolus surrounded by a "halo." This pattern gives the cell the appearance of "owl's eyes." Pathologists have puzzled over the cell of origin of the Reed-Sternberg cell since it was first described around 1900. At present, the true macro-

TABLE 52–14. HODGKIN'S DISEASE: PATHOLOGIC TYPES

SUBGROUP	RELATIVE FREQUENCY
Lymphocyte predominance	5–15%
Nodular sclerosis	40–75%
Mixed cellularity	20–40%
Lymphocyte depletion	5–15%

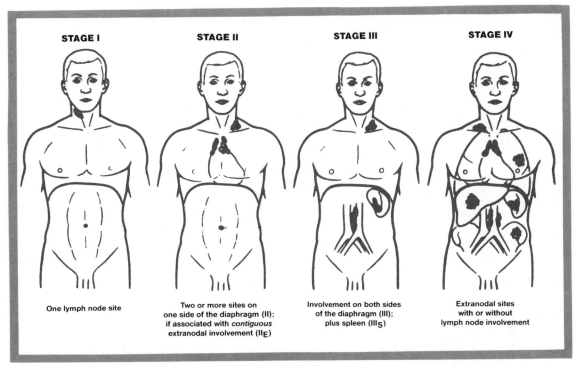

STAGE I — One lymph node site

STAGE II — Two or more sites on one side of the diaphragm (II); if associated with *contiguous* extranodal involvement (II$_E$)

STAGE III — Involvement on both sides of the diaphragm (III); plus spleen (III$_S$)

STAGE IV — Extranodal sites with or without lymph node involvement

FIGURE 52–5. Malignant lymphoma: Examples of stages I through IV. (Reprinted from Tindle BH: Teaching monograph: Malignant lymphomas. Am J Pathol 116:115, 1984, with permission.)

phage or histiocyte rather than a lymphocyte is considered the progenitor of the Reed-Sternberg cell.

Nodular sclerosis is the most common pathological subtype of Hodgkin's disease. Broad bands of fibrosis disrupt the lymph node architecture. "Lacunar" cells and scattered Reed-Sternberg cells are characteristic. This subtype of Hodgkin's disease typically presents as an asymptomatic mediastinal mass in a young woman. Hodgkin's disease of the mixed cellularity subtype demonstrates a pathological picture of a heterogeneous cellular background with lymphocytes, eosinophils, and plasma cells; the Reed-Sternberg cell is present. Young and middle-aged men rather than women are more likely to have this subtype. Lymphocyte-predominant Hodgkin's disease is an uncommon subtype. An asymptomatic young man presenting with an enlarged high cervical node would be a typical patient. The prognosis for this subtype is generally excellent. Lymphocyte-depleted Hodgkin's disease is also uncommon. An older patient with fever, night sweats, or weight loss would be most likely to have this subtype, and the prognosis is generally poor.

Cure of the patient with Hodgkin's disease is the goal of treatment. Treatment is planned once the extent of disease or the stage is known. The definition of stages I, II, III, and IV is outlined in Table 52–15. Figure 52–5 shows examples of the various stages. The presence or absence of systemic symptoms is also part of the staging criteria. The staging process is rigorous, and a basic outline of tests that should be done to establish the stage is shown in Table 52–16. Hodgkin's

disease tends to follow a logical anatomical progression of node involvement. For example, a patient with cervical adenopathy may have supraclavicular or mediastinal adenopathy but in the absence of supraclavicular or mediastinal adenopathy is unlikely to have pelvic adenopathy or liver involvement. This principle is important when considering how far to pursue a staging evaluation. For example, the patient with a high cervical node and no other adenopathy by CTT scan is very unlikely to have abdominal disease. An exploratory laparotomy with liver biopsy, multiple node biopsies, and splenectomy may be necessary to establish an accurate stage for a patient. A laparotomy

TABLE 52–15. ANN ARBOR STAGING CLASSIFICATION FOR HODGKIN'S DISEASE

Stage I:	Involvement of a single lymph node region (I) or a single extralymphatic site (I$_E$)
Stage II:	Involvement of two or more lymph node regions on the same side of the diaphragm (II) or a solitary extralymphatic site and one or more lymph node areas on the same side of the diaphragm (II$_E$)
Stage III:	Involvement of lymph node regions on both sides of the diaphragm (III), accompanied by spleen involvement (III$_S$), or solitary involvement of an extralymphatic organ or site (III$_E$) or both (III$_{SE}$)
Stage IV:	Diffuse involvement of extralymphatic sites with or without lymph node enlargement

In addition to above, presence or absence of symptoms (specifically, fever, night sweats, loss of 10% body weight) is designated by B (presence) or A (absence).

TABLE 52–16. STAGING EVALUATION FOR A PATIENT WITH LYMPHOMA

1. Complete history and physical examination
2. CBC, differential, platelet count, urinalysis
3. Screening blood chemistries
4. Chest x-ray, CAT scan of chest, abdomen, and pelvis
5. Bone marrow aspirate and biopsy
6. Consider lymphangiogram, gallium scan

NON-HODGKIN'S LYMPHOMA	HODGKIN'S DISEASE
Stage III or IV—Treat with chemotherapy	Stage IIIB or IV—Treat with chemotherapy
Stage I—Treat with radiotherapy	Stage IA—Treat with radiotherapy
Stage II—Treat with radiotherapy and/or chemotherapy	Stage IIA, IIB, IIIA—Consider exploratory laparotomy

should be considered in two situations: first, if the findings at laparotomy will alter the treatment plan; and, secondly, if abdominal or pelvic radiotherapy is being considered for a young woman of child-bearing age, the laparotomy would include transposing the ovaries out of the radiotherapy field. If a patient has clinical stage IIIB or stage IV Hodgkin's disease, the treatment is chemotherapy; laparotomy is not necessary because the findings will not change this recommendation. If a patient has a mediastinal mass and cervical node involvement but a lymphangiogram suggests pelvic node involvement, a laparotomy may be necessary to establish whether the patient has stage IIA or stage IIIA disease. Both these stages can be treated with radiotherapy, but the ports would differ according to the findings at laparotomy.

The treatment of Hodgkin's disease is radiotherapy, chemotherapy, and, in certain cases, both therapies (Table 52–16). Radiotherapy is the recommended

TABLE 52–17. CLASSIFICATION OF THE NON-HODGKIN'S LYMPHOMAS

INTERNATIONAL WORKING FORMULATION	RAPPAPORT CLASSIFICATION
I. Low-grade lymphoma	
a. Small lymphocytic cell	Diffuse lymphocytic, well-differentiated
b. Follicular, mixed cleaved cell	Nodular lymphocytic, poorly differentiated
c. Follicular, mixed small cleaved and large cell	Nodular mixed lymphocytic-histiocytic
II. Intermediate-grade lymphoma	
d. Follicular, large cell	Nodular histiocytic
e. Diffuse, small cleaved cell	Diffuse lymphocytic, poorly differentiated
f. Diffuse, mixed small cleaved cell	Diffuse mixed lymphocytic-histiocytic
g. Diffuse large cell	Diffuse histiocytic
III. High-grade lymphoma	
h. Large cell immunoblastic	Diffuse histiocytic
i. Lymphoblastic cell	Diffuse undifferentiated
j. Small noncleaved cell (Burkitt and non-Burkitt)	

treatment for patients with stages I and IIA. Some patients with stage II or IIIA will have such massive adenopathy that chemotherapy may be used initially to shrink the bulk of the disease before curative radiotherapy. Patients with stage IIB are a controversial group; because of a high relapse rate after radiotherapy alone, combined modality (i.e., radiotherapy and chemotherapy) may be recommended. Patients with stage IIIB or IV are considered to have widespread disease that cannot be cured by radiotherapy; curative chemotherapy is used in these patients.

Radiotherapy is delivered in tumoricidal doses to areas of known disease and to adjacent areas. For example, a patient with stage I Hodgkin's disease in a cervical node receives a "mantle" port designed to treat cervical, supraclavicular, axillary, mediastinal, and hilar lymph nodes. A patient with inguinal node involvement receives an "inverted Y" to encompass the para-aortic, iliac, and inguinal nodes. The immediate side effects of radiation depend on the field irradiated and include sore throat, dysphagia, nausea, and diarrhea. Delayed effects include radiation pneumonitis and hypothyroidism if the thyroid has been included in the field. Ovarian function will be suppressed unless the ovaries are surgically moved out of the radiation field prior to treatment.

A major advance in Hodgkin's disease has been the development of combination chemotherapy that can cure the majority of patients with stages IIIB and IV. The original program was the "MOPP" program (nitrogen-mustard, vincristine [oncovin], procarbazine, and prednisone). This program is still one of the best programs for advanced-stage Hodgkin's disease. The immediate side effects include nausea, vomiting, and bone marrow suppression. The delayed side effects include sterility and the potential for the late development of leukemia. The risk of leukemia increases if the patient is over 40 and also receives radiotherapy.

The long-term prognosis for patients with Hodgkin's disease is related to stage at diagnosis. Patients with stages IA and IIA disease have a five-year survival of over 90 per cent. Most patients with stage IIIA have a five-year survival of over 80 per cent. B symptoms decrease the survival figures at each stage. Stage IIIB and stage IV patients can expect a five-year survival of over 50 per cent. The five-year survival rates can translate to cure rates in most instances.

The risk of infection is a major problem in Hodgkin's disease. Immunological abnormalities, particularly reflecting T cell dysfunction, can be detected even before patients receive any treatment, a finding that explains the frequent occurrence of herpes zoster in Hodgkin's disease. These patients also are susceptible to fungal infections such as cryptococcosis. Bacterial infections, particularly pneumococcal and meningococcal, especially affect patients who have undergone laparotomy and splenectomy.

Non-Hodgkin's Lymphomas. These are a heterogeneous group of neoplasms that arise from a monoclonal proliferation of a malignant cell of lymphoid origin. As in Hodgkin's disease, the cause of lymphoma is not known. Viruses, radiation, immunosuppression (e.g., renal transplantation, AIDS), and certain genetic conditions have all been implicated. Burkitt's lymphoma, a rare monoclonal B cell neoplasm, has provided some clues about the pathogenesis of lymphoma. In Africa, there is a "lymphoma belt" in which the development of Burkitt's lymphoma mirrors the endemic area for malaria. This distribution, along with the finding of Epstein-Barr virus in the majority of cases of African Burkitt's lymphoma, suggests a viral pathogenesis. Chromosomal translocations in Burkitt's lymphoma involve chromosomes 8 and 14 and less commonly 2 and 22. These chromosomes carry the genes for the immunoglobulin heavy chains and light chains and their translocations produces immunoglobulin rearrangements. The translocations also occur at the chromosome site where a cellular oncogene (c-myc) is found. The relationship of the translocation at the site of a cellular oncogene and monoclonal proliferation of this malignant neoplasm is not yet understood.

Non-Hodgkin's lymphomas are classified by pathological subtype and clinical stage. The pathological subtype depends on the overall pattern of nodal architecture and on the morphology of the predominant cell in the neoplastic node. The malignant cells may replace the node in a diffuse pattern obliterating the germinal centers or follicles completely. This pattern defines a "diffuse" lymphoma. Alternatively, the malignant cells may form a pattern of nodules or follicles that defines the lymphoma as a nodular or follicular lymphoma. The predominant cell type further clas-

sifies the lymphoma. The major lymphoma cell types are the small, well-differentiated lymphocyte; the slightly larger, poorly differentiated lymphocyte with a cleaved nucleus; and the large lymphoid cell with characteristics of a histiocyte or lymphoblast. Two major lymphoma classification systems use these criteria, nodal architecture, and cell type to define the subtypes of lymphoma. Table 52–17 shows the International Formulation classification of lymphoma next to the classification of Rappaport. Both these systems have received wide acceptance because of their clarity and clinical applicability. These classifications are

TABLE 52–18. IMMUNOLOGICAL CLASSIFICATION OF THE NON-HODGKIN'S LYMPHOMAS

B-cell neoplasms	Low-grade lymphomas Intermediate-grade lymphomas (most) High-grade lymphomas (most)
T-cell neoplasms Thymic T cell	Lymphoblastic lymphoma (an aggressive lymphoma, particularly of young men, associated with mediastinal mass and CNS involvement)
Mature T cell	Peripheral T cell lymphoma HTVL-I–associated lymphoma (a virus-related lymphoma, clustered in South Japan and Caribbean) Mycosis fungoides (a "helper" T cell lymphoma of the skin, associated with circulating lymphoma cells, "Sézary cells")

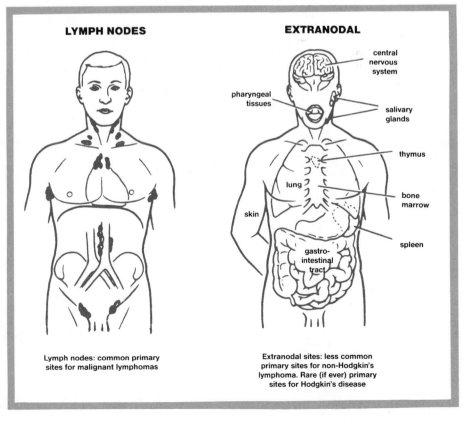

FIGURE 52–6. Malignant lymphomas: Examples of nodal and extranodal sites. (Reprinted from Tindle BN: Teaching monograph: Malignant lymphomas. Am J Pathol 116:115, 1984, with permission.)

LYMPH NODES

EXTRANODAL

central nervous system

pharyngeal tissues

salivary glands

thymus

lung

bone marrow

skin

spleen

gastro-intestinal tract

Lymph nodes: common primary sites for malignant lymphomas

Extranodal sites: less common primary sites for non-Hodgkin's lymphoma. Rare (if ever) primary sites for Hodgkin's disease morphologic and do not depend on immunological subtyping of the malignant cells. If lymph node biopsies are further subjected to studies of cell origin using surface immunoglobulin markers for B cells, erythrocyte rosettes for T cells, or more sophisticated monoclonal antibodies for B and T cells, most of the lymphomas are of B cell origin. Particularly aggressive B-cell lymphomas, refractory to therapy, occur in patients with acquired immunodeficiency syndromes. Some lymphomas are of T cell origin; in rare lymphomas, the cell of origin cannot be determined (Table 52–18).

Clinical staging of non-Hodgkin's lymphoma is defined by the same criteria as those for Hodgkin's disease (see Table 52–15). Two aspects of the staging process are different from Hodgkin's disease. First, the non-Hodgkin's lymphomas are more likely than Hodgkin's lymphomas to present in an extranodal site (Fig. 52–6). Secondly, the progression of the non-Hodgkin's lymphomas does not follow the orderly anatomical progression described above for Hodgkin's disease. Non-Hodgkin's lymphoma is much more likely to be disseminated at the time of diagnosis. True stage I or stage II non-Hodgkin's lymphomas are rare. The treatment and prognosis of the patient with non-Hodgkin's lymphoma depend on the clinical stage and the pathological classification. Patients with stage I or stage II disease may be treated with radiotherapy alone. The overall cure rate for these patients is less than 50 per cent. This suggests that there may be a role for adjuvant chemotherapy in the treatment of some of these patients. Patients with stage III or IV disease are treated primarily with chemotherapy. Curability in this group depends on the pathological subtype. Paradoxically, some patients with "high-grade" or "high-intermediate grade" lymphomas in whom the natural history would lead to survival of less than one or two years are now curable with aggressive combination chemotherapy programs incorporating drugs such as cyclophosphamide, adriamycin, vincristine, predni-

sone, and bleomycin. Patients with low-grade lymphomas are rarely curable by chemotherapy. The natural history of these lymphomas tends to be an indolent one, with median survivals of five years and sometimes longer. Treatment offers palliation but may not alter survival. Thus, observation alone, less aggressive chemotherapy, and palliative radiotherapy may be used in the management of the patient with an indolent lymphoma (Fig. 52–7).

PLASMA CELL DISORDERS

The plasma cell disorders include a group of neoplasms that arise from a clone of immunoglobulin-secreting cells and produce a monoclonal immunoglobulin (or part of an immunoglobulin). If the monoclonal immunoglobulin (Ig) is of the IgM class, the disease is Waldenström's macroglobulinemia and the malignant cells are plasmacytoid lymphocytes. If the monoclonal immunoglobulin is of the IgG, IgA, IgD, or rarely the IgE class, the disease is multiple myeloma and the malignant cells are plasma cells. Normal plasma cells represent the most specialized cells in the B cell lineage. Figure 52–3 illustrates one scheme of maturation proceeding from a pluripotent stem cell to an early B cell to a well-differentiated plasma cell. The figure also indicates the malignant diseases that can arise from neoplastic proliferation at each stage of B cell maturation.

Plasma cells normally secrete immunoglobulins and are responsible for maintaining humoral immunity. The basic structure of all immunoglobulins is the same and includes two heavy ("H") polypeptide chains and two light ("L") polypeptide chains, bound together by disulfide bonds. Both H chains and L chains have "constant" regions of amino acid sequence and "variable" regions that allow for antibody specificity. The five subclasses of immunoglobulin, immunoglobulin gamma (IgG), mu (IgM), alpha (IgA), delta (IgD), and epsilon (IgE) are determined by the constant region of their H chains. Light chains are of two types: kappa and lambda. Each antibody molecule has two identical H chains and two identical L chains; hybrid molecules are not synthesized. Table 52–19 outlines special properties of the five immunoglobulin classes. Protein electrophoresis provides the first step in detecting a monoclonal immunoglobulin in serum. Analysis of the protein "spike" by agar gel immunoelectrophoresis using specific antibodies (e.g., anti-human IgG, anti-kappa chains, etc.) further defines the exact type of monoclonal immunoglobulin.

Monoclonal immunoglobulin elevations can be found in conditions other than multiple myeloma or Waldenström's macroglobulinemia. Approximately 10 per cent of patients with chronic lymphocytic leukemia have monoclonal IgG or IgM spikes in their serum. In addition, a monoclonal spike on serum electrophoresis may be found in patients with no detectable associated disease. The "spike" is usually not large (i.e., is less than 2 gm/dl) and is accompanied by no other clinical or laboratory evidence of multiple myeloma or Waldenström's macroglobulinemia. This find-

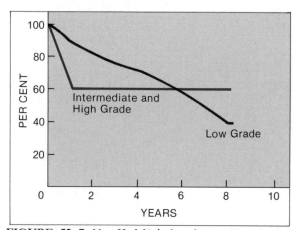

FIGURE 52–7. Non-Hodgkin's lymphoma: Hypothetical actuarial survival according to classification, based on 1985 data. (From Portlock CS: The non-Hodgkin's lymphomas. *In* Wyngaarden JB, Smith LH Jr (eds). Cecil Textbook of Medicine. 18th ed. Philadelphia, WB Saunders Co, 1988, p 1012.)

TABLE 52–19. SOME PROPERTIES OF NORMAL IMMUNOGLOBULINS

	IgG	IgA	IgM	IgD	IgE
Molecular weight	150,000	180,000	900,000 (a pentamer)	150,000	200,000
Plasma concentration (mg/ml)	7–15	2.0	1.0	0.03	trace
Biologic half-life (days)	20	6	5	3	–
Complement fixation	+	–	+	–	–
Crosses placenta	+	–	–	–	–
Special properties	4 subclasses (1–4)	Present in external secetions	Synthesized by lymphocytes	–	Important in hypersensitivity

ing, called "benign monoclonal gammopathy," is found in elderly patients (i.e., over 60); approximately 10 per cent of these patients later develop a true immunoproliferative disorder.

Multiple myeloma. This is a malignant disease of plasma cells that is characterized by the presence of monoclonal immunoglobulin or light chains in the serum and urine and bone destruction. The typical patient is over 50 and presents with back pain, mild anemia, and an elevated sedimentation rate. Initial bone x-rays may demonstrate only osteoporosis, although widespread lytic lesions are typical. Less frequently the patient will have hypercalcemia and renal disease ("light chain nephropathy") at the time of diagnosis. Serum immunoelectrophoresis generally demonstrates a monoclonal elevation of one immunoglobulin (e.g., IgG^k), with reciprocal depression of the other immunoglobulins (e.g., IgA and IgM). Free kappa or lambda light chains (Bence-Jones protein) are usually detected by a 24-hour urine immunoelectrophoresis. About 20 per cent of patients with multiple myeloma will not have a monoclonal serum spike but will have free light chains detectable in urine and serum ("light chain disease"); about 1 per cent of patients with multiple myeloma will have neither monoclonal nor free light chains detectable. These patients with "nonsecretory" myeloma can be shown to have a malignant clonal proliferation of plasma cells by immunofluorescent staining of the bone marrow. The plasma cells will be shown to stain with either the anti-kappa or anti-lambda antiserum, but not with both reagents.

Bone marrow aspiration is essential for the diagnosis of myeloma. Plasma cells usually make up less than 5 per cent of bone marrow cells; greater than 10 to 20 per cent plasma cells are required to make a bone marrow diagnosis of multiple myeloma. Some of the plasma cells may have bizarre morphology with binucleated and multinucleated plasma cells. The clinical manifestations of multiple myeloma center on the systemic effects of the monoclonal protein (the paraprotein) and the concomitant humoral immunodeficiency state, as well as the effects of the bone and bone marrow invasion by malignant cells. Table 52–20 outlines the common clinical syndromes associated with multiple myeloma. Despite high levels of paraprotein, syndromes of hyperviscosity are rare in myeloma.

The prognosis of multiple myeloma is a reflection of the tumor cell burden. A poor prognosis is associated with a high tumor cell burden, as reflected by anemia, decreased renal function, hypercalcemia, extensive bony involvement, and large monoclonal protein peaks. A patient without any of these poor prognostic criteria may have a median survival of five years; a patient in the poor prognosis category is likely to have a median survival of less than two years. The development of a staging system that correlates clinical criteria with the "measured" myeloma cell mass has been useful for predicting prognosis and selecting therapy (Table 52–21).

The treatment of a patient with multiple myeloma requires meticulous attention to supportive care as well as expertise in the administration of chemotherapy. Cautious exercise and ambulation are important to retard bone resorption. Bone lesions may require local radiotherapy to prevent a pathologic fracture. Adequate hydration and avoidance of intravenous dye injection (e.g., for intravenous pyelography) helps to prevent renal failure. Administration of pneumococcal vaccine and early detection and treatment of infections are important in these susceptible patients.

The current chemotherapy of multiple myeloma

TABLE 52–20. COMMON CLINICAL MANIFESTATIONS OF MULTIPLE MYELOMA

Bone involvement
  Malignant plasma cells may secrete osteoclast activating factor leading to:
    a. osteoporosis, pathologic fracture, and bone pain
    b. hypercalcemia
Anemia
  Decreased red cell production due to tumor inhibition of erythropoiesis and marrow invasion by plasma cells
Renal disease
  Calcium nephropathy
  Light chain nephropathy
  Uric acid nephropathy
  Amyloidosis (may develop in about 15% of patients)
Elevated sedimentation rate
  The paraprotein causes red cell rouleaux.
Infection
  Normal immunoglobulin production is suppressed.
  Pneumococcal disease is particularly prevalent.

TABLE 52–21. MYELOMA STAGING SYSTEM

STAGE	CRITERIA	MYELOMA CELL MASS*

I.	*All* of the following:
	1. Hemoglobin value >10 gm/dl
	2. Serum calcium value (≤12 mg/dl)
	3. On x-ray, normal bone structure (scale 0) or solitary bone plasmacytoma only
	4. Low M-component production rates
	  a. IgG value <5 gm/dl
	  b. IgA value <3 gm/dl
	  c. Urine L chain M-component on electrophoresis <4 gm/24 hr
		<0.6 (low)

II.
III.
	Fitting neither Stage I nor Stage III
	One or more of the following:
	1. Hemoglobin value <8.5 gm/dl
	2. Serum calcium value >12 mg/dl
	3. Advanced lytic bone lesions (scale 3)
	4. High M-component production rates
	  a. IgG value >7 gm/dl
	  b. IgA value >5 gm/dl
	  c. Urine L chain M-component on electrophoresis >12 gm/24 hr
		0.6–1.20 (intermediate)
		>1.20 (high)

Subclassification:
A = Relatively normal renal function (serum creatinine value <2.0 mg/dl)
B = Abnormal renal function (serum creatinine value ≥2.0 mg/dl)
Examples:
Stage IA = Low cell mass with normal renal function
Stage IIIB = High cell mass with abnormal renal function

Adapted from Durie BGM, Salmon SE: Cancer 36:842, 1975.
* Cells × 10^{12} per square meter body surface.

centers on the use of cell cycle-nonspecific cytotoxic drugs (alkylating agents, nitrosoureas, and anthracycline antibiotics) and corticosteroids. Improvement in symptoms ensues in the majority of patients. Clinical remission is associated with a decrease of less than one log of tumor cells (e.g., 10^{12} to 10^{11}). Eradication of all tumor cells and cure of multiple myeloma are not attainable with available therapy.

Waldenström's macroglobulinemia. This is a clonal disease of IgM-secreting plasmacytoid lymphocytes. It is a chronic disorder that usually affects older people. The patient commonly presents with anemia and symptoms due to the physical properties of the elevated monoclonal IgM. IgM is a large molecule and remains primarily in the intravascular space. If the IgM level is elevated, plasma viscosity may be high. Nosebleeds, retinal hemorrhages, mental confusion, and congestive heart failure are clinical presentations of the hyperviscosity syndrome. Some IgM molecules precipitate in the cold. The patient with this type of IgM may manifest the clinical picture of cryoglobulinemia. Blue (cyanotic) fingers, toes, nose, and ear-

lobes on exposure to cold are a typical presentation. Foot and leg ulcers may develop, and vascular occlusion with gangrene may ensue. Leukocytoclastic vasculitis is seen on biopsy of these skin lesions. Some IgM molecules may have activity directed against red cells, particularly the "I" antigen (see Hemolytic Anemias). This type of IgM, a cold agglutinin, agglutinates red cells at temperatures below 37°C (e.g., in the extremities). These patients present with Raynaud's phenomenon and a hemolytic anemia. Keeping patients with cryoglobulinemia or the cold agglutinin syndrome warm is a primary part of their treatment. Peripheral neuropathy is a rare presentation of Waldenström's macroglobulinemia. A few patients have been described in whom the IgM monoclonal protein had antimyelin activity. Splenomegaly and lymphadenopathy may develop during the course of Waldenström's macroglobulinemia but are rarely a major cause of disability. Bone pain and hypercalcemia rarely occur.

The treatment of Waldenström's macroglobulinemia is directed to relief of symptoms. If the symptoms are primarily due to the elevated IgM (e.g., hyperviscosity syndrome), plasmapheresis is a useful tool and may be combined with chemotherapy. If the IgM is a cold agglutinin or a cryoglobulin, the plasmapheresis must be done in a warm environment. Chemotherapy (e.g., alkylating agents) may be useful to decrease the lymphadenopathy and splenomegaly but does not alter the natural history of the disease. The median survival is about three years, although some patients may live ten or more years with indolent disease.

Rarely, a patient may present with *heavy chain disease*, a disorder that has some characteristics of myeloma or Waldenström's macroglobulinemia but behaves clinically more like lymphoma. Analysis of the serum reveals only the heavy chain of IgG, IgA, or IgM. Gamma chain disease is associated with lymphadenopathy and edema of the soft palate. Alpha chain disease ("Mediterranean lymphoma") is characterized by intestinal infiltration by lymphoma; mu chain disease is associated with chronic lymphocytic leukemia.

REFERENCES

Adamson JW, Fialkow PJ, Murphy S, et al: Polycythemia vera: Stem cell and probable clonal origin of the disease. N Engl J Med 295:913, 1976.

Bergsagel DE, Rider WD: Plasma cell neoplasms. *In* Devita VT, Hellman S, Rosenberg SA (eds): Cancer: Principles and Practice of Oncology. 2nd ed. Philadelphia, JB Lippincott Co, 1985.

Champlin RE, Gale RP: Review: Acute myelogenous leukemia: Recent advances in therapy. Blood 69:1551, 1987.

Champlin RE, Golde DW: Chronic myelogenous leukemia: Recent advances. Blood 65:1039, 1985.

Devita VT, Jaffe ES, Hellman S: Hodgkin's disease and the non-Hodgkin's lymphomas. *In* Devita VT, Hellman S, Rosenberg SA (eds): Cancer: Principles and Practice of Oncology. 2nd. ed. Philadelphia, JB Lippincott Co, 1985.

Gale RP, Foon KA: Chronic lymphocytic leukemia. Ann Intern Med 103:101, 1985.

Jacobs AD, Gale RP: Recent advances in the biology and treatment of acute lymphoblastic leukemia in adults. N Engl J Med 311:1219, 1984.

53
HEMOSTASIS

The arrest of bleeding after blood vessel injury involves a complex interaction among three responding systems: the blood vessel wall, the platelets, and the plasma coagulation proteins. This interaction results in normal *hemostasis*, but if pathologically exaggerated produces *thrombosis*. While hemostasis is initiated within a few seconds after blood vessel injury, it is not completed for minutes to about an hour.

Primary hemostasis involves constriction of the injured vessel, exposure of subendothelial collagen, and the adhesion and aggregation of blood platelets on the damaged surface to form a *primary hemostatic plug* that is completed within 3 to 7 minutes. This process also involves participation of von Willebrand factor (Factor VIII: von Willebrand Factor, Factor VIII: VWF), which mediates platelet adhesion and the release from platelets of vasoactive materials that augment aggregation. Clinical assessment of primary hemostasis is made with the bleeding time, which is a sensitive index of the adequacy of platelet function.

Secondary hemostasis represents the formation of a *fibrin clot* at the site of the initiating primary hemostatic plug. The surface of activated platelets catalyzes the formation of thrombin by its efficient assembly of coagulation factors involved in the prothrombinase complex in the presence of membrane phospholipid and calcium released upon platelet activation. Such localized thrombin activation in turn has several crucial effects. (1) Thrombin catalyzes fibrinogen conversion to fibrin, the fibrous protein that consolidates the platelet plug and entraps erythrocytes to provide bulk for the permanent clot. (2) Thrombin stimulates further platelet activation, prothrombin conversion, platelet release, and thromboxane production. (3) Thrombin activates coagulation Factor XIII, fibrin stabilizing factor, which covalently cross-links and stabilizes the fibrin clot. Measurement of secondary hemostasis is made with the whole blood clotting time, which averages 8 to 10 minutes.

The *third stage of coagulation* is clot retraction, a process in which the loose meshwork of platelet aggregates, fibrin strands, and trapped red cells is formed into a firm clot. This process involves the contraction within individual platelets of the smooth muscle protein, thrombosthenin, which compresses the clot. This stage may be evaluated in vitro and takes about one hour.

EVALUATION OF A BLEEDING TENDENCY

A clinically important bleeding tendency may result from defects in the blood vessels, the platelets, or the coagulation proteins. The defects may be qualitative or quantitative, and single or multiple. Inherited hemorrhagic disorders tend to result from single defects, whereas acquired disorders result from single or multiple deficiencies. Evaluation of a patient for a bleeding tendency is needed in three settings: (1) screening prior to surgery, (2) when prior episodes of spontaneous or traumatic bleeding are reported, and (3) during active bleeding unresponsive to simple measures (Table 53–1).

The personal and family history is essential in evaluation of a bleeding tendency. A positive family history of bleeding in males suggests one of the hemophilias, which make up 95 per cent of congenital coagulation deficiencies. Spontaneous bleeding or bruising or easy bruising and bleeding after minor trauma are important, especially if bruises are large or raised (hematomas). Excessive bleeding after prior surgery or dental extraction, events that stress the hemostatic process, may indicate a bleeding tendency in persons without spontaneous bleeding history. A history of menorrhagia or peripartum hemorrhage in a woman can also signify an underlying bleeding diathesis.

If bleeding has occurred, its timing, location, and clinical setting provide key clues to the type of defect. In platelet disorders, bleeding tends to be immediate and transient and involves mucous membranes or skin (e.g., epistaxes or bruising). In contrast, delayed bleeding after trauma or surgery, or bleeding into joints or muscles, is typical of coagulation disorders. The presence of systemic diseases such as liver disease, hematologic malignancy, or uremia may impair hemostasis. Drug ingestion is the single most common cause for acquired hemostatic defects; a careful drug history

TABLE 53–1. DIFFERENTIAL DIAGNOSIS OF BLEEDING DISORDERS

	COAGULATION DEFECT	PLATELET DEFECT	VASCULAR DEFECT
Family history	Usually positive	Rarely positive	Usually negative
Sex predominance	Males	Often females	Mainly females
Type of bleeding	"Deep" joint, muscle and visceral; spontaneous and post-traumatic	Mucosal skin, mucous membranes	Purpuric or GI
Time sequence	Delayed after trauma followed by prolonged oozing	Immediate, brief	Ecchymoses after trauma
Response to local pressure	Ineffective	Effective	Effective

TABLE 53-2. CLINICAL CLUES TO BLEEDING DISORDERS

CLINICAL SIGN	DISORDER
Lifelong history of easy bruising or bleeding	Congenital coagulopathy (factor deficiency)
	Von Willebrand's disease
Family history of bleeding in males only	Hemophilia A or B
Family history of bleeding in both sexes	Factor XI deficiency
	Von Willebrand's disease
Excessive bleeding at surgery	Mild coagulation factor deficiency
	Von Willebrand's disease
	Thrombocytopenia
Acquired bruising tendency	Aspirin or other drug ingestion
	Thrombocytopenia
Delayed bleeding after trauma or surgery	Factor XIII deficiency
Bleeding after dental extraction	If negative, a bleeding disorder is unlikely.
Bruising or bleeding starting during another illness	Drug ingestion
	Thrombocytopenia
	Acquired anticoagulant

should include direct questioning about ingestion of aspirin, nonsteroidal anti-inflammatory compounds, antibiotics, and anticoagulants as well as alcohol. All of these substances can cause bleeding or exacerbate an underlying bleeding disorder, as can profound nutritional impairment. Some specific bleeding disorders to be considered from the patient's history are listed in Table 53-2.

Pertinent aspects of the physical examination in evaluating possible bleeding disorders include examination of the skin, mucous membranes, and retina for petechiae, ecchymoses, or hematomas and examination of the abdomen for hepatosplenomegaly. Petechiae are pinpoint hemorrhages from microvessels in the skin and are associated with platelet disorders or thrombocytopenia. Because pressure can exacerbate petechial bleeding, these lesions are commonly found on the legs or in other areas of increased hydrostatic pressure (e.g., on the buttocks in a bedridden patient). Purpura (confluent petechiae) are also common in thrombocytopenia. Ecchymoses, especially if spontaneous or raised (hematomas), and hemarthroses suggest defects in plasma coagulation factors as in he-

mophilia. Hepatomegaly suggests liver disease, and splenomegaly is associated with thrombocytopenia or with hematological malignancy.

LABORATORY EVALUATION OF HEMOSTASIS

Basic screening for hemostatic integrity can be accomplished with a prothrombin time, partial thromboplastin time, platelet count, and bleeding time (Table 53-3). If all results from these tests are normal, a serious bleeding diathesis is unlikely. Any abnormalities indicate that further investigation for particular defects should be made. Levels of individual coagulation factors, the presence of circulating anticoagulants, the nature of thrombocytopenia, abnormal platelet function, and signs of intravascular consumption of procoagulants can all be assessed.

PLATELET DISORDERS

Normal platelet function and a platelet count greater than 100,000/μl in the peripheral blood are needed for normal primary hemostasis (Fig. 53-1). The platelet count represents the net balance between platelet production rate and the rate of loss or peripheral destruction of platelets. Since the bone marrow has the capacity to increase platelet production 8- to 10-fold, and platelets survive 8 to 10 days in the circulation, the platelet count can be maintained under most circumstances, even if loss or destruction is increased. Young platelets are more metabolically active and more hemostatically effective than older ones. Platelet adhesion, procoagulant activity, and aggregation and release of vasoactive substances must also be normal for hemostatic effectiveness. Impairment of one or several of these functions leads to a bleeding tendency characterized by mucosal and skin bleeding, purpura, and prolonged oozing of blood after trauma or surgery.

Thrombocytopenia

Platelet counts below 100,000/μl portend an increased bleeding risk, which correlates roughly with the depression of the platelet count. Counts above 50,000/μl are rarely associated with spontaneous bleed-

TABLE 53-3. SCREENING TESTS FOR BLEEDING DISORDERS

TEST	MECHANISM TESTED	NORMAL	WHERE ABNORMAL
Prothrombin time (PT)	Extrinsic and common pathways	<12 sec	Defect in vitamin K–dependent factors, liver disease, DIC, oral anticoagulants
Activated partial thromboplastin time (APTT)	Intrinsic and common pathways	25–40 sec	Hemophilia, von Willebrand's disease, heparin therapy, DIC; deficient XII, IX, IX circulating anticoagulant
Thrombin time (TT)	Fibrinogen-fibrin conversion	10–15 sec	Third-stage anticoagulant; fibrin split products, DIC; severe hypofibrinogenemia
Bleeding time (BT)	Primary hemostasis, platelet function	3–7 min	Platelet dysfunction, von Willebrand's disease, thrombocytopenia

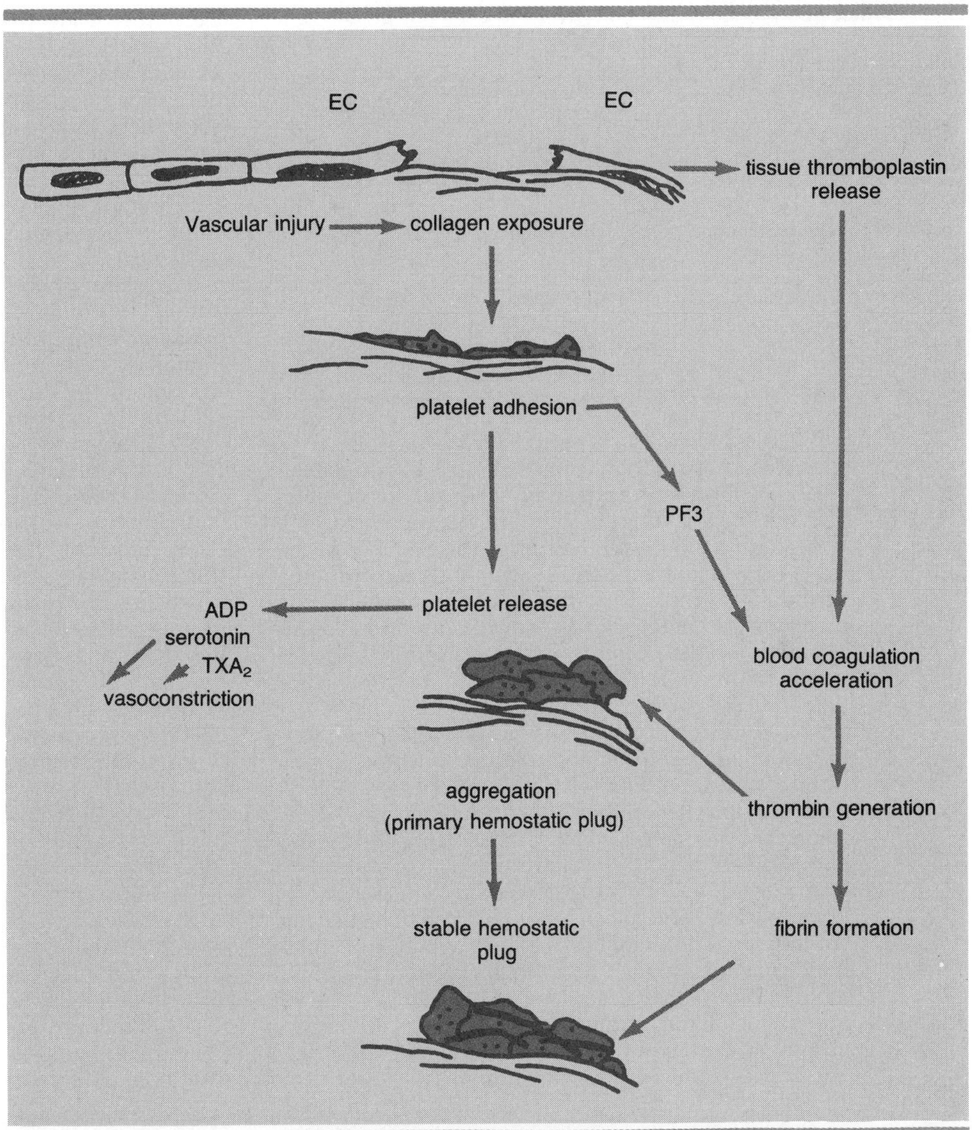

FIGURE 53-1. Hemostasis and platelet interactions with coagulation. Upon vascular injury, collagen fibrils underlying the endothelial cells (EC) are exposed when the endothelium is damaged. Adhesion of single platelets that flatten out and expose PF3 (procoagulant phospholipid) follows, then platelet release and primary aggregation to form a platelet plug. Release of ADP, serotonin, and TXA$_2$ induces vasoconstriction, while the PF3 accelerates blood coagulation, the formation of thrombin, and the generation of fibrin. Fibrin strands stabilize the hemostatic plug. Thrombin also promotes platelet aggregation and vasoconstriction.

ing, whereas counts below 20,000/μl are frequently associated with spontaneous bleeding, especially if the patient is febrile or anemic. Bleeding is observed more often in a thrombocytopenic patient with a rapidly falling platelet count than in a patient with a low, stable count. The mechanisms for severe thrombocytopenia include (1) decreased or ineffective platelet production, (2) increased peripheral destruction, (3) splenic sequestration, and (4) intravascular dilution (Table 53–4).

Decreased platelet production occurs with systemic infection, nutritional defects (folate or vitamin B$_{12}$), radiation, chemotherapy, or marrow replacement by fibrosis or tumor. Transient decreases in platelet production are common in viral infections and are the rule after radiation therapy to bone or after most types of cancer chemotherapy. Bone marrow megakaryo-

cytes may appear decreased or immature. Numerous drugs can inhibit megakaryocytopoiesis, including alcohol, anticonvulsants, and thiazides. Marrow hypoplasia as in aplastic anemia or Fanconi's syndrome also results in thrombocytopenia.

Increased platelet destruction is a common cause of thrombocytopenia and may be induced by commonly used drugs, including digitalis, quinidine, thiazides, imipramine, phenothiazines, sulfonamides, antibiotics (penicillins and cephalosporins), and gold salts. These agents usually produce thrombocytopenia by an immune mechanism in which a drug–antibody or drug–plasma protein complex adsorbs passively to the platelet surface ("innocent bystander") via the platelet Fc receptor, coating the platelets and resulting in their rapid removal from the circulation by the spleen. Other drugs may directly adsorb to the platelet sur-

TABLE 53—4. CAUSES OF THROMBOCYTOPENIA

Failure of platelet production	
Selective megakaryocyte depression	Drugs, viral infections
General bone marrow failure	Aplastic anemia, hematologic malignancy
	Myelophthisis
	Megaloblastic anemia
	Radiation
Increased platelet destruction	Drug-induced
	ITP
	Heparin
	DIC, TTP
Abnormal distribution	Hypersplenism
Dilutional	Massive transfusion of bank blood
	Extracorporeal circulation

face, resulting in neoantigens that provoke antiplatelet antibody formation. Stopping all drugs, if possible, and substituting drugs of different chemical structure if discontinuation is not possible is the first step in the evaluation and treatment of drug-induced immune thrombocytopenia. Unfortunately, direct tests of drug involvement are difficult to perform and often are insensitive, so that clinical assessment after drug discontinuation or switching is the main instrument for detecting drug-related thrombocytopenias.

Idiopathic (or autoimmune) thrombocytopenic purpura (ITP) represents immune thrombocytopenic purpura occurring without toxic or drug exposure. A polyclonal antiplatelet antibody has been demonstrated by transfer experiments. Platelet-associated IgG (and complement) may be elevated, large platelets circulate in the blood, and megakaryocytes are increased in the bone marrow. The spleen is not enlarged. The platelet survival is short. Acute ITP is mainly a disease of childhood, having a sudden onset following acute viral infection and resolving spontaneously in 80 per cent of affected children within a few weeks. In adults, chronic ITP is more common, has an insidious onset, and affects women more often than men. Fewer than 10 per cent of cases resolve spontaneously. In some cases an autoimmune hemolytic anemia is also present (Evan's syndrome). Adult ITP occurs alone or in association with diseases of disturbed immunity such as systemic lupus erythematosus, lymphoproliferative disorders, or AIDS. Homosexual patients with ITP are nearly all positive for HIV; because of increased risks of immunosuppression, therapy is withheld in mild cases. ITP can herald such diseases, appearing even years in advance of the full blown disease. Pregnant women with ITP can deliver thrombocytopenic infants, as the antiplatelet antibody is usually an IgG_1 or IgG_3 and thus crosses the placenta. The infant's platelet count does not correlate with the mother's count, so that a mother with ITP by history and a normal platelet count can deliver a thrombocytopenic infant.

Diagnosis of ITP is by exclusion. It is made in a patient with thrombocytopenia, increased megakaryocytes in the bone marrow, and increased platelet-associated IgG in the absence of drug exposure or toxic exposure. Aside from thrombocytopenia marked by large platelets, the blood count is otherwise normal. Platelet function may be entirely normal or may show diminished aggregation responses. Platelet survival is shortened, sometimes to hours compared to the normal survival of 8 to 10 days. Direct measurement of platelet survival can be made with ^{51}Cr or ^{112}In-labelled autologous platelets. This test, however, is not routinely performed because of expense and technical difficulty.

Treatment of both drug-induced thrombocytopenia and ITP is similar. Any suspected drug is stopped, and essential drugs are switched to substitutes of different chemical composition. All aspirin-like drugs are avoided. If the thrombocytopenia is severe, with purpura on the mucous membranes or retina, corticosteroids (1 to 2 mg/kg/day prednisolone) are given. Platelet transfusion should be avoided except for treatment of intracerebral bleeding because of the extremely short survival of transfused platelets. Plasmapheresis is generally not effective because of the IgG nature of the antiplatelet antibodies, which are inefficiently removed by this technique. In acute ITP of childhood or drug-induced thrombocytopenia, steroids can be tapered within a few weeks as platelet counts rise. In chronic ITP steroids should be administered for two to three months before tapering the dose or moving to alternative therapy, in order to achieve the maximum number of remissions and responses. In 70 per cent of patients the platelet count will rise toward normal within that period. Once a normal platelet count has been reached, the steroid dosage should be slowly tapered to avoid precipitating a relapse. The probable actions of steroids include inhibition of splenic reticuloendothelial phagocytic activity, decreased immune complex binding to platelets, decreased capillary fragility, and decreased immunoglobulin synthesis. When steroids are tapered following an initial increase in platelet count to the normal range, thrombocytopenia recurs in as many as 80 per cent of initially responding adult patients. Reinstitution of steroids may restore the platelet count, but many patients may require splenectomy for permanent remission. After splenectomy, 60 to 80 per cent of patients with ITP will maintain an adequate platelet count, while the remainder will require further therapy with steroids (at a lower dose) or with immunosuppressive drugs such as vincristine, cyclophosphamide, or azathioprine. For short-term therapy intravenous high-dose gamma globulin can transiently raise the platelet count in patients with refractory ITP (e.g., in preparation for emergency surgery), but adults do not respond well to repeated high-dose IgG therapy. Children with chronic ITP who are refractory to other therapy have been successfully managed with repeated infusion of high-dose intravenous IgG. Anabolic steroids such as danazol have also been reported to raise platelet counts in refractory ITP.

Other Causes of Immune Thrombocytopenia. *Post-transfusion purpura* is a rare syndrome that follows the administration of PL^{A1}-positive blood to patients who lack this common platelet antigen and who have developed anti-PL^{A1} antibodies after previous transfusion or pregnancy. An explosive thrombocytopenia develops five to eight days after transfusion (anamnestic response) which may require plasmapheresis and exchange transfusion with PL^{A1}-negative blood. The thrombocytopenia may persist a few weeks but is self-limited. Other platelet antigen systems are occasionally involved. *Neonatal purpura* may be seen in infants of PL^{A1}-negative mothers or mothers with ITP. In *systemic anaphylactic reactions* thrombocytopenia may result from sequestration of platelets coated with circulating antigen-antibody complexes. Thrombocytopenia may also result from platelet coating with anti-i cold antibodies that arise following viral infections such as rubella or infectious mononucleosis.

Platelet Consumption Syndromes. These include disseminated intravascular coagulation (DIC), thrombotic thrombocytopenia purpura, and the hemolytic uremic syndrome or can result from platelet damage during extracorporeal circulation. Intravascular activation of the coagulation mechanism is associated with sepsis, shock, exposure to toxins, or malignancies and may present with hemorrhage or thrombosis (see below). Thrombin-induced platelet aggregation or vascular damage that initiates platelet activation can cause thrombocytopenia. Vascular malformations such as cavernous hemangiomas (Kasabach-Merritt syndrome) sometimes produce localized DIC and platelet trapping, resulting in chronic thrombocytopenia.

Thrombotic thrombocytopenic purpura (Moschkowitz's syndrome) is an acute, relapsing disease affecting the microcirculation. There is a pentad of signs and symptoms including thrombocytopenia, microangiopathic hemolytic anemia, neurologic abnormalities, renal dysfunction, and fever. Two-thirds of affected persons are young women. There is often a history of preceding viral infection. The characteristic lesions are hyaline thrombi, consisting of platelet aggregates and fibrin, plugging small arterioles and capillaries. Endothelial proliferation may be seen, but vasculitis is not present. The blood smear shows schistocytes, increased reticulocytes, and normoblasts, reflecting the microangiopathic and hemolytic nature of the characteristic anemia; thrombocytopenia is usually severe, the serum lactic dehydrogenase and bilirubin are elevated, and the Coombs' test is negative. Early in the disease DIC is absent, but it appears as renal failure ensues. Abnormal forms of von Willebrand factor have been observed (released by injured endothelium), and some patients possess a plasma factor that promotes platelet activation. TTP is frequently fatal. Treatment by splenectomy, steroids, or platelet-inhibitory drugs such as aspirin and dipyridamole has had variable results. Exchange transfusion, plasmapheresis, and plasma infusion have more recently been used with greater success and represent the current approach of choice.

Hemolytic-uremic syndrome, usually seen in children, involves a Coombs-negative microangiopathic hemolytic anemia, thrombocytopenia, diarrhea, and acute renal failure. Unlike TTP, this disorder does not affect the brain to produce neurologic signs. DIC may be present. The major pathologic lesion consists of hyaline thrombi in the renal microcirculation, probably representing a form of immune complex disease. Renal dialysis is the mainstay of therapy. The role of plasmapheresis has not been defined.

Extracorporeal Circulation. Extracorporeal circulation frequently produces thrombocytopenia as the result of platelet activation, with subsequent adherence of platelets to the surface of the membrane oxygenator, dialyzer membrane, or other extracorporeal device. Platelet dysfunction induced by such contact may contribute to postoperative hemorrhage, over and above the contribution of thrombocytopenia.

Thrombocytopenia Produced by Platelet Sequestration. Normally the spleen contains about one third of the circulating pool of platelets. Increased splenic sequestration occurs with splenomegaly; very large spleens may sequester up to 90 per cent of the circulating platelets, resulting in a moderate thrombocytopenia of 50,000 to 100,000/cu mm. Platelet lifespan, however, is not shortened in hypersplenism, and severe hemorrhage is unusual.

Dilutional thrombocytopenia can follow massive transfusion of whole blood or plasma and lasts for several days. Platelet transfusions may be needed if the patient's residual platelets are dysfunctional or if bone marrow function is depressed and there is threatened or actual hemorrhage; the condition is transient in patients with normal marrow function.

Thrombocytosis

Elevation of the platelet count above 500,000/μl may be physiologic, secondary to bleeding, trauma, or infection, or can result from a primary bone marrow disease (thrombocythemia or other myeloproliferative disease). Transitory thrombocytosis follows stress or exercise and represents mobilization of platelets from the spleen or lung under the influence of epinephrine (Table 53–5).

Secondary, or reactive, *thrombocytosis* results from increased platelet production in response to hemorrhage, hemolysis, infection (such as tuberculosis), inflammatory disease, or malignancy. The platelets are normal in function and the platelet count may reach $10^6/\mu$l. A similar secondary thrombocytosis follows splenectomy and lasts for several weeks. In general, secondary thrombocytosis does not lead to hemorrhagic or thrombotic complications. Therapy to lower the platelet count or inhibit platelet function is not necessary. Treatment of the underlying disease usually results in a return of the platelet count to normal levels.

TABLE 53–5. CAUSES OF THROMBOCYTOSIS

Acute stress (release of splenic pool)
Secondary to inflammatory disease or infection: tuberculosis, rheumatoid arthritis, chronic inflammatory bowel disease, malignancy
Postsplenectomy
Myeloproliferative disease (primary thrombocytosis)

Primary thrombocytosis, or essential thrombocythemia, represents increased platelet production independent of normal regulatory control, except that the platelet count can increase further after hemorrhage. Platelet counts may exceed 1 to 2 × 10^6/μl. The platelets are large and bizarre in appearance, may appear in clumps on the blood smear, and are dysfunctional. The number of epinephrine receptors is decreased, and platelet aggregation responses to epinephrine are abnormal. The clinical picture of essential thrombocythemia is discussed in Chapter 52.

QUALITATIVE PLATELET DISORDERS

Inherited defects in platelet function are rare and produce mucosal bleeding when severe. Acquired defects in platelet function are common and are chiefly associated with drug ingestion—particularly of aspirin—or with underlying hematologic disease. They become clinically important if accompanied by another hemostatic defect, such as thrombocytopenia, or during therapy with anticoagulants. Acquired platelet function defects may also cause excessive bleeding at surgery. Evaluation of platelet disorders requires specialized testing (Table 53–6).

Congenital platelet disorders include *thrombasthenia* (Glanzmann's syndrome), characterized by a prolonged bleeding time, absent platelet aggregation despite normal platelet adhesion to collagen, and episodes of mucosal bleeding. The disorder is transmitted by an autosomal recessive gene. Thrombasthenic platelets lack two surface glycoproteins (IIb and IIIa) necessary for fibrinogen binding to the platelet membrane and for platelet aggregation. Bleeding may be life-threatening. The only therapy is transfusion of normal platelets. *Platelet-release defects* resulting in impaired platelet aggregation comprise several syndromes. First, a mild bleeding tendency results from an "aspirin-like" defect in which all platelet structures are normal, but normal activation does not take place when platelets are exposed to the usual agonists. The causes of this syndrome include defective phospholipase activation or a deficiency in enzymes of the prostaglandin pathway, such as cyclooxygenase or thromboxane synthase. Several types of *storage-pool deficiency* present with impaired platelet-release reactions, associated with poor platelet aggregation, a long bleeding time, and mucosal bleeding. The storage pool deficiencies are varied: they comprise defects in platelet granule storage of ADP or serotonin or abnormalities in platelet granule structure. In the *Hermansky-Pudlak syndrome*, platelet granule abnormalities are associated with albinism. An acquired storage pool defect occurs after exposure of blood to extracorporeal circulation and, rarely, in myeloproliferative disease. Since ADP release is necessary for normal platelet function, defective storage or release results in a hemorrhagic tendency. Bleeding episodes in affected patients are usually limited to trauma, surgery, or childbirth. Aspirin and nonsteroidal aspirin-like drugs should be avoided. As in thrombasthenia, platelet transfusion provides the only therapy.

Platelet adhesion is abnormal in two inherited bleeding disorders: von Willebrand's disease and the Bernard-Soulier syndrome. *Von Willebrand's disease* is a common bleeding disorder that affects both sexes and is transmitted as an autosomal recessive trait. In this condition, platelets are normal in structure and number but fail to adhere to the vascular subendothelium because of the lack of a plasma factor essential for platelet interaction with collagen in the vessel wall. The von Willebrand factor (VWF), which is synthesized in vascular endothelial cells and in megakaryocytes, normally circulates in a macromolecular complex with coagulation Factor VIII. In addition to decreased, absent, or abnormal VWF, patients with von Willebrand's disease also have decreased coagulation Factor VIII. In von Willebrand's disease, laboratory findings include a prolonged bleeding time, poor platelet adhesion, and normal platelet aggregation, but absent agglutination of platelets by the antibiotic ristocetin, which requires VWF. The clinical manifestations include mucosal bleeding, menorrhagia, and bruising. Both laboratory and clinical abnor-

TABLE 53–6. LABORATORY EVALUATION OF PLATELET DISORDERS: CBC, PLATELET COUNT, AND PERIPHERAL SMEAR EXAMINATION

Low Platelet Count
1. Bone marrow examination — Increased megas: ITP, immune purpura
   - Decreased megas: Drug, aplasia, infection
   - Sepsis, malignancy
2. Screen for DIC
3. Platelet associated IgG
4. Serum folate and vitamin B_{12}

Normal Platelet Count
1. Bleeding time — if prolonged: Thrombasthenia, uremia, drug ingestion (aspirin)
2. Platelet aggregation — if depressed: Aspirin, other drugs, uremia, DIC
3. Platelet agglutination with ristocetin — if depressed: von Willebrand's disease
4. Factor VIII: AHF and Factor VIII: VWF — if depressed: von Willebrand's disease
5. Platelet procoagulant activity — if decreased: Thrombocytopathy, uremia

High Platelet Count
1. Bone marrow examination — Myeloproliferative disease, malignancy
2. Platelet aggregation — if absent to epi: Myeloproliferative disease
3. Peripheral smear — if normal sized platelets: Secondary thrombocytosis
   - if giant platelets: Primary thrombocytosis is likely

malities are corrected by administration of VWF. Further discussion of von Willebrand's disease follows the discussion of hemophilia A.

In *Bernard-Soulier syndrome*, a very rare autosomal recessive disease, giant platelets are observed on the blood smear, the bleeding time is prolonged, and mucosal hemorrhage is common. A platelet membrane glycoprotein (Ib) that mediates VWF binding is absent. Plasma VWF is normal, but VWF cannot correct defective platelet adhesion in the absence of the platelet receptor. Treatment is limited to platelet transfusion.

The gray-platelet syndrome consists of a lack of platelet alpha granules containing VWF, fibronectin, and thrombospondin, the proteins necessary for normal platelet adhesion and aggregation. Their deficiency leads to a mild bleeding tendency, correctable by platelet transfusion.

Thrombocytopathy or impaired expression of platelet procoagulant activity, i.e., the acceleration of thrombin formation by the surface of activated platelets, produces a mild bleeding tendency mainly following trauma or surgery.

ACQUIRED DISORDERS OF PLATELET FUNCTION

Aspirin and other nonsteroidal anti-inflammatory drugs inhibit platelet cyclooxygenase, the key enzyme in transformation of platelet arachidonic acid to products that induce platelet aggregation, the cyclic endoperoxides and thromboxane A_2. These substances mediate the normal platelet release reaction initiated by platelet agonists such as ADP, epinephrine, or collagen. After contact with aspirin or similar drugs, platelets exhibit impaired aggregation and release, the bleeding time is moderately prolonged, and the number of microaggregates of platelets detectable in the blood is diminished. The duration of these platelet effects of the nonsteroidal anti-inflammatory drugs varies widely. Only aspirin, by virtue of covalent acetylation of cyclooxygenase at its active site, has a prolonged effect on platelet function (since platelets do not synthesize enzymes as they circulate, one dose of aspirin inhibits platelet function for up to a week); other nonsteroidal anti-inflammatory drugs have antiplatelet effects lasting less than 24 hours. Thrombin-induced platelet activation is unaffected by aspirin or similar drugs, accounting for the limited hemorrhagic tendency produced by these agents. However, when a second defect of hemostasis exists, such as hemophilia, thrombocytopenia, or anticoagulant therapy, ingestion of aspirin may lead to serious bleeding.

Acquired defects in platelet function can accompany several types of systemic diseases. *Uremia* produces a hemorrhagic tendency with epistaxes, ecchymosis, and gastrointestinal bleeding related to platelet dysfunction and often to thrombocytopenia. Platelet aggregation and platelet procoagulant activity are both abnormal and the bleeding time is prolonged. Accumulation of toxic metabolites in the plasma may be partly responsible for these dysfunctions, as may be an inadequate synthesis of thromboxane. Hemodialysis tends to improve platelet function. Infusion of cryoprecipitate, des-arginine vasopressin (DDAVP) or administration of estrogens has been reported to correct the hemostatic abnormalities. *Paraproteinemias* such as *multiple myeloma* can induce bleeding by coating the platelet surface with monoclonal immunoglobulin, which prevents platelet-platelet interaction, and by interfering with fibrin polymerization. In *leukemias* and *myeloproliferative syndromes*, defects in platelet function are common. In DIC, the presence of fibrin split products in the circulating blood also can impair platelet function (Table 53–6).

Laboratory findings distinguish *vascular purpuras* from purpuras directly involving the components of the hemostatic mechanism. The typical findings in vascular purpura include an abnormal tourniquet test (positive Rumpel-Leede test), indicating increased capillary fragility, and prolonged bleeding time in the presence of a normal platelet count, normal platelet function, and normal coagulation screen. Congenital vascular purpura is found in inherited diseases of connective tissue. Acquired vascular purpura can occur in paraproteinemias, scurvy, Cushing's disease, or corticosteroid treatment, in association with other drugs, or in old age. In children, *Henoch-Schönlein purpura* is an allergic-type vasculitis manifested by abdominal pain, hematuria and glomerulonephritis, hemorrhagic urticaria, and arthralgias.

Bleeding in *hereditary hemorrhagic telangiectasia* (Osler-Weber-Rendu disease) results from fragile, easily bleeding mucosal telangiectases. This disorder is inherited as an autosomal dominant trait in which the vascular abnormalities continue to form throughout life, becoming more prominent after puberty. All mucosal surfaces may be involved, with bleeding commonly originating from the nose and from the respiratory, gastrointestinal, and genitourinary tracts. Pulmonary arteriovenous fistulas are common (15 per cent). Telangiectases may or may not be present on the skin. The mainstays of treatment are cauterization of accessible lesions, vigorous iron replacement therapy to correct continual blood loss, and efforts at maintaining local hemostasis.

REFERENCES

Bachmann F: Diagnostic approach to mild bleeding disorders. Semin Hematol 17:292, 1980.
Colman RW, Hirsh J, Marder V, Salzman EW (eds): Hemostasis and Thrombosis: Basic Principles and Clinical Practice. 2nd ed. Philadelphia, JB Lippincott Co, 1987, pp 3–17.

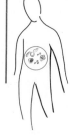

54

COAGULATION DISORDERS

THE BLOOD CLOTTING MECHANISM

Blood clotting involves the generation of a powerful serine protease, thrombin, which cleaves the soluble plasma protein fibrinogen so that an insoluble meshwork of fibrin strands develops, enmeshing red cells and platelets to form a stable clot (Table 54–1). This process is triggered by injury to the blood vessels and involves the rapid, highly controlled interaction of more than 20 different proteins to amplify initial activation of a few molecules to an appropriately sized, fully developed clot (see Fig. 53–1). Both the injured vessel wall and platelet aggregates provide specialized surfaces that localize and catalyze the coagulation reactions.

Blood coagulation proteins circulate as inactive zymogens in amounts far greater than required for blood clotting. Two activation pathways are recognized: an intrinsic pathway and an extrinsic pathway; the latter requires participation of a lipoprotein activity released from injured tissues: tissue factor (Fig. 54–1).

TABLE 54–1. BLOOD COAGULATION FACTORS

GROUP	HALF-LIFE (hours)	COMMENTS
Contact Factors		
XII (Hageman)	50	Deficiency does not produce bleeding tendency
XI	60	Do not require Ca^{++} to act
Prekallikrein		
High molecular weight kininogen		Do not require Vitamin K
		Stable, well preserved in plasma
Prothrombin Group		
II (prothrombin)	72	All vitamin K–dependent
VII	3–5	Require Ca^{++} for activity
IX (Christmas factor)	24	Not consumed in serum (except prothrombin)
X	40	Stable
Protein C		
Protein S		
Fibrinogen Group		
I (fibrinogen)	72–96	All interact with thrombin
V	15–30	Activity is lost on clotting
VIII	3–6	Increase in inflammation, pregnancy, birth control pill
XIII	>100	V, VIII unstable in stored plasma

These pathways converge in the activation of Factor X at the platelet surface. Most of the blood coagulation proteins are serine proteases that show a high degree of homology; others are cofactors without enzyme activity (Factors V and VIII).

The *intrinsic pathway of coagulation* begins by activation of Factor XII upon the altered vascular surface (endothelium, subendothelium) or another negatively charged surface such as glass. Cofactors or promoters of Factor XII activation include prekallikrein, high molecular weight kininogen (HMWK), and Factor XI. A surface-localized complex is formed which optimally activates Factor XII. Factor XIIa then converts complex-bound Factor XI to its active form XIa and prekallikrein to its active form, kallikrein, which then cleaves HMWK to form bradykinin. In turn, Factor XIa activates Factor IX but may also activate Factor VII (in the extrinsic coagulation pathway) as well as cleaving plasminogen to form plasmin, thus initiating fibrinolysis as well as coagulation.

Factor XIa requires calcium ions (Ca^{++}) to activate Factor IX, which binds to Factor VIII (antihemophilic factor). In the presence of Ca^{++} and phospholipid, IXa activates Factor X to Xa. This activation usually takes place at the plasma membrane of stimulated platelets but also may occur on the vascular endothelium.

In the *extrinsic pathway*, the release of tissue factor from injured tissues directly activates Factors VII, which then activates Factor X to Xa in the presence of Ca^{++}. In addition, the complex tissue factor–Factor VIII–Ca^{++} can activate Factor IX.

Assembly of the plasma prothrombinase complex on the surface of activated platelets in the presence of Factor V, another cofactor specifically bound to the platelet membrane, enhances the efficiency of prothrombin (Factor II) activation to thrombin on the platelet surface. Thrombin cleaves fibrinogen, a large, asymmetric, soluble protein (MW 340,000) consisting of three pairs of polypeptide chains: Aα, Bβ, and G. Thrombin first removes small peptides from the Aα chain of fibrinogen to form Fibrin I, which polymerizes end to end; further thrombin cleavage of small peptides from the Bβ chain leads to formation of Fibrin II molecules, which polymerize side to side and are then cross-linked via the plasma glutaminase (Factor XIII) to form an insoluble fibrin clot.

Thrombin has several different and critical actions during coagulation in addition to the cleavage of fibrinogen to fibrin. It activates platelets, exposing their procoagulant activity (e.g., binding sites for the prothrombinase complex) and inducing the release of platelet-aggregating substances such as thromboxane, Ca^{++}, ADP, von Willebrand factor, fibronectin, and thrombospondin. Thrombin cleaves Factors VIII and Va, augmenting clotting, and Factor XIII, promoting fibrin stabilization. Thrombin acts on the endothelium by binding to the surface protein thrombomo-

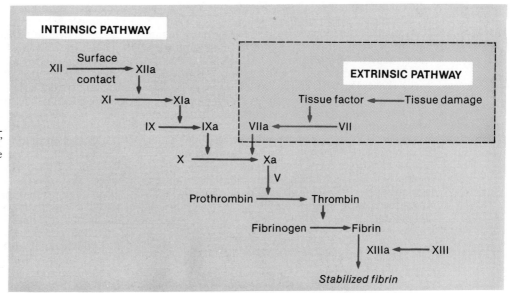

INTRINSIC PATHWAY

EXTRINSIC PATHWAY

FIGURE 54–1. Simplified pathways of blood coagulation. (The "a" denotes the activated form of the circulating inactive zymogen.)

dulin to activate protein C, a potent inactivator of Factors Va and VIIIa which also stimulate fibrinolysis. Thrombin also causes endothelial cell contraction. Conversely, endothelium can bind and inactivate thrombin, and in some cases can generate the vasodilatory substance prostacyclin in response to thrombin. Thus, thrombin activation contributes to the limitation as well as the initiation of clotting.

The final stage of the coagulation process is fibrinolysis, or clot resolution (Fig. 54–2). This process is initiated by the action of thrombin during clotting, including activation of protein C and the initiation of release of plasminogen activators from the blood vessel wall. Protein C, together with protein S, a promoter of its action, inhibits the coagulant activity of Factors Va and VIIIa. The circulating zymogen, plasminogen, is cleaved to the active protease, plasmin, by plasminogen activators. Plasmin then digests fibrin. The activity of tissue plasminogen activators is enhanced by their binding to fibrin, so that plasmin generation is localized to the clot. In addition the plasma protease inhibitors α_1-antitrypsin, α_2-plasmin inhibitor, and α_2-macroglobulin rapidly inactivate any circulating serine protease including thrombin and plasmin. Antithrombin III binds all the serine protease procoagulant proteins (Factor Xa as well as thrombin); its activity is enhanced by heparin or heparin-like substances. Complexes of antithrombin III and protease are rapidly cleared by the liver and the reticuloendothelial system.

The liver is the site of synthesis for most of the coagulation proteins. Factors II, VII, IX, and X and proteins C and S require vitamin K for their synthesis. In the absence of vitamin K, abnormal molecules lacking the γ-carboxyglutamate binding sites for Ca^{++} binding are produced. These abnormal molecules do not function in clotting. Fibrinogen, Factor V, and the protease inhibitors are also produced in the liver, and their levels may be depressed in liver disease. Vitamin

K is not required for their synthesis or function. Factor VIII is probably synthesized in the liver, but the precise location of its production is not known. Von Willebrand factor and tissue plasminogen activator are produced in the vascular endothelium. While von Willebrand factor and Factor VIII circulate together as a macromolecular complex, they are produced in different sites, are regulated by different genes, and are completely different in structure and function.

DISORDERS OF BLOOD COAGULATION: THE PATIENT WHO BLEEDS

A history of bleeding upon trauma or surgery, severe epistaxes, muscle or joint bleeding, or large ecchymoses arouse suspicion of a coagulation disorder. A family history of only affected males points to one of the hemophilias, whereas the other congenital coagulation disorders are transmitted as autosomal recessive traits. The most important screening tests are the prothrombin time and activated partial thromboplastin time (see Table 53–3); the bleeding time is generally

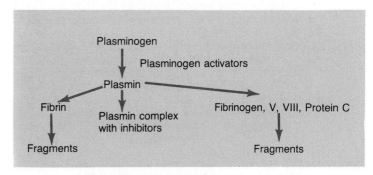

FIGURE 54–2. Fibrinolysis.

normal in plasma coagulation disorders except for von Willebrand's disease, in which the deficient factor affects platelet function, and therefore primary hemostasis is also impaired. The prothrombin time measures activity of Factors II, VII, IX, and X; the activated partial thromboplastin time measures Factors XII, XI, IX, VIII, and X. Both tests measure Factors V and II and fibrinogen. A history of delayed bleeding or rebleeding suggests Factor XIII deficiency, which requires specific testing of the stability of the fibrin clot (e.g., in 8M urea) for detection. The pattern of abnormalities and the ability of normal plasma or serum to correct them permits more specific identification of factor deficiencies or circulatory anticoagulants. Specific factor assays are available for confirmation and quantification of the various deficiencies.

INHERITED DISORDERS OF BLOOD COAGULATION

Hemophilia A

Classic hemophilia is the most common severe, inherited coagulation disorder. The gene for Factor VIII has recently been cloned and sequenced. It is an unusually large gene occupying 0.1 per cent of the length of the X chromosome. In 70 per cent of cases of hemophilia A a positive family history of affected males is obtained; the gene appears to have a high rate of spontaneous mutation, accounting for the remaining 30 per cent of cases. Because of the random inactivation of one X chromosome in females, the carrier mother of a hemophiliac has a 50 per cent (on the average) level of Factor VIII. Identification of the carrier state can frequently be made. Prenatal diagnosis can now be carried out in pregnancies at risk, and development of restriction polymorphism techniques for identifying hemophilic fetuses is now possible since the Factor VIII gene has been cloned. Laboratory results in hemophilia A show a normal PT, markedly prolonged APTT corrected by mixing with normal plasma, and a normal bleeding time. Specific assay for Factor VIII shows a deficient level of functional activity. Hemophilia A can represent both a quantitative deficiency and a dysfunctional molecule, so that both functional and immunological assays need to be combined. About half of affected patients have severe hemophilia with Factor VIII activity less than 1 per cent of normal; they have spontaneous and trauma-induced hemorrhage from infancy. Levels above 5 per cent are associated with a mild clinical course except with trauma or surgery, when supportive therapy is necessary. As the hemophilic child becomes physically active, bleeding into muscles and joints is common, and painful deformities follow. Bleeding is frequently spontaneous or may be related to stress or other illness. Any organ can be affected, and pressure on vital structures from deep hemorrhages can be life-threatening.

Replacement therapy with concentrates of Factor VIII to raise the plasma Factor VIII to hemostatic levels has become a mainstay of treatment. In home therapy programs, the hemophilic patient or his parent administers Factor VIII concentrate according to a preset schedule based on bleeding severity. This approach prevents delay in treatment following onset of bleeding and can reduce morbidity, cost of therapy, and emotional stress. Reconstructive joint surgery and dental care can also be undertaken with such replacement coverage. A high incidence of hepatitis, however, has accompanied extensive use of commercial Factor VIII concentrates. Moreover, transmission of AIDS to hemophilic patients receiving replacement therapy with Factor VIII concentrates (presumably carrying HLTV-3 virus) became common in the early 1980's. Improved testing for HIV in the blood and the availability of heat-inactivated and recombinant Factor VIII preparations have now greatly reduced or eliminated this danger.

Factor VIII has a short half-life (8 to 12 hours); infusion schedules are calculated according to the patient's plasma volume (40 ml/kg), the severity of the bleeding episode, and the per cent of normal Factor VIII level desired to control each type of bleeding. About 20 per cent of patients develop inhibitors to transfused Factor VIII and have accelerated destruction and decreased efficacy of the replacement therapy. Such inhibitory activity must also be taken into account when calculating Factor VIII replacement needs.

For milder hemophiliacs or during episodes of less severe hemorrhage, cryoprecipitate may suffice. Epsilon-aminocaproic acid, a potent inhibitor of fibrinolysis, diminishes bleeding after dental procedures. In addition to replacement of Factor VIII, local therapy such as joint immobilization and ice packs is helpful. For relief of pain, hemophiliacs should avoid aspirin and nonsteroidal anti-inflammatory drugs, which impair platelet function and worsen bleeding. Acetaminophen, codeine, or choline-magnesium salicylate should be used, as these analgesics do not affect platelets and thus preserve primary hemostasis.

The long-term complications of hemophilia include (1) hemorrhage; (2) progressive arthropathy; (3) development of inhibitor to Factor VIII; (4) hepatitis; (5) hypertension; and (6) AIDS. While in recent years the lifespan of hemophiliacs has markedly increased and morbidity lessened, hemorrhage still remains the major cause of death.

Von Willebrand's Disease (VWD)

This is one of the most common inherited bleeding disorders. It affects both sexes and is transmitted as an autosomal codominant or recessive trait. A double defect is observed in this disorder: abnormal platelet adhesion in combination with low Factor VIII procoagulant activity. Normal platelet adhesion to vascular subendothelium requires the presence of the plasma glycoprotein, von Willebrand factor (VWF). VWF circulates in the form of high molecular weight multimers (MW $>2 \times 10^6$) complexed with antihemophilic factor (Factor VIII:AHF). In VWD the level of VWF is decreased, absent, or present in a functionally abnormal form. The level of antihemophilic

TABLE 54–2. COMPARISON OF HEMOPHILIA A, HEMOPHILIA B, AND VON WILLEBRAND'S DISEASE

	HEMOPHILIA A	HEMOPHILIA B	VON WILLEBRAND'S DISEASE
Inheritance	X-linked	X-linked	autosomal dominant or recessive
Factor deficiency	VIII (coagulant) (= VIII:AHF)	IX	von Willebrand's factor and VIII:AHF
Bleeding sites	muscle, joints, surgical	muscle, joints, surgical	mucous membranes, skin, surgical
Prothrombin time (PT)	normal	normal	normal
Partial thromboplastin time (APTT)	prolonged	prolonged	prolonged or normal
Bleeding time	normal	normal	prolonged
Factor VIII coagulant activity	low	normal	low
Factor VIII antigen (VIII:VWF)	normal	normal	low
Factor IX	normal	low	normal
Platelet aggregation	normal	normal	normal
Ristocetin-induced platelet agglutination	normal	normal	impaired

factor may be mildly to severely depressed in VWD. This finding is reflected in the prolonged APTT in addition to the prolonged bleeding time (Table 54–2).

The clinical manifestations of VWD vary widely in the same patient at different times, in different affected members of the same family, and in different families. Mucosal bleeding, ecchymoses, epistaxis, gastrointestinal bleeding, and menorrhagia are common symptoms; severely affected persons may also have hemarthroses and behave like hemophiliacs, with the added complication of defective primary hemostasis. There are several subtypes of von Willebrand's disease. In 75 per cent of patients the bleeding time and APTT are prolonged, with an absolute decrease in the levels of both VWF and Factor VIII:AHF as measured by functional and immunological tests (Type I). Platelet agglutination to ristocetin is impaired but is restored by VWF or normal plasma. Other platelet aggregation responses are normal. All sizes of VWF multimers in plasma are decreased. Infusion of normal plasma (or hemophilic plasma) to Type I VWD patients results in a prolonged rise in VWF levels that is greater and longer lasting than expected from the amount of VWF infused or its half-life. Several variant types of VWD occur in which VWF is only slightly depressed by immunoassay despite a long bleeding time (Type IIA) or in which increased agglutination of platelets by ristocetin is observed and the large multimeric forms of plasma VWF are absent (Type IIB).

Treatment of von Willebrand's disease relies upon cryoprecipitate infusion for severe bleeding episodes and desmopressin for milder disease. The prolonged bleeding time and hemorrhagic diathesis are corrected by transfusion of normal plasma or cryoprecipitate (which is rich in VWF). In mild VWD, infusion of desmopressin (DDAVP, des-amino, des-argininine vasopressin) can raise VWF levels and correct the bleeding tendency. Desmopressin can be used before dental or other surgery in many cases. Most commercial Factor VIII concentrates contain low levels of VWF and are not effective therapy in VWD. In women with severe VWD, menorrhagia can be managed by hormonal suppression. The bleeding tendency may improve during pregnancy when the levels of VWF and

antihemophilic factor rise. Aspirin and similar drugs should be completely avoided by patients with VWD.

INHERITED DISORDERS OF OTHER COAGULATION FACTORS

Contact Factor Defects

Contact factor defects are rare disorders that produce prolongation of the APTT or clotting time without any clinical bleeding tendency, except for Factor XI deficiency. *Factor XII (Hageman factor) deficiency* is suspected when the clotting time or APTT is prolonged in an asymptomatic patient. This diagnosis is confirmed by mixing experiments, in which the patient's plasma is mixed with plasma from patients with known specific factor deficiencies to determine the type of defect (e.g., in Factor XII deficiency there is no correction of APTT upon mixing with known Factor XII deficient plasma, but the APTT becomes normal after mixing 1:1 with known Factor XI deficient plasma). *Prekallikrein deficiency (Fletcher trait)* and *high molecular weight kininogen deficiency (Fitzgerald trait)* are also asymptomatic, rare conditions. A bleeding tendency, however, does exist in persons with *Factor XI (or PTA) deficiency* when they undergo trauma, dental extraction, or surgery. This autosomal recessive trait is most common in persons of Jewish or Japanese origin. The APTT is prolonged, the PT normal. The bleeding tendency does not correlate well with the calculated deficiency of Factor XI, and some patients with low values have no bleeding problems. The half-life of Factor XI is about three days, so that treatment of bleeding or prophylaxis for surgery consists of daily infusion of fresh frozen plasma.

Defects in Vitamin K–Dependent Coagulation Factors

Defects of the vitamin K–dependent coagulation factors cause severe bleeding tendencies. The only common example is *Factor IX deficiency (hemophilia*

B, or Christmas disease), an X-linked recessive trait that is clinically similar to hemophilia A, producing muscle, joint, gastrointestinal, and central nervous system bleeding. A quantitative severe deficiency of Factor IX is the usual finding, but some families possess a functionally abnormal Factor IX molecule present in the blood in normal levels when measured by antigenic assay. Diagnosis of hemophilia B is suspected when a normal PT but prolonged APTT is observed and the APTT is corrected by normal serum but not by barium-adsorbed plasma (BaSO₄ adsorbs the vitamin K–dependent factors from plasma). The diagnosis is confirmed by specific factor assay. Fresh frozen plasma or prothrombin complex concentrates containing Factor IX correct the deficiency and are used to treat bleeding. The plasma half-life of 20 hours permits twice-daily infusion. Factor IX concentrates carry a high risk of transmitting hepatitis and are contaminated with activated coagulation factors. The latter can cause thromboembolism, so that use of prothrombin complex concentrates should be reserved for severe hemorrhage. Specific antibodies to transfused Factor IX develop in 10 to 15 per cent of patients and may complicate management, similarly to acquired Factor VIII inhibitors in hemophilia A.

Factor VII deficiency is a rare autosomal recessive defect, leading to a lifelong history of bleeding in homozygotes: mucous membrane and gastrointestinal bleeding, epistaxes, hemarthroses, and menorrhagia are observed. Individual patients show varied manifestations of bleeding over time. The PT is prolonged with a normal APTT. Since Factor VII is stable, the prolonged PT is corrected by stored plasma but not by BaSO₄-adsorbed plasma. Treatment is with plasma or prothrombin complex concentrates; the half-life of Factor VII is short (two to six hours), requiring frequent administration.

Factor X deficiency is another rare autosomal recessive trait that produces bleeding. Two types exist, a quantitative decrease in the factor or a dysfunctional molecule. Epistaxis, gastrointestinal bleeding, and occasionally joint or muscle hemorrhage result. Postpartum bleeding and menorrhagia may be severe in affected women. Both the PT and the APTT are prolonged; a specific factor assay establishes the diagnosis. Treatment is with fresh frozen plasma.

Afibrinogenemia or *congenital dysfibrinogenemia* represents a variety of disorders in which the plasma fibrinogen level is very low or abnormal fibrinogens are produced. The latter may lead to either hemorrhage or thrombosis. Both the PT and the APTT are abnormal in these disorders. Over 80 different types of dysfibrinogenemia have been described, varying widely in clinical effects. Current replacement therapy consists of cryoprecipitate, which is rich in fibrinogen, since formerly available fibrinogen concentrates carried a very high risk of transmitting hepatitis. The half-life of fibrinogen is four days, so that infusion to reach a normal plasma level of 150 mg/dl can be readily achieved.

Factor XIII deficiency is a rare, autosomal recessive trait in which only the homozygote shows a bleeding tendency, manifested by delayed bleeding after trauma and impaired wound healing. Affected persons usually have less than 1 per cent of the normal Factor XIII level; heterozygotes are asymptomatic. Absence of the fibrin-stabilizing factor also impairs cross-linking of fibronectin, the cell surface protein, and fibrin, which may contribute to poor wound healing. Since the initial formation of fibrin is unimpaired, PT, APTT, and thrombin time are normal. Dissolution of the patient's fibrin clot in 8M urea indicates a Factor XIII level of less than 1 per cent. Treatment is with fresh frozen plasma or cryoprecipitate to reach a Factor XIII level of 10 per cent. The prolonged half-life of the factor (21 days) makes infrequent replacement infusions (every three weeks) effective.

ACQUIRED DISORDERS OF BLOOD COAGULATION

Acquired coagulation abnormalities can result from several causes, including deficient production or increased consumption of clotting factors, production of functionally abnormal molecules, selective inhibition of factors by acquired anticoagulants, and selective inhibition or adsorption of factors, resulting in functional deficiency. The first three mechanisms are common complications of systemic disease, the last two are rare. For example, the adsorption of Factor X by vascular amyloid, producing a severe bleeding diathesis, has been reported in only a few cases.

Acquired Vitamin K Deficiency

Vitamin K–dependent clotting factors are a group of structurally closely related proteins synthesized in the liver, including prothrombin, Factors VII, IX, and X, and proteins C and S. Vitamin K is required for the post-translational gamma carboxylation of glutamyl residues at the amino terminal regions of these clotting factor zymogens, resulting in formation of calcium-binding sites important for normal hemostatic function. Calcium is required for the binding and activation of these factors from zymogen to active serine proteases on the surface of platelets. Vitamin K deficiency prevents the carboxylation of the glutamyl residues and results in functionally abnormal clotting factors. Because of its short half-life, Factor VII activity is the earliest to decrease in vitamin K deficiency or anticoagulation with vitamin K antagonists, followed by decreases in Factors IX and X and prothrombin.

As vitamin K is not stored in the body but is obtained from green vegetables in the diet and is a fat-soluble vitamin, a deficiency of vitamin K occurs in malabsorption or bile-salt deficiency, when dietary intake is poor, and when the gastrointestinal tract is sterilized by antibiotic therapy. Common clinical states producing vitamin K deficiency include (1) in newborn infants, especially premature infants, liver immaturity and lack of synthesis of vitamin K by intestinal bacteria until the gut is colonized; (2) malabsorption, including biliary tract disease; (3) prolonged parenteral feeding in combination with antibiotic therapy, especially bowel sterilization; and (4) ingestion of oral antico-agulants. Vitamin K absorption depends upon fat absorption, and any condition impairing that process (e.g., celiac disease, oral neomycin, cholestyramine, biliary obstruction, regional enteritis) can result in vitamin K deficiency. Mucosal or gastrointestinal bleeding may develop. Oral administration of vitamin K_1 (2 to 10 mg/day) can correct the vitamin deficiency, and 10 to 25 mg IM can correct an overt bleeding tendency.

Coumarin anticoagulants competitively inhibit the effects of vitamin K on gamma carboxylation of the vitamin K–dependent coagulation proteins and thus produce anticoagulation, which is monitored by the PT. The therapeutic goal is to maintain a PT 1.5 to 2 times greater than a normal control, achieved by administering 2.5 to 10 mg of Coumadin (warfarin) once daily. Since many drugs affect the action of coumarins, either directly enhancing or depressing their effect or altering their metabolic disposition, it is essential to monitor coumarin effects carefully during treatment with multiple drugs. Coumarin drugs possess a narrow toxic/therapeutic ratio. Administration of vitamin K can reverse the effects of coumadin anticoagulation within hours, and administration of fresh frozen plasma (or prothrombin concentrates) reverses anticoagulant effects even more rapidly. In emergency circumstances, such as with brain hemorrhage, severe gastrointestinal bleeding, or need for immediate surgery, anticoagulation can be reversed within minutes by Factor IX concentrates or prothrombin complex.

Liver Disease

In addition to the vitamin K–dependent coagulation factors, the liver synthesizes Factor V, fibrinogen, plasminogen, and Factors XII and XI. Patients with advanced liver disease commonly suffer bleeding tendencies. If these mainly involve deficiencies of vitamin K–dependent clotting factors, they are corrected by administering parenteral vitamin K. Bleeding in severe liver disease also results from dysfibrinogenemias, localized DIC, lack of Factor V, increased fibrinolysis, and thrombocytopenia. Treatment of these deficiencies employs fresh frozen plasma.

Renal Disease

Uremia is associated with mucous membrane, gastrointestinal, and skin bleeding. The cause of the bleeding tendency is complex. Thrombocytopenia may be present as part of depressed bone marrow function or may arise secondary to immunosuppressive drugs. Platelet dysfunction is typical and represents thrombocytopathy (impaired platelet procoagulant activity) with depressed platelet adhesion and aggregation, producing a prolonged bleeding time. In the nephrotic syndrome, urinary loss of plasma proteins may result in Factor IX deficiency. In patients undergoing hemodialysis, inaccurate reversal of heparinization at completion of dialysis may also contribute to uremic bleeding.

Disseminated Intravascular Coagulation

DIC represents the consumption of coagulation factors resulting from intravascular activation of the coagulation process with secondary activation of fibrinolysis. Depending upon the rates of these two processes, the compensatory synthesis of procoagulants, and the nature of the underlying disease, DIC may cause either thrombosis or hemorrhage. DIC is always secondary to another disease process and often resolves when the primary disease is controlled. Intravascular coagulation is initiated by release of procoagulant substances into the blood (amniotic fluid embolism, snakebite, abruptio placentae, malignancy, crush injury), by contact of blood with an abnormal surface (infections, burns, extracorporeal circulation, grafts), or by generation of procoagulants in the blood (promyelocytic leukemia, hemolytic transfusion reactions). The formation of microthrombi within the circulation secondarily activates fibrinolysis, as does the presence of injured endothelium. Circulating plasmin may further deplete Factors V and VIII and cleave fibrinogen. The degradation products of both fibrinogen and fibrin (formed by thrombin or plasmin action) act as circulating anticoagulants, delay fibrin polymerization, and impair platelet function.

Common clinical settings for DIC (Table 54–3) include sepsis, obstetric emergencies, burns, and liver disease. Chronic DIC is characteristic of Trousseau's syndrome, widespread visceral malignancy presenting as migrating superficial thrombophlebitis.

The diagnosis of DIC depends upon a pattern of laboratory test results (Table 54–4). No single test is diagnostic. In acute DIC the typical laboratory results include thrombocytopenia, a prolonged PT and PTT, decreased fibrinogen level, decreased Factors V and VIII, and increased fibrin split products. The thrombin time is also elevated because of the anticoagulant action of the fibrin split products. A microangiopathic hemolytic anemia may be present, resulting from shear damage to red cells passing intravascular fibrin strands. In chronic DIC, compensatory increases in synthesis of coagulation factors may produce normal levels of fibrinogen, Factors V and VIII, and platelets, and the PT and PTT may be normal or even short. However, fibrin split products are usually elevated.

TABLE 54–3. CLINICAL SETTINGS FOR DISSEMINATED INTRAVASCULAR COAGULATION

ACUTE	CHRONIC
1. Sepsis	1. Visceral malignancy
2. Obstetric emergencies Abruptio placentae Amniotic fluid embolism	2. Large arteriovenous malformations 3. Toxemia
3. Burns	4. Retained dead fetus
4. Heat stroke	5. Malignant hypertension
5. Shock	6. Severe liver cirrhosis
6. Snakebite	
7. Promyelocytic leukemia	
8. Hemolytic transfusion reactions	

TABLE 54—4. SCREENING LABORATORY TESTS FOR DIC

1. Prolonged prothrombin time
2. Prolonged partial thromboplastin time
3. Low fibrinogen
4. Thrombocytopenia
5. Presence of fibrin degradation products
6. Depressed Factors V and VIII

Microangiopathic hemolytic anemia is more likely to be present in chronic DIC. Localized DIC may occur in the liver in severe cirrhotic liver disease and in the kidney during malignant hypertension.

Therapy of DIC should be aimed at the underlying disease, for example, by treating sepsis in the infected patient or by emptying the uterus in the case of abruptio placentae. If the symptoms of bleeding or thrombosis are mild, no specific therapy is needed. If DIC produces significant bleeding, replacement of depleted clotting factors using fresh frozen plasma, cryoprecipitate, and platelets may be necessary. If thrombosis is the clinical problem, heparinization may be required (provided that the patient does not have central nervous system bleeding, is not hypertensive, and has not undergone surgery within the past few days). Replacement of fibrinogen and of antithrombin III (as plasma) may also be required. Heparin is generally reserved for cases that fail to respond to other measures. Special situations in which heparin is used include meningococcemia, acute promyelocytic leukemia, and Trousseau's syndrome. Oral anticoagulation cannot be substituted for heparin in the treatment of DIC.

Acquired Circulating Anticoagulants

Antibodies to procoagulants occur in hemophiliacs receiving replacement therapy (see above) as well as in states of disturbed immunity such as systemic lupus erythematosus, lymphoproliferative diseases, the postpartum period, and old age. Acquired inhibitors to Factor VIII:AHF can produce severe hemorrhagic disease. Several cases of inhibitors of von Willebrand's factor causing an acquired von Willebrand's disease have been reported in patients with lymphoma. Very rarely, a heparin-like anticoagulant molecule can circulate, producing a bleeding tendency.

In contrast to the above, the "lupus anticoagulant," which is the most common cause of a prolonged APTT in asymptomatic individuals, is rarely associated with a bleeding tendency unless combined with another hemostatic defect, such as thrombocytopenia. Only about half of "lupus anticoagulants" occur in patients with systemic lupus erythematosus. These antibodies are directed against membrane phospholipids or against the phosphodiester bond structure, which is a common chemical moiety in many diverse compounds including DNA, membrane phospholipids, and organic sugars. This circulating anticoagulant is associated with a tendency to thrombosis rather than hemorrhage. Antibodies to cardiolipin, in association with the lupus anticoagulant or alone, may also be associated with acute arterial or venous thrombosis in young adults who have no other predisposing factor. Some of these autoantibodies may alter normal endothelial functions to predispose toward thrombosis. Oral anticoagulation on a chronic basis is the treatment of choice in patients with these autoantibodies once a definite thrombotic episode has appeared.

DISORDERS OF BLOOD COAGULATION: THE PATIENT WHO CLOTS

Many clinical situations can disrupt the hemostatic balance and lead to excess clotting—thromboembolic disease. In order to pinpoint the reason for a prothrombotic or hypercoagulable state and to plan for appropriate therapy, one must consider the physiological pathways of thrombus formation and dissolution (see Chapter 53).

The history of the acute thrombotic event is critical for correct diagnosis and treatment. Is there an obvious systemic or local predisposing reason for a thrombosis? An increased tendency toward thrombosis accompanies surgery, many inflammatory disorders, malignancy, pregnancy, and vascular disorders and occurs following stasis. Inherited thrombotic tendencies, which are much rarer, are being increasingly recognized and include disorders of the protein C–protein S system, deficiencies of antithrombin III (AT III), dysfibrinogenemias, and disorders of the fibrinolytic system (Table 54–5).

Whereas the blood coagulation pathways involve a series of enzymatic activations of serine protease zymogens, down-regulation of blood clotting is influenced by several natural anticoagulant mechanisms, including AT III, the protein C–protein S system, and fibrinolysis. In addition, normal vascular endothelium promotes the activation of these anticoagulant mechanisms by acting as a source of (1) heparin-like substances that enhance AT III activation, (2) thrombomodulin, a cofactor in protein C activation, and (3) tissue plasminogen activators that initiate fibrinolysis.

Primary hypercoagulable states involve defects in the above three systems, in fibrinogen structure, or in abnormalities of endothelial function. The reader should recall that partial deficiencies of the natural anticoagulant systems (i.e., about 50 per cent of normal levels) are associated with excess thrombosis, in contrast to the severe deficiencies of procoagulants (i.e., less than 10 per cent of normal values and often less than 1 per cent) which are necessary to precipitate bleeding disorders.

Evaluation of hypercoagulable risk involves checking family history of thromboembolism, eliciting other systemic predisposing diseases or conditions that favor localized vascular stasis, such as prolonged immobilization, pregnancy or malignancy, and evaluating possible laboratory abnormalities such as thrombocytosis, elevated blood or plasma viscosity, and elevated plasma levels of coagulation factors or fibrin degradation products. The latter, as well as measurement of AT III, protein C, or protein S levels, should be tested judiciously and only when suspicion is high, since such abnormalities are uncommon compared to factors such as stasis or localized injury.

Antithrombin III Deficiency

AT III is a broadly acting inhibitor of serine proteases which blocks not only the potent coagulation enzyme, thrombin, but also other procoagulant proteins such as Factor X. AT III greatly potentiates the anticoagulant effect of heparin, which it binds. Heterozygous deficiency of AT III (levels 25 to 60 per cent of normal) is associated with venous thrombosis developing in young adults under the age of 40. Apparent resistance to heparin may be a clinical clue to this disorder, since AT III is necessary for full heparin efficacy. Inherited AT III deficiency varies clinically even within a single family; both functional and immunological tests may be needed to diagnose the condition, as immunologically reactive but functionally abnormal protein variants occur. Acquired deficiency of AT III can occur in liver disease, nephrotic syndrome (due to urinary loss of the factor), during thrombosis, accompanying disseminated intravascular coagulation, or during cancer chemotherapy with L-asparaginase.

Protein C and Protein S Deficiencies

Both protein C and protein S are vitamin K–dependent proteins that are central to the natural anticoagulant pathway involving activated protein C. This pathway not only inhibits blood coagulation but also stimulates fibrinolysis. In the presence of thrombomodulin on the endothelial surface, thrombin forms a complex in which its procoagulant activity is neutralized and its ability to activate protein C is enhanced. Activated protein C, with protein S as a cofactor, then inactivates Factors V and VIII, thereby blocking generation of more thrombin. Activated protein C also stimulates fibrinolysis, in part by neutralizing a major inhibitor of tissue plasminogen activator.

Familial venous thromboembolism can occur in patients with inherited deficiencies of either protein C or protein S. Heterozygotes with a partial protein C deficiency (autosomal dominant form) may present with thromboembolism as adolescents or young adults. In its autosomal recessive form, however, heterozygotes remain asymptomatic, but homozygous deficiency causes neonatal purpura fulminans, which is rapidly fatal without replacement plasma therapy combined with anticoagulants.

Protein S deficiency also leads to venous thromboembolism in heterozygotes. Here, the plasma level of free protein S is key, since the protein circulates partially bound to a plasma factor, C4b-binding protein, and the bound complex is biologically inactive. During pregnancy both increased plasma binding of protein S and decreased total protein S levels occur; these changes may contribute to the thrombotic tendency observed during pregnancy.

Treatment for protein C or protein S deficiency consists of the chronic use of oral anticoagulants. Because protein C has a short half-life, its level drops quickly after initiation of oral coumarin-type anticoagulants, the result leading to a coumarin-induced skin necrosis (actually a thrombotic necrosis). For this reason, initial therapy for protein C deficiency should include heparinization during the first few days.

TABLE 54–5. UNDERLYING CONSIDERATIONS IN THE PATIENT WHO CLOTS

Acquired Conditions
  Prolonged immobilization
  Obesity
  Medications (e.g., oral anticoagulants)
  DIC (e.g., underlying malignancy, sepsis)
  Myeloproliferative syndrome (e.g., polycythemia vera)
  Circulating anticoagulant (e.g., "lupus anticoagulant")
Inherited Conditions
  Protein C deficiency
  Protein S deficiency
  Antithrombin III deficiency
  Dysfibrinogenemia
  Homocystinuria

ANTITHROMBOTIC THERAPY

Four main types of therapy are used to prevent or treat thrombosis: antiplatelet agents, heparin, vitamin K antagonists, and thrombolytic agents. Each type of agent interferes with clotting at a different site in the coagulation pathway (Table 54–6).

In general, antiplatelet agents are used as prophylaxis against arterial thrombosis, since platelets are more important in initiating arterial than venous thrombi. Anticoagulants are used for both prevention and treatment of arterial and venous thrombosis. Heparin, which prevents the generation of thrombin as well as antagonizes thrombin's action, has an immediate anticoagulant effect; however, it must be administered parenterally. The coumarin anticoagulants prevent the synthesis of active coagulation factors and therefore have a slow onset of anticoagulant effect over several days. They are given orally; once the dose is established for an individual patient, they can provide a steady level of anticoagulation. The most recently developed category of antithrombotic drugs, the fibrinolytic agents, include activators of fibrinolysis (tissue plasminogen activator [TPA]) and fibrinolytic enzymes (streptokinase, urokinase) that directly activate plasmin. The fibrinolytic drugs are used to lyse freshly formed arterial and venous thrombi; fibrinolytic agents are not efficacious in dissolving thrombi that have been present for more than a few hours.

The major risk of antithrombotic therapy is bleeding, observed especially in patients who are predisposed to bleed easily because of a pre-existing defect in the coagulation pathway, such as alcoholism, uremia, thrombocytopenia, or the ingestion of aspirin. In general, the simultaneous use of two different types of these drugs (e.g., aspirin and warfarin) shold be avoided because of increased bleeding risk. Many drugs interact with antithrombotic therapy, and physicians should be aware of all other medications being taken by patients on anticoagulants, since they may either increase the sensitivity to the anticoagulant (e.g., estrogen blocks warfarin-albumin binding and increases effective warfarin levels) or decrease efficacy

TABLE 54–6. ANTICOAGULANT DRUGS

AGENTS	MECHANISM OF ACTION	LENGTH OF EFFECT	LABORATORY MEASUREMENT	ANTIDOTE
Aspirin	Irreversibly inhibits platelet cyclooxygenase	7 days	Bleeding time may be prolonged	Platelet transfusion
Heparin	Accelerates antithrombin III activity to inhibit thrombin generation	2–4 hours	Partial thromboplastin (maintain at 1.5 to 2 times control)	Protamine sulfate
Vitamin K antagonists (e.g., warfarin)	Interfere with hepatic synthesis of Factors II, VII, IX, and X and proteins C and S	~48 hours	Prothrombin time (PT) (maintain at 1.5 to 2 times control)	Vitamin K (reverses PT in 12–36 hours) Fresh frozen plasma (reverses PT immediately for 4–6 hours) Factor II, VII, IX, X concentrate (reverses PT immediately for 4–6 hours)
Thrombolytic agents: streptokinase (SK), urokinase (UK), tissue plasminogen activator (TPA)	Accelerate fibrinolysis	Minutes	SK, UK: thrombin time (should be 2 times control) TPA: no systemic effect	Fresh frozen plasma

(e.g., phenobarbital stimulates metabolism of warfarin).

Indications for Antithrombotic Therapy

Venous Thromboembolism. Although this is a major clinical problem, prophylaxis is not universally applied, because of varying risk and the cost of accurate predictive tests. Low-dose subcutaneous heparin is frequently used as prophylaxis against thromboembolism in surgical patients but is ineffective in those at highest risk, for example, after hip fracture. Warfarin reduces mortality from pulmonary embolism and can be given more safely to immobilized or postsurgical patients in low-dose or step-wise regimens. Once a venous thrombosis has developed, however, full-dose heparinization followed by full-dose warfarin therapy is necessary to prevent clot progression and/or pulmonary embolism. Treatment of pulmonary embolism with thrombolytic agents is promising but has not been sufficiently well evaluated to make it the current treatment of choice. Aspirin offers little value in treating venous thromboembolism and may promote bleeding risks if combined with anticoagulation.

Arterial Thrombosis. Intravenous thrombolytic therapy may act rapidly to re-establish the patency of thrombosed peripheral arteries if administered within a few hours after acute thrombosis. Similarly, thrombolysis is recognized as an important treatment of acute coronary artery thrombosis (see below). Such treatment should be followed by heparin and then oral anticoagulants to prevent further clot promulgation or recurrence, similar to the regimen used in follow-up treatment after surgical embolectomy.

The use of anticoagulants versus aspirin in the management of patients with transient ischemic attacks or threatened or acute stroke is discussed in Chapter 118.

Cardiovascular Disease. Currently recommended prophylaxis against acute myocardial infarction includes aspirin on a daily basis for men; no unequivocal advantage for women has been clearly established. Aspirin also appears to be beneficial in patients with crescendo angina to decrease the incidence of myocardial infarction or sudden death. In patients with a fresh coronary thrombosis, intravenous fibrinolytic therapy (e.g., with tissue plasminogen activator, streptokinase, or urokinase) can permit rapid reperfusion of the thrombosed coronary artery if the fibrinolytic agent is administered within a few hours of the onset of symptoms. Such treatment is immediately followed by anticoagulation, but optimal long-term therapy to prevent restenosis has not been established. Aspirin is not effective in this setting. Streptokinase and TPA have similar efficacy for acute recanalization. At the clinical doses needed, both of these agents cause significant fibrinogenolysis, despite the theoretically greater fibrin specificity of TPA. The systemic loss of fibrinogen and platelet dysfunction caused by the fibrinolytic agents engender a hemorrhagic tendency. Bleeding complications including cerebrovascular bleeding are usually at a low level, depend upon dose of the fibrinolytic agent as well as other therapies, and represent lysis of hemostatic plugs as well as the thrombosis being treated. Much effort is being devoted to the development of more fibrin-specific fibrinolytic drugs in order to diminish the hemorrhagic side effects of this therapy.

Following a myocardial infarction, acute anticoagulation is often given during the early period of patient immobility to prevent venous thromboembolism; "miniheparin" is a common regimen. However, chronic full anticoagulation following a myocardial infarction is no longer recommended (see Chapter 8).

REFERENCES

Marder VJ, Sherry S: Thrombolytic therapy: Current status. N Engl J Med 318:1512, 1585, 1988.
Prevention of venous thrombosis and pulmonary embolism. JAMA 256:744, 1986.

SECTION
VII
ONCOLOGY

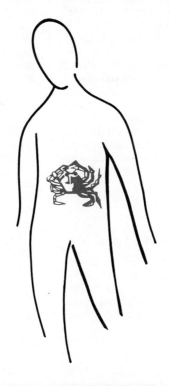

55

GENERAL CONSIDERATIONS

In the United States, cancer accounts for greater than 450,000 deaths annually, a toll second only to that from cardiovascular diseases. Current statistics suggest that approximately 30 per cent of Americans will develop cancer in their lifetime, of whom two thirds will die as a result of their disease. The leading sites of cancer are the lung in males, breast in females, and colorectal region in both sexes (Fig. 55–1). During the past 25 years, cancers of the skin, breast, pancreas, bladder, and testes have increased in incidence, while gastric and invasive cervical cancers have declined. Recently, lung cancer in men has declined in association with a decrease in smoking, but the drop is more than compensated for by an increase in women. Striking geographical differences exist in specific cancer rates. In Japan, for example, gastric and hepatocellular carcinomas are common, while breast and colon carcinomas are relatively rare. Presumably, the differences reflect environmental factors, as Japanese immigrants to the United States display American cancer rates within just one or two generations of residence.

ETIOLOGY

ENVIRONMENTAL CARCINOGENS

Carcinogenic stimuli in the environment include a variety of chemicals, radiation, and viruses (Table 55–1). Environmental carcinogenesis is thought to be a multistage process characterized by multiple exposures, some acting as initiators (true carcinogens) and others as promoters (cocarcinogens).

Although chemical carcinogens have widely diverse chemical structures, common principles govern their induction of carcinogenesis. These include covalent modification of host DNA, dose dependence, lack of a safe dose, and the existence of a lag period between exposure and malignant transformation. Occupational exposure to chemical carcinogens (e.g., asbestos, vinyl chloride) accounts for about 5 per cent of all cancers. Tobacco exposure strongly potentiates the effect of some agents, most notably asbestos, and itself contributes to 25 per cent of all cancer deaths, including cancers of the lung, head and neck, esophagus, and bladder, among others. Smokeless tobacco, increasingly popular among young adults in Southwestern United States, is associated with oropharyngeal carcinoma. Medications form another major category of chemical carcinogens, exemplified by the association of alkylating agents with acute myelogenous leukemia and the maternal ingestion of prenatal diethylstilbestrol with the later development of adenocarcinomas of the vagina and cervix in daughters exposed in utero.

Viruses have been linked to a number of human cancers. Examples include the association of HTLV-1 retrovirus with adult T-cell leukemia/lymphoma, papillomavirus (type 16) with cervical cancer, and hepatitis B with hepatoma.

Evidence derived from animal and epidemiological studies as well as from limited clinical trials suggests that diet plays an important causative and protective role in carcinogenesis. However, data regarding the carcinogenicity of specific dietary factors are largely inconclusive. Possible associations include high dietary fat intake with colon cancer and aflatoxin with liver cancer. Protective roles have been postulated for micronutrients and trace metals such as selenium, carotene, vitamins E and C, and calcium.

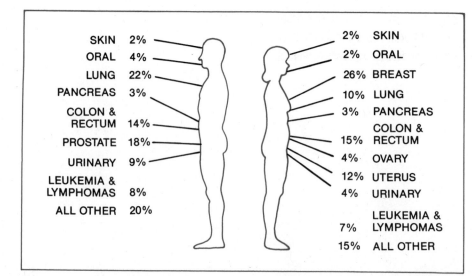

SKIN	2%	
ORAL	4%	
LUNG	22%	
PANCREAS	3%	
COLON & RECTUM	14%	
PROSTATE	18%	
URINARY	9%	
LEUKEMIA & LYMPHOMAS	8%	
ALL OTHER	20%	

2%	SKIN
2%	ORAL
26%	BREAST
10%	LUNG
3%	PANCREAS
15%	COLON & RECTUM
4%	OVARY
12%	UTERUS
4%	URINARY
7%	LEUKEMIA & LYMPHOMAS
15%	ALL OTHER

FIGURE 55–1. Estimated cancer incidence by site and sex, excluding nonmelanoma skin cancer and carcinoma in situ. The estimates of the incidence of cancer are based on data from the National Cancer Institute's Surveillance, Epidemiology and End Results (SEER) Program (1973–1979).

Radiation-induced carcinogenesis has been observed in atomic bomb survivors, patients receiving therapeutic irradiation for Hodgkin's disease and phosphorus-32 for polycythemia vera, children exposed to x-rays prenatally, and patients irradiated in the distant past for nonmalignant conditions such as thymus enlargement. Radiation exerts its carcinogenic effects in a dose-dependent manner and spares no organ, although bone marrow, breast, and thyroid are the most radiosensitive. The time lag varies: radiation-induced leukemia makes its advent at two to five years and peaks at six to eight years, whereas solid tumors develop after a latency period of at least five to ten years. Experts estimate that natural background irradiation (i.e., cosmic rays, radium, and other radionucleotides in the earth's crust) causes less than 2 per cent of all cancers. Exposure to ultraviolet irradiation, however, is the major risk factor for the development of melanoma and nonmelanoma skin cancers.

GENETIC SUSCEPTIBILITY

More than 200 single gene disorders have been linked to the development of neoplasms. Certain genes create a greater than 90 per cent risk of developing cancer (hereditary retinoblastoma, familial polyposis coli). Table 55–2 lists some hereditary neoplasms and preneoplastic syndromes. Most cancers demonstrate a minor familial component (two- to three-fold excess risk), exceptions being early and multifocal breast and colon cancers, in which familial risks increase to 20 to 30 times that of the general population. Appropriate management of hereditary cancers includes avoidance of environmental carcinogens (e.g., ultraviolet light in the dysplastic nevus syndrome), prophylactic treatment (e.g., colectomy in polyposis coli), early detection (e.g., thyrocalcitonin determinations in multiple endocrine neoplasia), and genetic counseling (e.g., retinoblastoma).

ONCOGENES

Recently, molecular biologists have discovered a class of genes termed proto-oncogenes which are highly conserved in vertebrate evolution and which may provide the substrate upon which the multitude of carcinogenic stimuli play. Over 20 proto-oncogenes have already been identified. They are normal constitutents of all cells and appear to be critically important in the regulation of normal cellular growth and differentiation. The products of proto-oncogenes assume specific cellular locations and can be divided into distinct functional families (Table 55–3). They include a growth factor and several growth factor receptors.

The conversion of a proto-oncogene, a vital normal cellular constituent, to an oncogene capable of transforming cells results from a mutation within the protooncogene or abnormal expression of the proto-oncogene. Chronic myelogenous leukemia (CML) exemplifies a malignancy characterized by a consistent and specific translocation of a proto-oncogene, c-abl, whose altered expression contributes to the pathogen-

TABLE 55–1. SOME ENVIRONMENTAL CAUSES OF CANCER

AGENT	SITE
Alcoholic beverages	Mouth, pharynx, esophagus, larynx, liver
Alkylating agents	Leukemia
Androgen-anabolic steroids	Liver
Aromatic amines	Bladder
Arsenic (inorganic)	Lung, skin, liver (angiosarcoma)
Asbestos	Lung, pleura, peritoneum, gastrointestinal
Benzene	Leukemia
Estrogens	
Synthetic (DES)	Vagina, cervix (adenocarcinoma)
Conjugated (Premarin)	Endometrium
Steroid contraceptives	Liver (benign)
Immunosuppressives	Histiocytic lymphoma, squamous carcinoma of skin, soft tissue sarcomas
Ionizing radiation	Nearly all sites
Mustard gas	Lung, larynx, nasal sinuses
Nickel dust	Lung, nasal sinuses
Phenacetin	Renal pelvis
Polycyclic hydrocarbons	Lung, squamous carcinoma of skin
Tobacco products	Mouth, lung, larynx, pharynx, esophagus, bladder, pancreas, kidney
Ultraviolet radiation	Skin (including melanoma)
Vinyl chloride	Liver (angiosarcoma)
Wood dusts	Nasal sinuses

Adapted from Fraumeni JF Jr: Epidemiology of cancer. In Wyngaarden JB, Smith LH Jr (eds): Cecil Textbook of Medicine. 18th ed. Philadelphia, WB Saunders Co, 1988, p 1093.

esis of the disease. The Philadelphia chromosome, resulting from a reciprocal translocation involving the long arms of chromosomes 9 and 22 (Fig. 55–2), exists in the hematopoietic cells of nearly all patients with CML. The c-abl proto-oncogene is localized to chromosome 9 near the breakpoint and is invariably trans-

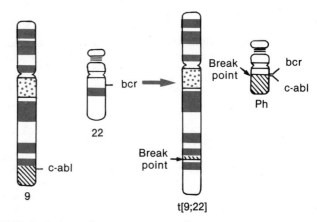

FIGURE 55–2. Reciprocal translocation resulting in the formation of the Ph chromosome pathognomonic of CML. The c-abl proto-oncogene on chromosome 9 is translocated to the breakpoint cluster region (bcr) on chromosome 22. A new bcr:abl fusion gene is created on the Ph chromosome which encodes a fusion protein, p210, likely to be important in the pathogenesis of CML. (Adapted from Champlin RE, Golde DW: Chronic myelogenous leukemia: Recent advances. Blood 65:1039, 1985.)

TABLE 55–2. SOME HEREDITARY NEOPLASMS AND PRENEOPLASTIC SYNDROMES

	INHERITANCE*	CLINICAL FEATURES
Hereditary Neoplasms		
Retinoblastoma	AD	Susceptibility to other cancers, particularly osteosarcoma; deletion in long arm of chromosome 13 in some cases
Multiple endocrine neoplasia I	AD	Adrenal, pancreatic, pituitary, parathyroid tumors; carcinoid tumors
Multiple endocrine neoplasia II	AD	Medullary thyroid carcinoma, pheochromocytoma; parathyroid tumors and neurofibromas in some
Polyposis coli	AD	Multiple adenomatous polyps; adenocarcinoma of large bowel
Dysplastic nevus syndrome	AD	Hereditary melanomas derived from nevi
Hereditary Preneoplastic Syndromes		
Neurofibromatosis	AD	Multiple neurofibromas; café au lait spots; some develop neurofibrosarcomas, gliomas, acoustic neuromas, leukemias
Xeroderma pigmentosum	AR	Skin cancers; defective repair of DNA damaged by UV light
Bloom's syndrome; Fanconi's anemia	AR	Acute leukemia; other malignancies; associated with chromosomal instability
X-linked lymphoproliferative syndrome	XR	Immunoblastic sarcoma; B cell lymphoma; associated with abnormal immune response to EBV

* AD = Autosomal dominant; AR = autosomal recessive; XR = X-linked recessive.

Adapted from Fraumeni JF Jr: Epidemiology of cancer. *In* Wyngaarden JB, Smith LH Jr (eds): Cecil Textbook of Medicine. 18th ed. Philadelphia, WB Saunders Co, pp 1095–1096.

located to chromosome 22, with the breakpoint on 22 occurring in a tightly restricted region called the "breakpoint cluster region (bcr)." The resulting bcr:c-abl fusion gene encodes a chimeric fusion protein, p210 (i.e., molecular weight of 210 Kd). Unlike the native c-abl gene product, p145, the fusion protein, p210, undergoes autophosphorylation of its tyrosine residues and possesses potent tyrosine kinase activity that may be fundamental to the pathogenesis of CML.

The cells of several human malignancies, including bladder cancer and acute myelogenous leukemia, contain ras oncogenes that result from point mutations in normal ras genes. Ras genes normally encode GTP binding proteins (Table 55–3); the mutated ras pro-

teins contain single amino acid substitutions and are capable of neoplastic transformation.

Amplification of proto-oncogene sequences has been detected in some tumors, e.g., N-myc in neuroblastoma and neu in breast cancer. In these cancers proto-oncogene amplification is associated with a poor prognosis, suggesting that its enhanced expression may be critically related to disease progression.

SCREENING FOR EARLY CANCER DETECTION

Periodic, thorough physical examinations as well as analyses of simple blood tests (i.e., a complete blood count and routine chemistries) and urine are critical for the early detection of malignancy. Rectal, breast, and testicular examinations are the most effective means of diagnosing early cancers of the prostate and rectum, breast, and testes, respectively. A microcytic anemia in a nonmenstruating patient should alert one to the possibility of an occult gastrointestinal malignancy. Similarly, microscopic hematuria in an asymptomatic patient should prompt a search for a bladder or kidney cancer.

More complex screening procedures must take into account cost-benefit ratios. Costs include not only the dollar cost to society, but the risk of the procedure to the individual. Costs can be reduced by using epidemiologically derived data to restrict screening to (1) individuals at highest risk of developing cancer and (2) cancers whose early detection and treatment lead to significantly increased survival.

The American Cancer Society recommends screening as detailed in Table 55–4. Only one of the recommendations results from controlled, randomized, prospective clinical trials: mammography in women over the age of 40 years. The basis for the remaining recommendations is less firm. The recommendations do not include chest radiographs and sputum cytologies even in populations at high risk for developing lung cancer, as several studies demonstrate that this approach fails to detect lung cancers at a resectable stage.

TUMOR MARKERS

Routine radiographs rarely detect tumor masses of less than 1 cu cm, a size that reflects approximately one billion tumor cells. This has prompted a search for tumor-specific products—tumor markers—in body fluids. A number of available tumor markers are useful as indices of response to treatment and early disease recurrence (Table 55–5). However, lack of sensitivity and specificity precludes their use as screening tests for asymptomatic populations.

PARANEOPLASTIC EFFECTS OF TUMORS

Even small, localized tumors can produce widespread systemic effects via biochemical, hormonal,

TABLE 55–3. PROTO-ONCOGENE FAMILIES

FAMILY	CARDINAL PROPERTIES	EXAMPLES
Tyrosine-specific protein kinase	Protein phosphorylation with specificity for tyrosine. Most kinases localize to the cell surface, and some members are bona fide receptors.	c-erbB (EGF-receptor) c-fms (CSF-1 receptor) c-abl c-scr
Serine-threonine	Protein phosphorylation with specificity for serine or threonine. Proteins are homologous to tyrosine kinase. Proteins localize to the cytosol.	c-mos c-raf
Receptor for thyroid hormone	Homology to steroid receptors	c-erbA
GTP-binding proteins	Bind guanine nucleotides and hydrolyze GTP. Are analogous to G proteins that modulate receptor signals, including transducin, Gi, Gs, and Go.	c-Ha-ras c-Ki-ras
Growth factor	Beta chain of platelet-derived growth factor	c-sis
Nuclear proteins	Generally short half-life and rapid inducibility, DNA binding	c-myc c-fos p53

From Nienhuis AW, Sherr CJ: Oncogenes in hematopoietic neoplasms. *In* HEMATOLOGY–1987. The Educational Program of the American Society of Hematology.

TABLE 55–4. AMERICAN CANCER SOCIETY RECOMMENDATIONS FOR SCREENING OF ASYMPTOMATIC INDIVIDUALS

TEST	SEX	AGE	FREQUENCY
Sigmoidoscopy	M & F	over 50	every 3–5 years after 2 negative exams 1 year apart
Stool guaiac test	M & F	over 50	every year
Digital rectal exam	M & F	over 40	every year
PAP test ⎫ ⎬ Pelvic exam ⎭	F	all women who have reached age 18 or have been sexually active	every year[1]
Endometrial tissue sample	F	at menopause if high risk[2]	at menopause as indicated
Breast self-exam	F	over 20	every month
Breast physical exam	F	20–40 over 40	every 3 years every year
Mammography	F	35–39 40–49 over 50	one baseline study every 1–2 years every year
Health counseling	M & F	over 20	every 3 years
Cancer check-up[3]	M & F	over 40	every year

[1] After three or more consecutive satisfactory normal annual exams, PAP test may be done less frequently at the discretion of the physician.
[2] History of infertility, obesity, failure of ovulation, abnormal uterine bleeding, or estrogen therapy
[3] To include examination for cancers of the thyroid, testicles, prostate, ovaries, lymph nodes, oral region, and skin

TABLE 55–5. TUMOR MARKERS USEFUL IN FOLLOWING KNOWN MALIGNANCIES

TUMOR MARKER	POSITIVE IN SOME	FALSE POSITIVES IN
Carcinoembryonic antigen (CEA)	GI, lung, breast cancers	Smokers, cirrhotics Inflammatory bowel disease Rectal polyps Pancreatitis
Alpha-fetoprotein (αFP)	Hepatocellular, gastric, pancreatic, colon, and lung cancers Nonseminomatous germ cell cancers	Pregnancy Alcoholic and viral hepatitis Cirrhosis
Human chorionic gonadotropin (beta subunit of hCG)	Trophoblastic tumors Germ cell neoplasms Adenocarcinomas of ovary Pancreatic, gastric, and hepatocellular cancers	Pregnancy (the alpha subunit cross-reacts with luteinizing hormone)
Acid phosphatase (prostate-specific)	Prostatic cancer (especially if bony metastases are present), myeloma, bony metastases from nonprostatic cancers	Benign prostatic hypertrophy, osteoporosis, hyperthyroidism, hyperparathyroidism
CA 125 (ovarian tumor marker)	80% of ovarian cancer 20% of nongynecologic cancers	1% healthy control, 5% benign diseases

and immunological mediators. These are called paraneoplastic syndromes.

ANOREXIA AND CACHEXIA

Complex factors act to produce tumor cachexia. They include anorexia due to aberrations in taste and smell, depression, and malaise; gastrointestinal dysfunction due to obstruction and the deleterious effects of chemotherapy, radiation, and surgery; and increased catabolism due to fever, tumor-induced alterations in protein and energy metabolism, and loss of protein into third spaces (e.g., ascites). Patients receiving effective oncologic therapy have higher response rates if they concomitantly receive nutritional support.

HEMATOLOGIC MANIFESTATIONS

Malignancy can cause prominent abnormalities in coagulation and all hematopoietic cell lines (Table 55–6). Most can be reversed only by successfully treating the underlying malignancy.

TABLE 55–6. HEMATOLOGIC MANIFESTATIONS OF MALIGNANCY

MANIFESTATION	ASSOCIATED TUMORS	CONTRIBUTING FACTORS
Anemia	About 50% of all advanced malignancies	Chronic disease; extrinsic blood loss; bone marrow invasion by tumor or suppression by therapy; autoimmune hemolytic anemia; disseminated intravascular coagulation (DIC); microangiopathic hemolytic anemia; erosion of the tumor into a blood vessel; splenic sequestration
Thrombocytopenia	Lymphoma, CLL, carcinoma	Immune thrombocytopenia
Erythrocytosis	Hepatoma, hypernephroma, cerebellar hemangioblastoma	Inappropriate production of erythropoietin
Leukemoid reaction	Carcinomas of lung, pancreas, stomach; hepatoma; lymphomas	Tumor necrosis; tumor elaboration of colony stimulating factors; marrow invasion by metastases
Eosinophilia	Lymphomas, especially Hodgkin's disease; melanoma; brain tumors	Tumor elaboration of eosinophilopoietin
Thrombocytosis	Carcinoma; lymphoma	
Bleeding diatheses	Myeloma; Waldenström's macroglobulinemia Myeloproliferative diseases	Platelet dysfunction; abnormal fibrin polymerization Platelet dysfunction

Hypercoagulability
  Migratory thrombophlebitis (Trousseau's syndrome)
  Disseminated intravascular coagulation
  Nonbacterial thrombotic endocarditis
	Mucin-secreting adenocarcinoma of GI tract; carcinomas of lung, breast, ovary, prostate	Tumor cell expression of tissue factor; mucin activation of factor X; prothrombinase-promoting tumor cell activity

ENDOCRINE MANIFESTATIONS

Some tumors develop a remarkable capacity to express one or another of the body's natural hormones (Table 55–7). Such hormone production is usually independent of normal regulatory mechanisms.

NEUROLOGICAL MANIFESTATIONS

Metastases to the brain, epidural space, and meninges constitute the major cause of neurological dysfunction in cancer patients. Neurological symptoms may also result from metabolic abnormalities, opportunistic infections of the CNS, and vascular disease due to hemorrhage (intraparenchymal, subdural, and subarachnoid) and infarction (thrombotic and embolic).

Table 121–2 lists some of the remote effects of cancer on the central nervous system; these can be the presenting signs of occult malignancy.

CUTANEOUS MANIFESTATIONS

Paraneoplastic skin lesions include a variety of erythemas (e.g., necrolytic migratory erythema), pigmented lesions (e.g., acanthosis nigricans), and miscellaneous lesions (e.g., dermatomyositis) (Table 55–8). They can occur before, concomitant with, or after the diagnosis of malignancy. Their association with malignancy may be specific (e.g., necrolytic migratory erythema and glucagonoma) or generalized (e.g., dermatomyositis).

RENAL MANIFESTATIONS

Etiologies of renal dysfunction in malignancy include direct tumor or amyloid infiltration, urinary tract obstruction, electrolyte imbalances (hypercalcemia, hyperuricemia, etc.) and the toxicities of chemotherapy. Glomerular lesions associated with the nephrotic syndrome constitute the primary paraneoplastic manifestation. In Hodgkin's disease, the malignancy most commonly associated with the nephrotic syndrome, the predominant renal lesion is lipoid nephrosis. In contrast, membranous glomerulonephritis is the most frequent glomerular lesion observed in patients with carcinoma.

REFERENCES

Bunn PA Jr, Minna JD: Paraneoplastic syndromes. In Devita VT, Hellman S, Rosenberg SA: Cancer: Principles and Practice of Oncology. 2nd ed. Philadelphia, JB Lippincott Co, 1985, pp 1797–1842.

Fraumeni JF Jr: Epidemiology of cancer. In Wyngaarden JB, Smith LH Jr (eds): Cecil Textbook of Medicine. 18th ed. Philadelphia, WB Saunders Co, 1988, pp 1092–1096.

Holt JT, Morton CC, Nienhuis AW, Leder P: Molecular mechanisms of hematologic neoplasms. In Stamatoyannopoulos G, Nienhuis P, Leder P, Majerus P (eds): Molecular Basis of Blood Diseases. Philadelphia, WB Saunders Co, 1986, pp 347–376.

TABLE 55–7. ECTOPIC HORMONES PRODUCED BY MALIGNANCY

HORMONE	MANIFESTATIONS	ASSOCIATED TUMORS
ACTH	Cushing's syndrome (psychosis, hyperglycemia, generalized weakness)	Lung (especially oat cell); thymus; pancreas, medullary thyroid, pheochromocytoma
Humoral hypercalcemia of malignancy (HHM)–factor (a recently identified parathyroid hormone-like peptide)	Hypercalcemia	Carcinomas of lung (especially epidermoid and large cell), kidney, head and neck, and ovary
Somatomedins (also called nonsuppressible insulin-like activity—NSLIA)	Hypoglycemia	Mesenchymal tumors (especially mesothelioma), hepatoma, adrenal carcinomas, GI tumors
Antidiuretic hormone (ADH)	Hyponatremia, hyperosmolar urine, high urinary sodium concentration	Small cell carcinoma of lung
Human chorionic gonadotropin (HCG)	Gynecomastia in men; oligomenorrhea in premenopausal women	Germ cell tumors, lung cancer

TABLE 55–8. SOME PARANEOPLASTIC CUTANEOUS SYNDROMES

LESION	DESCRIPTION	ASSOCIATED MALIGNANCIES
Dermatomyositis	"Heliotrope" erythema of face, eyelids, neck, and arms; raised papules over knuckles (Gottron's papules)	All cancers (especially breast and lung)
Acanthosis nigricans	Hyperkeratosis, hyperpigmentation of axillae, neck, anogenital region	Adenocarcinoma of GI tract (92%), particularly stomach (50–60%)
Necrolytic migratory erythema	Migratory bullous erythematous patches with central blister formation, then crusting; painful glossitis	Pathognomonic of glucagonoma
Tylosis	Hyperkeratosis of palms and soles	Hereditary disorder associated with esophageal carcinoma

56

PRINCIPLES OF CANCER THERAPY

The advent of effective chemotherapy, radiotherapy, and surgery has made many cancers curable or amenable to palliation. This chapter outlines the basic principles governing the use of these therapeutic modalities. Therapy of specific tumors is discussed in chapters related to diseases of the affected organ.

FORMING A TREATMENT PLAN

The first step in the evaluation of a patient diagnosed as having cancer is a thorough review of the diagnostic biopsy material with an experienced pathologist. Accurate classification of tumors and valuable prognostic information may be obtained by careful analysis of the following: morphology, histochemical stains, cell surface immune markers, hormone receptors, karyotype, oncogene expression, and electron microscopic appearance. Certain malignancies such as lymphomas, leukemias, and lung cancers require accurate subclassification, since prognosis and treatment are different and distinct for the various subtypes.

Determination of the extent and specific sites of neoplastic involvement is essential. This requires knowledge of the usual pattern of metastasis for the neoplasm in question. Staging procedures, particularly if invasive or costly, should be carried out only if the derived information will alter the therapeutic approach or significantly change prognosis. Low yield procedures, such as bone scans in asymptomatic patients with localized breast cancer, should be avoided.

The biological aggressiveness and curability of the tumor must be assessed. Patients with indolent malignancies such as early stage chronic lymphocytic leukemia and low-grade lymphomas are not curable with available chemotherapy and often can be safely followed without therapy for several years. In contrast, those with biologically aggressive high-grade lymphomas are eminently curable with combination chemotherapy and should generally be treated even in the absence of symptoms.

Patients with curable malignancies (e.g., Hodgkin's disease) should receive an optimal therapeutic regimen that is not compromised in any way, as the potential toxicities of treatment are generally justified. Even when curative therapy is available, however, patients with serious underlying medical conditions may not be suitable candidates.

In patients with incurable cancers, one often can achieve a significant prolongation of survival. In these instances, the physician must consider the probability of extending meaningful survival as well as the impact of the therapeutic program on the quality of the patient's remaining life. Ultimately, effective palliation of symptoms and improvement of the functional status and quality of life of the incurable cancer patient represent the physician's twin objectives. Effective palliation requires close observation for the development and treatment of the complications of malignancy, such as bony metastases, metabolic disturbances, visceral obstruction, persistent pain, and emotional distress.

PRINCIPLES OF ONCOLOGIC SURGERY

Definitive surgical resection with attainment of tumor-free margins is the treatment of choice for the majority of localized solid tumors. Since, however, most malignant tumors have already micrometastasized at the time of diagnosis, surgery is increasingly being integrated with other modalities to achieve local as well as distant disease control and to minimize the magnitude and morbidity of operative procedures. For example, conservative surgery, local radiotherapy, and adjuvant chemotherapy are widely applied to the treatment of localized breast cancer with positive regional lymph nodes as well as to childhood rhabdomyosarcoma. In rare circumstances, such as with solitary lung metastases in sarcoma patients and solitary hepatic metastases in colorectal cancer patients, resection of isolated metastases may be curative. Although not itself curative, cytoreductive or debulking surgery plays a role in the treatment of some cancers (e.g., ovarian), presumably by increasing the growth fraction of the remaining cells, thereby rendering them more susceptible to the effects of chemotherapy.

Regional lymph node dissection, as in axillary lymph node sampling for breast cancer, provides prognostic information about the likelihood of distant tumor recurrence and serves as a guide to the administration of adjuvant therapy.

Surgical intervention also can offer palliation of symptoms resulting from complications of cancer such as intestinal or biliary obstruction, hemorrhage (e.g., from gastric carcinoma), perforation (e.g., in the setting of chemotherapy for gastrointestinal lymphoma), and compression of vital structures (e.g., spinal cord compression). Surgery also figures prominently in the rehabilitation of treated cancer patients. Examples include breast reconstruction after mastectomy and lysis of radiation-induced contractures.

PRINCIPLES OF RADIATION THERAPY

Radiation exerts its biological effect by ejecting electrons from target molecules, a process called ionization. Ionizing radiation may interact with DNA directly or indirectly, the latter by generating free radicals. The biological end point is loss of cellular reproductive capacity.

Radiotherapy is delivered in the form of electromagnetic waves such as x-rays or gamma rays or as streams of particles such as electrons. High energy (megavoltage) beams in the form of gamma rays generated by radioactive isotopes (e.g., cobalt-60) or x-rays generated by linear accelerators are ideal for the treatment of visceral tumors, as they penetrate to great depths before reaching full intensity and thereby spare toxicity to skin. Electron beam irradiation is most useful in the treatment of superficial tumors, as energy is deposited at the skin and quickly dissipates, sparing toxicity to deeper tissues.

FRACTIONATION

Radiotherapy is generally administered in fractions of 180 to 250 rads/day, five days/week. Fractionation improves the therapeutic index (the margin of safety between therapeutic and toxic doses), presumably because sublethal radiation injury is repaired more effectively in normal tissues than in tumors. Weekend treatment breaks allow the patient to recover from acute toxicities and the tumor to regress and reoxygenate. Such improved oxygenation renders the tumor more susceptible to subsequent radiotherapy, since hypoxic cells at the center of poorly vascularized neoplasms are two to three times more radioresistant than their well-oxygenated counterparts.

CLINICAL CONSIDERATIONS

The goal of radiotherapy is to deliver a tumoricidal dose while sparing normal tissues. The probability of both achieving tumor control and producing toxicity in normal tissue increases with dose in a sigmoid-curve relationship (Fig. 56–1). Greater separation of these curves results in an improved therapeutic index. The tumoricidal dose depends on the inherent radiosensitivity of the neoplasm as well as its volume. The tumoricidal dose for lymphomas, for example, is 4000 to 4500 rads, while that for most solid tumors ranges from 5000 rads for microscopic disease to 7000 rads for 4-cm tumors. The normal tissue tolerance to radiation also varies considerably (Table 56–1). Cell renewal tissues requiring rapid, continued proliferation for their function—skin, bone marrow, and gastrointestinal mucosa—are most vulnerable to acute toxicities (stomatitis, diarrhea, cytopenias, etc.). Late toxicities such as fibrosis, necrosis, and nonhealing ulcerations are determined by the total radiation dose and fraction size rather than by the proliferative potential of the affected tissue.

Radiotherapy is preferable to surgery in the management of localized tumors such as laryngeal carcinomas or certain deep-lying malignant brain tumors whose resection would be associated with significant functional impairment or mutilation. Radiocurable tumors include Hodgkin's and non-Hodgkin's lymphomas, seminomas, and localized carcinomas of the larynx, cervix, and prostate.

Radiotherapy is frequently administered in an "adjuvant" setting with surgery, chemotherapy, or both.

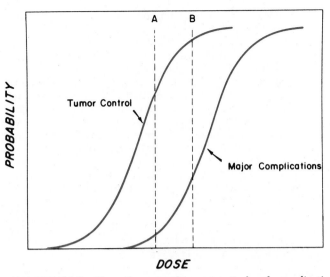

FIGURE 56–1. Sigmoid curves of tumor control and complications. A, Dose for tumor control with minimal complications. B, Maximum tumor dose with significant complications. (Reprinted with permission from Hellman S: Principles of radiation therapy. *In* Devita VT, Hellman S, Rosenberg SA (eds): Cancer: Principles and Practice of Oncology. 2nd ed. Philadelphia, JB Lippincott Co, 1985, p 242.)

Postoperative adjuvant radiotherapy may eradicate residual foci of microscopic tumor and decrease the likelihood of local recurrence. It may also permit a more conservative surgical approach, such as is attained by employing lumpectomy and radiation therapy rather than mastectomy for localized breast cancers. The addition of adjuvant chemotherapy in such a setting may further increase the likelihood of cure by eradicating occult distant micrometastases. Examples of this principle include the administration of adjuvant radiotherapy and chemotherapy after resection of localized breast and rectal carcinomas. Adjuvant radiotherapy to sanctuary sites, such as the central nervous system and testes which are not accessible to systemic chemotherapy, increases the likelihood of cure in malig-

TABLE 56–1. NORMAL TISSUE TOLERANCE TO RADIOTHERAPY*

ORGAN	TOXICITIES	DOSE LIMIT†
Bone marrow	Aplasia, pancytopenia	250
Liver	Acute and chronic hepatitis	2500
Stomach, intestine	Ulceration, diarrhea, hemorrhage	4500
Brain	Infarction, necrosis	6000
Spinal cord	Infarction, necrosis	4500
Heart	Pericarditis, pancarditis, coronary artery disease	4500
Lung	Pneumonitis, fibrosis	1500
Kidney	Nephrosclerosis	2000
Skin	Dermatitis, sclerosis	5500

* Assuming 200 rads/fraction, 5 fractions/week
† Dose for 5% injury in 5 years.

nancies such as acute lymphocytic leukemia and small cell lung cancer.

Chemotherapy and radiotherapy are combined in the primary treatment of a number of malignancies, including bulky Hodgkin's lymphoma, limited-stage small cell lung cancer, and anal carcinoma. In another dimension, chemoradiotherapy is administered in supralethal doses as a preparative regimen for bone marrow transplantation (discussed below).

Radiotherapy can be a potent palliative modality, as is illustrated in the treatment of painful bony metastases. It is also employed as the primary therapy for many oncologic emergencies, including the superior vena cava syndrome, spinal cord compression, and brain metastases.

PRINCIPLES OF CHEMOTHERAPY

Most cancers have established metastatic clones by the time they become clinically detectable. Systemic chemotherapy plays a major role in the management of the 60 per cent of cancer patients who are not curable by regional modalities. The advent of effective combination chemotherapy has produced cures in a number of advanced malignancies (Table 56–2) and meaningful remissions in many others (Table 56–3).

TUMOR KINETICS

Exponentially growing tumors double approximately 30 times before becoming clinically detectable (as a 10^9 cell or 1-cm mass). Each tumor has a characteristic doubling time ranging from two to five days for Burkitt's lymphoma to over 100 days for adenocarcinomas of the lung and breast. Tumor kinetics are best described by the Gompertz growth curve (Fig. 56–2)—over a short time, tumor growth appears exponential; with time, a progressively greater percentage of the cell population enters a nonproliferative pool by virtue of cell death, differentiation, and entry into the G_0 or resting phase of the cell cycle. Eventually a plateau is reached, where the rate of new cell production equals that of cell death. The exponential increase in the proportion of nonproliferating cells decreases the susceptibility of large tumors to antineoplastic agents, which are most active against rapidly dividing cells. This principle provides the rationale for "debulking" tumors (by surgery or irradiation) so as to recruit residual G_0 cells into an active proliferative state with an enhanced susceptibility to chemotherapy.

Most chemotherapeutic agents exploit kinetic differences between normal and malignant cells by acting preferentially on dividing cells. Such "cell cycle–specific" agents (e.g., cyclophosphamide, methotrexate, cytosine arabinoside) achieve a kill rate of certain lymphoproliferative tumor cells that is several thousand–fold greater than that of bone marrow stem cells that are partially in a resting phase. This results in rapidly reversible cytopenias but permanent tumor eradication.

TABLE 56–2. ADULT TUMORS CURABLE WITH CHEMOTHERAPY

TUMOR	LONG-TERM DISEASE-FREE SURVIVAL (%)
Choriocarcinoma	90
Burkitt's lymphoma (Stage I)	90
Testicular carcinoma	90
Diffuse large cell non-Hodgkin's lymphoma	50–60
Hodgkin's disease	60
Acute lymphocytic leukemia	35–45
Acute myelogenous leukemia	20
Ovarian carcinoma	10–20
Small cell lung carcinoma	10

TABLE 56–3. ADULT TUMORS RESPONSIVE TO CHEMOTHERAPY

TUMOR	PARTIAL OR COMPLETE RESPONSE (%)
Chronic lymphocytic leukemia	75
Chronic myeloproliferative disorders	80
Hairy cell leukemia	75
Multiple myeloma	75
Low- and intermediate-grade non-Hodgkin's lymphoma	80
Mycosis fungoides	75
Breast carcinoma	65
Bladder carcinoma	40–50
Gastric carcinoma	35
Head and neck carcinoma	65
Ovarian carcinoma	75
Prostate carcinoma	75
Islet cell tumors	50

MECHANISMS OF ACTION OF ANTINEOPLASTIC DRUGS

All chemotherapeutic agents act by interfering with cell division (Fig 56–3). Antimetabolites, acting as fraudulent analogues of vital physiological substrates, inhibit the synthesis of DNA or their nucleotide building blocks. Examples include methotrexate, a folic acid analogue; cytosine arabinoside, a pyrimidine analogue; and 6-mercaptopurine, a purine analogue. Alkylating agents such as cyclophosphamide chemically interact with DNA. They contain highly reactive alkyl groups that cause DNA breaks and cross-link complementary DNA strands that prevent replication. *Cis*-platinum, a heavy metal compound, achieves its cytotoxicity by a similar mechanism. Many of the antitumor antibiotics, such as the anthracyclines, daunomycin and doxorubicin, intercalate themselves between strands of the DNA double helix and thereby inhibit DNA, RNA, and ultimately protein synthesis. The vinca alkaloids, vincristine and vinblastine, are plant products that arrest cells in the metaphase of mitosis by binding to tubulin and thereby inhibit microtubular function. The enzyme L-asparaginase depletes cells of the nonessential amino acid asparagine. Most human tissues have the capacity to synthesize asparagine by the action of L-asparigine synthetase. Some tumor cells, particularly those of T-cell lineage, lack this enzyme. As a result, depletion of circulating pools of asparagine by L-asparaginase results in inhibition of protein synthesis and ultimately cytotoxicity.

TOXICITY

Safe administration of antineoplastic drugs, with their narrow therapeutic indices, requires knowledge of their routes of metabolism and elimination. Dose modification in the setting of renal or hepatic dysfunction minimizes toxicity. Major dose modifications of the anthracyclines and vinca alkaloids are required when hepatic dysfunction exists and of *cis*-platinum, methotrexate, streptozocin, bleomycin, and hydroxyurea when azotemia is present. The toxic manifestations of chemotherapy are legion and spare no organ. The patterns of toxicity of some commonly used drugs are outlined in Table 56–4.

DOSE INTENSITY

Most antineoplastic agents produce a steep dose-response curve. Dose intensity and dose rate (drug delivered per unit time) are powerful determinants of response to therapy and overall survival. The strong correlation between the dose and cure rates of chemosensitive malignancies such as Hodgkin's disease justifies the enhanced toxicity of aggressive treatment in these settings.

RESISTANCE TO CHEMOTHERAPY

The major cause of treatment failure is drug resistance. Although most neoplasms arise from a single clone, random mutations lead to marked cellular heterogeneity with regard to radiosensitivity and susceptibility to cytotoxic drugs. The probability of drug resistance within a tumor is proportional to the size of the neoplasm and the rate at which the drug-resistant gene mutates (Goldie-Coldman hypothesis). This principle explains the greater curability of small cancers with a low likelihood of drug resistance and the relative refractoriness of widely metastatic cancers that are likely to contain cells resistant to several drugs. Many solid tumors have long doubling times because of a high rate of cell loss; by the time they become clinically detectable (approximately 30 doublings), they have undergone numerous divisions and mutational events. This biological characteristic may account for their relative resistance to chemotherapy when compared with rapidly dividing lymphoproliferative malignancies such as high-grade lymphomas. The practice of giving adjuvant chemotherapy shortly after tumor resection when the systemic tumor burden is low derives from this principle. Such an approach

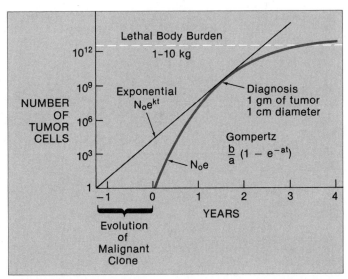

FIGURE 56–2. A schematic plot to describe models of exponential and Gompertzian growth curves. (From Laszlo J: Introduction to oncology. *In* Wyngaarden JB, Smith LH Jr (eds): Cecil Textbook of Medicine. 18th ed. Philadelphia, WB Saunders Co, 1988, p 1085.)

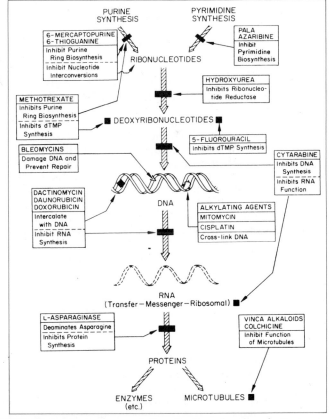

FIGURE 56–3. Mechanisms and sites of action of antineoplastic agents. (Reproduced with permission from Calabresi P, Parks RE Jr: Antiproliferative agents and drugs used for immunosuppression. *In* Gilman AG, Goodman LS, Rall TW, Murad F (eds): Goodman and Gilman's The Pharmacological Basis of Therapeutics. 7th ed. New York, Macmillan Publishing Co, 1985, p 1246.)

TABLE 56–4. MAJOR TOXICITIES OF COMMONLY USED ANTINEOPLASTIC DRUGS

DRUG	ALOPECIA	CARDIAC	CARCINOGENESIS	DERMATOLOGIC	DIARRHEA	GONADAL	HEPATIC	HYPERSENSITIVITY	LOCAL IRRITATION	MUCOSITIS	MYELOSUPPRESSION	NAUSEA/VOMITING	NEUROLOGIC	PULMONARY	RENAL	VASCULAR
Alkylating agents	•		•			•					•	•				
Nitrosoureas	•		•						•		•	•				
Mitomycin	•						•			•	•	•		•	•	
Methotrexate				•			•			•	•					
5-Fluorouracil	•			•	•					•		•				
Cytosine arabinoside							•			•	•		•			
6-Mercaptopurine							•			•	•					
Vincristine	•								•				•			
Vinblastine									•		•		•			
VP-16	•										•	•				
Adriamycin	•	•		•					•	•	•					
Bleomycin				•				•	•			•		•		•
Mithramycin							•			•	•					•
Cis-platinum										•	•	•	•		•	
L-asparaginase							•	•			•	•				

may bring a cure to patients with malignancies that have a propensity to recur such as breast and rectal carcinomas and osteogenic and soft tissue sarcomas.

Chemotherapy selectively eradicates sensitive tumor clones and permits the overgrowth of resistant cell populations. Mechanisms of drug resistance include impaired drug uptake or activation, enhanced drug inactivation, increased expression of the target enzyme by gene amplification, and altered target proteins. Some tumor cells develop pleiotropic (multidrug) resistance to several classes of drugs which are structurally and functionally distinct (vinca alkaloids, anthracyclines, dacarbazine). Such multidrug-resistant cells contain amplified gene sequences that encode a 170-kd protein, P-glycoprotein, involved in drug efflux. Overexpression of this protein results in decreased intracellular drug accumulation and clinical resistance.

COMBINATION CHEMOTHERAPY

The cure of advanced malignancies, when possible, has been achieved primarily with combination chemotherapy. The rationale for combination regimens stems from the fact that antineoplastic agents have diverse mechanisms of action. Hence, tumor cells resistant to one drug may still be sensitive to another. The most effective regimens consist of drugs that are individually effective against the neoplasm and have nonoverlapping toxicities, thereby permitting administration of full dosage of all drugs (e.g., mustard, Oncovin, procarbazine, prednisone (MOPP) for Hodgkin's disease). Proper scheduling of combination

regimens is integral to their efficacy. The administration of nonmyelosuppressive drugs such as bleomycin or methotrexate with leucovorin rescue between cycles of myelotoxic drugs such as the alkylating agents or anthracyclines allows the bone marrow to recover despite continued treatment. Treatment breaks of two to three weeks between cycles also permit recovery of sensitive normal tissues, such as gastrointestinal mucosa and bone marrow. Newer approaches include instituting alternating cycles of equally effective non–cross-resistant combinations and the early introduction of all effective drugs in an effort to prevent the emergence of resistance.

As mentioned above, combination chemotherapy has been successfully integrated with radiotherapy in the treatment of certain cancers such as bulky Hodgkin's disease. A regimen of high-dose chemotherapy and total body irradiation (TBI) followed by reconstitution with allogeneic or autologous bone marrow has been administered with varying degrees of success to patients with acute and chronic leukemias, refractory lymphomas, and a number of chemoradiosensitive solid tumors, including small cell lung, breast, ovarian, and testicular cancers. Allogeneic HLA-matched bone marrow transplantation has become the treatment of choice for younger patients with chronic myelogenous leukemia in chronic phase, acute lymphocytic leukemia in second remission, and acute myelogenous leukemia in relapse. Bone marrow transplantation as a treatment of refractory lymphomas and solid tumors is promising but remains experimental in view of its extreme toxicities, which include interstitial pneumonitis, graft-versus-host disease, opportunistic infections, and hepatic veno-occlusive disease.

HORMONAL THERAPY

A number of cancers, most notably breast and prostate, respond to manipulations of their hormonal milieu. Manipulation involves alteration in steroid hormone levels or their activity. Steroid hormones enter the cell and bind to cytoplasmic receptors. The hormone-receptor complex is translocated to the nucleus where it influences the transcription of messenger RNA for growth-inhibitory or stimulatory proteins.

Steroid antagonists, such as the antiestrogen tamoxifen used in the treatment of breast cancer, compete with endogenous hormones for binding to receptor sites. Hormone antagonist-receptor complexes fail to initiate transcriptional changes induced by the native hormone. Estrogen and progesterone receptor levels in breast cancer tissue correlate well with hormonal dependence and predict responsiveness to hormonal therapy.

Aminoglutethimide inhibits adrenal steroidogenesis by blocking the enzymatic conversion of cholesterol to pregnenolone as well as the aromatization in peripheral tissues of androgens to estrone, a major source of estrogen in postmenopausal women. This agent has almost entirely replaced surgical adrenalectomy in the treatment of breast cancer.

Estrogens such as diethylstilbesterol and analogues of luteinizing hormone–releasing hormone (LHRH), which are potent inhibitors of testosterone production, help to palliate prostate cancer.

Glucocorticoids are used extensively in the treatment of lymphomas, lymphocytic leukemias, multiple myeloma, and breast cancer.

BIOLOGICAL RESPONSE MODIFIERS

Human beings possess cellular and humoral antitumor capacity. Three classes of cytotoxic lymphocytes exist—lymphokine-activated killer (LAK) cells, natural killer cells, and natural cytotoxic cells. Biological substances such as interferons and interleukins potentiate the antitumor effects of lymphocytes. The reinfusion of LAK cells that are derived from patients with renal cell carcinoma and malignant melanoma and then expanded in vitro with exogenous interleukin-2 (IL-2) has produced significant regressions of these chemoresistant tumors. Broad application of this technique has been limited by its serious toxicities, which include a capillary leak syndrome, hypotension, and marked fluid retention.

Naturally occurring products of lymphocytes (lymphokines) such as interferons are antiproliferative and immunomodulatory and are endowed with direct antitumor activity. Alpha-interferon has been successfully used to treat hairy cell leukemia, chronic myelogenous leukemia, and low-grade non-Hodgkin's lymphomas. More modest responses have been observed with solid tumors such as renal cell carcinoma and Kaposi's sarcoma.

Monoclonal antibodies against specific tumor antigens have been utilized in purging autologous bone marrow from patients with B-cell lymphoma and acute lymphocytic leukemia. Similarly, T-cell antibodies have been used to purge allogeneic marrow of T lymphocytes in order to prevent graft-versus-host disease. The use of monoclonal antibodies against the idiotype of the immunoglobulin on the surface of B-cell lymphomas and leukemias has also been attempted but has met with limited success owing to the emergence of mutations within the idiotype.

REFERENCES

Carter SK, Livingston RB: Principles of cancer chemotherapy. *In* Carter SK, Glatstein E, Livingston RB (eds): Principles of Cancer Treatment. New York, McGraw-Hill Book Co, 1982, pp 95–110.

Chabner BA: Principles of cancer therapy. *In* Wyngaarden JB, Smith LH Jr (eds): Cecil Textbook of Medicine. 18th ed. Philadelphia, WB Saunders Co, 1988, pp 1113–1129.

Devita VT Jr: Principles of chemotherapy. *In* Devita VT Jr, Hellman S, Rosenberg SA (eds): Cancer: Principles and Practice. 2nd ed. Philadelphia, JB Lippincott Co, 1985, pp 257–285.

Hellman S: Principles of radiation therapy. *In* Devita VT Jr, Hellman S, Rosenberg SA (eds): Cancer: Principles and Practice. 2nd ed. Philadelphia, JB Lippincott Co, 1985, pp 227–255.

57

ONCOLOGIC EMERGENCIES

The natural history of malignancies leads to several types of medical emergencies. Many gastrointestinal and genitourinary tumors present with acute obstruction or hemorrhage. Bone marrow infiltrated by tumor or suppressed by chemotherapy can lead to life-threatening infection. Tumor erosion into a blood vessel and tumor- or treatment-induced thrombocytopenia can precipitate life-threatening hemorrhage. Other types of oncologic emergencies include those summarized in Table 57–1, a few of which are discussed in detail below.

HYPERCALCEMIA

Hypercalcemia occurs in 10 to 20 per cent of cancer patients. It is seen in association with solid tumors in the presence (e.g., breast cancer) or absence (e.g., renal cell and squamous cell lung cancers) of bone metastases as well as with hematologic malignancies (e.g., myeloma and adult T-cell lymphoma). Tumor cells in bone can directly stimulate bone resorption or induce bone resorption by secreting cytokines (interleukin-1, tumor necrosis factors) or prostaglandin E_2. Tumor-derived parathyroid hormone-like peptides and growth factors appear to be important humoral mediators of cancer-associated hypercalcemia.

Common presenting symptoms include an altered mental status (ranging from apathy to coma), generalized muscle weakness, nausea and vomiting, abdominal pain, polyuria (resulting from a reversible renal tubular defect in urine concentrating ability), and polydipsia. Clinical findings associated with hypercalcemia include an altered mental status, dehydration, renal insufficiency, hyporeflexia, pancreatitis, peptic ulcer, hypertension, cardiac arrhythmias, prolonged PR interval, shortened QT interval, and widening of the T wave on EKG.

Although definitive treatment of hypercalcemia requires tumor control, interim therapy should be aimed at enhancing calcium excretion and diminishing calcium resorption from bone.

Repleting intravascular volume is of primary importance in the management of hypercalcemia. This enhances the glomerular filtration rate and increases the clearance rates of sodium and calcium. Once the patient is euvolemic, a diuretic such as furosemide, which diminishes renal tubular reabsorption of sodium and calcium and promotes calciuresis, may be administered. During this time, fluid and electrolyte balance must be carefully monitored and congestive heart failure vigorously treated. Such therapy usually lowers serum calcium by 2 to 4 mg/dl within 24 hours.

Glucocorticoids are most useful in the treatment of hypercalcemia associated with hematologic malignancies and breast cancer, as they are effective antineoplastic agents in these diseases. Steroids also act by decreasing intestinal absorption and increasing renal excretion of calcium, as well as by blocking activation of osteoclasts by OAF's and reducing prostaglandin synthesis. Calcium levels decline only after several days of steroid therapy.

Refractory hypercalcemia may be treated with the antitumor antibiotic mithramycin, which directly inhibits bone resorption. Its effects are usually detectable within 24 to 48 hours and can last for a week or more. The adverse effects of mithramycin (including bone marrow suppression, postural hypotension, and hepatocellular and renal damage) limit its usefulness as a first-line agent.

Calcitonin, a polypeptide hormone secreted by thyroid parafollicular cells, is moderately effective in treating malignancy-associated hypercalcemia. Its hypocalcemic effect is due to inhibition of bone resorption and is manifest within hours of administration. Concomitant administration of steroids may prolong its hypocalcemic effect.

Diphosphonates, synthetic analogues of pyrophosphate, inhibit osteoclastic bone resorption and are effective in treating malignancy-associated hypercalcemia.

Oral phosphates can be used for chronic maintenance of normocalcemia, but their use should be limited to patients with normal renal function who are not hyperphosphatemic.

SPINAL CORD COMPRESSION

Extradural spinal cord compression (SCC) is found at autopsy in as many as 5 per cent of patients with cancer. Vertebral or occasionally paravertebral metastases from carcinomas of the lung, breast, and prostate, as well as lymphoma and myeloma, account for most cases.

Back pain, with or without a radicular component, is the presenting symptom in nearly all patients with SCC; the pain is frequently worse when supine. Later signs and symptoms include weakness, sensory loss, autonomic dysfunction, and ataxia.

Unless diagnosed and treated early, SCC leads to irreversible neurological deficits, making prompt diagnosis and initiation of appropriate treatment a crucial matter. A high index of suspicion must be employed in any older patient presenting with back pain of recent onset, especially if there is a history of malignancy. Once SCC enters into the differential diagnosis of neurological symptoms, diagnostic and therapeutic measures must be undertaken immediately. Interim medical management includes the use of high-dose steroid therapy in an attempt to decrease pressure on the cord.

Although plain films are likely to demonstrate extensive vertebral involvement or destruction by tumor,

TABLE 57–1. SOME ONCOLOGIC EMERGENCIES

	MOST COMMON MANIFESTATIONS	MOST COMMON ETIOLOGIES
Hemodynamic		
Superior vena cava syndrome	Superficial thoracic vein collaterals Neck vein distention Facial edema Tachypnea	Bronchogenic carcinoma Lymphoma
Pericardial tamponade	CHF-like symptoms Kussmaul's sign Pulsus paradoxus Distant heart sounds	Lung carcinoma Breast carcinoma Lymphoma
Hyperviscosity syndrome	Confusion, coma Stroke Hypervolemia Retinopathy	Waldenström's macroglobulinemia Myeloma
Thrombosis	Trousseau's syndrome (migratory thrombophlebitis) Nonbacterial thrombotic endocarditis (NBTE) Disseminated intravascular coagulation (DIC)	Mucinous adenocarcinomas Myeloproliferative disorders Prostatic carcinoma Acute promyelocytic leukemia
Neurologic		
Increased intracranial pressure	Mental status changes Seizures Signs of herniation	Brain metastases Primary brain tumors Carcinomatous or lymphomatous meningitis
Spinal cord compression	Pain (usually radicular) Weakness Autonomic dysfunction Sensory abnormalities	Carcinoma of lung, breast, prostate Lymphoma Myeloma
Metabolic		
Hypercalcemia	Anorexia, nausea, and vomiting Abdominal pain Apathy, coma Muscle weakness Polyuria, azotemia Cardiac conduction abnormalities	Carcinoma of breast, lung, kidney, head, and neck Myeloma
"Tumor lysis syndrome"	Acute renal failure	Undifferentiated lymphomas, (particularly Burkitt's and lymphoblastic lymphomas) Acute lymphoblastic leukemia Anaplastic small cell carcinoma
Hypoglycemia	Confusion, loss of consciousness	Insulinoma Mesenchymal tumors Hepatoma
Hyponatremia	Confusion, coma Seizures Anorexia	SIADH (usually small cell carcinoma)

myelography is required to diagnose SCC, to demonstrate the number of lesions, and to define the upper and lower margins of the blockage to free flow of spinal fluid. At the time of myelography, spinal fluid should be obtained for cell count and chemical and cytological analysis. In the rare case that myelography in contraindicated, CT scanning with contrast enhancement or magnetic resonance imaging (MRI) can be helpful.

Available treatment approaches include radiation therapy and surgical decompression with or without postoperative radiation. Surgery causes more morbidity and mortality and is usually reserved for (1) cases in which there has not been a previous diagnosis of malignancy and there is no more accessible site for biopsy, (2) lesions known to be radioresistant, and (3) tumors involving areas already treated with radiation. In certain instances, chemotherapy can be used as adjunct therapy but is not recommended as the primary mode of treatment.

In general, neurological prognosis (sphincter control and independence of ambulation) depends on the degree of impairment when treatment is initiated and on the radiosensitivity of the primary tumor.

INCREASED INTRACRANIAL PRESSURE

Patients with mass lesions or diffuse infiltrative processes such as lymphomatous or carcinomatous meningitis may present with signs and symptoms of increased intracranial pressure (ICP).

Early signs of increased ICP include headache, seizures, lethargy, confusion, and papilledema. Additional signs and symptoms of neurological dysfunction reflect the anatomical site of metastasis. The CT or MR scan has become the safest and most reliable diagnostic test and should be promptly obtained in all patients with suspected mass lesions in the brain. Prompt recognition of the cause of increased ICP and rapid institution of medical therapy (prior to definitive diagnosis and treatment of the precipitating cancer) are essential for preservation of cerebral function.

While definitive diagnostic and therapeutic measures are being planned and executed, medical therapy including pharmacological doses of intravenous steroids, diuretics, and fluid restriction can temporarily decrease ICP. Anticonvulsant therapy is not routinely administered except to patients presenting with seizures. Patients with elevated ICP, carcinomatous meningitis, and melanoma have seizures more frequently and should be considered for prophylactic anticonvulsant therapy.

Care must be taken to exclude nonmalignant intracranial masses, particularly in patients without a previous diagnosis of malignancy or widely disseminated cancer. For example, there is an increased incidence of benign meningioma in women with breast cancer. Similarly, brain abscesses occur more commonly in the immunocompromised cancer patient. Radiation-induced brain necrosis may be difficult to differentiate from recurrent tumor. Surgical intervention is indicated in these instances of uncertain diagnosis.

Once a diagnosis of brain metastasis is established, radiotherapy should be instituted promptly. Fifty to 75 per cent of patients so treated will demonstrate neurological improvement, although in many, tumors will eventually recur.

SUPERIOR VENA CAVA SYNDROME

The onset of a superior vena cava (SVC) syndrome creates a subacute or acute medical emergency whose diagnosis and treatment usually require the multidisciplinary efforts of the medical oncologist, surgeon, and radiation therapist. The SVC is the major venous channel for blood return from the head, neck and upper extremities, and thorax. A thin-walled vessel enclosed in a relatively unyielding compartment, its low intravascular pressures make it particularly vulnerable to extrinsic compression by an adjacent mass.

Common presenting symptoms include distended thoracic and neck veins, facial edema, tachypnea, cyanosis, upper extremity edema, Horner's syndrome, and vocal cord paralysis. Chest x-ray almost invariably shows a mass—usually in the right superior mediastinum. Lung carcinoma and lymphoma cause most cases of the SCV syndrome; fewer than 5 per cent result from benign causes such as thyroid goiter, pericardial constriction, idiopathic sclerosing mediastinitis, and thrombosis of the SVC.

Sputum cytology, bronchoscopy, mediastinoscopy, or lymph node biopsy will usually yield a tissue diagnosis, although a diagnostic thoracotomy may be required.

Radiotherapy is generally the therapeutic modality of choice, although chemotherapy may be equally efficacious in patients with small cell lung carcinoma. The vast majority of patients have prompt palliation of symptoms. Failure to respond usually signifies thrombotic obstruction of the SVC. Supportive medical therapy with steroids, diuretics, anticoagulation, and (in the case of SVC thrombosis) fibrinolytic therapy may help to ameliorate symptoms.

REFERENCES

Kornblith PL, Cassady JR: Central nervous system emergencies. In Devita VT Jr, Hellman S, Rosenberg SA (eds): Cancer: Principles and Practice. 2nd ed. Philadelphia, JB Lippincott Co, 1985, pp 1860–1866.

SECTION
VIII
METABOLIC DISEASES

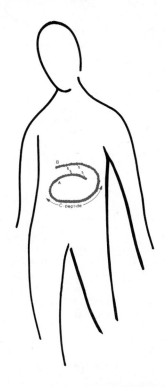

58

INTRODUCTION

A disorder is classified as a disease of metabolism when the fundamental pathogenic mechanism includes one of numerous chemical transformations that occur within living organisms. Such chemical reactions are divided into two large categories. Anabolic reactions are usually energy-requiring and generally result in the synthesis of molecules larger than those of the initial reactants. Catabolic reactions are energy-yielding processes that cause degradation of larger molecules into smaller products. Many diseases of metabolism involve specific enzyme defects that alter anabolic or catabolic processes. Defects that can be attributed to an underlying genetic abnormality are termed inborn errors of metabolism. Other metabolic diseases are acquired rather than hereditary.

The diseases discussed in this section are chiefly those whose manifestations are multisystemic or in which biochemical and genetic factors dominate the clinical presentation. A complete discussion of all known inborn errors of metabolism falls beyond the scope of this text. Many inborn errors are life-limiting, leading to death in infancy or early childhood. This section focuses upon the more common hereditary or acquired metabolic diseases encountered in adults.

59

EATING DISORDERS

OBESITY

Skinfold thickness is occasionally used to estimate body fat in clinical practice, but more precise measures (e.g., underwater weighing) are rarely employed. Clinicians most frequently use body weight or preferably the body mass index (weight (kg)/height (m)^2) to judge if a patient is "overweight." Very muscular individuals may be moderately overweight and not obese. Others with small frames and low muscle mass may be obese without fulfilling criteria for overweight. Nevertheless, most seriously overweight patients are also obese. An obesity classification scheme based on body mass index is presented in Table 59–1.

Pathogenesis. Obesity and overweight are largely genetically determined and are strongly conditioned by available palatable food and sedentariness. A child of two obese parents has about an 80 per cent chance of becoming obese, whereas the risk is only 15 per cent for the offspring of two normal-weight parents. Moreover, a correlation between parental and child body mass index is found across a broad spectrum of values, suggesting both polygenic inheritance of obesity and several contributing metabolic mechanisms. The precise causative mechanisms remain unknown.

Fat accounts for 25 to 40 per cent of the weight of middle-aged men and women (Table 59–2). Body fat cells vary from 10 to 200 μ in diameter or about 8000-fold in total volume. Their numbers may vary between 2×10^{10} and 16×10^{10}. Fat cell size generally increases (hypertrophy) with increasing adiposity until the body fat content is about 30 kg. There is little increase in size as more body fat accumulates. Fat cell number, in contrast, increases in a linear fashion (hyperplasia) as total body fat increases from 10 to 90 kg.

A remarkable feature of adiposity is its constancy. Small increases in adiposity occur regularly with age (Table 59–2), but these are slight relative to the differences in adiposity among individuals. The extent of adiposity is therefore carefully and unconsciously regulated. Intentional overfeeding to increase weight is very difficult for experimental subjects and is followed by spontaneous caloric restriction until body weight returns to baseline.

How then does obesity occur? Fat people do not generally eat more than lean people, and many eat less. Since mass and energy are conserved, it is clear that at some time in life the obese individual consumed more calories than he expended. This temporary imbalance between energy intake and expenditure could be due to several factors (Table 59–3) involving the central nervous system or the adipocyte itself. Reduced sympathetic activity manifested by lower

TABLE 59–1. OBESITY CLASSIFICATION BASED ON BODY MASS INDEX (KG/M^2)

	BMI
Underweight	<20
Normal	20–25
Overweight	25–30
Obese	30–40
Morbidly obese	>40

plasma norepinephrine and epinephrine levels, reduced fat mobilization, or low thermogenesis could reduce energy mobilization and expenditure. Enhanced parasympathetic activity, typical of ventromedial hypothalamic lesions, may augment food consumption. And, at least in theory, the brain may be insensitive to normal neural or humoral satiety signals.

Fat cells with enhanced lipoprotein lipase activity may have a competitive advantage in assimilating lipoprotein triglycerides. This occurs in the syndrome of multiple symmetric lipomatosis. The adipocyte itself may also resist lipolytic stimuli from nerves or circulating catecholamines. Gluteal fat in both men and women, for example, has a lower lipolytic response to α-adrenergic stimulation than does abdominal fat. Some fat depots may resist mobilization even when the rest of the body is starving, as in women with steatopygia who have massive accumulation of gluteal and femoral fat. Abdominal fat in men appears to have more α_2-adrenergic receptor function (antilipolytic) than abdominal fat in women, leading to more "beer bellies" in men. The fat cell may also fail to provide the brain with neural (afferent) or humoral (e.g., adipsin) signals indicating that peripheral fat stores are replete. Finally, when adipocytes of some individuals reach nearly maximal size they may trigger differentiation and replication of preadipocytes and thus perpetuate growth of adipose mass.

Irrespective of the basic mechanism, at least transient reductions in energy expenditure seem to be important in the pathogenesis of most obesities. Babies with low total energy expenditure are likely to gain more weight in the first year of life, and low energy expenditure is a risk factor for weight gain even in adulthood. Paradoxically, the very weight gain that causes obesity can lead to a normalization of energy expenditure. Caloric restriction to achieve weight loss, in contrast, is associated with reductions in energy expenditure to levels far below those in naturally lean individuals.

THE ANATOMY OF OBESITY

Regional patterns of body fat distribution may partially explain apparent inconsistencies in the epidemiology of obesity. It has been puzzling that obesity appears associated with risk factors for vascular disease, but in prospective studies obesity is poorly predictive of vascular disease. It appears that the form of obesity which characteristically occurs in men, called android or abdominal obesity, is closely associated with metabolic complications such as hypertension, insulin resistance, hyperuricemia, and dyslipoproteinemia. The typical female or gynecoid obesity, with fat deposited in hips and gluteal and femoral regions, has much less metabolic significance. The waist to hip circumference ratio has been used to distinguish these forms of obesity. In men a ratio above 1.0 and in women above 0.8 suggests the undesirable male obesity pattern. Thus, it is better to be shaped like a pear than like an apple.

TABLE 59–2. VARIATION OF FAT AND LEAN BODY MASS (LBM) WITH AGE

AGE	MEN		WOMEN	
	(% Body Weight)			
	LBM	FAT	LBM	FAT
25	81	19	68	32
45	74	26	58	42
65	65	35	51	49

TABLE 59–3. POSSIBLE CAUSES OF OBESITY

Neurological	Reduced sympathetic activity
	Increased parasympathetic activity
	Insensitivity to satiety signals
Adipocyte	Increased lipoprotein lipase activity
	Diminished fatty acid mobilization
	Reduced feedback to CNS
	Excessive cell replication
Other	Hyperinsulinemia

MEDICAL CONSEQUENCES OF OBESITY

Morbid Obesity. Subjects weighing 45 kg or 100 lbs (~60 per cent) more than desirable are designated morbidly obese. This corresponds to a weight of 240 lbs in a woman 63 inches tall or 260 lbs in a man of 68 inches. Cardiorespiratory problems present the greatest risk (Table 59–4). Chronic hypoventilation is common and leads to hypercapnia, pulmonary hypertension, and right heart failure. Left ventricular dysfunction also occurs and may be related to both hypertension and hypervolemia. Severe episodic hypoxia can cause arrhythmias, and sudden death is ten times more common in the morbidly obese. Most devastating, however, are the psychosocial consequences of the disorder. Self-esteem and body image are impaired, immobility greatly limits work and recreational activities, and humiliation is a daily experience when body size is too large for conventional scales, furniture, vehicles, and clothes.

Moderate Obesity. The health hazards of moderate overweight are less clear than those of morbid obesity. A weight more than 20 per cent above ideal poses increased risk of early mortality. Subjects more

TABLE 59–4. MEDICAL COMPLICATIONS OF MORBID OBESITY

Sudden death
Obstructive sleep apnea
Pickwickian syndrome: daytime hypoventilation, somnolence, polycythemia, and cor pulmonale
Congestive heart failure
Nephrotic syndrome/renal vein thrombosis
Immobility limiting daily activities

than 30 per cent overweight have about a 50 per cent greater mortality rate than those of average weight. Such naked statistics, however, can be deceiving. Overweight young adults (< 45 yrs), for example, appear at risk from complications of moderate obesity, whereas obesity is less of a risk factor in older people. Restated, obesity does not appear to be a major risk factor in the age range where mortality is greatest. Moreover, there has been a slight increase in obesity prevalence in the United States in the last two decades, whereas total mortality rates have fallen by 20 to 30 per cent.

Clear-cut associations with obesity include the following: Hypertension is more frequent in obese people than in those of normal weight. This may be due to sympathetic hyperactivity or to hyperinsulinemia, but neither mechanism is clearly established. Type II diabetes mellitus can be unmasked and aggravated by excess weight, and this may be the most important medical complication of moderate obesity. The cause appears to be insulin resistance, but it is not known why many obese individuals have normal glucose metabolism. Obesity is often associated with high triglycerides and low HDL concentrations, particularly when mild glucose intolerance is also present. Finally, obesity clearly increases risk of cholelithiasis and endometrial carcinoma.

TREATMENT OF OBESITY

Morbid Obesity. Severe caloric restriction (200 to 800 kcal/day), with or without anorectic drugs, should be tried first. A greater than 90 per cent failure rate is the rule. Subjects more than 100 pounds overweight who have failed medical treatment may be candidates for surgery (gastroplasty or gastric bypass) to reduce stomach size. Patients in general lose 40 to 50 per cent of excess weight within a year of gastric surgery, but some consume calorically dense liquids and regain weight. The long-term safety and efficacy of this surgery are not certain. The once common intestinal bypass surgery for morbid obesity has been abandoned because of unacceptable long-term complications.

Moderate to Severe Obesity. Low-calorie diets re-

TABLE 59–5. DIAGNOSTIC CRITERIA FOR ANOREXIA NERVOSA AND BULIMIA NERVOSA

Anorexia Nervosa
Intense fear of obesity undiminished with weight loss
Disturbed body image
Loss of 25% original body weight; if < 18 yrs, 25% less than original + projected weight gain
No identifiable illness accounting for weight loss
Refusal to maintain normal body weight

Bulimia Nervosa
Recurrent binge eating and at least three of following criteria:
Ingestion of high-calorie, easily ingested food during a binge
Termination of binge by abdominal pain, sleep, social interruption, or self-induced vomiting
Repeated weight loss attempts using severe diet restriction, induced vomiting, or cathartics or diuretics
Weight fluctuations > 4.5 kg due to binges and fasts

main the most widely advocated treatment for obesity. The recommendation to count calories and eat less of everything has intuitive appeal but little success. Behavioral modification techniques focusing on stimulus control, the obese eating style, group and spouse support, reinforcement procedures, and exercise are far more effective. More popular, but less successful, are innumerable eating plans based on marked diet imbalance (e.g., rice diet, ice cream diet, Fit-for-Life diet). These are only transiently helpful because a diet very low in either fat or carbohydrate rapidly becomes monotonous and unpalatable. Diets very low in carbohydrate are also ketogenic and inhibit appetite. Most dramatic in effect, but potentially hazardous, are the very low calorie diets that approximate a supplemented fast, rely on withdrawal of most conventional foods, and entail purchase and consumption of an expensive diet supplement. No diet calling for 800 or fewer calories should be undertaken without medical supervision. More than 50 deaths, some from documented ventricular tachycardia and fibrillation, occurred with the early "liquid protein" very low calorie diets.

No program consisting of caloric restriction alone has been generally successful beyond 12 to 18 months despite the enormous commercial success of diet books and systems.

Anorectic drugs are potentially addicting, often unsafe, and only marginally effective. Patients with any history of drug abuse should avoid any of the amphetamines. These agents may be useful in the short term when incorporated in a program that includes diet counseling, behavior modification, and close medical supervision.

When the pathophysiology of obesity is better defined, then more specific and effective measures should emerge.

ANOREXIA NERVOSA AND BULIMIA NERVOSA

These two psychiatric disorders are characterized by a distorted body image and abnormal eating patterns. Neither has a distinctive pathognomonic feature; the two disorders share some common features, and they may overlap (Table 59–5). Bulimia nervosa is not associated with cachexia, whereas this is the most prominent aspect of anorexia nervosa. The primary treatment of both disorders is psychiatric, although they may manifest important medical complications.

ANOREXIA NERVOSA

Prevalence. The overall prevalence of anorexia nervosa is not known but has apparently increased over the past decade. In amenorrhea clinics, between 5 and 15 per cent of patients may be affected, and in a London study the prevalence among girls 16 to 18 years old was about 1 per cent. The disorder affects girls at least ten times as often as boys, with typical onset in adolescence but occurrence as late as the menopause.

Pathogenesis and Clinical Features. Some individuals can recall life situations or events that triggered their preoccupation with thinness. The usual pubertal weight increase may be critical in most girls. The restriction of food intake is initially voluntary, and a compulsion to lose weight may lead to self-induced vomiting, abuse of purgatives and diuretics, and exhausting exercise. Patients view their own body dimensions as excessive, while their view of other people is not abnormal.

In typical cases, the diagnosis of anorexia nervosa presents little difficulty. In atypical cases (e.g., males, older women), individuals warrant careful evaluation for hyperthyroidism, malignancy, and malabsorption. Amenorrhea occurs early in the disorder. Weight loss, as in young female endurance athletes, is probably the cause of the amenorrhea. Hypothalamic dysfunction with markedly defective gonadotropin secretion appears to be the responsible mechanism. Other signs of hypothalamic dysfunction include abnormal thermoregulation in hot and cold environments and sometimes frank hypothermia, loss of cyclical pattern of ACTH secretion, reduced vasopressin secretion with mild diabetes insipidus, delayed TSH response after TRF, and abnormal growth hormone response to glucose or apomorphine infusion.

Physical examination reveals little subcutaneous fat with gaunt facies, atrophic breasts and buttocks, and often excessive growth of lanugo hair on neck and extremities. Hypotension may occur in association with hypovolemia (secondary to starvation and diabetes insipidus) and bradycardia (secondary to low T_3 levels due to reduced conversion of T_4). Psychiatric evaluation may reveal a major depressive disorder in up to 50 per cent of patients. Otherwise, patients are often well-behaved, perfectionistic, competitive, and achieving.

Treatment and Prognosis. There are no strict guidelines for treatment of anorexia nervosa. Patients should be evaluated by a psychologist or psychiatrist familiar with treatment of this disorder. Occasional patients may be successfully managed as outpatients. Most will benefit more from psychiatric hospitalization and intensive skilled nursing using positive and negative reinforcement, informational feedback, and supervised provision of 3000 to 5000 kcal/day. Weight gain of 0.2 kg/day is a reasonable expectation after the first seven to ten days of gradually increased food consumption. Acutely ill and cachectic patients may require short-term parenteral nutrition with careful avoidance of water intoxication and hyperkalemia. More than one hospitalization of 20 to 50 days is required in half the patients.

Hypothalamic and endocrine problems generally resolve when 85 per cent of normal body weight is restored. Amenorrhea may persist for several more months, but menses usually return without specific intervention.

Anorexia nervosa causes death in at least 5 per cent of patients because of the starvation-dehydration-hypokalemia syndrome or deliberate suicide. The illness may also be lifelong and appears less likely to remit when present for more than ten years. Overall, 40 to 60 per cent of individuals make a good physical and psychosocial recovery.

BULIMIA NERVOSA

Prevalence. Bulimia nervosa may affect as many as 1 to 3 per cent of female adolescents and young adults in North America. As in the case of anorexia nervosa, the prevalence in boys is only 10 per cent of that in girls.

Pathogenesis and Clinical Features. Patients with bulimia often have a family history of major affective disorder (depression or manic-depression). The increase in weight and adiposity at puberty is probably the stimulus for bulimia, just as for anorexia nervosa. A history of unsuccessful diet attempts often precedes the discovery that self-induced vomiting or purgatives can be used to control weight. The hallmark of bulimia, however, is not induced vomiting but binge eating; bulimia is synonymous with paroxysmal hyperphagia. Binges are planned, often center on "junk food," and are secretly conducted like an illicit addictive behavior. Binges leave the patient embarrassed, guilty, and focused again on maintaining weight below an arbitrary level. This end is achieved by prolonged fasting, self-induced vomiting, nonprescription anorectics, and use of substances like diuretics and laxatives. In marked contrast to patients with anorexia nervosa, bulimics generally feel out of control and often welcome help.

Since bulimics are not wasted, physical findings may be subtle or absent. Calluses or scratches on the dorsum of the hand may result from abrasion by teeth during induced gagging. Puffy cheeks from parotid or other salivary gland enlargement are present in up to 50 per cent of patients, and serum salivary amylase may be elevated. Erosions occur on the lingual, palatal, and posterior occlusal surfaces of the teeth from acid-induced enamel dissolution and decalcification.

The medical complications of bulimia nervosa are caused by the vomiting or other maneuvers to purge and induce weight loss. Frequent binge eating and vomiting may cause gastric or esophageal perforation or bleeding, pneumomediastinum, or subcutaneous emphysema. Heavy use of ipecac to induce vomiting may cause myopathic weakness and electrocardiographic abnormalities from emetine toxicity. Loss of gastric fluids can result in metabolic alkalosis with elevated CO_2 and hypochloremia. Diuretic abuse can produce both hypokalemia and hyponatremia. Menstrual irregularities are common, but amenorrhea is rare.

Treatment and Prognosis. Serious medical complications occasionally occur, but bulimics, in general, do not need psychiatric hospitalization. Depression and very abnormal beliefs about body weight and shape are typically present and underlie attitudes toward eating and weight control. Outpatient psychotherapy stresses self-monitoring and acquisition of a normal eating pattern, since fear of being out of control is intense. Issues of diet pills, laxatives, and diuretics must be directly dealt with, together with misconceptions about "fattening" foods. Most difficult is the restructuring of attitudes about body weight and shape. It is often necessary to accept the misconceptions as immutable while nonetheless encouraging adaptive behavior.

Anticonvulsants and antidepressants have been successfully employed by some therapists, although such agents are not necessary in the majority of patients. Phenytoin has appeared moderately effective and imipramine may be even more useful. Monoamine oxidase inhibitors have also reduced both depressive symptoms and binge eating. The natural history of bulimia nervosa is poorly defined, and it is not certain how often current therapeutic approaches result in cures as opposed to short-term remissions.

REFERENCES

Health and Public Policy Committee, American College of Physicians: Eating disorders: Anorexia nervosa and bulimia. Ann Intern Med 105:790–794, 1986.
Herzog DB, Copeland PM: Eating disorders. N Engl J Med 313:295–303, 1985.
Mitchell JE, Seim HC, Colon E, Pomeroy C: Medical complications and medical management of bulimia. Ann Intern Med 107:71–77, 1987.
Stunkard AJ, Stellar E (eds): Eating and Its Disorders. New York, Raven Press, 1984.

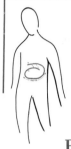

60

PRINCIPLES OF ALIMENTATION AND HYPERALIMENTATION

PRINCIPLES OF NUTRITION AND NUTRITIONAL ASSESSMENT

Good nutrition is a prerequisite not only for optimal resistance to illness, but also for optimal response to medical and surgical therapy. The recognition and treatment of malnutrition that accompanies illness play an important role in optimizing patient care. Energy needs vary with body size, age, sex, activity, and the presence or absence of disease. The use of recommended dietary allowances (RDA's) that have been established for most essential nutrients may not apply to sick or traumatized patients or to those with metabolic disorders. Increasingly, methods of nutritional assessment that have been used to assess the severity of malnutrition among populations in developing countries are being applied to hospitalized patients. New modes of delivering nutrients to sick patients by both the enteral and parenteral routes may improve morbidity and mortality by eliminating the role of malnutrition in the natural history of many diseases.

Protein, carbohydrate, and fat are the basic nutrients that provide energy in health and disease. Protein and carbohydrate supply about 4 kcal of energy per gram and fat 9 kcal per gram. Basal energy expenditure (BEE) is estimated from the oxygen consumed under resting conditions in healthy, nonobese subjects and usually approximates 25 kcal/kg/day. A number of calories are required in addition to the BEE depending on daily activity: 400 to 800 kcal for sedentary activity, 800 to 1200 kcal for light activity, 1200 to 1800 kcal for moderate activity, and up to 4500 kcal for strenuous exercise. Fasting and malnutrition reduce energy expenditure; however, the stress of illness increases caloric requirements. For example, in catabolic patients, an additional 50 to 100 per cent of the BEE may be required to prevent further tissue breakdown. In febrile patients, a 13 per cent increase in calories is required for each 1°C of fever.

Although carbohydrates comprise the main source of energy for most people in the world, there is no fixed requirement for this food group in the diet. Protein is needed to maintain body structure and function. The quality of dietary protein varies depending on the digestibility of the protein and its amino acid composition. High-quality proteins are easily absorbed and contain adequate amounts and proportions of the nine essential amino acids. The recommended allowance for dietary protein in healthy adults is 0.8 gm/kg/day. Catabolic patients may require 1.2 to 1.6 gm/kg/day. Dietary fat is a concentrated source of calories and a source of lipid-soluble vitamins. Essential fatty acids (i.e., linoleic acid, linolenic acid) are needed for membrane structure and integrity and serve as precursors for important eicosanoids. With the exception of neurons and erythrocytes, all body cells can utilize fatty acids as a direct source of energy. In addition to providing nutrients to match energy needs, the judicious diet must supply adequate amounts of water, essential minerals, and vitamins.

Nutritional assessment of hospitalized patients most often focuses on the recognition and treatment of the malnutrition that accompanies many illnesses. Protein-calorie malnutrition occurs whenever inadequate protein and/or calories are ingested to meet an individual's nutritional requirements (Table 60–1). The diagnosis of malnutrition is based on the dietary history, physical examination, anthropometric measurements, and laboratory studies. Dietary evaluation should include an assessment of the intake of major food groups and should focus on a history of recent weight loss, alterations in appetite, and symptoms of gastrointestinal disorders including problems with chewing or swallowing, diarrhea, constipation, nausea, vomiting, and early satiety. The social history is an important facet of the dietary evaluation because social isolation, old age, poverty, and depression increase the risk of malnutrition.

The most obvious physical manifestation of chronic malnutrition is loss of body weight. Most individuals can tolerate a loss of up to 10 per cent of body weight without significant consequences; however, losses greater than 40 per cent below ideal weight are almost always fatal. Temporal muscle wasting, edema, and depigmentation of hair are other signs of malnutrition that can be confirmed by anthropometric and laboratory measurements. "Ideal" body weights for each inch of height have been derived from life insurance actuarial data. Other commonly employed anthropometric parameters include measurements of triceps skinfold thickness (an estimate of body fat reserves) and midarm muscle area (an estimate of lean body or skeletal muscle mass). Direct measurement of mineral or vitamin concentrations in body fluids may identify specific nutrient deficiencies; more often, measurements of various serum proteins (e.g., hemoglobin, albumin, transferrin) are used in assessing a patient's overall nutritional status, recognizing that certain laboratory abnormalities that could reflect malnutrition may have a non-nutritional cause (e.g., hypoalbuminemia, anemia). Serum albumin values more than 20 per cent below the lower limit of the normal range generally are regarded as substandard and corroborate a diagnosis of malnutrition in the proper clinical setting. In malnourished patients, the number of circulating lymphocytes diminishes, and delayed hypersensitivity to common skin antigens is impaired. A lymphocyte count of fewer than $1200/\mu l$ is substandard.

PRINCIPLES OF NUTRITIONAL SUPPORT

Nutritional support of the hospitalized patient has become a complex system using alternate routes of metabolic support (enteral, peripheral venous, central venous) and multiple types of solutions. Decisions about the mode of nutritional support may be guided by the algorithm shown in Figure 60–1. The algorithm begins with a nutritional assessment based on the dietary history, physical examination, laboratory studies, and anthropometric measurements. If the diet is meeting requirements, no further therapy is needed. If the diet is inadequate, the decision to provide nutritional support is guided by the degree of nutritional depletion as assessed by body weight and by the anticipated duration of nutritional depletion. If body weight has declined by less than 5 per cent and the

TABLE 60–1. CAUSES OF PROTEIN-CALORIE MALNUTRITION IN HOSPITALIZED PATIENTS

Decreased Oral Intake	
Anorexia	Gastrointestinal obstruction
Nausea	Poor dentition
Dysphagia	
Increased Nutrient Losses	
Malabsorption	Fistula drainage
Diarrhea	Protein-losing enteropathy
Bleeding	Nephrotic syndrome
Increased Nutrient Requirements	
Fever	Trauma
Infection	Burns
Neoplasms	Surgery

anticipated duration of inadequate nutrition is less than seven days, nutritional supplements may not be necessary. If the degree of depletion is moderate (5 to 10 per cent) or severe (greater than 10 per cent) and the anticipated duration of illness is more than seven days, intensive therapy may be needed. Whether forced enteral feeding or parenteral nutrition is chosen depends on the availability and adequacy of the gastrointestinal tract.

Enteral nutritional therapy encompasses the use of nutritional supplements to provide part or all of daily requirements and the use of special diets that either restrict a particular element of the diet (e.g., fat, lactose) or add a nutrient (e.g., fiber, calcium, potassium) that may be required in larger amounts than are available in conventional diets. If requirements are not great and appetite is good, table foods can be recommended as protein and calorie supplements. Chronically ill patients with anorexia, those with chronic inflammatory disorders who have increased requirements, and those who are marginally nourished and preparing for surgery are candidates for oral supplementation with one of a variety of commercial products that are high in caloric density. Forced enteral feeding (via nasogastric tube or gastrostomy tube) typically is used for those patients who have moderate to severe anorexia, those who cannot maintain a caloric intake commensurate with their needs, or those with swallowing disorders. Nasoduodenal tubes are preferred in patients at high risk for aspiration. Feeding via a percutaneous gastrostomy tube is now used when the anticipated time for enteral supplementation is long (greater than six weeks) and the patient cannot swallow.

Parenteral nutrition provides protein and calories to partially meet, totally meet, or exceed daily nutritional requirements. Total parenteral nutrition (TPN) is indicated for two groups of patients: (1) those selected for nutritional support in whom the gastrointestinal tract is not usable for forced enteral feedings, and (2) those in whom a nothing-by-mouth regimen (i.e., "bowel rest") is deemed beneficial for a primary gastrointestinal disease. TPN solutions must provide a source of protein (amino acids) and energy. A combination of dextrose, amino acids, and water provides the base solution to which vitamins and minerals can

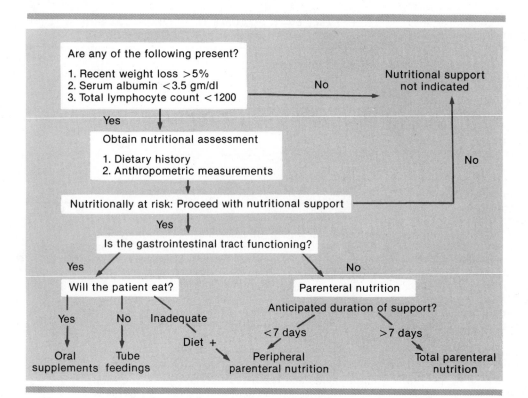

FIGURE 60–1. An algorithm for selecting nutritional therapy.

be added. The amino acid contents of standard commercial solutions are based largely on normal plasma amino acid concentrations; special formulas with an increased proportion of essential amino acids often are used in patients with renal failure to minimize the generation of urea. The monohydrate form of dextrose used in most commercial solutions provides 3.4 kcal/gm and can be used alone to achieve both positive energy balance and positive nitrogen balance as long as adequate amino acids are supplied. However, lipid emulsions of soybean or safflower oil are often added to provide up to 70 per cent of the daily caloric requirement, since they contain a concentrated source of calories, reduce the volume of fluid needed, and reduce the likelihood of hyperglycemia.

Parenteral solutions that provide all energy and protein requirements are hypertonic and must be administered through a central vein. Lesser concentrations of dextrose and amino acids (with a final osmolarity less than 600 mOsm/L) can be administered through a peripheral vein and often are employed as supplements to an inadequate enteral regimen. Isotonic lipid emulsions are regularly used as an energy source in peripheral vein parenteral nutrition because they reduce the osmolarity of the solution, thereby reducing the risk of thrombophlebitis.

REFERENCES

Frisancho AR: New standards of weight and body composition by frame size and height for assessment of nutritional status of adults and the elderly. Am J Clin Nutr 40:808, 1984.

Kaminski MV Jr (ed): Hyperalimentation: A Guide for Clinicians. New York, Marcel Dekker, 1985.

Siberman H, Eisenberg D: Parenteral and Enteral Nutrition for the Hospitalized Patient. E Norwalk, CT, Appleton-Century-Crofts, 1982.

61

HYPERURICEMIA AND GOUT

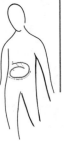

The term *gout* refers to a group of disorders characterized by a derangement in purine metabolism manifested by hyperuricemia, crystalline deposits of monosodium urate monohydrate in tissues (tophi), and recurrent episodes of acute arthritis. Hyperuricemia and gout may be classified as primary or secondary (Table 61–1). *Primary gout* results from inborn errors in the metabolism of purines or inherited defects in the renal tubular secretion of urate. *Secondary gout* occurs in disorders characterized by increased catabolism of nucleic acids or by acquired defects in the renal excretion of urate.

Pathogenesis

The biochemical hallmark of gout is an elevated serum urate, a metabolic end-product formed by the oxidation of both exogenous and endogenous purine bases. The concentration of uric acid in body fluids reflects the balance between rates of production and elimination. Approximately one third of uric acid produced on a daily basis (100 to 300 mg in the adult) is excreted in the gastrointestinal tract, where it is destroyed by bacteria. The remaining two thirds (300 to 600 mg) is excreted in the urine. Hyperuricemia may result from increased production of uric acid, decreased renal excretion, or some combination of these factors.

The risk of developing gout increases with the degree of hyperuricemia; however, the pathogenesis of gout is related more closely to the *solubility* of urate in various body fluids than to its absolute concentration. The solubility of urate is influenced by temper-

TABLE 61–1. CLASSIFICATION OF HYPERURICEMIA AND GOUT

Primary (presumably genetic)
I. Metabolic (overproduction)
  A. Idiopathic (10% of primary gout)
  B. Associated with specific enzyme defects (<1% of primary gout)
    1. PP-ribose-P synthetase overactivity
    2. Partial deficiency of hypoxanthine-guanine phosphoribosyl transferase
    3. "Complete" deficiency of hypoxanthine-guanine phosphoribosyl transferase
II. Renal (idiopathic underexcretion—90% of primary gout)
Secondary (acquired)
I. Metabolic
  A. Increased nucleic acid turnover (e.g., chronic hemolysis, lymphoproliferative or myeloproliferative disorders)
  B. Glucose-6-phosphatase deficiency (i.e., Type I glycogen storage disease)
II. Renal
  A. Acute or chronic renal failure
  B. Volume depletion
  C. Altered tubular handling by drugs or endogenous metabolic products

ature and pH. At 37°C and pH 7.40, the solubility of urate is 6.4 to 6.8 mg/dl. But solubility is considerably less at the lower temperatures of peripheral joints. A urate concentration of 7.0 mg/dl usually constitutes the physicochemical upper limit of normal beyond which supersaturation occurs and crystal formation increases. Virtually all patients with gout have serum urate levels above 7.0 mg/dl. Occasional patients exhibit lower levels during an acute attack, but hyperuricemia can almost always be demonstrated during quiescent periods.

Overproduction of uric acid, detected clinically by the urinary excretion of more than 600 mg of uric acid per day, accounts for less than 10 per cent of all cases of gout. Increased production of uric acid occurs as the result of an inherited enzyme defect, as the secondary consequence of a disorder in which nucleic acid turnover is increased, or as an idiopathic phenomenon probably representing as yet undetected enzyme defects. A review of purine metabolism will clarify the enzyme defects associated with primary gout (Fig. 61–1).

The purine nucleotides—adenylic acid (AMP), inosinic acid (IMP), and guanylic acid (GMP)—are products of purine biosynthesis ultimately utilized for the synthesis of nucleic acids, cyclic AMP, ATP, cyclic GMP, and various cofactors. Degradation of purine nucleotides occurs via intermediate purine nucleotide formation of uric acid. The intracellular concentration of 5-phosphoribosyl-1-pyrophosphate (PRPP) controls the rate of uric acid synthesis.

Increased activity of the enzyme PRPP synthetase (Fig. 61–1) results in increased concentrations of PRPP, accelerated purine biosynthesis, and increased production of uric acid. Hypoxanthine-guanine phosphoribosyl transferase (HPRT) catalyzes the salvage conversion of hypoxanthine to IMP and guanine to GMP (Fig. 61–1). Deficiency or reduced activity of HPRT leads to decreased consumption and increased accumulation of PRPP, thus accelerating the *de novo* synthesis of purines and uric acid. Approximately 10 per cent of patients with gout and overproduction of uric acid exhibit partial deficiency of HPRT. Complete or virtually complete deficiency of HPRT results in the Lesch-Nyhan syndrome, a rare infantile disorder characterized by hyperuricemia, gout, choreoathetosis, mental retardation, and self-mutilation. PRPP synthetase overactivity and HPRT deficiency are familial enzyme defects inherited as X-linked traits. Together these inborn errors of metabolism account for less than 15 per cent of all cases of gout associated with uric acid overproduction. In the majority of overproducers of uric acid with gout, the biochemical abnormalities remain undefined.

Uric acid is overproduced whenever there is increased turnover of nucleic acids due to rapid division or lysis of cells. Myeloproliferative and lymphoproliferative diseases, hemolytic anemias, and various hem-

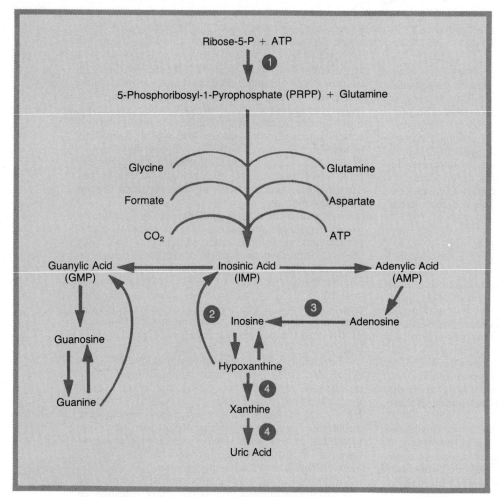

FIGURE 61–1. Purine biosynthetic pathway. (1) 5-Phosphoribosyl-1-pyrophosphate (PRPP) synthetase. (2) Hypoxanthine-guanine phosphoribosyl transferase (HPRT). (3) Adenosine deaminase. (4) Xanthine oxidase.

oglobinopathies are the most common disorders in which this occurs. Hyperuricemia is a prominent feature of the "tumor lysis syndrome" that may follow treatment of patients with lymphoma, myeloproliferative disorders, or carcinomatosis.

Underexcretion of uric acid accounts for more than 90 per cent of all cases of gout. Impaired excretion may result from (1) reduced glomerular filtration of uric acid, (2) enhanced renal tubular reabsorption, (3) reduced tubular secretion, or (4) a combination of defects in filtration and tubular handling. In most instances of primary renal gout the defect remains undefined.

A number of factors can secondarily reduce renal urate excretion and cause gout. In patients with acute or chronic renal failure, reductions in glomerular filtration rate lead to a decrease in the filtered load of uric acid. Although renal disease is a frequent cause of hyperuricemia, clinical gout seldom ensues, perhaps because uremia blunts the inflammatory response to urate crystals. Because renal tubular reabsorption of urate is linked to sodium reabsorption, hyperuricemia frequently accompanies disorders characterized by renal sodium avidity. Extracellular volume depletion of any etiology (e.g., hemorrhage,

gastrointestinal losses, adrenal insufficiency, diabetes insipidus) leads to decreased filtration and enhanced renal tubular reabsorption of uric acid. In clinical practice, diuretic therapy is probably the most common cause of secondary hyperuricemia and gout mediated by volume depletion. A number of other drugs can cause hyperuricemia by directly altering renal tubular handling of uric acid (Table 61–2). Some of these (e.g., thiazides, "loop" diuretics) are organic acids that may occupy uric acid secretory sites along the proximal nephron, thus impairing tubular secretion of urate. Competitive inhibition of uric acid secretion by *endogenous* organic acids accounts for hyperuricemia in patients with lactic acidosis and ketoacidosis.

Clinical Features

Gout is chiefly a disorder of adult males; only about 5 per cent of cases occur in women. The natural history encompasses four distinct clinical syndromes: (1) asymptomatic hyperuricemia, (2) acute gouty arthritis, (3) chronic tophaceous gout, and (4) nephrolithiasis. In most patients, these syndromes arise in roughly chronological order; however, nephrolithiasis may precede the development of arthritis in approximately 20 per cent of cases. Clinical gout is uncommon before

TABLE 61–2. SOME DRUGS THAT AFFECT SERUM URIC ACID CONCENTRATION

Drugs That Increase Serum Uric Acid
Thiazides
"Loop" diuretics (furosemide, ethacrynic acid)
Small doses of salicylate (< 2 gm per day)
Acetazolamide
Pyrazinamide
Ethambutol
Drugs That Decrease Serum Uric Acid
Increased renal excretion
Probenecid
Sulfinpyrazone
Phenylbutazone, oxyphenylbutazone
Large doses of salicylate (4-6 gm per day)
Decreased production
Allopurinol

the third decade of life; its peak age of onset in men is about 45 years, usually after 20 to 30 years of sustained hyperuricemia. *Asymptomatic hyperuricemia* refers to elevation of serum urate prior to the development of arthritic symptoms, tophi, or nephrolithiasis.

Acute Gouty Arthritis. The primary manifestation of gout is a painful arthritis, usually involving the lower extremities. Ninety per cent of initial attacks are monoarticular, and at least half involve the first metatarsophalangeal joint (podagra). Other initial sites of involvement, in order of frequency, include the ankles, heels, knees, wrists, fingers, and elbows. Acute gouty arthritis may be precipitated by events such as trauma, surgery, alcohol ingestion, or systemic infection. While the course of an untreated attack varies, initial episodes are usually self-limited. Over 50 per cent of patients, however, will experience recurrent arthritis within one year of the first attack. Later attacks tend to be more prolonged and severe and more commonly involve multiple joints.

A presumptive diagnosis of gout can be made if the patient is hyperuricemic and has the classic clinical features described above. Unfortunately, a substantial minority of patients with acute gout exhibit *normal* uric acid levels. A dramatic response to colchicine is highly suggestive but not pathognomonic of acute gout. When the diagnosis is in doubt, acute gouty arthritis can be confirmed by demonstration of negatively birefringent, needle-shaped urate crystals within the white blood cells of synovial fluid examined under a polarizing lens. Synovial fluid analysis otherwise exhibits nonspecific signs of acute inflammation. The leukocyte count ranges from 1000 to over 70,000/μl, with a predominance of polymorphonuclear cells. Concentrations of glucose and uric acid in synovial fluid are usually similar to those in serum.

Chronic Tophaceous Gout. In untreated patients, tophaceous deposits of monosodium urate ultimately appear in cartilage, tendons, bursae, soft tissues, and synovial membranes at a rate that parallels the degree and duration of hyperuricemia. Common sites include the external ear and pressure points such as the Achilles tendons and olecranon bursae. Gouty tophi may spontaneously ulcerate and extrude a pasty material consisting of pure urate. Although tophi themselves are painless, their presence in and around joints ultimately can limit joint mobility.

Nephrolithiasis. Two distinct renal syndromes are associated with hyperuricemia. (1) *Acute urate nephropathy* results from the precipitation of urate within renal tubules and occurs almost exclusively in patients with myeloproliferative or lymphoproliferative disorders with severe hyperuricemia (serum uric acid >25 mg/dl), especially following chemotherapy. Intratubular obstruction with uric acid may cause profound reductions of glomerular filtration rate and severe azotemia. (2) *Uric acid urolithiasis* occurs in approximately 20 per cent of patients with a history of gouty arthritis. Increased urinary excretion of uric acid is the main factor favoring the formation of uric acid stones. Both gouty and nongouty uric acid stone formers also exhibit inappropriate urine acidity that favors the precipitation of uric acid. Gouty subjects also have an increased incidence of calcium oxalate stones, perhaps because uric acid crystals serve as a nidus for calcium stone formation.

More than 90 per cent of patients with chronic tophaceous gout exhibit interstitial urate deposits. There is, however, no clear-cut evidence that chronic gout directly causes renal insufficiency. The observation that renal disease is a common cause of death in patients with gouty arthritis may be explained by the frequent occurrence of hyperuricemia in patients with hypertension and diabetes mellitus. In some patients, especially in younger adults, the concurrence of hyperuricemia and renal dysfunction may reflect underlying lead nephropathy.

Treatment

Management of Asymptomatic Hyperuricemia. Controversy surrounds the management of asymptomatic hyperuricemia. Because only 10 to 20 per cent of patients with asymptomatic hyperuricemia develop arthritis, treatment should be withheld unless the patient (1) has a strong family history of gout or uric acid nephrolithiasis, (2) is excreting greater than 1100 mg/day of uric acid, or (3) has a serum uric acid level greater than 11 mg/dl.

Treatment of Acute Gouty Arthritis. Acute gout is treated with one of three types of anti-inflammatory agents: colchicine, nonsteroidal anti-inflammatory drugs, or corticosteroids. Colchicine is the only therapeutic agent with specific diagnostic value in acute gout. An initial oral dose of 0.6 to 1.2 mg should be administered as soon as the diagnosis is suspected. The initial dose should be followed by 0.6 mg every hour until (1) symptoms of arthritis abate, (2) nausea, vomiting, or diarrhea develops, or (3) a maximum dose of 6 mg has been administered. When this regimen is initiated within 12 hours of the onset of symptoms, colchicine is effective in over 90 per cent of cases; however, gastrointestinal side effects preclude administration of optimal doses in a number of patients. Intravenous colchicine is advantageous when a rapid response is desired or when gastrointestinal side effects prohibit oral administration of the drug. Occasionally, intravenous colchicine is effective when the oral preparation is not. The initial intravenous dose of colchicine is 2 mg (injected over two to five minutes), followed by 0.5 mg every six hours until a daily satisfactory response is achieved. The total daily dose of intravenous colchicine should not exceed 4 mg.

Nonsteroidal anti-inflammatory drugs including indomethacin, phenylbutazone, naproxen, fenoprofen, and ibuprofen are also effective in the treatment of acute gouty arthritis. In general, these agents should initially be administered at nearly maximal doses, with gradual tapering as symptoms subside. For example, indomethacin may be given as an oral dose of 75 mg, followed by 50 mg every 8 hours for three doses, and then 25 mg every 8 hours for three doses.

Corticosteroids should be reserved for patients in whom full doses of colchicine or nonsteroidal agents are either contraindicated or ineffective. Intra-articular injections of steroids (e.g., 5 to 10 mg of triamcinolone) are effective in treating acute gout limited to a single joint. Alternatively, 40 to 80 mg of prednisone administered daily for three to four days may be effective, but rebound attacks of gout are common. Uricosuric agents and allopurinol are of no value in the treatment of acute gouty arthritis. Once an attack subsides, administration of small daily doses of colchicine (0.6 to 1.2 mg per day) is effective in preventing further attacks.

Prevention or Reversal of Urate Deposition and Nephrolithiasis. Antihyperuricemic drugs should be administered to patients with recurrent gouty arthritis, nephrolithiasis, or tophi. The goal is to maintain the serum urate level below 7.0 mg/dl. Reductions to these levels can be achieved by drugs that increase the renal excretion of uric acid or decrease uric acid production. While a number of drugs exhibit uricosuric properties (Table 61–2), only probenecid and sulfinpyrazone are widely employed specifically as antihyperuricemic agents. Uricosuric therapy is accompanied by a transient increase in uric acid excretion, which returns to pretreatment levels a few days later as the total body urate pool is depleted. To avoid overt nephrolithiasis during this transient hyperuricosuric phase, the uricosuric agents should be started at low doses and gradually increased. For example, probenecid is started in doses of 250 mg twice daily and increased over a period of several weeks to the dose necessary to achieve effective reversal of hyperuricemia. Sulfinpyrazone is begun at 50 mg twice daily and increased to maintenance levels of 300 to 400 mg per day in divided doses. In addition, maintaining an ample urine flow with adequate hydration reduces the likelihood of stone formation. Probenecid and sulfinpyrazone are ineffective in patients with impaired renal function (glomerular filtration rate <30 ml/min).

Hyperuricemia may also be controlled by allopurinol, a drug that decreases uric acid production by inhibiting xanthine oxidase, the enzyme that catalyzes the conversion of hypoxanthine to xanthine and xanthine to uric acid (Fig. 61–1). In most patients, 300 mg per day is effective, but the half-life of allopurinol is increased in patients with renal insufficiency so that a smaller dose (100 to 200 mg) may be sufficient. Although uncommon, adverse effects with allopurinol are more severe than with uricosuric drugs and include fever, dermatitis, elevation of hepatic enzymes, diarrhea, and occasional vasculitis. *Initiation of antihyperuricemic therapy with any agent may precipitate acute gouty arthritis, since acute gout may occur whenever there is a rapid change in the serum urate concentration.* It is prudent to begin prophylactic therapy with colchicine just prior to the initiation of antihyperuricemic drugs.

Acute urate nephropathy can be prevented by administration of allopurinol to patients with neoplastic disorders prior to administration of chemotherapy. For prophylaxis during treatment of lymphoproliferative or myeloproliferative disorders, treatment with 600 to 900 mg daily is advisable during the first few days of therapy; thereafter the dose is tapered to 300 mg per day, so long as the serum urate remains less than 7.0 mg/dl. A generous intake of fluids should be maintained to assure a high rate of urine flow. Urinary alkalinization also helps to prevent intrarenal precipitation of uric acid. The pKa of uric acid is 5.75. In urine at pH 5.0, only 15 per cent of uric acid exists in soluble, ionized form. The solubility increases more than tenfold at pH 7.0 and more than 100-fold at pH 8.0. Administration of sodium bicarbonate and/or the carbonic anhydrase inhibitor, acetazolamide, should be considered in patients at high risk for developing acute urate nephropathy.

OTHER DISORDERS OF PURINE METABOLISM

Xanthinuria is a rare genetic disorder, probably inherited as an autosomal recessive trait, that results from deficiency of the enzyme xanthine oxidase. Affected patients exhibit hypouricemia, increased urinary excretion of hypoxanthine and xanthine, and sometimes xanthine kidney stones. They are otherwise asymptomatic.

Immune dysfunction may be associated with certain enzyme deficiencies in the purine pathway. Patients with deficiency of adenosine deaminase, which normally catalyzes the deamination of adenosine to inosine (Fig. 61–1), have severe combined immune deficiency (i.e., severe dysfunction of cell-mediated immunity with milder abnormalities of humoral immunity). Deficiency of purine nucleoside phosphorylase, which catalyzes the conversion of inosine to hypoxanthine and guanosine to guanine, has also been associated with an inherited immune deficiency syndrome.

REFERENCES

Berger L, Yu TF: Renal function in gout. IV. An analysis of 624 gouty subjects including long-term follow-up studies. Am J Med 59:605, 1975.

Wyngaarden JB: Gout. *In* Wyngaarden JB, Smith LH Jr (eds): Cecil Textbook of Medicine. 18th ed. Philadelphia, WB Saunders Co, 1988, pp 1161–1170.

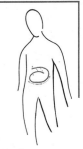

62

DISORDERS OF LIPID METABOLISM

PLASMA LIPOPROTEIN PHYSIOLOGY

The major properties of the plasma lipoproteins are summarized in Table 62–1. Normal men and women daily consume 80 to 120 gm of fat (triglyceride). Dietary fat is hydrolyzed by pancreatic lipase, absorbed by the intestinal mucosal cells, and secreted into the mesenteric lymphatics as chylomicrons (Fig. 62–1). One hundred grams of dietary fat mixed in an adult plasma volume of 25 dl can theoretically increase plasma triglycerides by 4000 mg/dl! The liver also transforms unneeded plasma free fatty acids and calories from any source into triglycerides and daily secretes an additional 10 to 30 gm of very low density lipoprotein (VLDL) triglyceride into the plasma. This potentially further increases triglycerides by 1000 mg/dl. Both chylomicrons and VLDL acquire a 9000 M.W. peptide called apolipoprotein C-II (apo C-II) from plasma high density lipoproteins (HDL). Apo C-II is a critical cofactor for lipoprotein lipase, which is located on the capillary endothelium of muscle and adipose tissue. After hydrolysis of chylomicron and VLDL triglycerides, excess phospholipid, cholesterol, and apoproteins transfer to HDL and increase HDL

TABLE 62–1. PROPERTIES OF LIPOPROTEINS

LIPOPROTEIN CLASS	ORIGIN	MAJOR APOPROTEIN GROUPS	MAJOR CORE LIPID
Chylomicrons	Intestine	B-48, C, E	Dietary triglycerides
VLDL	Liver	B-100, C, E	Hepatic triglycerides
LDL	VLDL catabolism	B-100	Cholesteryl esters
HDL	Liver, intestine	A, C	Cholesteryl esters

mass. The remnants remaining after hydrolysis of chylomicron triglycerides are cleared very rapidly by the liver and do not normally accumulate in plasma. This process is mediated by apolipoprotein E (apo E) on the chylomicron surface and the B,E receptor on the hepatocyte cell membrane.

Some VLDL remnants (10 to 30 per cent) are also cleared directly by the liver, but the majority are converted to intermediate density lipoproteins (IDL). IDL are normally short-lived and by the action of lipases

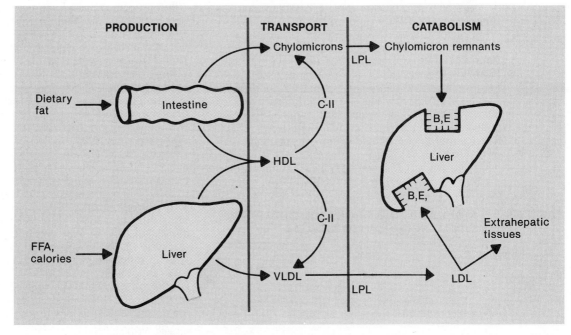

FIGURE 62–1. Normal metabolism of plasma lipoproteins. See text for details. FFA = Free fatty acids; HDL = high density lipoproteins; VLDL = very low density lipoproteins; LDL = low density lipoproteins; B,E = membrane receptor for lipoproteins containing apo B and apo E.

are converted to the final VLDL catabolic product, low density lipoproteins (LDL) (Fig. 62–1). In contrast to VLDL, which survive about 20 minutes in plasma, LDL circulate for three to five days. While LDL normally account for 70 per cent of the total plasma cholesterol, they are basically metabolic garbage. Most LDL clearance from plasma takes place when apo B on the LDL surface binds to the B,E receptor on membranes of many tissues, particularly the liver.

HDL are secreted into plasma by both intestine and liver. It is thought that HDL readily accept cholesterol from cells and other lipoproteins. This cholesterol initially is absorbed onto the HDL surface, where it is substrate for the plasma enzyme lecithin:cholesterol acyltransferase (LCAT). LCAT transfers a fatty acid from phosphatidyl choline to the 3-hydroxyl group of cholesterol. This produces cholesteryl esters that move from the hydrophilic HDL surface into the hydrophobic HDL core. The HDL surface is then free to accept more cholesterol from cells or other lipoproteins.

There are at least ten well-characterized apolipoproteins that are located on lipoprotein surfaces. These stabilize the lipoprotein micelle, are recognized by cell membrane receptors, and serve as enzyme cofactors. Their major lipoprotein associations are listed in Table 62–1. The usefulness of quantifying these apolipoproteins in clinical practice is uncertain.

EVALUATION OF SERUM LIPOPROTEIN CONCENTRATIONS

Every adult should have a total serum cholesterol determined during his/her third decade. A value less than 200 mg/dl at any time of day does not require retesting for five years. A level greater than 200 mg/dl should lead to measurement of total cholesterol, triglycerides, and HDL-cholesterol after a 14-hour fast. If triglycerides are over 500 mg/dl then specific treatment of hypertriglyceridemia should be undertaken. The highest total cholesterols commonly encountered (600 to 2000 mg/dl) are usually due to increases in chylomicrons and VLDL. Elevated cholesterols, therefore, cannot be interpreted without knowledge of triglyceride levels.

If triglycerides (TG) are less than 400 mg/dl, then the LDL-cholesterol (LDL$_C$) is calculated as follows:

$$LDL_C = Total\ C - (HDL_C + VLDL_C)$$

$$= Total\ C - (HDL_C + TG/5)$$

A therapeutic strategy based on LDL is indicated in Table 62–2.

Elevated HDL levels are thought to confer protection against coronary heart disease (CHD) and do not require treatment. Low HDL levels suggest increased CHD risk and justify aggressive modification of other factors, including even mild LDL elevations (>130 mg/dl).

ELEVATED CHYLOMICRONS, VLDL, AND IDL

Disorders Manifest in Childhood. The occurrence of eruptive xanthomata, lipemia retinalis, hepatosplenomegaly, and abdominal pain in an infant or small child suggests a primary defect in clearance of chylomicrons and VLDL. This may be due to a deficiency of lipoprotein lipase (assayed in plasma after heparin injection) or of apolipoprotein C-II, the cofactor for lipoprotein lipase. These abnormalities have a prevalence less than one or two in a million.

Disorders Manifest in Adulthood. Chylomicrons and VLDL are both catabolized by lipoprotein lipase, and the enzyme is saturable. The enzyme prefers chylomicrons, so VLDL usually accumulate first until triglycerides exceed 500 mg/dl. At higher levels, both VLDL and chylomicrons contribute to the hypertriglyceridemia. Testing to resolve the independent contribution of these two lipoproteins is rarely indicated, and tests for lipoprotein lipase and apolipoprotein C-II should be reserved for cases arising in childhood. Most hypertriglyceridemia in adults appears to be due to VLDL overproduction, although defective catabolism is responsible in a subset of patients.

Moderate to severe hypertriglyceridemia is relatively common in men and women older than 30 years. The disorder is usually genetic and is commonly associated with hypertension, hyperuricemia, and abnormal glucose tolerance. Hypertriglyceridemia may be aggravated by obesity, even moderate alcohol consumption, exogenous estrogens, and drugs such as diuretics and beta-adrenoreceptor blockers. Common secondary causes of hypertriglyceridemia are renal disease with proteinuria, both hyper- and hypothyroidism, exogenous and endogenous glucocorticoids, and Type II diabetes mellitus. A very severe form of hypertriglyceridemia (2000 to 6000 mg/dl) can occur in patients with chronic insulin deficiency and very mild acidosis. This abnormality is completely corrected by insulin administration. The hypertriglyceridemia occurring in acute diabetic ketoacidosis is usually milder (250 to 800 mg/dl) and also responds to insulin.

The importance of hypertriglyceridemia in vascular disease risk is controversial. An NIH consensus conference concluded that triglyceride levels under 250 mg/dl were normal, those 250 to 500 mg/dl were bor-

TABLE 62–2. APPROACH TO ELEVATED LDL-CHOLESTEROL LEVELS BASED ON CORONARY RISK STATUS*

LDL$_C$ LEVEL	TREATMENT
<130 mg/dl	None
130–160 mg/dl	Diet
160–190 mg/dl	Diet; consider drugs if two CHD risk factors present
>190 mg/dl	Diet and consider drugs if diet fails

*CHD risk factors include male sex, peripheral vascular disease, diabetes mellitus, hypertension, cigarette smoking, >30% overweight, low HDL (<35 mg/dl), and family history of CHD before 55 years.

derline, and only higher values were considered abnormal. Nevertheless, upper normal range triglycerides (120 to 250 mg/dl) are very prevalent in CHD populations, and within this range the inverse relationship between triglycerides and HDL-cholesterol is strongest. The association of hypertriglyceridemia with diabetes mellitus, obesity, and hypertension has further confounded efforts to define its independent role in vascular disease.

Dysbetalipoproteinemia. This disease is characterized by the accumulation of chylomicron remnants and IDL in plasma. It is caused by homozygosity for a species of apo E (E_2) which does not bind normally to the B,E receptor (Fig. 62–1). This leads to defective hepatic clearance of chylomicron remnants and ineffective catabolism of IDL to LDL.

Apo E_2 differs from normal apo E_3 and apo E_4 because of a point mutation causing a cysteine-for-arginine substitution. Homozygosity for apo E_2 occurs in 1 to 2 per cent of the population, but less than one in a thousand develops hyperlipidemia. Dysbetalipoproteinemia occurs only if the E_2 homozygote also has an additional disorder such as hypothyroidism or familial hypertriglyceridemia. This abnormality is suspected in individuals who have elevated levels of both cholesterol and triglycerides. Diagnosis requires demonstration of the apo E_2 homozygosity (not generally available) or unusual cholesterol enrichment of the VLDL. If the ratio of cholesterol to triglyceride in VLDL isolated by ultracentrifugation is higher than 0.40, then dysbetalipoproteinemia is likely. This form of hyperlipoproteinemia causes palmar and tuboeruptive xanthomata as well as coronary and peripheral vascular disease. The condition is worth identifying because it is exquisitely sensitive to weight reduction, cholesterol-lowering diets, and drugs such as clofibrate, gemfibrozil, lovastatin, and fenofibrate.

Familial Combined Hyperlipoproteinemia. This term has been used to describe families with a mixture of lipoprotein abnormalities that appear to segregate as an autosomal dominant trait. Affected members may have high VLDL levels, high LDL levels, or elevations of both VLDL and LDL. The basic abnormality is probably VLDL overproduction. Subjects who do not effectively catabolize VLDL show only hypertriglyceridemia. Those who are very efficient in VLDL catabolism manifest only increased cholesterol and LDL levels. Others show combined elevations of triglycerides (VLDL) and cholesterol (LDL). Family screening is required for a confident diagnosis, but the label is often loosely used to describe anyone with both VLDL and LDL elevations. The abnormality occurs frequently in patients with CHD, and affected patients often require diet and several lipid-lowering drugs to achieve normal lipid concentrations. This is one of the most difficult treatment problems.

TREATMENT OF HYPERTRIGLYCERIDEMIA

General Principles. The treatment of the hyperlipoproteinemias requires a systematic approach (Table 62–3). In general, the abnormality should be

TABLE 62–3. TREATMENT OF HYPERLIPOPROTEINEMIA

1. Document abnormality twice after a 14-hr fast while on typical American diet. Provisionally classify as cholesterol or triglyceride problem. Test total cholesterol, triglycerides, HDL_C.
2. Evaluate potential for control with diet modification—fish-vegetarian diet for three weeks; retest after two and three weeks.
3. Return to conventional lipid-lowering diet (special fat-restricted diet in severe hypertriglyceridemia) for four weeks; retest.
4. If target values are not achieved, add lipid-lowering medicine or food supplements. Retest four weeks after each change in regimen.

Maintenance

5. Patient keeps lipid record on flow sheet and has rapid access to test results.
6. Minimum follow-up test frequency is every four months.

documented twice before treatment is undertaken. About half of affected individuals will be sensitive to diet (>10 per cent reduction in lipids), and the extent of sensitivity should be defined by administering a very strict diet for two to three weeks (Table 62–4). Patients are retested once or preferably twice on this diet, and the results provide a point of reference for all future diet and drug interventions. If diet reduces lipids to target values—at or below the general population means—then it may be liberalized to give greater menu variety. Skinned, defatted fowl may substitute for some fish entrees and lean red meat may be consumed once each week. If target values are not achieved, then drug treatment is considered (Table 62–5). Compliance is best when patients chart their lipid levels, have ready access to test results, and have follow-up testing every three to four months. Assess-

TABLE 62–4. FISH-VEGETARIAN DIET

PERMISSIBLE FOODS/ BEVERAGES	FOODS TO BE OMITTED
Fish (including clams, oysters, lobster, shrimp, and scallops)	Meat (including fowl)
Bread	Baked goods (including desserts and "chips")
Pasta (with vegetable oil, tomato, or clam sauce if desired)	Dairy products (including eggs, butter, and cheese)
Potato	
Rice	**RESTAURANTS**
Vegetables (all)	None
Fruits (except avocado) and fruit juices	
Vegetable oils, margarine, and mayonnaise	**FAST FOODS**
Peanut butter	None
Nuts (except for coconut and macadamia)	
Cereal (except granola type "natural" cereals)	
Low-fat crackers (Matzo, Ry Krisp, Stoned Wheat Thins)	
Angel food cake (plain)	
Skimmed (not 1%) milk	
Coffee, tea, soda	
Alcohol	
Non-dairy creamers	
Coffee-Rich	
Poly-Rich	
Poly-Perx	

TABLE 62–5. DRUGS FOR HYPERLIPOPROTEINEMIA

CHOLESTEROL PROBLEMS	TRIGLYCERIDE PROBLEMS
Resins (cholestyramine, colestipol)	Fibrates (clofibrate, gemfibrozil, fenofibrate, etc.)
Niacin (regular or timed-release)	Niacin
Lovastatin	Fish oils
Combinations	Combinations
Others (probucol, fibrates)	

ment of drug effects takes no more than one to two months, and in general the efficacy of individual agents should be established before combinations are prescribed.

Diet. Reduced fat consumption is the only treatment for patients with lipoprotein lipase and apo C-II deficiency. The daily fat intake is limited to 25 gm by restricting all fat-enriched foods, including those made from vegetable oils. Adults with more common forms of hypertriglyceridemia and levels over 1000 mg/dl should also follow a low-fat diet until triglycerides have been reduced to less than 500 mg/dl. Subjects with milder triglyceride elevations benefit from a diet that is close to a fish-vegetarian diet (see Table 62–4). This very strict diet typically lowers cholesterol levels by 15 to 20 per cent and triglycerides by 30 to 40 per cent in hypertriglyceridemics. A second major objective of diet is to achieve leaner body mass. Most hypertriglyceridemics show marked improvement while actively losing weight, and a significant proportion are cured after weight reduction. Finally, alcohol should be restricted to one or two servings a week and in a major subset of hypertriglyceridemics this alone will correct the problem. If triglyceride levels of 300 mg/dl or less are not sustained by diet, then exercise programs or drugs are appropriate in many patients.

Exercise. Triglycerides are reduced after even a single exercise session, and exercise has been shown to augment lipoprotein lipase activity. The efficacy of regular aerobic exercise in mild to moderate hypertriglyceridemia has been repeatedly demonstrated, and exercise has great potential in promoting weight loss. The program goal should be 45 minutes of submaximal exercise on five days each week. The type of aerobics, duration, and intensity should be explicitly defined by the physician to promote compliance.

Drugs. The fibrate class of drugs (Table 62–5) enhances lipoprotein lipase activity and may have dramatic effects in severe hypertriglyceridemics requiring drug treatment. Fibrates are most effective in patients with dysbetalipoproteinemia and in others with high VLDL levels reflected by high total cholesterols (500 to 1000 mg/dl) as well as high triglycerides (1000 to 10,000 mg/dl). When hypertriglyceridemia is due primarily to chylomicronemia and the cholesterol is only modestly elevated (250 to 500 mg/dl), the fibrates are less effective than dietary fat restriction. Use of niacin in moderate hypertriglyceridemia (500 to 1000 mg/dl) can be gratifying but requires considerable patience by both physician and patient. The starting dose is 100

mg three times daily after meals, with very slow dose escalation to 1.5 to 4.5 gm/day. The user should be thoroughly familiar with niacin's side effects and their significance and control. Fish oils reduce hepatic VLDL production and are a popular but still experimental treatment for hypertriglyceridemia. The minimum effective dose is 12 to 16 gm/day (e.g., 4 gm with each meal and at bedtime), and triglycerides are usually reduced by 40 per cent in moderately severe hypertriglyceridemia (500 to 1500 mg/dl).

Fibrates and fish oils can considerably increase LDL levels while lowering VLDL and chylomicrons. Occasionally, LDL levels are raised above 160 mg/dl (see Table 62–2), and this undesirable effect must be weighed against the potential gain.

ELEVATED LDL

Polygenic Hypercholesterolemia. An individual's total cholesterol level is on average intermediate between that of his parents. About 60 to 70 per cent of a patient's cholesterol or LDL level is, therefore, genetically determined, with the remaining contribution from age, sex, diet, and other factors. The nature of these genetic effects is not defined. Subjects in the upper range of the normal distribution have increased CHD risk, and the upper 50 per cent contribute about 80 per cent of CHD cases. Those in the highest 25 per cent are generally considered targets for diet or even drug intervention.

Familial Monogenic Hypercholesterolemia. About 1 in 500 North Americans has a monogenic disorder producing an abnormality of the B,E receptor (Fig. 62–1). Affected individuals exhibit roughly half the normal number of receptors when their fibroblasts are grown in tissue culture. As a consequence, they generally have total cholesterols around 370 mg/dl and more than twice the average concentration of LDL. Increased LDL is manifest in the first year of life and is associated with early corneal arcus, xanthomata of the Achilles tendon and extensor tendons of the hands, and risk of CHD that is about 25 times that in unaffected relatives. Heterozygous men have a 50 per cent chance of myocardial infarction by 50 years of age, and the comparable risk in women is 10 to 20 per cent. Homozygotes or those heterozygotic for two abnormal alleles (compound heterozygotes) have cholesterol levels of 650 to 1000 mg/dl and severe xanthomatosis and typically die of cardiovascular disease before age 30.

TREATMENT OF HYPERCHOLESTEROLEMIA

General Principles. These are the same as defined for hypertriglyceridemia and as outlined in Table 62–3.

Diet. Limitation of dietary saturated fat is central to both cholesterol- and triglyceride-lowering diets. Carbohydrates are often substituted for the saturated fats, but high-carbohydrate diets may increase triglycerides and reduce HDL. Monounsaturated fats may prove better substitutes for saturated fat. Reduction of dietary cholesterol has a small additional LDL-lowering effect. In practice, the optimal diet approaches the fish-vegetarian diet used to establish diet sensitivity (see Table 62–4). The average hypercholesterolemic will lower total cholesterol by 12 per cent (range 0 to 40 per cent) on this diet. When diet responders show secondary failure, the usual cause is noncompliance. This can be identified by asking patients to complete a seven-day diet diary and reviewing the record with them. Subjects who travel extensively and eat frequently in restaurants have greatest trouble with diet prescriptions.

Exercise. Although trained endurance athletes have LDL levels about 10 per cent lower than those of controls, endurance training is generally not effective in reducing LDL concentrations. As noted above, exercise effects in hypertriglyceridemics are much more substantial.

Drugs. Several considerations govern choice of drugs for hypercholesterolemics not controlled by diet. The drugs are usually prescribed for years to decades and most are moderately expensive. The risk-benefit profile must be carefully assessed because any significant morbid or mortal effects can offset the modest potential gains. Annoying side effects limit compliance with some agents, and no drug has been shown to prolong life in populations at CHD risk.

The resins (Table 62–5) are safe and efficacious and are the only agents appropriate for children. The starting dose is 2 scoops or unit dose packets before supper; more than 6 unit doses a day is rarely worth the cost and inconvenience. A large bowl of wheat or corn bran cereal can prevent constipation during resin use, but many patients still feel bloated. Resins are contraindicated in the hypertriglyceridemias, and triglycerides should be reduced to under 300 mg/dl before resins are used in mixed or combined hyperlipidemics.

Niacin is efficacious in patients with LDL elevations, and the same precautions apply that were noted for niacin use in hypertriglyceridemia. The drug can cause fatty liver and cirrhosis, and the long-term safety is not established. Lovastatin is the first of a series of drugs that competitively inhibit hydroxymethyl glutaryl coenzyme A (HMG-CoA) reductase, the rate-limiting enzyme in cholesterol biosynthesis. This leads to an increase in hepatic B,E receptors, and LDL typically are lowered by 30 per cent. The efficacy of these agents in CHD prophylaxis has not been proven, and their long-term safety is unknown. Lovastatin and its cogeners now seem appropriate for hypercholesterolemics of any age who have established CHD and for moderately severe hypercholesterolemics (LDL >190 mg/dl) older than 40 years. Lovastatin is expensive but well tolerated, and compliance is excellent. Use in combination with fibrates or cyclosporine may cause myositis and even rhabdomyolysis.

The fibrates are not approved for simple hypercholesterolemia. They typically lower LDL levels by only 8 to 10 per cent but may produce dramatic results in some patients. Many patients, particularly those who have heterozygotic familial hypercholesterolemia, require two or three drugs to achieve adequate control. Resins plus niacin plus lovastatin or resins plus fibrates have been widely used. Resins plus fish oils are also effective in mixed hyperlipidemics. Familial monogenic hypercholesterolemia homozygotes are poorly responsive to diet and drugs and are considered candidates for liver transplantation.

Perspective

The National Cholesterol Education Program guidelines for treatment of elevated LDL concentrations (Table 62–2) are not age specific. It is recognized that almost half of all postmenopausal women have total cholesterol levels over 240 mg/dl and LDL$_C$ levels over 160 mg/dl. This presents a dilemma for both health professionals and patients. All agree that diet modification which does not radically reduce the quality of life is advisable for women in this category. The wisdom of prescribing cholesterol-lowering drugs in this population is more controversial. The Framingham Study failed to show a relationship between longevity and serum cholesterol levels in women over 50. Women, in addition, have not been subjects of intervention trials showing a favorable effect of cholesterol lowering on coronary heart disease risk. It may be reasonable to withhold drug treatment in postmenopausal women with cholesterol levels under 300 mg/dl unless other risk factors (Table 62–2) are present.

Among middle-aged and older men, about 25 to 30 per cent have mild to moderate simple hypercholesterolemia. As in women, cholesterol levels have not been linked to early mortality in men over 50. Unless evidence of a beneficial effect of cholesterol lowering in older men is obtained, it may not be advisable to treat mild hypercholesterolemia with cholesterol-lowering drugs.

REFERENCES

Brown MS, Goldstein JL: Drugs used in the treatment of hyperlipoproteinemia. *In* Gilman AG, Goodman LS, Rull TW, Murad F (eds): The Pharmacological Basis of Therapeutics. 7th ed. New York, Macmillan Publishing Co, 1985.

Brunzell JD: The hyperlipoproteinemias. *In* Wyngaarden JB, Smith LH Jr (eds): Cecil Textbook of Medicine. 18th ed. Philadelphia, WB Saunders Co, 1988, pp 1137–1144.

Report of the National Cholesterol Education Program Expert Panel on Detection, Evaluation, and Treatment of High Blood Cholesterol in Adults. Arch Intern Med 148:36–69, 1988.

Section VII, Chapters 44–51. *In* Scriver CR, Beaudet AL, Sly WS, Valle D (eds): The Metabolic Basis of Inherited Disease. 6th ed. New York, McGraw-Hill Book Co, 1989.

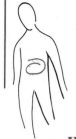

63

DISORDERS OF METALS AND METALLOPROTEINS

WILSON'S DISEASE (HEPATOLENTICULAR DEGENERATION)

Wilson's disease is a rare autosomal recessive disorder characterized by a defect in hepatic excretion of copper. Toxic levels accumulate in the liver, basal ganglia of the brain, and other tissues. The serum concentration of the copper-containing protein ceruloplasmin is low in 95 per cent of patients with Wilson's disease.

Pathogenesis. The primary genetic defect accounting for impaired biliary copper excretion in Wilson's disease is unknown. It is thought that hepatocytes of patients with this disorder contain an abnormal protein with an increased affinity for copper. Affected livers lack the ability to excrete copper that has been cleaved from circulating ceruloplasmin. This may cause a secondary deficiency of ceruloplasmin, because excess copper inhibits the formation of ceruloplasmin from apoceruloplasmin. The capacity of hepatocytes to store copper is eventually overwhelmed, resulting in release of the metal into blood and accumulation at extrahepatic sites. In the brain, copper is deposited in the pericapillary areas and astrocytes of the basal ganglia and frontal lobe, leading eventually to atrophy of those structures with cystic changes in the putamen.

Clinical Features. The age of onset and initial signs and symptoms of Wilson's disease are quite variable; clinical manifestations of copper excess are rare before the age of six. Approximately one third of patients present with symptoms of liver disease that may mimic acute viral hepatitis or cirrhosis with portal hypertension. More frequently, patients first present with extrahepatic manifestations of copper excess.

The early neurological signs of Wilson's disease include intellectual deterioration, tremor, loss of coordination of fine movements, an unsteady gait, and a slightly dystonic facies in which the upper lip is drawn tightly over the teeth. Dysarthria, muscle rigidity or contractures, and drooling are late features. Seizures are rare and sensory abnormalities absent. The neurological symptom complex includes personality changes and unstable behavior. The neurological manifestations begin usually between ages 11 and 25, occasionally as late as 40 years.

The intellectual deterioration, especially in adolescents, may be an isolated finding, not accompanied by movement disorders or other signs of Wilson's disease. Wilson's disease must therefore be considered in the differential diagnosis of any individuals under the age of 30 with unexplained decrease in intellectual ability (e.g., the high school student with an unexplained fall in academic achievement). This is a critical issue, because early treatment can arrest and sometimes reverse the intellectual impairment.

Other clinical features of Wilson's disease include Kayser-Fleischer corneal rings caused by copper deposition at the margins of the cornea. The rings, which may require slit-lamp detection, are uniformly present in patients with neurological symptoms, but may be absent in patients with isolated hepatic involvement. Like other heavy metals, copper may be nephrotoxic; renal deposition of copper is usually manifest by tubular dysfunction, including glycosuria, phosphaturia, aminoaciduria, renal tubular acidosis, or the complete Fanconi syndrome. Acute or chronic hemolytic anemia in Wilson's disease has been attributed to the release of copper from overloaded tissues, but the exact mechanisms have not been elucidated. As with intellectual dysfunction, the hemolytic anemia may precede the development of the more characteristic clinical manifestations of Wilson's disease.

The diagnosis of Wilson's disease is supported in suspected cases by (1) detection of Kayser-Fleischer rings, (2) a serum concentration of ceruloplasmin less than 20 mg/dl, (3) a concentration of copper in a liver biopsy sample greater than 250 μg/gm of dry weight, or (4) urinary excretion of more than 100 μg/day of copper. While none of these criteria is sufficiently sensitive or specific to make an unequivocal diagnosis of Wilson's disease, they serve to corroborate the diagnosis in patients with appropriate clinical signs and symptoms. Although the level of direct-reacting (non–ceruloplasmin-bound) copper in the serum is typically elevated, total levels are not consistently altered, so that measurement of serum copper levels serves little purpose in the diagnosis of this disorder.

Treatment. D-Penicillamine is the drug of choice. Daily doses of 1 to 2 gm increase urinary copper excretion more than five-fold over pretreatment levels and can prevent virtually every manifestation of Wilson's disease, provided that treatment is begun before major neurological impairment has occurred.

HEMOCHROMATOSIS

An increase in the quantity of storage iron in the body is called *hemosiderosis*. The term *hemochromatosis* refers to an increase in total body iron stores with iron deposition in parenchymal tissues that ultimately leads to functional impairment of the most severely affected organs. Acquired hemochromatosis results from exogenous iron overload due to excessive dietary iron ingestion or repeated blood transfusions. This section focuses on familial hemochromatosis, a genetically determined iron storage disorder that is linked to the HLA locus and is clinically manifest in roughly one in 5000 Caucasians in the United States. The clinical and pathological features of acquired and familial hemochromatosis can be identical.

Etiology, Genetics, and Pathogenesis. Normally the total body iron content of 3 to 4 gm is maintained by a balance between intestinal absorption and fecal excretion of iron. The amounts of iron absorbed and excreted daily are small, being approximately 1.0 mg in men and 1.5 mg in menstruating women. In familial hemochromatosis, intestinal iron absorption is inappropriately large, usually amounting to more than 3 mg per day. The progressive accumulation of iron produces an early elevation of plasma iron and an increased saturation of circulating transferrin. In advanced disease, total body iron content may exceed 20 gm.

The tendency to absorb iron excessively is inherited as an autosomal recessive trait. This is the most common recessive trait in the Caucasian population of the United States, occurring in 1 in 10 individuals. Homozygotes have large iron stores and may manifest the disease. Fortunately, only a minority of the homozygotes develop clinical manifestations of the disease. Heterozygotes exhibit minor derangements in iron metabolism but may rarely develop clinical manifestations when an added factor such as alcohol consumption or increased oral iron intake enhances the accumulation of iron in excess of their usual stores. Hemochromatosis is observed five to ten times more commonly in men than in women, presumably because menstrual blood losses protect against iron overload. The gene for hemochromatosis is located on the short arm of chromosome 6 and is linked to the HLA locus. Among families that include at least one affected homozygote, additional homozygotes as well as heterozygote carriers often can be identified by HLA testing using the principles of genetic linkage. Siblings with both HLA haplotypes identical to that of the affected patient will carry the linked hemochromatosis allele, are at high risk to develop iron overload, or may already be affected. Siblings who share only one HLA haplotype are heterozygotes.

Excess iron is deposited predominantly in parenchymal cells of the liver, heart, pancreas, and other endocrine organs. In early stages of the disease, deposits of iron in these organs consist of ferritin and hemosiderin stored within lysosomes. Tissue injury results from disruption of lysosomes and lipid peroxidation of subcellular organelles by iron. Varying degrees of fibrosis occur in affected organs. Cirrhosis of the liver is almost invariably present in symptomatic cases. Iron deposition in the liver is initially limited to lysosomes in the pericanalicular cytoplasm of hepatocytes. As the disease progresses, iron is also deposited in bile duct epithelium and in Kupffer cells. In the advanced stage, an irregular multilobular cirrhosis develops with a paucity of inflammatory cells and prominent bile duct proliferation.

Clinical Features. Signs and symptoms of hemochromatosis usually develop between the ages of 40 and 60. The early clinical manifestations are subtle and are often not attributed to hemochromatosis.

Constitutional symptoms include lassitude and weakness, but the most prominent symptoms relate to iron deposition in specific organs. The liver is usually the first organ to be affected. Although firm hepatomegaly is present in more than 95 per cent of cases at the time of diagnosis, liver function tests may remain normal during early stages of the disease. The spleen is enlarged in almost half of recognized cases, but other clinical manifestations of portal hypertension occur less commonly than in other forms of cirrhosis. Hepatocellular carcinoma develops as a sequel to cirrhosis in about 35 per cent of cases. Hepatocellular carcinoma and cirrhosis each account for about 25 per cent of deaths in treated patients.

About 90 per cent of patients exhibit excessive skin pigmentation, developing a characteristic metallic gray appearance from increased deposition of melanin and hemosiderin in the basal layer of the epidermis. Pigmentation is usually greatest on the face, neck, genitalia, and extensor surfaces of the extremities.

Insulin-dependent diabetes mellitus develops in approximately 80 per cent of cases from iron deposition in pancreatic islet cells. Vascular complications of diabetes such as retinopathy, peripheral neuropathy, and nephropathy may develop in long-term survivors.

Cardiac manifestations include congestive heart failure, a variety of ventricular and supraventricular arrhythmias, and conduction disturbances including heart block. Cardiac involvement is the presenting manifestation in about 15 per cent of cases. Congestive heart failure in hemochromatosis may be resistant to digitalis therapy. Cardiomyopathy accounts for about one third of deaths.

Loss of libido, sexual impotence, and testicular atrophy are present in more than 50 per cent of clinically recognized cases. Although hypogonadism may result in part from chronic liver disease, the symptoms more often are due to deficient production of trophic hormones by the anterior pituitary gland. Adrenal insufficiency and hypothyroidism rarely have been described.

About 25 per cent of patients develop acute attacks of synovitis due to synovial deposition of calcium pyrophosphate (i.e., chondrocalcinosis). In late stages, a progressive polyarthritis involving the hands, wrists, knees, and hips may develop. Radiographic findings include cystic changes in subchondral bone, loss of articular cartilage, and diffuse demineralization. The pathophysiological link between the rheumatological manifestations of hemochromatosis and the underlying disturbance in iron metabolism is unknown.

Hemochromatosis should be suggested by the above clinical features and confirmed by laboratory tests (Table 63–1). Measurements of the plasma iron concentration and the plasma iron-binding capacity provide the best screening tests. Plasma iron is usually greater than 200 μg/dl; total iron-binding capacity is normal or slightly decreased, but the transferrin saturation is greatly elevated, usually between 80 and 100 per cent. Other available measures of excessive parenchymal iron stores include the serum ferritin concentration and urinary iron excretion following administration of the chelating agent desferrioxamine.

TABLE 63–1. IRON INDICES IN NORMAL SUBJECTS AND IN PATIENTS WITH SYMPTOMATIC HEMOCHROMATOSIS

INDEX	NORMAL SUBJECTS	PATIENTS WITH HEMOCHROMATOSIS
Plasma iron (μg/dl)	50–150	180–300
Total iron binding capacity (μg/dl)	250–375	200–300
Per cent transferrin saturation	20–40	80–100
Serum ferritin (ng/ml)	10–200	900–6000
Urinary iron after 0.5 gm desferrioxamine	0–2	9–23
Liver iron (μg/100 mg dry weight)	30–140	600–1800

Because all of the above tests are limited in their sensitivity and specificity, the definitive test for hemochromatosis is liver biopsy; parenchymal hemosiderin deposits can be demonstrated histochemically and the actual content of iron can be estimated biochemically.

Treatment and Prognosis. Treatment consists of removing excess body iron and supportive treatment of complications such as diabetes mellitus and heart failure. Body iron is best removed by phlebotomy. Since 500 ml of blood contains 200 to 250 mg of iron, two to three years of weekly phlebotomies may be required to remove 20 gm of iron and to restore normal plasma iron concentrations. Once plasma iron levels return to normal, less frequent phlebotomies are continued to maintain a plasma concentration less than 150 μg/dl.

Phlebotomy is more effective and less expensive than administration of chelating agents, but the latter may be useful when anemia precludes frequent venisections. Daily intramuscular injection of 0.5 to 1.0 gm of desferrioxamine removes 10 to 20 mg of iron per day—one tenth or less of the amount mobilized by weekly phlebotomy.

Without treatment, hemochromatosis offers an average life expectancy of four and one-half years following development of clinical symptoms. Life expectancy is extended to more than 15 years by removal of excessive iron stores. Therapy improves carbohydrate

intolerance in almost half of cases, but established cirrhosis is irreversible.

Early detection and treatment prevent the clinical manifestations of hemochromatosis. If adequate treatment is initiated *before* the development of cirrhosis, a nearly normal life expectancy can be anticipated. Blood relatives of affected patients should undergo HLA testing. Siblings who share all HLA determinants with the index case are homozygotes and should have measurements of iron indices. Testing of siblings should be initiated at puberty for males and after the age of 20 for females. HLA-identical male sibs found to have normal iron stores should be restudied every two to three years, females less frequently.

PORPHYRIA

The porphyrias are a group of heterogeneous disorders resulting from inherited or acquired disturbances in heme biosynthesis. Porphyrins are pigments that serve as intermediates in this synthetic pathway. Heme, the ferrous iron complex of protoporphyrin IX, serves as a prosthetic group for a number of hemoproteins, including hemoglobin and mitochondrial cytochromes. Each of the porphyrias results from a deficiency of a specific enzyme in the heme biosynthetic pathway and is characterized by a unique pattern of overproduction and accumulation of porphyrin intermediates (Table 63–2). The porphyrias are usually categorized into two main groups, erythropoietic and hepatic, according to the major site at which the metabolic error is expressed.

Pathogenesis. Porphyrins are "side-products" of intermediates in the heme biosynthetic pathway, schematically outlined in Figure 63–1. The precursors glycine and succinyl coenzyme A are converted to aminolevulinic acid (ALA) in a reaction catalyzed by ALA-synthetase. This reaction is the rate-limiting step in heme biosynthesis, subject to feedback regulation by heme, the end product of the pathway. Two moles of ALA combine to form porphobilinogen. Only protoporphyrin is utilized in heme synthesis. The other porphyrins (i.e., uroporphyrin, coproporphyrin) have no

TABLE 63–2. CLASSIFICATION AND CHARACTERISTICS OF THE PORPHYRIAS: HEME PRECURSORS PRESENT IN ABNORMAL AMOUNTS

TYPE	URINE	PLASMA	ENZYME DEFECT
Erythropoietic			
Congenital erythropoietic porphyria	URO ≫ COPRO	URO	UROgen III cosynthetase
Erythrohepatic			
Protoporphyria	—	PROTO	Ferrochelatase
Hepatic			
Acute intermittent porphyria	ALA < PBG ≫ URO	ALA, PBG	PBG deaminase
Hereditary coproporphyria	ALA < PBG < URO < COPRO	COPRO	COPROgen oxidase
Variegate porphyria	ALA < PBG < URO < COPRO	COPRO, PROTO	PROTOgen oxidase
Porphyria cutanea tarda	URO ≫ COPRO	URO	UROgen decarboxylase

ALA = δ-aminolevulinic acid; PBG = porphobilinogen; URO = uroporphyrin; COPRO = coproporphyrin; PROTO = protoporphyrin.

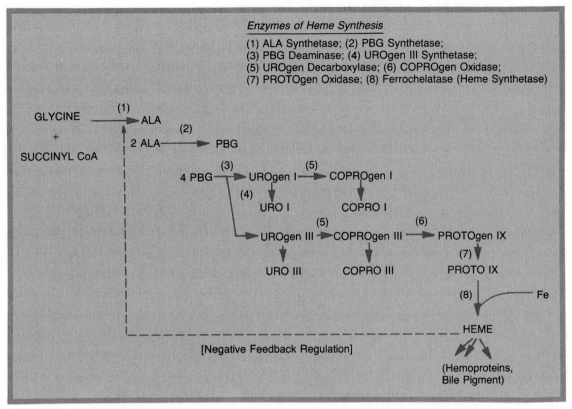

Enzymes of Heme Synthesis
(1) ALA Synthetase; (2) PBG Synthetase;
(3) PBG Deaminase; (4) UROgen III Synthetase;
(5) UROgen Decarboxylase; (6) COPROgen Oxidase;
(7) PROTOgen Oxidase; (8) Ferrochelatase (Heme Synthetase)

FIGURE 63–1. Pathway of heme biosynthesis. ALA = δ-aminolevulinic acid; URO = uroporphyrin; COPRO = coproporphyrin; PROTO = protoporphyrin; PBG = porphobilinogen. (Adapted from Bissell DM: Porphyria. *In* Wyngaarden JB, Smith LH Jr (eds): Cecil Textbook of Medicine. 18th ed. Philadelphia, WB Saunders Co, 1988, p 1183.)

physiological function and must be excreted; their fluorescent properties account for the diagnostic appearance of the urine in some patients.

Clinical Features. Congenital *erythropoietic porphyria* is a very rare disorder manifested by massive overproduction of uroporphyrinogen III and secondary accumulation of uroporphyrin and coproporphyrin, suggesting a defect in the activity of uroporphyrinogen III cosynthetase. Fewer than 100 cases have been described. Patients exhibit hemolytic anemia and severe photosensitivity, with mutilating bullous lesions on light-exposed skin. Treatment relies on avoidance of sunlight.

Protoporphyria results from partial deficiency of ferrochelatase, the final enzyme in heme biosynthesis that catalyzes the conversion of protoporphyrin to heme. The disease is characterized by excess protoporphyrin IX in erythrocytes, plasma, and feces. Cutaneous photosensitivity is the major clinical manifestation. About 10 per cent of patients develop protoporphyrin-containing gallstones, and some develop mild liver disease. Treatment includes avoidance of sunlight and administration of beta-carotene, which blocks light- and porphyrin-induced cutaneous injury.

The three variants of *hepatic porphyria* can be considered together, since their clinical manifestations and treatments are similar. Acute intermittent por-

phyria results from partial deficiency of porphobilinogen deaminase, leading to accumulation and excess urinary excretion of porphobilinogen and ALA. Hereditary coproporphyria is characterized by excess excretion of ALA, porphobilinogen, uroporphyrin, and coproporphyrin due to partial deficiency of coproporphyrinogen oxidase. Partial deficiency of protoporphyrinogen oxidase underlies variegate porphyria and leads to excess excretion of the entire series of heme precursors.

Clinical manifestations are protean, and the physician must consider acute hepatic porphyria in the differential diagnosis of a wide variety of symptoms, ranging from acute abdominal pain to delirium tremens. Focal or generalized seizures or severe motor polyneuropathies may be the presenting features. Intense abdominal pain during the first 24 to 48 hours of an attack may suggest acute cholecystitis, appendicitis, or other surgical diagnoses and may provoke unnecessary surgery. Psychiatric disturbances include personality changes and acute delirious reactions, with signs and symptoms resembling delirium tremens. Attacks may be precipitated by a variety of drugs (Table 63–3), especially those such as barbiturates that increase the demand for heme synthesis by induction of cytochrome P-450. Attacks are rare prior to puberty and are more common in women than in men, sug-

TABLE 63–3. DRUGS THAT MAY PRECIPITATE ACUTE ATTACKS IN HEPATIC PORPHYRIA

Barbiturates	Estrogens
Ethanol	Ergot preparations
Chlordiazepoxide	Methyldopa
Imipramide	Chloroquine
Meprobamate	Griseofulvin
Glutethimide	
Chlorpropamide	

gesting that endogenous hormones may play a role. Infection and fasting may also precipitate attacks. Because urinary porphobilinogen is increased in each of these porphyrias, the diagnosis is suspected by qualitative detection of porphobilinogen with the Watson-Schwartz test. Quantification of urinary and fecal porphyrins identifies the specific variant of porphyria. Treatment includes elimination of possible precipitating drugs, administration of carbohydrate to reverse fasting, analgesia, and supportive management of seizures, delirium, and other neurological complications. Hematin, a commercial preparation of ferriprotoporphyrin IX, has been administered to patients with prolonged attacks that do not respond to conservative therapy, but its efficacy remains unproven.

Porphyria cutanea tarda is another variant of porphyria. The condition results from partial deficiency of uroporphyrinogen decarboxylase, leading to increased urinary excretion of uroporphyrin and modest increments of urinary coproporphyrin. Mechanical fragility and photosensitivity of the skin are the primary clinical manifestations. Most affected patients give a history of ethanol abuse and/or chronic liver disease. The liver abnormalities are nonspecific but include increase in stainable iron and fluorescence resulting from the high content of uroporphyrin. Treatment includes avoidance of alcohol and phlebotomy to remove hepatic iron when clinically overt liver disease is present. Beta-carotene offers little or no protection against light-induced injury in this disorder.

REFERENCES

Bissell DM: Heme metabolism and the porphyrias. *In* Wright R, Alberti KGMM, Karran S, Millward-Sadler GH (eds): Liver and Biliary Disease. 2nd ed. London, WB Saunders Co, 1986.

Cartwright GE: Diagnosis of treatable Wilson's disease. N Engl J Med 298:1347, 1978.

Fairbanks VF, Baldus WP: Hemochromatosis: The neglected diagnosis. Mayo Clin Proc 61:296, 1986.

Stein JA, Tschudy DP: Acute intermittent porphyria. A clinical and biochemical study of 46 patients. Medicine 49:1, 1970.

Strickland T, Len ML: Wilson's disease: Clinical and laboratory manifestations in 40 patients. Medicine 54:113, 1975.

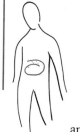

64

DISORDERS OF AMINO ACID METABOLISM

Defects in the membrane transport or catabolism of amino acids account for more than 70 inherited or acquired "aminoacidopathies." Each of these disorders is rare, but collectively they occur in approximately 1 in 1000 live births. This section describes selected disorders that illustrate the problems posed by aminoacidopathies.

HYPERAMINOACIDURIA (MEMBRANE TRANSPORT DEFECTS)

Although most of the body's 20 amino acids are contained within various polypeptides and proteins, a small but critical pool of *free* amino acids circulates in extracellular fluid. Most amino acids are freely filtered by renal glomeruli, but more than 95 per cent of the filtered load is actively and specifically reabsorbed in the proximal renal tubule via receptors that recognize and transport individual amino acids or groups of structurally related ones. Aminoaciduria results from either an acquired or a hereditary disturbance of cellular metabolism or when the transport of amino acids is impaired by (1) saturation of the receptor sites, (2) competition for the receptor sites by other substrates, or (3) a defect in the function or structural integrity of the receptor. Defects in membrane transport may affect a single amino acid, a group of structurally related amino acids, or all amino acids (Table 64–1).

Cystinuria, the most common inborn error of amino acid transport, results from an inherited defect in the membrane receptor for the dibasic amino acids lysine, arginine, ornithine, and cystine. The disorder is inherited as an autosomal recessive trait. Cystine is the least soluble of all amino acids, and its excessive excretion in urine predisposes to the formation of calculi. Normally, the maximum solubility of cystine in urine is about 300 mg/L. Affected homozygotes regularly excrete 600 to 1800 mg of cystine per day.

Signs and symptoms of cystinuria are those of urolithiasis: renal colic, hematuria, obstructive uropathy, and secondary infection, usually beginning during the second or third decade of life. Recurrent episodes of urolithiasis and infection can lead to progressive renal insufficiency.

The diagnosis of cystinuria requires either demonstration of the characteristic aminoaciduria by chromatography or electrophoresis or the detection of cystine in a urinary tract calculus. As many as 50 per cent of stones excreted by cystinuric patients, however, have a mixed composition. Urinary cystine crystals have a characteristic hexagonal shape; their discovery in the urine of a patient with signs and symptoms of urolithiasis is often the first clue to the diagnosis of cystinuria.

Treatment of cystinuria consists of efforts to reduce the urinary concentration of cystine. Vigorous hydration, with fluid ingestion of 4 to 8 L per day, is the most important aspect of medical management. Because the solubility of cystine increases sharply as urine pH rises above 7.5, urinary alkalinization may be effective in preventing stone formation; however, vigorous administration of sodium bicarbonate and/or acetazolamide is required to maintain a persistently alkaline urine. Administration of D-penicillamine in doses of 1 to 3 gm per day effectively lowers the urinary concentration of free cystine, prevents new stone formation, and promotes the dissolution of existing calculi. The drug undergoes sulfhydryl-disulfide exchange with cystine to form a mixed penicillamine-cysteine disulfide that is 50 times more soluble than cystine. D-Penicillamine, however, has a number of serious side effects (e.g., exfoliative dermatitis, heavy proteinuria, bone marrow depression), and should be reserved for patients who fail to respond to more conservative measures.

Generalized aminoaciduria reflects a generalized defect in the renal tubular reabsorption of all filtered amino acids and is characteristic of patients with Fanconi's syndrome. The renal loss of amino acids in Fanconi's syndrome is usually outweighed by other disturbances of proximal tubular function, including glycosuria, phosphaturia, bicarbonaturia, and uric aciduria. Presenting manifestations of this disorder may include hypophosphatemic rickets in children, osteomalacia in adults, proximal renal tubular acidosis, or hypouricemia. Fanconi's syndrome may be acquired or associated with an inherited enzymatic disorder (e.g., hereditary fructose intolerance). In addition, a primary hereditary disorder (idiopathic Fanconi's syndrome) has been identified. The common causes of acquired Fanconi's syndrome are listed in Table 64–2.

AMINO ACID STORAGE DISEASES

Cystinosis is a rare idiopathic disorder characterized by the accumulation of cystine crystals in various tissues, including the cornea, bone marrow, lymph

TABLE 64–1. CLASSIFICATION OF MAJOR HYPERAMINOACIDURIAS

	TRAIT	SUBSTANCE(S) AFFECTED
Substrate-specific	Histidinuria	Histidine
	Hypercystinuria	Cystine
Group-specific	Cystinuria	Lysine, ornithine, arginine, cystine
	Hartnup disease	Neutral amino acids
	Iminoglycinuria	Proline, glycine, hydrocyproline
	Dicarboxylic aminoaciduria	Glutamic acid, aspartic acid
	Hyperdibasic aminoaciduria	Lysine, ornithine, arginine
Generalized	Idiopathic Fanconi's syndrome	Generalized effect on all amino acids, solutes, and water
	Acquired Fanconi's syndrome	Generalized effect on all amino acids, solutes, and water

TABLE 64–2. SOME DISORDERS ASSOCIATED WITH ACQUIRED FANCONI'S SYNDROME

1. Systemic or Hereditary Diseases
   Multiple myeloma   Wilson's disease
   Amyloidosis   Hereditary fructose intolerance
   Sjögren's syndrome   Galactosemia
   Cystinosis
2. Heavy Metal Poisonings
   Mercury   Uranium
   Lead   Strontium
   Cadmium
3. Drugs
   6-Mercaptopurine

nodes, and kidneys. Three clinical forms exist: (1) *infantile cystinosis*, characterized by the Fanconi syndrome and progressive renal failure, occurs during the first decade of life; (2) in *juvenile cystinosis*, renal failure does not occur until the second decade; (3) *adult cystinosis* is a relatively benign disorder in which cystine accumulation is usually limited to the cornea, resulting in photophobia or mild irritation of the eyes.

Adult cystinosis requires no treatment. Treatment of nephropathic cystinosis consists of supportive management of progressive renal failure; D-penicillamine is ineffective. Renal transplantation has been performed successfully in patients with cystinosis and end-stage renal failure, but reaccumulation of cystine can occur in the transplanted allograft after many years.

Alcaptonuria, a rare disorder of tyrosine catabolism resulting from hereditary deficiency of homogentisic acid oxidase, is associated with the excretion of large amounts of homogentisic acid in the urine and the accumulation of oxidized homogentisic acid in connective tissues. *Ochronosis*, a bluish-gray pigmentation, occurs when homogentisic acid and its oxidized polymers bind to collagen. The earliest clinical manifestations of alcaptonuria include slight pigmentation of the sclerae and external ears during the second and third decades. The urine tends to darken on standing, a finding that frequently goes unnoticed. Most patients develop degenerative joint disease by the fourth or fifth decade, ankylosis of the lumbar spine being a common late finding. The diagnosis is suggested by the triad of degenerative arthritis, ochronotic pigmentation, and the detection of urine that blackens on standing and is confirmed by measurement of urinary homogentisic acid. There is no known specific treatment.

OTHER DISORDERS OF AMINO ACID METABOLISM MEDIATED BY ENZYMATIC DEFECTS

Phenylketonuria is an autosomal recessive disorder resulting from impaired conversion of the essential amino acid phenylalanine to tyrosine due to deficient activity of the enzyme phenylalanine dehydroxylase. This disorder is manifested by accumulation of phenylalanine and its minor metabolites and by severe mental retardation. Infants with phenylketonuria are usually normal at birth, but signs of mental and psychomotor retardation, hyperactivity, tremors, or seizures usually develop within the first year of life. Early recognition of this disorder is imperative, since its devastating consequences can be prevented completely if dietary restriction of phenylalanine is instituted within the first 30 days of life. Most newborns in the United States are screened for this disorder by determinations of blood phenylalanine concentrations using a bacterial inhibition assay. Quantitative chromatographic assays are employed for definitive diagnosis in infants with abnormal screening results. Treatment of phenylketonuria consists of a diet in which the bulk of protein is replaced by an amino acid mixture low in phenylalanine. Although scrupulous adherence to such a dietary regimen is of critical importance during the early months of life, it is probably wise to continue dietary therapy at least through the first decade of life. Phenylalanine ingestion must also be monitored carefully in the pregnant woman with phenylketonuria to prevent central nervous system damage in the fetus.

The term *homocystinuria* refers to a group of biochemically and clinically distinct disorders characterized by accumulation of the sulfur-containing amino acid, homocystine, in blood and urine. Homocystine is the disulfide oxidation product formed by two molecules of homocysteine. Accumulation of homocystine results in impaired collagen formation, a phenomenon that accounts for many of the clinical manifestations of this disorder. The most common variant of homocystinuria results from deficiency of cystathionine β-synthase, resulting in a failure of homocysteine to react with serine to form cystathionine. Deficiency of this enzyme is inherited as an autosomal recessive trait. Patients with homocystinuria and cystathionine β-synthase deficiency exhibit dislocated optic lenses, lax ligaments, and sparse fine hair. They may resemble patients with Marfan's syndrome. Mental retardation occurs in approximately 50 per cent of cases. Thromboembolic disease is the major cause of morbidity and mortality and may be initiated by damage to vascular endothelium.

REFERENCES

Scriver CR: Inborn errors of amino acid metabolism. *In* Wyngaarden JB, Smith LH Jr (eds): Cecil Textbook of Medicine. 18th ed. Philadelphia, WB Saunders Co, 1988, pp 1149–1160.

Wellner D, Meister A: A survey of inborn errors of amino acid metabolism and transport in man. Annu Rev Biochem 50:911, 1981.

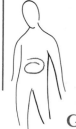

65

DISORDERS OF CARBOHYDRATE METABOLISM

GALACTOSEMIA

Two inherited enzyme deficiencies impair the metabolic conversion of galactose to glucose and cause accumulation of galactose in the body, or galactosemia. *Classic galactosemia* results from deficient activity of the enzyme galactose-1-phosphate uradyl transferase; a less common form of galactosemia results from *galactokinase deficiency*. Accumulation of galactose in the ocular lens produces excessive hydration, precipitation of lens protein, and formation of cataracts. Classic galactosemia also features liver disease, mental retardation, and failure to thrive, untreated infants surviving only a few days to weeks. Further details regarding the clinical features of these neonatal disorders can be found in pediatric textbooks.

THE GLYCOGEN STORAGE DISEASES

Glycogen is present in virtually all animal cells and constitutes the principal storage form of carbohydrate. In contrast to starch, the storage form of carbohydrate in plants, glycogen has a highly branched structure that enhances its solubility. A variety of inherited enzyme defects adversely affect the synthesis and degradation of glycogen. In general, such defects produce either an elevated tissue concentration of glycogen or an abnormality in the structure of the carbohydrate. As specific enzyme defects were recognized, the glycogen storage diseases were numbered or assigned eponyms. The diseases are grouped as either hepatic or muscular disorders, according to the major site affected by the metabolic error. The enzyme deficiencies, clinical manifestations, and laboratory findings of the glycogen storage diseases are shown in Table 65–1. Hepatic variants are largely disorders of children and frequently cause death early in life. Clinical features of the muscle glycogen storage diseases are discussed elsewhere in this text.

PRIMARY HYPEROXALURIA

Primary hyperoxaluria results from either of two rare autosomal recessive genetic disorders, each of which results in excessive synthesis and urinary excretion of oxalic acid. The two variants of this disorder can be distinguished by characteristic excretion of oxalate metabolites in the urine. *Type I primary hyperoxaluria* results from a defect in the enzyme alanine: glyoxalate aminotransferase with resultant increased urinary concentrations of oxalate and glycolate. In *Type II hyperoxaluria*, there is a defect in the enzyme D-glyceric dehydrogenase, resulting in increased urinary excretion of oxalate and L-glycerate. Each of these disorders is characterized by recurrent calcium oxalate nephrolithiasis and/or nephrocalcinosis during childhood, resulting in renal failure and death in patients not supported by dialysis. Once renal failure supervenes, the diagnosis may be difficult to establish because urinary excretion of oxalate metabolites declines as the glomerular filtration rate falls. Calcium oxalate deposition also occurs in other tissues, including the liver, spleen, testes, and bone marrow. Deposition of calcium oxalate in the walls of blood vessels may result in severe peripheral vascular insufficiency. Milder forms of primary hyperoxaluria have been described in adults with calcium oxalate kidney stones. The vast majority of patients with calcium oxalate nephrolithiasis have normal oxalate metabolism.

There is no specific treatment for primary hyperoxaluria. Phosphate or magnesium supplementation and forced diuresis have been variably successful in decreasing urinary stone formation. High doses of pyr-

TABLE 65–1. THE GLYCOGEN STORAGE DISEASES

NUMERIC TYPE	EPONYM	ENZYME DEFICIENCY	CLINICAL MANIFESTATIONS	LABORATORY FINDINGS	DIAGNOSIS
Hepatic Forms					
I	Von Gierke's	Glucose-6-phosphatase	Massive hepatomegaly, short stature, failure to thrive, severe hypoglycemia, retinal lesions	↑ lactate, pyruvate, triglycerides, cholesterol, uric acid	↓ enzyme activity or ↑ glycogen on liver biopsy
III	Cori's	Debrancher	Similar to Type I, but less severe; myopathy in adults	Normal lactate and uric acid, cholesterol, triglycerides	Enzyme assay on liver, muscle, WBC's, or RBC's
IV	Anderson's	Brancher	Cirrhosis, hepatosplenomegaly, ascites, early death from liver failure	↑ Transaminase, normal glucose tolerance	Normal liver glycogen
VI	Hers'	Liver phosphorylase	Mild hepatomegaly, mild hypoglycemia	Minimal	Enzyme assay on liver, ↑ liver glycogen
VIII	None	Phosphorylase β-kinase	Marked hepatomegaly, sex-linked disorder	Minimal	Enzyme assay on liver or WBC's
Muscle Forms					
II	Pompe's	α-1,4-glucosidase (acid maltase)	Massive cardiomegaly, hypotonia, early death from cardiorespiratory failure. Milder form in adults	↑ CPK	Enzyme assay on WBC's
V	McArdle's	Muscle phosphorylase	Exercise-induced muscle pain and cramps, rhabdomyolysis	↑ CPK with episodes; no blood lactate with exercise	↑ glycogen and ↓ enzyme activity on muscle biopsy

idoxine (200 to 400 mg/day) may reduce oxalate excretion in Type I hyperoxaluria. More physiological doses of pyridoxine (2 to 10 mg) may be effective in some patients. Patients with end-stage renal disease can be maintained on chronic dialysis. Successful renal transplantation has been hampered by rapid deposition of calcium oxalate in the transplanted kidney; however, intensive daily hemodialysis in the early post-transplant period may reduce plasma oxalate levels to sufficiently low levels to minimize renal oxalate deposition.

REFERENCES

Howell RR: The glycogen storage diseases. *In* Wyngaarden JB, Smith LH Jr (eds): Cecil Textbook of Medicine. 18th ed. Philadelphia, WB Saunders Co, 1988, pp 1133–1135.
Segal S: Disorders of galactose in metabolism. *In* Stanbury JB, Wyngaarden JB, Frederickson DS, et al (eds): The Metabolic Basis of Inherited Disease. 5th ed. New York, McGraw-Hill Book Co, 1982.
Yendt ER, Cohanim M: Response to a physiological dose of pyridoxine in type I primary oxaluria. New Engl J Med 312:953, 1985.

66

INHERITED DISORDERS OF CONNECTIVE TISSUE

The genetically transmitted disorders discussed in this section are characterized by histologically or ultramicroscopically demonstrable structural changes in the integumentary system. They are neither inflammatory nor immunological in origin and must be distinguished from acquired immunological diseases such as systemic lupus erythematosus, scleroderma, rheumatoid arthritis, and polymyositis, which have been improperly termed connective tissue diseases.

THE MUCOPOLYSACCHARIDOSES

The mucopolysaccharidoses are a group of disorders resulting from deficiencies of specific lysosomal enzymes involved in the degradation of the glycosaminoglycans, including chondroitin sulfate, dermatan sulfate, heparan sulfate, and keratan sulfate. Clinical manifestations derive from the accumulation of partially degraded glycosaminoglycans in connective tissues, heart, bony skeleton, and central nervous system. Features common to most of the mucopolysaccharidoses include onset in childhood, coarse facial features, corneal clouding, hepatosplenomegaly, joint stiffness, and a tendency to develop inguinal and umbilical hernias. Changes in the body skeleton, collectively referred to as dysostosis multiplex, include short stature, impaired growth of long bones, short, stubby hands, and a variety of cranial abnormalities. Enzyme deficiencies and clinical manifestations of the more common mucopolysaccharidoses are summarized in Table 66–1.

MARFAN'S SYNDROME

Marfan's syndrome is inherited as an autosomal dominant trait with ocular, skeletal, and cardiovascular manifestations. Approximately 15 per cent of cases represent new mutations. The exact nature of the molecular defect is unknown. The clinical expression of Marfan's syndrome varies greatly among affected family members, some patients having findings limited to one or two organ systems. The typical patient is tall and thin with long extremities: the arm span measures greater than the height, and the floor-to-pubis measurement exceeds the distance from pubis to crown. The fingers are long, thin, and hyperextensible (arachnodactyly). Kyphoscoliosis, asymmetry of the thoracic cage, and sternal deformities are common. The palate is high and arched, the facies is long and narrow, and the anterior teeth are crowded. Ligamentous weakness may lead to loose- or double-jointedness, and skeletal muscles often are poorly developed and hypotonic. Inguinal and femoral hernias are common, as are recurrent joint dislocations. Weakness and redundancy of the supporting tissues of the ocular lens lead to subluxation, most frequently in an upward and outward direction. Myopia and flattened corneas are common.

About 80 to 90 per cent of patients with Marfan's syndrome develop aortic disease, the most common cause of death. Medial degeneration leads to dilatation or dissection of the proximal aorta and aortic valvular insufficiency. Mitral valve prolapse is also common; either valvular lesion can be complicated by bacterial endocarditis. Surgical repair of aortic lesions has been

TABLE 66–1. THE MUCOPOLYSACCHARIDOSES

ABBREVI-ATION	EPONYM	ENZYME DEFICIENCY	MAJOR STORAGE PRODUCT	INHERI-TANCE	CLINICAL FEATURES
MPS-IH	Hurler's	α-L-Iduronidase	DS + HS	AR	Onset 6–12 months, dysostosis multiplex, progressive mental retardation, cardiac disease, death by age 10
MPS-IS	Scheie's	α-L-Iduronidase	DS + HS	AR	Onset 5–15 years, dysostosis multiplex, normal intelligence, long survival
MPS-II	Hunter's	L-Sulfoiduronate sulfatase	HS + DS	X-linked	May be mild or severe. If severe, similar to MPS-IH, death by age 15. If mild, survival to 30's–60's, depending on cardiac involvement
MPS-III	Sanfilippo's	4 types	HS	AR	Onset 2–6 years, dysostosis multiplex, rapidly progressive mental retardation, death at end of puberty
MPS-IV	Morquio's	N-acetylgalactosamine-6-sulfatase	KS + CS	AR	Severe, distinctive skeletal dysplasia, odontoid hypoplasia, aortic insufficiency, normal intelligence, death in 20's
MPS-VI	Maroteaux-Lamy	N-acetylgalactosamine-4-sulfatase (arylsulfatase B)	DS + ?CS	AR	Onset 2–4 years, dysostosis multiplex, aortic valve disease, normal intelligence, death in 20's (severe) or long survival (mild)
MPS-VII	None	β-glucuronidase	HS, DS, CS	AR	Onset 1–2 years, dysostosis multiplex, granulocyte inclusions, vascular involvement very rare

DS = dermatan sulfate; HS = heparan sulfate; KS = keratan sulfate; CS = chondroitin sulfate; AR = autosomal recessive.

variably successful. Propranolol has been recommended to decrease myocardial contractility and diminish the stress on the aorta, but results have not been encouraging. Isometric exercises and pregnancy increase the risk of cardiovascular catastrophe in patients with aortic disease.

EHLERS-DANLOS SYNDROME

The Ehlers-Danlos syndrome, a group of inherited connective tissue diseases, causes hyperextensible skin and joints, easy bruisability, friability of tissues, and poor wound healing. Eight variants of Ehlers-Danlos syndrome have been distinguished on the basis of clinical manifestations and purported alterations in collagen biosynthesis. Ehlers-Danlos syndrome Type I is the prototype with the most severe clinical manifestations. The skin is unusually soft, velvety, and hyperextensible, having a rubber-like quality allowing it to be stretched away from the underlying structures, promptly returning to its original position upon release. With aging, the skin may sag and become redundant, particularly over the elbows. Extreme fragility affects the skin so that minor trauma may produce gaping wounds. Minor injuries may also produce large hematomas that may organize into tumor-like calcified masses. Hyperextensibility of the joints allows affected patients to perform unusual contortions. Chronic or recurrent joint dislocations are common, particularly affecting the hips, knees, shoulders, and temporomandibular joints. Many patients suffer inguinal, hiatal, and umbilical hernias as well as gastrointestinal or genitourinary diverticula. Ophthalmologic changes include blue sclerae, myopia, microcorneas, dislocated lenses, retinal detachment, and the appearance of widely spaced eyes. Cardiovascular manifestations include mitral valve prolapse, myocardial conduction abnormalities, and a variety of congenital cardiac anomalies. Catastrophic cardiovascular complications including rupture of large arteries occur most commonly in Ehlers-Danlos syndrome Type IV. Weakness of blood vessel walls or abnormal interaction of platelets with collagen often leads to a hemorrhagic diathesis.

The diagnosis of Ehlers-Danlos syndrome is usually suggested by the combination of hyperextensible skin and hypermobile joints. Additional clinical features and a family history of similar manifestations help in establishing the genetic type. Loose joints may also occur in Marfan's syndrome, several of the chondrodystrophies, and osteogenesis imperfecta. No specific treatment is available. Protection of the skin and joints from trauma is important, and surgery should be undertaken with extreme caution. Pregnancy carries a great risk.

REFERENCES

Hollister D, Byers PH, Holbrook KA: Genetic disorders of collagen metabolism. Adv Hum Genet 12:1, 1982.

Sly WS: The mucopolysaccharidoses. *In* Wyngaarden JB, Smith LH Jr (eds): Cecil Textbook of Medicine. 18th ed. Philadelphia, WB Saunders Co, 1988, pp 1174–1177.

SECTION
IX
ENDOCRINE DISEASES

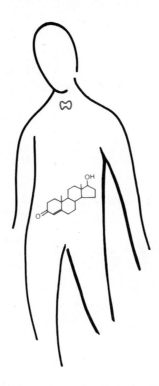

67

HYPOTHALAMIC-PITUITARY AXIS

The pituitary gland is a complex endocrine organ located in a bony fossa, the sella turcica, at the base of the brain. It consists of two distinct portions: the anterior pituitary (adenohypophysis) or glandular portion, derived from Rathke's pouch, and the posterior pituitary (neurohypophysis), which is an anatomical extension of the hypothalamus, derived from the dien-

cephalon. Hormonal secretion by both portions of the pituitary gland is under the control of the central nervous system: the posterior lobe by a direct neurosecretory pathway from the anterior hypothalamus; the anterior lobe by a neuroendocrine system in which peptide and monoamine products of cells of the ventral hypothalamus are transported to the anterior pituitary via the hypothalamic-hypophyseal portal system. Owing to its unique location and intimate relationship with the central nervous system, the pituitary gland or, more appropriately, the hypothalamic-pituitary axis, is often referred to as the master gland of the endocrine system.

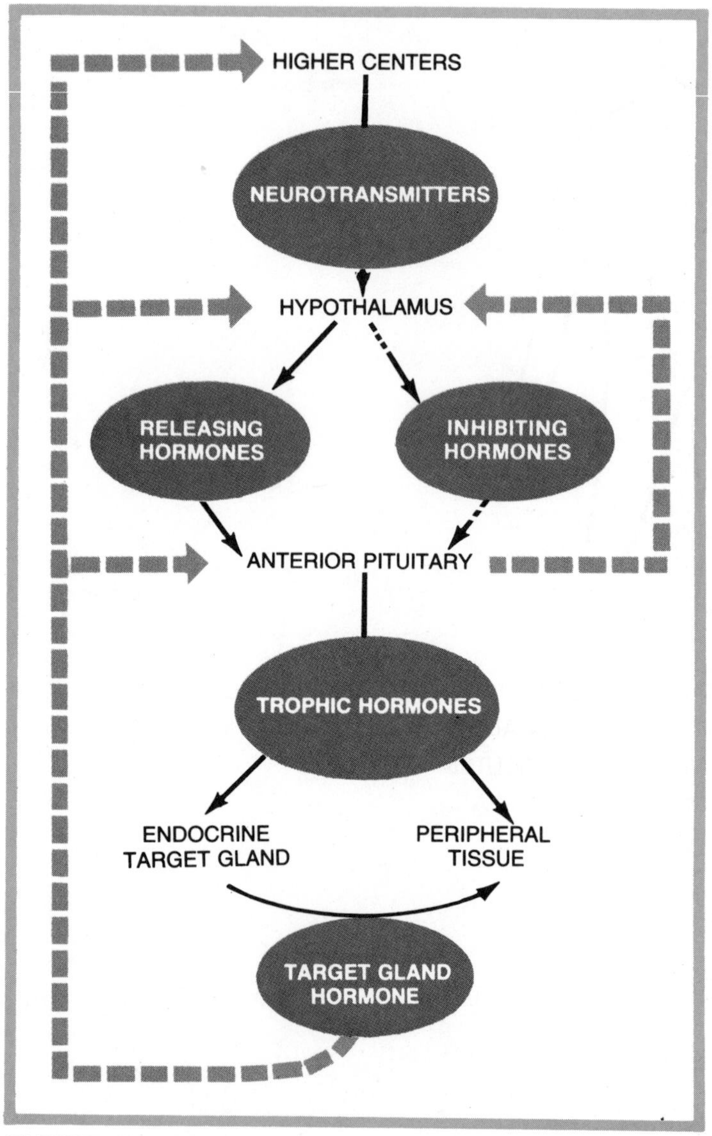

HYPOTHALAMIC HORMONES

Hypothalamic peptides stimulate the secretion of the anterior pituitary hormones. As an exception dopamine, a monoamine, provides tonic inhibition of prolactin secretion. Releasing hormones for thyrotropin (thyrotropin-releasing hormone or TRH), gonadotropin (GnRH), corticotropin (CRF), and growth hormone (GRF), and an inhibitory hormone for growth hormone secretion (somatostatin, or SRIF) have been sequenced and synthesized. In addition to their roles in regulation of anterior pituitary function, several of these peptides and amines are found elsewhere in the brain and even outside of the central nervous system, particularly in the gut, where they may have neurotransmitter and other regulatory functions.

Hypothalamic hormones are secreted under neural regulation involving a variety of neurotransmitters (e.g., biogenic amines such as catecholamines and serotonin) (Fig. 67-1). Their secretion is also regulated by a blood-borne (closed-loop) feedback system involving the secretory products of pituitary and endocrine target cell origin. The hypothalamic hormones enter the hypophyseal portal system in complex mixtures, but the selectivity of their effects is assured by the presence of highly specific receptors on the various subtypes of endocrine cells in the anterior pituitary gland.

ANTERIOR PITUITARY HORMONES

The anterior pituitary gland contains several cell types, each of which is capable of synthesizing, storing, and releasing specific hormonal products. Six major and distinct secretory products have been recognized, which can be further subdivided into three classes of hormones: somatomammotropins, corticotropin and related peptides, and glycoproteins.

FIGURE 67-1. Neural regulation and feedback control of the hypothalamic-pituitary axis. Solid lines indicate positive and broken lines indicate negative regulation.

The *somatomammotropins* include growth hormone and prolactin as well as a placental secretory product known as chorionic somatomammotropin. These structurally similar hormones have primarily lactogenic and growth-promoting effects. The somatomammotropins differ from the other hormonal products of the anterior pituitary in that they do not have a single classic endocrine target organ through which their effects are mediated. Many actions of growth hormone are mediated by a peptide, somatomedin C or insulin-like growth factor I (IGF-I), that is synthesized in the liver and other tissues. Prolactin acts directly on the breast to promote synthesis of constituents of breast milk, but it is not responsible for breast development or milk release. The release of breast milk is regulated by oxytocin, a peptide that is released from the posterior pituitary.

Corticotropin (ACTH) is a 39 amino acid peptide that is part of a larger precursor molecule, proopiomelanocortin, which is the actual secretory product of the corticotrope. The larger molecule contains a number of biologically active peptides, including β-lipotropin, β-endorphin, melanocyte-stimulating hormone (MSH), and a large N-terminal fragment containing peptides that may have natriuretic properties of uncertain physiological significance. The mechanism controlling the differential release of these various fragments is unclear. ACTH stimulates secretion of glucocorticoid (and to a lesser extent mineralocorticoid hormones) by the adrenal cortex. ACTH also has extra-adrenal effects such as stimulation of lipolysis in adipose tissue.

The pituitary glycoprotein hormones—thyroid stimulating hormone (TSH), follicle-stimulating hormone (FSH), and luteinizing hormone (LH)—contain an α and a β subunit. The α units are identical, whereas the β units differ and confer thereby the specificity of the biological effects of each of these substances. A gonadotropin of chorionic origin, similar in structure to the glycoproteins of pituitary origin, also possesses an identical α subunit. The glycoprotein hormones exert their biological effects via the secretory products of their respective target organs: TSH modulates secretion of thyroxine and triiodothyronine by the thyroid gland; FSH and LH in women regulate ovulation and secretion of the steroid products of the ovary, whereas in men these gonadotropins regulate development of the seminiferous tubules and production of testosterone by the Leydig cells.

TESTS OF ANTERIOR PITUITARY FUNCTION

Radioimmunoassays for all of the major secretory products of the anterior pituitary gland are currently available in most clinical laboratories. When measurements of these hormones are used in conjunction with the appropriate physiological maneuvers and pharmacological probes, a precise characterization of states of anterior pituitary hypo- and hyperfunction is generally possible.

ACTH

Levels of plasma ACTH may be undetectable in normal individuals when obtained under basal conditions. Demonstration of ACTH deficiency therefore requires the use of a stimulatory maneuver such as induction of hypoglycemia with insulin (0.1 U/kg intravenously) or of hypocortisolism with the 11β-hydroxylase inhibitor, metyrapone (750 mg orally every six hours for four doses). If ACTH assays are not available, ACTH reserve can be evaluated indirectly by measuring the response of plasma cortisol to the former and of 11-deoxycortisol to the latter stimulus; this approach presupposes that adrenal function is intact. The use of corticotropin-releasing factor (CRF) to determine ACTH secretory reserve may soon be available for general use. When used in conjunction with indirect stimuli such as insulin hypoglycemia, CRF testing may identify patients with hypothalamic lesions causing ACTH deficiency (e.g., a positive CRF test but a negative response to hypoglycemia).

In states of suspected ACTH excess, suppression tests using exogenous glucocorticoid hormones such as dexamethasone are generally employed (see Chapter 69). Administration of CRF may also prove to be of value in this setting, particularly in distinguishing pituitary from ectopic sources of ACTH.

TSH

In patients with hypothyroidism and normal or undetectable levels of TSH, distinction between hypothalamic and pituitary abnormalities can be made using thyrotropin-releasing hormone (TRH). In this procedure, TSH levels are obtained before and 15 to 30 minutes after administration of TRH, 500 μg intravenously. Normally, TSH levels will increase to values of up to 15 μU/ml in response to this stimulus. Patients with pituitary hypothyroidism have a flat response, whereas TSH levels increase in those with hypothalamic hypothyroidism, although the response may be delayed. A flat TSH response to TRH may also be found in hyperthyroidism, acromegaly, renal insufficiency, and depression and during steroid therapy.

Gonadotropins

Administration of gonadotropin-releasing hormone (GnRH), 100 μg intravenously, can frequently distinguish between pituitary and hypothalamic etiologies of gonadotropin deficiency. Normally, the response of LH is greater than that of FSH, averaging three to five times the control value. Repeated injections may be required to elicit normal responses in some patients with hypothalamic disorders. In children the pattern of response also differs depending on the age of the patient, and, in particular, the stage of pubertal development. The estrogen antagonist, clomiphene, can stimulate LH and FSH secretion in patients with hypothalamic hypogonadism and may be used as a therapeutic as well as diagnostic agent in this setting.

Prolactin

Prolactin secretory reserve can be evaluated by administration of dopamine antagonists such as metoclopramide. For evaluation of hyperprolactinemia, tests of suppressibility with L-dopa or water loading are employed. However, the failure of these latter procedures to distinguish readily between prolactin-secreting adenomas and other causes of hyperprolactinemia has reduced their usefulness.

Growth Hormone

Growth hormone secretory reserve can be evaluated as its response to insulin-induced hypoglycemia (0.1 U insulin/kg intravenously), to growth-hormone releasing factor (1 μg/kg intravenously), during a 30-minute infusion of arginine (0.5 gm/kg), or as its response to L-dopa (0.5 gm orally). Autonomy of growth hormone secretion can be evaluated by oral glucose loading, a maneuver that normally suppresses growth hormone secretion.

ANTERIOR PITUITARY HYPOFUNCTION: HYPOPITUITARISM (Table 67–1)

Etiology

Hypopituitarism, an endocrine deficiency state characterized by diminished or absent secretion of the hormones of the anterior pituitary gland, results either from a primary disorder of the secretory cells of the anterior pituitary gland or as a secondary consequence of reduced stimulation by the releasing hormones of the hypothalamus. When the deficiency of anterior pituitary hormones is generalized, the condition is referred to as panhypopituitarism.

Hypopituitarism can be caused by destruction of the pituitary by tumors or granulomas or by hemorrhagic necrosis of a hypertrophied pituitary gland in preg-

TABLE 67–1.   CAUSES OF HYPOPITUITARISM

Neoplasms
  1. Pituitary tumors
  2. Hypothalamic tumors, e.g., craniopharyngioma
  3. Metastatic tumors, lymphoma, etc.
Infections or Granulomas
  1. Tuberculosis
  2. Sarcoidosis
  3. Meningitis
  4. Syphilis
Vascular
  1. Postpartum necrosis (Sheehan's syndrome)
  2. Hemorrhagic infarction of a pituitary tumor
  3. Aneurysm of the carotid artery
Infiltrative
  1. Histiocytosis X
  2. Hemochromatosis
Physical Injury
  1. Head trauma
  2. Surgery
  3. Radiation therapy
Isolated or Combined Hypothalamic-Releasing Hormone Deficiencies

nancy as a complication of postpartum hemorrhage and shock (Sheehan's syndrome). Secondary hypopituitarism can result from lesions of the hypothalamus per se, from destruction of the pituitary stalk, or from a deficiency of one or more of the specific hypothalamic-releasing hormones that regulate secretion of the anterior pituitary gland. Isolated growth hormone deficiency in children is a typical example of a secondary form of anterior pituitary deficiency presumed to be due to a selective deficiency of growth hormone–releasing factor.

Clinical Features

The clinical manifestations of hypopituitarism depend upon the rapidity with which the hormonal deficiencies occur, the specific hormones that are deficient, the sex of the patient, and the age at the time of onset of the disease. Often pituitary insufficiency occurs insidiously, and the complaints are vague and nonspecific. Much less commonly, the onset of hypopituitarism occurs with dramatic suddenness in association with acute infarction of a pituitary tumor, a condition referred to as pituitary apoplexy.

In prepubertal children, the deficiencies of growth hormone and gonadotropins result in short stature and delayed puberty. In adults, growth hormone deficiency is of little clinical consequence, so that the predominant clinical features depend upon which of the other anterior pituitary hormones are deficient. Deficiency of ACTH results in findings similar to those of primary adrenocortical insufficiency (Addison's disease), including weakness, malaise, nausea, vomiting, and eventual collapse (see Chapter 69). These manifestations of glucocorticoid deficiency, however, are generally of lesser severity than in primary adrenal insufficiency. In contrast to Addison's disease, hyperpigmentation is absent and severe sodium depletion is rare, since aldosterone secretion is maintained at normal or nearly normal levels. Hyponatremia can occur, however, as a consequence of impaired water excretion secondary to cortisol deficiency. Deficiency of TSH results in many of the typical findings of thyroid hormone deficiency, but the severity is generally less than that seen in primary hypothyroidism, and true myxedema is rare. Gonadotropin deficiency results in amenorrhea and atrophy of the breasts in women, testicular atrophy in men, and diminished libido and the absence of pubic and axillary hair in both sexes. Additional findings include a waxy character and color of the skin and a fine wrinkling in the periorbital area that suggests premature aging. Hypothermia, hypotension, and hypoglycemia may also occur.

Diagnosis

Once suspected, the diagnosis of hypopituitarism can usually be established without difficulty, although care must be taken to distinguish the multiple deficiencies of target organ hormone production due to pituitary insufficiency from those due to primary polyglandular deficiency states resulting from autoimmune processes (e.g., Schmidt's syndrome). Demonstration of deficiency of the major target organ products (cortisol, thyroxine, testosterone, estrogen) together with an absence of compensatory increases in levels of the trophic hormones of pituitary origin (ACTH, TSH, FSH, LH) establishes that the abnormality resides in the hypothalamic-pituitary axis.

In patients with hypopituitarism, the finding of increased levels of prolactin, which is normally under tonic inhibition by the hypothalamus, suggests that the lesion is in the hypothalamus or pituitary stalk. Distinction between primary pituitary abnormalities and secondary deficiencies due to impaired hypothalamic function can also be made using the specific hypothalamic-releasing hormones as outlined above.

Treatment

Treatment of patients with panhypopituitarism consists of replacement of the specific hormone deficiencies with glucocorticoid, thyroxine, and the appropriate gonadal steroid. Growth hormone replacement is indicated in children who have not reached adult stature. Growth hormone and prolactin deficiencies in adults require no specific therapy. Restoration of fertility is theoretically possible with a combination of human menopausal gonadotropin and chorionic gonadotropin and by GnRH therapy in cases in which the lesion is in the hypothalamus or pituitary stalk.

Special precautions are required when initiating hormonal replacement therapy in patients with panhypopituitarism. Administration of thyroxine in patients who have concomitant ACTH deficiency can result in an increase in the metabolic clearance rate of glucocorticoid hormones and the sudden precipitation of an Addisonian crisis. Accordingly, such patients should always receive glucocorticoid therapy at the same time or preceding the onset of thyroid hormone replacement. Initiation of therapy with glucocorticoid hormones and thyroxine can unmask co-existing diabetes insipidus by improving free water clearance in patients with combined anterior and posterior pituitary insufficiency. Such patients may require concomitant treatment with antidiuretic hormone, as discussed in a subsequent section.

SYNDROMES OF ANTERIOR PITUITARY HYPERFUNCTION: THE PITUITARY ADENOMA

Adenomas of the pituitary gland may be nonfunctioning or they may secrete any of the trophic hormones normally produced by the gland. Hypersecretion of prolactin, growth hormone, or ACTH occurs commonly, resulting in the syndromes of amenorrhea-galactorrhea, acromegaly, and Cushing's syndrome, respectively. Hypersecretion of TSH or of gonadotropins from a pituitary adenoma is extremely rare. Whether or not hyperfunction of the anterior pituitary represents a primary disorder or is secondary to increased stimulation by hypothalamic releasing factors has not been resolved. Even the demonstration of a microadenoma and reversal of the clinical abnormalities with removal of the neoplasm does not exclude the latter possibility, since long-term follow-up is necessary to assure that the disease will not recur. In the following sections we will discuss the management of pituitary tumors in general as well as the pathogenesis, clinical features, and management of the specific syndromes produced by excess secretion of prolactin and growth hormone. For a discussion of Cushing's syndrome the reader is referred to Chapter 69.

PITUITARY NEOPLASMS: GENERAL CONSIDERATIONS

Pituitary neoplasms are usually benign and slow growing and may remain undetected for many years. Neurologic symptoms, principally headache and visual disturbances, may be the first manifestations, or the patient may present with findings consistent with pituitary insufficiency or with excessive secretion of any of the anterior pituitary hormones. Not infrequently, the presence of a pituitary neoplasm may be discovered in an asymptomatic patient in whom a skull radiograph is obtained for unrelated reasons.

Because of the close proximity of the optic nerves and optic chiasm, visual field defects are often the principal neurologic findings when a pituitary tumor extends beyond the confines of the sella turcica. Typically, this is manifested as bitemporal hemianopsia, often beginning in the upper quadrants of the visual field. Extraocular nerve palsies can also occur when the tumor enlarges laterally into the cavernous sinus. Headache, due in some cases to increased intracranial pressure secondary to obstruction of outflow of cerebrospinal fluid from the third ventricle, may also be a prominent complaint with large tumors. Headache is also common with smaller tumors due to stretching of the diaphragma sella and overlying dura.

Decisions regarding the management of pituitary tumors should be made in collaboration with a neurosurgeon. The optimal approach usually depends upon the size, location, and whether or not the tumor is endocrinologically active. Large tumors that impinge on extrasellar structures usually require surgical management whether or not they are secretory. Smaller tumors that are actively secreting anterior pituitary hormones, such as prolactinomas, as well as large tumors that are surgically incurable, can often be managed medically with bromocriptine (see below).

An enlarged sella turcica does not of itself indicate the presence of a pituitary tumor. Many patients with an enlarged sella, particularly obese women, have the so-called empty sella syndrome, in which the pituitary gland is displaced by cerebrospinal fluid that enters the sella via a defect in the diaphragm above the sella. These patients rarely have endocrinologic abnormalities. Distinction from pituitary tumor is usually possible with magnetic resonance imaging or high-resolution CT scans.

HYPERPROLACTINEMIA: GALACTORRHEA-AMENORRHEA SYNDROME

Etiology (Table 67–2)

Prolactin is under chronic inhibitory control by a hypothalamic factor (presumably dopamine). Any

TABLE 67–2. CAUSES OF HYPERPROLACTINEMIA

Physiological
1. Pregnancy and lactation
2. Breast stimulation
3. Estrogen therapy
4. Stress
5. Newborn

Hypothalamic-Pituitary Lesions
1. Prolactinoma
2. Stalk section
3. Hypothalamic disorders—craniopharyngioma, granulomas
4. Empty sella syndrome

Metabolic Disorders
1. Hypothyroidism
2. Renal failure

Chest Wall Injury

Drugs
1. Phenothiazines, haloperidol
2. Alpha methyldopa
3. Reserpine
4. Metoclopramide
5. Opiates

pharmacologic agent or lesion of the hypothalamus or pituitary stalk that interferes with dopamine secretion or its action can result in hyperprolactinemia. In view of the wide clinical use of pharmacologic agents that interfere with dopaminergic action, such as the phenothiazines, it is not surprising that the majority of patients with hyperprolactinemia do not harbor a pituitary adenoma. Once the use of such an agent can be excluded, however, and mechanical or neurogenic factors eliminated, the frequency with which a pituitary microadenoma is found is quite high. The most common pituitary tumor, chromophobe adenoma, once thought to be nonfunctioning and endocrinologically silent, is frequently a prolactin-secreting adenoma (prolactinoma).

Clinical Manifestations

The clinical manifestations of hyperprolactinemia depend upon the hormone level, the sex of the patient, and individual sensitivity to the lactogenic and mammotropic effects of the hormone. In women, hyperprolactinemia results in the so-called galactorrhea-amenorrhea syndrome. Persistent lactation, unprovoked by breast stimulation, and amenorrhea are the classic features. The syndrome may appear following pregnancy or may be unrelated to pregnancy. In men, galactorrhea can occur, but impotence and loss of libido are more frequent complaints.

Diagnosis

The diagnosis of hyperprolactinemia should be considered in patients with any of the previously described clinical manifestations, i.e., galactorrhea, secondary amenorrhea, and impotence. Serum prolactin determinations are required to establish a diagnosis of hyperprolactinemia. If levels are markedly elevated (>150 ng/dl, normal <20), the presence of a prolactin-

secreting adenoma is highly likely. With lower levels a greater degree of overlap with non-neoplastic causes of hyperprolactinemia occurs. Some overlap may occur with physiologically elevated levels in response to stress. Prolactin levels may also vary widely as a consequence of intermittent secretory bursts in patients with tumors. For these reasons, multiple levels should be obtained to establish the presence of pathological hyperprolactinemia. Galactorrhea can occur with persistently normal serum prolactin levels, presumably as a consequence of increased sensitivity to the hormone.

Treatment

For tumors located in the sella, or with minimal suprasellar extension, many centers now prefer an initial trial of medical therapy. Bromocriptine, a dopamine agonist, at doses of 10 to 15 mg daily will usually result in cessation of lactation, resumption of menses and fertility, and restoration of libido and potency. Bromocriptine may also result in regression of the tumor per se, although surgical therapy is probably indicated in patients with tumors large enough to produce neurologic symptoms. The surgical procedure of choice is transsphenoidal microsurgery. This procedure preserves the surrounding normal pituitary tissue and rarely results in hypopituitarism. Pituitary irradiation, using either conventional sources or heavy particle beams, is also frequently successful, but the incidence of hypopituitarism is greater than in patients treated with transsphenoidal hypophysectomy. This may be a very important consideration in women in the childbearing years or in children who have not yet achieved adult height.

GIGANTISM AND ACROMEGALY

Clinical Manifestations (Table 67–3)

The manifestations of excess growth hormone production are critically dependent on the age of the patient at the time that the abnormality first occurs. If growth hormone is present in excess before the epiphyses close, the increase in linear skeletal growth results in gigantism. After closure of the epiphyses, growth hormone excess results in acromegaly, a disorder characterized by physical changes in the bones and soft tissues as well as metabolic abnormalities reflecting the physiologic actions of this polypeptide.

The typical physical changes of acromegaly result from enlargement of the skeleton and soft tissues and thickening of the skin (Fig. 67–2). Enlargement of the acral parts (fingers and toes), coarsening and enlargement of the facial features, prognathism, frontal bossing, enlargement of the tongue, and deepening of the voice are characteristic findings. Since these changes may occur insidiously, comparisons of pictures of the patient taken serially over the years is often very helpful in recognizing their appearance. An increase in shoe size, hat size, or ring size may be noted by the patient. Additional complaints include headache, weakness, increased perspiration, paresthesias, and bilateral carpal tunnel syndrome. Enlargement of the viscera, hypertension, and congestive heart failure can also occur.

In addition to the physical changes that result from excess growth hormone secretion, a variety of metabolic abnormalities may also occur. Impaired glucose tolerance is present in more than half the cases, but frank diabetes mellitus is not evident unless pancreatic insulin secretion is incapable of responding to the counter-regulatory effect of growth hormone. An increase in glomerular filtration rate and in renal tubular reabsorption of phosphate may also be observed, the latter causing the typical finding of hyperphosphatemia.

Diagnosis

In fully developed acromegaly the physical findings are so characteristic as to provide an unmistakable diagnosis. Confirmation of this diagnosis as well as determination of whether or not the disease is in an active phase requires measurement of growth hormone. Levels of growth hormone obtained under basal conditions generally exceed the upper limit of normal (5 ng/ml) and typically cannot be suppressed by a physiological maneuver such as administration of glucose. A paradoxical increase in growth hormone levels in response to administration of glucose occurs in some patients with acromegaly, whereas administration of

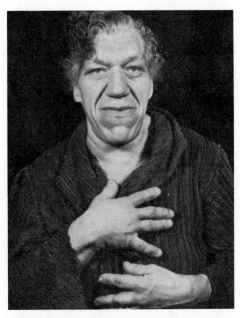

FIGURE 67-2. Typical physical appearance of a 52-year-old woman with end-stage acromegaly. Note the coarsening and enlargement of the facial features, prognathism, and enlargement of the hands. (From Mendeloff AI, Smith DE (eds): Acromegaly, diabetes, hypermetabolism, proteinuria and heart failure. Clinical pathological conference. Am J Med 20:133, 1956.)

TABLE 67-3. CLINICAL MANIFESTATIONS OF ACROMEGALY IN 100 PATIENTS

Manifestations of GH Excess	
Acral enlargement	100*
Soft tissue overgrowth	100
Hyperhidrosis	88
Lethargy or fatigue	87
Weight gain	73
Paresthesias	70
Joint pain	69
Photophobia	46
Papillomas	45
Hypertrichosis	33
Goiter	32
Acanthosis nigricans	29
Hypertension	24
Cardiomegaly	16
Renal calculi	11
Disturbance of Other Endocrine Functions	
Hyperinsulinemia	70
Glucose intolerance	50
Irregular or absent menses	60
Decreased libido or impotence	46
Hypothyroidism	13
Galactorrhea	13
Gynecomastia	8
Hypoadrenalism	4
Local Manifestations	
Enlarged sella	90
Headache	65
Visual deficit	20

* Percentage of patients in whom these features were present.
From Findling JW, Tyrrell JB: Anterior pituitary and somatomedins: I. Anterior pituitary. In Greenspan FS, Forsham PH (eds): Basic and Clinical Endocrinology. Los Altos, CA, Lange Medical Publishers, 1983, p 77.

L-dopa, which normally stimulates secretion of growth hormone, usually reduces the levels in acromegaly. Both TRH and GnRH, which normally have no effect on growth hormone, may cause a paradoxical rise in growth hormone levels in patients with acromegaly. Measurement of plasma concentrations of somatomedin C may also be useful, inasmuch as plasma levels of this mediator of growth hormone action fluctuate less than those of growth hormone and are thought to reflect more accurately the state of disease activity.

Treatment

Treatment of acromegaly depends partially on the size of the tumor, particularly whether or not the mass extends beyond the sella and whether or not the optic nerves are involved. Surgical results are often not as gratifying as with other pituitary neoplasms, presumably because the secretory cells are more widely dispersed and therefore are not entirely removed with the microsurgical technique. External radiation using either standard cobalt or proton beams generally results in a slow decrease in elevated growth hormone levels and eventually arrests the progress of the disease, but at the cost of a high incidence of hypopituitarism. A somatostatin analogue has been effective in reducing growth hormone levels in some patients with acromegaly and in decreasing tumor size in a few. Bromocriptine has been far less effective in the treatment of acromegaly than in the treatment of the amenorrhea-galactorrhea syndrome.

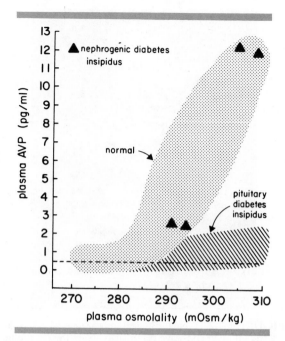

FIGURE 67–3. The relations between plasma AVP concentrations and plasma osmolality. Patients with nephrogenic diabetes insipidus (triangles) respond normally to increases in plasma osmolality. (From Reeves WB, Andreoli TE: Nephrogenic diabetes insipidus. *In* Schriver CR, Baudet AL, Sly WS, et al (eds): The Metabolic Basis of Inherited Disease. 6th ed. New York, McGraw-Hill Book Co, 1989.)

DISORDERS OF THE POSTERIOR PITUITARY

The posterior lobe of the pituitary gland (neurohypophysis) is an anatomical extension of the hypothalamus, containing the axons and axon terminals of neurons whose nuclei originate in the supraoptic and paraventricular areas of the hypothalamus. Two pep-

TABLE 67–4. NONOSMOTIC STIMULI OF VASOPRESSIN RELEASE

Neural
1. Stress—pain, fright
2. Coitus
3. Suckling

Diminished Effective Extracellular Fluid Volume
1. Hemorrhage
2. Decreased cardiac output
3. Hypoalbuminemia
4. Prolonged quiet standing

Drugs
1. Morphine
2. Barbiturates
3. Acetylcholine
4. Nicotine
5. Clofibrate
6. Vincristine
7. Carbamazepine

Hypoxemia

tide hormones, arginine vasopressin and oxytocin, and their carrier proteins, the neurophysins, are synthesized in the cell bodies of these neurons. These peptides and their carrier proteins travel down the axons to the nerve terminals from which they are released in response to a variety of physiological stimuli.

Oxytocin causes release of breast milk and may promote uterine contractions during labor. There is no known function for this peptide hormone in men. Arginine vasopressin (also known as antidiuretic hormone [ADH]) is the principal hormonal factor regulating water metabolism. Deficiency of ADH or impaired action in its major target organ, the kidney, results in a polyuric state known as diabetes insipidus. Excessive and physiologically inappropriate secretion of ADH results in hyponatremia (the syndrome of inappropriate ADH secretion), as discussed elsewhere in this volume (Chapter 27). Arginine vasopressin, as the name implies, also has pressor activity, the physiological relevance of which is unknown.

PHYSIOLOGICAL REGULATION OF ADH SECRETION

Variations in secretion of ADH by the posterior pituitary occur primarily in response to changes in body osmolality. Normally, osmolality averages approximately 285 mOsm/kg body water. An increase in body osmolality as small as 1 per cent (3 mOsm/kg), such as occurs after 10 to 12 hours of water deprivation, will normally increase ADH secretion (Fig. 67–3). Conversely, reduction in osmolality following administration of an oral water load causes dilution of body fluids and a prompt suppression of ADH secretion. Concomitant stimulation and suppression of the hypothalamic thirst center in response to hypertonicity and hypotonicity, respectively, provides a parallel physiological mechanism for regulating body osmolality.

In addition to osmotic regulation, several nonosmotic factors (Table 67–4) can influence ADH secretion. Most notable among these is the state of the so-called effective extracellular fluid (ECF) volume, perceived by high-pressure baroreceptors in the aorta and by low-pressure volume receptors in the left atrium. Hypotension and/or decreased effective ECF volume result in stimulation of ADH secretion via adrenergically mediated signals to the hypothalamus. Although minute-by-minute regulation of ADH secretion is probably through its osmotic control mechanism, nonosmotic factors will predominate in situations in which there is diversion of the two stimuli (e.g., hypovolemia in a hypotonic individual).

ADH acts primarily on the distal nephron to induce an increase in osmotic water permeability of the collecting tubule and collecting duct. Permeability to urea is also increased in response to ADH. The hormone acts through a classic cyclic AMP–dependent mechanism that is initiated by binding to a receptor on the basolateral surface of the target cell. This process is modulated by a number of factors, including calcium, prostaglandins, adrenal corticosteroids, and a variety of adrenergic agents.

DIABETES INSIPIDUS

Etiology

In diabetes insipidus the urinary concentrating mechanism is impaired either as a consequence of a failure to secrete adequate amounts of vasopressin (central diabetes insipidus) or as a consequence of failure of the distal tubule and collecting duct to respond normally to the hormone (nephrogenic diabetes insipidus). Central diabetes insipidus is usually caused by head trauma, surgical hypophysectomy, granulomatous diseases, histiocytosis X, primary or metastatic neoplasms, or following anoxic brain damage or meningoencephalitis. In at least one third of patients no pathological cause is evident. Diabetes insipidus following surgery or head trauma may occur transiently, may be followed by a transient period of hyponatremia due to inappropriate release of ADH from the damaged pituitary tissue, and then may resolve completely or progress to a permanent ADH-deficient state. Rarely central diabetes insipidus is familial, presumably due to hypoplasia of the secretory cells in the hypothalamus. Nephrogenic diabetes insipidus can occur as an inherited disorder, predominantly affecting males, or can be an acquired condition due to a variety of renal diseases, electrolyte disorders (hypokalemia, hypercalcemia), or drug therapies (e.g., lithium).

Diagnosis

In both central and nephrogenic diabetes insipidus the principal findings are polyuria and polydypsia with urinary volumes generally in excess of 3 L per day, and occasionally, depending upon the concomitant water intake, exceeding 5 to 10 L per day. The diagnosis is generally suspected in patients who excrete large quantities of a dilute urine in which the specific gravity is less than 1.010 or osmolality is less than 300 mOsm/kg. The major diagnostic challenge is to distinguish diabetes insipidus of either type from compulsive water drinking (psychogenic polydipsia), in which maximal urinary concentrating ability may be impaired as a consequence of "washout" of the normally hypertonic medulla by continuous excretion of a dilute urine. Demonstration of frank hypertonicity (serum osmolality >295 mOsm/kg) will exclude primary polydypsia, but usually a protocol employing water deprivation (overnight dehydration) followed by administration of aqueous pitressin is required to distinguish between these three polyuric states. In this procedure, water is withheld until the osmolality of hourly voided urine samples reaches a plateau. In patients with primary polydipsia, urine osmolality is generally much greater than plasma osmolality and increases minimally in response to the subsequent administration of aqueous vasopressin, 5 units subcutaneously. In patients with severe central diabetes insipidus, urine osmolality is usually much less than plasma osmolality and increases by at least 50 per cent in response to vasopressin. Those with nephrogenic diabetes insipidus are distinguished by the failure of a low urine osmolality to respond normally to vasopressin. Occasionally, patients with partial defects in ADH secretion will require further investigation using hypertonic saline infusion or more elaborate water deprivation tests.

Treatment

Treatment of central diabetes insipidus depends to a large extent on the severity of the hormone deficiency. In patients in whom the deficiency is only partial, chlorpropamide will potentiate the effect of ADH on the renal tubule. However, hypoglycemia may result, particularly if the dose of chlorpropamide exceeds 250 mg per day. Patients with more complete hormone deficiency require ADH replacement therapy using a synthetic analogue, 1-desamino-8-D-arginine vasopressin (DDAVP). Devoid of significant pressor activity, DDAVP can be conveniently administered by nasal insufflation in doses of 5 to 10 μg every 12 to 24 hours or intramuscularly if necessary. No specific treatment is available for patients with nephrogenic diabetes insipidus, but reduction of solute load by salt restriction and administration of thiazide diuretics will reduce the polyuria.

REFERENCES

Andreoli TE: The posterior pituitary. *In* Wyngaarden JB, Smith LH Jr (eds): Cecil Textbook of Medicine. 18th ed. Philadelphia, WB Saunders Co, 1988, pp 1305–1313.

Cook DM: Pituitary tumors. Diagnosis and therapy. CA 33:215, 1983.

Frohman LA: The anterior pituitary. *In* Wyngaarden JB, Smith LH Jr (eds): Cecil Textbook of Medicine. 18th ed. Philadelphia, WB Saunders Co, 1988, pp 1290–1305.

Lufkin EG, Kao PC, O'Fallon WM, et al: Combined testing of anterior pituitary gland with insulin, thyrotropin-releasing hormone, and luteinizing hormone-releasing hormone. Am J Med 75:471, 1983.

Miller M, Dalakos T, Moses AM, et al: Recognition of partial defects in antidiuretic hormone secretion. Ann Intern Med 73:721, 1970.

Robertson GL, Mahr EA, Athar S, et al: Development and clinical application of a new method for the radioimmunoassay of arginine vasopressin in human plasma. J Clin Invest 52:2340, 1973.

Robertson GL: Vasopressin in osmotic regulation in man. Ann Rev Med 25:315, 1974.

Wollesen F, Andersen T, Karle A: Size reduction of extrasellar pituitary tumors during bromocriptine treatment: Quantitation of effect on different types of tumors. Ann Intern Med 96:281, 1982.

68

THE THYROID

Dysfunction of the thyroid gland causes some of the most common endocrine disorders seen by the physician. Thyrotoxicosis (hyperthyroidism) is a consequence of excess thyroid hormone; a deficiency of thyroid hormone causes hypothyroidism (myxedema). Thyroid dysfunction is frequently manifested clinically by a swelling (enlargement) of the gland, a condition referred to as goiter formation.

The thyroid gland arises embryologically from the fourth pharyngeal pouch. The lateral components combine to develop the easily palpable, butterfly-shaped mature thyroid gland (20 gm). The lateral lobes (2 × 3 cm), partially hidden by the sternocleidomastoid muscles, are connected by the isthmus, which sits just below the cricoid cartilage. A pyramidal lobe is present in about 30 per cent; it extends upward from the isthmus lateral to the trachea. The gland consists of spherical follicles (acini) lined by epithelial tissue and filled with colloid. This substance consists of thyroglobulin, the storage form of T_4 (thyroxine), T_3 (3,5,3'-triiodothyronine), and the precursors MIT (monoiodothyronine) and DIT (diiodothyronine). Other functioning cells of neural crest origin located in the parafollicular area of the thyroid (C cells) secrete calcitonin.

THYROID PHYSIOLOGY

Iodide, a substrate for thyroid hormone synthesis, also plays an autoregulatory role in the metabolism of the thyroid gland. The normal gland contains approximately 10,000 μg of iodine, which is predominantly organically bound. The minimal daily requirement of iodide is only about 200 μg (renal loss replacement). Iodide deficiency is a rare occurrence in the iodide-replete western world but remains the most common cause of goiter (endemic goiter) in the world. Many patients with endemic goiter are mentally deficient owing to hypothyroidism dating from birth (cretinism) or suffer from retarded musculoskeletal development owing to thyroid hormone deficiency during childhood.

The thyroid gland concentrates iodide through a unique trapping mechanism to maintain a cell-to-plasma iodide ratio of about 50 to 1. Trapped iodide is rapidly oxidized by peroxidase to iodine and subsequently undergoes organification by iodinating tyrosine residues on thyroglobulin to form MIT and DIT. Coupling of these compounds results in the formation of T_3 and T_4. The secretory process is initiated by pinocytosis of thyroglobulin from the follicular lumen followed by the release of T_4 and T_3 from their storage form by proteolysis induced by lysosomal enzymes. The active hormones T_4 and T_3 are then secreted into the circulation. The thyroid gland is the only source for T_4, whereas it contributes only about 20 per cent of the T_3 produced daily.

A number of chemicals interfere with thyroid gland metabolism. These effects have been exploited for therapeutic purposes in the case of propylthiouracil (PTU) and methimazole. Both drugs effectively block thyroid hormone synthesis and are utilized clinically in the treatment of hyperthyroidism. Agents that are preferentially trapped by the thyroid (iodide, pertechnetate) are used diagnostically for gland imaging. Pharmacologic amounts of iodide will also inhibit thyroid gland synthesis and release of hormones. This inhibitory effect is generally of short duration in normal people, but if sustained it can lead to hypothyroidism and compensatory goiter formation. Lithium has a similar effect to that of iodide. Its extensive use in manic-depressive illness has led to a significant problem with hypothyroidism in this patient group.

Thyroid hormones circulate in two forms, protein-bound and free. Thyroxine-binding globulin (TBG), the principal carrier, binds about 70 per cent of the thyroid hormones under normal conditions. Other carrier proteins, thyroxine-binding pre-albumin (TBPA) and albumin, play a lesser role. A small but very important quantity of T_4 (0.03 per cent) and T_3 (0.3 per cent) is free and remains in rapid equilibrium with the protein-bound fraction. The metabolic state of the patient correlates with the free component rather than the total (bound) thyroid hormone level. Alterations in serum TBG concentration are common and account for the majority of changes in serum total T_4 not attributable to hyper- or hypothyroidism (Table 68–1). These changes in serum total T_4 levels are not accompanied by changes in the free T_4 concentration. Thus a measurement of free T_4 or an index of free T_4 is obligatory under these conditions in order to interpret accurately the significance of a change in the total hormone value.

TABLE 68–1. ALTERATIONS IN THYROXINE-BINDING GLOBULIN (TBG) CONCENTRATION

TBG Increased (Total $T_4 \uparrow$, $FT_4 \rightarrow$)
  Newborn
  Pregnancy (estrogen effect)
  Acute hepatitis
  Acute intermittent porphyria
  Genetic TBG excess
  Oral contraceptives (estrogens)
  Heroin and/or methadone abuse
  Clofibrate or 5-fluorouracil use
TBG Decreased (Total $T_4 \downarrow$, $FT_4 \rightarrow$)
  Cirrhosis
  Nephrotic syndrome
  Severe nonthyroidal illness
  Genetic TBG deficiency
  Anabolic steroids (androgens)
  Glucocorticoids

T_4 = Serum thyroxine level; FT_4 = serum level of free (unbound) thyroxine; TBG = thyroxine-binding globulin.

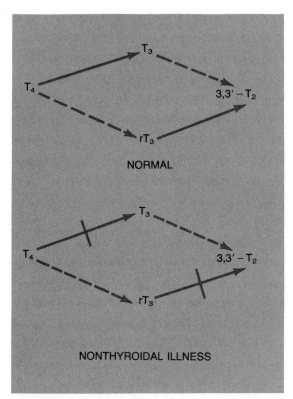

FIGURE 68–1. Sequential deiodination of thyroxine (T₄) to 3,3'-diiodothyronine (3,3'-T₂) via 3,5,3'-triiodothyronine (T₃) and 3,3',5'-triiodothyronine (reverse-T₃, rT₃), in the normal subject and in a patient with nonthyroidal illness. The solid arrows reflect outer-ring deiodination. The dashed arrows reflect inner-ring deiodination. The changes in serum T₃ and rT₃ associated with nonthyroidal illness are consequent to the indicated lesions in deiodination.

The thyroid gland is the only endogenous source of T₄. Although the thyroid also secretes T₃, 80 per cent of the daily T₃ produced is derived from extrathyroidal T₄ deiodination. Since T₃ is biologically the most active thyroid hormone, this process is regarded as an activation step. In addition, T₄ can be deiodinated to 3,5',3'-triiodothyronine (reverse-T₃, rT₃). This pathway inactivates T₄, as rT₃ is calorigenically inactive. These balanced pathways for T₄ deiodination are frequently disturbed during acute illness (Fig. 68–1). This results in an impairment in T₃ neogenesis (low T₃ syndrome) and increased levels of serum rT₃. Despite these alterations such patients are currently considered euthyroid, and T₃ replacement is not indicated. Should the low T₃ state persist, however, such patients may become hypothyroid.

The integrated control of thyroid hormone metabolism is regulated by the hypothalamic-pituitary-thyroid axis (Fig. 68–2). Thyrotropin-releasing hormone (TRH) secreted by the hypothalamus controls the synthesis and secretion of pituitary thyroid-stimulating hormone (TSH). The set point for the pituitary TSH response to TRH is regulated by the feedback inhibitory effect of the thyroid hormones. TSH stimulates all aspects of the synthesis and secretion of thyroid hormone.

The metabolic effects of thyroid hormone are mediated through a variety of mechanisms. Thyroid hormones regulate protein synthesis by binding to specific nuclear receptors. They enhance mitochondrial oxidation and regulate the activity of membrane-bound enzymes. Normal brain maturation during fetal and infant development is dependent on adequate quantities of thyroid hormone. Irreversible mental retardation develops in the absence of thyroid hormone (cretinism). During childhood, deficiency of thyroid hormone results in delay of somatic growth and development. In the geriatric population reversible dementia consequent to hypothyroidism is not an uncommon problem.

THYROID FUNCTION TESTS

Serum Thyroid Hormone Concentration. No one test can specifically determine thyroid status. Thus a variety of tests have been developed. These must be interpreted in an integrated fashion, keeping the patient's clinical presentation clearly in mind. Measurement of serum total T₄ (5 to 11 µg/dl) and free T₄ concentration (1.5 to 3.5 ng/dl) (or the free T₄ index)

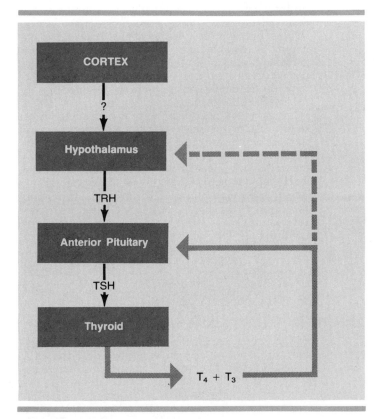

FIGURE 68–2. The normal hypothalamic-pituitary-thyroid axis. Both T₄ and T₃ feed back negatively on the pituitary and inhibit the secretion of thyroid-stimulating hormone (TSH). A similar process may regulate the hypothalamic secretion of thyrotropin-releasing hormone (TRH).

is the best current initial screening for the determination of thyroid dysfunction. Since the serum total T_4 can be altered by changes in carrier-protein concentration as well as by changes in thyroid function, its value must be evaluated in conjunction with a measurement of serum free T_4 or an indirect index of free T_4. Direct measurement of serum free T_4 is preferable. Many centers, however, continue to use indirect methods and derive a "free T_4 index" (0.5 to 1.5) from a combination of serum total T_4 and a thyroid hormone binding ratio (THBR). The latter procedure allows an estimation of changes in serum TBG. The patient's serum, a trace amount of radioiodine-labeled T_3, and a solid matrix (resin, charcoal, talc, or antibody) are co-incubated. The matrix-bound T_3 is measured and expressed as a percentage of the residual serum protein bound counts (25 to 35 per cent). Values correlate inversely with the concentration of unsaturated TBG. Generally, a parallel increase or decrease in both total T_4 and THBR indicates hyperthyroidism or hypothyroidism, whereas opposite changes suggest alterations in TBG binding. The derivation of the free T_4 index from the total T_4 and THBR generally gives a normal value in the setting of alterations in TBG. The free T_4 index or absolute free T_4 concentration is high or low in the hyperthyroid or hypothyroid subject, respectively. Occasionally free T_4 values may be misleadingly low in patients with severe nonthyroidal illness, "euthyroid sick syndrome." Serial analysis of thyroid function tests will generally resolve this dilemma. Measurement of total and free T_3 values is clinically useful only when T_3-thyrotoxicosis is suspected. In this setting T_4 values are normal and the hyperthyroidism will be missed in the absence of a T_3 measurement. Measurement of serum rT_3 has limited value as a routine clinical test. A measurement of serum TSH is the single best test to detect primary thyroid failure, since the value is invariably elevated in primary hypothyroidism owing to loss of the inhibitory feedback effect of thyroid hormone. The new TSH immunometric assays (TSH-IMA) can differentiate between a normal TSH (0.5–5.0 μU/ml) and the suppressed value (<0.1 μU/ml) found in hyperthyroidism. These assays may eliminate the need for confirmatory TRH testing in patients with suspected hyperthyroidism. However, it is premature to use these assays (TSH-IMA) as a screening test for thyroid dsyfunction.

The TSH response to TRH remains a very useful test. The normal TSH response ranges between a serum level of 15 and 30 μU/ml at 20 minutes after 500 μg of intravenous TRH. An incremental TSH rise of 5 μU above baseline in response to TRH is consistent with a normal axis. In hyperthyroidism the TSH response is flat. The mildly hypothyroid patient with a borderline high serum TSH value will have an exaggerated response to TRH.

Thyroid Radioiodide Uptake (RAIU) Test. The accumulation of tracer iodide (^{123}I, ^{131}I) in the thyroid can be quantitated at standard intervals (6 to 24 hours) to assess thyroid activity. Owing to the enrichment of western diets with iodide, this procedure is of no value in the differentiation between a normal and a hypoactive gland. In addition the uptake value may be normal in many hyperthyroid patients (approximately 30 per cent), especially with multinodular goiter and with T_3 thyrotoxicosis. Consequently a normal RAIU test does not exclude hyperthyroidism. In patients with thyrotoxicosis associated with thyroiditis, low (<3 per cent) uptake values are usually found in contrast to normal or high values in Graves' disease. A low uptake value is also a feature of thyrotoxicosis consequent to excess thyroid hormone medication.

Immunologic Tests. Autoimmune thyroid disease (Hashimoto's thyroiditis and Graves' disease) is associated with positive tests for antibodies to specific thyroid antigens (antimicrosomal and antithyroglobulin), which are useful in the detection of these autoimmune disorders. A biological assay for thyroid-stimulating immunoglobulin (TSI), a specific marker for Graves' disease, has helped in both the diagnosis and the management of this common disorder. A reduction in TSI level during therapy with antithyroid drugs is a good indicator that a remission has been induced and that therapy can be modified or withdrawn.

SCINTISCAN. The RAIU test provides useful information on the anatomy of the thyroid. A scan at 6 hours demonstrates a homogeneous distribution of ^{123}I in the normal gland, whereas ^{123}I activity will be heterogeneous in Hashimoto's thyroiditis and multinodular goiter. Furthermore, this procedure will differentiate a functioning (benign) from a nonfunctioning (possible carcinoma) thyroid nodule. Functioning nodules demonstrate normal (warm) to increased (hot) ^{123}I activity, whereas nonfunctioning nodules fail to concentrate ^{123}I (cold).

SONOGRAPHY. Ultrasound imaging will decisively differentiate whether a nonfunctioning nodule on ^{123}I scan (cold nodule) is cystic or solid. In addition, this noninvasive procedure is very helpful in the serial sizing of the thyroid nodule and provides an objective basis for the evaluation of T_4 suppressive therapy.

NEEDLE BIOPSY. Fine needle aspiration biopsy with cytological analysis of the tissue has now become the best test in the evaluation of a thyroid nodule. The specificity and sensitivity of this procedure are now so reliable that most centers will use needle biopsy as the first step in the evaluation of a thyroid nodule, even before scintiscanning.

THYROTOXICOSIS (HYPERTHYROIDISM)

Thyrotoxicosis, a common clinical condition consequent to excess thyroid hormone, can be caused by a number of different disorders; these should be differentiated in the individual patient for proper management (Table 68–2). Graves' disease is the most common cause of thyrotoxicosis. Toxic nodular goiter is most prevalent in the elderly. Transient thyrotoxicosis is frequently associated with thyroiditis. Also exposure to iodide (contrast studies) and iodine-containing drugs (e.g., amiodarone) has become a relatively common cause of thyrotoxicosis. The other conditions listed are relatively rare.

Graves' Disease

This complex autoimmune disorder consists of toxic goiter, ophthalmopathy, and rarely (< 1 per cent) dermopathy, which may occur together or separately. The abnormal immunoglobulin(s) (TSH receptor antibodies—TRAb) responsible for the hyperthyroidism can now be measured by bioassay. Thyroid-stimulating immunoglobulins (TSI) are antibodies to the normal thyroid gland TSH receptor site. They have powerful agonist action and consequently induce hyperthyroidism. The initiating factors in the development of TRAb and the role of TRAb in the development of the ophthalmopathy or dermopathy have not been elucidated.

Clinical Features. The clinical presentation of the thyrotoxic patient is extremely variable (Table 68–3). The actual features relate to the age at onset, the duration of the condition, and the degree of hormone excess. The patient most frequently presents with a history of nervousness, heat intolerance, sweating, palpitations, tremor, and weight loss. In addition a change in collar size (goiter formation) and eye discomfort (Graves' ophthalmopathy) may be noted.

More prolonged disease is associated with features of chronic catabolism. Skeletal muscle wasting, especially of the limb girdles, induces a proximal myopathy. Patients may experience difficulty in climbing stairs or getting up from the sitting position. Although dyspnea in the absence of cardiac failure is common, more severe disease can be manifested by a severe cardiomyopathy and congestive failure, especially in the elderly.

The mental changes are characterized by anxiety, irritability, poor concentration, restlessness, and emotional lability. In addition, insomnia and forgetfulness may be disturbing features.

Physical Findings (Table 68–3). The majority of young patients with hyperthyroidism have an enlarged thyroid (goiter). Diffuse symmetrical enlargement of the thyroid is characteristic of Graves' disease, whereas asymmetric changes occur in toxic nodular goiter. A bruit over the thyroid indicates extreme vascularity and is generally found only in Graves' disease. In addition, the finding of a palpable pyramidal lobe in a hyperthyroid patient is suggestive of Graves' disease.

The eye changes may be due to excess thyroid hormone or to the ophthalmopathy of Graves' disease. Enhanced sympathetic tone due to excess thyroid hormone causes the characteristic widening of the palpebral fissure (stare) and failure of the upper lid to closely follow globe movement (lag). Proptosis (exophthalmos), forward protrusion of the globe due to retro-orbital deposition of fat, mucopolysaccharides, and lymphocytes, are the cardinal features of Graves' ophthalmopathy. In addition, extraocular muscle weakness may limit eye movement and result in diplopia.

Smooth, shiny, silky, warm skin is frequently noted in hyperthyroidism. Thinning and loss of hair may be

TABLE 68–2. CAUSES OF THYROTOXICOSIS

Graves' disease
Toxic multinodular goiter
Toxic adenoma
Thyroiditis
Iodide-induced hyperthyroidism
Factitious thyrotoxicosis
Thyrotoxicosis due to excess TSH
Toxic thyroid carcinoma
Toxic struma ovarii

TABLE 68–3. CLINICAL FEATURES OF THYROTOXICOSIS

SYMPTOMS	SIGNS
Nervousness	Thyroid enlargement
Heat intolerance (sweating)	Eyestare and lid lag
Palpitations	*Proptosis and ophthalmoplegia
Tremulousness	Warm smooth skin
Weight loss (good appetite)	*Pretibial myxedema
Muscle weakness	Fine tremor
Emotional lability	Brisk reflexes
Hyperdefecation	Onycholysis
	Tachycardia or atrial fibrillation

* Graves' disease only

particularly worrisome for women. Hyperpigmentation over extensor surfaces and clubbing (thyroid acropachy) are rare features. Onycholysis, separation of the distal portion of the nail from the nailbed (Plummer's nails), fine tremor of the outstretched hands, and brisk reflexes are commonly noted. Pretibial myxedema may occasionally be seen in Graves' disease.

A spectrum of cardiovascular abnormalities may be detected on physical examination. Sinus tachycardia with a wide pulse pressure may progress to atrial fibrillation and congestive heart failure. Systolic flow murmurs and a forceful apical pulse are common features.

Diagnosis. A typical case of Graves' disease is easily diagnosed. In many instances, however, the typical eye features are minimal, goiter may be moderate (especially in the elderly), and systemic features may be few. Thus the condition may go unrecognized for years. In the majority of cases serum total and free T_4 levels will be high. If normal, a serum total T_3 must be performed, as T_3 toxicosis occurs in 5 to 10 per cent of cases. If all other tests are equivocal, the TSH response to TRH should be flat if the patient is indeed hyperthyroid. Measurement of basal TSH by TSH-IMA may replace the need for a TRH test.

The recognition of hyperthyroidism in the elderly is frequently delayed owing to the insidious nature of the disease. These patients have been classically described as "apathetic" owing to the paucity of features of sympathetic overactivity. The dominant features may be reflected in other systems such as the cardiovascular system. Patients present with atrial fibrillation and congestive failure. In the absence of ophthalmopathy and goiter the hyperthyroid state is generally missed.

All elderly patients presenting with new-onset cardio-vascular disorders should be screened for hyperthyroidism. Beware, however, that patients with nonthyroidal systemic disorders may have a transient rise in serum total and free T_4 values as a byproduct of their disease and require close monitoring with serial thyroid function tests in order to elucidate their thyroid status.

Anxiety neurosis may be difficult to differentiate clinically from hyperthyroidism. These patients may present with tremor, tachycardia, irritability, and fatigue. Typical anxiety neurosis is generally associated with depression, weight loss accompanied by anorexia, cold moist hands, and a normal resting (sleeping) pulse. If the clinical suspicion for hyperthyroidism remains, a baseline screening test with total and free T_4 should clarify the diagnosis. Some patients with psychiatric disorders (10 per cent) have a transient elevation in serum total and free T_4 levels, such that serial analyses may be needed or further detailed testing may be indicated to exclude hyperthyroidism.

Graves' ophthalmopathy may occur in a euthyroid or even a hypothyroid patient. Other diseases of the orbit or retro-orbital space must be considered as a cause of exophthalmos. Orbital pseudotumor may display similar extraocular muscle swelling on CT scan or sonogram. When the ophthalmopathy is bilateral and the TRH test and TSI analysis are positive, the diagnosis of Graves' disease can generally be made. Other features of the disease eventually become evident in most cases.

Hyperthyroidism in the absence of goiter suggests factitious thyrotoxicosis or thyroiditis (or very rarely struma ovarii). In both conditions the RAIU test is suppressed. Serum thyroglobulin is high in thyroiditis but reduced in subjects taking exogenous thyroid hormone.

Therapy. Graves' disease is a self-limiting disease; 30 per cent of cases will go into spontaneous remission within one to two years. Antithyroid drugs can be used for the temporary control of symptoms, or the gland can be ablated with ^{131}I or surgery. The choice of therapy is usually dictated by the patient's age, the size of gland, and the severity of the disease.

DRUGS. The thionamides propylthiouracil (PTU) and methimazole (Tapazole) will control the features of hyperthyroidism in almost all cases. These drugs inhibit the synthesis of thyroid hormone and will restore a euthyroid state in four to eight weeks. The initial dose recommended is 150 to 300 mg every 8 hours for PTU or 10 to 15 mg every 12 hours for methimazole. Once achieved, euthyroidism can generally be maintained by smaller doses of PTU (50 to 100 mg twice daily) or methimazole (5 to 10 mg once daily). Antithyroid drugs are preferred for children, young adults, and the pregnant patient. They are also used in the adult and elderly patient to induce euthyroidism prior to definitive therapy with ^{131}I or surgery. Antithyroid drugs will induce a permanent remission in about 30 per cent of patients with Graves' disease, usually within three to six months of therapy. A reduction in TSI during therapy generally indicates that a remission has occurred and consequently is a good guide for the discontinuation of therapy.

Transient dermatitis, the most common side effect of antithyroid drugs, is not dose-related and generally disappears despite continued therapy. Urticaria and pruritus may also occur. Dose-related leukopenia, myalgia, arthralgia, and elevated serum alkaline phosphatase may occur in patients during therapy with PTU. Generally these abnormalities can be controlled by dose adjustment. The most serious side effect (agranulocytosis) is not dose-related. A routine blood count is of no value as a predictor, since this complication occurs acutely. Thus patients should be advised to watch for fever and sore throats and to report such developments immediately to their physician. Fortunately the majority of patients recover from agranulocytosis once the drug is stopped.

Sympathetic overactivity can be controlled with beta-adrenergic blockade. Such therapy with propranolol (40 mg every 6 hours) is indicated for severe agitation, tremor, sweating, and tachycardia. Beta-blockers should not be used in the patient with severe thyrotoxic heart disease.

Radioactive iodine therapy with ^{131}I is the preferred form of therapy for the majority of patients with Graves' disease. An appropriate dose (7 to 12 mCi ^{131}I) will induce euthyroidism in most patients. This form of therapy is inexpensive and easy to administer. Since the gonadal exposure is extremely low (less than a diagnostic radiograph), genetic effects are unlikely. Thus ^{131}I can be used in all adult patients. ^{131}I is contraindicated during pregnancy; thus a pregnancy test should be performed prior to therapy, or the dose should be given during the first half of the menstrual cycle. Long-term hypothyroidism (70 per cent at 10 years) is the major disadvantage of ^{131}I therapy. In addition, dose-related hypothyroidism occurs acutely after therapy (in six months) in a number of subjects. These complications are currently unavoidable, since lower doses may fail to induce euthyroidism.

SURGERY. Surgical ablation is still preferred for children who cannot be controlled with antithyroid drugs and possibly for young adults with extremely large glands. The procedure, subtotal thyroidectomy, should be performed only by an experienced surgeon. In the proper hands it is very effective therapy associated with minimal morbidity. Recurrent laryngeal nerve damage with vocal cord paralysis, permanent hypoparathyroidism, and hypothyroidism may be significant postoperative problems. Long-term hypothyroidism (40 per cent at 10 years) occurs despite the best of surgery, and immediate postoperative hypothyroidism may occur in 5 to 10 per cent of patients. Furthermore, recurrent hyperthyroidism also occurs in about 5 to 10 per cent of cases and should always be treated with ^{131}I therapy, since reoperation is more frequently accompanied by major complications.

Hyperthyroidism During Pregnancy. Graves' disease is responsible for the majority of cases of thyrotoxicosis associated with pregnancy. It should always be treated with antithyroid drugs. Surgery is rarely indicated and ^{131}I therapy should never be used. The dose of antithyroid drug used should be the minimum needed to restore euthyroidism. These drugs freely cross the placenta; thus hypothyroidism and goiter can be induced in the fetus with inappropriate high dosage. In general propylthiouracil is the drug of choice in the pregnant patient needing thionamide therapy, since aplasia cutis has been described in fetuses following methimazole therapy. The maternal thyroid status should be monitored with free T_4 determinations, since the total T_4 concentration is normally elevated during pregnancy because of the estrogen-induced high serum TBG level. The physician caring for the newborn infant of a Graves' mother should carefully monitor for neonatal Graves' disease. Passive transfer of TSI occurs and may produce transient neonatal hyperthyroidism. The cord blood TSI level may predict the infant at risk.

Toxic Nodular Goiter

This common cause of hyperthyroidism in the elderly generally occurs in patients with a long history of nodular goiter, but only a few patients with nodular goiter develop hyperthyroidism. It is not clear why these few nodular goiters progress to the toxic state and become autonomous in function. These patients generally present with symptoms and signs referable to the cerebrovascular, cardiovascular, musculoskeletal, or gastrointestinal system. Their hyperthyroidism is frequently masked by the nonthyroidal manifestations so that the true diagnosis is often delayed. Elderly patients with nodular goiter should be screened for thyroid dysfunction whenever they present with features of a new illness. The majority of these hyperthyroid patients will have an unequivocal increase in serum total and free T_4 values. Since 10 to 15 per cent may have normal T_4 values but a high serum T_3 concentration (T_3 toxicosis), the latter measurement should always be included when hyperthyroidism is clinically suspected in the elderly patient.

The majority of these patients can be treated with ^{131}I, but the effective dose generally ranges from 15 to 30 mCi. Hypothyroidism follows less frequently than in Graves' disease. It is preferable to induce a euthyroid state with antithyroid drugs prior to definitive therapy in order to avoid aggravation of the thyrotoxicosis. Surgery may be indicated in individuals with very large goiters (>100 gm) and in those patients who have pressure complications from goiter.

Thyroiditis

Transient thyrotoxicosis may be a feature of subacute granulomatous and lymphocytic thyroiditis. Subacute granulomatous thyroiditis is viral in origin, whereas lymphocytic thyroiditis probably results from autoimmune injury. The thyrotoxicosis associated with subacute granulomatous thyroiditis is generally mild, and symptomatic therapy is rarely needed. However, patients with subacute lymphocytic thyroiditis may need therapy for more prolonged and severe thyrotoxicosis. The latter condition is estimated to cause 15 to 20 per cent of thyrotoxicosis in adults and is also a common cause of postpartum thyroiditis. Both forms of thyroiditis are characterized by low RAIU tests. It is important to differentiate thyroiditis from Graves' disease, since therapy with ^{131}I or surgery is not indicated and antithyroid drugs (PTU or methimazole) are not effective. These patients are treated symptomatically with beta-blockers (propranolol) until remission occurs.

Hyperthyroxinemia of Acute Illness

Both serum total and free T_4 values may be elevated transiently during acute systemic (nonthyroidal) illness, especially in the elderly. This does not represent true hyperthyroidism. Serum T_3 concentrations are usually normal or low, and the TSH response to TRH is usually normal or slightly blunted. Hyperthyroidism can generally be excluded by demonstrating that the T_4 values return to normal during the recovery from the acute disorder. A similar phenomenon can be associated with acute psychiatric illness. It is important not to confuse these features of nonthyroidal illness with the diagnosis of true hyperthyroidism.

Familial Dysalbuminemic Hyperthyroxinemia (FDH)

This autosomal dominant condition may be a relatively common and misleading cause for an elevated total T_4 and free T_4 index. These subjects possess an abnormal albumin that has a high affinity for T_4, resulting in a high serum total T_4. Furthermore, the free T_4 index when derived from the T_3 uptake method is also high because the abnormal albumin does not have a high affinity for T_3. Thus an incorrect diagnosis of hyperthyroidism may be made. The serum free T_4 concentration and the total T_3 level are normal in these subjects. Thus in the absence of clinical features of thyrotoxicosis a high free T_4 index should suggest FDH as a differential possibility.

Thyrotoxic Crisis

This medical emergency is due to stress-induced exaggeration of the features of thyrotoxicosis. Additional clinical features include mental disorientation, fever, disproportionate tachycardia, and jaundice. Patients may rapidly deteriorate with shock and coma. The mortality of thyrotoxic crisis (thyroid storm) remains high. The diagnosis is made clinically, as time generally does not permit the laboratory confirmation of hyperthyroidism. Treatment should be initiated based on clinical suspicion.

Supportive measures are as important as specific therapy. Hyperpyrexia is controlled with a cooling blanket and acetaminophen (aspirin is contraindicated), and the hypotension is reversed by volume expansion and vasopressor agents. During the extreme catabolic phase, adequate attention to nutritional support is mandatory. Other therapy includes glucocorticoids (hydrocortisone 100 mg t.i.d.), to cover the severe stress and purported relative adrenal insufficiency. Specific therapy includes propylthiouracil (200 mg q4h), and propranolol (40 mg q6h) and iodide (500 mg b.i.d.). Iodide is given as a specific blocker of thyroid hormone secretion. It is preferable to give PTU

TABLE 68—4. CAUSES OF HYPOTHYROIDISM

Primary

Autoimmune	Hashimoto's thyroiditis
	Idiopathic myxedema
Iatrogenic	^{131}I therapy for hyperthyroidism
	Subtotal thyroidectomy
Drug-induced	Iodide deficiency or excess
	Lithium, amiodarone
	Antithyroid drugs
Congenital	Synthetic enzyme defect
	Thyroid dysgenesis or agenesis

Secondary

Hypothalamic dysfunction	Therapeutic irradiation
	Granulomatous disease
	Neoplasms
Pituitary dysfunction	Therapeutic irradiation
	Pituitary surgery
	Idiopathic hypopituitarism
	Neoplasms
	Postpartum pituitary necrosis

before iodide or at the same time. Cardiac decompensation should be treated with conventional doses of digoxin and diuretics. If cardiac failure is the dominant component of the crisis, beta-blockade may be contraindicated. This combined therapeutic approach should provide an effective amelioration of the thyrotoxic crisis within a few days.

HYPOTHYROIDISM

Deficiency of thyroid hormone may occur as a primary thyroid defect or more rarely may be due to pituitary or hypothalamic disease (secondary hypothyroidism). Primary thyroid failure is a common disorder (prevalence 0.8 per cent) whose clinical features range from mild hypothyroidism to severe myxedema. The latter condition develops in the setting of prolonged severe hypothyroidism and is due to the deposition of mucopolysaccharides in the skin and other tissues.

Two acquired and possibly related autoimmune disorders, atrophic (idiopathic) and Hashimoto's thyroiditis, are responsible for most cases of hypothyroidism (Table 68–4). Iatrogenic hypothyroidism consequent

TABLE 68—5. CLINICAL FEATURES OF HYPOTHYROIDISM

SYMPTOMS	SIGNS
Weakness	Dry, coarse, cold skin
Lethargy, fatigue	Periorbital and peripheral edema
Memory impairment	Coarse, thin hair
Cold intolerance	Pallor of skin
Weight gain (anorexia)	Thick tongue
Constipation	Slow speech
Loss of hair	Decreased reflexes
Hoarseness	Hypertension
Deafness	Bradycardia
Dyspnea	Pleural, pericardial effusions
Myalgia, arthralgia	Ascites
Paresthesias	Vitiligo
Precordial pain	
Menstrual irregularity	

to definitive therapy (^{131}I or surgery) for hyperthyroidism constitutes a second major group. More recently drugs (iodide, lithium, and amiodarone) have become increasingly common causes of hypothyroidism in the hospital setting. The congenital causes are rare and generally present in childhood. Secondary causes induce hypothyroidism infrequently (approximately 1 per cent).

Clinical Features (Table 68–5)

The spectrum of clinical presentation depends on the degree, severity, and age at onset of the hypothyroidism. Cretinism, irreversible mental and motor retardation, presents within six months after delivery in the hypothyroid infant. Mass screening at birth should help to eliminate this correctable metabolic deficiency, since prompt replacement therapy with thyroid hormone can prevent or minimize this serious condition. Congenital hypothyroidism occurs in 1 in 5000 newborns. The development of hypothyroidism in childhood is associated with growth retardation and delayed puberty. Bone age is delayed relative to chronological age. In the adult the insidious nature of hypothyroidism may result in its being undetected for years. Symptoms are nonspecific, and in the absence of goiter the primary thyroid defect is frequently overlooked. Fatigue, lethargy, tiredness, cold intolerance, myalgias, and arthralgias are generally the earliest symptoms. The skin is dry and scaly, and hair loss is frequent. Facial puffiness and periorbital edema are characteristic features. The voice becomes hoarse and rough. In older subjects mental changes, confusion, paranoia, depression, and dementia are often attributed to aging per se. Nerve entrapment syndromes are common, such as deafness and hand paresthesia (median nerve distribution) due to the carpal tunnel syndrome.

In severe hypothyroidism (myxedema) the above features are exaggerated and characteristic clinical features develop. Extensive scaling of the skin leads to exfoliation, and diffuse subcutaneous infiltration with mucopolysaccharides gives the skin a thickened or doughy feeling. The edematous change is characteristically nonpitting except when hypoproteinemia develops. Deposition of carotene gives the skin a yellow-orange appearance. Sinus bradycardia may progress to variable degrees of heart block. This in conjunction with myocardial dilatation may lead to decompensation and congestive heart failure. More commonly the heart appears enlarged owing to pericardial effusion. Pleural effusions and ascites may also be prominent.

Deep tendon reflexes show the characteristic delayed relaxation phase (hung-up reflexes). Slow mentation progressing to confusion, disorientation, and coma is not uncommon. Rarely marked cerebellar ataxia occurs.

Myxedema Coma. This severe form of myxedema is frequently fatal. Decompensation is frequently precipitated by stress such as infection, alcohol (drugs), or cold exposure. Severe respiratory failure (CO_2 narcosis), hypothermia, and sluggish cerebral perfusion all contribute to the development of coma. The diagnosis is based on the clinical presentation. Therapy must be instituted before the clinical suspicions are substantiated by laboratory tests, since delay may lead to a fatal outcome in this medical emergency.

Laboratory Findings

Primary thyroid failure can be definitely diagnosed with the demonstration of low serum total T_4 and free T_4 values combined with a high serum TSH level. Measurement of serum T_3 is of no value in the diagnosis of hypothyroidism. Occasionally when the serum TSH value is borderline, the exaggerated TSH response to TRH will substantiate the diagnosis of primary hypothyroidism. Secondary hypothyroidism is associated with an inappropriately low serum TSH level. The finding of other features of pituitary or hypothalamic disease generally confirms the diagnosis.

In addition to the definitive diagnostic tests noted above, hypothyroidism is associated with other abnormal laboratory tests. Muscle enzymes, especially creatine phosphokinase (CPK), are frequently elevated. In fact CPK isoenzyme analysis may show a modest increase in MB bands (cardiac). This in conjunction with myalgias and arthralgias, especially of the anterior chest wall, should not be mistaken for myocardial infarction. Hyponatremia, consequent to a relative excess of antidiuretic hormone (ADH) and impaired free water clearance, may be difficult to differentiate from the syndrome of inappropriate ADH secretion (SIADH).

Anemia in hypothyroidism is generally normochromic normocytic but may be macrocytic (vitamin B_{12} deficiency due to pernicious anemia) or microcytic because of poor nutrition or blood loss in women (menorrhagia). The combination of Hashimoto's disease, pernicious anemia, and type I diabetes mellitus is called Schmidt's syndrome.

The electrocardiogram classically demonstrates bradycardia and low voltage. In addition, variable degrees of heart block may be found, and nonspecific ST/T changes can occur. Blood gas analyses will demonstrate moderate to severe hypoxia and hypercapnia consequent to hypoventilation.

Differential Diagnosis

A clinical awareness of the wide spectrum of presentation and a high index of suspicion for hypothyroidism will generally detect most cases. A number of clinical states may mimic hypothyroidism, e.g., nephrotic syndrome and cirrhosis, including an associated reduction in serum TBG and consequent low serum total T_4 value. However, the serum free T_4 is generally normal. The diagnosis of hypothyroidism during acute illness is complicated by the finding of a low serum total T_4 and free T_4 index in many (10 to 20 per cent) of these patients. Serum T_3 is also low and serum TSH is generally within the normal range. The serum TSH response to TRH is either normal or blunted. These patients do not have primary thyroid failure but appear to have a stress-related form of secondary hypothyroidism. They are currently considered euthyroid ("euthyroid sick syndrome"), and T_4 replacement therapy is not warranted. In the majority of these patients the serum free T_4 concentration is normal and serum rT_3 is elevated. Furthermore, should clinically relevant primary hypothyroidism be present, the serum TSH will be unequivocally elevated ($>20 \mu U/ml$) despite their acute illness.

Treatment

Hypothyroidism should be treated with a synthetic preparation of L-thyroxine. In young healthy individuals with hypothyroidism of recent onset and without cardiac disease, thyroxine replacement may be initiated at full dosage. Elderly subjects with heart disease or a history of pre-existing heart troubles should be slowly corrected to euthyroidism by incremental dose adjustments over several months in order to reduce the risk of cardiac complications. The average full replacement dose of L-thyroxine in the healthy adult ranges between 75 and 100 μg daily. In the elderly patient, thyroxine therapy should begin at 25 to 50 μg daily, with an incremental dose of 25 μg every two to four weeks. The therapeutic response should be monitored clinically and with serial serum T_4 and TSH analyses.

In a patient with myxedema coma, a large dose of thyroxine (300 to 500 μg) is given parenterally as a bolus and followed by 100 μg daily over the succeeding five days. Even elderly subjects with cardiac disorders tolerate these doses under this condition. The underlying stressful, precipitating event (e.g., infection) must obviously be corrected. Furthermore, standard supportive therapy for the comatose patient must be promptly introduced. This is especially important with respect to respiratory support. Many of these patients need mechanical ventilatory assistance, which may persist for some period after improvement in mental status. In addition, because of the associated relative adrenal insufficiency, these patients are treated with glucocorticoids. With proper therapy patients with myxedema coma should improve clinically within 24 to 36 hours. If this does not occur, the clinical diagnosis may not have been correct or the underlying aggravating medical illness may have persisted or advanced. The expected mortality from myxedema coma with adequate therapy remains around 25 per cent.

GOITER

This most common thyroid abnormality means basically an enlargement of the thyroid gland. Patients suffering from goiter are predominantly euthyroid (simple goiter) but may be hyperthyroid (toxic goiter) or hypothyroid. In areas where iodine deficiency is still prevalent, goiter formation is said to be endemic. The development of euthyroid simple colloid goiter, termed sporadic goiter, in an iodide-replete location is predominantly due to congenital defects in thyroid hormone synthesis. Dietary goitrogens such as the thiocarbamides found in cabbage, turnips, and soybeans may also induce sporadic goiter. Thyroid enlargement may be symmetrical and diffuse (simple goiter, Graves', Hashimoto's) or may be asymmetrical and nodular (nodular goiter, Hashimoto's).

Goiter formation is generally a TSH-mediated compensatory enlargement of the thyroid gland that ensures sufficient synthesis and secretion of thyroid hormone and prevents hypothyroidism. In addition, goiter formation may be consequent to an autoimmune process, as in Hashimoto's thyroiditis and Graves' disease.

Pain is unusual with a goiter except in the course of subacute thyroiditis, or consequent to cystic or hemorrhagic degeneration. Most frequently patients with nontoxic goiter present because of the neck swelling or features of obstruction. A large goiter can cause dysphagia, respiratory distress, or hoarseness. The latter symptom generally indicates recurrent laryngeal nerve invasion and most likely thyroid cancer rather than a benign simple goiter. The neck swelling can be readily confirmed as due to enlargement of the thyroid gland by either radioiodine scan or sonogram. In addition, the functional activity of the goiter can be determined from the radioiodine scan.

Most simple nontoxic goiters can be treated with continuous T_4 suppression of TSH, which should prevent further enlargement and eventually induce regression. It is important to determine that the gland is suppressible, since hyperthyroidism may develop from exogenous hormone therapy if the gland is autonomous. Autonomous function is frequent in patients with nontoxic multinodular goiter and patients with euthyroid Graves' disease. Thus a careful monitoring of the serum T_4 response to T_4 suppression is mandatory. If serum T_4 increases inappropriately during standard suppression therapy (75 to 150 μg L-thyroxine daily), the gland is probably autonomous and the dose should be reduced accordingly.

A diffusely enlarged gland should regress in 6 to 12 months, but long-standing multinodular goiter may take several years to respond. Therapy may be continued indefinitely or terminated when appropriate. Permanent loss of TSH secretion never occurs, even after years of T_4 suppression. Recovery will take place within six to eight weeks following the withdrawal of therapy. Goiters that fail to suppress, that are associated with pressure features, or that are large enough to be cosmetically embarrassing should be surgically removed.

The Solitary Thyroid Nodule

Thyroid nodules occur in approximately 5 per cent of the population. A nodule is a focal area of gland enlargement. It can be caused by a number of factors, but solitary nodules are predominantly adenomatous and benign (Table 68–6). Since a small percentage are carcinomatous, a practical clinical approach must be pursued to detect these patients. A number of factors from the clinical history, examination, and specific evaluations are helpful in the differentiation of benign from malignant lesions (Table 68–7). These relate to patient age and sex and whether the nodule is single or part of a multinodular gland. A young man presenting with a single dominant nodule associated with hoarseness and lymph node enlargement has a high possibility of malignancy. Any individual who presents with a nodule and a past history of head-neck irradiation should be referred for thyroidectomy, as these lesions are frequently malignant (~ 30 per cent).

The traditional approach is to perform a RAIU study initially to determine the functional status of the nodule. Scanning with ^{123}I will demonstrate no accumulation ("cold nodule"), equal isotope trapping ("warm nodule"), or greater accumulation ("hot nodule") when compared with the rest of the gland. Warm and hot nodules are overwhelmingly benign (99.8 per cent). Cold nodules are also predominantly benign (90 per cent). Patients with hot nodules may be hyperthyroid (toxic adenoma). These can be treated effectively with ^{131}I therapy or surgery. Generally, however, they are not currently hyperthyroid, but they should be followed carefully, since approximately 30 per cent will eventually become hyperthyroid.

Most solitary nodules are "cold" (80 per cent). A definitive pathological diagnosis can be made in most of these subjects (80 per cent) by cytological examination of tissue specimen obtained by fine needle aspiration biopsy (FNA). In fact, most centers will perform FNA as the initial procedure. Benign lesions (75 per cent) such as benign thyroid nodules, multinodular goiter, and thyroiditis can be identified by the *expert* cytologist. In addition, malignant lesions (5 per cent), such as papillary, anaplastic, and medullary car-

TABLE 68–6. PATHOGENESIS OF THYROID NODULES

LESIONS*	PREVALENCE (%)
Benign thyroid nodule	40
Multinodular goiter	20
Cyst	12
Thyroiditis	10
Follicular adenoma	12
Carcinoma	6

* Data are representative of findings on fine needle aspiration followed by surgical excision in indicated cases.

TABLE 68–7. HIGH RISK FACTORS FOR CANCER IN A THYROID NODULE

History	Childhood therapeutic irradiations (low dose <500 rads) of head or neck
	Hoarseness
	Rapid growth
	Pain
Clinical Features	Children, young adults, men
	Solitary, firm, dominant nodule
	Associated lymphadenopathy
	Vocal cord paralysis
	Distant metastasis
Serum Factors	Elevated serum calcitonin
Scanning Techniques	
Pattern on [123]I	"Cold" nodule
ECHO scan	Solid lesion
Thyroxine Therapy	No regression

cinoma, can be specifically diagnosed. Follicular neoplasms (20 per cent), however, cannot be identified as benign or malignant by this technique and require examination of tissue specimens obtained by surgical excision. Despite the lack of sensitivity in the analysis of the follicular neoplasm, FNA has proved to be a powerful diagnostic procedure in the evaluation of the thyroid nodule. The ability to make a definitive diagnosis through the application of this safe and simple technique has markedly reduced the need for diagnostic thyroid surgery. The therapy for a malignant nodule is considered in the section on thyroid carcinoma. Benign lesions are treated with T_4 suppression therapy. Regression of the nodule may occur during a six-month course. Generally, long-standing nodules remain stable and do not progress. If the nodule increases in size, it should be re-evaluated and the appropriate therapy instituted.

THYROID CARCINOMA

Thyroid cancer is a relatively rare disorder. Furthermore, most varieties of thyroid cancer are of low-grade malignancy. Papillary or follicular carcinomas constitute about 90 per cent of all thyroid cancers. Anaplastic and medullary carcinoma accounts for the remainder.

Papillary carcinoma generally presents as a thyroid nodule that may be associated with local invasion and lymph node spread. The size of the initial lesion (>4.0 cm) and the presence of lymph node involvement adversely influence the recurrence rate and long-term prognosis. Follicular carcinoma is more aggressive and frequently presents with metastases, especially to the lung, bone, or brain. The size of the initial lesion does not influence prognosis. In many cases the small thyroid primary is overlooked and is diagnosed in retrospect following examination of the metastatic tissue. Both of these cancers have a low recurrence rate and a relatively good prognosis.

Primary therapy entails total thyroidectomy with nodal dissection followed in most cases (six weeks postoperatively) by ^{131}I ablative therapy for any remnant tissue. Lobectomy and isthmectomy with no radiation are adequate for small (<2.5 cm), noninvasive papillary lesions. Both surgical and radioactive ablative therapies are followed with T_4 suppression of TSH. Measurement of serum thyroglobulin has no pretherapeutic diagnostic value. It is, however, an excellent way to determine the effect of treatment and to monitor for recurrence.

Anaplastic carcinoma predominantly affects older individuals (>50 years). It is very aggressive and rapidly induces pain and symptoms related to local pressure (dysphagia, hoarseness). Death generally occurs within 12 months, but surgically resectable disease may have a better prognosis, with a five-year survival of approximately 30 per cent.

Medullary carcinoma, which develops in the parafollicular cells (C cells), may be sporadic or familial (autosomal dominant). When familial, it is frequently a component of a multiple endocrine neoplasia syndrome (MEN type II). This tumor produces calcitonin; measurement of basal serum calcitonin can substantiate its presence. Provocative testing with calcium or pentagastin (calcitonin response) may detect early C-cell hyperplasia in subjects at risk (MEN type II families). Surgical excision of the primary lesion in the absence of nodal involvement produces an excellent prognosis (90 per cent survival at 10 years). In contrast, patients with nodal disease have only a 40 per cent survival at 10 years.

One of the most important factors in the evaluation of a patient with suspected thyroid cancer is a history of low-dose irradiation (<500 rads) to the head or neck area during childhood. Such individuals are at high risk for thyroid cancer. Careful investigation of such patients will detect follicular or papillary carcinoma in about 30 per cent of cases. It is now recommended that these patients have a thyroid (clinical) examination at two-year intervals. In the absence of palpable disease, laboratory evaluation is not warranted. Post-irradiated patients with a palpable dominant nodule should receive total thyroidectomy with removal of nodes if there is metastatic disease. If invasive carcinoma is present, postoperative remnant ablation with ^{131}I should be carried out at six weeks. Suppressive therapy with T_4 will be necessary for life.

THYROIDITIS

In subacute granulomatous (de Quervain's) thyroiditis, a common disorder, the thyroid gland is painful and tender, and symptoms may be preceded by or associated with fever. Clinical hyperthyroidism may occur during the early phase (5 per cent), followed by transient hypothyroidism and then eventual recovery. The elevated serum total and free T_4 values are associated with a depressed RAIU test. Antithyroid antibodies are rarely detected. The erythrocyte sedimentation rate is characteristically high.

Therapy is symptomatic; the symptoms of thyroid pain and tenderness generally respond to aspirin. However, a small percentage of patients may need a short course of prednisone (20 mg b.i.d.) for relief. Symptomatic hyperthyroidism should be treated with propranolol (40 mg t.i.d.). Since both the hyper- and hypothyroid phases are self-limiting (total disease course 8 to 12 weeks), patient reassurance is generally all that is needed.

Subacute lymphocytic thyroiditis (silent thyroiditis) is currently considered to be an autoimmune disorder that is responsible for 20 to 30 per cent of all cases of thyrotoxicosis, with a high prevalence during the postpartum period. This condition was discussed in the section on hyperthyroidism. Chronic lymphocytic thyroiditis (Hashimoto's disease) is probably the most common cause of goiter in the western world. High titers of antithyroid antibodies are present in 90 per cent of cases. It is frequently complicated by hypothyroidism and was discussed in that section. Acute suppurative thyroiditis, an unusual disorder, generally follows bacteremia rather than being a primary infection.

REFERENCES

Chopra IJ, Hershman JM, Pardridge WM, et al: Thyroid function in nonthyroidal illness. Ann Intern Med 98:946, 1983.

Cooper DS: Antithyroid drugs. N Engl J Med 311(21):1353, 1984.

Gavin LA: The diagnostic dilemmas of hyperthyroxinemia and hypothyroxinemia. Adv Intern Med 33:185, 1988.

Klee G, Hay ID: Assessment of sensitive thyrotropin assays for an expanded role in thyroid function testing: Proposed criteria for analytic performance and clinical utility. J Clin Endocrinol Metab 64:461, 1987.

Larsen PR: The thyroid. In Wyngaarden JB, Smith LH Jr (eds): Cecil Textbook of Medicine. 18th ed, Philadelphia, WB Saunders Co, 1988, pp. 1315–1340.

Van Herle AJ, Rich P, Ljung BM, et al: The thyroid nodule. Ann Intern Med 96:221, 1982.

Weetman AP, McGregor AM: Autoimmune thyroid disease: Developments in our understanding. Endocr Rev 5:309, 1984.

69

ADRENAL GLAND

The adrenal glands, paired structures located retroperitoneally at the upper pole of each kidney, include two distinct endocrine organs: an outer cortex that secretes steroid hormones and an inner medulla that, as part of the sympathetic nervous system, secretes catecholamines (epinephrine and norepinephrine). The cortex consists of three zones: the outer zona glomerulosa, which secretes a potent mineralocorticoid hormone, and the inner zonae fasciculata and reticularis, which secrete glucocorticoids, androgens, and minute quantities of estrogens. Each of these steroid hormones as well as the catecholamines causes striking effects when produced in excess. In contrast, only glucocorticoid and mineralocorticoid hormones, which are secreted exclusively by the adrenal gland, are physiologically important products. The gonadal production of androgens in men and estrogens in women and the secretion of norepinephrine by sympathetic ganglia are quantitatively more important sources of these hormones and neurotransmitters.

MAJOR HORMONES OF THE ADRENAL GLAND

Cortisol is the major glucocorticoid secreted by the adrenal cortex. Glucocorticoids are involved in multiple biological processes, affecting carbohydrate, protein, lipid, and water metabolism. Cortisol secretion is under the control of adrenocorticotropin (ACTH), which in turn is regulated by the secretion of corticotropin-releasing hormone (CRF) (Fig. 69–1A). Secretion of ACTH and cortisol is pulsatile, manifests a diurnal circadian rhythm, and is under negative feedback control. Stress in a variety of forms can override the diurnal rhythm as well as the negative feedback relationship of the system.

Aldosterone is the principal mineralocorticoid hormone secreted by the adrenal cortex. Normally, the renin-angiotensin system is the major factor controlling aldosterone secretion (Fig. 69–2). Renin is released from the juxtaglomerular cells of the kidney in response to a reduction in renal perfusion pressure, a decrease in effective circulating volume, or sympathetic stimulation. Renin enzymatically cleaves the hepatic renin substrate (angiotensinogen) to liberate a decapeptide, angiotensin I. Removal of the carboxy terminal dipeptide by an endothelial converting enzyme produces the octapeptide angiotensin II. Angiotensin II stimulates the zona glomerulosa of the adrenal gland directly to increase aldosterone secretion. Aldosterone increases transepithelial transport of sodium by the kidney, and the resultant sodium retention tends to ameliorate the initial stimulus for renin secretion. Increases in plasma K^+ concentration normally increase aldosterone secretion, whereas hypokalemia suppresses it. Inasmuch as aldosterone promotes K^+ secretion by the kidney, this provides a second feedback mechanism regulating aldosterone secretion. When stimulation by the renin-angiotensin system is reduced during periods of recumbency, plasma aldosterone concentration correlates with the pulsatile release of cortisol, implying that ACTH also plays a role in the physiological regulation of aldosterone secretion.

The clinical disorders of the adrenal glands discussed in this chapter result in some of the most striking syndromes in clinical medicine and, not infrequently, are considered in the differential diagnosis of many clinical disorders. When suspected, the diagnosis can be established using biochemical measurements that are readily available in clinical laboratories and, in most instances, the response to appropriate therapy is dramatic and rewarding.

SYNDROMES OF ADRENOCORTICAL HYPOFUNCTION (Table 69–1)

Hypofunction of the adrenal cortex occurs either from primary adrenal disorders or from disordered

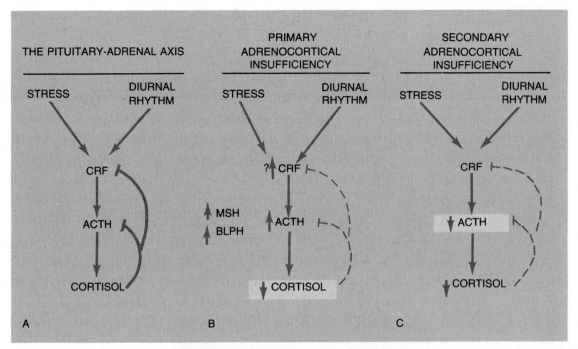

FIGURE 69–1. The hypothalamic-pituitary-adrenal axis. Secretion of corticotropin-releasing hormone (CRF) normally regulates secretion of ACTH, which in turn controls cortisol production (A). The system is subject to negative feedback control: Reduced levels of cortisol result in diminished feedback regulation (dashed lines) and marked increases in ACTH levels as in primary adrenocortical insufficiency. Levels of melanocyte-stimulating hormone (MSH) and lipotropin (BLPH) also increase, resulting in hyperpigmentation (B). Hypothalamic-pituitary disorders that diminish ACTH secretion result in secondary adrenocortical insufficiency (C).

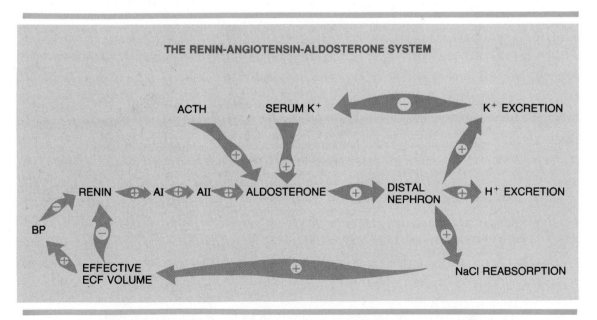

FIGURE 69–2. The renin-angiotensin-aldosterone system. Aldosterone secretion is principally regulated by the renin-angiotensin system. Potassium (K^+) and ACTH also stimulate aldosterone secretion, whereas sodium and dopamine (not shown) may inhibit it. Negative feedback control occurs by virtue of mineralocorticoid-induced kaliuresis and sodium retention, which reduce levels of K^+ and angiotensin II (AII), respectively. ⊕ = increases; ⊖ = decreases.

TABLE 69–1. SYNDROMES OF ADRENOCORTICAL HYPOFUNCTION

I. **Primary Adrenal Disorders**
   A. Combined Mineralocorticoid and Glucocorticoid Deficiency
      1. Acquired adrenal injury (Addison's disease)—over 90% due to autoimmune injury
      2. Bilateral adrenalectomy
      3. Adrenal enzyme deficiency states
   B. Aldosterone Deficiency Without Glucocorticoid Deficiency
      1. Corticosterone methyl oxidase deficiency
      2. Isolated zona glomerulosa defect
      3. Critically ill patients
      4. Heparin therapy
      5. Converting enzyme inhibitors
II. **Secondary Adrenal Disorders**
   A. Secondary Adrenal Insufficiency
      1. Panhypopituitarism
      2. Selective deficiency of ACTH
      3. Exogenous glucocorticoids
   B. Hyporeninemic Hypoaldosteronism
      1. Injury to the juxtaglomerular apparatus
      2. Autonomic neuropathy
      3. Extracellular volume expansion
      4. Impaired conversion of prorenin to active renin
      5. Impaired renal prostaglandin production caused by nonsteroidal anti-inflammatory drugs

extra-adrenal regulation of adrenal steroid biosynthesis and secretion. Clinical manifestations vary depending upon the relative dysfunction of mineralocorticoid, glucocorticoid, or androgen/estrogen secretion. Table 69–1 lists the most common disorders.

GENERALIZED ADRENOCORTICAL INSUFFICIENCY

Pathophysiology

Generalized adrenocortical insufficiency (Addison's disease) occurs when adrenocortical tissue injury, bilateral adrenalectomy, or inherited disorders of steroid biosynthesis reduce secretion rates of both mineralocorticoid and glucocorticoid hormones below physiological needs. If untreated, such panhypoadrenocorticoidism is often fatal.

Cortisol deficiency results in anorexia, weight loss, weakness, apathy, hypotension, and inability to withstand "stress" (Table 69–2). Because cortisol normally inhibits ACTH secretion, levels of ACTH are characteristically elevated (Fig. 69–1B). Increased levels of ACTH or related proopiomelanocortin-derived peptides (lipotropin, melanocortin) cause hyperpigmentation. Mineralocorticoid deficiency results in impaired renal Na^+ conservation and impaired K^+ and H^+ secretion. If NaCl intake is sufficiently large, extracellular fluid volume and plasma K^+ and bicarbonate levels can be maintained at nearly normal levels. If NaCl intake is low, however, or if extrarenal losses of Na^+ occur, impaired Na^+ conservation results in marked Na^+ deficits, hyponatremia, hyperkalemia, acidosis, hypovolemia, and increased plasma renin

levels. Glucocorticoid deficiency may exacerbate hypovolemia by redistributing fluid between vascular and extravascular compartments and may exacerbate hyponatremia by impairing renal solute-free water excretion.

A variety of pathological processes can result in generalized adrenocortical insufficiency: tuberculosis, histoplasmosis and other fungal diseases, metastatic carcinoma, amyloidosis, and bilateral adrenal hemorrhage. At present, Addison's disease appears to occur most frequently as a component of an autoimmune process that results in selective atrophy of the adrenal cortex ("idiopathic" adrenal insufficiency), usually sparing the adrenal medulla. Patients so affected often manifest evidence of other autoimmune injury affecting the thyroid, islet cells, gonads, or other tissues.

Combined glucocorticoid and mineralocorticoid deficiency also occurs in several inherited disorders characterized by diffuse bilateral enlargement of the adrenal cortex and collectively termed "congenital adrenal hyperplasia." In these disorders abnormalities of specific biosynthetic enzymes lead to reduced secretion of adrenal steroids and secondarily through release of feedback inhibition, to increased circulating levels of adrenotropic hormones (ACTH and/or angiotensin). The latter hormones induce adrenal hyperplasia in an attempt to increase the rate of secretion of the steroids by the defective gland.

In the most common form of congenital adrenal hyperplasia, that resulting from defective 21-hydroxylation, secretion of all glucocorticoid and mineralocorticoid hormones (21-hydroxylated steroids) is subnormal, whereas secretion of progesterone and 17-hydroxyprogesterone (the normal substrates for 21-hydroxylation) is increased. Manifestations of combined glucocorticoid and mineralocorticoid deficiency are common but not invariable. Increased levels of 17-hydroxyprogesterone result in overproduction of androgens, causing virilization (female pseudohermaphroditism, male precocious puberty), differing greatly in severity among patients. Increased circulating levels of 17-hydroxyprogesterone and progesterone contribute to clinical hypomineralocorticoidism inasmuch as those steroids are mineralocorticoid recep-

TABLE 69–2. CLINICAL FEATURES OF CHRONIC PRIMARY ADRENOCORTICAL INSUFFICIENCY

SIGNS AND SYMPTOMS	PER CENT
Weakness and fatigue	100
Weight loss	100
Anorexia	100
Hyperpigmentation	92
Hypotension	88
Gastrointestinal symptoms	56
Salt craving	19
Postural symptoms	12

Adapted from Baxter JD, Tyrrell JB: The adrenal cortex. *In* Felig P, Baxter JD, Broadus AH, et al (eds): Endocrinology and Metabolism. 2nd ed. New York, McGraw-Hill Book Co, 1987, p 587.

tor antagonists that inhibit the renal action of aldosterone.

Diagnosis and Treatment (Fig. 69–3)

The diagnosis of generalized adrenocortical insufficiency is confirmed by the finding of subnormal plasma levels of cortisol and aldosterone and by reduced urinary excretion of their major metabolites, the urinary 17-hydroxycorticoids and aldosterone-18-glucuronide, respectively. The primary abnormality resides in the adrenal cortex; plasma levels of ACTH and renin are elevated concomitantly. Inasmuch as plasma ACTH assays are not always available and special precautions are required for handling plasma samples, the primary nature of the adrenal disorder is frequently demonstrated by measurement of cortisol levels following either acute or chronic stimulation by exogenous ACTH. A subnormal cortisol response suggests a primary adrenal abnormality. Aldosterone levels also fail to increase normally in such patients. Prolonged administration of ACTH may be required in certain circumstances to distinguish primary from secondary syndromes of adrenocortical deficiency.

Generalized adrenocortical insufficiency often presents as a medical emergency; therapy should never be withheld pending laboratory results that establish the disagnosis. When the diagnosis of adrenal insufficiency is suspected in a critically ill patient, it is prudent to obtain plasma samples in which cortisol, aldosterone, ACTH, and renin activity can be measured subsequently. Intravenous administration of $^{1-24}$ACTH (Cortrosyn, 25 U) given as a bolus followed by a second plasma sample one hour later, is an additional useful step in diagnosis. If delay of therapy for even one hour is deemed inadvisable, glucocorticoid therapy can be initiated with dexamethasone, a potent synthetic glucocorticoid that will not interfere with the subsequent measurement of plasma cortisol. In adrenal crisis glucocorticoids should be administered in doses that reflect the levels normally secreted by the adrenal cortex under maximal stress, usually 200 to 300 mg of hydrocortisone per day or its equivalent. The manifestations of associated mineralocorticoid deficiency are best treated in such circumstances with parenteral fluids and salt replacement rather than with mineralocorticoid hormones.

Life-long treatment with hydrocortisone (usually 20 to 30 mg/day) or an equivalent glucocorticoid is required. Doses should be increased at times of stress (e.g., surgery, severe medical illnesses). Because aldosterone secretion is reduced, mineralocorticoid replacement may be needed, but many patients can be maintained on a high NaCl intake without mineralocorticoid. The need for mineralocorticoid replacement therapy is best assessed by clinical indexes (orthostatic hypotension, hyperkalemia, hyponatremia). Plasma renin activity provides a sensitive index of extracellular volume but is not a practical or necessary guide to treatment. The usual therapeutic mineralocorticoid is the orally effective steroid, fludrocortisone.

Administration of fludrocortisone in adrenal insufficiency requires special attention. With fixed exoge-

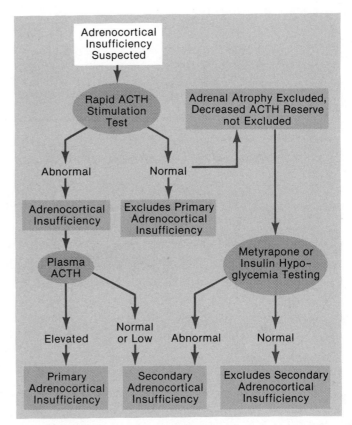

FIGURE 69–3. Evaluation of suspected primary and secondary adrenocortical insufficiency. Boxes enclose clinical decisions and ovals enclose diagnostic tests. (Reprinted from Baxter JD, Tyrrell JB: The adrenal cortex. *In* Felig P, Baxter JD, Broadus AE, et al (eds): Endocrinology and Metabolism. 2nd ed. New York, McGraw-Hill Book Company, 1987, p. 593.)

nous administration, circulating mineralocorticoid levels cannot vary inversely with potentially large erratic variations in dietary NaCl intake, as can endogenous aldosterone in normal subjects. If dietary NaCl increases, abnormal renal NaCl retention and K$^+$ secretion can result in hypervolemia, hypertension, cardiac decompensation, and hypokalemia, because mineralocorticoid levels are inappropriately high. If dietary NaCl decreases, or extrarenal (sweating, diarrhea) NaCl losses occur, hypovolemia and hyperkalemia may supervene, because mineralocorticoid levels are inappropriately low. Thus patients must be carefully monitored.

ALDOSTERONE DEFICIENCY WITHOUT GLUCOCORTICOID DEFICIENCY

Aldosterone deficiency in the absence of glucocorticoid deficiency is most commonly the result of deficient secretion of renin, so-called hyporeninemic hypoaldosteronism (see below). Rarely, isolated deficiency of aldosterone may result from a primary abnormality of the adrenal cortex, either as a conse-

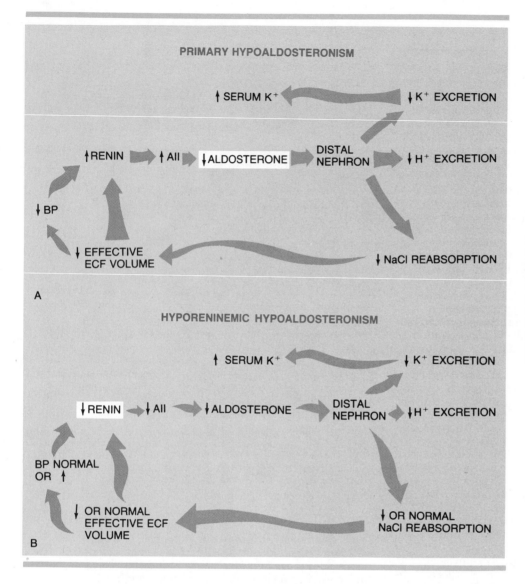

PRIMARY HYPOALDOSTERONISM

HYPORENINEMIC HYPOALDOSTERONISM

FIGURE 69–4. Perturbations of the renin-angiotensin-aldosterone system in primary hypoaldosteronism (*A*) and in hyporeninemic hypoaldosteronism (*B*). Hypoaldosteronism in primary adrenal disorders can occur as an isolated defect or as a component of generalized adrenocortical deficiency. In the latter, ACTH levels are also increased as a consequence of cortisol deficiency (see Fig. 69–1*B*).

quence of an inherited deficiency of the enzyme responsible for the final step of aldosterone biosynthesis (corticosterone methyloxidase) or as a manifestation of rare acquired disorders that selectively impair zona glomerulosa function. In primary isolated aldosterone deficiency, plasma renin activity is increased (Fig. 69–4).

Acquired lesions that selectively destroy the zona glomerulosa include a chronic autoimmune process in which antibodies are directed only against cells of the zona glomerulosa, or as the initial phase of a pathological process that eventually leads to generalized adrenocortical insufficiency. Mineralocorticoid replacement is given as in other primary adrenal disorders. Hypoaldosteronism that occurs in critically ill patients or in those on heparin therapy rarely results in clinically significant electrolyte disorders, and thus mineralocorticoid therapy may not be indicated. Administration of converting enzyme inhibitors may

cause significant hyperkalemia, particularly in patients with underlying renal insufficiency. In such patients hyperreninemic hypoaldosteronism is present as a consequence of reduced angiotensin II levels and does not imply the presence of a primary adrenal abnormality. Mineralocorticoid therapy will correct the electrolyte abnormalities, but the usual approach is to discontinue the agent.

SECONDARY ADRENAL INSUFFICIENCY

In secondary adrenal insufficiency, glucocorticoid deficiency results from inadequate stimulation of the adrenal cortex by ACTH. Causes include destructive lesions in the hypothalamic-pituitary axis, isolated defects of ACTH secretion, and prolonged suppression of the pituitary-adrenal axis by exogenous glucocorticoids. Mineralocorticoid deficiency is rare in those cases because aldosterone secretion is not regulated primarily or chronically by ACTH.

The clinical findings are similar to those of primary glucocorticoid deficiency, with several important differences. Hyperpigmentation is absent because plasma levels of ACTH and related proopiomelanocortin-derived peptides are not increased (Fig. 69–1C). Because mineralocorticoid levels are normal, hyperkalemia and metabolic acidosis also do not occur, but hyponatremia can occur as a consequence of the impaired water excretion that accompanies glucocorticoid deficiency. In primary pituitary diseases, the clinical manifestations may be complicated also by hypothyroidism and hypogonadism (see Chapter 67).

Prior administration of glucocorticoids is a common cause of secondary adrenocortical insufficiency. Suppression of the hypothalamic-pituitary axis by glucocorticoids occurs rapidly, to a degree that depends upon the duration and dose of the therapy. The use of alternate-day therapy with glucocorticoids when feasible reduces the frequency and severity of this complication. Three potential problems occur when glucocorticoids are withdrawn: (1) exacerbation of the underlying inflammatory disease being treated; (2) clinical manifestations suggesting adrenal insufficiency despite glucocorticoid levels still in the normal range; and (3) true adenal insufficiency that occurs when the doses of glucocorticoid are reduced below maintenance levels. Recovery of adrenal function may take up to a year; resumption of normal ACTH secretion must occur first. Recovery is hastened if the patient can tolerate total withdrawal of glucocorticoid therapy, but glucocorticoids should be given without hesitation in the event of intercurrent medical or surgical illness.

HYPORENINEMIC HYPOALDOSTERONISM

Pathophysiology

Mineralocorticoid deficiency occurs in numerous renal and extrarenal disorders that cause diminished renal secretion of renin. Under ordinary physiological conditions, the product of renin's action, angiotensin II, provides the major tonic stimulatory effect on aldosterone secretion. With diminished renin secretion, hypoangiotensinemia leads to a clinically significant state of mineralocorticoid deficiency: hyporeninemic hypoaldosteronism. Diabetes mellitus and chronic renal tubulointerstitial diseases are the most common underlying disorders.

Mineralocorticoid deficiency manifests usually as hyperkalemia and commonly as hyperchloremic metabolic acidosis. Sodium depletion and renal sodium wasting are not invariably present. In some patients, total body sodium and extracellular fluid volume are supernormal, suggesting that deficient renin secretion is a functional consequence of reduced renal clearance of sodium chloride.

The pathogenesis of the hyporeninemia is probably multifactorial. Renin secretory impairment may result from renal injury (e.g., sclerosis of the juxtaglomerular apparatus), and from functional impairment of renin secretion (e.g., subnormal stimulation by the sympathetic nervous system as in the autonomic insufficiency of diabetics). Impaired conversion of prorenin to active renin occurs in some affected individuals. Administration of certain pharmacological agents such as nonsteroidal anti-inflammatory agents, inhibitors of angiotensin-converting enzyme, and beta-adrenergic receptor antagonists can produce a clinical syndrome similar to that which occurs spontaneously.

Treatment

Patients with this syndrome are usually asymptomatic. Nevertheless, marked hyperkalemia can potentiate life-threatening arrhythmias, and protracted metabolic acidosis can adversely affect bone mineralization and other cellular functions. Administration of fludrocortisone in doses from 100 to 300 µg/day generally results in a prompt increase in renal potassium and hydrogen ion excretion and amelioration of hyperkalemia and metabolic acidosis. Patients with renal insufficiency may be more resistant to the renal effect of mineralocorticoids.

Fludrocortisone treatment, however, is not always effective and safe, particularly in patients who are hypertensive and have pretreatment increases in extracellular volume and body sodium. By increasing renal reabsorption of sodium chloride, fludrocortisone can exacerbate hypertension and other deleterious consequences of extracellular fluid volume expansion. Furosemide, in doses of 40 to 120 mg daily, increases potassium and net acid excretion and ameliorates the hyperkalemia and metabolic acidosis in such patients. With severe hypoaldosteronism, the ameliorative effect of furosemide is attenuated, so that pretreatment with small doses of fludrocortisone increases its effectiveness. Combined therapy with fludrocortisone and furosemide offers the advantages of mutual potentiation of kaliuretic and acid-excretory effects and countervailing natriuretic and chloruretic effects. The combination reduces hyperkalemia and acidosis and, concomitantly, through adjustment of relative doses, allows control of body content of sodium chloride.

SYNDROMES OF ADRENOCORTICAL HYPERFUNCTION (Table 69–3)

The major clinical manifestations of adrenocortical hyperfunction vary depending upon the predominant steroid produced in excess. Hypersecretion of glucocorticoid hormone results in Cushing's syndrome, a metabolic disorder affecting carbohydrate, protein, and lipid metabolism. Hypersecretion of aldosterone and related mineralocorticoid hormones results in a disturbance of electrolyte and blood pressure homeostasis.

CUSHING'S SYNDROME

Pathophysiology

Cushing's syndrome, the consequence of chronic exposure to excessive amounts of glucocorticoid hor-

TABLE 69–3. SYNDROMES OF ADRENOCORTICAL HYPERFUNCTION

I. **Syndromes of Glucocorticoid Excess (Cushing's Syndrome)**
  A. Secondary to Increased ACTH Stimulation
    1. Hypothalamic-pituitary abnormality (Cushing's disease)
    2. Ectopic ACTH secretion
  B. Primary Adrenal Abnormality
    1. Adenoma
    2. Carcinoma
  C. Exogenous Glucocorticoid Therapy
II. **Syndromes of Mineralocorticoid Excess**
  A. Primary Aldosteronism
    1. Aldosterone-producing adenoma
    2. Bilateral adrenal hyperplasia (idiopathic hyperaldosteronism)
    3. Adrenal carcinoma
  B. Adrenal Enzyme Defects
    1. 11β-hydroxylase deficiency
    2. 17α-hydroxylase deficiency
  C. Exogenous Mineralocorticoids
    1. Licorice
    2. Carbenoxolone
  D. Secondary Aldosteronism
    1. Nonhypertensive disorders
    2. Hypertensive disorders

mone, occurs as a consequence of increased endogenous production of cortisol (Fig. 69–5) or, more commonly, as the result of prolonged exposure to glucocorticoid therapy administered in superphysiological doses. Of the endogenous causes, the most common in adults is bilateral adrenal hyperplasia due to excessive pituitary secretion of ACTH, a condition referred to as Cushing's disease (Fig. 69–5A). Bilateral adrenal hyperplasia can also result from ectopic production of ACTH by a variety of neoplasms (Fig. 69–5B). Primary adrenal tumors, either adenomas or carcinomas, account for the remaining cases (Fig. 69–5C).

In Cushing's disease the hypersecretion of ACTH by the pituitary gland is due to the presence of an adenoma in approximately 90 per cent of cases. These are frequently small (microadenomas) and basophilic. Whether such an adenoma arises spontaneously or as a secondary consequence of excessive secretion of corticotropin-releasing hormone has not been resolved. This disorder is much more common in women (female to male ratio, 5:1), typically occurs during the childbearing years and, as a consequence of an insidious onset, may go undetected for many years.

In patients with bilateral adrenal hyperplasia due to ectopic ACTH secretion, the level of cortisol may be several times higher than in Cushing's disease, yet the clinical manifestations are often less striking. This difference is presumably due to the more rapid progression of the disease, as a consequence of the underlying neoplasm. In addition to marked increases in cortisol production, such patients may have greatly increased levels of deoxycorticosterone (DOC), a potent mineralocorticoid that can result in severe hypertension and hypokalemic metabolic alkalosis. Small cell carcinoma of the lung, bronchial carcinoid, and medullary carcinoma of the thyroid are among the neoplasms reported to secrete ACTH ectopically. Ectopic ACTH syndrome occurs more frequently in men, and the age of onset is typically later than in Cushing's disease.

The primary adrenal neoplasms that result in Cushing's syndrome may also be associated with severe hypokalemic metabolic alkalosis and hypertension as a consequence of marked increases in mineralocorticoid hormone secretion. Such tumors may also present

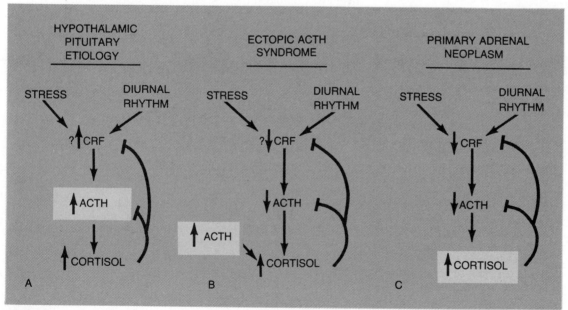

FIGURE 69–5. Perturbations of the hypothalamic-pituitary-adrenal axis that result in Cushing's syndrome.

TABLE 69–4. COMMON CLINICAL FEATURES OF CUSHING'S SYNDROME

FEATURE	INCIDENCE (%)
Obesity	94
Facial plethora	84
Hirsutism	82
Menstrual disorders	76
Hypertension	72
Muscular weakness	58
Back pain	58
Striae	52
Acne	40
Psychological symptoms	40
Bruising	36

Modified from Plotz CM, et al: Am J Med 13:597, 1952, and Ross EJ, et al: Q J Med 35:149, 1966.

with findings reflecting predominant secretion of androgens or estrogens, causing virilization or feminization in women and men, respectively. Adrenal carcinomas are the most frequent cause of Cushing's syndrome in children.

Clinical Manifestations

The clinical manifestations of Cushing's disease are very diverse (Table 69–4). Regardless of the etiology, hypercortisolism results in obesity, carbohydrate intolerance, muscle wasting, and osteoporosis. Obesity is centripedal, manifested typically by a "buffalo hump," increased supraclavicular fat pads, and moon facies. Easy bruisability and abdominal striae may be noted. Mild hypertension is common. Depression occurs commonly and, rarely, patients may be frankly psychotic. An increase in adrenal androgen production can result in hirsutism, acne, and menstrual disorders in women. Men may complain of impotence and loss of libido.

Diagnosis (Fig. 69–6)

The diagnostic approach in patients who are suspected of having Cushing's syndrome consists of two phases. In the first, the presence of hypercortisolism is established to separate those with Cushing's syndrome from patients who may have certain clinical features that suggest the diagnosis but in whom glucocorticoid excess is not present. Once hypercortisolism is established, the challenge is to differentiate among the causes discussed above.

Does the patient have Cushing's syndrome? Although surreptitious administration of glucocorticoids may occur rarely, one is generally able to exclude an exogenous cause of Cushing's syndrome by the medical history. Endogenous Cushing's syndrome is relatively uncommon. In view of the severity of the untreated illness, the diagnosis should be considered in all patients who manifest typical clinical features. Since many of these abnormalities (e.g., obesity, hirsutism, hypertension, acne) occur in patients who do not have Cushing's syndrome, a reliable means of differentiating among such individuals is necessary.

Endogenous Cushing's syndrome is characterized by varying degrees of autonomous production of cortisol, resulting in an overall net increase in steroid production. Inasmuch as cortisol secretion is normally pulsatile, only distinctly elevated random measurements of plasma cortisol help in establishing the diagnosis. A more reliable index of the integrated plasma concentration can be obtained by measurement of the 24-hour urinary excretion of cortisol. Measurement of a urinary metabolite of cortisol (such as 17-hydroxycorticoids) can also be performed, but values often overlap normal levels, limiting the usefulness of this procedure.

One of the most reliable means of detecting Cushing's syndrome is the overnight dexamethasone suppression test. Dexamethasone, 1 mg, is administered orally between 11:00 PM and midnight and the plasma cortisol is obtained at approximately 8:00 AM the following morning. A value of plasma cortisol of less than 5 μg/dl excludes the diagnosis of Cushing's syndrome. False-negative results are unusual. False-positive results can occur in patients with depression or other stressful situations and with ingestion of drugs such as phenytoin and estrogens. In patients in whom this screening test suggests the diagnosis of Cushing's syndrome, confirmation should be sought by other means, such as measurement of urinary free cortisol.

If Cushing's syndrome is present, what is its cause?

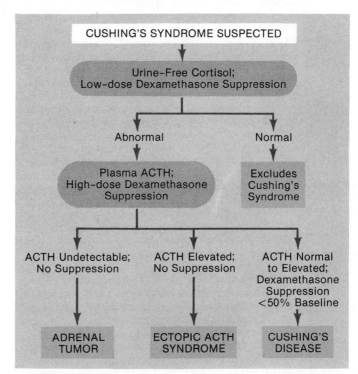

FIGURE 69–6. Evaluation of Cushing's syndrome. Boxes enclose clinical decisions and ovals enclose diagnostic tests. See the text for details and the potential for false-positive and false-negative results. (Reprinted from Baxter JD, Tyrrell JB: The adrenal cortex. *In* Felig P, Baxter JD, Broadus AE, et al (eds): Endocrinology and Metabolism. 2nd ed. New York, McGraw-Hill Book Company, 1987, p. 609.)

Once the diagnosis of Cushing's syndrome is established, additional procedures are required to identify the underlying etiology (see Table 69–3). The high-dose dexamethasone suppression test should distinguish between patients with Cushing's disease and those with ectopic ACTH secretion or a primary adrenal neoplasm. In this test dexamethasone, 2 mg q6h, is administered orally for two consecutive days or as a single "overnight" dose of 8 mg. Suppressibility of endogenous cortisol production is evaluated either by a plasma cortisol measurement at the end of this period or by measurement of urinary free cortisol or 17-hydroxycorticoid excretion on the second day of dexamethasone administration. Patients with Cushing's disease, in whom cortisol production is not entirely autonomous, will usually manifest a 50 per cent or greater suppression of cortisol levels in response to these large doses of dexamethasone. In contrast, cortisol production in patients with adrenal neoplasms or ectopic ACTH syndrome is usually more autonomous, so that little or no change in the cortisol level occurs during this procedure. Some patients with ectopic tumors, however, particularly those with a bronchial carcinoid or an adenoma, will undergo at least partial suppression and may appear therefore to have Cushing's disease. Also, some patients with Cushing's disease do not adequately suppress with dexamethasone. Despite these relatively uncommon exceptions, the high-dose dexamethasone suppression test remains one of the most reliable means of distinguishing among the causes of Cushing's syndrome.

Measurement of the plasma ACTH level, when available, is also helpful in differentiating among subtypes of Cushing's syndrome. Plasma ACTH levels are normal to only modestly increased in patients with Cushing's disease, are usually markedly elevated in those with ectopic ACTH secretion, and are generally undetectable in patients with primary adrenal neoplasms. Additional procedures that can help to localize the primary abnormality and to confirm the etiologic diagnosis include magnetic resonance imaging and high-resolution contrast-enhanced CT scans of the pituitary and CT scans of the adrenal to localize a primary adrenal neoplasm. An apparently normal pituitary fossa does not exclude an adenoma, however, since these tumors are frequently small and may be detected only at the time of surgery.

Treatment

Treatment of Cushing's syndrome depends on its cause. Pituitary microsurgery employing the transsphenoidal approach is now the treatment of choice for patients with suspected pituitary adenomas. In experienced hands an adenoma may be localized in 90 per cent of patients and removed with a low morbidity. This approach has the advantage of preserving the surrounding pituitary tissue so that hypopituitarism is a rare complication. Pituitary irradiation using either conventional sources or heavy particle beams is also successful in many cases, but the incidence of hypopituitarism is higher than with transsphenoidal hypophysectomy. This may be an important consideration in women in the childbearing years or in children who have not yet achieved adult height. Bilateral adrenalectomy, once performed commonly, is associated with a high incidence of subsequent enlargement of the pituitary neoplasm and hyperpigmentation (Nelson's syndrome) and should be reserved for patients who do not respond to the other approaches. Treatment of patients with primary adrenal neoplasms generally consists of surgical removal of the affected adrenal gland. Even those with carcinoma in whom cure is rare should have the tumor removed in an effort to control the hypercortisolism. Surgery is also recommended in patients with ectopic ACTH syndrome due to well-localized ACTH-secreting tumors. In those with benign ACTH-secreting tumors such as bronchial carcinoid, pheochromocytoma, or thymoma, such an operation is frequently curative. In patients with ectopic malignancies that are already metastatic as well as in those who have inoperable adrenal carcinoma, medical inhibition of adrenal cortisol secretion by drugs such as mitotane, aminoglutethimide, and metyrapone may be helpful.

PRIMARY ALDOSTERONISM

Pathophysiology

Hypersecretion of aldosterone can occur as a primary adrenal disorder or in response to increased stimulation by the renin-angiotensin system or ACTH. Primary aldosteronism is an adrenal disorder characterized by autonomous production of mineralocorticoid hormone (Fig. 69–7). Secondary aldosteronism results from the overstimulation of an otherwise normal adrenal gland by the renin-angiotensin system. The latter disorders are pathophysiologically and clinically distinct from primary aldosteronism and will be considered in a separate section.

Primary overproduction of aldosterone results in increased sodium reabsorption in the distal nephron. As a consequence, the extracellular fluid volume is expanded until approximately 1.5 to 2.5 kg of excess fluid has been retained. At this point, proximal tubular sodium reabsorption becomes markedly reduced. The resultant increased delivery of sodium to the distal tubule overwhelms the increased capacity for distal sodium reabsorption so that a new steady state of sodium balance is achieved. This phenomenon is referred to as "mineralocorticoid escape." Further expansion of extracellular fluid volume does not occur despite continued hypersecretion of mineralocorticoid hormone. Affected subjects actually excrete an administered sodium load more rapidly than do normals. Two of the cardinal findings of the syndrome of primary aldosteronism, hypertension and suppressed plasma renin activity, probably result from this expansion of extracellular fluid volume.

The mineralocorticoid hormone–enhanced sodium reabsorption in the distal tubule and collecting duct results in increased secretion of potassium and hydrogen ion in these portions of the nephron. Even when the renal escape mechanism allows a new steady state of sodium balance to develop, mineralocorticoid-dependent potassium secretion and hydrogen ion se-

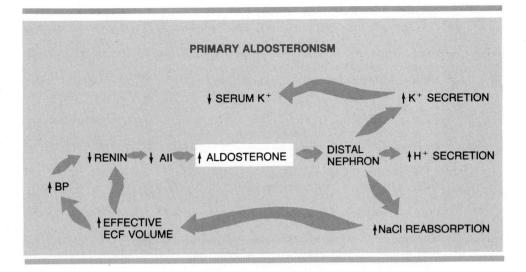

FIGURE 69–7. Perturbations of the renin-angiotensin-aldosterone system in primary aldosteronism. By tending to suppress aldosterone secretion, hypokalemia mitigates hyperaldosteronemia.

cretion continue. The increased delivery of sodium to the distal nephron may actually augment the potassium secretion.

In the syndrome of primary aldosteronism, autonomous overproduction of aldosterone by the adrenal gland can be due to a benign adenoma, a carcinoma, or diffuse bilateral nodular hyperplasia, with adenomas accounting for 75 to 85 per cent of cases. Less than 1 per cent are due to a functioning carcinoma, and the remaining 15 to 25 per cent result from bilateral hyperplasia. The extremely rare cases of so-called glucocorticoid-remediable hyperaldosteronism are believed to result from excessive stimulation of the adrenal cortex by ACTH. The patterns of mineralocorticoid secretion and the degree of autonomy from the renin-angiotensin system vary between the different entities.

Clinical Manifestations

The major clinical manifestations of primary aldosteronism are hypertension and hypokalemia. In addition, hypernatremia and metabolic alkalosis are characteristically found. A dilute urine may be present because hypokalemia impairs the renal concentrating mechanism. The severity of the presenting symptoms depends on the degree of potassium depletion. Mildly hypokalemic patients complain of muscle weakness, polyuria (especially nocturia), polydipsia, and paresthesias. Patients with more severe hypokalemia experience intermittent paralysis of the legs and arms or even tetany. Patients with marked hypokalemia sometimes experience autonomic dysfunction with orthostatic hypotension occurring without reflex tachycardia.

Diagnosis and Treatment

Recognition of primary aldosteronism, usually during evaluation of hypertension, is important because it is a potentially curable form of hypertension. Less than 1 per cent of unselected hypertensive patients have this disorder, which is found in women more often than in men by a 2:1 margin. The patients are usually between 30 and 50 years of age.

Hyperaldosteronism can be documented by showing an increased secretion rate, an increased excretion rate, or an elevated plasma concentration of the hormone. Single measurements of plasma aldosterone concentration may be misleading because even patients with markedly increased secretion rates show diurnal variations in plasma levels that can obscure recognition of hyperaldosteronism. The measurement of the 24-hour urinary excretion of the 18-glucuronide metabolite of aldosterone reflects aldosterone production accurately. The urine should be collected while the patient consumes a normal sodium intake (120 to 180 mEq/day).

Demonstration of suppressed and nonstimulable plasma renin activity in a patient with elevated plasma or urinary aldosterone levels establishes the diagnosis of primary aldosteronism. Autonomy of aldosterone production can be confirmed by demonstrating failure of suppression of the hormone levels by maneuvers that normally suppress the renin-angiotensin-aldosterone system, such as administration of mineralocorticoid hormones (DOCA, fludrocortisone) or intravenous infusion of normal saline.

The principal reason for attempting to differentiate between aldosterone-producing adenoma and bilateral hyperplasia is to select the most appropriate therapy. Unilateral adrenalectomy cures approximately 70 per cent of cases due to an adenoma, whereas even bilateral adrenalectomy does not ameliorate the hypertension in most cases of hyperplasia. Several biochemical determinations have been proposed to differentiate adenoma from hyperplasia. Patients with an adenoma generally have lower plasma renin activity values and plasma potassium concentrations with higher basal plasma aldosterone and 18-hydroxycorticosterone concentrations than patients with hyperplasia. Plasma aldosterone levels in patients with adenoma fail to increase with upright posture, in contrast to a two- to three-fold increase in those with hyperplasia. Specific techniques for localizing an adenoma (iodocholesterol scan, CT scan, adrenal venous catheterization) also aid in differentiating those with tumor from those with bilateral hyperplasia.

ADRENAL ENZYME DEFECTS

Genetically transmitted deficiencies of the enzymes required for adrenal steroid biosynthesis lead to distinct clinical syndromes of disturbed mineralocorticoid production. In two such enzyme deficiency states, 11β- and 17α-hydroxylase deficiency, impaired cortisol production results in increased ACTH secretion and secondary increased production of DOC, which produces a typical syndrome of mineralocorticoid excess. In 11β-hydroxylase deficiency, conversion of DOC to corticosterone and its derivatives is impaired, and thus corticosterone, 18-hydroxycorticosterone, and/or aldosterone may be deficient. In 17α-hydroxylase deficiency, conversion of DOC to its derivatives is not enzymatically blocked; hence corticosterone levels are markedly elevated and may contribute to the hypermineralocorticoid state. Despite the intact enzymatic pathway to aldosterone, aldosterone production is generally subnormal, presumably as a consequence of the reduced plasma renin activity and the hypokalemia that occur due to the hypermineralocorticoid state.

These two syndromes can be readily distinguished clinically by their different effects on sexual development. In the 17α-hydroxylase deficiency syndrome, biosynthesis of adrenal and gonadal androgen and estrogen is impaired, inhibiting normal sexual maturation. Genotypic female patients fail to undergo menarchy or to develop secondary sexual characteristics. Genotypic male patients become pseudohermaphrodites as a consequence of androgen deficiency in utero. In the 11β-hydroxylase deficiency syndrome, the enzymatic steps required for the synthesis of adrenal sex steroids are unimpaired. The increased ACTH level stimulates increased production of adrenal androgen, frequently causing virilism. In both syndromes, glucocorticoid hormone replacement therapy inhibits both ACTH secretion and the resultant excess mineralocorticoid production and therefore ameliorates the hypermineralocorticoid state. In treated patients with the 11β-hydroxylase deficiency syndrome, androgen production diminishes and signs of virilization tend to disappear.

SECONDARY ALDOSTERONISM
(Table 69–3)

Aldosterone is secreted as a physiological response to reduced effective arterial blood volume owing to activation of the renin-angiotensin system. The resultant increase in plasma aldosterone concentration stimulates renal tubular reabsorption of Na^+ and Cl^- and thereby tends to restore normal "effective" blood volume. When hypovolemia is of extrarenal origin (vomiting, diarrhea, and hemorrhage) and renal tubular reabsorption of Na^+ and Cl^- is not specifically impaired, the Na^+-retaining effect of hypermineralocorticoidism is manifested by reduced urinary excretion rates of Na^+ that persist until effective arterial blood volume is restored. Provision of adequate amounts of dietary NaCl may normalize the effective arterial blood volume. The Na^+-retaining effect of hypermineralocorticoidism does not reduce excretion rates of Na^+ when hypovolemia is caused predominantly by impaired renal tubular reabsorption of Na^+ and Cl^- (e.g., diuretic administration, Bartter's syndrome, and some types of renal tubular acidosis). When the reduction in effective arterial blood volume is due to congestive heart failure, cirrhosis, or the nephrotic syndrome, provision of dietary NaCl leads to progressive expansion of extracellular fluid volume and edema without restoration of effective blood volume.

Hyperaldosteronism secondary to activation of the renin-angiotensin system also occurs in patients with accelerated hypertension, renovascular or segmental renal lesions, and, rarely, renin-secreting neoplasms. Activation of the renin-angiotensin-aldosterone system in the absence of hypovolemia results in hypertension.

The exact contribution of excess mineralocorticoid production to the pathophysiology observed in states of secondary hyperaldosteronism is not always clear. Hypertension persists despite adrenalectomy in patients with a renin-secreting tumor and in animals with experimental renovascular hypertension. Reduction of Na^+ excretion and edema formation can occur in patients with cardiac, renal, or hepatic disease without increased aldosterone secretion. Potassium wasting persists despite sustained correction of secondary hyperaldosteronism in some patients with type 1 renal tubular acidosis and in some patients with Bartter's syndrome. In these disorders, it seems likely that the secondary aldosteronism serves to amplify the consequences of the primary defect causing renal potassium wasting.

ADRENAL MEDULLARY HYPERFUNCTION

The adrenal medulla synthesizes and releases biologically active amines derived from the amino acid tyrosine. Norepinephrine, the major product of this biosynthetic pathway, is also synthesized in the central nervous system and sympathetic postganglionic neurons, whereas epinephrine originates nearly entirely from the adrenal gland. A third catecholamine, dopamine, which acts as a neurotransmitter in the central nervous system, has a less clearly defined role as a circulating hormone, although dopamine may normally inhibit aldosterone secretion.

Catecholamines have a variety of potent hemodynamic and metabolic effects depending upon their relative abilities to serve as agonists for the alpha- and beta-adrenergic receptors. Epinephrine acts chiefly on beta receptors, having a positive chronotropic and inotropic effect on the heart and producing vasodilatation in most vascular beds. Epinephrine also increases plasma glucose concentration by inhibiting insulin secretion and stimulating glycogenolysis in the liver. Epinephrine is released from the medulla in response to a variety of stresses, including hypoglycemia. Norepinephrine has predominant alpha-agonist effects, causing vasoconstriction with relatively little metabolic action. Inasmuch as norepinephrine is secreted widely throughout the sympathetic nervous system, the contribution by the adrenal medulla is relatively small. Bilateral adrenalectomy results in little if any measurable change in the levels of norepinephrine, although epinephrine levels are markedly reduced. Thus, adrenal medullary hypofunction has little or no physiological impact, whereas hypersecretion of catecholamines produces a dramatic clinical syndrome, namely pheochromocytoma.

Pheochromocytoma

Pathophysiology

Pheochromocytoma, an uncommon but important tumor of chromaffin cells, can occur in any sympathetic ganglion in the body. More than 90 per cent of such tumors, however, arise from the adrenal medulla. The majority of extra-adrenal pheochromocytomas are associated with sympathetic ganglia in the mediastinum or abdomen. Bilateral adrenal pheochromocytomas or multiple tumors may be present in 5 to 10 per cent of cases. Such patients may also have medullary carcinoma of the thyroid and other manifestations of the multiple endocrine neoplasia syndrome, type 2 (Sipple's syndrome). Pheochromocytoma should always be considered in patients with this syndrome, in which there is also a familial tendency to develop tumors of the C cells of the thyroid (medullary carcinoma) and of the parathyroid glands.

Clinical Manifestations

The clinical manifestations of pheochromocytoma depend upon the predominant catecholamine secreted by the tumor. Since most tumors secrete norepinephrine as the principal product, hypertension is the most common finding. Superimposed on sustained hypertension are classic paroxysms in which a sudden release of catecholamines results in exacerbation of hypertension, accompanied by palpitation, headache, pallor, sweating, flushing, and anxiety. Such attacks can be provoked by ingestion of tyramine-containing foods, particularly in patients taking monoamine oxidase inhibitors. Occasionally, patients with pheochromocytoma may not exhibit hypertension at all and in fact may become hypotensive during paroxysms. Such patients usually have epinephrine-secreting tumors or tumors whose principal product is dopamine. Orthostatic hypotension is common in patients with pheochromocytoma, even in those who have sustained supine hypertension.

Diagnosis and Treatment

The diagnosis of pheochromocytoma can be difficult, since the symptoms are relatively nonspecific, often resembling those of simple anxiety. In addition, because secretion may be episodic in some patients, plasma and urinary levels of catecholamines may be intermittently normal. The diagnosis should be established by demonstrating increased plasma levels or urinary excretion of catecholamines or their major metabolites, the metanephrines and vanillylmandelic acid (VMA). Of these, urinary metanephrines may be the most sensitive index. Epinephrine is present only in the adrenal medulla and the organ of Zuckerkandl; norepinephrine is the sole product of tumors arising in sympathetic ganglia outside of these sites. In addition, norepinephrine is the major secretory product of adrenal pheochromocytoma. Catecholamines can be measured in plasma for the diagnosis of pheochromocytoma, but meticulous attention must be given to the technique of specimen collection and caution must be exercised in interpreting borderline elevated levels in stressed individuals. Clonidine suppresses catecholamine levels in normal subjects, but fails to do so in patients with pheochromocytoma. This test can be used as a means of evaluating patients with only borderline biochemical abnormalities.

Pheochromocytomas, particularly those arising from the adrenal medulla, are usually several centimeters in diameter by the time symptoms develop and can be readily visualized on abdominal CT scans. In the absence of an obvious adrenal tumor, localization of the tumor in the sympathetic ganglia may be difficult. Catheterization of the inferior vena cava with sampling of multiple sites for catecholamine measurements may help to localize the tumor preoperatively. An isotope scan technique utilizing ^{131}I-metaiodobenzylguanidine can often localize small neoplasms effectively. The possibility of multiple pheochromocytomas should be considered, particularly in patients with family histories of other endocrine neoplasms.

Pheochromocytomas should be surgically removed if possible. Preoperative adrenergic blockade has markedly improved the once formidable surgical morbidity and mortality. In patients with norepinephrine-secreting lesions, alpha blockade should be effected first, using either phenoxybenzamine, dibenzyline, or prazosin in sufficient doses and for a sufficient period of time to prevent episodes of hypertension and to allow expansion of the effective extracellular fluid volume. Beta-adrenergic blockade may also be useful, particularly in those who develop tachycardia on alpha blockers. Careful preoperative planning among an experienced anesthesiologist, an endocrinologist, and a surgeon usually assures a good outcome.

In patients with inoperable tumors or with metastatic pheochromocytoma, pharmacological therapy may be continued on a chronic basis. In addition, alpha-methyltyrosine may be of some benefit in reducing catecholamine secretion by the neoplastic tissue.

REFERENCES

Baxter JD, Perloff D, Hsueh W, et al: The endocrinology of hypertension. *In* Felig P, Baxter JD, Broadus A, et al: (eds): Endocrinology and Metabolism (2nd ed.). New York, McGraw-Hill Book Co, 1987, pp 693–788.

Crapo L: Cushing's syndrome: A review of diagnostic tests. Metabolism 28:955, 1979.

DeFronzo RA: Hyperkalemia and hyporeninemic hypoaldosteronism. Kidney Int 17:118, 1980.

Kannan CR: Diseases of the adrenal cortex. DM 34:603, 1988.

Mampalam TJ, Tyrrell JB, Wilson CB: Transsphenoidal microsurgery for Cushing Disease. A report of 216 cases. Ann Intern Med 109:487, 1988.

Tyrrell JB, Baxter JD: Disorders of the adrenal cortex. *In* Wyngaarden JB, Smith LH Jr (eds): Cecil Textbook of Medicine. 18th ed. Philadelphia, WB Saunders Co, 1988, pp 1340–1359.

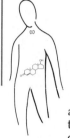

70

FEMALE ENDOCRINOLOGY

Each adult ovary (approximately 4 × 3 × 1 cm) is attached to the lateral pelvic wall and to the uterus by the ovarian ligament. The follicle in its different stages of maturation is the critical structural and functional component of the ovary. Both steroidogenesis and gametogenesis depend on the follicle complex. The primary components of the follicle are the oocyte, granulosa cells, and interstitial cells (theca cells).

SEXUAL DEVELOPMENT AND DIFFERENTIATION

Normal sexual development and differentiation depend on a full complex of sex and autosomal chromosomes. The genital ridge develops at approximately three weeks' gestation. Subsequently germ cells migrate to the genital ridge from the yolk sac. Undifferentiated gonads consisting of both müllerian and wolffian ducts are present by six weeks' gestation. Differentiation of the female gonad proceeds in the absence of müllerian-inhibiting factor and androgens, facilitating the development of female ducts and the regression of male ducts. Appropriate female genitalia develop consequent to the lack of androgen secretion. The genes determining ovarian formation have not been identified.

Normal ovarian function requires the integrated action of the hypothalamic-pituitary-ovarian axis (Fig. 70–1). Follicular growth, steroid hormone production (secretion), ovulation, and atresia are gonadotropin-dependent (follicle stimulating hormone, FSH; luteinizing hormone, LH). Subsequent to synthesis (Fig. 70–2) and secretion, ovarian sex steroid hormones (estrogens, androgens, progestins) mediate their effects locally on the ovary and the genital tract (uterus, cervix, and vagina) and systemically to coordinate functions of the hypothalamic-pituitary complex. Measurement of serum estradiol, progesterone, FSH, and LH levels with specific radioimmunoassays provides accurate information on the integrity of the hypothalamic-pituitary-ovarian axis in health and disease. In addition, the biological activity of the sex steroids on target organs can be reliably evaluated by analyzing cellular morphology and mucus characteristics. Estrogens increase the quantity, viscosity, and elasticity ("spinnbarkeit") of the cervical mucus as well as the tendency of the electrolytes to crystallize in a "ferning" pattern. Progesterone inhibits these changes in mucus. In addition, the endometrium undergoes characteristic changes during the menstrual cycle. The follicular phase is associated with proliferation of the endometrial glands under the influence of estrogen. During the luteal phase progesterone induces the glands to become secretory. Endometrial biopsies are used to date the stage of the cycle and to assess the tissue response to gonadal steroids.

ABNORMAL SEXUAL DIFFERENTIATION

Chromosomal

Turner's syndrome, the most common disorder of gonadal differentiation in the female, results from a 45XO chromosomal abnormality. It has an incidence of 1 in 3000 newborn females. These patients have nonfunctioning streak gonads (gonadal dysgenesis) and unambiguous female external genitalia and internal ducts and may exhibit many or all of the following abnormalities: sexual infantilism, short stature, musculoskeletal abnormalities (webbed neck, low hairline, shield chest, cubitus valgus, short digits), hypertension, coarctation of the aorta, renal disorders, and deafness. Patients with a mosaic karyotype present fewer stigmata, and gonadal function may be normal. The short stature can be treated with anabolic steroids and growth hormone between 10 and 14 years. Feminization can be induced with estrogen replacement.

Enzymatic

Pseudohermaphrodites are females with a normal 46XX karyotype and internal sexual organs but masculinized external genitalia (male phenotype) due to

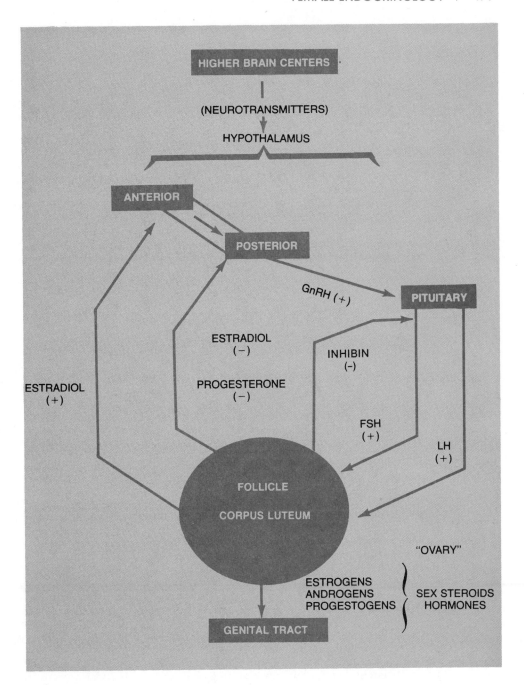

FIGURE 70–1. Hypothalamic-pituitary-ovarian axis. Gonadotropin-releasing hormone (GnRH) stimulates the pituitary gland to synthesize and secrete the gonadotropins FSH (follicle-stimulating hormone) and LH (luteinizing hormone). These hormones stimulate sequential ovarian follicle development and differentiation. The sex steroid hormones secreted by the ovary regulate genital tract changes and modulate hypothalamic GnRH secretion. In addition, inhibin secreted by the follicle specifically inhibits the release of FSH.

excess androgens. The extent of the virilization and the degree of ambiguity in genital development depend on the timing and severity of the androgen exposure. The most common cause of female pseudohermaphroditism is *congenital adrenal hyperplasia* (CAH). This syndrome has a wide spectrum of clinical presentations due to the variable involvement of specific enzymes necessary for cortisol synthesis by the adrenal cortex (Fig. 70–2). This syndrome complex is inherited in an autosomal recessive manner and expresses itself only in the homozygous offspring. It has

a prevalence of 1 per 60,000 births. The cortisol deficiency results in increased ACTH secretion and consequent adrenal hyperplasia. The most frequent lesion involves a deficiency of 21-hydroxylase. The hyperplastic glands secrete androgens in excess, which masculinize the female fetus. Furthermore, the excess secretion of 17-hydroxyprogesterone causes salt wasting. In the 11-hydroxylase form, masculinization also occurs, but salt retention and hypertension develop because of the excess production of 11-deoxycorticosterone. Congenital adrenal hyperplasia can be

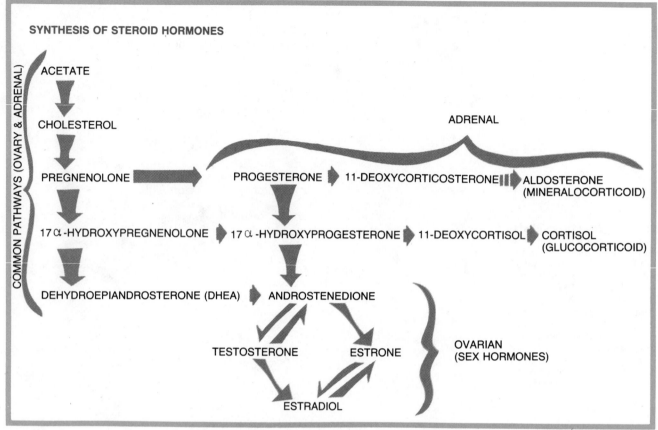

FIGURE 70–2. Synthetic pathways for steroid hormone production by the ovary and adrenal gland.

successfully treated with a glucocorticoid (hydrocortisone); this is supplemented with a mineralocorticoid (fludrocortisone) in the salt-wasting form of the syndrome. Surgical correction of the external genitalia, if necessary, should be performed before the age of three years.

PUBERTY

The adolescent or pubescent phase of development provides the individual with reproductive capacity. In the female somatic growth accelerates, the breasts develop (thelarche), pubic hair appears (pubarche), and finally the menarche occurs. This process generally begins between 8 and 14 years of age with full development over a three-year period. The order of appearance of pubertal features varies greatly.

The age of onset of puberty is variable and influenced by genetic factors, socioeconomic conditions, and general health. Prepubertal girls have low serum levels of gonadotropins and sex steroid hormones. During the progression of puberty the characteristic inhibitory effect of estrogens on gonadotropin (FSH, LH) secretion declines and in the case of LH a positive feedback process develops (see Fig. 70–1). An early feature of the pubescent girl is the nocturnal pulsatile secretion of LH. Enhanced LH activity stimulates the ovary to secrete increasing amounts of estrogens, and secondary sex characteristics subsequently develop.

PRECOCIOUS PUBERTY

Isosexual precocious puberty relates to the premature (less than age eight years) development of adult genitalia consistent with the chromosomal sex of the child. In girls the majority of cases (80 per cent) are idiopathic, with both gonadotropins (FSH and LH) and sex steroid hormones (estradiol and progesterone) in the normal adult range. Isosexual precocious puberty also occurs in the McCune-Albright syndrome (polyostotic fibrous dysplasia). High gonadotropin levels should suggest an intracranial lesion or a human chorionic gonadotropin (HCG) secreting tumor. Hypothyroidism can also be associated with precocious puberty due to increased secretion of gonadotropins. Precocious puberty associated with low levels of gonadotropins should suggest an ovarian or adrenal tumor. Adrenal tumors generally secrete large amounts of steroids that can be detected as urinary 17-ketosteroids. Ovarian tumors can usually be detected on physical examination.

In heterosexual precocious puberty, pubertal changes occur that are consistent with the opposite sex of the child. This occurs most frequently in congenital adrenal hyperplasia (CAH) or due to androgen-secreting tumors of the adrenal cortex or ovary. High serum levels of 17-hydroxyprogesterone are typically found in congenital adrenal hyperplasia.

Treatment. Gonadal and adrenocortical tumors should be removed surgically. Intracranial tumors may be treated surgically, by radiation, and/or by chemotherapy. The progression of idiopathic precocious puberty can be delayed by medical intervention. This avoids psychosocial problems in the young child and may avoid premature closure of the epiphyses with permanent short stature. Depomedroxyprogesterone acetate (200 to 300 mg IM weekly) will stop breast development and menstruation. However, adult short stature may remain a problem. Analogues of GnRH will also effectively stop the progression of precocious puberty. Patients with congenital adrenal hyperplasia must receive replacement therapy with a glucocorticoid preparation.

Incomplete Sexual Precocity

Isolated premature breast development (thelarche) and pubic hair growth (pubarche or adrenarche) are benign conditions that rarely warrant specific therapy. Bone age may be slightly advanced in association with either of these forms of incomplete precocious puberty.

DELAYED PUBERTY

Girls who have not displayed breast growth by age 14 years are considered delayed developers. The majority of these cases are constitutional and will eventually undergo puberty spontaneously. Understandably these delays create psychological problems and parental anxiety. Thus reassurance can only be provided once other lesions have been excluded. Delayed puberty is also associated with excessive exercise (endurance training), nutritional disorders such as anorexia nervosa, chronic systemic illnesses (especially those involving the gastrointestinal tract), and hypothyroidism. Rarely, delayed puberty is due to hypogonadotropic hypogonadism (hypothalamic-pituitary disorders) or primary gonadal failure (gonadal dysgenesis), with increased levels of gonadotropins. If indicated, secondary sexual characteristics can be induced with estrogens (e.g., ethinylestradiol 20 μg orally daily) over a six-month period. Spontaneous progression of puberty frequently develops during or subsequent to therapy.

MENSTRUAL CYCLE

The onset of menarche (initiation of regular menstrual cycles) indicates the near completion of normal sexual development. Menarche occurs at a mean age of 12.6 years, with a standard deviation of 1.2 years. The current age range of menarche in the United States is 9 to 16 years. Early (<9 years) and delayed (>16 years) menarche warrants evaluation.

The menstrual cycle is conveniently divided into three phases—the follicular, the ovulatory, and the luteal phases (Fig. 70–3). Menstruation conventionally marks the beginning of a new cycle. Plasma FSH increases at the completion of the luteal phase of the previous cycle and initiates maturation of the follicle. During this phase the developing follicle secretes increasing amounts of estradiol, reaching a peak secretion about 12 hours before the LH ovulatory surge. This sudden increase in estradiol triggers the LH/FSH spike through a positive feedback process on the anterior hypothalamus. The mid-cycle surge in gonadotropins induces ovulation. Following ovulation the ruptured follicle is transformed into the corpus luteum. A rapid decrease in serum estradiol and increase in serum progesterone occur during the early part of the luteal phase. Subsequently the developing corpus luteum secretes increasing amounts of progesterone and estradiol and serum levels peak at about seven days postovulation. The corpus luteum then regresses, with a consequent decrease in serum hormone levels. At day 28 of the cycle, serum estradiol and progesterone are at their nadir, menstruation occurs, and a new cycle begins.

DYSMENORRHEA

Dysmenorrhea (pain just prior to and during menstruation) affects about half of all women. Primary dysmenorrhea is due to prostaglandin-induced uterine contractions. Systemic features may include headache, nausea, diarrhea, and emotional disturbances. Endometriosis is the most common cause of secondary dysmenorrhea. Inhibitors of prostaglandin synthesis generally relieve primary dysmenorrhea. If it persists or remains severe, the addition of an oral contraceptive is generally effective. Endometriosis should be treated medically, with additional surgery deferred until indicated by infertility or severe pain resistant to medication. Continuous suppression with an oral contraceptive agent or danazol for six months should give relief. Subsequent to a course of therapy, an oral contraceptive agent should be prescribed until fertility is desired.

THE PREMENSTRUAL SYNDROME

This common clinical entity affects about 70 per cent of women. Many women will experience some of the following symptoms before menses—bloating and weight gain, emotional lability, headaches (migraine), breast congestion, acne, and arthralgias. For most women these symptoms are merely a nuisance; about 20 per cent of patients, however, may experience severe problems from the time of ovulation to menstruation such that normal daily activities may be interrupted.

The cause of the premenstrual syndrome is not understood. Water retention, estrogen excess, and possibly dopamine deficiency in the central nervous system have been postulated as pathogenetic factors. These patients should be advised to restrict salt intake and exercise regularly to decrease fluid retention.

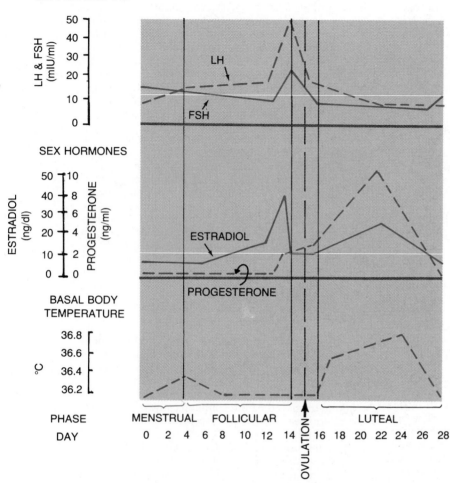

GONADOTROPINS

SEX HORMONES

BASAL BODY
TEMPERATURE

PHASE — MENSTRUAL FOLLICULAR OVULATION LUTEAL

DAY — 0 2 4 6 8 10 12 14 16 18 20 22 24 26 28

FIGURE 70–3. Normal menstrual cycle. The sequential changes that occur in serum gonadotropins (LH and FSH), estradiol, and progesterone during the various phases of the cycle are outlined. Day 0 correlates to the first day of menstruation. A typical basal body temperature chart is also depicted.

Women with severe symptoms may benefit from diuretic therapy during the second half of the menstrual cycle. Oral pyridoxine (50 mg orally daily) may be effective in some patients with a severe premenstrual syndrome. Pyridoxine is a cofactor in dopamine synthesis.

AMENORRHEA

Absence of menses for three months or longer defines amenorrhea. Failure of menarche to occur during adolescent development is primary amenorrhea, whereas the discontinuation of menses after the onset of menarche is secondary amenorrhea. Physiological amenorrhea occurs during pregnancy and after menopause. Approximately 5 per cent of women suffer from nonphysiological amenorrhea. Amenorrhea is a sign of any of several disorders involving different organ systems. Although traditionally the evaluation of amenorrhea is approached by focusing on the primary and secondary presentation, it is important to note the overlap in the etiologies (Tables 70–1 and 70–2).

Primary Amenorrhea

Primary amenorrhea always calls for a detailed history and physical examination. It may occur in association with normal, decreased, or increased sex steroid hormone production (Table 70–1). Women with normal secondary sex characteristics may have an abnormality of the outflow tract (vaginal aplasia or imperforate hymen) and retain the menstrual effluent. This may lead to endometriosis and cyclic abdominal pain but absent menstruation.

Incorrect gender assignment to genetic males (male pseudohermaphroditism) in the neonatal period accounts for about 50 per cent of cases of primary amenorrhea. The phenotypic females develop consequent to deficient testosterone synthesis and various androgen-resistant syndromes.

A spectrum of sexual immaturity may occur consequent to hypofunction of the hypothalamic-pituitary complex (hypogonadotropic hypogonadism). Secondary sexual characteristics do not develop and menses do not occur. Kallman's syndrome is a familial disorder characterized by anosmia or hyposmia, various midline defects (hair lip, cleft palate) and sexual immaturity due to low gonadotropin levels. Acquired forms may result from pituitary tumors, craniopharyngiomas and other parapituitary lesions. Psychogenic and stressful systemic disorders may also interfere with hypothalamic-pituitary function and delay sexual maturation and menarche.

A relatively common cause of primary amenorrhea without secondary sexual characteristics is gonadal dysgenesis (Turner's syndrome). This syndrome, characterized by streak gonads, elevated serum gonadotropin levels, short stature, and various other abnormalities, was described earlier.

Congenital adrenal hyperplasia (adrenogenital syndrome) may cause primary amenorrhea if not detected and treated. Mild forms with minimal genital ambiguity are often not detected until puberty. These patients are usually of short stature owing to androgen-induced premature closure of epiphyses. Primary amenorrhea can rarely be associated with polycystic ovaries or with androgen-secreting tumors.

Secondary Amenorrhea

Secondary amenorrhea is not a disease entity but a signal that function has been compromised at some level in the hypothalamic-pituitary-ovarian-uterine axis. Absence of menses for three to six months in a previously normally menstruating woman establishes the diagnosis of secondary amenorrhea. The most common cause of secondary amenorrhea is pregnancy. Thus such a patient should be considered pregnant until proven otherwise with a sensitive pregnancy test.

Secondary amenorrhea also occurs in association with normal, decreased, or increased sex steroid hormone production (Table 70–2). Amenorrhea associated with normal cyclic changes in the secretion of ovarian steroid hormones is a frequent finding in women with damaged endometrium. This may occur consequent to repeated uterine curettage following delivery or abortion or following infection (e.g., tuberculosis). Surgical or medical correction of these lesions generally leads to a resumption of menses.

Primary ovarian failure may develop following abdominal irradiation, chemotherapy, or surgery. However, premature ovarian failure probably occurs most commonly secondary to autoimmune injury. Serum gonadotropin levels are high. Destructive lesions of the hypothalamus and pituitary, such as surgery, irradiation, chemotherapy, infection, infarction, or tumor, may result in secondary ovarian failure. Pituitary tumors secreting prolactin account for about 30 per cent of cases with secondary amenorrhea. Most of these lesions can be detected by CT scanning. These patients have high serum prolactin levels and low serum levels of gonadotropins. Many cases of secondary amenorrhea are due to hypothalamic-pituitary dysfunction resulting from severe emotional stress or systemic disease. Thus amenorrhea may occur in association with anorexia nervosa, intensive exercise, endocrine disease (thyroid, adrenal, diabetes), and medications (postpill amenorrhea). Ovarian tumors may produce excess sex steroids (androgens), which

TABLE 70–1. CAUSES OF PRIMARY AMENORRHEA

1. Normal Sex Hormone Production
   Müllerian dysgenesis
   Amenorrhea traumatica
2. Decreased Sex Hormone Production
   A. Male pseudohermaphroditism due to an absolute or relative deficiency of testosterone
   B. Gonadal dysgenesis (Turner's syndrome)
   C. Hypothalamic-pituitary disease
      Familial hypogonadotropic hypogonadism (Kallman's syndrome)
   C. Pituitary and parapituitary tumors
      Anorexia nervosa
   D. Systemic diseases
3. Increased Sex Hormone Production
   Congenital adrenal hyperplasia
   Polycystic ovarian disease (Stein-Leventhal syndrome)
   Androgen-secreting ovarian and adrenal tumors

TABLE 70–2. CAUSES OF SECONDARY AMENORRHEA

1. Normal Sex Hormone Production
   Amenorrhea traumatica
      Postinfectious
      Postoperative
2. Decreased Sex Hormone Production
   A. Primary ovarian failure (high serum gonadotropins)
      Postsurgery, irradiation, chemotherapy, or toxins
      Autoimmune premature ovarian failure
      Gonadal dysgenesis
   B. Secondary ovarian failure (low serum gonadotropins)
      Hypothalamic-pituitary dysfunction
      Postsurgery, irradiation, infection, infarction
      Pituitary tumor with normal prolactin
      Empty sella syndrome
      Pituitary tumor with hyperprolactinemia
      Postpartum or postpill amenorrhea
      Psychogenic
      Anorexia nervosa
      Endocrine disorders—thyroid, adrenal, diabetes
      Systemic disorders
3. Increased Sex Hormone Production
   A. Polycystic ovarian disease
   B. Androgen-secreting ovarian or adrenal tumor

suppress gonadotropins and cause amenorrhea. A frequent cause of secondary amenorrhea consequent to increased ovarian production of androgens (androstenedione) is polycystic ovaries (Stein-Leventhal syndrome). An elevated LH/FSH ratio is very characteristic of this disorder. The etiology of polycystic ovaries is not known in most cases. These patients present with amenorrhea (anovulation), hirsutism, obesity, and bilaterally enlarged ovaries.

DIAGNOSIS AND TREATMENT

In a patient with amenorrhea the physician should first exclude pregnancy, pituitary tumor, and premature menopause. Pregnancy can be easily detected by measuring the serum level of the beta subunit of human chorionic gonadotropin. A normal serum FSH level rules out premature menopause. Pituitary microadenoma can generally be detected by sella turcica CT scanning. A positive finding in conjunction with high serum prolactin and low gonadotropin levels documents the presence of a pituitary tumor (see Chapter 67). Additional studies should focus on specific disorders of the central nervous system, thyroid, adrenal, pancreas (diabetes), ovary, uterus, and vagina.

In the absence of clinically detectable disease, very valuable information concerning the cause of amenorrhea can be obtained by proceeding through the following diagnostic steps. In most cases the need for expensive laboratory tests can be avoided.

A normal estrogen effect (sex steroid hormone production) can generally be deduced from a healthy vaginal mucosa and copious amounts of clear cervical mucus. A progesterone withdrawal (medroxyprogesterone acetate 10 mg daily for five days) screening test may be performed to test the integrity of the reproductive axis. Menstrual bleeding following this short course of progesterone indicates that the axis is functional and that the amenorrhea most likely is due to anovulation. If bleeding does not occur, a course of conjugated estrogens (Premarin 1.25 mg daily for 21 days) should be administered and followed by the progesterone withdrawal test. Failure to bleed following this regimen indicates target organ (endometrium) or outflow tract failure. The patient should be referred to a gynecologist for further investigations. A positive withdrawal test should be followed by measurement of gonadotropins and prolactin levels. High gonadotropin levels are consistent with primary ovarian disease, whereas low values indicate hypothalamic-pituitary dysfunction or failure. Individuals with high levels should have a karyotype performed to detect Turner's syndrome (XO) or male pseudohermaphroditism (female phenotype).

The approach to therapy for each specific cause of amenorrhea should be dictated by the lesion and the patient's wishes. If no clearly detectable lesion is evident, reassurance and follow-up are appropriate. A desire for regular menstrual cycles can be fulfilled by medication with a cyclic estrogen-progesterone preparation.

Amenorrhea associated with hyperprolactinemia can be treated surgically or medically, depending on the size of the pituitary tumor. Pituitary microadenomas (less than 10 mm) can be treated with bromocriptine (orally 2.5 mg b.i.d.). This restores regular cycles and fertility in the majority of patients. Premature ovarian failure should usually be treated with estrogen replacement (e.g., Premarin, 0.625 to 1.25 mg daily).

ABNORMAL UTERINE BLEEDING

The causes of abnormal uterine bleeding during the reproductive years include complications from the use of oral contraceptives, pregnancy (threatened, incomplete, or missed abortion), coagulation disorder, uterine polyps, leiomyomas, and tumors of the cervix and vagina. A history of diethylstilbestrol (DES) exposure would place the patient at a low but increased risk for adenocarcinoma of the vagina or cervix. Abnormal bleeding may also be a feature of trauma, endocrinopathies (diabetes mellitus, thyroid disorders, and adrenal disease), or other systemic diseases.

Dysfunctional uterine bleeding (DUB), defined as abnormal uterine bleeding that cannot be attributed to an organic lesion, is the most common cause (75 per cent) of abnormal uterine bleeding. The majority of these cases are associated with anovulation and occur at each end of the reproductive years, as postmenarcheal adolescent bleeding secondary to hypothalamic immaturity or as premenopausal bleeding consequent to imminent ovarian failure. Most cases of anovulatory bleeding are examples of estrogen withdrawal or estrogen breakthrough bleeding. Unopposed estrogen induces a progressive endometrial hyperplasia. In the absence of growth-limiting progesterone and natural periodic menstruation, the endometrium achieves an abnormal height without the necessary structural support. This fragile tissue will intermittently undergo spontaneous necrosis, and bleeding results. The classic presentation is one of a pale, frightened teenager who has bled excessively for weeks or an older woman with prolonged bleeding who is concerned about the development of a possible neoplasm. It is important to exclude the organic causes listed above before attributing abnormal uterine bleeding to DUB.

Therapy attempts to control the acute bleeding and to prevent recurrent bleeding. Acute hemostasis can be accomplished rapidly (less than 24 hours) with a high dose of a progesterone-estrogen combination birth control pill. Therapy is administered as one pill q.i.d. for seven days. These patients must be warned that a heavy flow associated with severe cramping will probably occur two to four days after stopping therapy. This initial withdrawal bleeding should be followed with three cycles of therapy using a low-dose combined contraceptive pill. The three months of therapy will restore the endometrium to its normal height. Each patient should subsequently be followed closely in order to document normal ovulatory cycles.

HIRSUTISM

Excessive growth of body hair in women is called hirsutism. An abnormal pattern of body hair growth, such as terminal hair on the upper abdomen, shoulders, back, and face, may be a sign of disease. In the majority of patients, however, no underlying disease can be found.

Hirsutism is predominantly an androgen-dependent process, except when associated with specific drugs (phenytoin, steroids, minoxidil), malnutrition (anorexia nervosa), or rare genetic disorders. Because androgens in women are secreted only by the ovaries or adrenal glands, a disorder of one or the other must be the source of any excess androgens (Table 70–3). Thus excessive secretion of testosterone or of its immediate

TABLE 70–3. HIRSUTISM

1. Ovarian Causes
   Idiopathic hirsutism
   Polycystic ovarian disease
   Ovarian tumors secreting excess androgens
2. Adrenal Disorders
   Congenital adrenal hyperplasia
   Virilizing adrenal tumors
3. Medications
   Minoxidil, phenytoin, diazoxide
   Androgens, glucocorticoids

precursors androstenedione and dehydroepiandrosterone, which are subsequently converted to testosterone in peripheral tissues, can cause abnormal terminal hair growth.

Clinical hirsutism may be associated with acne, temporal balding, increased muscle strength, altered libido, and, in virilized patients, clitoral enlargement and deepening of the voice. There may be generally defeminization with amenorrhea, decrease in breast size, and an alteration in the female body habitus. However, the two most common causes of hirsutism, idiopathic hirsutism and polycystic ovarian disease, are rarely associated with virilization or deepening of the voice. The hair growth is generally first noted in the peripubertal period and tends to stabilize after progressing for a few years. Adrenal and ovarian tumors generally present in adults. Most ovarian tumors are palpable on physical examination. Overt virilization occurs with most of the androgen-secreting ovarian tumors but rarely consequent to the weak androgens secreted by adrenal tumors. Congenital adrenal hyperplasia usually becomes clinically apparent at birth or during childhood. It is characterized by rapid growth, heterosexual precocious puberty in girls, and occasionally hypertension. However, it may not become apparent until later life in a small percentage of patients.

The etiology of most cases of hirsutism can be determined by measuring serum total testosterone and dehydroepiandrosterone sulfate (DHEA sulfate). Increased levels of plasma testosterone (values in excess of 200 ng/dl) are rarely associated with idiopathic hirsutism or polycystic ovarian syndrome but are frequently present in patients with ovarian tumors. Adrenal lesions (CAH or tumor) will have high plasma DHEA sulfate levels. In the benign process (CAH) DHEA sulfate will suppress after three days of dexamethasone (0.5 mg q.i.d.), whereas the secretion of DHEA sulfate will not suppress in cases with tumor. Furthermore, the high testosterone level associated with the polycystic ovarian syndrome will normalize on a "pill" (estrogen-progesterone) suppression test, in contrast to the lack of suppression in a patient with an ovarian tumor. However, since some tumors may suppress, the final diagnosis must be carefully assessed.

Ovarian and adrenal tumors are treated surgically. Congenital adrenal hyperplasia is suppressed with glucocorticoid replacement. Hirsutism associated with idiopathic hirsutism and polycystic ovarian disease is generally stable and rarely progresses to virilization. Thus, the abnormal hair growth is primarily a cosmetic and psychological problem. In this group, which consists of the majority of cases of hirsutism, the risks of suppressive therapy with either contraceptives, glucocorticoids, or antiandrogens (cyproterone is unavailable in the United States) and spironolactone must be carefully evaluated. These hormonal approaches have had mixed success.

GALACTORRHEA

Nonpuerperal lactation (galactorrhea) is of benign significance in about 30 per cent of patients. This is termed idiopathic and is associated with regular menses. If associated with amenorrhea, however, galactorrhea often indicates the presence of a serious condition such as a pituitary tumor (30 per cent). Table 70–4 outlines the relative frequency of disorders causing galactorrhea. The measurement of basal serum prolactin is very helpful in the evaluation of a patient with galactorrhea. The serum prolactin level is normal in the majority (85 per cent) of patients with idiopathic galactorrhea associated with continued menstruation. Thus a normal prolactin level generally indicates a benign disorder. Hyperprolactinemia is present in most (70 per cent) patients with galactorrhea associated with amenorrhea. This is the most common presentation of a pituitary tumor secreting prolactin in women. A patient presenting with a serum prolactin greater than 300 ng/ml invariably has a prolactinoma. Hyperprolactinemia of lesser magnitude (<300 ng/ml) may be associated with a prolactinoma or more frequently a spectrum of other causes (Table 70–4.) Galactorrhea in this latter group may be idiopathic (with amenorrhea), postpartum, postpill, or associated with endocrine disease (hypothyroidism, acromegaly, Cushing's syndrome) or drug therapy (phenothiazines, benzodiazepines, alpha methyldopa, reserpine). Rarely galactorrhea may be due to the empty sella syndrome or hypothalamic disease.

The suspected presence of a pituitary tumor can generally be documented by a plain skull radiograph of the sella turcica (macroadenoma, serum prolactin greater than 300 ng/ml) or a CT scan of the sella for a microadenoma (tumor less than 10 mm).

TABLE 70–4. GALACTORRHEA

CAUSES	FREQUENCY
Idiopathic with menses	32%
Idiopathic with amenorrhea	9%
Pituitary tumor	18%
Postpartum or postabortion	8%
Postpill or pill-related	10%
Drugs (phenothizides, etc.)	8%
Hypothyroidism	4%
Empty sella syndrome	2%
Miscellaneous	9%
	100%

Treatment of galactorrhea depends upon the primary disorder. Hypothyroidism, acromegaly, and Cushing's syndrome can be effectively corrected. Offending drugs should be stopped. Hyperprolactinemia due to a pituitary microadenoma or idiopathic hyperprolactinemia can be successfully treated with bromocriptine, a dopamine agonist. Macroadenomas may also respond successfully to bromocriptine therapy, and this is an acceptable form of treatment in the absence of local pituitary erosion or suprasellar extension. Large sellar tumors are generally treated definitively by transsphenoidal surgery and/or radiotherapy.

INFERTILITY

Infertility can be defined as involuntary inability to conceive. Sterility is total inability to reproduce. The problem may or may not be correctable for each particular couple. About 10 per cent of couples seek medical evaluation for infertility. In approximately 40 per cent of cases, the infertility is caused by the male. This may be due to decreased production of spermatozoa, ductal obstruction, inability to deliver sperm to the vagina, or abnormal semen. Female infertility is most commonly due to fallopian tube pathology, amenorrhea (anovulation), cervical or uterine polyps, systemic disorders, vaginal factors, and immunological disorders. Infertility remains idiopathic in about 10 per cent of couples.

Assessment involves a detailed history and physical examination of both subjects. Separate interviews may reveal significant information. Evaluation includes (1) semen analysis, (2) documentation of ovulation by basal body temperature records, timed serum progesterone determination, or endometrial biopsy, and (3) hysterosalpingography. Basal levels of prolactin and thyroid hormones should be measured. If all the tests are normal, laparoscopy with tubal dye instillation should be performed, as endometriosis or tubal disease is common (30 to 50 per cent). Treatment is determined by the findings on the infertility evaluation.

MENOPAUSE

The menopause refers to the cessation of menses. The mean age of spontaneous menopause is currently 50 years, although generally there is a transitional phase of ovarian failure over 6 to 18 months during the perimenopausal period. Pituitary gonadotropins are secreted excessively as progressive ovarian (follicular) failure reduces estrogen secretion. Measurement of serum follicle-stimulating hormone (FSH) is the single best test to detect ovarian failure (FSH > 50 mIU/ml).

The majority (85 per cent) of women experience some feature of estrogen deficiency at menopause. Breasts atrophy, thermoregulatory dysfunction begins (hot flushes, sweats), vaginal epithelium thins, vaginal and cervical secretions decline (dyspareunia may be experienced), the endometrium atrophies, and osteoporotic changes in bone accelerate (see Chapter 78). These alterations become sufficiently severe to warrant estrogen replacement in about 25 per cent of postmenopausal women.

Estrogen replacement will generally control hot flushes. The minimal effective dose should be given for as short a time as required for the relief of symptoms. The generally effective dose of conjugated estrogens (Premarin) ranges from 0.625 to 1.25 mg per day. These preparations can be administered on a cyclic basis, 25 days each month. This approach, when combined with a progestin (Provera, 5 to 10 mg orally q.d.) during the second half of each month, may reduce even further the low risk for uterine cancer. Local estrogen creams may be used to treat vaginal atrophy and the frequently associated dyspareunia. These estrogens are absorbed systemically, however, and the accepted contraindications to estrogen use also apply to such preparations. Long-term estrogen use at low doses will retard the accelerated bone loss associated with menopause and may possibly prevent the related fractures (see Chapter 78).

Estrogen use is contraindicated in patients with a history of thromboembolic disorders and vascular problems, including thrombophlebitis and cerebral vascular disorders. Estrogen therapy does not cause hypertension in postmenopausal women and may decrease the risk of cardiovascular disease. Estrogens should not be prescribed for patients with breast carcinoma or other estrogen-dependent neoplasias such as endometrial cancer. The presence of significant diffuse liver disease or benign or malignant liver tumors also prohibits the use of estrogens. Obviously all women taking estrogen preparations need constant surveillance to detect the onset of these disorders.

REFERENCES

Judd H, Meldrum D, Deftos L, et al: Estrogen replacement therapy: Indications and complications. Ann Intern Med 98:195, 1983.

Rebar RW: The ovaries. In Wyngaarden JB, Smith LH Jr (eds): Cecil Textbook of Medicine. 18th ed. Philadelphia, WB Saunders Co, 1988, pp 1425–1446.

Styne DM, Grumbach MM: Puberty in male and female: Its physiology and disorders. In Yen SSC, Jaffe RB (eds): Reproductive Endocrinology. Philadelphia, WB Saunders Co, 1978, p 189.

71

CANCER OF THE BREAST, UTERUS, AND OVARY

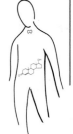

CANCER OF THE BREAST

In the United States cancer of the breast is the leading cause of death from cancer in women, followed closely by cancer of the lung. More than 120,000 women (and less than 10,000 men) receive this diagnosis annually. This represents a lifetime risk of approximately 8 per cent for white women, with a lesser incidence for other racial groups (as low as 2.5 per cent for Native American women). Only 15 per cent of cases occur before age 40; approximately two thirds occur after menopause.

Etiology. In the absence of specific knowledge about etiology, cancer of the breast can only be described in terms of risk factors (Table 71–1). The importance of family history is reflected in the nine-fold greater risk if a first-degree relative has had bilateral premenopausal breast cancer. Prolonged estrogen stimulation may be of importance (early menarche, late menopause, postmenopausal obesity), but the use of birth control pills or of small doses of estrogens for the prevention of osteoporosis has not clearly increased the risk of breast cancer. Furthermore, early pregnancy seems to have a protective effect, despite its characteristic hyperestrinism.

Classification. The most common breast malignancy is infiltrating ductal carcinoma (70 to 80 per cent). Less frequent are infiltrating lobular carcinoma (5 to 6 per cent) and noninvasive (intraepithelial) carcinomas that are still confined within the ductal basement membrane. Rarely other histological forms of breast cancer are found (medullary, colloid, etc.).

Clinical Presentation. The most frequent symptoms and signs of breast cancer are summarized in Table 71–2. The presentation is commonly that of an asymptomatic postmenopausal woman who becomes aware of a painless breast mass, usually through self-examination. The other listed signs and symptoms are distinctly uncommon (<6%) at the time of diagnosis. In the course of the patient's illness the late manifestations may occur. Breast cancer metastasizes to the lymph nodes, lung, bone, liver, and adrenal in order of descending frequency but may involve the central nervous system and virtually any other site as well. Of the systemic manifestations hypercalcemia is particularly notable, since (a) it may produce symptoms that are mistaken for those of advanced malignancy per se (weakness, nausea, vomiting, reduced mental activity), and (b) it can often be successfully treated.

Screening. Cure of breast cancer depends on its detection at an asymptomatic stage. The earliest possible detection of a breast mass is therefore of central importance. All adult women should be taught the techniques and importance of self-examination of the breasts. Examination of the breasts by a physician should ideally be carried out at least every three years, although this level of surveillance is difficult to attain for the public at large. The most effective screening test is that of routine radiographic mammography, best carried out according to the guidelines listed in Table 71–3. Routine use of screening mammography may reduce the number of deaths from breast cancer by one half to two thirds owing to early detection of lesions.

Diagnosis. The diagnosis of breast cancer usually depends upon differentiating between a benign and a malignant mass in the breast. This distinction can be made reliably only by examining the tissue histologically after fine needle aspiration, percutaneous needle biopsy, or open biopsy (incisional or excisional). Prior

---

TABLE 71–1. RISK FACTORS FOR CANCER OF THE BREAST

Age
Country of residence (North America, Europe)
History of breast cancer (especially premenopausal) in a first-degree relative
Upper socioeconomic class
Nulliparity
Early menarche
Late menopause
Obesity (in postmenopausal women)
History of fibrocystic disease (particularly lesions with dysplasia)
Radiation to the chest
Previous cancer in one breast, or primary endometrial or ovarian cancer
Consumption of alcohol? (needs further confirmation)

TABLE 71–2. SYMPTOMS AND SIGNS OF BREAST CANCER

1. **Initial**
   A. Palpable mass (75%)
   B. Rare (<6% each)
        pain in the breast
        nipple discharge, retraction, or erosion
        skin dimpling, edema, or erythema
        axillary tumor
2. **Late**
   A. Local or axillary
        inflammation
        ulceration
        fixation to the chest wall
        swelling of the left arm
   B. Metastatic
        lung—nodules, lymphangitic spread, pleural involvement
        bone—pain, fractures
        liver—hepatomegaly, usually asymptomatic
        brain—localizing symptoms and signs
   C. Systemic (Chapter 55)
        tumor cachexia
        hypercalcemia

TABLE 71–3. SUGGESTED GUIDELINES FOR SCREENING OF WOMEN BY MAMMOGRAPHY (American Cancer Society)

1. Baseline mammogram for all women aged 35 to 40
2. Mammography every one to two years from age 40 to 49
3. Mammography annually for women aged 50 or older

to biopsy, mammography of both breasts should be carried out to rule out the presence of a second lesion.

If the diagnosis of breast cancer is established, it is important to measure the level of estrogen and progesterone receptor proteins in the tumor tissue. This may serve as a guide to future hormonal therapy.

Staging. The diagnosis of breast cancer is incomplete unless followed by staging as a guide to therapy (Table 71–4). In addition to bilateral mammograms, all patients should receive a chest radiograph and blood chemistries to include alkaline phosphatase, carcinoembryonic antigen (CEA), and γ-glutamyl transpeptidase. Of patients with Stage I or Stage II disease, only those with Stage II disease with histologically positive lymph nodes or those with bone pain or an elevated alkaline phosphatase usually require initial radionuclide bone and liver scans.

Therapy. Since the therapy of breast cancer is complex and changing, it will not be described in detail here. Therapy may vary with clinical staging (Table 71–4), the presence or absence of histological axillary node involvement by the tumor, the age of the patient (pre- or postmenopausal), the presence or absence of hormone receptor proteins in the tumor, the preference of the patient, and the personal experience of the physician.

For Stage I and Stage II disease, radical mastectomy has been the standard therapy. Increasingly in selected patients the alternative of simple tumor resection ("lumpectomy") with axillary dissection and postop-

erative local irradiation is being carried out. For patients with positive axillary nodes but with no other evidence of metastatic disease, some form of adjuvant drug therapy (chemotherapeutic or hormonal) is usually recommended as well, in order to reduce the risk of recurrence.

For premenopausal patients with metastatic disease who are hormone receptor protein–positive (RP-positive), an attempt is made to reduce estrogenic stimulation by oophorectomy, followed by various combinations or sequences of tamoxifen, progestins, adrenalectomy, or androgens, as the clinical response, or lack thereof, requires. For postmenopausal patients who are RP-positive, tamoxifen is usually the first drug of choice. For patients who are RP-negative, for those who no longer respond to hormonal manipulations, or for those who have extensive metastatic disease, chemotherapy with various described multiagent protocols is indicated. The prognosis varies with the stage at which the initial diagnosis is made and therapy is instituted (Table 71–4).

CANCER OF THE UTERUS

Cancer of the uterus ranks fourth among the malignancies affecting women, following only carcinoma of the breast, lung, and large bowel. The incidence of endometrial cancer (about 40,000 cases per year in the United States) is approximately twice that of cancer of the ovary or cervix and increases with age. Less than 5 per cent of cases occur before age 40; more than 75 per cent occur postmenopausally.

Etiology. In the absence of direct information concerning the cause of cancer of the uterus, one can only describe statistical associations. The incidence of uterine malignancy is increased in association with obesity, nulliparity, late menopause, polycystic ovary disease, breast cancer, diabetes mellitus, and estrogen therapy in the absence of progestins. One common

TABLE 71–4. TNM CLASSIFICATION OF BREAST CANCER

	CLINICAL STAGE	TREATMENT OPTIONS	FIVE-YEAR SURVIVAL
Stage I	Tumor <2 cm Negative nodes No distant metastases	Modified radical mastectomy and axillary node dissection or "Lumpectomy" with axillary node dissection and postoperative radiation therapy	85%
Stage II	Tumor >2 <5 cm Positive nodes, not fixed No distant metastases	Modified radical mastectomy and axillary node dissection or "Lumpectomy" with axillary node dissection and postoperative radiation therapy	65%
Stage III	Tumor >5 cm or skin or chest wall involvement Positive supraclavicular nodes No distant metastases	Hormonal manipulation or Combination chemotherapy and local treatment with surgery and/or radiation	40%
Stage IV	Distant metastases	Hormonal manipulation or Combination chemotherapy Palliative radiation therapy	10%

element may be excessive and/or prolonged estrogenic stimulation of the endometrium without adequate progestational balancing.

Classification. More than 95 per cent of malignant uterine tumors are endometrial in origin; various types of sarcomas account for 3 to 5 per cent. Approximately 60 per cent are adenocarcinomas, followed in frequency by adenoacanthomas, adenosquamous carcinomas, clear cell carcinomas, and papillary carcinomas. Each tumor may present with differing degrees of differentiation.

Clinical Presentation. The hallmark of endometrial cancer is abnormal uterine bleeding—menometrorrhagia or, more frequently, postmenopausal bleeding. Much more rarely pelvic discomfort, urinary frequency, or the sense of a mass may be early complaints. Recurrence of vaginal bleeding after the menopause should always be considered to represent endometrial cancer until proven otherwise. Cancer may spread through the myometrium into the peritoneal cavity and ovaries and metastasize to the vagina or via the bloodstream and lymphatics throughout the body.

Diagnosis. The diagnosis depends upon the examination of biopsy material of the endometrium obtained by dilation and curettage. The Papanicolaou test is positive in less than half of the cases.

Staging. A commonly used staging system, summarized in Table 71–5, is based on the initial clinical and biopsy evaluation. It should be noted, however, that 10 per cent of those classified as Stage I may have nodal involvement at the time of surgery.

Therapy. Standard therapy for endometrial cancer is abdominal hysterectomy and bilateral salpingo-oophorectomy with cytological examination of peritoneal washings obtained at surgery. With more malignant grades of tumors, selective lymphadenectomy is often carried out as well. The tumor is examined for estrogen and progestin receptors as a guide for subsequent treatment with progestins if the tumor recurs. Various protocols for irradiation and/or chemotherapy have been developed, but their description is beyond the scope of this brief review. The approximate five-year survival of patients treated for endometrial cancer based on initial staging is shown in Table 71–5.

CANCER OF THE OVARY

Approximately 70 per cent of all ovarian tumors are benign. Nevertheless, the ovary is the eighth most common site of malignancy in women. It is estimated

TABLE 71–5. CLASSIFICATION OF ENDOMETRIAL CANCER*

STAGE	DEFINITION	FIVE-YEAR SURVIVAL
Stage I	Cancer confined to the corpus	75–80%
Stage II	Cancer involves the corpus and cervix	60%
Stage III	Cancer extends beyond the corpus but not outside the true pelvis	30%
Stage IV	Cancer involves the bladder or rectum or extends beyond outside the pelvis	10%

The tumors are also graded 1, 2, or 3 from well-differentiated adenocarcinoma to predominantly solid or undifferentiated carcinoma.

* Modified from the classification of the International Federation of Gynecology and Obstetrics.

that one out of each 70 newborn girls will develop an ovarian malignancy. Currently about 20,000 cases are diagnosed annually in the United States. Malignant ovarian tumors are rare in childhood, but their incidence increases progressively with age.

Etiology. The cause of carcinoma of the ovary is unknown. There seems to be an increased incidence with nulliparity, early menopause, irradiation of pelvic organs, a high fat diet, and a higher socioeconomic status.

Classification. As a complex organ, the ovary may be host to a large variety of malignant tumors. A partial listing of these tumors is shown in Table 71–6. Approximately 85 per cent of malignant ovarian tumors arise from the ovarian epithelium (serous cystadenocarcinoma being most frequent); many are bilateral. Fewer than 5 per cent are hormonally active. The ovary is not infrequently the site of metastases, most frequently from the gastrointestinal tract, breast, and thyroid.

Clinical Manifestations. Ovarian cancer is relatively silent clinically in its early stages. As the unfortunate result, most patients are at Stage III or Stage IV at the time of diagnosis. Early nonspecific symptoms include vague abdominal discomfort, loss of appetite, "indigestion," and anorexia. Lower abdominal pain may occur early from torsion or rupture of the tumor; when it occurs late it is more likely to be related to local invasion of pelvic organs. Later the patient may become aware of an abdominal mass or of diffuse abdominal swelling (ascites). At this stage nausea and vomiting may also be prominent owing to intestinal obstruction.

TABLE 71–6. OVARIAN TUMOR HISTOLOGY

EPITHELIAL (85%)	GONADAL STROMAL TUMORS (10%)	GERM CELL TUMORS (5%)
Serous cystadenocarcinoma (40%)	Sertoli-Leydig cell	Dysgerminoma
Endometroid carcinoma (15%)	Granulosa-stromal cell	Endodermal sinus
Mucinous cystadenocarcinoma (12%)	Androblastoma	Embryonal carcinoma
Clear cell (13%)		Choriocarcinoma
Undifferentiated (5%)		Teratoma

TABLE 71–7. STAGING OF OVARIAN CARCINOMA*

STAGE	DESCRIPTION
I	Growth limited to the ovaries
A	Growth limited to one ovary
B	Growth limited to both ovaries
C	IA or IB plus ascites or positive peritoneal washings
II	Ovarian involvement with pelvic extension
A	Involvement of uterus and/or tubes
B	Involvement of other pelvic structures
C	IIA or IIB plus ascites or positive peritoneal washings
III	Intraperitoneal metastases outside the pelvis, or positive retroperitoneal nodes, or both
IV	Distant metastases (liver, bone, lung, etc.)

Rarely a tumor secretes excessive estrogens (granulosa cell tumors) with precocious puberty, dysfunctional uterine bleeding, or postmenopausal uterine bleeding, depending upon the age of the patient. Even more rarely the tumor may secrete androgens with resulting virilization. Carcinoma of the ovary has been the source of a number of the systemic syndromes associated with cancer (Chapter 55), including neuropathy, hypercalcemia, hypoglycemia, Cushing's syndrome, and thyrotoxicosis.

Diagnosis. The early diagnosis of ovarian carcinoma is often a fortuitous occurrence, because the symptoms are usually so nonspecific. This diagnosis should always be considered in a woman over age 40 with gastrointestinal complaints for which no explanation is apparent. The diagnosis usually depends upon the demonstration of an enlarged ovary (or ovaries) by pelvic examination, or by ultrasonography, CT, or MRI, followed by surgical exploration. The "postmenopausal palpable ovary syndrome" refers to the fact that even seemingly normal-sized ovaries in this age group may be abnormal and require careful follow-up. Very rarely hormonal aberrations may direct attention to this ovary at a time when it is not clinically enlarged. Serum markers, such as the carcinoembryonic antigen, the Regan isoenzyme of alkaline phosphatase, and the CA 125 antigen, have proven to be more useful in following the course of the disease than in its diagnosis.

Staging. The most frequently used staging system for carcinoma of the ovary is presented in Table 71–7. As noted, approximately two thirds of patients are at Stage III or IV at the time of diagnosis.

Therapy. The primary purpose of surgery is to remove as much of the malignant tissue as possible, usually by bilateral salpingo-oophorectomy, a complete abdominal hysterectomy, and omentectomy. This procedure may be curative for the few patients who are diagnosed at Stage I or Stage II. Occasionally unilateral salpingo-oophorectomy may be indicated for a younger patient with a low-grade malignancy in order to preserve fertility. In view of the significant incidence of ovarian carcinoma, some physicians advocate elective oophorectomy in all women who have a hysterectomy after the age of 40. For patients with Stage III or IV disease, various multi-agent chemotherapeutic protocols have been advocated, most frequently using combinations of cyclophosphamide, doxorubicin, and cisplatin. Radiation has generally not been as effective as chemotherapy. Occasionally widespread peritoneal spread of ovarian carcinoma with ascites has responded dramatically to intraperitoneal chemotherapy. Overall about one third of patients survive five years after the diagnosis of ovarian carcinoma.

REFERENCES

Barber HRK: Ovarian cancer. CA 36:149, 1986.

Herbst AL: Neoplastic diseases of the uterus. *In* Droegemueller W, Herbst AL, Mishell DR, et al (eds): Comprehensive Gynecology. St Louis, The CV Mosby Co, 1987.

Kemp GM: The corpus uteri. *In* Rosenwaks Z, Benjamin F, Stone ML (eds): Gynecology, Principles and Practice. New York, Macmillan Publishing Co, 1987, p 489.

Lewis BJ: Breast cancer. *In* Wyngaarden JB, Smith LH Jr (eds): Cecil Textbook of Medicine. 18th ed. Philadelphia, WB Saunders Co, 1988, p 1452.

Lippman ME, Lichter AS, Danforth DN Jr (eds): Diagnosis and Management of Breast Cancer. Philadelphia, WB Saunders Co, 1988.

Zaloudek C, Tavassoli FA, Kurman RJ: Lesions of the ovary: Malignant lesions. *In* Danforth DN, Scott JR (eds): Obstetrics and Gynecology. 5th ed. Philadelphia, JB Lippincott Co, 1986, p 1132.

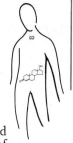

72

TESTICULAR AND BREAST DISORDERS IN MALES

Hypogonadism can refer to either (1) the failure of the testes to produce adequate testosterone, resulting in the signs and symptoms of androgen deficiency, or (2) impaired spermatogenesis, resulting in infertility. Impaired spermatogenesis and infertility may be present with normal testosterone production, but testosterone production is necessary for normal spermatogenesis. Normal adult males produce approximately 7 mg of testosterone per day and normal serum plasma concentrations are 3 to 10 ng/ml. Testosterone production is dependent on an intact hypothalamus, pituitary gland, and Leydig cells in the testis (Fig. 72–1). Spermatogenesis requires both intact pituitary and Leydig cell function. The 5α-reduced derivative of testosterone, 5α-dihydrotestosterone, is an active form of the hormone and is responsible for inducing growth and differentiation of the male secondary sex structures.

The causes of hypogonadism can be divided into two major categories (Table 72–1): (1) *Primary hypogo-nadism* is due to testicular disorders and is associated with elevated serum gonadotropin levels as a result of a diminished negative feedback. (2) *Secondary hypogonadism* results from hypothalamic pituitary disease and is associated with low or low-normal serum gonadotropin levels. In primary hypogonadism when testosterone levels are low, serum LH levels are increased, and when spermatogenesis is impaired, serum FSH levels are elevated.

ANDROGEN DEFICIENCY

The signs and symptoms of androgen deficiency depend upon the age of onset and the severity of the deficiency. If androgen deficiency occurs prior to puberty, the usual changes associated with puberty do not occur and the patient will develop the features of eunuchoidism (Table 72–2). Disproportionate growth of long bones occurs owing to the delay in epiphyseal closure. If testosterone secretion fails after sexual maturity, the signs of androgen deficiency are much less

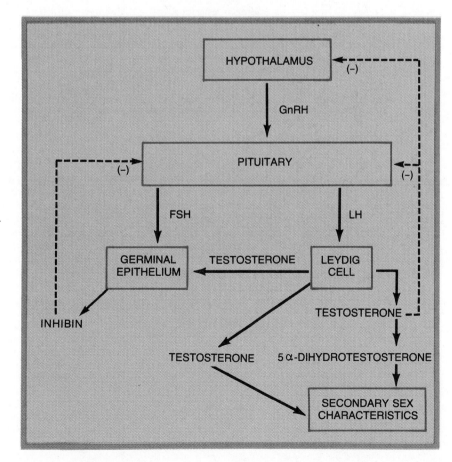

FIGURE 72–1. Pathway of production of testosterone.

TABLE 72–1. CLASSIFICATION OF THE CAUSES OF ABNORMALITIES IN TESTICULAR FUNCTION

	ANDROGEN DEFICIENCY AND INFERTILITY	INFERTILITY ONLY
Primary Hypogonadism		
1. Developmental and genetic disorders	Klinefelter's syndrome Noonan syndrome	Sertoli cell only syndrome Kartagener's syndrome Cryptorchidism
2. Structural defects	Anorchia	Varicocele
3. Acquired defects	Viral or bacterial orchitis Trauma Radiation Polyendocrine autoimmune failure Granulomatous disease Drugs—spironolactone, alcohol, marijuana Ischemia (torsion)	Radiation Drugs—alkylating agents and antimetabolites
4. Associated with systemic disease	Liver disease Renal disease Sickle cell disease	Myotonic dystrophy Paraplegia Febrile illness
Secondary Hypogonadism	Panhypopituitarism Hyperprolactinemia Kallman's syndrome Malnutrition Cushing's syndrome Hemochromatosis	Isolated FSH deficiency Congenital adrenal hyperplasia Exogenous sex steroid use
Other	Androgen resistance	Absence or obstruction of the vas deferens (cystic fibrosis)

overt (Table 72–2). The most common symptoms and signs are a reduction in prostate size, decreased rate of growth of beard and body hair, the appearance of fine wrinkles around the eyes, decreased semen volume, decreased libido, and impotence. Occasionally libido and potency will persist despite androgen deficiency.

When androgen deficiency is suspected, serum testosterone levels should be measured. If the serum testosterone concentration is low, serum LH and FSH levels should be determined next. Elevated LH and FSH concentrations indicate primary hypogonadism, whereas low or normal LH and FSH levels are most consistent with secondary hypogonadism.

TABLE 72–2. CLINICAL FEATURES OF EUNUCHOIDISM AND HYPOGONADISM

Eunuchoidism
Increased height and a span more than 2 inches greater than height
Lack of adult hair distribution
High-pitched voice
Small penis, testes, and scrotum
Decreased muscle mass
Hypogonadism Beginning After Puberty
Decreased prostate size
Diminished rate of growth of beard and body hair
Fine wrinkles around eyes
Decreased potency and libido

Androgen deficiency regardless of etiology is treated by administering testosterone. Testosterone may be given orally, sublingually, buccally, or intramuscularly via injections. In general, androgen replacement is most effective when long-acting testosterone preparations are administered intramuscularly. Undesirable effects of androgen replacement include edema secondary to sodium retention, erythremia, acne, gynecomastia, and premature closure of the epiphyses (if given during or before puberty). Methyltestosterone and other oral androgens will occasionally cause intrahepatic cholestatic jaundice. The most serious complication of oral androgens is hepatoma or peliosis hepatis (blood-filled cysts in the liver). Androgen therapy is contraindicated in patients with prostatic carcinoma and on occasion can precipitate urinary retention secondary to prostatic hypertrophy. Exogenous androgen therapy will not restore fertility.

The use of androgens by male athletes in the belief that performance will be improved is widespread. Currently there is no objective evidence that androgens enhance athletic performance even when given in very high doses. The commonly observed increase in body weight is secondary to the retention of salt and water. In women androgens do have a positive effect on nitrogen retention, but there are distressing virilizing side effects. Because of the potential of toxicity, the use of androgens has been barred by most athletic organizations.

INFERTILITY

About 15 per cent of married couples have fertility problems and in 30 per cent of these cases the male is the major cause of the infertility. The initial diagnostic procedure in evaluating a male for the many possible causes of infertility is a semen analysis. The test is considered abnormal if (1) the total sperm count is less than 60 million, (2) less than 60 per cent of the sperm are actively motile, or (3) more than 60 per cent of the sperm have an abnormal morphology. There is considerable variability in the sperm count for a given individual, so several counts over a period of time should be done if the count is borderline. Abnormalities in semen do not preclude fertility; many men with low sperm counts have fathered children. Fertility in the male is dependent on his female partner's fertility; i.e., a male with a relatively low sperm count may father a child with a partner of relatively high fertility.

If the semen analysis is abnormal, serum testosterone and FSH levels should be measured next. If a patient has azoospermia with a normal testosterone and FSH level, an obstructive disorder is a likely diagnostic possibility. Normal testosterone levels and elevated FSH concentrations indicate a primary testicular disorder of spermatogenesis as the basis for the infertility.

PRIMARY HYPOGONADISM

Klinefelter's Syndrome. Klinefelter's syndrome and its variants are important causes of male infertility and occur in approximately 1 in 500 newborn males. This syndrome is characterized by more than one X chromosome, most commonly a 47XXY karyotype, but occasionally 48XXYY, 48XXXY, or 49XXXXY karyotype has been described.

The classic features of this disorder are small, firm testes (usually less than 2 cm in length), azoospermia, gynecomastia, decreased signs of androgenicity, and elevated gonadotropin levels. Patients with this disorder are often tall, but the span-to-height ratio is frequently less than 1, suggesting that the increased height is not simply due to eunuchoidism. In some patients a mild degree of mental retardation is present, and poor social adaptation is not uncommon. Chronic pulmonary disease and varicose veins have been described as being more common in patients with Klinefelter's syndrome.

The manifestations of Klinefelter's syndrome may vary and may be minimal in some patients. Sex chromosome mosaicism, in which at least two populations of cells have different chromosomal complexes (example XY in one cell type and XXY in another), perhaps accounts for this remarkable variability in severity. In fact, fertility has been documented in rare individuals with this disorder.

Serum testosterone levels in patients with Klinefelter's syndrome vary from very low to low-normal. FSH levels are invariably elevated, but LH levels may be within the normal range, especially in those individuals with adequate testosterone levels. Buccal smears will frequently detect the condensed X chromosome (Barr bodies), but karyotyping of various cell types is the most definitive diagnostic procedure.

The treatment of this disorder is by testosterone replacement if there is evidence of androgen deficiency.

Myotonic Muscular Dystrophy. This syndrome is characterized by muscle wasting, myotonia, frontal baldness, cataracts, diabetes, and testicular atrophy, which occurs in the third to fourth decade. Androgen deficiency and gynecomastia occur in only a small percentage of these patients.

Sertoli Cell Only Syndrome (Germ Cell Aplasia). This syndrome is characterized by fully developed secondary sex characteristics and azoospermia. FSH levels are increased, and testosterone and LH levels are within the normal range. Testicular biopsy reveals seminiferous tubules that do not contain germinal cells and are lined only with Sertoli cells.

Kartagener's Syndrome. This genetic syndrome includes situs inversus, chronic sinusitis, bronchiectasis, and infertility secondary to nonmotile sperm. The immotility of the sperm and the respiratory difficulties are due to the absence of the protein dynein, a constituent of both the tail of the sperm and the cilia of the respiratory tract mucosa.

Anorchia. Absence of both testes in a phenotypically normal male is very rare. It is important to distinguish bilateral abdominal cryptorchidism from anorchia because of the increased incidence of malignancy in cryptorchidism. Low testosterone levels that fail to rise following HCG stimulation suggest anorchia, but the final diagnosis depends on surgical exploration. Unilateral anorchia is more common and may result from developmental disturbances or following surgical procedures such as orchiopexy or herniorrhaphy.

Acquired Hypogonadism. Numerous chemical and physical factors can affect gonadal function and result in either transient or permanent dysfunction. Germ cells are sensitive to ischemia, and testicular torsion if not rapidly corrected can irreversibly damage the testes. In adults, mumps is complicated by orchitis in 15 to 25 per cent of patients, and the affected testes may sustain permanent damage. Mumps orchitis is usually unilateral and typically does not affect testosterone production. Other viruses and bacterial infections can also cause orchitis and result in hypogonadism. Many chemicals and drugs are directly toxic to spermatogenesis or affect the androgen-to-estrogen ratio and thus may result in oligospermia or azoospermia. Many of the alkylating agents and antimetabolites that are commonly used in cancer chemotherapy adversely affect spermatogenesis. Ionizing radiation primarily inhibits spermatogenesis. Testicular failure occurs rarely as part of the polyendocrine failure syndrome secondary to an autoimmune process. Lastly, systemic disorders such as hepatic or renal failure can result in hypogonadism.

SECONDARY HYPOGONADISM

Secondary hypogonadism, due to the decreased secretion of gonadotropins by the pituitary gland, may result from any disorder that adversely affects pituitary or hypothalamic function (see Table 72–1). Gonadotropins may be decreased as an isolated deficiency or in association with deficiency of other pituitary hormones. A functional and reversible suppression of gonadotropin secretion occurs in malnutrition and in disorders that cause hyperprolactinemia. High serum concentrations of either androgens or estrogens can also inhibit gonadotropin secretion. The hypogonadism that occurs in patients with liver disease, for example, is partially due to increased levels of estrogen. Exogenous sex steroid intake by athletes also will lead to infertility.

Kallmann's syndrome, a familial disorder characterized by hypogonadotropic hypogonadism, occurs in association with anosmia or hyposmia. The hypogonadism is due to an abnormality in the secretion of gonadotropin-releasing factor by the hypothalamus.

Fertility can occasionally be restored in individuals with secondary hypogonadism by treatment with Pergonal (FSH activity) and human chorionic gonadotropin (LH activity).

CRYPTORCHIDISM

Cryptorchidism refers to a testis that has never descended into the scrotum. Unilateral cryptorchidism is approximately four times as common as bilateral cryptorchidism. Undescended testes are found at birth

TABLE 72–3. CLASSIFICATION OF THE CAUSES OF IMPOTENCE

Psychogenic
Endocrine
   Hypogonadism
   Hyperprolactinemia
Chronic Illness
   Cirrhosis
   Uremia
   Malignancy
   Cardiac disease
Neurologic
   Spinal cord lesions
   Diabetes mellitus
   Tabes dorsalis
   Polyneuropathies
   Parasympathetic nerve damage following surgical procedure such as prostatectomy, aortic bypass, or rectosigmoid operation
   Temporal lobe disorders
Vascular Disease
Drugs
   Antihypertensives—clonidine, methyldopa, propranolol, reserpine, spironolactone, thiazides
   Antihistamines—cimetidine, diphenhydramine
   Antidepressants—doxepin, amitriptyline
   Antipsychotics—chlorpromazine, haloperidol
   Tranquilizers—diazepam, barbiturates, chlordiazepoxide
   Anticholinergics
   Addicting drugs—alcohol, heroin, methadone
Penile Disease
   Priapism
   Peyronie's disease

in 3 to 4 per cent of male infants but by one year of age only 0.5 per cent have an undescended testis. In adult males approximately 0.2 to 0.4 per cent have either unilateral or bilateral cryptorchidism.

It is important to distinguish an undescended testis from the more common retractile testes of childhood. Repeated examinations in a warm room with the patient standing, squatting, recumbent, or performing a Valsalva maneuver are necessary. Careful questioning to determine if the testis has ever been in the scrotum is mandatory. Absence of the testis in the scrotum historically and on repeated physical examination suggests that the testis is truly undescended.

Adult men with bilateral cryptorchidism are sterile. However, the age at which these testes become infertile is uncertain. Abnormalities in testicular histology have been noted as early as six years of age, but the significance of these changes is uncertain. After puberty the undescended testis shows degenerative changes that eventually progress to atrophy. Even when cryptorchid testes are placed in the scrotum, degenerative changes occur in approximately 50 per cent, suggesting that intrinsic abnormalities of the organ account for the failure of normal descent. Even when unilateral cryptorchidism is corrected many patients have abnormal spermatogenesis, suggesting that the testicular abnormality is bilateral. Thus in many cases the degenerative changes are due to a testicular abnormality that orchiopexy will not correct. The incidence of malignancy in an undescended testis is 30 to 50 times greater than in the normal testis.

Cryptorchidism is treated by orchiopexy, although some clinicians first administer HCG followed by orchiopexy if the testis does not descend. The age when therapy should be initiated is uncertain, but it certainly should be prior to the onset of puberty. Many experts recommend treatment between five and seven years of age.

IMPOTENCE

Impotence is a common problem that can occur secondary to a wide variety of causes (Table 72–3). While impotence that is psychogenic in origin is not uncommon, a specific etiology can frequently be identified. Patients with psychogenic impotence have morning erections and/or erections that are associated with REM sleep, whereas in patients with physiological impotence erections at these times are either impaired or absent. The measurement of nocturnal penile tumescence by a variety of different procedures can therefore be helpful in the evaluation of impotent men. A very careful drug history is also indicated in all patients. The physical examination should search thoroughly for the signs of peripheral vascular disease or neuropathies. On occasion hyperprolactinemia may be the cause of the impotence, and lowering the prolactin level can restore potency. If the cause of the impotence cannot be corrected, many men will benefit by the implantation of a penile prosthesis.

GYNECOMASTIA

Gynecomastia, the enlargement of the male breast, may occur unilaterally or bilaterally. Gynecomastia is very commonly observed during the newborn period and puberty and in senescence. For example, approximately 50 per cent of normal boys at puberty and 40 per cent of elderly men have been noted to have gynecomastia. If gynecomastia develops between late puberty and male senescence, one should search carefully for an underlying disorder that can account for the breast enlargement (Table 72–4).

Estrogens stimulate while androgens inhibit breast development, and therefore disorders that alter the usual ratio of estrogens to androgens can result in gynecomastia. Increased estrogen production secondary to adrenal carcinoma, testicular tumors, and some types of congenital adrenal hyperplasia will lead to breast development. Similarly, the increased conversion of androgens to estrogens which occurs in liver disease, thyrotoxicosis, obesity, and refeeding after starvation will also result in gynecomastia. Conversely, the decreased production of androgens in primary or secondary testicular failure or insensitivity to the cellular effects of testosterone can also result in breast enlargement. Lastly, gynecomastia occurs in association with the use of a wide variety of drugs. Estrogen treatment will lead to gynecomastia; androgen administration may also on occasion result in breast development because of the biotransformation of androgens to estrogens. Some drugs, such as HCG, will increase endogenous estrogen production, and other drugs such as digitalis or marijuana have an estrogen-like effect. Additionally, drugs can block testosterone synthesis (chemotherapeutic agents, high doses of spironolactone) or interfere with the action of testosterone (cyproterone, low doses of spironolactone), resulting in gynecomastia.

It is essential to be sure that "true" gynecomastia is present. The most frequent error is to confuse the fatty breast of the obese patient, which lacks the glandular elements, with gynecomastia. The diagnosis of gynecomastia is based on the palpation of subareolar glandular tissue. Particular attention should be paid to the testes, as either small testes or a testicular mass will suggest the likely mechanism for the gynecomastia. Additionally, a careful search for signs of liver disease, thyrotoxicosis, other evidence of feminization, and galactorrhea is indicated. Lastly, in all patients with gynecomastia a complete drug history (including illicit drugs) is essential.

Many laboratory studies can be useful in the evaluation of gynecomastia when judiciously selected on the basis of history and physical examination. In the pubertal boy, for example, laboratory studies are not usually indicated. Liver function tests, serum estrogen, testosterone, LH and HCG concentrations, and adrenal androgen levels are sometimes useful in the evaluation of patients with gynecomastia.

Regression or significant improvement in gynecomastia occurs in a substantial number of patients. Gynecomastia usually improves after stopping an offending drug or after correcting a hormonal deficiency or excess. Pubertal gynecomastia will spontaneously regress and drug therapy is not indicated. Long-standing cases of gynecomastia or large breasts will rarely regress entirely after the causal disorder has been corrected. In these instances cosmetic mastectomy may be very helpful. The risk of breast cancer in men is proportional to the amount of breast tissue present and therefore is increased in patients with substantial gynecomastia.

TABLE 72–4. CLASSIFICATION OF THE CAUSES OF GYNECOMASTIA

Physiological—Newborn, Puberty, Senescence
Pathological
  Increased Estrogen Secretion
    Adrenal carcinoma
    Testicular tumors
    HCG secreting tumors (lung, liver, etc.)
    Congenital adrenal hyperplasia
    Hermaphroditism
  Increased Conversion of Androgens to Estrogens
    Liver disease
    Adrenal disease
    Nutritional (refeeding after starvation)
    Thyrotoxicosis
  Decreased Androgen Secretion
    Primary hypogonadism
    Secondary hypogonadism
  Androgen Resistance
    Testicular feminization
    Reifenstein's syndrome
Drugs
  Hormones—estrogens, androgens, HCG
  Antihypertensives—reserpine, methyldopa, spironolactone
  Psychotropics—phenothiazine, butyrophenone, marijuana, methadone, heroin, tricyclic antidepressants, diazepam
  Cardiac—digitalis
  Gastrointestinal—cimetidine, metoclopramide
  Cytotoxic—cyclophosphamide, vincristine, mitotane
  Miscellaneous—penicillamine

TUMORS OF THE TESTIS

Tumors of the testis are uncommon (6 per 100,000 males annually), and the peak age of incidence is 20 to 35 years. The most significant risk factor for developing testicular cancer is cryptorchidism. In unilateral cryptorchidism both the undescended and normally descended testis have an increased risk of malignancy. Whether orchiopexy reduces the risk of cancer is unresolved.

The vast majority of testicular tumors are malignant (95 per cent) and are derived from germ cells. Germ cell cancers may be subdivided into two groups: seminomas and nonseminomas (embryonal cell carcinoma, choriocarcinoma, and teratoma). The presence of any nonseminomatous element indicates that the tumor should be classified as a nonseminoma.

Patients with germ cell tumors usually present with a painless testicular mass. Pain or a sudden increase in tumor size is usually due to bleeding into the tumor.

Other symptoms include back or abdominal pain secondary to retroperitoneal lymphadenopathy, supraclavicular lymphadenopathy, shortness of breath due to pulmonary metastases, gynecomastia, or ureteral obstruction.

Nonseminous tumors may secrete biological markers: alpha-fetoprotein by embryonal cell cancers; HCG by choriocarcinomas or embryonal cell cancers. Increased HCG levels may lead to gynecomastia. Pure seminomas never produce alpha-fetoprotein and only rarely secrete HCG. Both alpha-fetoprotein and HCG levels are useful in monitoring the response to therapy, and increasing levels can be an early indicator of tumor recurrence.

Seminomas usually metastasize via the lymphatics, resulting in retroperitoneal, mediastinal, and supraclavicular lymph node invasion. Seminomas are very sensitive to radiation, and therefore the combination of surgical orchiectomy and radiotherapy has resulted in cure rates of 80 to 95 per cent. Nonseminomatous cancers, which metastasize by both the lymphatic and hematogenous routes, are radioresistant. Multiple drug chemotherapy has resulted in long-term remissions in approximately 40 per cent.

Non–germ cell tumors are rare (5 per cent of testicular tumors) and usually benign (90 per cent). They are composed of Leydig and Sertoli cells, which may secrete estrogens or androgens and thereby result in feminization or virilization. Gynecomastia is present in 30 per cent of patients with non–germ cell tumors. In children, non–germ cell tumors may result in precocious puberty.

REFERENCES

Lipsett MB: Physiology and pathology of the Leydig cell. N Engl J Med 303:682, 1980.

Matsumoto AM: The testis. In Wyngaarden JB, Smith LH Jr (eds): Cecil Textbook of Medicine. 18th ed. Philadelphia, WB Saunders Co, 1988, pp 1404–1421.

Schiavi RC: Male erectile disorders. Annu Rev Med 32:509, 1981.

Tolis G: Nonmalignant diseases of the breast. In Wyngaarden JB, Smith LH Jr (eds): Cecil Textbook of Medicine. 18th ed. Philadelphia, WB Saunders Co, 1988, pp 1449–1452.

Wilson JD, Himan J, MacDonald PC: The pathogenesis of gynecomastia. Adv Intern Med 25:1, 1980.

73

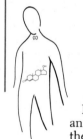

DIABETES MELLITUS

Diabetes mellitus is a very common disorder with an estimated prevalence between 2 and 4 per cent in the United States. The complications of diabetes account for over 25 per cent of all new cases of end-stage renal failure and over 50 per cent of all lower extremity amputations, and diabetes is the leading cause of blindness, with approximately 5,000 new cases per year. Additionally, diabetic patients account for 10 per cent of all acute care hospital days.

DIAGNOSIS

A patient is considered to have diabetes mellitus if any of the three criteria shown in Table 73–1 are met. Nearly all patients who are diabetic according to oral glucose tolerance test criteria also have fasting plasma glucose levels greater than 140 mg/dl. Routine screening of patients with glucose tolerance tests is therefore not usually indicated. An oral glucose tolerance test may be indicated in individuals with normal fasting blood glucose levels if there is a strong suspicion of diabetes, such as the presence of complications possibly secondary to diabetes, an extensive family history of diabetes, or certain genetic syndromes. In general, the diagnosis of diabetes mellitus should rarely be made in the absence of fasting hyperglycemia.

"Impaired glucose tolerance" exists if the fasting plasma glucose is less than 140 mg/dl and during glucose tolerance testing, the 30-, 60-, or 90-minute plasma glucose level exceeds 200 mg/dl, with a two-

TABLE 73–1. CRITERIA FOR THE DIAGNOSIS OF DIABETES IN NONPREGNANT ADULTS

Any one of the following are considered diagnostic of diabetes:
A. Presence of the classic symptoms of diabetes, such as polyuria, polydipsia, ketonuria, and rapid weight loss, together with gross and unequivocal elevation of plasma glucose.
B. Elevated fasting glucose concentration on more than one occasion, venous plasma glucose ≥ 140 mg/dl (7.8 mmol/L).
C. Fasting glucose concentration less than that which is diagnostic of diabetes (B), but sustained elevation of glucose concentration during the oral glucose tolerance test* on more than one occasion. Both the two-hour sample and some other sample taken between the administration of the oral 75-gm glucose dose and the two-hour sample must meet the following criteria, venous plasma glucose ≥ 200 mg/dl (11.1 mmol/L).

* O.G.T.T. should be performed in the morning after at least three days of unrestricted diet (≥150 gm carbohydrate) and physical activity. The subject should have fasted at least 10 hours and should remain seated throughout the study. (These guidelines were taken from the National Diabetes Data Group. Diabetes 28:1039, 1979.)

hour value between 140 and 200 mg/dl. Many individuals with impaired glucose tolerance do not progress to diabetes, and the specific microvascular complications associated with diabetes occur infrequently. The clinical significance of impaired glucose tolerance is unclear.

CLASSIFICATION OF DIABETES (Tables 73–2 and 73–3)

Type I Insulin-Dependent Diabetes Mellitus (IDDM)

Type I diabetes is characterized by little or no endogenous insulin secretion. Because of the marked hypoinsulinemia, patients with this disorder usually present with the acute complications of diabetes mellitus such as polyuria, polydipsia, polyphagia, and ketoacidosis. In order to prevent ketoacidosis and death, these patients require exogenous insulin replacement. After the onset of diabetes, patients occasionally enter a "honeymoon phase" that may last several weeks or months during which time endogenous insulin secretion is restored and glucose metabolism may approach normal. Unfortunately, the disease invariably relapses and lifelong insulin therapy is required.

The peak age of onset of IDDM is between 11 and 13 years, coinciding with the onset of puberty, but type I diabetes can begin at any age, including in the elderly. Patients with this disorder are usually of normal weight or thin. Specific HLA phenotypes (DR3, DR4) occur at a much greater frequency in patients with IDDM than in the general population. There is less than a 50 per cent concordance rate for diabetes in identical twins with IDDM (i.e., less than 50 per cent of identical twins both have diabetes), suggesting the importance of both genetic and environmental factors.

The etiology of IDDM is unknown. A leading hypothesis is that a viral illness or another yet unspecified initiating event may damage the beta cells of the pancreas, followed by a slow autoimmune destruction of the remaining beta cells in susceptible individuals. Anti–islet cell and anti-insulin antibodies may be detected in individuals several years prior to the onset of diabetes, followed by a slow deterioration in glucose tolerance which finally results in the abrupt onset of clinical diabetes. Soon after the onset of the disease, antibodies against the islet cells of the pancreas are present in as high as 90 per cent of type I diabetic patients, but they diminish in frequency to 5 to 10 per cent after 20 years. This autoimmune hypothesis would also account for the increased risk of developing diabetes in individuals with certain HLA genes, because the genes that control the immune response are located on the sixth chromosome close to the HLA loci.

Based on the presumed autoimmune origin of IDDM, studies are being carried out on the acute treatment of these patients with immunosuppressive agents. Some initial success in preventing permanent diabetes has been reported, but at the cost of contin-

TABLE 73–2. CLASSIFICATION OF DIABETES

Type I—Insulin-Dependent Diabetes
Type II—Non–Insulin-Dependent Diabetes
Secondary Diabetes
    Pancreatic disease
    Hormonal
    Drug-induced
    Insulin receptor abnormalities
    Specific genetic syndromes
    Gestational diabetes
    Genetic defects of the insulin receptor (rare)

TABLE 73–3. COMPARISON OF TYPE I AND TYPE II DIABETES

	TYPE I	TYPE II
Synonym	IDDM	NIDDM
	Juvenile onset	Adult onset
Age of onset	Usually <30	Usually >40
Ketosis	Common	Uncommon
Body weight	Nonobese	Obese (50–90%)
Endogenous insulin secretion	Severe deficiency	Moderate deficiency
Insulin resistance	Occasional	Almost always
HLA association	DR3, DR4	None
Identical twins	<50% concordant	Almost 100% concordant
Islet cell antibodies	Frequent	Absent
Association with other autoimmune disease	Frequent	No
Treatment with insulin	Always necessary	Usually not required

ued immunosuppression. Whether this aggressive early treatment of IDDM is warranted has not been established.

Type II Non–Insulin-Dependent Diabetes Mellitus (NIDDM)

Type II diabetes is much more common than IDDM (approximately 10 cases of type II diabetes for every case of type I) and usually has its onset after age 40. Between 50 and 90 per cent of the patients with NIDDM are overweight. Some patients are asymptomatic and an elevated plasma glucose is noted on routine laboratory study. In other patients, polyuria, polydipsia, weakness, fatigue, or weight loss brings the patient to the attention of the physician. More rarely, patients with NIDDM first seek medical care because of the complications of long-standing diabetes.

Plasma insulin levels are relatively decreased in patients with NIDDM but are not as severely reduced as in type I diabetics. In some individuals, plasma insulin levels may be within the normal range or even elevated. Patients with NIDDM almost always secrete decreased amounts of insulin, however, following oral glucose challenge. Because insulin deficiency is not marked, ketoacidosis rarely occurs in NIDDM unless a stressful event such as a myocardial infarction or infection is superimposed.

In addition to the abnormalities of insulin secretion, patients with NIDDM are also resistant to the action of insulin. This insulin resistance is due both to a decrease in insulin binding to its plasma membrane receptor and to postreceptor defects in insulin action. Thus, both a decrease in insulin secretion and impaired insulin action contribute to the hyperglycemia observed in NIDDM. At this time, the relative importance of these abnormalities in producing the impaired glucose metabolism is unclear.

Identical twins are almost 100 per cent concordant for NIDDM, suggesting a very strong genetic component to this disorder.

While this classification is convenient and useful, there are some patients who are difficult to place in a specific category. Additionally, patients will, on occasion, progress from a type II form of diabetes to a type I. It is likely that within each category, there are multiple subtypes that have not yet been recognized and defined.

Secondary Diabetes

Diabetes that is secondary to an identifiable condition is comparatively rare. For example, destruction of the pancreas secondary to pancreatitis will impair insulin secretion and result in diabetes. In certain endocrine disorders such as Cushing's syndrome, acromegaly, pheochromocytoma, and glucagonoma, the increased secretion of hormones that counteract the effect of insulin can also result in hyperglycemia. By a variety of mechanisms, a number of commonly used drugs such as diuretics, corticosteroids, propranolol, phenytoin, and adrenergic agents also cause or exacerbate diabetes.

Acanthosis nigricans may be associated with severe insulin resistance, resulting in diabetes by two distinct mechanisms: (1) Type A—the insulin resistance is due to a marked decrease in the number of cellular insulin receptors. These patients are usually young females with hirsutism and polycystic ovaries. (2) Type B—the insulin resistance is due to autoantibodies against the insulin receptor as part of a more generalized autoimmune process manifested by proteinuria, leukopenia, and antinuclear antibodies.

Genetic Defects of the Insulin Receptor

With the elucidation of the structure of the insulin receptor on cell membranes, several families have been recently discovered in whom diabetes and hyperinsulinemia have been associated with specific abnormalities of the receptor. This work is being rapidly extended, but it seems unlikely that this type of genetic defect accounts for more than a very small proportion of patients with glucose intolerance or clinical diabetes.

GENETICS

Diabetes has a strong familial tendency. Genetic factors are clearly important in the development of both type I and type II diabetes, but the mode of inheritance of both disorders is unknown. The direct transmission of clinical diabetes from a single parent with the disorder to offspring is relatively low: only 2 to 5 per cent for IDDM and 10 to 15 per cent for NIDDM. If a nonidentical sibling has either IDDM or NIDDM, the chance of an individual having diabetes is only approximately 10 per cent. However, in IDDM, if the siblings are identical for HLA phenotypes, the chances of being concordant for diabetes are greatly increased, whereas if all HLA phenotypes are different, the chances of concordance are greatly reduced. Recognizing these low rates of transmission from parent to sibling and the low incidence of concordance between siblings is important in counseling and reassuring patients.

ACUTE SYMPTOMS OF DIABETES

Hyperglycemia can result in a wide variety of symptoms (Table 73–4). When plasma glucose concentration exceeds the renal threshold for glucose reabsorption (approximately 180 mg/dl plasma glucose), glycosuria occurs and results in an osmotic diuresis. The resulting symptoms of nocturia and polyuria are directly attributed to this osmotic diuresis. The osmotic diuresis tends to lead to dehydration and hyperosmolality, which stimulate thirst and polydipsia. Each gram of urinary glucose represents approximately 4.5 calories. A poorly controlled diabetic who spills 100 gm of glucose per day in the urine, for example, loses 450 calories per day, enough to result in weight loss and stimulation of food intake (polyphagia). Thus, the polyuria, polyphagia, polydipsia, and weight loss, which are the cardinal signs of poorly controlled diabetics, are all attributable to increased urinary loss of glucose.

In addition to the above symptoms, transient visual blurring secondary to osmotic swelling of the lens is a common complaint of a poorly controlled diabetic and should not be confused with diabetic retinopathy. *Candida* vaginitis, thrush, or balanitis are occasionally observed and frequently do not respond to appropriate antibiotics until the plasma glucose concentration is lowered and the urine becomes glucose-free. Lastly, generalized fatigue is a common complaint in diabetic patients with persistent hyperglycemia.

TABLE 73–4. SYMPTOMS OF HYPERGLYCEMIA

Polyuria
Polydipsia
Polyphagia
Weight loss
Fatigue
Candida infections
Blurred vision
Vulvovaginitis

THERAPY

GENERAL PRINCIPLES

The initial goal of treatment in all diabetic patients is the elimination of the symptoms that occur secondary to hyperglycemia. A second goal of therapy is the prevention of the long-term complications of diabetes. At this time, there is no *definitive* evidence that a reduction in blood glucose levels will prevent the long-term complications of diabetes. Nevertheless, there is substantial clinical and experimental evidence that elevated blood glucose levels may be detrimental. It seems worthwhile, therefore, to attempt to normalize blood glucose levels in diabetic patients. Hypoglycemia is a serious and potentially fatal complication of therapy, and therefore the physician must balance the possible benefits of "tight" glucose control with the risks of inducing hypoglycemia.

Factors that predispose to serious hypoglycemia, such as end-stage liver or kidney disease, adrenal or pituitary insufficiency, autonomic insufficiency, ethanol abuse, and psychiatric disturbances, are strong contraindications to "tight" control.

In patients with cerebral vascular disease or coronary artery disease, the potential complications of hypoglycemia are more severe, and therefore aggressive therapy should also not be undertaken lightly. The goal of "tight" metabolic control is to prevent complications; if a patient already has severe diabetic complications, there is little evidence to suggest that aggressive therapy will be beneficial. The complications of diabetes usually take 10 to 20 years to develop and therefore in a patient whose life expectancy is greatly reduced due to other medical disorders, "tight" control is not usually indicated. Success in normalizing blood glucose levels requires a patient who is willing and able to undertake the responsibility of extensive self-care.

In a patient who is capable of undertaking the responsibilities of extensive self-care and who has no contraindications to aggressive metabolic control, an attempt should be made to control blood glucose in the range of a fasting plasma glucose concentration between 100 to 140 mg/dl and a two-hour postprandial plasma glucose level between 100 to 200 mg/dl.

TREATMENT OF TYPE I DIABETES

By definition, type I diabetics require insulin therapy. Nevertheless, dietary treatment is also an important part of the management of IDDM.

Diet

Dietary therapy for type I diabetics attempts to maintain consistency in the timing and caloric content of meals and to furnish a diet that will diminish the risks of vascular disease. In patients treated with intermediate or long-acting insulin, the timing of meals must be coordinated with the action of insulin. If meals are delayed or missed or are substantially smaller than usual, the chances of hypoglycemia are increased. Conversely, meals much larger than usual can result in hyperglycemia. Consistency in the timing and caloric content of meals allows an insulin regimen to be tailored to suit the particular patient's lifestyle. If consistency in meal patterns is impossible, the goal of good control will not be achievable using intermediate or long-acting insulins alone, but may require additional rapid-acting insulin prior to and proportional to the meal.

To diminish the risk of vascular disease, all diabetic patients should be placed on a diet low in fat (less than 30 per cent of the total caloric content should be lipids) with a polyunsaturated-to-saturated fat ratio of at least 1:1 and with a low cholesterol content (less than 350 mg/day). Therefore, the recommended "diabetic" diet is between 25 and 30 per cent lipid, 50 and 60 per cent carbohydrate, and 10 and 20 per cent protein. Diets containing this percentage of carbohydrate are no longer believed to be detrimental to diabetic control. It is hoped that such a diet will reduce blood lipid levels and thereby decrease the risk of macrovascular disease.

The role of dietary fiber in the diabetic diet is unresolved. Large quantities of dietary fiber tend to slow the rate of carbohydrate absorption and lower serum lipid levels. Patients should be encouraged, therefore, to incorporate foods with a high fiber content into their diets.

The effect of simple sugars and complex carbohydrates on blood glucose levels is currently being re-evaluated. Simple sugars ingested with meals do not, as previously thought, adversely affect blood glucose levels. All complex carbohydrates cannot be grouped together, because the glycemic response to different starches varies greatly. When incorporated into meals, various complex carbohydrates may also have significantly different effects on blood glucose levels. As a result, definitive recommendations regarding simple and complex carbohydrates must await further data.

Insulin

The various insulins currently in use differ in their time course of action, degree of purity, and source (Table 73–5). The time of the peak effect of insulin and the duration of action of insulin may vary a great deal from patient to patient. Even in a particular patient the absorption of subcutaneous insulin can vary

TABLE 73–5. INSULIN PREPARATIONS

TYPE	PROTEIN ADDITIVE	PEAK ACTION (hours)	DURATION OF ACTION (hours)
Rapid			
Regular	None	2–4	6–8
Semilente	None	2–6	10–12
Intermediate			
NPH	Protamine	6–12	18–24
Lente	None	6–12	18–24
Long-acting			
Protamine zinc	Protamine	14–24	36
Ultralente	None	18–24	36

from site to site and from day to day. For example, exercise of an extremity injected with insulin can increase the speed of insulin absorption and contribute to exercise-induced hypoglycemia. Most insulin-dependent patients require between 20 and 60 units of insulin per day. A requirement of greater than 200 units of insulin per day indicates insulin resistance, which can be due to a variety of factors, including circulating antibodies that bind insulin.

The indications for highly purified insulins or human insulin in the treatment of diabetes are currently unresolved. Insulin resistance secondary to antibodies, allergic reactions to insulin, and lipodystrophy should be treated with either highly purified pork insulin or human insulin. Some physicians believe that all patients who are going to be intermittently treated with insulin should be treated with human insulin to decrease the possibility of the future development of antibodies. Additionally, some physicians start all new patients on either human or purified pork insulin, but the clinical advantage for this practice has not yet been shown.

Rather than using rigid recipes, it is far better to tailor the insulin regimen for each individual patient. The degree of glycemic control desired, the time of insulin action, the timing and size of meals, and the preferences of the individual patient are all factors that will determine the appropriate insulin regimen.

As one approach, patients of normal weight who have IDDM can be started on a single morning dose of intermediate insulin (approximately 20 to 25 units 30 to 45 minutes before breakfast) with close following of their plasma glucose levels. If glucose values are uniformly elevated, the morning insulin dose can be slowly increased (approximately 5 units every other day) until glucose levels are lowered. In the occasional patient in whom plasma glucose levels measured at 7 AM, 11 AM, 4 PM, and 9 PM are all within an acceptable range, this single daily dose of intermediate insulin suffices. More commonly, glucose levels are decreased only for a particular portion of the day and more complex insulin regimens are required. If glucose levels are high early in the day but are in an acceptable range later in the day (late-acting insulin), a short-acting insulin should be added in the morning. Conversely, if control is reasonable early in the day but glucose levels are not acceptable later in the day (early-acting insulin), a second injection of intermediate insulin is indicated in the afternoon. Further refinements in the insulin regimen can be carried out based on additional glucose measurements.

The type, dose, and timing of the insulin given should be based on the patient's response and not on a preconceived ideal. Furthermore, an insulin regimen established for a particular patient is not fixed and will in all likelihood need adjustments with time. Changes in physical activity, growth status, or meal content and the use of other drugs or the advent of intercurrent illnesses or stresses will require adjustments in the insulin regimen. The physician and patient must constantly monitor the diabetic control and be prepared to make changes as indicated.

Intensive insulin treatment programs are sometimes used. The administration of regular insulin delivered via an insulin pump in carefully selected patients has resulted in excellent control. In this regimen, continuous regular insulin is given subcutaneously at a basal rate, supplemented by an additional bolus of regular insulin prior to meals. Another intensive treatment regimen involves the use of very long-acting ultralente insulin (basal insulin delivery) and injections of regular insulin prior to each meal. This regimen can also result in the normalization of blood glucose levels. Success with either of these regimens requires a highly motivated and educated patient who is dedicated to the achievement of excellent control. Ultimately it may be possible to transplant functioning islet cells or whole pancreas and thereby ameliorate the diabetic state. Currently this approach remains promising but experimental.

Complications of Insulin Therapy. The major complication of insulin therapy is hypoglycemia. The symptoms and signs of hypoglycemia are listed in Table 74–1. Occasional mild episodes of hypoglycemia, especially if due to an identifiable cause such as increased exercise or delaying a meal, are not indications for altering the insulin regimen. However, frequent mild hypoglycemic reactions or a severe reaction is unacceptable and requires an alteration in insulin treatment. The ability of some diabetics to recover from hypoglycemia is seriously impaired. In normal individuals, the secretion of glucagon is chiefly responsible for the recovery from hypoglycemia. In the absence of glucagon the secretion of epinephrine can result in a relatively normal recovery. In some diabetics, especially those with long-standing diabetes and autonomic insufficiency, the release of these two counter-regulatory hormones is impaired and recovery from hypoglycemia is absent or sluggish.

Hypoglycemia will occasionally result in rebound hyperglycemia, perhaps due to excessive secretion of counter-regulatory hormones (the Somogyi phenomenon). Characteristically, unrecognized nocturnal hypoglycemia may result in morning hyperglycemia. If the insulin dose is increased, the frequency of hypoglycemia is increased, resulting in a paradoxical worsening of the morning hyperglycemia. The appropriate therapy is to decrease the insulin dose. The Somogyi phenomenon should be considered in a poorly controlled diabetic.

A variety of local and systemic allergic reactions occur occasionally with insulin administration, but the frequency of these reactions has decreased with the use of purified insulins. Similarly, lipoatrophy at the injection site is only rarely observed with purified insulin. Lipohypertrophy secondary to the lipogenic effects of insulin occasionally occurs, but it can be prevented by rotating injection sites.

TREATMENT OF TYPE II DIABETES

In patients with NIDDM, diet therapy is of greatest importance. If diet does not satisfactorily control blood glucose levels, the use of oral hypoglycemic agents or insulin is indicated. The choice of an oral hypoglycemic drug or insulin will depend on many factors, including the degree of hyperglycemia, the social and economic situation, the relative risks and dangers of hypoglycemia, and the personal preferences of the patient and physician.

Diet

The majority of type II patients are obese; the main goal of diet therapy is therefore weight loss. A diet restricted in calories usually results in a marked amelioration of the patient's hyperglycemia. This effect on blood glucose levels can occur even before significant weight loss is achieved. In some cases, a reduction in caloric intake will result in a normalization of fasting plasma glucose concentrations.

A wide variety of different diets has been advocated for inducing weight loss. The success rate of long-term weight loss is very poor in both the general population and in patients with NIDDM. It is crucial that the physician stress to the patient the important relationship between food intake and diabetic control. Occasionally, a short hospitalization with strict dietary supervision will convince the patient that caloric restriction can greatly improve their metabolic control. In thin, type II patients calories should not be restricted. The diet of all patients with NIDDM should be limited in fat and cholesterol, with an increased ratio of polyunsaturated to saturated fats.

Oral Hypoglycemic Drugs

A substantial number of patients with type II diabetes do not attain successful metabolic control with dietary therapy alone. In these patients, the use of an oral hypoglycemic agent in conjunction with diet is the next therapeutic step. There are several different oral hypoglycemic agents available in this country (Table 73–6). The main difference between these sulfonylureas is their duration of action and the mode by which they are metabolized and excreted. While they exhibit a wide range of potency, no specific sulfonylurea, including the "second generation" drugs, has been shown to be any more effective in lowering blood glucose levels. The sulfonylureas lower blood glucose levels by enhancing insulin secretion by the beta cells of the pancreas and/or by increasing the sensitivity of tissues to the metabolic effects of insulin.

The major complication of oral hypoglycemic drug therapy is hypoglycemia, most frequently observed with long-acting agents such as chlorpropamide. Elderly patients, those who abuse ethanol, and those with either renal or hepatic disease are most likely to become hypoglycemic. Some diabetics, especially those receiving chlorpropamide, develop an antabuse-like intolerance to alcohol, with flushing. Idiosyncratic reactions may occur with gastrointestinal symptoms, diffuse skin rashes, cholestatic jaundice, agranulocytosis, and aplastic anemia, but these adverse reactions are very rare. Chlorpropamide potentiates the secretion and/or the action of ADH and therefore can result in water retention and hyponatremia, especially in patients with congestive heart failure or cirrhosis.

Insulin

Some patients with NIDDM require insulin therapy. Acceptable metabolic control may not be achievable with oral hypoglycemic agents (primary failure) or a patient who initially responded to oral agents may, with time, no longer achieve adequate control (secondary failure). Additionally, in some type II diabetic patients who are thin and have had very high blood glucose levels, it may be preferable to treat initially with insulin because these patients, in general, do not do well with other treatments. In fact, some such patients may really have type I diabetes as evidenced by the presence of islet cell or insulin antibodies prior to their having received insulin therapy.

The use of insulin in type II diabetes is similar to that described in type I patients above, except that because of the presence of insulin resistance, higher doses of insulin are frequently required. Additionally, because of some residual endogenous insulin secretion, NIDDM patients are more likely to be well-controlled on simpler regimens, such as a single daily dose of an intermediate insulin, than are patients with IDDM.

MONITORING DIABETIC CONTROL

Traditionally, diabetic control has been monitored by measuring urine glucose concentration at various times throughout the day. The concentration of glucose in the urine is dependent on the renal threshold for glucose excretion (quite variable in the diabetic patient), the renal blood flow, and the urine volume.

TABLE 73–6.   ORAL HYPOGLYCEMIC DRUGS

GENERIC NAME	BRAND NAME	DAILY DOSE (mg)	DOSES/DAY	DURATION OF EFFECT (hours)
Tolbutamide	Orinase	500–3000	2–3	6–12
Chlorpropamide	Diabinese	100–500	1	60
Acetohexamide	Dymelor	250–1500	1–2	12–24
Tolazamide	Tolinase	100–1000	1–2	10–18
Glyburide	Micronase Diabeta	2.5–20	1–2	10–30
Glipizide	Glucotrol	5–40	1–2	18–30

As a result, the correlation between urine glucose values and blood glucose measurements has generally been poor. Additionally, because the renal threshold for plasma glucose is approximately 180 mg/dl, urinary glucose measurements are negative when the plasma glucose is less than 180 mg/dl and, therefore, one cannot determine the degree of control in the glucose range that is most important.

Home blood glucose monitoring, employing a variety of different techniques, is the method of choice for monitoring diabetic control. Patients are instructed to measure their blood glucose levels at various times throughout the day as a basis for therapy. The accurate and routine measurement of home blood glucose levels is an essential ingredient in any intensive treatment regimen.

The measurement of glycosylated hemoglobin is very useful in assessing the degree of control over the preceding several months. Nonenzymatic glycosylation of hemoglobin is proportional to and therefore reflects average blood glucose experienced by the red blood cell during its lifespan. In normals, approximately 5 to 8 per cent of the hemoglobin is glycosylated, whereas in diabetics, as much as 20 per cent is in the glycosylated form. With tight control, the percentage of hemoglobin that is glycosylated will decrease and approach that in normal subjects. Glycosylated hemoglobin measurements, while useful in giving an overall picture of metabolic control, are *not* helpful in making specific adjustments in insulin therapy.

Lastly, quantitative measurement of glucose in 24-hour urine samples has been used to assess diabetic control. The excretion of less than 10 gm of glucose per day is indicative of excellent control.

ACUTE COMPLICATIONS

Diabetic Ketoacidosis

Pathophysiology. Diabetic ketoacidosis is characterized by hyperglycemia, acidosis (pH < 7.2, $HCO_3^- < 15$ mEq/L), and elevated plasma ketone concentrations. The hyperglycemia is secondary to insulin deficiency, which leads to both an increase in hepatic glucose production and a decrease in peripheral glucose utilization. Hyperglycemia produces an osmotic diuresis that can result in volume depletion and urinary loss of electrolytes.

Plasma ketone levels rise because of their overproduction by the liver. In the insulin-deficient state, especially if there is an increased secretion of catecholamines, excessive amounts of free fatty acids are released from the adipose tissue and transported to the liver. In the liver, free fatty acids can either be re-esterified or enter the mitochondria and be oxidized to ketones. In patients with hypoinsulinemia and hyperglucagonemia, fatty acids preferentially enter the mitochondria at an accelerated rate, resulting in an increased production of ketones. Thus, ketosis requires both an increased delivery of free fatty acids to the liver and a liver that is primed to transport them

into the mitochondria. Low plasma insulin levels, in conjunction with elevations in glucagon and other hormones, can result in both of these conditions and thus account for the ketosis. The accompanying acidosis results from the accumulation of β-hydroxybutyrate and acetoacetate, and is associated with low serum bicarbonate levels and an anion gap.

Clinical and Laboratory Presentation. Patients with diabetic ketoacidosis usually present after several days of polyuria and polydipsia with associated progressive nausea, vomiting, anorexia, and occasionally abdominal pain. The abdominal pain can sometimes mimic an acute abdominal condition. Diabetic ketoacidosis occurs in both young and old diabetic patients and may be the presenting manifestation of the disease. Infections, trauma, cardiovascular events, emotional stress, and omission of insulin are common precipitating causes, but in some cases there is no obvious etiology for the diabetic ketoacidosis. In all patients with diabetic ketoacidosis a careful search for the precipitating factor is required.

Patients with diabetic ketoacidosis typically exhibit tachypnea, dehydration, acetone halitosis (a fruity odor on the breath), and an altered mental status ranging from disorientation to coma. The alteration in mental status correlates directly with elevations in the serum osmolality. Kussmaul respirations are usually present when the acidosis is severe.

The clinical diagnosis of diabetic ketoacidosis should be confirmed by demonstrating elevations in blood glucose levels, ketones in the blood or urine, and acidosis. The blood glucose levels can be quite variable, ranging from 200 mg/dl to values greater than 1000 mg/dl. Blood and urine ketones are usually measured semiquantitatively by using Keto-Diastix or Ace-test tablets. Both of these methods detect primarily acetoacetate (the nitroprusside reaction). In ketoacidosis, β-hydroxybutyrate levels are higher than the acetoacetate levels, and thus the actual degree of ketosis is not accurately measured by the nitroprusside reaction. In patients with concomitant lactic acidosis or ethanol intake, β-hydroxybutyrate levels are much higher than acetoacetate levels, and the routine tests for ketosis can be falsely low. Additionally, during the course of treatment of diabetic ketoacidosis, β-hydroxybutyrate may be converted to acetoacetate, giving the false impression that the diabetic ketoacidosis is worsening.

Treatment. In the treatment of diabetic ketoacidosis the clinical status must be frequently and carefully assessed. A complete flow sheet, including fluids, electrolytes, and insulin administered, as well as laboratory data, is mandatory in monitoring therapy.

Many insulin regimens have been successfully used in the treatment of diabetic ketoacidosis, varying from continuous intravenous insulin to intermittent boluses of intramuscular or subcutaneous insulin. In the majority of patients, 5 to 10 units of regular insulin/hour given by a continuous intravenous infusion or by intermittent intramuscular or subcutaneous injections are adequate to correct the metabolic disturbance. In patients who are hypotensive, intravenous administration of the insulin is desirable because the absorption of the insulin may be impaired by poor tissue perfusion. Regardless of the route of administration and dosage, it is important to follow closely the decline in blood glucose levels. If the blood glucose concentrations are not decreasing, one should increase the insulin dosage and strongly consider employing the intravenous route.

Patients with diabetic ketoacidosis are virtually always dehydrated and hypovolemic. The average fluid deficit in adults is approximately 6 liters. Rapid volume expansion is usually required; this is best begun by administering normal saline at a rate of 1 liter/hour. In patients with cardiovascular or renal disease, slower rates of administration may be necessary. After the delivery of 2 liters of normal saline, if there are no signs of orthostatic hypotension, the rate of fluid administration can be decreased and the solution switched to half-normal saline. The remainder of the fluid deficit should be replaced over the next 12 to 24 hours.

On initial evaluation, many patients with diabetic ketoacidosis are hyperkalemic because of acidosis, dehydration, and hypoinsulinemia, but total body potassium stores are usually depleted. With correction of the acidosis and dehydration and the administration of insulin, plasma potassium concentrations will decrease. To prevent hypokalemia, it is very important to administer potassium in the intravenous fluids (20 to 40 mEq KCl per liter) as soon as urine flow is established and renal function is adequate. This is even more important if the patient presents with normal or low levels of serum potassium.

Phosphate depletion also occurs in diabetic ketoacidosis, but its replacement has not been shown to have a beneficial clinical effect. Therefore, the routine administration of phosphate is not indicated unless an additional disorder that also depletes body phosphate stores is present. Bicarbonate replacement also should not routinely be administered to patients with diabetic ketoacidosis unless the patient is severely acidotic (pH < 6.9).

Once the plasma glucose is in the range of 250 mg/dl, glucose should be included in the intravenous fluids to prevent hypoglycemia. Insulin administration should not be discontinued when the glucose falls because this will result in the recurrence of diabetic ketoacidosis. When the acidosis has cleared, the dehydration has been corrected, and the patient is eating, it is possible to return to the usual diabetic treatment schedules.

The major complications of the treatment of diabetic ketoacidosis are (1) hypoglycemia, (2) hypokalemia, and (3) cerebral edema. Both the hypoglycemia and hypokalemia can be prevented by careful management. Cerebral edema is very rare, is usually observed in children, and may occur because of the too-rapid correction of the metabolic disturbance.

Nonketotic Hyperosmolar Syndrome

This disorder occurs primarily in type II diabetics who present with dehydration, hypovolemia, and cerebral symptoms ranging from confusion to coma.

Blood glucose levels are markedly elevated (600 to 2000 mg/dl), but ketosis and acidosis are usually not present. The absence of significant ketosis may be secondary to residual insulin secretion sufficient to suppress lipolysis. The symptoms of poorly controlled diabetes have frequently been present for several days to weeks prior to presentation, and the acute decompensation is often secondary to an inability to consume adequate quantities of water, which may be precipitated by infection, stroke, myocardial infarction, abdominal disorder, etc. In the absence of sufficient water replacement, the hyperglycemia-induced osmotic diuresis results in dehydration, hypovolemia, impaired renal function, and decreased renal glucose excretion, which further increases plasma glucose levels. The decreased renal function associated with aging, especially in the diabetic, makes these patients more susceptible to develop the syndrome.

Similar to diabetic ketoacidosis, the alterations in mental status are believed to be secondary to the high serum osmolality. Stupor and coma occur only when the effective serum osmolality is greater than 340 mOsm/liter [effective serum osmolality = 2(Na + K) + glucose/18]. If the effective serum osmolality is not in this range, another etiology for the change in mental status should be sought.

The therapy of the hyperosmolar syndrome is very similar to that for diabetic ketoacidosis, with the administration of insulin, fluids, and potassium being the chief priorities. Patients with the hyperosmolar syndrome have a substantial mortality that is usually secondary to concomitant medical disorders such as myocardial infarction, stroke, infection, pulmonary emboli, etc.

CHRONIC COMPLICATIONS
(Table 73–7)

The chronic complications of diabetes can be divided into three main categories: (1) Microvascular dis-

TABLE 73–7. CHRONIC COMPLICATIONS OF DIABETES

Microvascular Disease
  Retinopathy
  Nephropathy
Macrovascular Disease
  Coronary artery disease
  Cerebrovascular disease
  Peripheral vascular disease
Neuropathic
  Peripheral symmetrical polyneuropathy
  Mononeuropathies
  Autonomic neuropathies
  Diabetic amyotrophy
Foot Ulcers
Dermopathies
Infections
  Gingival
  Dermal
  Vulvovaginal

ease, which is specific for diabetes, involves small blood vessels and is clinically manifested by eye and kidney disease. (2) Macrovascular disease, which involves the large blood vessels and is clinically manifested by coronary, cerebral, and peripheral vascular disease. The macrovascular disease is similar to that observed in nondiabetics but with a greater tendency to affect the extremities, especially the legs and feet. (3) Neuropathy, which can affect motor, sensory, cranial, and autonomic nerves. The diabetic is also particularly susceptible to develop foot ulcers as well as certain skin lesions especially of the legs, known as necrobiosis lipoidica diabeticorum, and diabetic dermopathy.

DIABETIC MICROANGIOPATHY

Eye

Diabetic retinopathy can be classified as *nonproliferative retinopathy* (background) or *proliferative retinopathy*. Nonproliferative retinopathy is characterized by microaneurysms, hard waxy exudates, cotton-wool or soft exudates, and retinal hemorrhages. Nonproliferative retinopathy is very common, and its frequency increases with the duration of diabetes. By 10 years, approximately 50 per cent and by 20 years, approximately 90 per cent of diabetics have nonproliferative retinopathy. Nonproliferative retinopathy usually does not impair vision and, in many diabetics, remains relatively stable.

In a small percentage of diabetics, nonproliferative retinopathy progresses to proliferative retinopathy. Proliferative retinopathy is characterized by neovascularization (new vessel formation), which can result in vitreous hemorrhages and traction retinal detachments that lead to severe visual loss or blindness. The incidence of proliferative retinopathy increases with the duration of diabetes. Approximately 25 per cent of type I diabetics develop proliferative retinopathy after 20 years of disease. Laser photocoagulation, the main treatment of proliferative retinopathy, can greatly decrease the incidence of visual loss.

Macular edema, which is due to the accumulation of intraretinal fluid secondary to breakdown of the blood/brain barrier, can result in a marked impairment of central vision. Macular edema is a common cause of visual loss in elderly diabetics. Laser therapy is also beneficial in the treatment of this type of diabetic eye disease.

Other nonmicroangiopathic disorders, such as cataracts and glaucoma, occur more frequently in patients with diabetes and can adversely affect visual acuity.

Kidney Disease

Diabetic nephropathy usually occurs between 15 and 20 years after the onset of diabetes in approximately 50 per cent of insulin-dependent diabetics. In non–insulin-dependent diabetics nephropathy occurs more rarely. The clinical manifestations and treatment of diabetic nephropathy are discussed in detail in Chapter 31.

The diagnosis of diabetic nephropathy is usually ob-vious; renal biopsy is rarely required. An active urinary sediment, the absence of retinopathy, or an atypical clinical course are indications for renal biopsy. Contrast studies, such as intravenous pyelography, should not be routinely conducted without clear indications, since rapid deterioration of renal function has been observed in azotemic diabetic patients following such studies. When a contrast study is necessary, diabetic patients should be well-hydrated prior to the procedure.

In any diabetic with renal failure, it is important to consider other factors that could be contributing to the renal dysfunction. The possibility of a neurogenic bladder secondary to diabetic neuropathy, urinary tract infections, uncontrolled hypertension, or renal papillary necrosis needs to be considered. Renal failure, regardless of etiology, tends to decrease the daily insulin requirement, and therefore the treatment regimen may need to be adjusted.

MACROVASCULAR DISEASE

Arteriosclerosis is a common problem in diabetics and occurs more extensively and earlier than in the general population. The etiology of the accelerated atherosclerosis in diabetics is unknown, but the causes are probably multifactorial. Because of the high risk of atherosclerosis, the usual risk factors for vascular disease must be aggressively treated. Diabetic patients should be strongly encouraged to stop smoking, and hypertension, if present, should be carefully treated. Elevated plasma lipid levels are frequently observed in diabetic patients, and efforts should be made to reduce them. Plasma lipid levels will frequently improve with control of the hyperglycemia. In populations such as Japan, with a low incidence of atherosclerosis, the incidence of vascular disease in diabetic patients is much lower than in the United States, suggesting that the amelioration of other risk factors will be very beneficial.

Atherosclerotic vascular disease in diabetic patients affects the coronary, cerebral, and peripheral vessels, and the manifestations of vascular disease are similar to those observed in nondiabetics. There is a tendency for the vascular disease to be more diffuse in diabetics, making vascular reconstructive surgery more difficult. Nevertheless, the indications for vascular surgery and the success of vascular surgery are not significantly different than in the nondiabetic population.

NEUROPATHY

Diabetic neuropathy is a common disabling complication of diabetes, resulting in a great deal of morbidity and a reduced quality of life. Diabetic neuropathy may be classified into four main categories:

Symmetrical Distal Polyneuropathy

This form of neuropathy is the most common and usually presents with a loss of sensation in a "stocking-glove" distribution that is most commonly observed bilaterally in the distal lower extremities but can also affect the upper extremities. The decreased sensory perception may result in neuropathic foot ulcers or Charcot joints. Rarely, proprioception can be so severely diminished that patients have difficulty walking in the dark. Frequently, in addition to the lack of sensation, there is associated numbness, tingling, a "pins-and-needles" sensation, burning, cramping, or shooting pains. The pain and discomfort that occur in association with diabetic neuropathy can be very disabling and are often worse at night. In most instances, the pain spontaneously disappears in six months to one year. The pain associated with neuropathy has been treated with variable success with phenytoin, carbamazepine, or a combination of amitriptyline and fluphenazine. In addition to sensory nerve dysfunction, symmetrical motor nerve abnormalities can occur and are often manifested by bilateral wasting of the interosseous muscles of the hand. This polyneuropathy and the autonomic neuropathies described below are thought to be secondary to the metabolic abnormalities of diabetes.

Autonomic Neuropathy

Diabetic autonomic neuropathy has a wide variety of clinical manifestations affecting a number of different organs. Most patients with significant autonomic neuropathies also have symmetrical distal polyneuropathies.

Impotence is a common manifestation of autonomic neuropathy but, of course, is often due to other etiologies, such as vascular insufficiency, psychological causes, or endocrinological dysfunction. A neurogenic bladder with associated urinary retention and urinary tract infections is another very troublesome complication. Orthostatic hypotension occurs secondary to autonomic neuropathies and can be disabling if severe. The entire gastrointestinal tract can be affected by autonomic nerve dysfunction, resulting in dysphagia, gastroparesis, intermittent diarrhea, especially with postprandial and nocturnal discharge, constipation, and anal incontinence. Gastroparesis can result in poor diabetic control because of the erratic food absorption. Abnormal sweating, manifested by anhidrosis or hyperhidrosis, is also sometimes observed.

Asymmetrical Neuropathy

While the polyneuropathies usually appear late in the course of established diabetes, mononeuropathies often occur in mild diabetes or prior to the diagnosis of diabetes. Diabetic mononeuropathies can involve cranial nerves III, IV, or VI, resulting in extraocular muscle paralysis with diplopia. The most common syndrome is a third nerve palsy with sparing of the pupillary reflex, which distinguishes this condition from compressive neuropathies of the oculomotor nerve such as that caused by a carotid aneurysm. The onset is usually abrupt, and pain around the eye frequently occurs. Findings are occasionally bilateral, and more than one cranial nerve can be involved. Spontaneous recovery generally occurs in 3 to 12 months, but recurrences are not uncommon.

Peripheral nerve mononeuropathies usually occur at sites of external pressure and can result in wrist or foot drop. Mononeuropathies can also affect sensory nerves and result in painful dysesthesias and hypesthesias localized to the anatomical distribution of the nerve. Similar to the mononeuropathies affecting the cranial nerves, these neuropathies frequently remit spontaneously in several weeks to months. These mononeuropathies are thought to be due to a vascular insult.

Diabetic Amyotrophy

Diabetic amyotrophy is a type of neuropathy that occurs mainly in elderly men and most commonly presents with unilateral atrophy and weakness of the large muscle groups of the upper leg and pelvic girdle. Pain localized to the involved muscle groups may be present and the patellar reflex may be lost. The neuropathy on occasion can be bilateral and/or affect the upper extremity. In addition to the neuropathy, marked weight loss and depression are frequently observed. In the majority of cases, recovery occurs spontaneously in 6 to 12 months.

FOOT ULCERS

Foot ulcers can occur in diabetic patients secondary to large vessel atherosclerosis, microangiopathy, neuropathy, or a combination of these factors. Ulcers secondary to large vessel disease characteristically occur on the tip of the toes, whereas those secondary to neuropathy occur in areas of weight-bearing and pressure (plantar surface).

The best therapy of diabetic foot ulcers is prevention. Patients with diabetes should be instructed to examine their feet daily for calluses, blisters, or inflammation, and their feet should be kept clean and dry. In addition, the shoes of a diabetic should be properly fitted and patients should be instructed to wear new shoes for short periods of time until well broken-in. Walking barefoot is dangerous and should be strongly discouraged. Meticulous foot care can decrease the incidence of ulcers and gangrene and prevent amputations. If an ulcer occurs, treatment includes bed rest, elevation of the foot, and debridement. If there is evidence of infection, cultures, including anaerobic cultures, should be obtained. Initial antibiotic therapy needs to be effective against gram-positive, gram-negative, and anaerobic bacteria, with further therapy guided by the culture results.

REFERENCES

Brownlee M, Cerami A, Vlassara H: Advanced glycosylation end products in tissue and the biochemical basis of diabetic complications. N Engl J Med 318:1315, 1988.

Feingold KR: Hypoglycemia: A pitfall of insulin therapy. West J Med 139;688, 1983.

Foster DW, McGarry JD: The metabolic derangements and treatment of diabetic ketoacidosis. N Engl J Med 309:159, 1983.

National Diabetes Data Group. Classification and diagnosis of diabetes mellitus and other categories of glucose intolerance. Diabetes 28:1039, 1979.

Nutall FQ: Diet and the diabetic patient. Diabetes Care 6:197, 1983.

Olefsky JM: Diabetes mellitus. In Wyngaarden JB, Smith LH Jr (eds): Cecil Textbook of Medicine. 18th ed. Philadelphia, WB Saunders Co, 1988, pp 1360–1381.

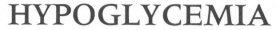

74

HYPOGLYCEMIA

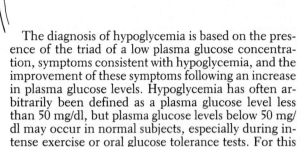

The diagnosis of hypoglycemia is based on the presence of the triad of a low plasma glucose concentration, symptoms consistent with hypoglycemia, and the improvement of these symptoms following an increase in plasma glucose levels. Hypoglycemia has often arbitrarily been defined as a plasma glucose level less than 50 mg/dl, but plasma glucose levels below 50 mg/dl may occur in normal subjects, especially during intense exercise or oral glucose tolerance tests. For this reason, oral glucose tolerance tests are not an appropriate procedure for the diagnosis of hypoglycemia. Furthermore, in a significant percentage of healthy young women (but rarely in men) a 24-hour fast also results in a plasma glucose level below 50 mg/dl. Therefore, in men a *fasting* plasma glucose less than 45 to 50 mg/dl is highly suspicious of significant hypoglycemia, whereas in women the fasting plasma glucose may be below 45 mg/dl after a prolonged fast.

Plasma glucose levels should be interpreted in relation to a patient's symptoms. During a 5-hour oral glucose tolerance test at least 10 per cent of normal individuals have plasma glucose levels less than 50 mg/dl, but few are symptomatic. Conversely, many patients have symptoms resembling those observed with hypoglycemia, even though the plasma glucose level is not below the "normal" range. Additionally, it is important to demonstrate that the symptoms, presumed to be secondary to hypoglycemia, improve or disappear soon after increases in plasma glucose following carbohydrate ingestion. Therefore *the triad of a low plasma glucose, symptoms consistent with hypoglycemia, and the improvement of these symptoms following an increase of plasma glucose concentration is necessary to confirm the diagnosis of hypoglycemia* (Whipple's triad).

TABLE 74–1. SYMPTOMS AND SIGNS OF HYPOGLYCEMIA

Secondary to Catecholamine Release (Adrenergic)

Sweating	Tremor
Shakiness	Hunger
Anxiety	Faintness
Palpitations	Tachycardia
Weakness	

Secondary to CNS Dysfunction (Neuroglucopenic)

Confusion	Diplopia
Irritability	Inappropriate affect
Headaches	Motor incoordination
Abnormal behavior	Convulsions
Weakness	Coma

Nocturnal Hypoglycemia (usually due to excessive insulin therapy)

Morning headaches	Difficulty in waking
Lassitude	Psychological changes
Night sweats	Restlessness during sleep
Nightmares	Loud respirations

(Symptoms do not usually awaken the patient.)

TABLE 74–2. CAUSES OF HYPOGLYCEMIA

Fasting
 Insulinoma
 Extrapancreatic tumors
 Hormonal deficiency—glucocorticoids, growth hormone, and epinephrine
 Chronic renal failure
 Extensive hepatic dysfunction
 Starvation
 Sepsis
 Drugs—insulin, oral hypoglycemic agents, ethanol, salicylates, propranolol, pentamidine, disopyramide, and quinine when used to treat malaria
 Disorders of childhood—glycogen storage diseases
 Immune disease with antibodies that bind insulin
 Antibodies that bind to insulin receptor
Postprandial
 Alimentary hypoglycemia
 Idiopathic reactive hypoglycemia
 Genetic disorders—galactosemia, fructose intolerance
Artifactual
 Leukemia
 Polycythemia

CLINICAL MANIFESTATIONS

The symptoms of hypoglycemia result from catecholamine release, from impaired CNS function, or both (Table 74–1). The degree of hypoglycemia that produces symptoms and the clinical manifestations produced are quite variable from individual to individual and from time to time. In a particular individual, the symptoms induced by hypoglycemia tend to be reproducible. The adrenergic symptoms may predominate when plasma glucose concentrations fall rapidly, whereas the cerebral manifestations of hypoglycemia may appear without the adrenergic warning when the decrease in plasma glucose levels occurs slowly or when hypoglycemia is a chronic problem. The symptoms and signs of hypoglycemia usually are rapidly reversible with treatment, but permanent brain damage can result from prolonged severe hypoglycemia.

CAUSES OF HYPOGLYCEMIA
(Table 74–2)

The classification of the causes of hypoglycemia is based on whether symptoms occur in the fasting state or following food intake (postprandial). An approach to the evaluation of patients suspected of having hypoglycemia is shown in Figure 74–1.

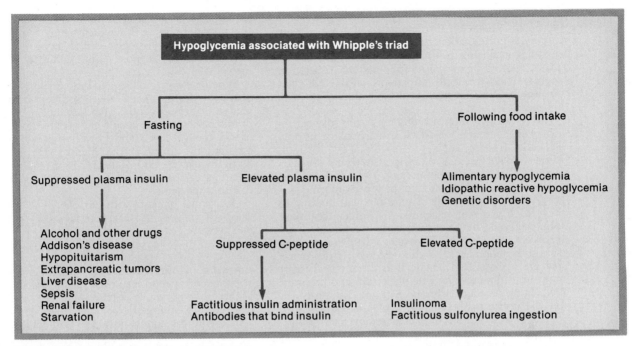

FIGURE 74–1. Evaluation of hypoglycemia.

FASTING HYPOGLYCEMIA

Insulinoma

Insulinomas are relatively rare tumors that occur most commonly between the ages of 40 and 70 years. Approximately 60 per cent of patients with an insulinoma are women. Between 5 and 10 per cent of insulinomas are malignant; in 10 per cent of cases multiple benign tumors are present. In patients with the multiple endocrine neoplasia type I (MEN I) syndrome, insulinomas occur at an earlier age and multiple benign tumors are very common. In these individuals a family history of other endocrine tumors is usually present.

The symptoms of hypoglycemia may be present for many years prior to the diagnosis of an insulinoma because the symptoms of chronic hypoglycemia are nonspecific and not initially attributed to hypoglycemia. Often the patients are thought to have a psychiatric or neurological disorder prior to the correct diagnosis. Patients sometimes increase their food consumption to prevent symptoms and, therefore, weight gain is occasionally observed.

The diagnosis of an insulinoma is based on the demonstration of a low plasma glucose level in the presence of an inappropriately high plasma insulin concentration. The most reliable test is a prolonged *supervised fast*. In normal individuals, fasting results in a decline in both plasma glucose and insulin levels. In the majority of patients with an insulinoma hypoglycemia occurs within 24 hours, but in a small number of patients a fast lasting 72 hours with or without exercise will be required to induce hypoglycemia. Plasma for insulin measurements should be obtained at the time the patient is hypoglycemic. In patients with an insulinoma, plasma insulin levels are inappropriately elevated. During the fast a patient suspected of harboring an insulinoma must be closely observed for symptoms of hypoglycemia, and if symptoms occur the plasma glucose must be rapidly determined and the fast terminated if the patient is hypoglycemic. Additionally, it is important to measure plasma glucose levels every four to six hours because patients with hypoglycemia may at times be asymptomatic.

In addition to determining plasma insulin levels, it is also helpful to measure plasma C-peptide concentrations during the fast to eliminate the possibility of self administration of insulin as the etiology of the hypoglycemia. In individuals who surreptitiously administer insulin, plasma C-peptide levels will be very low; in patients with an insulinoma, plasma C-peptide levels are elevated in parallel with insulin, reflecting its rate of secretion.

In the past many provocative maneuvers such as the use of glucagon, tolbutamide, leucine, or calcium were employed to diagnose patients with insulinomas. Currently, because of the high frequency of false-positive and false-negative results, these tests are only rarely used for this purpose.

Once the diagnosis of an insulinoma is firmly established, additional studies may be helpful in localizing the tumor within the pancreas. CT scans, ultrasonography, and pancreatic angiography have all been employed to localize the tumor. During angiography the tumors appear as vascular masses. Nevertheless, in some patients with insulinomas radiographic studies do not localize the insulinoma. In some centers percutaneous transhepatic portal venography with selective blood sampling for insulin measurement may be useful in the localization of insulinomas. However, failure to localize an insulinoma should not obviate surgery, since experienced surgeons are usually successful in localizing the tumor intraoperatively. Serum levels of HCG or one of its subunits are elevated in approximately two thirds of patients with a malignant insulinoma, but not in individuals with benign insulinomas.

The treatment of an insulinoma is the surgical removal of the tumor, which will usually restore normal glycemia. In approximately 5 to 10 per cent of individuals, hypoglycemia will persist following surgery, owing to metastatic insulinomas, islet cell hypertrophy, or a tumor that could not be located during surgery. These patients will require medical therapy to prevent hypoglycemic episodes. Initial treatment should include frequent high carbohydrate feedings. If this is not successful, diazoxide, a drug that inhibits insulin secretion, can be administered. Other drugs that are occasionally beneficial in the medical treatment of insulinomas include phenytoin and propranolol. Streptozotocin with or without 5-fluorouracil may be useful in the treatment of malignant insulinomas that cannot be completely removed surgically.

Extrapancreatic Tumors

Hypoglycemia also occurs secondary to a wide variety of neoplasms. Mesenchymal tumors or sarcomas located in the retroperitoneal spaces of the chest and abdomen are the tumors most commonly implicated and are usually very large and easily detectable. Hypoglycemia has also been described in association with hematologic malignancies, hepatomas, and adrenocortical, gastrointestinal, and pancreatic carcinomas.

The mechanism by which tumors cause hypoglycemia is unresolved and probably varies depending upon tumor type. Plasma insulin levels are low during hypoglycemia, indicating that ectopic insulin production by the tumor is not the cause of the hypoglycemia. In some instances, elevated levels of a substance that resembles nonsuppressible insulin-like activity (insulin-like growth factors) have been found, and it is possible that the production by the tumor of such hormones could account for the hypoglycemia. Other possible mechanisms for tumor-induced hypoglycemia include increased utilization of glucose by the tumor when there is a very large tumor burden; metastatic destruction of the liver, adrenals, or pituitary glands; the production of substances that inhibit hepatic glucose production; and generalized cachexia. Total or partial surgical removal of the tumor is the ideal treatment and usually results in the amelioration of the hypoglycemia. However, most of the tumors associated with hypoglycemia cannot be resected and, therefore, management must be directed toward increasing plasma glucose levels through frequent feedings, glucose infusions, and prednisone therapy.

Hepatic, Renal, and Endocrine Disease

Hypoglycemia secondary to liver disease, other than that due to hepatomas, is rare and is usually associated with massive hepatic necrosis. In order for hypoglycemia to occur as a result of liver disease, approximately 80 to 90 per cent of the liver must be dysfunctional, and therefore the hypoglycemia is frequently a premorbid event. Hypoglycemia that occurs in the setting of cirrhosis is most commonly due to ethanol ingestion.

In patients with Addison's disease hypoglycemia will occur with fasting. Adequate cortisol replacement prevents the hypoglycemia. Hypopituitarism, regardless of etiology, may also result in hypoglycemia because of low cortisol levels and impaired growth hormone production. Cortisol replacement prevents symptomatic hypoglycemia in adults, but in children hypoglycemia can still occur despite apparently adequate cortisol replacement.

Occasional patients with chronic renal failure develop hypoglycemia; this complication is observed most commonly in cachectic individuals.

Drug-Induced Hypoglycemia

Insulin. Insulin-induced hypoglycemia is a frequent occurrence in insulin-requiring diabetics. Most of these hypoglycemic reactions are mild and rapidly relieved by food ingestion. However, severe hypoglycemia requiring admission to the hospital is not infrequent. Moreover, death due to hypoglycemia occurs in approximately 2 to 7 per cent of insulin-dependent diabetics.

On rare occasions, a nondiabetic will surreptitiously take insulin and induce hypoglycemia. Most of these individuals are women who have been associated with the health professions. The presence of insulin antibodies in the plasma of a nondiabetic patient being evaluated for hypoglycemia is very suggestive of surreptitious insulin usage. The presence of antibodies to insulin will result in an artifactual elevation in plasma insulin levels when assayed in most radioimmunoassays. Additionally, as discussed earlier, the presence of hypoglycemia, high insulin levels, and a low C-peptide level indicates exogenous insulin administration as the etiology of hypoglycemia.

Oral Hypoglycemic Drugs. Hypoglycemia in diabetics on oral hypoglycemic drugs is much less common than in insulin-treated diabetic patients. Long-acting oral hypoglycemic agents such as chlorpropamide are more frequently associated with hypoglycemia than are short-acting agents such as tolbutamide. Severe hypoglycemia secondary to oral hypoglycemic agents occurs most commonly in elderly patients or in those who abuse ethanol or have renal or hepatic disease.

The surreptitious use of oral hypoglycemic agents can induce hypoglycemia in nondiabetics. In these cases, the insulin and C-peptide measurements are identical to those seen in patients with insulinomas. When oral agents are suspected as the cause of hypoglycemia in nondiabetics, either blood or urine should be assayed for the presence of these drugs.

Ethanol Ingestion. The syndrome of ethanol-induced hypoglycemia is most prevalent in chronically malnourished alcoholic males and occurs because ethanol inhibits hepatic gluconeogenesis. Nonalcoholics are also susceptible to ethanol-induced fasting hypoglycemia, which can occur with moderate ethanol intake in individuals who have missed one or two meals. Diabetics using insulin or oral hypoglycemics are particularly at risk for ethanol-induced hypoglycemia.

POSTPRANDIAL HYPOGLYCEMIA (*Reactive Hypoglycemia*)

True postprandial hypoglycemia is most commonly observed in patients who have undergone gastric surgery (alimentary hypoglycemia). The presumed mechanism is rapid gastric emptying with brisk glucose absorption and secretion of gastrointestinal hormones leading to excessive insulin release. Glucose is metabolized rapidly, but the insulin levels remain high, resulting in hypoglycemia approximately one to two hours postprandially. Very rarely alimentary hypoglycemia is present in patients who have not undergone gastric surgery. The elimination of simple sugars, especially beverages, from the diet and frequent small feedings usually results in an improvement of symptoms.

Diabetes mellitus in its earliest phases is frequently listed as a cause of reactive hypoglycemia, but this is not well-documented. Symptomatic hypoglycemia as a premonitory symptom of diabetes occurs very rarely, if at all.

Idiopathic postprandial hypoglycemia is a rare syndrome whose mechanism is unknown. Much more common are patients with "nonhypoglycemia," who have a wide variety of nonspecific symptoms that occur two to five hours after a meal. The lay press and misinformed physicians have often attributed these nonspecific symptoms to hypoglycemia. In some of these patients, oral glucose tolerance tests are performed and, just as in normal individuals without symptoms, occasionally low blood glucose levels are observed. Because of the high frequency in normal individuals of plasma glucose concentrations below 50 mg/dl during oral glucose tolerance tests, this procedure is not very helpful in attempting to diagnose postprandial hypoglycemia. It is far better to measure plasma glucose levels after meals that are similar to those that caused the symptoms in the individual under study. After these more typical test meals, hypoglycemia is not consistently observed in the majority of patients. Rarely, one will observe a patient in whom both symptoms and low plasma glucose levels occur simultaneously and consistently after a test meal. In these individuals idiopathic postprandial hypoglycemia is a reasonable diagnosis, and they should be treated with frequent small meals that are low in carbohydrate and high in protein. Much more commonly the symptoms attributed to hypoglycemia occur after the test meal but the plasma glucose levels are within the normal range. The explanation for these patients' symptoms may be related to adrenergic stimulation, but the symptoms should not be attributed to hypoglycemia.

TREATMENT OF SEVERE HYPOGLYCEMIA

In every unconscious patient hypoglycemia should be considered and blood should be obtained first for a glucose determination. The initial treatment of a confused or comatose patient is to infuse a bolus of 50 ml of 50 per cent glucose intravenously, after a sample for measuring glucose levels has been obtained. The bolus of glucose should be followed by the continuous infusion of 10 per cent glucose at a rate sufficient to keep the plasma glucose greater than 100 mg/dl. When the patient is capable of eating, a diet with a minimum of 300 gm/day of carbohydrates should be supplied. In many situations, especially following long-acting insulin or oral hypoglycemic drugs, the hypoglycemia will last for an extended period of time. It is very important to continue treatment and close observation for an extended period to prevent a relapse.

REFERENCES

Fajans SS, Floyd JC Jr: Diagnosis and medical management of insulinomas. Annu Rev Med 30:313, 1979.

Gastineau CF: Is reactive hypoglycemia a clinical entity? Mayo Clin Proc 58:545, 1983.

Merimee TJ: Spontaneous hypoglycemia in man. Adv Intern Med 22:301, 1977.

Nelson RL: Hypoglycemia: Fact or fiction. Mayo Clin Proc 60:844, 1985.

Service FJ: Hypoglycemic disorders. *In* Wyngaarden JB, Smith LH Jr (eds): Cecil Textbook of Medicine. 18th ed. Philadelphia, WB Saunders Co, 1988, pp 1381–1387.

DISEASES OF BONE AND BONE MINERAL METABOLISM

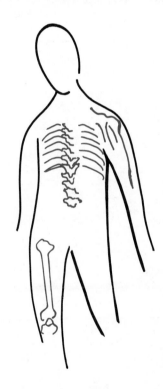

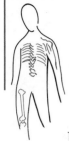

75

NORMAL PHYSIOLOGY OF BONE AND BONE MINERALS

BONE STRUCTURE AND METABOLISM

One of the largest organs in the body, bone is a living tissue that is superbly constructed to carry out the following vital functions: (1) to provide the necessary support to maintain the structures of the body, including the integrity of such specialized "containers" as the thorax and the cranium; (2) to allow for movement by providing levers, articulations, and points of attachment for muscles; (3) to provide a reservoir of simple but essential elements such as calcium, magnesium, phosphorus, and sodium; (4) to surround and protect the hematopoietic system.

Bone is about two thirds mineral, largely hydroxyapatite with the approximate formula $Ca_{10}(PO_4)_6(OH)_2$. This mineral phase is deposited with high specificity at certain sites in type I collagen, the major organic component of bone. In addition, bone contains water, various proteoglycans, and other noncollagenous proteins including osteocalcin, which contains a distinctive calcium-binding amino acid, γ-carboxyglutamic acid.

Bone Cells. At least three specialized cells in bone are necessary for the synthesis, modeling, and remodeling of this largely extracellular tissue (Fig. 75–1):

OSTEOBLASTS. These mesenchymal cells secrete the three chains that make up type I collagen to form

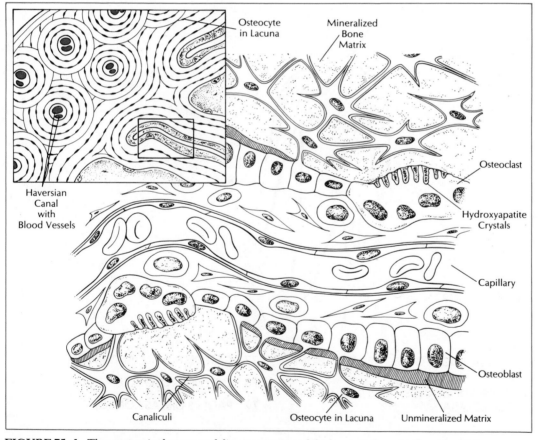

FIGURE 75–1. The most active bone remodeling occurs around the haversian canals, through which capillaries run. Osteoclasts and osteoblasts in all stages of development are found in greatest density in these areas. Larger-scale inset drawing depicts the syncytium-like layer of osteoblasts, connected with lacunar osteocytes via canaliculi, across which substances are exchanged between the modified bone interstitial fluid and the systemic ECF. (From Levine MM, Kleeman CR: Hypercalcemia: Pathophysiology and treatment. Hosp Pract 22:75, 1987.)

osteoid, the uncalcified precursor of bone, at the surface sites of growth or remodeling. It is probable that osteoblasts also influence the local availability of calcium and/or phosphate necessary for mineralization. Osteoblasts contain alkaline phosphatase, the function of which is not clear. It may serve to hydrolyze pyrophosphate locally, a potent inhibitor of mineralization. With increased activity of osteoblasts the level of serum alkaline phosphatase rises; the increase of the bone isozyme of alkaline phosphatase is used clinically as a marker for osteoblastic activity.

OSTEOCYTES. Osteocytes are thought to be relatively quiescent osteoblasts that have become entrapped within the structure of bone. They appear to communicate with one another and with surface osteoblasts as a network through bone canaliculi. They probably play a role in mobilizing bone minerals ("osteocytic osteolysis"), although the mechanisms involved are obscure.

OSTEOCLASTS. These multinucleated giant cells, derived from mononuclear phagocytic cells of hematopoietic origin, destroy bone as part of its continuous remodeling process. This complex process of destruction requires the removal of bone minerals followed by the action of collagenases and other proteolytic enzymes. Osteoclastic function is normally stimulated by parathyroid hormone (PTH) and probably by other factors as well: e.g., lymphokines (interleukin 1, tumor necrosis factor, transforming growth factor β) and prostaglandins of the E series. Heparin can also stimulate osteoclasts. Deficiency of osteoclastic activity results in osteopetrosis (marble bone disease), a serious disorder of increased bone density.

Types of Bone. Bone is complex and heterogeneous in structure and is designed to give maximal strength with minimal mass. In general there are two kinds of bone in the adult. *Cortical bone* is densely packed with concentric parallel layers of mineralized collagen surrounding its central vascular supply to form a unit known as an osteon or a haversian system (Fig. 75–1). This type of bone is predominant in the cortex of long bones. Cortical bone serves principally for support. *Trabecular bone*, also called cancellous bone, forms a more open, spongy pattern and is predominant in the axial skeleton. Both types of bone serve as calcium buffers for calcium homeostasis.

Bone Turnover. Even in the adult, bone is constantly being shaped and remodeled at its surfaces owing to the coordinated activities of osteoblasts, osteoclasts, and osteocytes, acting presumably under the influence of a number of exogenous factors, both known and unknown. As much as one fifth of bone calcium turns over annually, yet the destruction and formation of bone are normally closely coordinated. Bone biopsies demonstrate that in remodeling, destruction and synthesis occur simultaneously but at distinct sites. The balance between bone destruction and synthesis, which determines bone density, is influenced by stress on the bone through unknown mechanisms as well as by hormones.

Clinical Studies. Several techniques are available to study patients suspected of having generalized (metabolic) bone diseases:

1. Measurement of serum calcium, phosphorus, and alkaline phosphatase. The patterns of abnormalities discovered may give considerable information about the type of disorder, as will be documented later in the discussion of specific entities.

2. Measurement of parathyroid hormone and/or vitamin D, usually 25-OH-D. These measurements are usually obtained if abnormalities are noted in the tests mentioned above.

3. Studies of bone density. Routine radiographs of bone are notoriously insensitive for detecting generalized osteopenia but may demonstrate vertebral compression fractures in osteoporosis or pseudofractures (see below) in osteomalacia. More accurate methods for measuring bone density are quantitative CT scans of vertebral trabecular bone, dual photon absorptiometry (used primarily for axial skeleton), and single photon absorptiometry (used primarily for the study of peripheral cortical bone).

4. Studies of bone turnover. Examination of sections of undemineralized bone obtained by transiliac biopsy may demonstrate the relative activities of bone formation and destruction, especially when combined with the use of tetracycline given orally in advance at timed intervals. Tetracycline binds to recently mineralized bone, so the distance between bands is an indication of the rate of osteogenesis. As a research technique bone turnover can also be studied with isotopes such as $^{47}Ca^{++}$.

CALCIUM METABOLISM

A normal adult usually has 20 to 25 gm of calcium/kg of body weight, over 98 per cent of which is in the skeleton. Although our emphasis in this discussion is on bone formation, ionized calcium is also of great importance in many other functions, such as neuromuscular excitability, blood coagulation, and integrity of membranes, and as an intracellular second messenger for hormone action. Because of these various and important functions, the level of ionized calcium in extracellular fluid is carefully maintained in homeostasis.

Normal Plasma Calcium. Calcium circulates in plasma in three forms: (a) ionized as Ca^{++}, approximately 46 per cent, (b) protein-bound, approximately 46 per cent, largely to albumin, (c) diffusible but complexed, approximately 8 per cent (Fig. 75–2). Serum calcium is usually reported in the United States as its total concentration with a normal range of 8.9 to 10.1 mg/dl (2.2 to 2.5 mmol/L), rather than as a measurement of its biologically active ionized fraction. The bound fraction will vary as a percentage of total serum calcium based on the protein concentration and is often estimated as:

Per cent protein-bound calcium = 8 × albumin (gm/dl) + 2 × globulin (gm/dl) + 3

As a shorthand estimate, the serum calcium can be

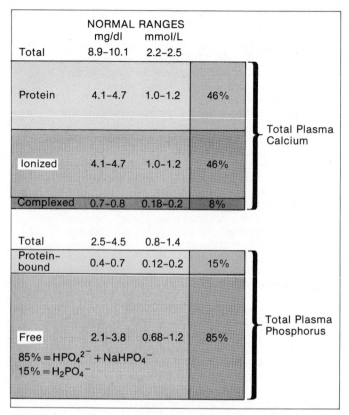

NORMAL RANGES			
	mg/dl	mmol/L	
Total	8.9–10.1	2.2–2.5	
Protein	4.1–4.7	1.0–1.2	46%
Ionized	4.1–4.7	1.0–1.2	46%
Complexed	0.7–0.8	0.18–0.2	8%
Total	2.5–4.5	0.8–1.4	
Protein-bound	0.4–0.7	0.12–0.2	15%
Free	2.1–3.8	0.68–1.2	85%

Total Plasma Calcium

Total Plasma Phosphorus

$85\% = HPO_4^{2-} + NaHPO_4^{-}$
$15\% = H_2PO_4^{-}$

FIGURE 75–2. Distribution and normal ranges of calcium and phosphorus in the plasma. (From Arnaud CD: Mineral and bone homeostasis. *In* Wyngaarden JB, Smith LH Jr (eds): Cecil Textbook of Medicine. 18th ed. Philadelphia, WB Saunders Co, 1988, p 1471.)

adjusted downward by 0.8 mg/dl for each 1 gm/dl decrease in serum albumin.

Absorption of Dietary Calcium. The average diet of an adult in the United States contains 600 to 1000 mg of calcium, in considerable measure derived from dairy products (milk has approximately 1 mg/ml). Usually there is a net absorption of 150 to 300 mg of calcium per day, in part by active transport in the proximal small intestine stimulated by 1,25-dihydroxycholecalciferol (Fig. 75–3). Calcium is present in all intestinal secretions (bile, pancreatic and gastric juices included), so that there is a fecal loss of about 100 mg of endogenous calcium per day. In general, calcium absorption is diminished in many generalized malabsorptive states (see Chapter 34C) as well as by hypovitaminosis D and dietary phytates. Absorption is increased by 1,25-dihydroxycholecalciferol, with excessive calcium ingestion (the "milk-alkali syndrome"), and in absorptive idiopathic hypercalciuria.

Excretion of Calcium. As noted, some endogenous calcium is secreted into the gut with a net fecal loss of about 100 mg. The primary route of excretion, however, is via the kidney. Over 50 per cent of plasma calcium (that fraction not bound to protein) is filterable by the glomerulus, representing 7 to 10 gm in the

glomerular filtrate per day. Only 100 to 250 mg of calcium are normally excreted in the urine, less than 4 mg/kg/24 hr, reflecting a net tubular reabsorption of about 98 per cent. Renal tubular reabsorption is enhanced by PTH, phosphate, metabolic alkalosis, thiazide diuretics, and enhanced reabsorption of sodium. Hypercalciuria may be caused by reduced PTH, metabolic acidosis, hypermagnesemia, loop diuretics, saline diuresis, and other variables.

Calcium Balance. The level of ionized calcium in the extracellular fluid and the integrity of bone mineral content are homeostatically maintained over years of varied calcium ingestion by an effective balance of bone formation, bone destruction, calcium absorption, and calcium excretion (Fig. 75–3). Some of the control mechanisms are known and will be described briefly below in separate sections (PTH, vitamin D, calcitonin); others are not. For convenience the symptoms and signs of hypercalcemia and hypocalcemia will be described in the chapter on the parathyroid glands (Chapter 76).

PHOSPHORUS METABOLISM

A normal adult usually has about 10 to 13 gm of phosphorus/kg of body weight (700 to 900 gm), of which about 80 to 85 per cent is in the skeleton and 10 per cent is in muscle. Phosphorus in the form of phosphate is necessary for a wide variety of structural and metabolic functions in addition to its role in bone mineralization: e.g., phospholipids in internal and external cell membranes, high-energy phosphate in energy capture and transfer ($\sim$P), as a second messenger in the endocrine system (cAMP), and as the backbone of DNA and RNA. Abnormalities of phosphorus metabolism can therefore lead to many manifestations.

Normal Plasma Phosphorus. In plasma the normal concentration of phosphorus is 2.5 to 4.5 mg/dl (0.8 to 1.4 mM). This is conventionally expressed as elemental P because the amount of P in its different forms ($H_2PO_4^{-}$, $HPO_4^{=}$) varies with pH. In contrast to calcium, 85 per cent is free and only 15 per cent is protein-bound (Fig. 75–2). The normal range of plasma P varies much more than that of calcium, including variation with age (higher in children). Plasma P is transiently reduced following carbohydrate ingestion, by insulin (because of the formation of intracellular phosphate esters), and by acute respiratory alkalosis.

Absorption of Dietary Phosphate. The average diet of an adult in the United States contains about 1000 mg of P, most of which (70 to 90 per cent) is absorbed by active transport. Deficiency of dietary phosphate or an abnormality of absorption is rarely a cause of phosphate deficiency except in alcoholics or in patients taking large amounts of antacids, such as aluminum hydroxide, which bind phosphate in the intestine and prevent its absorption. The control of phosphate balance is largely in its excretion.

Excretion of Phosphate. Being non–protein-bound, most plasma phosphate is filtered by the glomerulus, following which about 70 to 90 per cent is

FIGURE 75–3. The vitamin D endocrine system. Vitamin D is made available to the body by photogenesis in the skin and absorption from the intestine. Vitamin D is then hydroxylated in the liver to 25OHD, then in the kidney to 1,25(OH)₂D and 24,25(OH)₂D. The active vitamin D metabolites act on different tissues to produce a variety of responses. The three target tissues principally responsible for calcium (Ca) and phosphate (Pi) homeostasis are kidney, bone, and intestine. Endocrine tissues such as the parathyroid gland (PTG) and anterior pituitary are also target tissues. Their hormones, parathyroid hormone (PTH), prolactin (PRL), and growth hormone (GH), help regulate vitamin D metabolism in the kidney. In addition, PTH has a direct effect on bone and kidney regulation of calcium and phosphate homeostasis. (Reproduced with permission from Bikle DD: The vitamin D endocrine system. *In* Stollerman GH, et al (eds): Advances in Internal Medicine, Volume 27. Copyright © 1982 by Year Book Medical Publishers, Inc., Chicago.)

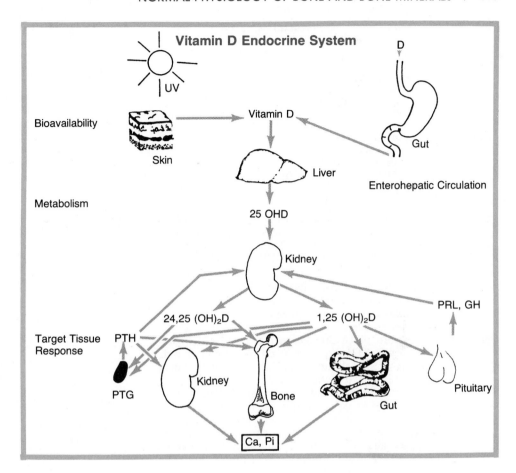

TABLE 75–1. CAUSES OF HYPOPHOSPHATEMIA*

I. **Moderate hypophosphatemia** (P 1.0 to 2.5 mg/dl)
   Hyperparathyroidism
   Osteomalacia (usually with hyperparathyroidism), malabsorption, deficiency of vitamin D, familial hypophosphatemic rickets, vitamin D–dependent rickets, oncogenic rickets
   Carbohydrate administration or ingestion or enhanced metabolism—glucose, fructose, glycerol, lactate, insulin administration
   Hypomagnesemia
   ECF volume expansion
   Acute alkalosis—bicarbonate infusion or moderate hyperventilation
   Hemodialysis

II. **Severe hypophosphatemia** (P less than 1.0 mg/dl)
   Chronic alcoholism and alcoholic withdrawal
   Diabetic ketoacidosis, recovery phase
   Enteric phosphate binding—excessive use of agents binding phosphate in the gut
   Hyperalimentation
   Nutritional recovery syndrome

* From Smith LH Jr: Phosphorus deficiency and hypophosphatemia. *In* Wyngaarden JB, Smith LH Jr (eds): Cecil Textbook of Medicine. 18th ed. Philadelphia, WB Saunders Co, 1988, p 1193. Modified from Knochel JP: West J Med 134:15, 1981.

actively reabsorbed, largely in the proximal tubule. Proximal tubular reabsorption of phosphate is increased by phosphate depletion, hypoparathyroidism, volume contraction, growth hormone, and hypocalcemia. Reabsorption is diminished (and renal clearance therefore increased) by phosphate loading, PTH, volume expansion, hypercalcemia, carbonic anhydrase inhibitors, thiazides, and furosemide.

Hyperphosphatemia. Hyperphosphatemia is usually encountered only in renal insufficiency (acute or chronic), hypoparathyroidism, acromegaly, rhabdomyolysis, or acute tumor lysis (e.g., chemotherapy of lymphoma). As noted, serum P is normally elevated over the usual adult range in growing children. The acute effects of elevating serum P are usually those of secondary hypocalcemia with tetany and/or seizures. Acute or chronic elevation of serum P may be associated with metastatic calcification.

Hypophosphatemia. The causes of hypophosphatemia most frequently encountered clinically are listed in Table 75–1. The long-term effects of phosphate depletion are commonly those of osteomalacia or rickets, to be described later (see Chapter 77). The acute effects are more likely to be metabolic (Table 75–2). Phosphate depletion may be associated with a reduction in erythrocytic 2,3-diphosphoglycerate

TABLE 75–2. CONSEQUENCES OF SEVERE HYPOPHOSPHATEMIA*

I. Acute—"metabolic"
    Hematologic
        Red cell dysfunction and hemolysis
        Leukocyte dysfunction
        Platelet dysfunction
    Muscle
        Weakness
        Rhabdomyolysis
        Myocardial dysfunction
    Central nervous system dysfunction
    Hepatic dysfunction
II. Chronic—"structural"
    Osteomalacia or rickets

* From Smith LH Jr: Phosphorus deficiency and hypophosphatemia. *In* Wyngaarden JB, Smith LH Jr (eds): Cecil Textbook of Medicine. 18th ed. Philadelphia, WB Saunders Co, 1988, p 1193.

(2,3-DPG), a molecule that normally affects the dissociation curve of oxyhemoglobin to enhance tissue availability of oxygen. In phosphate deficiency, therefore, tissue delivery of oxygen may be impaired. In very severe phosphate deficiency (P < 1.0 mg/dl), erythrocytic ATP may be reduced low enough that the integrity of the cell membrane cannot be maintained, with resulting hemolytic anemia. Leukocyte and platelet dysfunction are less well-established. Patients may be generally weak; severe phosphate deficiency may lead to rhabdomyolysis, perhaps comparable in mechanism to hemolytic anemia. Central nervous system function may be impaired, with symptoms varying from fatigue and irritability to metabolic encephalopathy with coma. The metabolic abnormalities associated with hypophosphatemia and phosphate depletion are rapidly reversible with phosphate therapy. The structural changes in bone require months or even years of replacement therapy.

MAGNESIUM METABOLISM

An adult normally has about 0.35 gm of magnesium/kg of body weight (a total of 25 gm or 100 mmol), of which about 50 to 60 per cent is in bone. In addition to its structural role in bone crystals, magnesium is an important cofactor in a large number of enzymatic reactions, especially those involving ATP.

Magnesium Balance. The normal serum level of magnesium is 1.6 to 2.1 mEq/L (0.8 to 1.05 mmol/L), of which about 30 per cent is protein-bound. About one third of ingested magnesium (the average diet contains about 500 mg) is absorbed in the intestine. This is balanced by its renal excretion, which reflects both filtration and active tubular reabsorption. Magnesium metabolism has a close interaction with that of calcium: (1) these cations are competitive for renal tubular reabsorption; (2) magnesium and calcium are physiological antagonists in the central nervous system; (3) magnesium is necessary for the release of parathyroid hormone by the parathyroid glands and for the action of the hormone on its target tissues.

Magnesium balance is usually assessed by its serum level, although this may not parallel tissue levels precisely. This assessment can be extended by measuring the amount of Mg excreted in the urine after its intravenous infusion (the Thoren test). Retention is presumed to reflect depleted stores. When dietary Mg is restricted, the normal kidney can reduce urinary loss to less than 1 mEq/day.

Hypomagnesemia. The most common causes of hypomagnesemia are summarized in Table 75–3. In clinical practice magnesium deficiency is encountered most frequently in alcoholics (poor dietary intake, vomiting, diminished absorption, increased renal excretion) and in patients with malabsorption. Significant depletion of magnesium may result in any or all of the abnormalities listed in Table 75–4. Many of these manifestations are relatively nonspecific, and magnesium deficiency rarely occurs as a pure entity without other nutritional and metabolic abnormalities. Its most characteristic presentation is that of hypocalcemia (irritability, tetany, positive Chvostek and Trousseau signs) because of the failure of normal secretion and action of parathyroid hormone. In effect Mg deficiency leads to a combination of functional hypoparathyroidism and pseudohypoparathyroidism (see Chapter 76). This form of hypocalcemia responds rapidly to Mg replacement therapy. Mg deficiency is not a recognized cause of metabolic bone disease. Treatment of magnesium deficiency is rarely an emergency. When it is urgent, approximately 1 mEq/kg/24 hr can be given by intravenous infusion. Long-term oral replacement can be carried out with various magnesium preparations, with careful attention to dosage in order not to induce diarrhea.

Hypermagnesemia. Hypermagnesemia rarely occurs. With normal renal function excess Mg is readily

TABLE 75–3. CAUSES OF HYPOMAGNESEMIA (SEEN MOST FREQUENTLY CLINICALLY IN ALCOHOLISM AND MALABSORPTION)*

I. Decreased absorption from dietary sources
    Diet poor in magnesium
    Parenteral feeding without magnesium
    Ethanol effect on absorption
    Malabsorption syndromes
    Uremia
    Selective intestinal defect for magnesium absorption (rare)
II. Increased loss of magnesium from the body
    Gastrointestinal tract
    Kidney
        Primary renal tubular defects
        Secondary—diuretics, Ca^{++}, ethanol, expansion of ECF, diabetes mellitus, treatment with gentamicin, cisplatin, or amphotericin B
        Breast—lactation hypomagnesemia (mostly in cattle, rarely in humans)
III. Internal redistribution
    Acute pancreatitis
    Increased loss into bone ("hungry bone syndrome")

* From Smith LH Jr: Disorders of magnesium metabolism. *In* Wyngaarden JB, Smith LH Jr (eds): Cecil Textbook of Medicine. 18th ed. Philadelphia, WB Saunders Co, 1988, p 1195.

excreted. In a patient with impaired renal function the excessive use of magnesium-containing antacids may produce hypermagnesemia, or it may occur with injudicious use of intravenous Mg in the acute treatment of hypertension. Hypermagnesemia may result in depression of central nervous system function, vasodilatation with hypotension and depression of the cardiac conduction system, ultimately leading to cardiac arrest in diastole. Discontinuation of magnesium infusion or ingestion usually suffices for treatment. Calcium is an antagonist of Mg in the central nervous system and can be used by intravenous injection if magnesium toxicity is acute.

VITAMIN D

Vitamin D is more properly a hormone than a vitamin: (1) When there is sufficient exposure to ultraviolet light no dietary source is required. (2) "Vitamin" D undergoes successive modifications in the body under hormonal and metabolic control, and then functions as a hormone-like agent in the metabolism of bone and bone salts.

Synthesis of Vitamin D (Fig. 75–3). The active form of vitamin D is synthesized in three sequential steps: (1) the dermal phase, (2) the hepatic phase, and (3) the renal phase. Ultraviolet light (approximately 290 to 320 nm wavelength) converts epidermal 7-dehydrocholesterol to an unstable previtamin D_3. The latter slowly converts nonenzymatically to vitamin D_3 (cholecalciferol) by a molecular rearrangement over the subsequent 24 to 48 hours. Vitamin D_3, bound to a specific vitamin D–binding protein (DBP), is then transported to the liver, where it is enzymatically hydroxylated to 25-hydroxyvitamin D (25-OH-D). This activation step, catalyzed by a cytochrome P450 mixed function oxidase in hepatocytes, is not under tight homeostatic control. The product, 25-OH-D (also called calcifediol), is not the most biologically potent form of vitamin D, but its circulating level furnishes a good index of the bioavailability of vitamin D.

25-OH-D, bound to DBP, is then transported to the kidney. In the renal parenchyma it may undergo one of two competing metabolic transformations:

1. FORMATION OF 1,25-DIHYDROXYCHOLECALCIFEROL (CALCITRIOL).   The 25-OH-D from the liver is further hydroxylated enzymatically at the 1 position to yield $1\alpha,25$-$(OH)_2D$, the most active hormonal form of the vitamin. This hydroxylation, which is normally highly specific for the kidney and the placenta, is under tight metabolic control. Activity of this 1-hydroxylase is increased by PTH, hypocalcemia, hypophosphatemia, and low levels of 1,25-$(OH)_2D$. Conversely, synthesis of 1,25-$(OH)_2D$ is diminished by reductions in PTH, hypercalcemia (independent of PTH), hyperphosphatemia, high levels of 1,25-$(OH)_2D$, and severe renal disease.

2. FORMATION OF 24,25-DIHYDROXYCHOLECALCIFEROL.   The kidney may alternatively hydroxylate 25-OH-D in the 24 position, catalyzed by a separate hydroxylase, to produce 24,25-$(OH)_2D$. Less is known about the control or purpose of this pathway, but high

levels of 1,25-$(OH)_2D$, calcium and phosphate tend to divert 25-OH-D into the 24,25-$(OH)_2D$ pathway.

Other pathways of vitamin D metabolism have been described, but their physiological roles, if any, remain to be demonstrated.

Absorption of Vitamin D.   Ingested vitamin D bypasses the dermal step in the activation process. The usual dietary source is vitamin D_2 (ergocalciferol) formed from the irradiation of ergosterol, a plant sterol. This differs in the structure of the side chain from vitamin D_3 (cholecalciferol) but is equal in potency, undergoes the same biotransformations, and is measured by the same commonly employed competitive protein-binding assays.

The dietary requirement of vitamin D is difficult to establish owing to the vagaries of endogenous synthesis. In the absence of better information, the suggested dietary requirement for an adult in the United States is about 10 μg (400 International Units) of vitamin D_2 or vitamin D_3 daily. As a fat-soluble molecule, vitamin D depends for its absorption on the complex series of events described for the absorption of fat in Chapter 34C. Chronic malabsorption of fat in the absence of adequate exposure to ultraviolet light can lead to hypovitaminosis D.

Assessment of Vitamin D Metabolism.   In the past the demonstration of rickets or osteomalacia for which no other cause was apparent and which was responsive to vitamin D was used for the diagnosis of hypovitaminosis D. Similarly, hypercalcemia, with a history of excessive ingestion of the vitamin, was necessary for the diagnosis of hypervitaminosis D. Currently assay methods are available using natural binding proteins, immunoassays, or a bioassay based on resorption of cultured bone in vitro. Values vary from laboratory to laboratory, but the most frequently measured products are 25-OH-D, 10 to 50 ng/ml, and 1,25-$(OH)_2D$, 15 to 55 pg/ml.

Function of Vitamin D.   Vitamin D acts with PTH to maintain the level of ionized calcium in extracel-

TABLE 75–4. CONSEQUENCES OF MAGNESIUM DEFICIENCY*

I. **Neuromuscular**
   Lethargy, weakness, fatigue, decreased mentation
   Neuromuscular irritability, in part due to associated hypocalcemia
   Hyaline and vacuolar degeneration of myofibers with segmental necrosis
II. **Gastrointestinal**
   Anorexia, nausea, vomiting
   Paralytic ileus
III. **Cardiovascular**
   Increased sensitivity to digitalis glycosides
   Possible cause of tachyarrhythmias
IV. **Metabolic**
   Hypocalcemia—probably due to the combined result of decreased PTH secretion and decreased end organ responsiveness to PTH
   Hypokalemia—tendency toward renal potassium wasting

* From Smith LH Jr: Disorders of magnesium metabolism. *In* Wyngaarden JB, Smith LH Jr (eds): Cecil Textbook of Medicine. 18th ed. Philadelphia, WB Saunders Co, 1988, p 1195.

lular fluid and to enhance calcification of osteoid by actions on the intestine, on bone, and, to a lesser extent, on the kidney.

Vitamin D, largely as 1,25-$(OH)_2$D, enhances the intestinal absorption of calcium through complex mechanisms, including the synthesis of a cytosolic calcium-binding protein. It also enhances phosphate absorption. In its effect on the absorption of calcium and phosphate it enhances the mineralization potential of extracellular fluid (the calcium × phosphate product). In its direct action on bone in vitro, 1,25-$(OH)_2$D stimulates bone resorption. There is some evidence, however, that 24,25-$(OH)_2$D may stimulate bone formation rather than bone resorption. In vivo the vitamin D metabolites are clearly necessary for normal bone formation. Vitamin D may enhance renal tubular reabsorption of calcium, but such a direct effect has been difficult to separate from its interaction with PTH and phosphate.

Hypervitaminosis D. Hypervitaminosis D occurs from the excessive ingestion of vitamin D or one of its active metabolites or from the abnormal conversion of 25-OH-D to 1,25-$(OH)_2$D at sites not subject to tight metabolic regulation. The former occurs usually in the therapy of hypoparathyroidism, osteomalacia, or osteoporosis. The latter occurs in certain granulomatous diseases, notably sarcoidosis, and in certain T-cell lymphomas in which the 1-hydroxylase is pathologically expressed in the abnormal tissue.

The clinical picture of hypervitaminosis D is that of hypercalcemia (see Chapter 76) and metastatic calcification. The hypercalcemia is probably due in larger measure to the osteolytic effects of vitamin D than to its effect on calcium absorption. For a given level of serum calcium, patients with this syndrome are more likely to have metastatic calcification (especially calcium nephropathy, band keratopathy, and calcifications in bursae and around joints) than are patients with hyperparathyroidism, since the level of PTH is suppressed and serum phosphate levels are higher. Treatment is by discontinuation of vitamin D, the usual acute treatment of hypercalcemia if indicated (Chapter 76), and the use of prednisone.

Hypovitaminosis D. The clinical picture of hypovitaminosis D is that of rickets or osteomalacia, to be described in Chapter 77. Hypovitaminosis D is also one component of the complex entity, renal osteodystrophy.

CALCITONIN

Calcitonin, a small polypeptide hormone, is secreted by the parafollicular C cells in the thyroid gland in response to a rise in the level of ionized calcium. As a physiological antagonist of parathyroid hormone, calcitonin inhibits bone resorption and increases the renal excretion of calcium and phosphate, tending to return the level of calcium toward normal. Whether it plays a significant role in normal calcium homeostasis in man has not been established.

Hypocalcitoninemia. No deficiency syndrome for calcitonin has been clearly established. Patients with total thyroidectomy do not require replacement with this hormone, do not develop hypercalcemia, and do not have a greater incidence of osteoporosis.

Hypercalcitoninemia. Excessive secretion of calcitonin usually reflects a medullary carcinoma of the thyroid gland, a malignancy of the parafollicular cells. Elevated serum levels of calcitonin may also be found with its ectopic secretion by other tumors and in uremia and pregnancy.

The excessive secretion of calcitonin by medullary carcinomas does not usually lead to any bone disease or to any change in the serum calcium, phosphorus, or alkaline phosphatase. Sporadic medullary carcinoma usually presents with a hard thyroid mass. Familial medullary carcinoma may present with some other features of the associated polyendocrine syndrome. These tumors are often versatile in their secretory capabilities, producing ACTH (with Cushing's syndrome), prostaglandins, nerve growth factor, serotonin, histaminase, vasoactive intestinal peptide, and prolactin. Some patients have an associated secretory diarrhea that remits with the removal of the tumor.

Familial Medullary Carcinoma. Medullary carcinoma may occur sporadically; it is also found in two distinct patterns of familial multiple endocrine neoplasia (MEN) syndrome, both of which are transmitted as autosomal, dominant traits:

MEN Type II (also called IIA) (Sipple's syndrome). In this syndrome familial parafollicular C-cell hyperplasia evolving into medullary carcinoma is linked with pheochromocytomas (20 to 30 per cent) and chief cell hyperplasia of the parathyroid glands (20 to 30 per cent). The pheochromocytomas tend to be bilateral and benign. Only about 10 per cent of patients exhibit hypercalcemia with its associated symptoms.

MEN Type III (also called Type IIB). This syndrome resembles type II in the linkage of medullary carcinoma and pheochromocyomas but differs in that the parathyroid glands are rarely involved. In addition there tends to be a distinct body habitus resembling the Marfan syndrome, and patients uniformly develop visible, sometimes disfiguring, benign ganglioneuromas of the lips, tongue, and buccal mucosa.

In addition, medullary carcinoma can occur as a familial disorder without being associated with other endocrine disorders. In all about 10 per cent of medullary carcinomas are familial and approximately 5 to 10 per cent of all thyroid carcinomas are medullary.

DIAGNOSIS AND TREATMENT. The diagnosis of medullary carcinoma (or of familial C-cell hyperplasia) is best established by measuring serum immunoreactive calcitonin before and after a provocative test with the infusion of calcium or of pentagastrin. Treatment is total thyroidectomy for familial cases, since the tumor is usually multicentric.

REFERENCES

Bone

Arnaud CD: Mineral and bone homeostasis. *In* Wyngaarden JB, Smith LH Jr (eds): Cecil Textbook of Medicine. 18th ed. Philadelphia, WB Saunders Co, 1988, p 1469.

Krane SM, Neer RM: Connective tissue. *In* Smith LH Jr, Thier SO (eds): Pathophysiology, The Biological Principles of Disease. 2nd ed. Philadelphia, WB Saunders Co, 1985, p 611.

Calcium

Levine MM, Kleeman CR: Hypercalcemia: Pathophysiology and treatment. Hosp Pract 22:73, 1987.
Slatopolsky E, Klahr S: Disorders of phosphorus, calcium, and magnesium metabolism. *In* Schrier RW, Gottschalk CW (eds.): Diseases of the Kidney. 4th ed. Boston, Little, Brown and Co, 1988, p. 2865.

Phosphorus

Knochel JP: The clinical status of hypophosphatemia: An update. N Engl J Med 313:447, 1985.
Smith LH Jr: Phosphorus deficiency and hypophosphatemia. *In* Wyngaarden JB, Smith LH Jr (eds): Cecil Textbook of Medicine. 18th ed. Philadelphia, WB Saunders Co, 1988, p 1193.

Magnesium

Elin RJ: Magnesium metabolism in health and disease. DM 34:166, 1988.
Smith LH Jr: Disorders of magnesium metabolism. *In* Wyngaarden JB, Smith LH Jr (eds): Cecil Textbook of Medicine. 18th ed. Philadelphia, WB Saunders Co, 1988, p 1195.

Vitamin D

Audran M, Kumar R: The physiology and pathophysiology of vitamin D. Mayo Clin Proc, 60:851, 1985.
Avioli LV, Haddad JG: The vitamin D family revisited. N Engl J Med 311:47, 1984.

Calcitonin

Arnaud CD: The ultimobranchial cells and calcitonin. *In* Wyngaarden JB, Smith LH Jr (eds): Cecil Textbook of Medicine. 18th ed. Philadelphia, WB Saunders Co, 1988, p 1505.
Austin L, Heath H III: Calcitonin: Physiology and pathophysiology. N Engl J Med 304:269, 1981.
Loeb JN: Polyglandular disorders. *In* Wyngaarden JB, Smith LH Jr (eds): Cecil Textbook of Medicine. 18th ed. Philadelphia, WB Saunders Co, 1988, p 1458.

76

THE PARATHYROID GLANDS, HYPERCALCEMIA, AND HYPOCALCEMIA

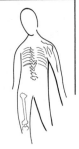

NORMAL PHYSIOLOGY

The parathyroid glands, usually four in number, normally weigh only about 120 mg. They are usually found in close association with the thyroid gland, but not infrequently one or both of the lower glands may be found in the superior mediastinum.

Secretion of PTH. Parathyroid hormone (PTH) is an 84-amino acid linear polypeptide (molecular weight 9500) whose main function is the control of the level of ionized calcium in extracellular fluid. When the level of ionized calcium falls, PTH secretion is stimulated; when ionized calcium rises above the normal set point, the secretion of PTH is suppressed. When ionized calcium is reduced over long periods of time, as for example in uremia, the parathyroid glands are capable of undergoing massive hyperplasia in order to enhance their secretory capacity. A normal or nearly normal level of ionized magnesium in extracellular fluid is necessary for normal secretion of PTH.

Actions of PTH (Fig. 76–1). The main function of PTH is to defend against hypocalcemia. In this defense it acts in a number of ways, both direct and indirect. All of these actions depend upon binding to specific receptors on the cell membrane and probably upon the subsequent intracellular release of cyclic AMP.

1. PTH stimulates osteolysis by osteoclasts that release calcium and phosphate into extracellular fluid. This action on bone, through mechanisms that are not well understood, is partially impaired when there is deficiency of calcitriol or of extracellular magnesium.

2. PTH *increases* the renal tubular reabsorption of calcium (and magnesium), reducing urinary loss of that which has been filtered.

3. PTH *decreases* the renal tubular reabsorption of phosphate and of bicarbonate, enhancing their urinary loss. This helps to get rid of the phosphate released from bone, which might otherwise tend to reduce ionized calcium. The loss of bicarbonate produces a form of renal tubular acidosis; this has a secondary effect of diminishing protein binding of calcium.

4. PTH increases the synthesis of the active form of vitamin D, calcitriol, from 25-OH-D through activation of the specific 1-hydroxylase in the kidney (see Chapter 75). It therefore indirectly enhances the intestinal absorption of calcium.

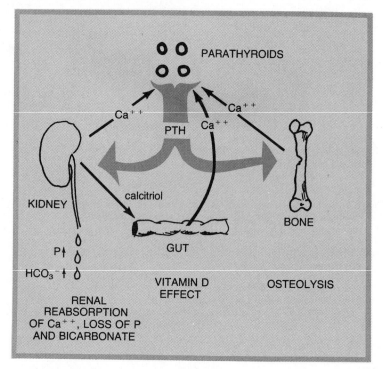

FIGURE 76–1. Actions of parathyroid hormone (PTH) in calcium homeostasis.

Many of the actions of PTH are upon the kidney. This is indirectly reflected in the amount of cyclic AMP of nephrogenous origin excreted in the urine.

Measurement of PTH. PTH can be measured directly using radioimmunoassay procedures. There are inherent difficulties with most current assays, however, because of two variables: (1) "Immunoreactive PTH" (iPTH) does not circulate as a single entity. In plasma there are a number of fragments of the active hormone. Most of the immunological activity measured by assay is not in fact the active hormone. (2) The antibodies used are multivalent and heterogeneous, recognizing different parts of the PTH linear peptide. Fortunately, newer assays that are capable of selectively measuring the intact PTH molecule are now available. In vitro cytochemical assays for active PTH are also used in some centers, but the new two-site immunoradiometric assays of the intact hormone make these less attractive. Measurement of the excretion of nephrogenous cAMP can also be used to reflect PTH action on the kidney.

PRIMARY HYPERPARATHYROIDISM

In primary hyperparathyroidism, a relatively common endocrine disorder, PTH continues to be secreted inappropriately despite an elevation in the level of ionized calcium in extracellular fluid. The disorder is more common in women than in men (two to four times greater), is very rare before the age of puberty,

and increases in incidence with age. Population surveys have found the prevalence of primary hyperparathyroidism in adults to be as high as 1 in 200 to 1 in 800. The average annual age-adjusted incidence of primary hyperparathyroidism is approximately 25 per 100,000.

Etiology. Primary hyperparathyroidism results from the development through unknown mechanisms of autonomous parathyroid tissue. In fact autonomy is seldom complete, since PTH secretion is usually partially suppressed at higher levels of ionized calcium. A single parathyroid adenoma accounts for 80 to 85 per cent of cases; most other patients with primary hyperparathyroidism have hyperplasia of all four glands. Carcinoma of the parathyroids is rare (less than 2 per cent of cases) and is usually not very malignant. Although most patients represent sporadic cases, primary hyperparathyroidism can occur in various patterns as a familial disorder, usually with hyperplasia and with a dominant mode of transmission: (1) familial hyperparathyroidism alone; (2) multiple endocrine neoplasia type I (Wermer's syndrome)—hyperparathyroidism, islet cell tumors, pituitary tumors; (3) multiple endocrine neoplasia type II (Sipple's syndrome)—medullary carcinoma of the thyroid, pheochromocytoma, hyperparathyroidism. Hyperparathyroidism is rare in multiple endocrine neoplasia type IIB or III—medullary carcinoma of the thyroid, pheochromocytoma, mucosal neuromas, and marfanoid body habitus.

Symptoms and Signs. Many patients are now discovered by measurement of serum calcium to have hyperparathyroidism when they are asymptomatic. When symptoms do occur, they most frequently result from hypercalcemia (Table 76–1). They may vary from easy fatigability to coma, but generally hypercalcemia is modest (11.0 to 12.5 mg/dl) and symptoms are mild. Some population surveys have found most patients to have serum calcium levels less than 11.0 mg/dl. Symptoms may also result from hypercalciuria, since kidney stones occur in about 10 per cent of patients with hyperparathyroidism. Approximately 5 per cent of patients with kidney stones are found to have hyperparathyroidism. More rarely bone pain due to osteitis fibrosa cystica (the bony lesion caused by excess PTH) may dominate the symptomatology, and very rarely there may be a pathological fracture at the site of a bone cyst. Physical findings of hyperparathyroidism are usually absent. A nodule felt in the neck is more likely to be in the thyroid gland than to be the offending parathyroid adenoma.

Laboratory and Radiographic Manifestations. Serum calcium levels are elevated and serum phosphorus levels tend to be low in primary hyperparathyroidism. Occasionally the total serum calcium is at the upper normal range but with ionized calcium increased. Serum alkaline phosphatase is elevated in the minority of patients in whom there is significant osteitis fibrosa cystica; its elevation reflects reparative osteoblastic activity. Urinary calcium may be normal or elevated. Its measurement is of greatest use in the diagnosis of familial benign hypercalcemia (see below), but marked hypercalciuria may suggest a non–PTH-related hypercalcemia. Because of the effect of PTH on bicarbonate excretion, the serum chloride is often elevated (> 105 mEq/L) and the serum bicarbonate somewhat reduced. Immunoassay of PTH should show an inappropriately high level of the hormone (and its related peptides) for the level of serum calcium (Fig. 76–2).

Most patients with primary hyperparathyroidism show no radiographic evidence of bone disease. When bone disease is found, it is most readily demonstrated as subperiosteal resorption of the cortex in the phalanges (Fig. 76–3). In addition, there may be generalized osteopenia and, in more advanced cases, resorption of the distal ends of the clavicle and of distal phalangeal tufts and a characteristic "salt-and-pepper" mottling of the skull.

Diagnosis. The diagnosis of primary hyperparathyroidism in the past was primarily based on finding hypercalcemia, usually with hypophosphatemia, in the absence of any other detectable cause of this abnormality (Table 76–2). That same differential diagnosis exists today, but the diagnosis can now be made with greater assurance using an immunoassay of high specificity for the intact PTH molecule (Fig. 75–2). In all other causes of hypercalcemia the level of PTH should be suppressed by an elevation of ionized calcium. Most of the other causes of hypercalcemia listed in Table 76–2 can be readily identified by other clinical manifestations or by laboratory studies.

The diagnosis of hyperparathyroidism can also be strengthened if subperiosteal bone reabsorption is present (Fig. 76–3), if nephrogenous cAMP is elevated in the urine, and if an enlarged parathyroid gland is found by ultrasonography. Two entities continue to be troublesome in the differential diagnosis:

1. HYPERCALCEMIA OF MALIGNANCY. Hypercalcemia occurs frequently with malignant tumors with or without metastases to bone. Osteolytic factors associated with malignant tumors fall into three classes: (a) lymphokines and monokines (interleukin 1, tumor necrosis factor, transforming growth factor β); (b) a recently described PTH-like protein with similar activities and limited sequence homology to PTH; and (c) 1,25-dihydroxyvitamin D. The PTH-like protein probably accounts for most of the hypercalcemia associated with nonhematological malignancies (lung, kidney, etc.). Contrary to previous concepts, PTH itself or prostaglandins of the E_2 series are rarely if ever the cause of human hypercalcemia of malignancy. The PTH level is therefore lower for the level of serum calcium in malignancy than in primary hyperparathyroidism (Fig. 76–2).

2. FAMILIAL BENIGN HYPERCALCEMIA (also called familial hypocalciuric hypercalcemia). This genetic disorder, transmitted as a dominant trait, is characterized by modest hypercalcemia, either normal urinary calcium or hypocalciuria, and no symptoms. There is no evidence of bone disease and, as expected, no stone diathesis. The PTH levels by immunoassay are usually normal. The diagnosis is important, since surgery is contraindicated. To rule out this disorder,

TABLE 76–1. SYMPTOMS AND SIGNS OF PRIMARY HYPERPARATHYROIDISM*

I. Related to hypercalcemia per se
 Central nervous system
  lethargy — altered mental function
  drowsiness — stupor
  depression — coma
 Neuromuscular
  fatigue — proximal myopathy
  weakness — hypotonia
 Cardiovascular
  hypertension — short Q-T interval
  bradycardia — potentiation of digitalis intoxication
 Renal
  polyuria
  calcium nephropathy—nephrocalcinosis
 Gastrointestinal
  nausea — dyspepsia
  vomiting — increased peptic ulcer ?
  constipation — pancreatitis
 Metastatic calcification (usually requires P to be elevated as well)
  band keratopathy
  pruritus

II. Related to hypercalciuria
 Kidney stone diathesis (10 per cent)

III. Related to PTH effect on bone and joints
 Bone pain from osteitis fibrosa cystica
 Bone cysts—rarely with fracture
 Epulis—a brown tumor (osteoclastic) of the jaw
 Arthralgias
 Increased incidence of gout and pseudogout

* The majority of patients are now discovered at a time when they have few or any symptoms, through measurement of the serum calcium.

urine calcium should be measured in patients with asymptomatic hypercalcemia, and serum calcium levels should be measured in the relatives of those with hypocalciuria. Clues to this diagnosis include young age, male sex, a family history of hypercalcemia or

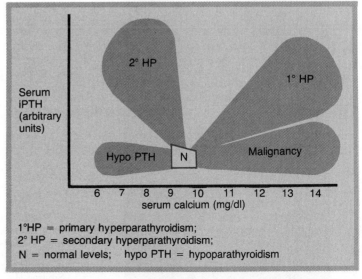

1°HP = primary hyperparathyroidism;
2° HP = secondary hyperparathyroidism;
N = normal levels; hypo PTH = hypoparathyroidism

FIGURE 76–2. Relation of iPTH and serum calcium in various disorders.

TABLE 76–2. DIFFERENTIAL DIAGNOSIS OF HYPERCALCEMIA

Due to increased PTH
  Primary hyperparathyroidism
  Hypercalcemia of malignancy (very few if any)
Without increased PTH (PTH usually suppressed)
  Hypercalcemia of malignancy
    malignant hematologic disorders (especially multiple myeloma)—often due to lymphokines and monokines
    nonhematologic malignancies—PTH-like factors, PGE_2, possibly other factors
  Vitamin D excess
    excessive ingestion
    excessive activation—sarcoidosis, berylliosis, some lymphomas
  Milk-alkali syndrome—excessive ingestion
  Use of thiazide diuretics
  Familial benign hypercalcemia (familial hypocalciuric hypercalcemia)
  Immobilization (especially with Paget's disease or paraplegia)
  Hyperthyroidism
  Miscellaneous—Addison's disease, vitamin A excess, hyperproteinemia states (increased bound calcium), idiopathic hypercalcemia of infancy

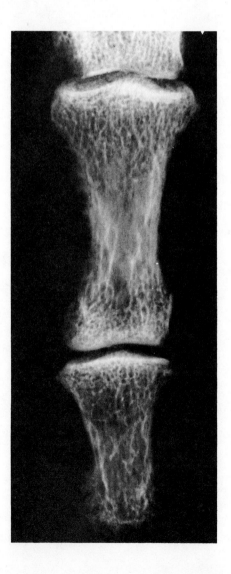

FIGURE 76–3. Magnified x-ray of an index finger on fine-grain industrial film, showing classic subperiosteal resorption in a patient with severe primary hyperparathyroidism. (Courtesy of Professor H. Genant, University of California, San Francisco, Department of Radiology.) (From Arnaud CD: The parathyroid glands, hypercalcemia, and hypocalcemia. *In* Wyngaarden JB, Smith LH Jr (eds): Cecil Textbook of Medicine. 18th ed. Philadelphia, WB Saunders Co, 1988, p 1486.)

neck surgery, a normal serum PTH, and a urinary calcium excretion of less than 100 mg/24 hr.

Treatment. The treatment of choice for primary hyperparathyroidism is surgical removal of the abnormal gland or glands. With hyperplasia subtotal (3½ glands) parathyroidectomy is carried out. In some patients with slight elevations of serum calcium (<11.0 mg/dl) or in those with contraindications to surgery, it is justifiable to follow the patient medically, maintaining adequate hydration and increased phosphate intake (if there is hypophosphatemia) and withholding thiazide diuretics or excessive dietary calcium.

HYPERCALCEMIA

Normal calcium metabolism was discussed in Chapter 75. For convenience hypercalcemia is being considered with the discussion of primary hyperparathyroidism.

Clinical Manifestations. The clinical manifestations of hypercalcemia are summarized in Table 76–1. In general, the severity of these manifestations tends to parallel the level of ionized calcium in extracellular fluid, but there are wide variations in the manner in which individual patients exhibit these various symptoms. Most frequently now elevations of serum calcium are found on routine chemical determinations. These tests should be repeated several times, since false elevations may be reported.

Differential Diagnosis. The differential diagnosis of hypercalcemia is presented in Table 76–2. These specific entities will not be discussed further here. An algorithm for a logical approach to the differential diagnosis of hypercalcemia is presented in Figure 76–4.

Treatment. Obviously the treatment of hypercalcemia should be directed toward reversal of the pathogenetic mechanisms responsible for it whenever possible. For example, primary hyperparathyroidism is usually treated by surgery. Successful treatment of malignancy may reverse or diminish its associated hypercalcemia, at least temporarily. The slight hypercalcemia found with hyperthyroidism or with Addison's disease is readily reversed by the treatment of those endocrine disorders. We shall discuss here the medical treatment of acute severe hypercalcemia (>13 to 14 mg/dl). The following approaches, presented briefly, are available and may be used in sequence, or many of them can be used concurrently if indicated by the severity of the patient's illness:

HYDRATION. Urinary excretion of calcium tends to parallel that of sodium. Patients should be vigorously hydrated, usually with normal saline, in order to enhance excretion.

FIGURE 76–4. Etiologic diagnosis in true hypercalcemia. (From Levine MM, Kleeman CR: Hypercalcemia: Pathophysiology and treatment. Hosp Pract 22:73, 1987.)

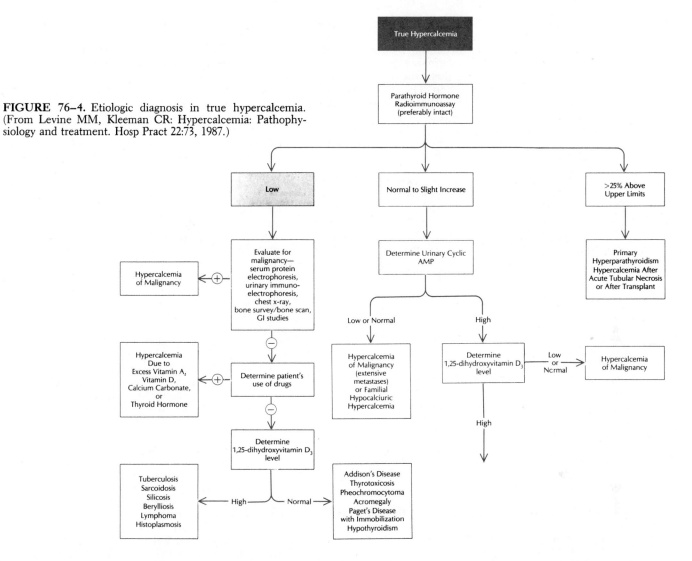

FUROSEMIDE (OR ETHACRYNIC ACID). Large doses of furosemide increase further the urinary excretion of calcium. Since excretion of potassium and magnesium is also increased, their serum levels must be closely followed and the amount lost in the urine replaced.

GLUCOCORTICOIDS. High doses of glucocorticoids (prednisone 50 to 100 mg per day or the equivalent of another agent) may lower serum calcium, especially in sarcoidosis, vitamin D poisoning, multiple myeloma, or other hematopoietic malignancies.

CALCITONIN. Calcitonin (usually as salmon calcitonin) given intramuscularly (4IU/kg q12h) may diminish the release of calcium from bone (see Chapter 75).

MITHRAMYCIN. This agent diminishes osteoclastic activity when given intravenously (25 μg/kg body weight) by slow infusion over 3 to 6 hours.

PHOSPHATE. Orthophosphate must be given with great care in the treatment of severe hypercalcemia because of the danger of metastatic calcification. In the presence of hypophosphatemia and good renal function, oral phosphate can be given in amounts sufficient to return its serum level to normal.

DIPHOSPHONATES. Etidronate disodium (Didronel) may be effective in the temporary control of the hypercalcemia of malignancy, when given intravenously 7.5 mg/kg/day for three to five days.

DIALYSIS. Very rarely, especially when there is acute hypercalcemia and renal insufficiency, dialysis may be required for the treatment of hypercalcemia.

These measures are usually successful in controlling acute hypercalcemia. The most difficult problems usually arise in the long-term treatment of the hypercalcemia of inoperable malignancy.

SECONDARY HYPERPARATHYROIDISM

Whenever the level of ionized calcium in extracellular fluid falls, the parathyroid glands are stimulated to secrete PTH. If the tendency toward hypocalcemia is sustained, the glands become hyperplastic and secrete increasing amounts of PTH, a condition known as secondary hyperparathyroidism. By definition the serum calcium level is low-normal or low in secondary hyperparathyroidism, since this is the driving force for hyperplasia and hypersecretion. The serum phosphorus will usually be low if renal function is intact. Osteitis fibrosa cystica may be present as noted by bone pain, subperiosteal bone resorption (Fig. 76–3), or elevation of serum alkaline phosphatase. The most frequent causes of secondary hyperparathyroidism are chronic renal failure (renal osteodystrophy), malabsorption of calcium (rickets, osteomalacia), and pseudohypoparathyroidism. The term "tertiary hyperparathyroidism" is sometimes used to describe hypercalcemia arising in the setting of severe secondary hyperparathyroidism in which chronic stimulation is thought to produce relatively autonomous parathyroid tissue.

HYPOPARATHYROIDISM

In contrast to hyperparathyroidism, hypoparathyroidism is rare. In this section hypocalcemia in general will be discussed.

Etiology. The causes of hypoparathyroidism (Table 76–3) range from surgical removal of the glands to resistance to the action of PTH at the tissue level. Magnesium deficiency was discussed in Chapter 75, and pseudohypoparathyroidism will be discussed subsequently. DiGeorge's syndrome is a very rare congenital abnormality representing absence of embryological formation of the parathyroids and of the thymus, both products of the third and fourth branchial

TABLE 76–3. ETIOLOGY OF HYPOPARATHYROIDISM

Surgical removal of the parathyroids
Impaired secretion of PTH—Mg deficiency
Inherited forms of hypoparathyroidism
  DiGeorge's syndrome—congenital absence of parathyroids and thymus
  Multiple endocrine deficiency—autoimmune—candidiasis (MEDAC) syndrome
Sporadic, idiopathic hypoparathyroidism
Pseudohypoparathyroidism—target organ resistance
  acquired—Mg deficiency
  inherited—various subtypes noted

TABLE 76–4. SYMPTOMS AND SIGNS OF HYPOCALCEMIA

Enhanced neuromuscular irritability
  Paresthesias (numbness, tingling), especially around mouth and tips of fingers
  Tetany—positive Chvostek's and Trousseau's sign
  Grand mal seizures
Lenticular cataracts—decreased vision
Basal ganglia calcification—rarely extrapyramidal abnormalities
Papilledema and increased intracranial pressure
Intestinal malabsorption (which may further exacerbate hypocalcemia)
Trophic changes in skin, fingernails, and developing teeth
Prolonged Q-T interval; rarely heart block and congestive heart failure

clefts. These children usually die of immunodeficiency (T-cell dysfunction) in early life. The MEDAC syndrome (Table 76–3) is characterized by chronic mucocutaneous candidiasis and autoimmune injury of various endocrine glands, especially of the parathyroids and the adrenal cortex (producing Addison's disease).

Symptoms and Signs (Table 76–4). Symptomatology varies not only with the level of ionized calcium but also with the rate at which hypocalcemia has developed and its total duration. A rapid fall in ionized calcium is more likely to produce symptoms. The symptoms associated with hypoparathyroidism largely relate to the neuromuscular consequences of hypocalcemia. They can vary from a vague sense of anxiety with paresthesias to recurrent grand mal seizures, erroneously treated with phenytoin. Most of the other symptoms and signs listed in Table 76–4 occur only after years of hypocalcemia. Physical findings are those of neuromuscular irritability (positive Chvostek's and/or Trousseau's sign) and sometimes cataracts, basal ganglia signs, dry dystrophic skin and nails, or rarely associated findings such as candidiasis, signs of Addison's disease, a scar from a previous thyroidectomy, or the physical findings of pseudohypoparathyroidism to be noted below.

Laboratory and Radiographic Manifestations. Hypoparathyroidism is characterized by hypocalcemia and hyperphosphatemia. Serum bicarbonate tends to be slightly elevated and serum iPTH is undetectable or markedly reduced, except in pseudohypoparathyroidism (Fig. 76–2). There are no radiographic changes in bone, but calcification of basal ganglia may be noted. Skeletal changes of pseudohypoparathyroidism are noted below. The ECG usually shows a long Q-T interval and may exhibit heart block.

Diagnosis. The diagnosis of hypoparathyroidism is relatively simple once it is considered or when hypocalcemia is discovered. The triad of hypocalcemia, hyperphosphatemia, and normal renal function is virtually diagnostic of the disorder. Hypomagnesemia should be ruled out. Measurement of iPTH should readily confirm the diagnosis and rule out pseudohypoparathyroidism (in which condition it should be elevated).

Other causes of hypocalcemia are readily excluded: hypoproteinemia, acute pancreatitis, azotemia, and malabsorption of calcium. In the latter condition there is secondary hyperparathyroidism, so that the serum phosphorus should be low and the level of iPTH high.

Treatment. Patients are usually treated with a regimen of a high calcium diet and a vitamin D preparation along with phosphate binders (Al(OH)$_3$). Dihydrotachysterol has been used most frequently, but calcitriol has some theoretical advantages. Care must be taken to avoid hypercalcemia, since metastatic calcification and calcium nephropathy are special dangers with elevated levels of serum P. In the absence of PTH, normocalcemic hypercalciuria may increase the tendency to kidney stone formation. Acute tetany may require use of an intravenous preparation of calcium, such as calcium gluconate, to raise levels of ionized calcium to the normal level.

PSEUDOHYPOPARATHYROIDISM

This rare group of disorders has elicited more interest than its prevalence would warrant, in considerable measure because pseudohypoparathyroidism was the first clear-cut demonstration of an endocrine deficiency syndrome caused by unresponsiveness of a target organ. As would be expected, the clinical manifestations of hypocalcemia are the same in these patients as in those with other forms of hypoparathyroidism (Table 76–4). The laboratory findings are also similar except for the fact that the serum level of iPTH is elevated, since the persistent hypocalcemia tends to drive parathyroid secretion. Pseudohypoparathyroidism differs from other forms of hypoparathyroidism in two general ways:

1. There are a number of dominantly inherited developmental and skeletal abnormalities that may be associated with the disorder. These include short stature, shortening of the metacarpal and metatarsal bones (especially the fourth and fifth bones), thickening of the calvarium, exostoses, and frequently mental deficiency. The appearance is often typical, with short stature, a round face, obesity, and a short neck, together with the bony abnormalities above. When these findings occur in the absence of hypoparathyroidism, the condition is termed "pseudopseudohypoparathyroidism."

2. End-organ resistance to PTH can be demonstrated in a number of ways and occurs in various patterns. For patients with the skeletal anomalies described above, the molecular defect thought to cause PTH resistance is a 50 per cent decrease in the membrane protein that couples the PTH receptor to adenylate cyclase. Other possibilities for end-organ resistance include a structurally abnormal hormone or an inhibitor of hormone action. Resistance is usually demonstrated by an impaired effect of administered PTH on the kidney, as judged by phosphaturia or nephrogenous cAMP. Rarely cAMP may be elevated but no phosphaturia results. Suitable preparations of PTH for this test are not currently available commercially. Rarely PTH may be effective on bone but not on the kidney, producing osteitis fibrosa cystica in the presence of functional hypoparathyroidism.

Treatment of pseudohypoparathyroidism is similar to that for other forms of hypoparathyroidism.

REFERENCES

Arnaud C: The parathyroid glands, hypercalcemia, and hypocalcemia. *In* Wyngaarden JB, Smith LH Jr (eds): Cecil Textbook of Medicine. 18th ed. Philadelphia, WB Saunders Co, 1988, p 1486.

Heath H III, Hodgson SF, Kennedy MA: Primary hyperparathyroidism: Incidence, morbidity and potential economic impact in a community. N Engl J Med 302:189, 1980.

Juan D: Hypocalcemia: Differential diagnosis and mechanisms. Arch Intern Med 139:1166, 1979.

Law WM Jr, Heath H III: Familial benign hypercalcemia (hypocalciuric hypercalcemia). Ann Intern Med 102:511, 1985.

Levine MM, Kleeman CR: Hypercalcemia: Pathophysiology and treatment. Hosp Pract 22:73, 1987.

Mundy GR. The hypercalcemia of malignancy. Kidney Int 31:142, 1987.

77

OSTEOMALACIA AND RICKETS

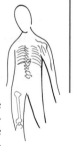

Osteomalacia and rickets represent the same metabolic bone disease characterized by inadequate calcification of osteoid on trabecular surfaces or in newly formed haversian systems. In rickets there is also an abnormality in the zone of provisional calcification related to endochondral skeletal growth at the open epiphyses.

Pathogenesis

The normal structure of bone was reviewed briefly in Chapter 75. In the process of new bone formation in growth or in remodeling, osteoid is laid down in an appositional fashion by the osteoblasts. Soon thereafter bone salts are deposited in the osteoid to form bone, a process of mineralization that is still incompletely understood but that depends on a normal ion product of ionized calcium and phosphate, on alkaline phosphatase (probably necessary to remove the inhibitor pyrophosphate), and probably on several of the metabolites ($1,25$-$(OH)_2D$ and $24,25$-$(OH)_2D$) of vitamin D. Other factors may normally influence this process; mineralization can be impeded by inhibitors such as aluminum or diphosphonates.

In osteomalacia and in rickets, mineralization of osteoid (and of cartilage in rickets) does not keep pace with osteoid formation. As a result the osteoid seams are much wider and are found more extensively throughout bone. The bones are therefore weaker (osteomalacia means bone softening); in children the epiphyseal plate is widened, flared, and irregular. These changes are potentially reversible as normal mineralization is restored.

Specific Causes

The conditions in which osteomalacia and rickets are most frequently found are listed in Table 77–1. It has not been firmly established whether a pure deficiency of calcium results in osteomalacia. The major categories are those of inadequate bioavailability of the active metabolites of vitamin D, chronic phosphate depletion, abnormal inhibition of mineralization, and hypophosphatasia. These will be commented upon very briefly. A full discussion of these entities is beyond the scope of this introductory book.

Reduced Bioavailability of Active Forms of Vitamin D. The metabolic cycle in which vitamin D is successively converted to its active hormonal form is described in Chapter 75 and illustrated in Figure 75–3. As might be expected, and as summarized in Table 77–1, a wide variety of disorders may interfere with the formation of sufficient 1,25-$(OH)_2$D for its action on the gut and its action (or that of 24,25-$(OH)_2$D) on bone. These vary from malabsorption of the vitamin, especially if there is inadequate sunlight for endogenous synthesis of precursors, impaired activation in the liver and kidney, increased catabolism or excretion, and failure of tissue responsiveness (e.g., diffuse disease or shortening of the bowel). In vitamin D–dependent rickets type II, there do not seem to be sufficient normal receptors for 1,25-$(OH)_2$D.

TABLE 77–1. CAUSES OF OSTEOMALACIA OR RICKETS OR BOTH*

1. Vitamin D deficiency—dietary lack, too little sunshine, neonatal rickets
2. Vitamin D malabsorption—sprue, postgastrectomy, bile salt deficiency, pancreatic insufficiency, small bowel disease, bypass or resection
3. Impaired activation of vitamin D
   a. 25-Hydroxylation (liver)—immaturity, cirrhosis of liver ± alcoholism
   b. 1-Hydroxylation (kidney)—chronic renal failure, genetic enzyme defect (vitamin D dependency), parathyroid hormone deficiency or "resistance," ? hyperphosphatemia
4. Increased catabolism or excretion of vitamin D and its metabolites
   a. Hepatic microsomal enzyme induction—anticonvulsants (phenytoin, barbiturates)
   b. Renal excretion—nephrotic syndrome, biliary cirrhosis
5. Phosphate depletion and hypophosphatemia
   a. Complicating 1 through 4 above owing to PTH excess or lack of vitamin D metabolites or both
   b. Negative phosphate balance—malabsorption, phosphate-binding antacids, hemodialysis
   c. Primary hypophosphatemia (vitamin D refractory)—vitamin D-resistant rickets (VDRR), several types; oncogenic rickets and osteomalacia, neurofibromatosis
   d. Metabolic acidosis—distal renal tubular acidosis, ureterocolostomy
   e. Fanconi's syndrome—cystinosis, Wilson's disease, etc.
6. Inhibitors of mineralization—diphosphonates, fluoride, chronic renal failure, aluminum
7. Miscellaneous or unclassified—hypophosphatasia, "axial" osteomalacia, fibrogenesis imperfecta ossium

* From Avioli LV: Osteomalacia and rickets. *In* Wyngaarden JB, Smith LH Jr (eds): Cecil Textbook of Medicine. 16th ed. Philadelphia, WB Saunders Co, 1982, p 1337. Modified from Frame B, Parfitt AM: Osteomalacia: Current concepts. Ann Intern Med 89:966, 1978.

Chronic Depletion of Phosphate. Normal metabolism of phosphate and the metabolic consequences of phosphate depletion are summarized in Chapter 75 (see Tables 75–1 and 75–2). Chronic phosphate depletion may lead to osteomalacia or rickets, depending upon the patient's age. As noted, the causes of hypophosphatemia are many and range from enteric binding of phosphate with antacids to renal tubular wasting of phosphate (e.g., as a specific renal tubular disorder, due to secondary hyperparathyroidism, or as part of the Fanconi syndrome). Whatever the cause, the resulting hypophosphatemia may reduce the mineralization potential of bone salts below the critical level for normal deposition in osteoid.

Inhibitors of Mineralization. The use of aluminum-containing antacids in the presence of azotemia or the use of dialysis fluid high in aluminum may result in aluminum levels sufficient to inhibit mineralization, as may the use of diphosphonates in the treatment of Paget's disease. Chronic renal failure itself may inhibit normal mineralization.

Hypophosphatasia. In this rare genetic disorder, transmitted as an autosomal recessive trait, tissue and serum levels of alkaline phosphatase are low. The disease varies in severity from severe, deforming rickets to mild osteomalacia in adults.

Clinical Manifestations

In the adult the manifestations of osteomalacia are often subtle. They may consist of aching in bones, tenderness over bones, and muscle weakness, especially of proximal and pelvic girdle muscles. As a result there may be a waddling gait. Bones may fracture more easily than normal.

The clinical manifestations of rickets are more striking and characteristic. The child is usually listless and hypotonic and fails to grow normally. The epiphyses are enlarged and tender, and the long bones are often bowed. The chondrocostal junctions are enlarged and prominent to produce the "rachitic rosary." The pull of the diaphragm on the softened rib cage may produce an indentation known as Harrison's groove. Rachitic bones are easily fractured. Dentition is delayed and poor.

Laboratory and Radiographic Abnormalities

The laboratory findings depend to a considerable degree on the specific cause of the defect in mineralization (Table 77–1). In the absence of renal failure the most typical finding would be slight hypocalcemia, more significant hypophosphatemia, an elevated serum alkaline phosphatase, and an elevated level of iPTH, representing secondary hyperparathyroidism. Osteomalacia can exist in the absence of any of these findings, however. A comparison of these laboratory findings with those expected in two other causes of diffuse osteopenia, primary hyperparathyroidism with bone disease (osteitis fibrosa) and osteoporosis, is given in Table 77–2.

The radiographic findings in osteomalacia are most often nonspecific and show only osteopenia, which cannot readily be differentiated from osteoporosis.

Pseudofractures (also known as Looser's zones) occasionally occur and when found are virtually pathognomonic for osteomalacia or rickets. These appear as ribbon-like clear zones, often bilaterally and symmetrically, and most characteristically in the pubic and ischial rami, the femoral neck, the ribs, and the axillary margins of the scapulae (Fig. 77–1).

TABLE 77–2. TYPICAL LABORATORY FINDINGS IN SERUM IN METABOLIC BONE DISEASE

	Ca^{++}	P	ALK. P'TASE	iPTH
1. Osteomalacia	N or ↓	↓	↑	↑
2. Primary hyperparathyroidism with osteitis fibrosa cystica	↑	↓	↑	↑
3. Osteoporosis	N	N	N	N

iPTH = Immunoreactive parathyroid hormone; alk. p'tase = alkaline phosphatase; N = normal. The changes in osteomalacia are to a large extent due to secondary hyperparathyroidism.

Diagnosis

The diagnosis of rickets is rarely difficult because of the characteristic clinical and radiographic findings. The diagnosis of osteomalacia may be more difficult, especially if there are no demonstrable pseudofractures. The diagnosis is best established by use of a transcortical bone biopsy (most frequently taken from the iliac crest) with careful histological study of the undecalcified specimen for widened osteoid seams. The biopsy is more definitive when it follows the use of timed tetracycline to determine the rate of bone formation (depressed in osteomalacia), as noted in Chapter 75.

Treatment

It is difficult to generalize about the treatment of a condition with such diverse pathogenetic mechanisms. Most frequently calcium and vitamin D are given; in some patients large supplements of phosphate may be required as well (e.g., X-linked hypophosphatemia). The reader is referred to discussions of the specific disorders in Table 77–1 for a summary of their respective modes of therapy.

REFERENCES

Bikle DD: Osteomalacia and rickets. *In* Wyngaarden JB, Smith LH Jr (eds): Cecil Textbook of Medicine. 18th ed. Philadelphia, WB Saunders Co, 1988, p 1479.

Marel GM, McKenna MJ, Frame B: Osteomalacia. *In* Bone Mineral Research, Vol 4. Amsterdam, Elsevier, 1986, pp 335–412.

Tieder M, Modai D, Samuel R, et al: Hereditary hypophosphatemic rickets with hypercalciuria. N Engl J Med 312:611, 1985.

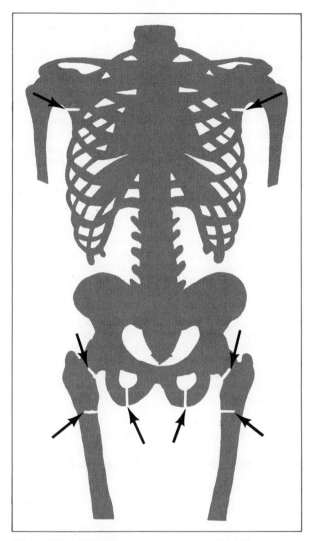

Figure 77–1. Most frequent locations of pseudofractures (Looser's zones) in osteomalacia.

78

OSTEOPOROSIS

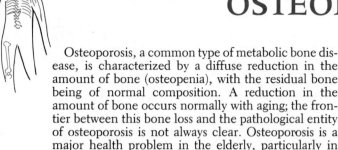

Osteoporosis, a common type of metabolic bone disease, is characterized by a diffuse reduction in the amount of bone (osteopenia), with the residual bone being of normal composition. A reduction in the amount of bone occurs normally with aging; the frontier between this bone loss and the pathological entity of osteoporosis is not always clear. Osteoporosis is a major health problem in the elderly, particularly in elderly women, with increased susceptibility to serious fractures, disability, and death.

Pathology

In osteoporosis there is too little bone, but that which is present is normally composed of osteoid and bone minerals. Osteoporosis can be localized to the bones of one extremity, as in disuse atrophy with immobilization in a cast, but usually it is generalized. Different types may be most markedly manifested in the trabecular bone of the axial skeleton or in both trabecular and cortical bone.

Etiology and Pathogenesis

As noted in Chapter 75, bone is a living tissue that undergoes remodeling throughout life, with balanced processes of destruction (osteolysis) and repair (osteogenesis). Osteopenia must result from increased destruction, decreased formation, or a combination of the two. Although all combinations of these factors have been described in the osteoporotic syndromes, a relative increase in the rate of destruction is most commonly found in the osteoporosis of the elderly. It is not always possible to determine a specific cause of osteoporosis in a given individual. In this brief discussion certain general risk factors will be described, as well as a listing of the clinical conditions in which osteoporosis is most frequently manifested. The risk factors include the following:

Decreased Estrogen. Osteoporosis, more common by far in women than in men, occurs most frequently in the postmenopausal period. Bone loss is accelerated with reduction of ovarian function by either spontaneous or surgically induced menopause. The rate of bone loss varies markedly among women, but bone loss can largely be prevented by the continued administration of exogenous estrogens. The link between estrogen deficiency and increased bone destruction is not clear. Possibly there is enhanced sensitivity to parathyroid hormone or some effect on local mediators of bone metabolism. This type of involutional osteoporosis is sometimes described as "type I," or postmenopausal, and is most marked in trabecular bone, resulting in vertebral fractures.

Starting Level of Bone Density. Over a normal life span a woman loses about half of her bone mass and a man about a quarter of his bone mass from that present in young adulthood. Whether the residual level is reduced enough to be considered pathological osteoporosis with enhanced danger of fracture depends in part on the starting level. Blacks, for example, in general have more initial bone and therefore rarely develop clinical osteoporosis. Small, slender women of northern European extraction have lighter bones and are more prone to develop osteoporosis.

Ingestion and Absorption of Calcium. If absorbed calcium is insufficient to replace its obligatory loss in urine and stool (150 to 250 mg/day), it will be mobilized from the skeleton under the influence of PTH. Since dietary calcium is often marginal, particularly so with the decreased efficiency of its absorption in the aged, this may contribute to loss of bone mass.

Aging. Beyond the hormonal effects of estrogen deficiency, there is age-related loss of bone in both men and women, especially after the age of 75, sometimes referred to as "type II" involutional osteoporosis. There is usually a balanced loss of both trabecular and cortical bone, and therefore fractures occur in the hip, pelvis, and long bones as well as in the trabecular bone of the vertebral bodies. Type II osteoporosis is thought to result from decreased bone formation as well as from a secondary increase in PTH secretion because of reduced calcium absorption.

Other risk factors are known, as shown in Table 78–1, such as excess glucocorticoids, alcoholism, immobilization, certain rare genetic abnormalities of connective tissue, heparin (either administered or associated with mastocytosis), multiple myeloma, and a number of gastrointestinal disorders associated with impaired bioavailability of calcium. In addition, severe transient osteoporosis of unknown cause may occur in children or young adults.

Clinical Manifestations

Osteoporosis is usually asymptomatic unless it results in a fracture—a vertebral compression fracture or a fracture of the hip, pelvis, humerus, or any other bone. The most typical symptom is the sudden onset of back pain associated with vertebral compression caused by a modest stress (e.g., picking up an object, leaning over). This may be associated with muscle spasms and ileus but usually improves over some weeks. With a series of such axial fractures, usually with anterior wedging, there is telescoping with loss of height and the development of kyphosis. Compression of the vertebral bodies may occur gradually without acute episodes of pain and produce the characteristic dorsal kyphosis with cervical lordosis, sometimes known as the "dowager's hump." Fractures of the hip may occur with modest trauma or even spontaneously and carry a mortality rate of 15 per cent as well as resulting in severe disability and long-term care for many of those who survive.

Diagnosis

The diagnosis of osteoporosis can usually be established by the presence of typical radiographic changes (see below) in a patient in whom the disease might be anticipated (e.g., a white woman 10 to 20 years post-menopausal) and in the absence of evidence for any other cause of diffuse osteopenia. Serum calcium, phosphorus, and alkaline phosphatase levels are usually normal, although the alkaline phosphatase level may rise slightly after a fracture. The conditions in Table 78–1 should be carefully considered. It is especially important to rule out multiple myeloma, which can closely mimic involutional osteoporosis. If osteomalacia is considered to be a possibility, a bone biopsy may be warranted, since the therapy would be very different (see Chapter 77).

Radiographic Findings

The most characteristic radiographic findings of osteoporosis are in the spine, illustrated diagrammatically in Figure 78–1. With the loss of trabecular bone, the end plates of the vertebral bodies stand out, and the washed-out radiolucent bodies tend to show fine vertical striations because of preferential loss of horizontal trabeculae. The intervertebral discs expand into concavities within the vertebral bodies and may rupture into the body (Schmorl's nodules). There is loss of height with compression fractures producing anterior wedging.

Treatment

The treatment of osteoporosis will depend on its cause and the stage of the illness. For example, if there is Cushing's syndrome, multiple myeloma, or thyrotoxicosis, the treatment differs from that of either type I or type II involutional osteoporosis. During the acute phase of a vertebral compression, attention is directed toward relief of pain (analgesics, heat, massage, rest), but early ambulation and careful exercises of back muscles should be encouraged. Most patients with symptomatic osteoporosis are elderly women. An approach to the treatment of this group of patients is directed toward the prevention of further loss of bone.

Estrogens. Small doses of estrogens (the equivalent of 0.625 to 1.25 mg of estrone sulfate daily) can

TABLE 78–1. CLASSIFICATION OF CAUSES OF OSTEOPOROSIS*

Primary osteoporosis
  Juvenile
  Idiopathic (young adults)
  Involutional osteoporosis
Endocrine diseases
  Hypogonadism
  Ovarian agenesis
  Hyperadrenocortisolism
  Hyperthyroidism
  Hyperparathyroidism
  Diabetes mellitus (?)
Gastrointestinal diseases
  Subtotal gastrectomy
  Malabsorption syndromes
  Chronic obstructive jaundice
  Primary biliary cirrhosis
  Severe malnutrition
  Alactasia
Bone marrow disorders
  Multiple myeloma and related disorders
  Systemic mastocytosis
  Disseminated carcinoma
Connective tissue diseases
  Osteogenesis imperfecta
  Homocystinuria
  Ehlers-Danlos syndrome
  Marfan's syndrome
Miscellaneous causes
  Immobilization
  Chronic obstructive pulmonary disease
  Chronic alcoholism
  Chronic heparin administration
  Rheumatoid arthritis (?)
  Anticonvulsant drugs (?)

* From Riggs BL: Osteoporosis. *In* Wyngaarden JB, Smith LH Jr (eds): Cecil Textbook of Medicine. 18th ed. Philadelphia, WB Saunders Co, 1988, p 1510.

reduce the loss of bone in postmenopausal women. This should be given cyclically with a progestin added during the last 10 days of the cycle to reduce the danger of endometrial carcinoma.

Calcium. Supplement of the diet by 1.0 to 1.5 gm of calcium may enhance absorption sufficiently to reduce bone loss, particularly by reducing secondary hyperparathyroidism. If the patient has a malabsorptive syndrome, supplementary vitamin D may also be useful, but it should be used cautiously in order to prevent hypercalcemia.

Experimental forms of therapy include the use of calcitonin to reduce bone destruction and the use of sodium fluoride (together with calcium supplementation) to stimulate osteoblastic formation of trabecular bone in the axial skeleton. Response to all forms of treatment can be followed by careful measurement of the patient's height over time as an index of compression of vertebral bones or more accurately and

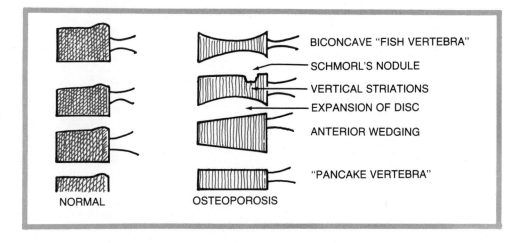

Figure 78–1. Vertebral changes in osteoporosis.

expensively by use of quantitative computed tomography of the vertebral bodies or photon absorptiometry of peripheral cortical bone.

REFERENCES

Mundy GR: Osteopenia. DM 33:540, 1987.

Raisz LG: Local and systemic factors in the pathogenesis of osteoporosis. N Engl J Med 318:818, 1988.
Riggs BL: Osteoporosis. In Wyngaarden JB, Smith LH Jr (eds): Cecil Textbook of Medicine. 18th ed. Philadelphia, WB Saunders Co, 1988, p 1510.
Riggs BL, Melton LJ III: Involutional osteoporosis. N Engl J Med 314:1676, 1986.

79

PAGET'S DISEASE OF BONE

Paget's disease of bone, also called osteitis deformans, is characterized by chronic, localized areas of bone destruction complicated by concurrent exuberant bone repair. Approximately 3 per cent of adults over age 40 have histological evidence of Paget's disease at autopsy, the prevalence increasing with age. Less than 1 per cent have radiographic evidence of the disease.

Etiology

The etiology of Paget's disease has not been established. Strictly speaking it is not a metabolic bone disease, since it is localized (although many bones may be involved); a primary abnormality of endocrine function or of mineral metabolism seems highly unlikely. It is provocative that inclusion bodies resembling certain viral nucleocapsids can be demonstrated in pagetic osteoclasts, and these inclusions have shown immunological reactivity to antisera to the measles virus and to the respiratory syncytial virus.

TABLE 79–1. CLINICAL MANIFESTATIONS OF PAGET'S DISEASE

Musculoskeletal pain
Skeletal deformity
Pathological fractures
Enlarged skull
  leontiasis ossea
  deafness, tinnitus
Platybasia—spinal cord and brain stem compression
Erythema and heat over pagetic areas
Increased cardiac output—rarely congestive failure
Angioid streaks in retina
Osteogenic sarcoma
Reparative granuloma
Characteristic radiographs
Serum alkaline phosphatase increased
Urinary hydroxyproline increased
Hypercalciuria and hypercalcemia during immobilization (decreased reparative osteogenesis)
Hyperuricemia—not uncommon, sometimes with gout

Pathology and Pathophysiology

The primary process in Paget's disease is localized osteolysis, which seems to result from an enhanced number and activity of osteoclasts. This chronic destructive process occurs in the setting of continued reparative osteogenesis by osteoblasts, the products of which may also undergo simultaneous or subsequent destruction. The result is usually thickened but weakened bone without the normal pattern of cortical or trabecular bone. The resulting random mix of cement lines is generally described as a "mosaic pattern." The weakened bone may fracture or bend under stress. For example, the base of the skull may flatten with basilar invagination (platybasia); cortical infractions may occur on the convex surfaces of bowed long bones, particularly with the characteristic lateral bowing of the femur and anterior bowing of the tibia.

Repair usually matches destruction, so that serum calcium and phosphorus are usually normal despite a remarkably enhanced bone turnover rate. Serum alkaline phosphatase may be markedly elevated, reflecting osteoblastic activity, and urinary hydroxyproline is usually increased, reflecting increased osteoclastic activity.

Clinical Picture (Table 79–1)

Most patients with Paget's disease have no symptoms, the disorder being discovered by radiographs taken for some other purpose or during investigation of the source of an elevated alkaline phosphatase. The most common symptom is pain in the area of bone involvement, which occurs most frequently in the sacrum, pelvis, and spine. Sudden onset of pain may result from a fracture or an infraction of a long bone. More rarely the patient may note painless deformity of the skull or of the long bones of the leg. Involvement of the skull may result in headaches, deafness, tinnitus, or vertigo. With platybasia, compression of the spinal cord and brain stem may result in serious neurological complications. Osteogenic sarcoma occurs in

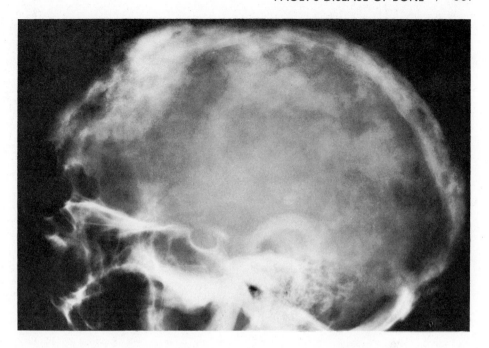

Figure 79–1. "Cottonwool" appearance of the skull in the osteoblastic phase of Paget's disease. (From Kelley WN, Harris ED Jr, Ruddy S, et al (eds): Textbook of Rheumatology. 2nd ed. Philadelphia, WB Saunders Co, 1985, p 1677.)

a small number of pagetic patients, especially those with polyostotic involvement of long duration.

The physical examination may show an enlarged skull, typical bowing of the long bones of the legs, redness and heat from vasodilatation over the areas of bone involvement, and angioid streaks in the optic fundi. Very rarely the increased cardiac output to the involved bone may result in high-output congestive failure. Other clinical and laboratory findings are listed in Table 79–1.

Diagnosis

The diagnosis can usually be established by the clinical picture and the characteristic radiographic findings (Fig. 79–1). Very rarely bone biopsy may be indicated to exclude the presence of osteoblastic metastases.

Treatment

Most patients do not require therapy, or else their pain responds adequately to full doses of salicylates or indomethacin. If pain persists, or in the face of neurological syndromes, increasing deformity or high output cardiac failure, an attempt to control the activity of the disease is indicated. Three approaches have been used with some success in reducing the activity of the disease, as measured by serum alkaline phosphatase or osteocalcin, or by the urinary excretion of hydroxyproline-containing (collagen-derived) peptides:

Calcitonin. This hormone is given parenterally, usually as salmon calcitonin, to inhibit osteoclastic activity. Human calcitonin is also available.

Diphosphonates. Oral disodium etidronate may be effective in inhibiting bone resorption but in large doses may inhibit mineralization as well, producing osteomalacia.

Mithramycin. This potent cytotoxic agent seems to have particular activity against the osteoclast, and its use parenterally may cause a remission of disease activity.

In addition, patients may benefit from orthopedic surgery to reduce deformities, replace a degenerative hip, or relieve neurological compression.

REFERENCES

Rebel A: Symposium: Paget's disease. Clin Orth Rel Res 217:2, 1987.

Singer FR: Paget's disease of bone (osteitis deformans). *In* Wyngaarden JB, Smith LH Jr (eds): Cecil Textbook of Medicine. 18th ed. Philadelphia, WB Saunders Co, 1988, p 1515.

SECTION
XI

INFECTIOUS DISEASES

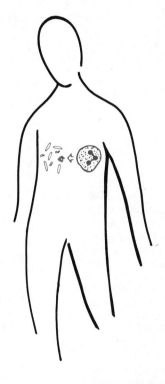

80

ORGANISMS THAT INFECT HUMANS

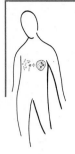

Of diseases afflicting humans, the great majority of those that are curable and preventable are caused by infectious agents. The infectious diseases that capture the attentions of physicians and the public periodically shift, for example from syphilis to tuberculosis to AIDS, but the challenges of dealing with these processes endure. To the student, understanding of infectious diseases offers insights into medicine as a whole. Osler's adage (with updating) remains relevant. "He (or she) who knows syphilis (AIDS), knows medicine."

VIRUSES

Viruses produce a wide variety of clinical illnesses. A virus consists of either DNA or RNA wrapped within a protein nucleocapsid. The nucleocapsid may be covered by an envelope composed of glycoproteins and lipids. Viral genes can code for only a limited number of proteins, and viruses possess no metabolic machinery. They are entirely dependent upon host cells for protein synthesis and replication and are therefore obligate intracellular parasites. Some viruses are dependent upon other viruses to produce active infection. Such is the case with the delta agent, which produces disease only in the presence of hepatitis B infection. All must attach to "receptors" on the host cell and achieve entry into the cell through host-derived mechanisms, usually pinocytosis. Once within the cells, the virus uncoats, allowing its nucleic acid to utilize host cellular machinery to reproduce (productive infection) or to integrate into the host cell (latent infection). Some viruses, such as influenza virus, cause disease by lysis of infected cells. Others such as hepatitis B virus do not directly cause cell destruction but may involve the host immune responses in the pathogenesis of disease. Still others such as the human T lymphotropic viruses types I and II promote neoplastic transformation of infected cells.

Viruses have developed several mechanisms of evading host defense mechanisms. By multiplying within host cells, viruses can avoid cytotoxic antibodies and other extracellular host defenses. Some viruses can spread to uninfected cells by intercellular bridges. Some viruses, especially the herpes group, are capable of persisting without multiplication in a metabolically inactive form within host cells for prolonged periods (latency). The influenza virus is capable of extensive gene rearrangements, resulting in significant changes in surface antigen structure. This allows new strains to evade host antibody responses directed at earlier strains.

CHLAMYDIA

Chlamydia are also obligate intracellular parasites, but unlike viruses they contain both DNA and RNA, divide by binary fission (rather than multiplying by assembly), can synthesize proteins, and contain ribosomes. They are unable to synthesize ATP and thus depend on energy from the host cell to survive. The three chlamydial species known to cause disease in man are *Chlamydia trachomatis*, *Chlamydia psittaci* and the TWAR agent. *C. trachomatis* causes trachoma, the major cause of blindness in the developing world, and a variety of sexually transmitted genitourinary disorders including urethritis, salpingitis, and lymphogranuloma venereum. *C. psittaci*, a common infectious disease of birds, can produce a serious systemic illness, with prominent pulmonary manifestations, in man. The TWAR agent is a recently described cause of pneumonia. These organisms are susceptible to tetracycline and erythromycin.

RICKETTSIA

Rickettsia are small bacterial organisms that, like chlamydia, are obligate intracellular parasites. Rickettsia are animal pathogens that generally produce disease in man through the bite of an insect vector such as a tick, flea, louse, or mite. The organisms specifically infect vascular endothelial cells. With the exception of Q fever, rash due to vasculitis is a prominent manifestation of these often disabling febrile illnesses. These organisms are susceptible to tetracyclines and chloramphenicol.

MYCOPLASMAS

Mycoplasmas are the smallest free-living organisms. In contrast to viruses, chlamydia, and rickettsia, mycoplasmas can grow on cell-free media and produce disease without intracellular penetration. Like other bacteria, these organisms have a membrane but, unlike other bacteria, they have no cell walls. Thus, antibiotics that are active against bacterial cell walls have no effect on mycoplasmas. Three major species of mycoplasmas cause disease in man: *Mycoplasma pneumoniae* is an agent of pharyngitis and pneumonia, whereas *Mycoplasma hominis* and *Ureaplasma urealyticum* are agents of genitourinary disease. Mycoplasmas are sensitive to erythromycin or tetracycline or both.

BACTERIA

Bacteria are a tremendously varied group of organisms that are generally capable of cell-free growth, although some produce disease as intracellular parasites. There are numerous ways of classifying bacteria, including morphology, ability to retain certain dyes, growth in different physical conditions, ability to metabolize various substrates, and antibiotic sensitivities. Although combinations of these methods are used to identify bacteria in hospital bacteriology laboratories, relatedness for taxonomic purposes is established by DNA homology.

SPIROCHETES

Spirochetes are slender, motile, spiral-shaped organisms that are not readily seen under the microscope unless stained with silver or viewed under darkfield illumination. Many of these organisms cannot yet be cultured on artificial media or in cell culture. There are four genera of spirochetes that cause disease in man. *Treponema* include the pathogens of syphilis and the nonvenereal endemic syphilis-like illnesses of yaws, pinta, and bejel. The illnesses caused by these organisms are chronic and characterized by prolonged latency in the host. Penicillin is active against *Treponema*. *Leptospira* species are the causative agents of leptospirosis, an acute or subacute febrile illness occasionally resulting in aseptic meningitis, jaundice, and (rarely) renal insufficiency. *Borrelia* species are arthropod-borne spirochetes that are the causative agents of Lyme disease (see Chapter 84) and relapsing fever. During afebrile periods in relapsing fever, these organisms reside within host cells and emerge with modified cell surface antigens. These modifications may permit the bacterium to evade host immune responses and produce relapsing fever and recurrent bacteremia. *Spirillum minor* is one of the causative agents of rat-bite fever.

ANAEROBIC BACTERIA

Anaerobes are organisms that cannot grow in atmospheric oxygen tensions. Some are killed by very low oxygen concentrations, whereas others are relatively aerotolerant. As a general rule, anaerobes that are pathogens for man are not as sensitive to oxygen as nonpathogens. Anaerobic bacteria are primarily commensals. They inhabit the skin, gut, and mucosal surfaces of all healthy individuals. In fact, the presence of anaerobes may inhibit colonization of the gut by virulent, potentially pathogenic bacteria. Anaerobic infections generally occur in two circumstances: (1) contamination of otherwise sterile sites with anaerobe-laden contents. Examples include (a) aspiration of oral anaerobes into the bronchial tree, producing anaerobic necrotizing pneumonia; (b) peritonitis and intra-abdominal abscesses following bowel perforation; (c) fasciitis and osteomyelitis following periodon-

tal infections or oral surgery. (2) Infections of tissue with lowered redox potential as the result of a compromised vascular supply. Examples include (a) foot infections in diabetic patients, in whom vascular disease may produce poor tissue oxygenation; and (b) infections of pressure sores, in which perianal anaerobic flora gain access to tissue whose vascular supply is compromised by pressure. The pathogenesis of anaerobic infections, i.e., soilage by a complex flora, generally results in polymicrobial infections. Thus, the demonstration of one anaerobe in an infected site generally implies the presence of others. Often facultative organisms (organisms capable of anaerobic and aerobic growths) coexist with anaerobes. Certain anaerobes such as *Clostridium* produce toxins that cause well-defined illnesses such as food poisoning, tetanus, and botulism. Other toxins may play a role in the soft tissue infections—cellulitis, fasciitis, and myonecrosis—occasionally produced by *Clostridium* species. *Bacteroides fragilis*, the most numerous bacterial pathogen in the normal human colon, has a polysaccharide capsule that inhibits phagocytosis and promotes abscess formation. Clues to the presence of anaerobic infection include (a) a foul odor (the diagnosis of anaerobic pneumonia can, on occasion, be made from across the room); (b) the presence of gas, which may be seen radiographically or manifested by crepitus on examination (however, not all gas-forming infections are anaerobic); and (c) the presence of mixed gram-positive and gram-negative flora on a Gram's stain of purulent exudate, especially when there is little or no growth on plates cultured aerobically. Most anaerobes are sensitive to penicillin. Exceptions are strains of *Bacteroides fragilis* (usually sensitive to metronidazole, clindamycin, or chloramphenicol) and *Clostridium difficile*, which is almost always sensitive to metronidazole and vancomycin. Strains of *Fusobacterium* may also be relatively resistant to penicillin. As a general rule, infections caused by anaerobes originating from sites above the diaphragm are penicillin-sensitive, whereas infections below the diaphragm are often caused by penicillin-resistant organisms, notably *Bacteroides fragilis*.

GRAM-NEGATIVE BACTERIA

The cell walls of these bacteria, which appear pink on a properly prepared Gram's stain, contain lipopolysaccharide, a potent inducer of endogenous pyrogen release and fever. These organisms cause a wide variety of illnesses. Gram-negative bacteria are the most common cause of cystitis and pyelonephritis. *Haemophilus* species organisms are common pathogens of the respiratory tract causing otitis media, sinusitis, tracheobronchitis, and pneumonia. Lower respiratory tract infections due to these organisms are particularly common in adults with chronic obstructive pulmonary disease. *Haemophilus* is also an important cause of meningitis, particularly in children. Excepting *Haemophilus* species, gram-negative bacteria are uncommon causes of community-acquired pneumonia but common causes of nosocomial pneumonia. Excepting the peculiar risk of *Pseudomonas* infection in I.V. drug abusers, gram-negative organisms are rare causes of endocarditis on natural heart valves but occasional pathogens on prosthetic valves. The Enterobacteriaceae include *Escherichia coli*, *Klebsiella*, *Enterobacter*, *Serratia*, *Salmonella*, *Shigella*, and *Proteus*. These are large gram-negative rods. Except for the occasional presence of a clear space surrounding some *Klebsiella* (representing a large capsule), these organisms are not readily distinguished from each other on Gram's stain. The Enterobacteriaceae can be thought of as gut-related or genitourinary pathogens. *Salmonella*, a relatively common cause of enteritis, may occasionally infect atherosclerotic plaques or aneurysms. *Shigella* is an agent of bacterial dysentery. *Proteus* species, which split urea, are the agents associated with staghorn calculi of the ureters and urinary collecting system.

GRAM-POSITIVE BACTERIA

Although these organisms (which appear deep purple on Gram's stain) lack endotoxin, infections with gram-positive bacteria also produce fever and cannot be reliably distinguished, on clinical grounds, from infections caused by gram-negative bacteria.

GRAM-POSITIVE RODS

Infections due to gram-positive rods are relatively uncommon outside certain specific settings. Diphtheria is rare but other corynebacteria produce infections in the immunocompromised host and on prosthetic valves and shunts. Because corynebacteria are regular skin colonizers, they often contaminate blood cultures; in the appropriate setting, however, they must be considered potential pathogens. *Listeria monocytogenes* resembles *Corynebacterium* on initial isolation and is an important cause of meningitis and bacteremia in the immunocompromised patient. *Bacillus cereus* is a recognized cause of food poisoning. Serious infections due to this and other *Bacillus* species occur among I.V. drug abusers. *Clostridium* species are gram-positive rods. Infections due to these organisms are discussed under anaerobes (see above).

GRAM-POSITIVE COCCI

Staphylococcus aureus is a common pathogen that produces a wide spectrum of disease in humans. Staphylococci can infect any organ system. They are common causes of bacteremia and sepsis. The organism often colonizes the anterior nares, particularly among diabetics, hemodialysis patients, and I.V. drug abusers; these populations also have a greater frequency of infections due to this organism. Hospital workers colonized with *Staphylococcus aureus* have also been responsible for hospital epidemics of staphylococcal disease.

Generally protected by an antiphagocytic polysaccharide capsule, staphylococci also possess catalase, which inactivates hydrogen peroxide—a mediator of bacterial killing by neutrophils. Staphylococci tend to form abscesses; the low pH within an abscess cavity also limits the effectiveness of host defense cells. Staphylococci elaborate several toxins that mediate certain manifestations of disease. A staphylococcal enterotoxin is responsible for staphylococcal food poisoning. Staphylococcal toxins also mediate the scalded skin syndrome and the multisystem manifestations of toxic shock syndrome. Most staphylococci are penicillinase-producing and some are resistant to penicillinase-resistant penicillin analogues as well. Vancomycin is active almost against all strains. Some staphylococci are "tolerant" to cell wall–active antibiotics such as penicillins or vancomycin; such organisms are inhibited but not killed by these agents. The clinical significance of tolerance is not certain. Other staphylococci are distinguished from *Staphylococcus aureus* primarily by their inability to produce coagulase. Some of these coagulase-negative staphylococci produce urinary tract infection (*Staphylococcus saprophyticus*). Another, *Staphylococcus epidermidis*, is part of the normal skin flora and an important cause of infection on foreign bodies such as prosthetic heart valves, ventriculoatrial shunts, and intravascular catheters. Like *Corynebacterium*, *Staphylococcus epidermidis* may be a contaminant of blood cultures but in the appropriate setting should be considered a potential pathogen. *Staphylococcus saprophyticus* is sensitive to a variety of antibiotics used in the treatment of urinary tract infection; *Staphylococcus epidermidis* is often resistant to most antimicrobials but is usually sensitive to vancomycin.

Streptococci are a group of organisms whose classifications humble the internist and embarrass the microbiologist. Streptococci are classified into groups according to the presence of serologically defined carbohydrate capsules (Lancefield typing). Group A streptococci produce skin infections and pharyngitis. These organisms are also associated with the immunologically mediated post-streptococcal disorders—glomerulonephritis and acute rheumatic fever. Group D streptococci include enterococci, which are unique among the streptococci in their uniform resistance to penicillin. Streptococci can be classified according to the pattern of hemolysis on blood agar—alpha for incomplete hemolysis (producing a green discoloration on the agar), beta for complete hemolysis, and gamma for nonhemolytic strains. Most Lancefield group strains are beta-hemolytic. An important alpha-hemolytic strain is *Streptococcus pneumoniae* (pneumococcus), the most common cause of bacterial pneumonia and an important cause of meningitis and otitis media. A heterogeneous group of streptococci, often improperly referred to as viridans streptococci (these organisms show alpha- or gamma-hemolysis) includes several species of streptococci that are common oral or gut flora and are important agents of bacterial endocarditis, abscesses, and odontogenic infections.

MYCOBACTERIA

Mycobacteria are a group of rod-shaped bacilli that stain weakly gram-positive. These organisms are rich in lipid content and are recognized in tissue specimens by their ability to retain dye after washing with acid-alcohol (acid-fast). These bacteria are generally slow-growing (some require up to six weeks to demonstrate growth on solid media) obligate aerobes. They generally produce chronic disease and manage to survive for years as intracellular parasites of mononuclear phagocytes. Some escape intracellular killing mechanisms by disrupting the phagosome. Almost all provoke cell-mediated immune responses in the host, and clinical disease expression may be related in large part to the nature of the host immune response. Tuberculosis is caused by *Mycobacterium tuberculosis*. Other mycobacteria—nontuberculous mycobacteria—can produce diseases resembling tuberculosis. Certain rapid-growing mycobacteria cause infections following surgery or implantations of prostheses, and *Mycobacterium avium* has been implicated as an important cause of disseminated infection among patients with the acquired immunodeficiency syndrome. Leprosy is a mycobacterial disease of skin and peripheral nerves caused by *M. leprae*.

"HIGHER BACTERIA"

Nocardia and *Actinomyces* are weakly gram-positive filamentous structures. *Nocardia* is acid-fast and aerobic; *Actinomyces* is anaerobic and not acid-fast. *Actinomyces* inhabits the mouth, gut, and vagina and produces cervicofacial osteomyelitis and abscess, pneumonia with empyema, and intra-abdominal and pelvic abscess, the latter generally associated with intrauterine contraceptive devices. *Nocardia* most commonly produces pneumonia and brain abscess. Approximately half of patients with *Nocardia* infection have underlying impairments in cell-mediated immunity. Infections with either of these organisms require long-term treatment. *Actinomyces* is relatively sensitive to most antibiotics; penicillin is the treatment of choice. *Nocardia* infections are treated with high doses of sulfonamides.

FUNGI

Fungi are larger than bacteria. Unlike bacteria, they have rigid cell walls that contain chitin as well as polysaccharides. They regrow and proliferate by budding, by elongation of hyphal forms, and/or by spore formation. Excepting *Candida* and related species, fungi are rarely visible on Gram's stained preparations but can be stained with Gomori methenamine silver stain. They are also resistant to potassium hydroxide and can often be visualized on wet mounts of scrapings or secretions to which several drops of 10 per cent solution of potassium hydroxide has been added. Fungi are resistant to antibiotics used in the treatment of bacterial infections and must be treated with drugs active against their unusual cell wall. Most fungi can exist in a yeast form—round to ovoid cells that may reproduce by budding—and a mold form—a complex of tubular structures (hyphae) that grow by branching or extension.

Candida species are oval yeasts that often colonize the mouth, gastrointestinal tract, and vagina of healthy individuals. They may produce disease by overgrowth and/or invasion. *Candida* stomatitis (thrush) often occurs in individuals who are receiving antibiotic or corticosteroid therapy or who have impairments of cell-mediated immunity. Vulvovaginitis due to *Candida* may occur in these same settings but is also seen among women with diabetes mellitus or with no apparent predisposing factors. *Candida* can also colonize and infect the urinary tract, particularly in the presence of an indwelling urinary catheter. Occasionally *Candida* species may gain entry into the blood stream and produce sepsis. This may occur in the setting of neutropenia and chemotherapy, where the portal of entry is the gastrointestinal tract, or in individuals receiving intravenous feedings, in whom the catheter is the source of the infection. Mucosal candidiasis can be treated with topical (clotrimazole) or systemic (ketoconazole) imidazole drugs; systemic candidiasis is generally treated with amphotericin B.

Histoplasma capsulatum is a fungus, endemic to the Ohio and Mississippi River valleys, which produces a mild febrile syndrome in most individuals and a self-limited pneumonia in some. Occasionally patients develop potentially fatal disseminated disease. Some individuals with chronic pulmonary disease may develop chronic pneumonia due to this yeast. Systemic or progressive disease is treated with amphotericin B; ketoconazole may also be effective in some cases.

Coccidioides immitis is endemic in the Southwestern United States and, like *Histoplasma capsulatum*, produces a self-limited respiratory infection or pneumonia in most individuals. Some individuals, particularly blacks and patients of Philippine descent, may be at greater risk for fatal systemic dissemination. Amphotericin B is used for progressive or extrapulmonary disease.

Cryptococcus neoformans is a yeast with a large polysaccharide capsule. It produces a self-limited or chronic pneumonia, but the most common clinical manifestation of infection with this fungus is a chronic meningitis. Although patients with impairment in cell-mediated immunity are at risk for cryptococcal meningitis, some patients with this syndrome have no identifiable immunodeficiency. Treatment is with amphotericin B combined with flucytosine.

Blastomyces dermatitidis is a yeast also endemic in the Ohio and Mississippi River basins. Acute self-limited pulmonary infection is followed rarely by disseminated disease. Skin disease is most common, but bones and genitourinary tract may be involved as well. Amphotericin B is used for systemic disease.

Aspergillus is a mold that produces several different clinical illnesses in man. Acute bronchopulmonary aspergillosis is an IgE-mediated hypersensitivity to *Aspergillus* colonization of the respiratory tract. This produces wheezing and fleeting pulmonary infiltrates in patients with asthma. Occasionally, *Aspergillus* will colonize a pre-existent pulmonary cavity and produce a mycetoma or fungus ball. Hemoptysis is the most serious complication of such infection. Invasive pul-

TABLE 80–1. SOME PROTOZOAN DISEASES OF MAN

PROTOZOAN	CLINICAL ILLNESS	TRANSMISSION	DIAGNOSIS
Plasmodium	Malaria: fever, hemolysis	Mosquito, transfusion	Peripheral blood smear
Babesia microti	Fever, hemolysis	Tick, transfusion	Peripheral blood smear
Trichomonas vaginalis	Vaginitis	Sexual contact	Vaginal smear
Toxoplasma gondii	Fever, lymph node enlargement. Encephalitis, brain abscess in compromised host	Raw meat, cat feces	Serologies, tissue biopsy
Pneumocystis carinii	Pneumonia in immuno-compromised host	?Airborne*	Lung biopsy, bronchial lavage
Entamoeba histolytica	Colitis, hepatic abscess	Fecal-oral	Stool smear, serologies
Giardia lamblia	Diarrhea, malabsorption	Fecal-oral	Stool smear, small bowel aspirate
Cryptosporidium	Diarrhea	?Fecal-oral	Sugar flotation, acid-fast stain of stool

* *Primary* infection is presumably airborne, but clinical disease usually results from multiplication of resident microorganisms in an immunocompromised host. Respiratory isolation is not indicated.

monary aspergillosis rarely is a chronic illness of otherwise healthy or marginally compromised hosts, but more often it is a cause of acute pneumonia in patients with neutropenia or recipients of organ transplants. Amphotericin B is the drug of choice for invasive aspergillosis.

The zygomycetes (Mucorales) are molds with ribbon-shaped hyphae that produce disease in patients with poorly controlled diabetes mellitus or hematologic malignancy and among recipients of organ transplantation. Invasive disease of the palate and nasal sinuses, producing venous thrombosis and infarcts in the brain, is the most common presentation, but pneumonia may be seen as well. These infections are generally treated with surgical excision plus amphotericin B.

PROTOZOANS

In contrast to the pathogens listed above, these single-cell organisms are animals, not plants. With the exception of *Plasmodium*, the pathogens listed on Table 80–1 are all transmitted within the United States.

HELMINTHS

Diseases due to helminths are among the most prevalent diseases in the developing world but are uncommon causes of illness in North America.

REFERENCE

Gardner P, Provine HT: Manual of Acute Bacterial Infections. Boston, Little, Brown & Co, 1975.

81

HOST DEFENSES AGAINST INFECTION

Both nonspecific and specific host defense mechanisms contribute to the prevention of infectious diseases. The integument, mucous membranes, and epithelial surfaces provide a vital mechanical barrier to infection. The indigenous flora of these surfaces, particularly the anaerobic bacteria, prevent colonization with virulent organisms by competing for nutrients and receptor sites on host cells and by producing factors, termed bacteriocins, that are toxic to other bacteria. The local milieu, chiefly the pH and redox potential, provides an additional barrier to colonization and infection with certain pathogenic organisms. Gastric acid reduces bacterial counts by 10- to 10,000-fold. The normal flow of mucus and other secretions helps to eliminate microorganisms from mucosal surfaces. The mucociliary blanket, for example, transports organisms away from the lungs. In addition, locally produced and active antimicrobial substances prevent infection. Lactoperoxidase, lysozyme, and lactoferrin in salivary and vaginal secretions and milk have microbicidal activity. Secretory IgA has a particularly important role in this respect, opsonizing organisms and thereby blocking their ability to adhere to epithelial surfaces and colonize the mucosa.

The elements of the systemic host resistance to infection are best considered in terms of the components of the immune system and nonspecific effector cell responses. Effective resistance requires interaction of these elements, however, as indicated by the overlapping of host defenses active against certain infectious agents.

COMPONENTS OF THE IMMUNE SYSTEM

The principal cells of the immune system are bone-marrow derived (B) and thymus-dependent (T) lymphocytes and mononuclear phagocytes. They are organized as a recirculating pool of lymphocytes and monocytes, bone marrow cells, and organized lymphoid tissue (lymph nodes, spleen, Peyer's patches, and the thymus).

The primary function of the immune system is to destroy foreign organisms and clear foreign antigens without damaging host tissues. Immunity also is important in maintaining certain infectious agents in a latent stage and may play a role in destroying virally infected cells or cells that have undergone malignant transformation. The immune response is characterized by three features—immunologic memory, specificity, and systemic action. The functional organization of the immune response can be considered in six sequential steps: encounter, recognition, activation, deployment, discrimination, and regulation.

ENCOUNTER

Microbes and soluble antigens encounter antigen-presenting cells (APC) in the tissues and are ingested and catabolized. Monocytes, macrophages, dendritic cells, and Langerhan's cells are examples of APC. The physical form of the antigen and the site of exposure or breaching of tissue determine which type of APC is relevant. Particulates are more readily ingested by active phagocytes such as macrophages; dendritic cells may be critical to the handling of soluble protein antigens. The gastrointestinal and respiratory tract, important sites for interface of the immune system with the environment, possess well-differentiated APC in submucosal areas. Some microbes elicit a neutrophilic inflammatory response and are phagocytosed and degraded by neutrophils, thereby bypassing traditional APCs and eliciting inflammation but little or no immune response. The disposition of soluble antigen is determined by the likelihood of uptake by APC; an aggregated form of antigen or antigen bound by specific antibody in immune complexes favors uptake by APC. Following ingestion by APC, the foreign antigen is degraded in acidic vesicles and reprocessed to the surface of the cell, where, in close approximation to determinants encoded by the Class II major histocompatibility complex (MHC), it is accessible to lymphocytes. APCs also produce cytokines such as interleukin-1 (IL-1) which amplify immune induction (Fig. 81–1).

RECOGNITION

The immune system has the capability of responding to virtually any antigen. It appears that B cells and T cells utilize similar mechanisms to generate and express the diversity required for such a broad range of specific antigenic responses.

Five classes of antibodies (isotypes) are recognized (Table 81–1). An IgG1 antibody (Fig. 81–2) consists of two light (kappa or lambda) and two heavy chains.

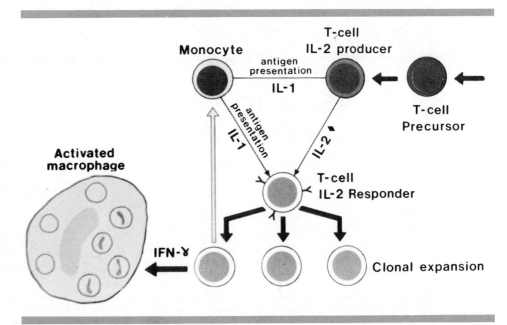

FIGURE 81–1. The cytokine cascade. The monocyte or other antigen-presenting cell ingests and degrades microbes, presents antigen to T cells, and produces the amplifying cytokine interleukin-1 (IL-1). T cells are activated to express surface receptors for the lymphokine interleukin-2 (IL-2) and to produce IL-2. The binding of IL-2 to its receptor leads to clonal expansion and enhances production of interferon-γ (IFN-γ). IFN-γ has major macrophage activating factor activity and promotes destruction of intracellular parasites such as the tubercle bacillus. IL-2 and IFN-γ also are required for the differentiation of cytotoxic T lymphocytes (not shown). IL-2 and IFN-γ are available in recombinant form and are undergoing evaluation for the treatment of AIDS and drug-resistant mycobacterial infections.

TABLE 81–1. PROPERTIES OF HUMAN IMMUNOGLOBULINS

	IgG	IgA	IgM	IgD	IgE
H chain class	γ	α	μ	δ	ϵ
Molecular weight (approximate)	150,000	160,000	900,000	180,000	190,000
Complement fixation (classic)	+	0	+ +	0	0
Serum concentration (approximate; mg/dl)	1,000	200	120	3	0.05
Serum half-life (days)	23	6	5	2–8	1–5

Adapted from Goodman JW: Immunoglobulins, I. *In* Stites DP, Stobo JD, Fudenberg HH, et al (eds): Basic and Clinical Immunology. Los Altos, Lange Medical Publications, 1982, p 34.

Each antibody has constant regions, which are identical in structure to all antibodies of that class, and also distinctive antigen recognition sites whose structures are quite variable. An IgG1 molecule has two such antigen-combining sites. The variable regions consist of the approximately 110 N-terminal amino acids of each chain. There are three short, hypervariable regions in each of the light and the heavy chains. The six hypervariable regions form the combining site.

The generation of antibody diversity is understood at the molecular level. The variable portion of the heavy chain is encoded by three different genes—V, D, and J; there are 500 to 1000 different V genes, 10 D genes, and 4 J genes. The variable portions of the

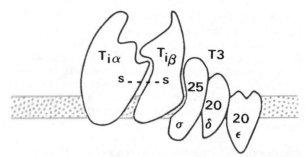

FIGURE 81–3. Structure of the human T-cell receptor and its subunits. This diagram shows subunit composition of the human T-cell receptor. The Tiα and Tiβ subunits are held together by S-S bonds and are anchored in the cell membrane with their transmembrane segments. The T_1 protein of the T cell receptor is most closely associated with the 25-kd γ chain of the T3 molecule. The T3 complex includes two additional subunits (δ and ϵ), with molecular weights of 20,000. (From Nossal GJV: Current concepts: Immunology. The basic components of the immune system. N Engl J Med 36:1320, 1987.)

light chains are encoded by V and J genes; there are 200 possible V and 6 J genes. During the differentiation of B cells, somatic translocations randomly select the V, D, and J heavy chain genes and the V and J light chain genes that will be transcribed in that cell. The diversity achieved by these means is enormous. Somatic mutations in B cells allow the possibility of improving the fit between antibody and antigen; repeated or sustained exposure to antigen selects B cells capable of producing antibody with the highest binding affinity. These circulate as memory cells.

The T-cell receptor for antigen is a heterodimer of two polypeptide chains, designated alpha and beta (Fig. 81–3). The variable portion is composed of the approximately 100 N-terminal amino acids. The generation of diversity is by translocation of V, D, and J genes, as is the case for B lymphocytes. The T-cell receptor is directed at a foreign antigen associated with MHC determinants. Class I MHC products are recognized by CD8 suppressor/cytotoxic T cells, and Class II by CD4 helper T cells.

ACTIVATION OF LYMPHOCYTES

CD4 helper T cells are activated when the T-cell receptors are occupied and effectively cross-linked by the antigen-Class II MHC complex on the surface of an APC. Activation of the T cell is promoted by IL-1 released as a consequence of the cellular interactions. The helper T cell enlarges, secretes a variety of lymphokines, and divides to form a clone. The antigen molecule may also form a bridge between T cells and B cells, permitting the targeted delivery of B-cell growth and differentiation factors from T cell to B cell. The B cell, which is activated by a combination of signals provided by binding of antigen and T cells, enlarges, divides, and differentiates into an antibody-producing cell. T-cell products also promote an isotype switch from IgM to production of IgG, IgA, or IgE.

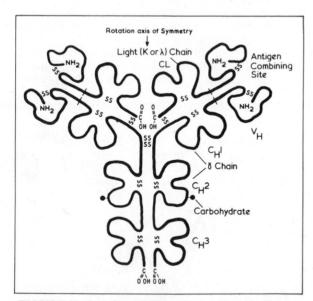

FIGURE 81–2. Schematic diagram of a molecule of human IgG, showing the two light (κ or λ) chains and two heavy (γ) chains held together by disulfide bonds. The constant regions of the light (CL) and heavy (C_H1, C_H2, and C_H3) chains and the variable region of the heavy chain (V_H) are indicated. Loops in the peptide chain formed by intrachain disulfide bonds (C_H1, and so forth) comprise separate functional domains. (From Nossal GJV: Current concepts: Immunology. The basic components of the immune system. N Engl J Med 316:1320, 1987.)

Initial exposure of humans to microbial antigens leads to proliferation of B cells recognizing the antigen and differentiation into antibody-forming plasma cells. T-cell help is required for responses to most antigens, although bacterial polysaccharides may directly elicit antibody production. Following the first exposure to an antigen, IgM is the main antibody class or isotype produced. An isotype switch then occurs such that IgG predominates. On any re-exposure to the antigen, production of IgG antibody is accelerated and antibody is produced in high titer and with high avidity for the antigen. Secretory IgA is found in tears, saliva, and bronchial, nasal, vaginal, prostatic, and intestinal secretions. Its primary role is to prevent organisms and antigens from attaching to and breaching mucosal barriers.

IgM accounts for 10 per cent of normal immunoglobulins and is the antibody isotype most efficient at complement fixation. Both IgM and IgG can neutralize the infectivity of viruses and lyse bacteria through complement fixation. Mononuclear phagocytes, neutrophils, and some lymphocytes possess surface receptors for the Fc fragment of IgG and/or the third component of complement. Therefore, IgG antibody or complement can bind to and opsonize bacteria, facilitating their phagocytosis (Fig. 81–4), and IgG antibody can arm host effector cells for preferential destruction of selected targets by the process of antibody-dependent cellular cytotoxicity.

APC and CD4 cells acting in concert are required for activation of CD8 cells for cytotoxic and suppressor cell activity. The activated CD4 cell also secretes a number of factors important in hematopoiesis, mobilization of bone marrow precursor cells, chemotaxis of mononuclear and other cells to areas of inflammation, and expression of the cellular immune response.

DEPLOYMENT

The events thus far discussed are required for activation of antigen-specific lymphocytes. Neither antibody nor activated lymphocytes are capable of directly destroying pathogenic organisms. Rather, they act in concert with antigen-nonspecific components of the immune response including phagocytes and the complement and other molecular systems. For example, one of the key cytokines produced by activated CD4 cells is interferon-gamma; the interferon activates mononuclear phagocytes and thus renders them capable of killing intracellular parasites and tumors (see Fig. 81–1).

The mobility of lymphocytes is central to the memory and systemic function of the immune response. Some progeny of activated B and T cells return to the resting stage, leaving the peripheral lymphoid tissue to traffic as memory cells in the recirculating pool. These lymphocytes perfuse the tissues of the body and can re-enter the lymph nodes. Reinfection or re-exposure to an antigen at any site can lead to activation of memory lymphocytes.

DISCRIMINATION

Tolerance of self-antigens prevents autoimmune disease. Several mechanisms contribute to tolerance. Early in ontogeny, exposure to antigen leads to refractoriness to that antigen. This process has been termed "clonal anergy." Suppressor T cells are activated when soluble antigen is injected intravenously without adjuvant; this resembles exposure to most self-antigens. Moreover, self-antigens are not presented to reactive CD4 cells in combination with Class II MHC determinants so that immune induction fails to occur. The breakdown of tolerance and autoimmune disease may result from a combination of factors: tissue damage exposing new antigens to the immune system and genetic factors that regulate the response to self-antigens and determine end-organ susceptibility to damage.

REGULATION

The immune response must be appropriate to the challenging event; too little may permit unchecked infection, whereas too great a response may damage tissue. Regulatory mechanisms amplify or mute an immune response and may be specific or nonspecific.

Antigen itself regulates the immune response. As antigen is cleared, a process enhanced by specific antibody, only lymphocytes bearing the highest affinity receptors are activated. Once antigen is cleared entirely, the immune response diminishes, although memory cells continue to provide surveillance for re-exposure to the antigen. Antibody has an additional role in immunoregulation, since immune complexes may directly modulate the response of specific lymphocytes. Antibody also may be directed at the antigen-combining site of antibody itself. Such "anti-idiotypic antibodies" are activated by the immune response and may suppress further production of the relevant antibody.

Activation of the immune response also induces cellular regulatory mechanisms. For example, the activated CD4 cell is an important stimulus for induction of suppression by CD8 cells and mononuclear phagocytes.

NONSPECIFIC EFFECTOR MECHANISMS

Complement. Complement activity results from the sequential interaction of a large number (25 are recognized) of plasma and cell-membrane interactive proteins. The classic complement pathway is activated by antibody-coated targets or antigen-antibody complexes. The alternative pathway is activated by bacterial polysaccharides. Complement binds to bacteria, facilitating their attachment by C3b receptors on phagocytes, thus constituting the heat-labile opsonic system (Fig. 81–4); it directly damages certain bacteria and viruses, and it induces inflammation through chemotactically active fragments.

Neutrophils. The neutrophil ingests bacteria and kills them through its production of toxic oxygen metabolites and halogenation of proteins via myeloperoxidase.

Mononuclear Phagocytes. Macrophages have immunoregulatory and secretory properties in addition to their role as effector cells of cell-mediated immunity. Macrophages degrade and kill bacteria directly and in antibody-dependent reactions. Macrophages must be activated by T cell products (e.g., interferon gamma) in order to kill facultative intracellular pathogens such as *Mycobacterium tuberculosis*.

Natural Killer Cells. These lymphocytes are defined by their ability to lyse certain tumor targets and may be involved in tumor surveillance. However, natural killer cells and cytotoxic T cells also are important in antiviral immunity; they kill virus-infected cells.

Integration of the various host defense mechanisms is apparent as one examines resistance to specific representative infectious agents.

RESISTANCE TO EXTRACELLULAR BACTERIA

Encapsulated Organisms

Streptococcus pneumoniae. The type-specific polysaccharide capsule is a major virulence factor because of its antiphagocytic properties. Antibody to the polysaccharide is itself capable of preventing pneumococcal disease, as reflected by experimental studies and the efficacy of pneumococcal polysaccharide vaccines.

In the absence of immunity, pneumococci reaching the alveoli are not effectively contained by the host. Their phagocytosis by neutrophils is inefficient, since organisms must be trapped against a surface to be ingested ("surface phagocytosis"—Fig. 81–4). The pneumococcus does, however, elicit a neutrophilic inflammatory response. The organism activates complement by the alternative pathway and interactions of C-reactive protein in serum with pneumococcal C-polysaccharide. Activated complement fragments (C3a, C5a, C567) and bacterial oligopeptides are chemotactic for neutrophils. Opsonic complement fragments (C3b) coating pneumococci favor their attachment to neutrophils but are less effective in promoting phagocytosis and killing than is specific antibody. Clinical observations also directly support the primal role of antibody in immunity. It is the development of specific antibody on days five to nine of untreated pneumococcal pneumonia that produces a clinical "crisis" with dramatic resolution of symptoms.

Neisseria meningitidis. Capsular polysaccharide also represents an important virulence factor for meningococci. In addition, pathogenic *Neisseria* species produce an IgA protease that dissociates the Fc fragment from the Fab portion of secretory and serum IgA, thus interfering with effector properties of the antibody molecule. Antibody-dependent complement-mediated bacterial killing is the critical host defense against meningococci. Illustrating this principle, the incidence of meningococcal meningitis during the first 12 years of life is inversely proportional to the age-related frequency of serum bactericidal antibody directed against capsular and cell wall bacterial antigens. Therefore, the presence of bactericidal antibody is associated with protection against the meningococcus. In epidemic situations, 40 per cent of individuals who

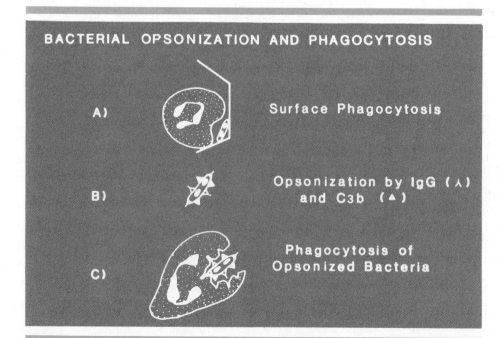

BACTERIAL OPSONIZATION AND PHAGOCYTOSIS

A) Surface Phagocytosis

B) Opsonization by IgG (⅄) and C3b (▲)

C) Phagocytosis of Opsonized Bacteria

FIGURE 81–4. Ingestion of pneumococci by the neutrophil. In the absence of opsonins, the slippery pneumococcus must be forced against an alveolar surface to be ingested, the inefficient process of surface phagocytosis. Bacteria are opsonized by C3b and IgG, which interact with receptors on the neutrophil, thereby facilitating phagocytosis.

become colonized with the epidemic strain but lack bactericidal antibodies develop disease. Protective serum antibody is elicited by colonization with (1) non-encapsulated and encapsulated strains of meningococci of low virulence which elicit antibodies cross-reactive with virulent strains, and (2) *E. coli* and *Bacillus* species with cross-reacting capsular polysaccharides. The lack of bactericidal activity in the serum of adolescents and adults manifesting susceptibility to *N. meningitidis* may be due to blocking IgA antibody. Susceptibility of patients lacking C6, C7, or C8 to meningococcal infection provides important evidence that the dominant protective mechanism against this organism involves complement-mediated bacteriolysis. Evaluation of children developing meningococcal disease in a nonepidemic setting reveals that a sizable proportion do have underlying abnormalities of the complement system.

Exotoxin-Producing Organisms

Clostridium tetani. All disease manifestations produced by this organism can be ascribed to the tetanus toxin, tetanospasmin. Antibody to toxin is protective. Survival from tetanus does not, however, lead to immunity to subsequent infection, because the toxin is sufficiently potent to cause disease at subimmunogenic concentrations.

RESISTANCE TO OBLIGATE INTRACELLULAR PARASITES: VIRUSES

The host directs several defenses against viral infection. The same humoral and cellular mechanisms that destroy bacteria serve to clear extracellular viruses. However, the host immune response also is effective against intracellular replicative stages of viruses and may destroy infected host cells that express viral antigens on their surfaces. Clinical and experimental observations indicate the respective roles of humoral and cellular immunity in resistance against certain viruses. In Hodgkin's disease and in T lymphocyte-deficient experimental models, selective defects in cellular immunity lead to reactivation of certain latent Herpetoviridae: herpes simplex, varicella-zoster, and cytomegalovirus. The prominent role for cellular immunity against these agents is biologically advantageous because virions spread intercellularly via desmosomes or intercellular bridges; viruses thereby avoid exposure to the antibody-rich extracellular milieu. Destruction of virus-infected cells by specific cytotoxic T cells becomes an essential first step in host defense by allowing extracellular mechanisms to mop up free viral particles.

In contrast, antibody-dependent mechanisms assume major importance against viruses that themselves lyse host cells and spread by extracellular means; for these agents, passive transfer of antibody confers protection. Nevertheless, the absence of greatly increased susceptibility of hypogammaglobulinemic patients to measles and influenza implies the continued contribution of cellular immunity in protection against these agents and indicates important overlap in antiviral host effector mechanisms.

The major antiviral defenses include humoral immune mechanisms, cellular immunity, and interferons.

Humoral Defenses

Complement-Independent Neutralization. Specific IgG, IgM, and IgA neutralize infectivity of viruses. The respective antibodies first combine with proteins of the virus coat. Resultant conformational changes may prevent adsorption of viruses to cells and cellular penetration; sometimes antibody coating of extracellular virus interferes with subsequent intracellular events such as uncoating. Alternatively, antibody may physically aggregate viral particles.

IgA is the key defender against viruses that begin in or are confined to respiratory epithelium. For infections such as polio, measles, and rubella, which begin on a mucosal surface and then disseminate hematogenously, local IgA antibody prevents infection, whereas serum IgG antibody prevents disease.

Complement-Facilitated Neutralization. Complement neutralizes some enveloped viruses by direct or antibody-dependent steric changes or aggregation. Infected host cells expressing surface virus antigens also are susceptible to lysis by mechanisms involving the alternate complement pathway and further enhanced by antibody.

Opsonization of extracellular viruses by complement and IgG antibody facilitates phagocytosis by neutrophils and macrophages. This process destroys some viruses (enteroviruses) but aids cellular penetration and replication of others (arboviruses).

Enzyme Inhibition. Antibody may interfere with release of progeny influenza virus by blocking viral neuraminidase. Replication is thereby limited, although the virion is not neutralized.

Cellular Immunity

Cellular Cytotoxicity. These defenses are of chief relevance for viruses that spread by intercellular means.

Cytotoxic T lymphocytes (CTL). These cells appear early in viral infection and are specific for viral antigens expressed on the surface of parasitized cells.

Antibody-Dependent Cellular Cytotoxicity (ADCC). Virus-infected cells that display surface viral antigens are opsonized by IgG antibodies and lysed by ADCC. The effector cells are lymphocytes (killer cells), macrophages, and neutrophils; all bear surface Fc receptors.

Natural Killer (NK) Cells. NK cells spontaneously lyse virally infected cells; this effector mechanism is activated by interferon and interleukin-2.

Interferons

The antiviral action of interferons provides a major host defense against viruses. Interferons are a family of proteins produced by lymphocytes, fibroblasts, epithelial cells, and macrophages early in the course of viral infection before specific antibody develops. Exposure of cells to interferon induces their synthesis of proteins that, in turn, selectively inhibit the production of viral proteins. The immunoregulatory effects of gamma-interferon also may contribute indirectly to antiviral immunity by activating effector cells.

RESISTANCE TO FACULTATIVE INTRACELLULAR PARASITES: MYCOBACTERIUM TUBERCULOSIS

Activation of host phagocytes provides the critical defense mechanism against *M. tuberculosis*. Primary infection progresses locally in the nonhypersensitive host, since ingested organisms persist and multiply within mononuclear phagocytes. The bacteria escape intracellular digestion by virtue of constituents (sulfatides, suramin, poly-D-glutamic acid) that inhibit phagolysosomal fusion. Antibody-coated mycobacteria do not evade phagolysosomal fusion but nonetheless resist degradation, probably because of shielding provided by their rich lipid content. The development of cellular immunity leads to T lymphocyte-dependent macrophage activation and to the killing of the intracellular tubercle bacillus organism. The lesions of primary tuberculosis regress. However, latent foci persist, and delayed reactivation remains a threat throughout the lifetime of the host.

REFERENCES

Nossal GJV: Current concepts: Immunology. The basic components of the immune system. N Engl J Med 316:1320, 1987.
Root RF: The compromised host. *In* Wyngaarden JB, Smith LH Jr (eds): Cecil Textbook of Medicine. 18th ed. Philadelphia, WB Saunders Co, 1988, pp 1529–1538.

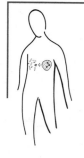

82

LABORATORY DIAGNOSIS OF INFECTIOUS DISEASES

Four basic laboratory techniques can be used in the diagnosis of infectious diseases: (1) direct visualization of the organism; (2) detection of microbial antigen; (3) a search for "clues" produced by the host immune response to specific microorganisms; and (4) isolation of the organism in culture. Each technique has its use and each its pitfalls. The laboratory can usually provide the clinician with prompt, accurate and, if used judiciously, inexpensive diagnosis.

DIAGNOSIS BY DIRECT VISUALIZATION OF THE ORGANISM

In many infectious diseases, pathogenic organisms can be directly visualized by microscopic examination of readily available tissue fluids such as sputum, urine, pus, and pleural, peritoneal, or cerebrospinal fluid. Using Gram's or acid-fast stains, bacteria, mycobacteria, and *Candida* can be readily identified. An India ink preparation can often identify *Cryptococcus*, and potassium hydroxide (KOH) preparations can occasionally identify other fungal pathogens.

Preparation of Specimens for Staining

Sputum and pus are often thick, and thinning is necessary to obtain a helpful preparation. A drop of sputum or pus is placed on a clean glass slide and another slide is pressed on top of the specimen and pulled away. This step can be repeated as often as necessary (using a clean slide each time) until the specimen has been thinned sufficiently to allow newsprint to be read through it. Unless grossly purulent, fluids such as cerebrospinal fluid (CSF) must be centrifuged to concentrate the organisms and the pellet used for staining. In examining unspun CSF, if no organisms are seen, the pellet must then be examined. To prevent the specimen from washing away during the staining procedure, a drop of CSF may be mixed with a drop of fresh serum or other sterile protein source. The specimen is allowed to air dry and is then gently fixed by passing it quickly through a flame.

Gram's Stain
1. Flood the slide with crystal violet—15 sec.
2. Rinse with water.
3. Flood with Gram's iodine—15 sec.
4. Rinse with water.

5. Decolorize with 95 per cent ethyl alcohol. This step is critical. Rinse with alcohol until blue stain just disappears from the rinse.
6. Immediately rinse with water.
7. Flood with safranin—15 sec.
8. Rinse with water.
9. Air dry.
10. Examine using oil immersion lens.

Proper decolorization is crucial. A good Gram's stain should show neutrophil nuclei as deep pink in all but the most dense regions, where they may have a touch of blue. Interpretation of the staining of organisms should be based on inspection of the areas in which transition of the coloration of neutrophil nuclei is present; i.e., some nuclei show minimal blue or purple staining. This will avoid areas which are over- or underdecolorized.

Acid-Fast Stain

1. Flood slide with Kinyoun carbol fuchsin—5 min.
2. Wash repeatedly with acid alcohol until wash is clear.
3. Rinse with water.
4. Counterstain with brilliant green or methylene blue—1 min.

Examine for at least 10 minutes using oil immersion lens. Mycobacteria will appear pink, often beaded, and slightly curved. Other bacteria will not retain pink dye. (Exceptions: *Nocardia* and the Pittsburgh agent [*Legionella micdadii*] may also appear acid-fast.) Experience is necessary to distinguish acid-fast bacilli that may be slightly refractile from debris and other artifacts that may be highly refractile.

India Ink Preparation. A drop of centrifuged cerebrospinal fluid is placed on a microscope slide next to a drop of artist's India ink. A coverslip is placed over the drops, and the area of mixing of CSF and India ink is examined at 100× magnification. Cryptococci are identified by their large capsules that exclude the India ink (Fig. 82–1). The entire slide should be examined.

KOH Preparation. A drop of sputum, skin scraping, or a smear of vaginal or oral exudate is placed on a slide together with one drop of 5 to 40 per cent KOH. A coverslip is placed on the specimen and the slide is heated for two to five seconds above a flame. The condenser of the microscope is lowered and the specimen is examined at 100× magnification when searching for elastin fibers (whose presence in sputum suggests a necrotizing pneumonia) or 400× when looking for fungal forms. The KOH will dissolve host cells and bacteria, sparing fungi and elastin fibers.

Tzanck Preparation. A vesicle suspected to harbor herpesvirus (zoster or simplex) is unroofed with a scalpel and the base is gently scraped. The scrapings are placed on a glass slide, air-dried and stained with Wright's stain, Giemsa stain, or a rapid stain such as methylene blue. The slide is then examined at low (100×) power for the presence of multinucleated giant cells; their characteristic appearance is then confirmed at high (400×) power. This technique is diagnostic for herpesvirus infection.

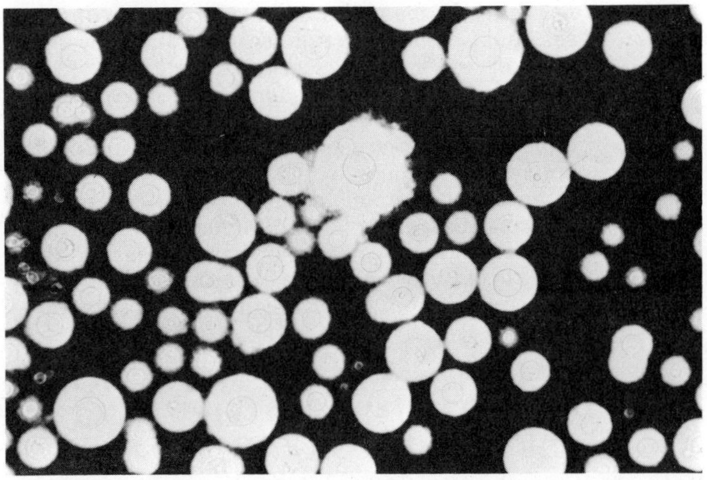

FIGURE 82–1. India ink preparation of cerebrospinal fluid revealing encapsulated cryptococci. Note the large capsules surrounding the smaller organisms.

These simple bedside techniques can provide rapid and inexpensive diagnosis of many infectious disease processes. There are other techniques that directly visualize pathogens, but they require more sophisticated techniques. Silver staining using the Gomori methenamine technique can identify most fungi and *Pneumocystis carinii*. Experienced microscopists also can identify *Pneumocystis carinii* on Giemsa-stained specimens of induced sputum. Immunofluorescence techniques using antibodies directed against the organisms rapidly identify pathogens such as *Legionella pneumophila* and *Bordetella pertussis* in clinical specimens. Darkfield microscopy can identify *Treponema pallidum*, and electron microscopy can often detect viral particles in infected cells.

DIAGNOSIS BY DETECTION OF MICROBIAL ANTIGENS

Certain pathogens can be detected by examination of specimens for microbial antigens (Table 82–1). These studies can be performed rapidly—often within one hour. The diagnosis of meningitis due to *Pneu-*

TABLE 82–1. DISEASES OFTEN DIAGNOSED BY DETECTION OF MICROBIAL ANTIGENS

DISEASE	· ASSAY
Meningitis	
Pneumococcus	CIE*, latex agglutination
Haemophilus	CIE, latex agglutination
Meningococcus	CIE, latex agglutination
Cryptococcus	Latex agglutination
Hepatitis B	Hepatitis B surface antigen (radioimmunoassay)
Human immunodeficiency virus	ELISA for p24 antigen detection

*Counterimmunoelectrophoresis

mococcus, *Haemophilus*, some strains of *Meningococcus*, and *Cryptococcus* can be made rapidly by detection of specific polysaccharide antigen in the cerebrospinal fluid using counterimmunoelectrophoresis (CIE) or latex agglutination. The demonstration of hepatitis B surface antigen in blood establishes the presence of infection by this virus. Cultures of blood of immunocompromised patients with disseminated candidiasis or aspergillosis are often negative. Detection of fungal antigens in blood and other fluids may prove to be more rapid and more sensitive than culture in this setting, but the techniques are experimental.

DIAGNOSIS BY EXAMINATION OF HOST IMMUNE OR INFLAMMATORY RESPONSES

Histopathologic examination of biopsied or excised tissue often reveals patterns of the host inflammatory response that can narrow down diagnostic possibilities. As a general rule, a polymorphonuclear leukocytic infiltrate is compatible with acute infection and suggests a bacterial process. A lymphocytic infiltrate is compatible with a more chronic process and is seen in viral, mycobacterial, fungal, and other nonbacterial infections. Eosinophilia is often seen in parasitic infestations. Granuloma formation suggests mycobacterial and certain fungal infections. Some diseases such as syphilis (obliterative endarteritis), cat-scratch disease (mixed granulomatous, suppurative and lymphoid hyperplastic changes), and lymphogranuloma venereum (stellate abscesses) have fairly characteristic histological features. Several viral infections produce characteristic changes in host cells; these may be detected by cytological examination. Skin or respiratory infection due to herpesviruses, or pneumonia due to cytomegalovirus or measles virus, for example, can be diagnosed with reasonable accuracy by cytological examination. Similarly, examination of cells and chemistries in infected fluids such as cerebrospinal fluid will provide clues to the etiology of the infection. Bacterial infections generally provoke a polymorphonuclear leukocytosis with elevated protein and depressed glucose concentrations. Viral infections most often provoke a lymphocytic pleocytosis; protein elevations are less marked and glucose levels are usually but not always normal.

Host cell–mediated immune responses can be used to help make certain diagnoses. A positive skin test for delayed-type hypersensitivity to mycobacterial or fungal antigens indicates active or previous infection with these agents. A negative skin test may be seen despite active infection in anergic patients. Therefore, control skin tests using commonly encountered antigens (e.g., mumps, *Trichophyton*) must also be applied to ascertain if the patient can mount a delayed-type hypersensitivity response. Occasionally the response to disease-related antigens is depressed selectively.

Host humoral responses may be used to diagnose certain infections, particularly those due to organisms whose cultivation is difficult or expensive to perform

TABLE 82–2. DISEASES OFTEN DIAGNOSED BY MEASUREMENT OF HOST HUMORAL RESPONSES (ANTIBODY LEVELS)

Many viral infections
Mycoplasma pneumonia
Rickettsial infections
Chlamydial infections
Lyme disease
Syphilis
Leptospirosis
Rheumatic fever
Legionnaire's disease
Tularemia
Brucellosis
Histoplasmosis
Coccidioidomycosis
Amebiasis

or hazardous to laboratory personnel (Table 82–2). In general, two sera are obtained at intervals of at least two weeks. A four-fold or greater rise (or fall) in antibody titer generally suggests a recent infection. Antibodies of the IgM class also suggest recent infection.

DIAGNOSIS BY ISOLATION OF THE ORGANISM IN CULTURE

Isolation of a single microbe from an infected site is generally considered evidence that the infection is due to this organism. Information obtained from the culture must, however, be interpreted according to the clinical setting. For example, cultures obtained from ordinarily contaminated sites (e.g., vagina, pharynx) may be overgrown with nonpathogenic commensals, and fastidious organisms such as *Neisseria gonorrhoeae* will be difficult to recognize unless cultured on medium that selects for their growth. Similarly, cultures of expectorated "sputum" may also be uninterpretable if heavily contaminated with saliva. The culture of an organism from an infected but ordinarily sterile site is reasonable evidence for infection due to that organism. On the other hand, the failure to culture an organism may simply result from inadequate culture conditions (e.g., "sterile" pus from brain abscess cultured only on aerobic media. Most brain abscesses are caused by anaerobic bacteria that do not grow under the aerobic conditions most commonly utilized.) Thus, when submitting samples for culture, the physician must alert the laboratory to likely pathogens.

Gram's stains of specimens submitted for culture are often invaluable aids to the interpretation of culture results. A Gram's stain of "sputum" will readily detect contamination by saliva if squamous epithelial cells are seen. On the other hand, a Gram's stain revealing bacteria despite negative cultures suggests infection by fastidious organisms. The presence of an organism in high density and within neutrophils also suggests that the corresponding bacterial isolate is causing disease rather than colonizing the patient or contaminating the specimen.

Viral Isolation. Since all viral pathogens that can be cultured require eukaryotic cells in which to grow, virus isolation is expensive and often laborious. Throat washings, stool samples, or cultures of infected sites should be transported immediately to the laboratory, or if this is not possible, placed in virus transport medium—usually an isotonic salt solution containing antibiotics and protein—and refrigerated overnight until they can be cultured in the laboratory. Notifying the laboratory of the suspected pathogens allows selection of the best cell lines for culture. The clinician must be aware of the viruses that the hospital's laboratory can isolate. As the antiviral armamentarium expands, cultivation of viruses will become more routine. A fourfold rise in titer of antibody to the isolated virus suggests that it is causing disease rather than simply colonizing the area sampled.

Isolation of Rickettsia, Chlamydia, and Mycoplasma. Rickettsia are cultivated primarily in reference laboratories. Diagnosis of rickettsial illness is generally made on clinical grounds and confirmed serologically. Chlamydia can be propagated in cell cultures used in most hospital virology laboratories. Mycoplasma will grow on selective media; the prolonged period of incubation required results in little advantage over serologic diagnosis.

Bacterial Isolation. Isolation of common bacterial pathogens is achieved readily by most hospital laboratories. Specimens should be carried promptly to the laboratory or, in certain instances, placed directly onto the culture medium with careful attention to sterile technique. The specimen is placed onto the culture plate. A loop is sterilized in a flame until it is red, then allowed to cool. The specimen is then streaked on bacteriologic medium. This allows separation of different bacterial colonies and rough quantitation of bacterial growth. Choice of agar plates and culture conditions for bedside culture are shown in Table 82–3.

Isolation of anaerobic bacteria is often critically important for clinical diagnosis. When anaerobes are suspected, the specimen, if pus or liquid, can be drawn into a syringe, the air expelled, and the syringe capped before transport to the laboratory. Otherwise, specimens must be taken immediately to the laboratory or placed in an anaerobic transport medium appropriate for survival of pathogens. Alternatively, the specimen may be placed in a vial containing thioglycollate broth. This will permit anaerobic growth but will not allow quantification of growth. Because of contamination by oral anaerobes, sputum should not be cultured anaerobically unless the sample was obtained by transtracheal or percutaneous lung aspiration.

Isolation of Fungi and Mycobacteria. Specimens for fungal and mycobacterial culture must be processed and cultured by the microbiology laboratory. Although some fungi and rapid-growing mycobacteria will grow readily on standard agars used for routine isolation of bacteria, others such as *Mycobacterium tuberculosis*, and *Histoplasma capsulatum*, must be cultured on special media for as long as several weeks.

TABLE 82–3. CHOICE OF MEDIA FOR BEDSIDE BACTERIAL CULTURES

SOURCE	PLATE	CONDITIONS
Throat	BAP[1]	37°C candle jar
Sputum	BAP + CHOC	37°C candle jar
CSF	BAP + CHOC	37°C candle jar
Urine	BAP + EMB or MAC	37°C
Suspected gonorrhea	TM[3]	37°C candle jar
Pus	BAP + EMB or MAC[4]	37°C[4]
Stool[2]		

[1]BAP = blood agar; CHOC = chocolate agar; EMB = eosin methylene blue; MAC = MacConkey; TM = Thayer Martin. EMB and MAC plates inhibit growth of gram-positive bacteria and have an indicator that detects lactose-fermenting bacteria. TM contains antibiotics that inhibit growth of most bacteria except pathogenic *Neisseria*.

[2]Stool cultures should be processed by the clinical laboratory immediately because of the variety of media and conditions needed to isolate stool pathogens.

[3]TM should be used only when culturing contaminated sites (e.g., pharynx, urethra, rectum, cervix). When *N. gonorrhoeae* is suspected elsewhere (e.g., joint space), the specimen should be placed on chocolate agar. This is because TM will also inhibit the growth of 3 per cent of pathogenic *Neisseria*.

[4]Use CHOC plus candle jar if respiratory pathogens are suspected. Pus also should be cultured anaerobically (see text).

Note: A candle jar provides increased tension of carbon dioxide but does not provide anaerobic conditions.

REFERENCES

Finegold SM, Martin WJ, Scott EG (eds): Bailey & Scott's Diagnostic Microbiology. 1978. St. Louis, The CV Mosby Co, 1978.

Menegus MA, Douglas RG: Viruses, rickettsia, chlamydia and mycoplasmas. *In* Mandell GL, Douglas RG, Bennett JE (eds): Principles and Practice of Infectious Diseases. 2nd ed. New York, John Wiley & Sons, 1984.

Washington JA: Bacteria, fungi and parasites. *In* Mandell GL, Douglas RG, Bennett JE (eds): Principles and Practice of Infectious Diseases. 2nd ed. New York, John Wiley & Sons, 1984.

83

ANTIMICROBIAL THERAPY

The advent of antimicrobial therapy has been the most dramatic advance in medical practice in this century. Antimicrobials are agents that interfere with microbial metabolism, resulting in inhibition of growth or death of the organism. Some, like penicillin, are natural products of other microbes. Others, such as sulfa drugs, are chemical agents synthesized in the laboratory. Still others are semisynthetic—chemical modifications of naturally occurring substances which result in enhanced activity (e.g., nafcillin) and/or diminished toxicity.

The most effective antimicrobials are characterized by their relatively selective activity against microbes. Some, such as penicillins and amphotericin B, interfere with the synthesis of microbial cell walls that are absent in human cells. Others, such as trimethoprim and sulfa drugs, inhibit obligate microbial synthesis of essential nucleic acid intermediates, pathways not required by human cells. Still others, such as acyclovir, an antiviral agent, are relatively inactive until metabolized by pathogen-derived enzymes. Nonetheless, these agents, although relatively selective in activity against microbes, have variable degrees of toxicity for human cells. Thus, monitoring for toxicity during antimicrobial therapy is often very important.

In the selection of an antimicrobial agent for a patient, the following factors are important:

THE PATHOGEN

If the pathogen has been clearly identified by culture or histopathologic techniques (Chapter 82), a drug with a narrow spectrum of activity (i.e., highly selective for the particular pathogen) is usually the most reasonable choice. If the pathogen responsible for the patient's illness has not been identified, then the physician must choose a drug or combination of drugs active against the most likely pathogens in the specific setting. In either instance, the physician must be guided by patterns of antimicrobial resistance common in the community and in the specific hospital. Some pathogens (e.g., pneumococcus, group A *Streptococcus*) are almost always sensitive to narrow-spectrum antimicrobials such as penicillin. Other pathogens such as *Staphylococcus* are variably resistant to penicillins but almost always susceptible to vancomycin. Resistance patterns, particularly among hospital-acquired bacteria, may vary widely and are important in devising antimicrobial strategies. Broad-spectrum antimicrobial coverage for all febrile patients ("shotgunning") must not be substituted for carefully evaluating the clinical problem and pinpointing therapy toward the most likely pathogen(s). Widespread use of broad-spectrum antimicrobials almost invariably leads to emergence of resistant strains. On the other hand, the sicker a patient appears and the less

certain the physician is of the responsible pathogen, the more important initial empirical broad-spectrum coverage becomes. Initial empirical treatment is also frequently indicated in the immunocompromised febrile patient (e.g., the patient with severe neutropenia secondary to chemotherapy). Once the pathogen is isolated and its antimicrobial sensitivities are known, empirical therapy must be scaled down to a definitive regimen with narrow and optimal activity against the specific microorganism.

SITE OF INFECTION

The location of the infection is also important in determining selection and dosage of an antimicrobial. Deep-seated infections and bacteremic infections generally require higher doses of antimicrobials than, for example, superficial infections of the skin, upper respiratory tract, or lower urinary tract. Penetration of various antimicrobials into sites such as meninges, eye, and prostate is quite variable. Thus treatment of infections at these sites involves selection of an antimicrobial agent that penetrates these tissues in concentrations sufficient to inhibit or kill the pathogen. The meninges are relatively resistant to penetration by most antimicrobials; inflammation renders the meninges somewhat more permeable. Thus high doses of antibiotics are the rule when treating meningitis. Infections of certain sites such as the heart valves must be treated with antimicrobials that kill the microbe (bactericidal) as opposed to simply inhibiting its growth (bacteriostatic). This is because local host defenses at these sites are inadequate to rid the host of infecting organisms. Infections involving foreign bodies are often difficult to eradicate without removing the foreign material.

Antimicrobials alone are often insufficient in the treatment of large abscesses. Although many drugs achieve reasonable concentrations in abscess walls, the low pH antagonizes the activity of some drugs (e.g., aminoglycosides) and some drugs bind to and are inactivated by white blood cells or their products. The large number of organisms, their depressed metabolism in this unfavorable milieu, and the frequent polymicrobial nature of certain abscesses increase the likelihood that some organisms present may be resistant. Most large abscesses should be drained whenever anatomically possible.

CHARACTERISTICS OF THE ANTIMICROBIAL

The physician must know the pharmacokinetics of the drug (i.e., its absorption, penetration into various sites, its metabolism and excretion) and its toxicity as

TABLE 83–1.   CHARACTERISTICS OF COMMONLY USED ANTIMICROBIAL AGENTS

DRUG CLASS	SITE OF ACTION	CNS PENETRATION	EXCRETION	USES/ACTIVITY
Antibacterials				
Aminoglycosides	Ribosome	−	Renal	Gram-negative bacilli; no activity in anaerobic conditions
Cephalosporins	Cell wall	1st genertion − 3rd generation +	Renal	Broad-spectrum, including some anaerobes
Chloramphenicol	Ribosome	+	Hepatic metabolism Renal excretion	Broad spectrum: especially useful for *Salmonella*, anaerobes, *Rickettsia*
Clindamycin	Ribosome	−	Hepatic metabolism Renal excretion	Anaerobes; gram-positive cocci
Erythromycin	Ribosome	−	Hepatic metabolism	Gram-positive cocci, *Legionella*, *Mycoplasma*
Metronidazole	DNA disruption	+	Hepatic metabolism	Anaerobes, *Clostridium difficile*, amoebae, *Trichomonas*
Penicillins	Cell wall	+/−	Renal	Streptococci, *Neisseria*, oral anaerobes
Quinolones	DNA gyrase	+	Some hepatic metabolism Renal excretion	Very broad spectrum
Rifampin	Transcription	+	Hepatic metabolism Renal excretion	*M. tuberculosis*; meningococcal and *Haemophilus influenzae* prophylaxis
Sulfonamides/ trimethoprim	Inhibit nucleic acid synthesis	+	Renal	Gram-negative bacilli, *Salmonella*, *Pneumocystis carinii*, *Nocardia*
Tetracyclines	Ribosome	+/−	Renal excretion Hepatic metabolism	Broad spectrum; especially useful for spirochetes, *Rickettsia*
Vancomycin	Cell wall	+/−	Renal	Coagulase-positive and negative staphylococci, other gram-positive bacteria
Antifungals				
Polyenes				
Amphotericin B	Binds membrane ergosterol	−	?	Most fungi
Flucytosine	Blocks DNA synthesis	−	Renal	Candidiasis; *Cryptococcus* with amphotericin B
Nystatin	Binds membrane ergosterol	−	Fecal	Mucosal candidiasis
Imidazoles				
Ketoconazole	Blocks membrane biosynthesis	−	Hepatic/fecal	Mucosal candidiasis, nonmeningeal histoplasmosis, blastomycosis
Antivirals				
Acyclovir	Inhibits DNA polymerase	+	Renal	Herpes simplex, including encephalitis; herpes zoster in immunosuppressed hosts
Amantidine/ rimantidine	? Inhibits uncoating	+	Renal	Influenza A treatment and prophylaxis
Vidarabine	Inhibits DNA polymerase	+	Renal	Neonatal herpes simplex
Zidovudine	Inhibits reverse transcriptase	+	Hepatic gluco-oxidation Renal excretion	Human immunodeficiency virus

well as its spectrum of antimicrobial activity before selecting it for use (Table 83–1).

Distribution and Excretion.   Lipid-soluble drugs such as chloramphenicol and rifampin penetrate most membranes, including the meninges, more readily than more ionized compounds such as the aminoglycosides. The physician must be certain that the achievable drug concentration at the site of infection is sufficient to inhibit or kill the pathogen. Understanding a drug's distribution, metabolism, and route of excretion is essential in selecting the appropriate drug and dose. Drugs excreted unchanged in the urine may be particularly good for the treatment of lower urinary tract infection or for treatment of systemic infection in the presence of renal insufficiency. Some antimicrobials are metabolized in the liver and must be adjusted appropriately in the presence of hepatic insufficiency.

Activity of the Drug. The physician must understand both the spectrum of activity of the drug against microbial isolates and the mechanism of activity of the agent and whether it is bactericidal or bacteriostatic in achievable concentrations. As a general rule, cell wall–active drugs are likely to be bactericidal. Bactericidal drugs are necessary for treatment of infections sequestered from an effective host inflammatory response such as meningitis and endocarditis. With the exception of aminoglycosides, agents inhibiting protein synthesis at ribosomal sites are generally bacteriostatic.

Toxicity of the Drug. The physician must have a thorough understanding of the contraindications of the drug, as well as the major toxicities of the drug and their general frequency. This will help in evaluating the risks of treatment and also will assist in advising the patient about the drug's effects and anticipating possible adverse reactions. History of drug hypersensitivity must be sought before prescribing any antimicrobials. The presence or absence of previous reactions to penicillin should be documented for every patient. Patients with a history suggestive of immediate hypersensitivity to penicillin, e.g., hives, wheezing, hypotension, laryngospasm, or angioedema at any site, must be considered at risk for anaphylaxis. These patients should not receive penicillins or related drugs (cephalosporins) if adequate alternatives are available. The major and minor determinants of penicillin allergy (breakdown products that bind to serum proteins to form haptens) detect most persons at risk for serious immediate hypersensitivity. If skin test reactivity to these determinants is present and there are no reasonable alternatives to therapy with a penicillin or related compound, these patients may be desensitized to penicillin using a graduated protocol of intracutaneous penicillin administration. Patients with a history of an uncomplicated morbilliform or delayed rash after penicillin therapy are not likely to be at risk for immediate hypersensitivity and may be treated with cephalosporins, for which the risk of cross-hypersensitivity to penicillins is likely to be in the range of 5 per cent.

ROUTE OF ADMINISTRATION

Oral administration of antimicrobials can often avoid the morbidity and expense associated with parenteral administration (intravenously or intramuscularly). Although some antimicrobials (e.g., amoxicillin) are very well absorbed after oral administration, most patients hospitalized with severe infections should, at least initially, be treated with intravenous antibiotics. Gut absorption of antimicrobials can be unpredictable, and the intravenous route often permits administration of greater amounts of drug than can be tolerated orally. Intramuscular administration of some antimicrobials can result in excellent drug absorption but should be avoided in the presence of hypotension (erratic absorption) and coagulation disorders (hematomas). Repeated intramuscular injections are uncomfortable and also can result in the formation of sterile abscesses (e.g., pentamidine).

Duration of Therapy. Antimicrobial therapy should be initiated as part of a treatment plan of defined duration. In some settings the duration of optimal antimicrobial therapy is established (e.g., ten days but not seven days of oral penicillin will prevent rheumatic fever after streptococcal pharyngitis); in most others the duration of treatment is empirical and sometimes can be based on the clinical and bacteriological course. Blood stream infections without endocarditis or other focal infections can generally be treated for 10 to 14 days. Pneumococcal pneumonia can be effectively treated in 7 to 10 days. The duration of therapy for endocarditis is largely dictated by the characteristics of the culpable microorganism, but generally is at least four weeks.

Combinations. Combinations of antimicrobials are indicated in serious infection when they provide more effective activity against a pathogen than any single agent. In some instances, combinations of drugs are used to prevent the emergence of resistance (e.g., infections due to *Mycobacterium tuberculosis*). In others, combinations are used because they provide synergistic action against the pathogen (e.g., penicillin, a cell-wall activity antibiotic, facilitates uptake of aminoglycosides by enterococci). In still other instances, drug combinations are used in empirical therapies to cover a wide spectrum of potential pathogens when the causative agent is unidentified or when infection is likely to be due to a mixture of organisms (e.g., fecal soilage of the peritoneum). Use of more than one drug increases the likelihood of toxicity, increases costs, and often increases the risk of superinfection.

MONITORING OF ANTIMICROBIAL THERAPY

The physician (and patient) should be alert to potential toxicities and be prepared to halt the drug in the event of serious toxicity. For some antimicrobials, such as aminoglycosides, the ratio of effective to toxic drug levels is narrow. Thus, serum levels of the drug must be monitored to assure appropriate dosing. For some infections (e.g., infective endocarditis due to relatively resistant organisms), monitoring of antimicrobial activity in serum shortly after (peak) and just before (trough) drug administration may help guide antimicrobial choices and usage. Although these techniques are not well-standardized, clinicans often adjust drugs and doses to maintain serum bactericidal titers of at least 1:8 in treating certain forms of endocarditis (e.g., enterococcal) in which the antimicrobial resistance pattern of the microorganism may be quite variable.

REFERENCES

Murray BE, Moellering RC: Patterns and mechanisms of antibiotic resistance. Med Clin North Am 62:899, 1978.
Young LS: Antimicrobial therapy. *In* Wyngaarden JB, Smith LH Jr (eds): Cecil Textbook of Medicine. 18th ed. Philadelphia, WB Saunders Co, 1988, pp 112–124.

84

FEVER AND FEBRILE SYNDROMES

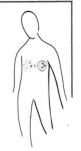

REGULATION OF BODY TEMPERATURE

Although "normal" body temperature ranges vary considerably, oral temperature readings in excess of 37.8°C (100.2°F) are generally abnormal. In healthy humans, core body temperature is maintained within a narrow range so that for each individual, daily temperature variations greater than 1 to 1.5°C are distinctly unusual. This homeostasis is controlled by hypothalamic nuclei that establish "set points" for body temperature. This is effected by a complex balance between heat-generating and heat-conserving mechanisms that raise body temperature on the one hand and mechanisms that dissipate heat and lower body temperature on the other (Table 84–1). Heat is regularly generated as a by-product of obligate energy utilization (e.g., cellular metabolism, myocardial contraction, breathing). When an increase in body temperature is needed, shivering—nondirected muscular contraction—generates large amounts of heat. Peripheral vessels vasoconstrict to diminish heat lost to the environment. At the same time, the person feels cold; this heat preference promotes heat-conserving behavior such as wrapping up in a blanket.

Obligate heat loss to the environment occurs through the skin and by evaporation of water through sweat and respiration. When the body must cool down, heat loss is promoted. Vasodilation flushes the skin capillaries, temporarily raising skin temperature but ultimately lowering core body temperature by increasing heat loss through the skin to the cooler environment. Sweating promotes rapid heat loss via evaporation, and, at the same time, the subject feels warm and sheds blankets to promote heat loss.

TABLE 84–1. MECHANISMS OF HEAT REGULATION

To raise body temperature
  Heat generation
    Obligate heat production
    Muscular work
    Shivering
  Heat conservation
    Vasoconstriction
    Heat preference
To lower body temperature
  Heat loss
    Obligate heat loss
    Vasodilatation
    Sweating
    Cold preference

FEVER AND HYPERTHERMIA

Fever is an elevated body temperature that is mediated by an increase in the hypothalamic heat-regulating set point. Thus, although fever may be precipitated by exogenous substances such as bacterial products, the increase in body temperature is achieved through physiological mechanisms. In contrast, hyperthermia is an increase in body temperature that overrides or bypasses the normal homeostatic mechanisms. As a general rule, body temperatures in excess of 41°C are rarely physiologically mediated and suggest hyperthermia. Hyperthermia may be seen after vigorous exercise, in patients with heatstroke, as a heritable reaction to anesthetics (malignant hyperthermia), as a response to phenothiazines (neuroleptic malignant syndrome), and occasionally in patients with central nervous system disorders such as paraplegia (see also Chapter 115). Some patients with severe dermatoses are also unable to dissipate heat and therefore experience hyperthermia.

Fever usually is a physiological response to infection or inflammation. Monocytes or tissue macrophages are activated by various stimuli to liberate various cytokines with pyrogenic activity (Fig. 84–1). Interleukin-1 is also an essential cofactor in initiation of the immune response. Another pyrogenic cytokine, tumor necrosis factor, or cachectin, activates lipoprotein lipase and also may play a role in immune cytolysis. A third, alpha-interferon, has antiviral activity (see Chapter 81). Endogenous pyrogens activate the anterior preoptic nuclei of the hypothalamus to raise the set point for body temperature by the mechanisms shown in Table 84–1. A list of classes of disorders that can cause fever is shown on Table 84–2. Infection by all types of microorganisms can be associated with fever. Tissue injury with resultant inflammation, such as seen in myocardial or pulmonary infarction or after trauma, can produce fever. Certain malignancies such as lymphoma, renal carcinoma, and hepatic carcinoma are also associated with fever; in some instances this is related to liberation of endogenous pyrogen by monocytes in the inflammatory response surrounding the tumor; in other cases, the malignant cell may release an endogenous pyrogen. Many immunologically mediated disorders such as connective tissue diseases, serum sickness, and some drug reactions are characterized by fever. In most cases of drug-induced fevers, the mechanisms of fever are unknown. Virtually any disorder associated with an inflammatory response (for example, gouty arthritis) can be associated with fever. Certain endocrine disorders such as thyrotoxicosis, adrenal insufficiency, and pheochromocytoma can also produce fever.

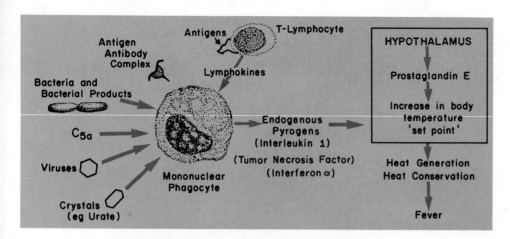

FIGURE 84–1. Pathogenesis of fever.

The association of fever with infections or inflammatory disorders raises the question of whether fever is beneficial to the host. Interleukin-1 (an endogenous pyrogen) is critical for initiation of the immune response, certain in vitro immune responses are marginally enhanced by elevated temperatures, and some organisms prefer cooler temperatures. It is not certain, however, that fever is helpful to the host in any infectious disease with the exception of neurosyphilis. Fever is deleterious in certain situations. Among individuals with underlying brain disease, and even in the healthy elderly, fever can produce disorientation and confusion. In young children, fever can result in seizures. Fever should be controlled if the patient is particularly uncomfortable or whenever it poses a specific risk to the patient. Children with a history of febrile seizures and patients with severe congestive heart failure or recent myocardial infarction should have fever treated with antipyretics such as salicylates or acetaminophen. Acetaminophen is preferred for children because of the association of salicylates with Reye's syndrome.

Heat stroke almost always results from prolonged exposure to high environmental temperature and humidity, usually associated, in otherwise healthy individuals, with strenuous exercise. It is characterized by a body temperature greater than 40.6°C associated with altered sensorium or coma and with cessation of sweating. Rapid cooling is critical to the patients' survival. Immersion in cool water (11°C) until core temperature reaches 39°C is the most effective initial therapeutic approach and should be followed by intravenous infusions of fluids appropriate to correct the antecedent fluid and electrolyte losses.

TABLE 84–2. CAUSES OF FEVER

Infection
Tissue injury—infarction, trauma
Malignancy
Drugs
Immune-mediated disorders
Other inflammatory disorders
Endocrine disorders

Fever Patterns. The normal diurnal variation in body temperature results in a peak temperature in the late afternoon or early evening. This variation often persists when patients have fever. In certain instances, fever patterns may be helpful in suggesting the cause of fever. Rigors—true shaking chills—often herald a bacterial infection, although they may occur in cases of viral infection, as well as in drug or transfusion reactions. Hectic fevers characterized by wide swings in temperature may indicate the presence of an abscess. Patients with malaria may have a relapsing fever with episodes of shaking chills and high fever, separated by one to three days of normal body temperature and relative well-being. Patients with tuberculosis may be relatively comfortable and unaware of a markedly elevated body temperature. Patients with uremia or diabetic ketoacidosis generally have a lowered body temperature, and "normal" temperature readings in these settings may indicate infection. Similarly, elderly patients with infection often fail to mount a febrile response and may present instead with loss of appetite, confusion, or even hypotension without fever. The administration of antiinflammatory drugs (aspirin, nonsteroidal antiinflammatory drugs, corticosteroids) also blunts or ablates the febrile response.

ACUTE FEBRILE SYNDROMES

Fever is one of the most common complaints that bring patients to a physician. The challenge is in discerning the few individuals who require specific therapy from among the many with self-limited benign illness. The approach is simplified by considering patients in three groups: (a) fever without localizing symptoms and signs, (b) fever and rash, and (c) fever and lymphadenopathy.

FEVER ONLY

Most patients with fever as their sole complaint defervesce spontaneously or present with localizing clinical or laboratory findings within two to three weeks of illness (Table 84–3). Beyond three weeks, the patient can be considered to have a fever of unex-

TABLE 84–3. INFECTIONS PRESENTING AS FEVER WITHOUT LOCALIZING SIGNS OR SYMPTOMS

INFECTIOUS AGENT	EPIDEMIOLOGY/ EXPOSURE HISTORY	DISTINCTIVE CLINICAL AND LABORATORY FINDINGS	DIAGNOSIS
Viral			
Rhinovirus, adenovirus, parainfluenzae	None (adenovirus in epidemics)	Often URI symptoms	Throat and rectal cultures, serologies
Enterovirus, ECHO virus	Summer, epidemic	Occas. aseptic meningitis, rash, pleurodynia, herpangina	Throat and rectal cultures, serologies
Influenza	Winter, epidemic	Headache, myalgias, arthralgias	Throat cultures, serologies
Epstein-Barr virus, cytomegalovirus	(see text)		
Colorado tick fever	Southwest, Northwest, tick exposure	Biphasic illness, leukopenia	Blood, CSF cultures, erythrocyte-associated viral antigen (indirect immunofluorescence)
Bacterial			
Staphylococcus aureus	IV drug users, patients with intravenous plastic cannulas, hemodialysis, dermatitis	Must exclude endocarditis	Blood cultures
Listeria monocytogenes	Depressed cell-mediated immunity	One half have meningitis	Blood, CSF cultures
Salmonella typhi, S. paratyphi	Food or water contaminated by carrier or patient	Headache, myalgias, diarrhea or constipation, transient rose spots	Early blood, bone marrow cultures; late stool culture
Streptococcus viridans	Valvular heart disease	Low grade fever, fatigue, anemia	Blood cultures
Fever Post–Animal Exposure			
Coxiella burnetti (Q fever)	Infected livestock	Retrobulbar headache, occas. pneumonitis, hepatitis. Culture-negative endocarditis	Serologies
Leptospires	Water contaminated by urine from dogs, cats, rodents, small mammals	Headache, myalgias, conjunctival suffusion Biphasic illness Aseptic meningitis	Serologies
Brucella sp.	Exposure to cattle or contaminated dairy products	Occas. epididymitis	Blood cultures, serologies
Granulomatous Infection			
Mycobacterium tuberculosis	Exposure to patient with tuberculosis, known positive tuberculin skin test	Back pain, sterile pyuria or hematuria suggests vertebral, renal infection	Liver, bone marrow histology, cultures
Histoplasma capsulatum	Mississippi and Ohio River valley	Pneumonitis, oropharyngeal lesions	Serologies. Liver, bone marrow, oral lesions histology and cultures

plained origin, a designation with its own circumscribed group of management considerations, as discussed below.

Viral Infection

In young healthy individuals, acute febrile illnesses generally represent viral infections. The causative agent is rarely established. Rhinovirus, parainfluenza, or adenovirus infections usually, but not invariably, are associated with symptoms of coryza or upper respiratory tract infection (rhinorrhea, sore throat, cough, hoarseness). Enterovirus and ECHO virus infections occur predominantly in summer, usually in an epidemic setting. Undifferentiated febrile syndromes account for the majority of enteroviral infections, but the etiology is more likely to be established definitively when macular rash, aseptic meningitis, or a characteristic syndrome, such as herpangina (vesicular pharyngitis due to coxsackievirus A) or acute pleurodynia (fever, chest wall pain, and tenderness due to coxsackievirus B) is present. Serological surveys also indicate that many arthropod-borne viruses (California encephalitis virus; Eastern, Western, and Venezuelan equine encephalitis; St. Louis encephalitis) usually produce mild, self-limited febrile illnesses. Influenza causes myalgias, arthralgias, and headache in addition to fever. It is unusual, however, for fever to persist beyond five days in uncomplicated influenza.

The mononucleosis syndromes caused by Epstein-Barr virus, cytomegalovirus, and *Toxoplasma gondii* may present in a typhoidal manner—that is, with fever but little or no lymphadenopathy. Diagnosis and management are discussed below under "Fever with Generalized Lymphadenopathy," the more typical presentation of these processes.

Colorado tick fever is a disease caused by arbovirus and transmitted by tick bite. Viremia is prolonged, lasting about four weeks. The illness is biphasic—two to three days of fever followed by a similar period of remission, then a second febrile episode. Some patients have rash, pericarditis, or aseptic meningitis.

The above syndromes are self-limited and untreatable. The impetus for establishing a specific diagnosis, therefore, is small. The differentiation between viral and other causes of febrile illnesses is, on the other hand, of critical importance. Some of the features that distinguish viral and bacterial infection are shown in Table 84–4. Viral cultures of throat and rectum and virus-specific antibodies in acute and convalescent serum samples may allow retrospective diagnosis of viral etiology. Usually, however, the fever is gone long before results of serologies become available.

Bacterial Infections

Bacterial disease may cause septicemia, which dominates the clinical presentation (see Chapter 85). *Staphylococcus aureus* frequently causes sepsis, sometimes without an obvious primary site of infection. Fever may be the predominant clinical manifestation of the illness. *S. aureus* sepsis should be considered in patients undergoing intravenous therapy with a plastic cannula, hemodialysis patients, intravenous drug users, and patients with severe chronic dermatoses. In the patient with *S. aureus* bacteremia, the question of whether intravascular infection exists is key in determining length of therapy. The following are more typical of endocarditis: community-acquired infection, long duration of symptoms, absence of removable focus of infection (e.g., IV cannula, soft tissue abscess), metastatic sites of infection (e.g., septic pulmonary emboli, arthritis, meningitis), and new heart murmur. *L. monocytogenes* septicemia is seen predominantly in patients with depressed cell-mediated immunity. One half of patients with *Listeria* sepsis have meningitis. Occasionally a relatively indolent clinical syndrome belies the bacterial etiology of *S. aureus* and *L. monocytogenes* bacteremia.

Enteric fevers also may present in a subacute fashion despite presence of bacteremia. The major species producing this syndrome are *Salmonella typhi*, which has a human reservoir, and *S. paratyphi* A, B, and C. The paratyphoid strains also have their major reservoir in humans and produce less severe disease than *S. typhi*. *S. typhi* is acquired by ingestion of food or water contaminated with fecal material from a chronic carrier or patient with typhoid fever. A large number of bacteria (10^6 to 10^8) must be ingested to cause disease in the normal host. Major host risk factors are achlorhydria, malnutrition, malignancy (particularly lymphomas and leukemias), sickle cell anemia, and other defects in cellular and humoral immunity. Major protective mechanisms are gastric acidity and fatty acid products of bacteria composing the normal gut flora. *Salmonella typhi* penetrates the gut wall and enters the lymphoid follicles (Peyer's patches), where it multiplies within mononuclear phagocytes and produces local ulceration. Primary bacteremia occurs with spread to the reticuloendothelial system (liver, spleen, and bone marrow). After further multiplication at those sites a secondary bacteremia occurs which can localize to lesions such as tumors, aneurysms, and bone infarcts. Infection of the gallbladder, particularly in the presence of gallstones, leads to the chronic carrier state. Approximately two weeks after exposure, patients develop prolonged fever with chills, headache, and myalgias. Diarrhea or constipation may be present but usually does not dominate the clinical picture. Crops of rose spots (2- to 4-mm erythematous maculopapular lesions) appear on the upper abdomen but are evanescent. Untreated, typhoid fever usually resolves in about one month. However, complication rates are high owing to bowel perforation, metastatic infection, and general debility of patients. *Salmonella typhi* must be isolated from blood or stool to confirm the diagnosis. Culture of the bone marrow is often positive early in the course of disease. Typhoid fever should be treated with chloramphenicol, 50 mg/kg/day intravenously or orally, for two weeks. Chloramphenicol-resistant strains of *S. typhi* have appeared in Mexico, India, and Vietnam and should be treated with ampicillin, 100 mg/kg/day intravenously or orally, or trimethoprim, 320 to 640 mg per day, with sulfamethoxazole, 1600 to 3200 mg/day. Ampicillin becomes the drug of choice in endocarditis or infected aneurysms (because of its bactericidal activity) and in patients with sickle cell anemia in whom the dose-related bone marrow suppression by chloramphenicol is unacceptable.

TABLE 84–4. FEATURES HELPFUL IN DISTINGUISHING VIRAL AND BACTERIAL INFECTION

	VIRAL	BACTERIAL
Epidemiology	During epidemic, close contacts with similar illness	Sporadic. Often elderly, significant underlying disease(s)
Symptoms	Associated coryza, upper respiratory tract infection	Shaking chills, fever
Signs	Relatively well appearing	Toxic appearing, confused.
	Temperature-pulse dissociation	Tachycardia, tachypnea.
Laboratory	Leukopenia or slight leukocytosis	Leukocytosis, shift to left (immature neutrophils), vacuolated neutrophils

Localized bacterial infection can be clinically occult and present as an undifferentiated febrile syndrome. Intra-abdominal abscess, vertebral osteomyelitis due to *S. aureus* or *Pseudomonas aeruginosa*, streptococcal pharyngitis, urinary tract infection, infective endocarditis, and early pneumonia may all cause fever with surprisingly few clinical clues to the location of the infection. Therefore, urinalysis, throat and blood cultures, and chest radiography should be performed in the febrile patient presenting with features suggestive of a bacterial infection (Table 84–4).

Febrile Syndromes Associated with Animal Exposure

Q fever, brucellosis, and leptospirosis are diseases associated with exposure to fluids from infected animals and may have similar clinical presentations.

Q Fever. Q fever is an underrecognized cause of acute febrile illness. *Coxiella burnetii*, the causative agent, produces mild infection in livestock. Humans are infected by inhalation of aerosolized particles or by contact with placental and amniotic fluids from infected animals. The source of animal exposure may go unnoticed. For example, in an outbreak of Q fever at the University of Colorado Medical School, 70 per cent of infected individuals lacked direct exposure to infected sheep.

Q fever characteristically begins explosively with severe, often retrobulbar headache, high fever, chills, and myalgias. Pneumonitis and hepatitis may occur but are seldom severe. Diagnosis usually is based on a fourfold rise in titer of complement-fixing antibodies. Untreated, Q fever lasts 2 to 14 days. *C. burnetii* is sensitive to tetracycline, which should be used in its treatment (2 gm/day orally for 14 days). Q fever may cause endocarditis, apparently as a form of reactivation of infection. The occurrence of hepatomegaly and thrombocytopenia in a patient with apparently culture-negative endocarditis may be a clue to this diagnosis.

Leptospirosis. Humans are infected with leptospires by exposure to urine from infected dogs, cats, wild mammals, and rodents. Exposure on the farm, in the slaughterhouse, on camping trips, or during swims in contaminated water is frequent. After an incubation period of about one week, patients develop chills, high fever, headache, and myalgias. The illness often pursues a biphasic course. During the second phase of illness, fever is less prominent, but headache and myalgias are excruciating, and nausea, vomiting, and abdominal pain become prominent complaints. Aseptic meningitis is the most important manifestation of the second or immune phase of the illness. Suffusion of the bulbar conjunctivae is a useful early sign, suggesting the diagnosis of leptospirosis. Lymphadenopathy, hepatomegaly, and splenomegaly may occur. Leptospirosis also may pursue a more severe clinical course characterized by renal and hepatic dysfunction and hemorrhagic diathesis. Although dark-field examination will reveal leptospires in body fluids, most laboratories do not have the expertise to identify the organisms. The diagnosis is made, rather, by a fourfold rise in indirect hemagglutination antibody titer. Antibiotic treatment shortens the duration of fever and may reduce complications. However, to be effective, antibiotics must be initiated presumptively, before serological confirmation. Penicillin G, 2.4 to 3.6 million units per day, or tetracycline, 2.0 gm orally per day, is effective therapy.

Brucellosis. Brucella infect the genitourinary tract of cattle (*Brucella abortus*), pigs (*B. suis*) and goats (*B. mellitensis*). Humans are exposed occupationally or by ingestion of contaminated dairy products. Acute disease is characterized by chills, fever, headache, arthralgias, and sometimes lymphadenopathy, hepatomegaly, and splenomegaly. During the associated bacteremia, any organ may be seeded. Epididymo-orchitis is one of the more characteristic findings. With or without antibiotic treatment of the acute infection, brucellosis may relapse or enter a chronic phase. Brucella species can be isolated from blood or other normally sterile fluids. However, the laboratory should be alerted to the suspicion of this infection, since the organism requires special conditions for growth. Otherwise, diagnosis must be made serologically. Treatment consists of tetracycline, 2 gm orally per day for 21 days, and streptomycin, 1.0 gm IM per day for 14 days. Trimethoprim, 480 mg per day, with sulfamethoxazole, 2400 mg orally per day, is an acceptable alternative regimen.

Granulomatous Infection

Tuberculosis. Extrapulmonary and miliary tuberculosis may present as febrile syndromes. In disseminated tuberculosis, initial chest radiographs may be normal, and tuberculin skin tests often are nonreactive. Protracted fevers should always suggest this possibility. Liver biopsy and bone marrow biopsy should be performed and have a high yield in miliary disease. Genitourinary and vertebral tuberculosis may present as unexplained fever. However, careful history, urinalysis, intravenous pyelography, and radiographs of the spine should reveal the site of tissue involvement. Extrapulmonary tuberculosis should be treated with isoniazid, 300 mg orally, rifampin 600 mg orally, and ethambutol 15 mg/kg orally per day for at least nine months. The ethambutol can be discontinued once the organism is shown to be sensitive to isoniazid. Corticosteroids may be a useful adjunctive measure in the patient with severe systemic toxicity; steroids should be tapered as soon as the patient shows symptomatic improvement.

Histoplasmosis. Most individuals living in endemic areas in the Mississippi and Ohio River valleys have a subclinical, self-limited febrile illness as a manifestation of acute pulmonary histoplasmosis. Although patients may complain of chest pain or cough, physical examination of the chest usually is unremarkable despite radiographic findings of infiltrates and mediastinal and hilar adenopathy. Therefore, in the absence of chest radiographs, the lower respiratory tract component of the illness is easily overlooked. A complement fixation titer of at least 1:32 or a fourfold rise in titer is suggestive of the diagnosis of acute histoplasmosis. Although spontaneous resolution of symptoms is the norm, unusually prolonged illness (more than two to three weeks) may require antifungal treatment with amphotericin B or ketoconazole.

Progressive disseminated histoplasmosis may occur as a consequence of reactivation of latent infection in immunosuppressed individuals or may reflect an uncontained or poorly contained primary infection. The febrile illness in such patients is protracted, and the differential diagnosis is that of fever of unknown origin (FUO). Oropharyngeal nodules and ulcerative lesions are commonly found in disseminated histoplasmosis. Biopsy of such lesions permits rapid diagnosis. Serologies are less helpful in disseminated histoplasmosis, as they are positive in only one third of cases; cultures and methenamine silver stains of bone marrow biopsy specimens, however, should establish the diagnosis. Disseminated histoplasmosis is treated with amphotericin B, 0.5 to 0.6 mg/kg/day intravenously for a total dose of 2 to 3 gm.

Other. Malaria produces febrile paroxysms that in some cases occur every 48 to 72 hours. The diagnosis should be suspected in travellers who have returned from endemic areas, intravenous drug users, and recipients of blood transfusions. *Plasmodium falciparum* causes a high level of parasitemia and is associated with a high mortality rate unless recognized and treated promptly. Daily fevers may be seen early in the course of this form of malaria. Although *P. vivax* and *P. malariae* may relapse long after primary infection owing to latent extraerythrocytic infection, the course is milder. Demonstration of parasites in blood smears establishes the diagnosis of malaria.

Many, if not most, infectious diseases may present with fever as an early finding, with subclinical or eventual clinical involvement of specific organ systems. Examples include cryptococcosis, coccidioidomycosis, psittacosis, *Legionella* sp. and *Mycoplasma pneumoniae* infections. Pulmonary involvement by these infectious agents tends to produce few signs on physical examination; chest radiographs often reveal more prominent abnormalities than are suspected clinically.

FEVER AND RASH

Some of the febrile syndromes already discussed may occasionally be associated with a skin rash (Table 84–5). However, this section considers diseases in which rash is a prominent feature of the presentation.

Bacterial Diseases

Petechial lesions, purpura, and ecthyma gangrenosum are lesions associated with bacteremia (see Chapter 85). Disseminated gonococcemia causes sparse vesiculopustular, hemorrhagic, or necrotic lesions on an erythematous base, typically on the extremities, particularly their dorsal surfaces (see Chapter 96). Meningococcemia is also an important cause of fever and a petechial skin rash that may be sparse.

Bacterial toxins produce characteristic clinical syndromes. Pharyngitis or other infections with an erythrogenic toxin-producing *Streptococcus* may lead to scarlet fever. Diffuse erythema begins on the upper chest and spreads rapidly, although sparing palms and soles. Small red petechial lesions are found on the palate, and the skin has a sandpaper texture owing to occlusion of sweat glands. The tongue at first shows yellowish coating and then becomes beefy red. The rash of scarlet fever heals with desquamation. *Corynebacterium hemolyticum* also produces pharyngitis and skin rash.

Toxic shock syndrome (TSS) was first recognized as a distinct entity in 1978 and became epidemic in 1980 and 1981, probably because of the marketing of hyperabsorbable tampons. *Staphylococcus aureus* strains producing toxic shock syndrome toxin (TSST-1) or other closely related exotoxins cause the syndrome. TSST-1 is a potent stimulus of interleukin-1 production by mononuclear phagocytes and enhances the effects of endotoxin; these properties may be important in the pathogenesis of this syndrome. Most cases have occurred in 15- to 25-year-old females using tampons. Other settings include prolonged use of contraceptive diaphragms, vaginal or cesarean deliveries, and nasal surgery. TSS in males usually is caused by superficial staphylococcal infections and abscesses. Patients with toxic shock syndrome develop the abrupt onset of high fever (temperature >40°C), hypotension, nausea and vomiting, severe watery diarrhea and myalgias, fol-

---

TABLE 84–5. DIFFERENTIAL DIAGNOSIS OF INFECTIOUS AGENTS PRODUCING FEVER AND RASH

Maculopapular Erythematous
 Enterovirus
 Epstein-Barr virus, cytomegalovirus, *Toxoplasma gondii*
 Human immunodeficiency virus
 Colorado tick fever virus
 Salmonella typhi
 Leptospires
 Measles virus
 Rubella virus
 Hepatitis B virus
 Treponema pallidum
Vesicular
 Varicella zoster
 Herpes simplex virus
 Coxsackie virus A
Cutaneous Petechiae
 Neisseria gonorrhoeae
 Neisseria meningitidis
 Rickettsia rickettsii (RMSF)
 Rickettsia typhi (murine typhus)
 Viridans streptococci (endocarditis)
Diffuse Erythroderma
 Streptococcus sp. (scarlet fever)
 Staphylococcus aureus (toxic shock syndrome)
Distinctive Rash
 Ecthyma gangrenosum—*Pseudomonas aeruginosa*
 Erythema chronicum migrans—Lyme disease
Mucous Membrane Lesions
 Vesicular pharyngitis—Coxsackie virus A
 Palatal petechiae—rubella, Epstein-Barr virus, scarlet fever (Group A streptococci)
 Erythema—toxic shock syndrome (*Staphylococcus aureus*)
 Ulceronodular oral—*Histoplasma capsulatum*
 Koplik's spots—Measles virus

lowed by confusion and oliguria. Characteristically, diffuse erythroderma (a sunburn-like rash) is apparent with erythematous mucosal surfaces. Later, intense scaling and desquamation of skin, particularly of the palms and soles, occurs. Laboratory abnormalities include elevated liver and muscle enzymes, thrombocytopenia, and hypocalcemia. Diagnosis is based on the clinical findings and requires specific exclusion of Rocky Mountain spotted fever, meningococcemia, leptospirosis, and measles. Management of the patient consists of restoration of an adequate circulatory blood volume by administration of intravenous fluids, removal of tampons if present, and treatment of the staphylococcal infection with nafcillin, 12 gm/day intravenously. Patients must be advised against using tampons in the future, as toxic shock syndrome often recurs within four months of the initial episode if tampon use continues.

Viral Infection (Table 84–6)

The rashes associated with viral infections may be so typical as to establish unequivocally the cause of the febrile syndrome. Varicella-zoster requires special consideration because of the availability of an effective antiviral drug, acyclovir. In the normal host, neither chickenpox nor herpes zoster confined within specific dermatomes requires treatment with antiviral agents. Ophthalmic zoster demands antiviral treatment, since it is associated with potentially severe complications, including orbital compression syndromes and intracranial extension. Acyclovir also has beneficial effects on chickenpox in immunocompromised children and on extradermatomal spread of zoster in immunocompromised adults.

Rickettsial Diseases

In the United States, three rickettsial diseases are endemic: Rocky Mountain spotted fever (RMSF), Q fever, and murine typhus. Rash is not a characteristic of Q fever. RMSF is a misnomer, as most cases occur in the southeastern United States. The causative organism, *Rickettsia rickettsii*, is transmitted from dogs (or small wild animals) to ticks to humans. Infection occurs primarily during warmer months, periods of greatest tick activity. About two thirds of patients cite a history of tick exposure. After 2 to 14 days, there is the fulminant onset of severe frontal headache, chills, fever, myalgias, conjunctivitis, and, in one fourth, cough and shortness of breath. At this point, the diagnosis may be particularly obscure. Rash characteristically begins on the third to fifth day of illness as 1- to 4-mm erythematous macules on hands, wrists, feet, and ankles. Palms and soles may be involved. The rash spreads to the trunk and may become petechial. Intravascular coagulopathy develops in some severely ill patients. Diagnosis and institution of appropriate therapy should be based on the clinical findings. The specific complement fixation test shows a rise in titers and allows retrospective confirmation of the diagnosis. Treatment is with chloramphenicol, 50 mg/kg orally or parenterally, or tetracycline, 25 to 50 mg/kg day orally for seven days.

TABLE 84–6. FEVER AND RASH IN VIRAL INFECTION

Coxsackie/ECHO virus	*Maculopapular "rubelliform."* 1–3 mm faint pink, begins on face, spreading to chest and extremities. *"Herpetiform."* Vesicular stomatitis with peripheral exanthem (papules and clear vesicles on an erythematous base), including palms and soles (hand, foot, and mouth disease).	Summertime, no itching or lymphadenopathy. Multiple cases in household or community-wide epidemic. Mostly diseases of children.
Measles	Erythematous, maculopapular rash begins on upper face and spreads down to involve extremities, including palms and soles. Koplik's spots are bluish-grey specks on a red base found on buccal mucosa near second molars. Atypical measles occurs in individuals who received killed vaccine, then are exposed to measles. The rash begins peripherally and is urticarial, vesicular, or hemorrhagic.	Incubation period 10 to 14 days. First, severe upper respiratory symptoms, coryza, cough, conjunctivitis. Then Koplik's spots, then rash.
Rubella	Maculopapular rash beginning on face and moving down. Petechiae on soft palate.	Incubation 12 to 23 days. Adenopathy: posterior auricular, posterior cervical, and suboccipital.
Varicella	Generalized vesicular eruption. Lesions in different stages from erythematous macules to vesicles to crusted. Spread from trunk centrifugally. Zoster—see text.	Incubation 14 to 15 days. Late winter, early spring.
Herpes simplex virus	Oral primary: small vesicles on pharynx, oral mucosa which ulcerate. Painful and tender. Recurrent: vermillion border, one or few lesions. Genital: See Chapter 96.	Incubation 2 to 12 days.
Hepatitis B	Prodrome in one fifth. Erythematous maculopapular rash, urticaria.	Arthralgias, arthritis. Abnormal liver function tests. Hepatitis B antigenemia.
Epstein-Barr virus	Erythematous, maculopapular rash on trunk and proximal extremities. Occasionally urticarial or hemorrhagic.	Transiently occurs in 5 to 10% of patients during first week of illness.
Human immunodeficiency virus	Maculopapular truncal rash may occur as early manifestation of infection.	Associated fever, sore throat and lymph node enlargement may persist for 2 or more weeks.

Lyme Disease

Lyme disease is a spirochetal infection caused by *Borrelia burgdorferi* and transmitted by the tick *Ixodes dammini*. Cases occur in several major foci (the Northeast, Wisconsin and Minnesota, California and Oregon), but sporadic cases occur elsewhere as well. Three to 32 days after tick bite, patients develop a febrile illness, usually associated with headache, stiff neck, myalgias, arthralgias, and erythema chronicum migrans (ECM). ECM begins as a red macule or papule at the site of the tick bite; the surrounding bright red patch expands to a diameter of up to 15 cm. Partial central clearing often is seen. The centers of lesions may become indurated, vesicular, or necrotic. Several red rings may be found within the outer border. Smaller secondary lesions may appear within several days. Lesions are warm but nontender. Enlargement of regional lymph nodes is common. The skin rash usually fades in about one month. Several weeks after onset of symptoms, neurologic involvement develops in 15 per cent of patients. Most characteristic is meningoencephalitis with cranial nerve involvement and peripheral radiculoneuropathy. CSF at this time shows about 100 lymphocytes per milliliter. Heart involvement also may become manifest as atrioventricular block, myopericarditis, or cardiomegaly. Joint involvement occurs in 60 per cent of patients. Early in the course, arthralgias and myalgias may be quite severe; however, months later, arthritis develops with marked swelling and little pain in one or two large joints, typically the knee. Episodes of arthritis may recur for months or years; in about 10 per cent of patients the arthritis becomes chronic and erosion of cartilage and bone occurs. Diagnosis is suspected on clinical grounds and confirmed by demonstration of IgM antibody to the spirochete which peaks by the third to sixth week. Total serum IgM is increased, as are IgM-containing immune complexes and cryoglobulins. The level of IgM is reflective of disease activity and predictive of neurologic, cardiac, and joint involvement. Synovial fluid contains an average of 25,000 cells per milliliter, most of them neutrophils.

Treatment with tetracycline, 1.0 gm orally per day for 10 days, usually prevents late complications. Meningitis, cardiac involvement, or arthritis should be treated with aqueous penicillin G, 20 million units or ceftriaxone 4 g intravenously per day for 10 days. Repeated courses may be necessary if relapses occur.

FEVER AND LYMPHADENOPATHY

Many infectious diseases are associated with some degree of lymphadenopathy (Table 84–7). However,

TABLE 84–7. INFECTIOUS DISEASES ASSOCIATED WITH GENERALIZED LYMPHADENOPATHY BUT OTHER DOMINANT FEATURES

Viral—measles, rubella, hepatitis B
Bacterial—scarlet fever, brucellosis, leptospirosis, tuberculosis, syphilis, Lyme disease

in some, lymphadenopathy is a major manifestation of the disease. These can be further divided according to whether lymphadenopathy is generalized or regional.

GENERALIZED LYMPHADENOPATHY

The mononucleosis syndromes are important causes of fever and generalized lymphadenopathy.

Mononucleosis Syndromes

Epstein-Barr Virus (EBV). Approximately 90 per cent of American adults have serological evidence of EBV infection; most infections are subclinical and occur before the age of five years or midway through adolescence.

Clinically manifest infectious mononucleosis usually develops late in adolescence after intimate contact with asymptomatic oropharyngeal shedders of EBV. Patients develop sore throat, fever, and generalized lymphadenopathy and sometimes experience headache and myalgias. Five to 10 per cent of patients has a transient rash that may be macular, petechial, or urticarial. Palatal petechiae often are present, as is pharyngitis, which may be exudative. Cervical lymphadenopathy, particularly involving the posterior lymphatic chains, is prominent, although some involvement elsewhere is common. The spleen is minimally enlarged in about 50 per cent of patients. Although rare, autoimmune hemolytic anemia, thrombocytopenia, encephalitis or aseptic meningitis, Guillain-Barré syndrome, hepatitis, or splenic rupture may dominate the clinical presentation. Three fourths of patients present with an absolute lymphocytosis. At least one third of their lymphocytes are atypical in appearance: large, with vacuolated basophilic cytoplasm, rolled edges often deformed by contact with other cells, and lobulated, eccentric nuclei. Immunologic studies indicate that some circulating B cells are infected with EBV and that the cells involved in the lymphocytosis are mainly cytotoxic T cells capable of damaging EBV-containing lymphocytes. Atypical lymphocytes are not restricted to infectious mononucleosis but may be seen in other viral illnesses.

B-cell infection with EBV is a stimulus to production of polyclonal antibodies. Antibodies to foreign red cells (heterophile) are helpful in diagnosis. The finding of sheep red cell agglutinins with differential absorption characteristics at a titer of at least 1:40 is good evidence for infectious mononucleosis. Rapid diagnostic tests, such as the Monospot test, have largely replaced the need for heterophile determination. The Monospot test is sensitive and specific; false-positive results occur rarely in patients with lymphoma or hepatitis. Some patients with EBV infection show delayed development of heterophile antibodies. Recourse to determination of antibodies to EBV is necessary only in atypical, heterophile-negative cases. The presence of IgM antibody to viral capsid antigen is diagnostic of acute infectious mononucleosis. The appearance of

TABLE 84–8. DIFFERENTIAL DIAGNOSIS OF HETEROPHILE-NEGATIVE MONONUCLEOSIS

Epstein-Barr virus mononucleosis (particularly in children)
Cytomegalovirus
Acute toxoplasmosis
Streptococcal pharyngitis
Hepatitis B
Acute HIV infection

antibody to EBV nuclear antigen also is indicative of EBV infection.

Infectious mononucleosis pursues a surprisingly benign course even in patients with neurological involvement. The fever resolves after one to two weeks, although residual fatigue may be protracted. Occasional patients have a persistent or recurrent syndrome with fever, headaches, pharyngitis, lymphadenopathy, arthralgias, and serological evidence for chronic active EBV infection. Patients should be managed symptomatically. Acetaminophen may be useful for sore throat. Antibiotics, particularly ampicillin, should be avoided. The use of ampicillin is associated with skin rash in almost all patients with EBV infection. Corticosteroids are indicated in the rare individual with serious hematological involvement (i.e., thrombocytopenia, hemolytic anemia).

Acute bacterial superinfections of the pharynx and peritonsillar abscesses should be considered when the course is unusually septic.

The differential diagnosis of heterophile-negative mononucleosis is shown in Table 84–8.

Cytomegalovirus (CMV). Serological surveys indicate that most adults have been infected with CMV. The ages of peak incidence of CMV infection are in the perinatal period (transmission by breast milk) and during the second to fourth decades. CMV shares with the other Herpetoviridae the propensity to reactivate, particularly in immunosuppressed patients.

Two modes of transmission of CMV are particularly important in the development of lymphadenopathy in otherwise healthy adults. CMV can be transmitted sexually. Semen is an excellent source for viral isolation. The frequency of antibody to CMV and active viral excretion is particularly high in male homosexuals. Blood transfusions carry a risk of approximately 3 per cent per unit of blood for transmitting CMV infection. This risk becomes substantial in the setting of open-heart surgery or multiple transfusions for other indications.

Primary infection with CMV causes about 50 per cent of heterophile-negative mononucleosis. The distinction between CMV and EBV may be impossible on clinical grounds alone. However, CMV tends to involve older patients (mean age 29), produce milder disease, and may be typhoidal in its presentation, that is, fever with little or no adenopathy. The infrequent but serious forms of neurological and hematological involvement which occur in EBV infection also can occur with CMV. Additionally, pneumonitis and hep-

atitis (which may be granulomatous) may be found. Isolation of CMV from urine or semen and demonstration of conversion of serologies (indirect fluorescent antibody test or complement fixation) from negative to positive are useful in establishing etiology. However, in groups such as male homosexuals, in whom asymptomatic excretion of CMV is found frequently, viral isolation alone is inadequate for determining the etiology of lymphadenopathy. CMV mononucleosis is a self-limited disease that does not require or respond to specific therapy.

Acute Acquired Toxoplasmosis. *Toxoplasma gondii* is acquired by ingesting oocysts contaminating meat and other foods or by exposure to cat feces. In certain geographic areas, such as France, 90 per cent of individuals have serological evidence of *Toxoplasma* infection. In the United States, the figure is close to 50 per cent by age 50. Ten to 20 per cent of infections in normal adult hosts are symptomatic. Presentation may take the form of a mononucleosis-like syndrome, although maculopapular skin rash, abdominal pain due to mesenteric and retroperitoneal lymphadenopathy, and chorioretinitis also may occur. Striking lymph node enlargement and involvement of unusual chains (occipital, lumbar) may necessitate lymph node biopsy to exclude lymphoma. Histologically, focal distention of sinuses with mononuclear phagocytes, histiocytes blurring the margins of germinal centers, and reactive follicular hyperplasia indicate *Toxoplasma* infection. Acute acquired toxoplasmosis is suggested by conversion of the indirect fluorescent antibody test from negative to positive or a fourfold increase in titer. Usually the titer is greater than 1:1000 and is associated with increased specific IgM antibody. Acute acquired toxoplasmosis generally is self-limited and does not require specific therapy. Significant involvement of the eye is an indication for treatment with pyrimethamine plus sulfadiazine.

Granulomatous Disease. Disseminated tuberculosis, histoplasmosis, and sarcoidosis may be associated with generalized lymphadenopathy, although involvement of certain lymph node chains can predominate. Lymph node biopsy shows granulomas or nonspecific hyperplasia.

Persistent Generalized Lymphadenopathy (PGL). Patients infected by the human immunodeficiency virus (HIV) (see Chapter 97) may develop lymph node enlargement in at least two extrainguinal sites, persisting for at least three months, thereby fulfilling the standard diagnostic criteria for PGL. Additional symptoms such as fever, night sweats, fatigue, diarrhea, and weight loss may develop as the severity of immunodeficiency increases. Among male homosexuals, intravenous drug users, and other individuals belonging to groups at increased risk for AIDS, the presence of generalized lymphadenopathy also could represent Kaposi's sarcoma, cytomegalovirus infection, toxoplasmosis, tuberculosis, cryptococcosis, B-cell lymphoma, or syphilis. Lymph node biopsy in a patient with HIV-related PGL is usually unnecessary. A serum VDRL should be performed to exclude secondary syphilis. A tuberculin skin test should also be done.

REGIONAL LYMPHADENOPATHY

Pyogenic Infection. *Staphylococcus aureus* and group A streptococcal infections produce acute suppurative lymphadenitis. The most frequently affected lymph nodes are submandibular, cervical, inguinal, and axillary, in that order. Involved nodes are large (>3 cm), tender, and firm or fluctuant. Pyoderma, pharyngitis, or periodontal infection may be present and the presumed primary site of infection. Patients are febrile and have a leukocytosis. Fluctuant nodes should be aspirated. Otherwise, antibiotic therapy should be directed toward the most common pathogens. Penicillin G therapy is appropriate if pharyngeal or periodontal origin implicates a streptococcal infection. Skin involvement suggests possible staphylococcal infection and is an indication for nafcillin (or dicloxacillin) therapy. The dosage and route of administration of the drug should be determined by the severity of the infection.

Tuberculosis. Scrofula, or tuberculous cervical adenitis, presents in a subacute to chronic fashion. Fever, if present, is low-grade. A large mass of matted lymph nodes is palpable in the neck. If *Mycobacterium tuberculosis* is the causative organism, other sites of active infection usually are present. The most common causative agent in children in the United States is *M. scrofulaceum*. Infection with this and other drug-resistant nontuberculous mycobacteria requires surgical excision.

Cat-Scratch Disease. Chronic regional lymphadenopathy following cat exposure or cat scratch should suggest the diagnosis. Histopathological studies indicate a gram-negative bacterial origin of this syndrome. About one week after contact with the cat, a local papule or pustule may develop. One week later regional adenopathy appears. Lymph nodes may be tender (sometimes exquisitely so) or just enlarged (1 to 7 cm). Fever is low-grade if present at all. Lymph node enlargement usually persists for several months. Lymph node biopsy shows necrotic granulomas with giant cells and stellate abscesses surrounded by epithelial cells. The diagnosis can usually be established on clinical grounds. The course usually is self-limited and benign.

Ulceroglandular Fever. Tularemia is the classic cause of ulceroglandular fever. The syndrome is acquired by contact with tissues or fluids from an infected rabbit or the bite of an infected tick. Patients have chills, fever, an ulcerated skin lesion at the site of inoculation, and painful regional adenopathy. When infection is acquired by contact with rabbits, the skin lesion usually is on the fingers or hand, and lymph node involvement is epitrochlear or axillary. In tick-borne transmission, the ulcer is on the lower extremities, perianal region, or trunk, and the adenopathy is inguinal or femoral. Most cases are diagnosed serologically, as Gram's stained preparations usually are negative, and culture of the causative organism, *Francisella tularensis*, is hazardous. A fourfold rise in agglutination titer is diagnostic. Patients should be treated presumptively with streptomycin, 15 to 20 mg/kg/day for 7 to 10 days.

Oculoglandular Fever. Conjunctivitis with preauricular lymphadenopathy can occur in tularemia, cat-scratch disease, sporotrichosis, lymphogranuloma venereum infection, listeriosis, and epidemic keratoconjunctivitis due to adenovirus.

Inguinal Lymphadenopathy. Inguinal lymphadenopathy associated with sexually transmitted diseases (see Chapter 96) may be bilateral or unilateral. In primary syphilis, enlarged nodes are discrete, firm, and nontender. Early lymphogranuloma venereum causes tender lymphadenopathy with later matting of involved nodes, and sometimes fixation to overlying skin, which assumes a purplish hue. The lymphadenopathy of chancroid is very painful and composed of fused lymph nodes. Tender inguinal lymphadenopathy also occurs in primary genital herpes simplex virus infection.

Plague. Bubonic plague usually presents as fever, headache, and a large mat of inguinal or axillary lymph nodes which go on to suppurate and drain spontaneously. Plague is an important consideration in the acutely ill patient with possible exposure to fleas and rodents in the western United States. If plague is suspected, blood cultures and aspirates of the buboes should be obtained and tetracycline, 30 to 50 mg/kg/day, plus streptomycin, 30 mg/kg/day, instituted. Gram's stained preparations of the aspirate reveal gram-negative rods in two thirds of cases. A fluorescent antibody test allows rapid specific diagnosis and is available through the Centers for Disease Control.

FEVER OF UNDETERMINED ORIGIN (FUO)

Fever of undetermined origin is the term applied to febrile illnesses with temperatures exceeding 101°F which are of at least three weeks' duration and remain undiagnosed after one week in hospital. The evaluation of an FUO remains among the most challenging problems facing the physician. The majority of illnesses that cause FUO are treatable, making pursuit of the diagnosis particularly rewarding. There is no substitute for a meticulous history and physical examination. These should be repeated frequently during the patient's hospital course, as frequent patient questioning may jar an important historical clue from the patient, and important physical findings may develop while the patient is in the hospital. These clues may direct the next series of diagnostic studies. Directed biopsies of lesions should be stained and cultured for pathogenic microbes. In many instances, however, localizing clues are not present or fail to yield rewarding information. In these cases, bone marrow biopsy can reveal granulomatous or neoplastic disease, even in the absence of clinical evidence of bone marrow involvement. Similarly, liver biopsy may also reveal the etiology of an FUO, but seldom in the absence of any clinical or laboratory evidence of liver disease. Exploratory laparotomy is generally not helpful unless signs, symptoms, or laboratory data point to abdominal pathology. Recent refinements in computerized tomography may assist in determining the need for

TABLE 84–9. FEVER OF UNDETERMINED ORIGIN*

Infections		
Intra-abdominal abscesses	11	
Subphrenic		3
Splenic		2
Diverticular		2
Liver and biliary tract		3
Pelvic		1
Mycobacterial	5	
Cytomegalovirus	4	
Infection of the urinary tract	3	
Sinusitis	2	
Osteomyelitis	2	
Catheter infections	2	
Other infections	3	
TOTAL	32	
Neoplastic diseases		
Hematologic neoplasms	22	
Non-Hodgkin's lymphoma		7
Leukemia		5
Hodgkin's disease		4
Other		6
Solid tumors	11	
TOTAL	33	
Collagen diseases	9	
Granulomatous diseases	8	
Miscellaneous	7	
Factitious fever	3	
Undiagnosed	13	
GRAND TOTAL	105	

*Adapted from Larson EB, Featherstone HJ, Petersdorf RG: Fever of undetermined origin: Diagnosis and follow-up of 105 cases, 1970–1980. Medicine 61:269–292, 1982.

laparotomy in cases of FUO. If tuberculosis remains a possibility after careful work-up fails to establish a diagnosis, an empirical trial of antituberculous drugs may be initiated while awaiting results of bone marrow, liver, and urine cultures.

The final diagnoses of 105 cases fulfilling criteria for FUO seen between 1970 and 1980 are shown in Table 84–9. Infectious diseases were the cause of about one third of these cases; another third were due to neoplasms; the remainder were due to connective tissue disorders, granulomatous diseases, and other illnesses.

CAUSES OF FUO

Infections

Abscesses account for as many as one third of infectious causes of FUO. Most of these abscesses are intra-abdominal or pelvic, as abscesses elsewhere (e.g., lung, brain, or superficial abscesses) are readily identifiable radiographically or as a result of the signs or symptoms they produce.

Intra-abdominal abscesses generally occur as a complication of surgery or leakage of visceral contents, as might be seen with perforation of a colonic diverticulum. Surprisingly, large abdominal abscesses may be present with few localizing symptoms. Abscesses of the liver (see Chapter 91) occur as a consequence of inflammatory disease of the biliary tract or of the bowel; in the latter instance bacteria reach the liver via portal blood flow. Occasionally blunt trauma predisposes to abscesses of the liver or spleen. Hepatic, splenic, or subdiaphragmatic abscesses are generally readily detected by ultrasound or CT scan. Diagnosis of intra-abdominal abscess may, however, be challenging, since even large abscesses in the pericolonic spaces may be difficult to distinguish from fluid-filled loops of bowel on CT scan. Gallium scanning, ultrasonography, or barium enemas may assist if the diagnosis is suspected and CT scans are not definitive.

Endovascular infections (infective endocarditis, mycotic aneurysms, infected atherosclerotic plaques) are uncommon causes of FUO, since blood cultures are generally positive. Infections of intravascular catheter sites generally are also associated with bacteremia unless the infection is limited to the insertion site. Diagnosis of endovascular infection is more difficult to make when blood cultures are negative and infection is due to slow growing or fastidious organisms such as *Brucella* species, *Coxiella burnetii* (Q fever), or *Haemophilus* species. It is especially difficult among patients who have been treated with antimicrobials. If endocarditis is suspected, blood cultures should be repeated for at least one week after antimicrobials are discontinued, the bacteriology laboratory should be alerted to the possibility of infection due to a fastidious organism, and evidence of valvular vegetations should be sought by two-dimensional echocardiography. Occasionally the suspicion of valvular infection is strong enough to warrant empirical antibiotic treatment of a presumed culture-negative endocarditis.

Although most patients with osteomyelitis have pain at the site of infection, occasionally localizing symptoms are absent and patients present only with fever. Technetium pyrophosphate bone scans and gallium scans demonstrate uptake at sites of osteomyelitis, but positive scans are not always diagnostic of infection.

Mycobacterial infections, generally due to *M. tuberculosis*, are important causes of FUO. Patients with impaired cell-mediated immunity are at particular risk for disseminated tuberculosis, and occult infection with this organism is seen with particular frequency among patients with renal failure undergoing hemodialysis. Fever may be the only sign of this infection. Both among immunocompromised patients and previously well persons with disseminated tuberculosis, PPD skin tests are often negative. In some patients, careful review of chest radiographs reveals apical calcifications or upper lobe scars suggestive of remote tuberculous infection. A diffuse, often subtle, radiographic pattern of "millet seed" densities, best appreciated on the lateral chest views, is highly suggestive of disseminated tuberculosis. In this setting lung biopsy will establish the diagnosis. Similar radiographic patterns may be seen in sarcoidosis, disseminated fungal infection (e.g., histoplasmosis), and some malignancies. Bone marrow or liver biopsy often reveals granulomas, and cultures of these sites are positive in 50 to 90 per cent of disseminated tuberculosis.

Viral infections such as cytomegalovirus or Epstein-Barr virus can produce prolonged fevers. Both infections may be seen in young healthy adults. Recipients of blood are at risk for acute post-transfusion CMV infection. Recipients of organ transplantation and other immunosuppressed patients may experience reactivation of latent CMV infection producing fever, leukopenia, and pulmonary and hepatic disease. Lymph nodes are often enlarged in EBV infection, and peripheral blood smear usually reveals a lymphocytosis with increased numbers of atypical lymphocytes. Occasionally the atypical lymphocytosis is delayed several weeks after the onset of fever. Unexplained fever may be a complication of infection with the human immunodeficiency virus; most such fevers are attributable to complicating opportunistic pathogens (see Chapter 97).

Simple lower urinary tract infections are readily diagnosed by symptoms and urinalysis. Complicated infections such as perirenal or prostatic abscess may be occult and present as FUO. Generally there is a history of antecedent urinary tract infection or disorder of the urinary tract. In prostatic abscess the prostate is usually tender on rectal exam. In suspected cases of perirenal and prostatic abscess, the urinalysis should be repeated if it is initially normal, as abnormalities of the sediment may be intermittent. Ultrasound or CT scan will detect most of these lesions.

Although most patients with sinusitis have localizing symptoms, occasionally infections of the paranasal sinuses may present with fever only, particularly among hospitalized patients who have had nasotracheal and/or nasogastric intubation. Sinus films reveal fluid in the sinuses. Infection of the sphenoid sinus may be difficult to detect unless special views or CT scans are obtained.

Neoplastic Diseases.

Neoplasms account for approximately one third of cases of FUO. Some tumors, particularly those of hematologic origin and hypernephromas, release endogenous pyrogens. In others the mechanism of fever is less clear but may result from pyrogen release by infiltrating or surrounding inflammatory cells. Lymphomas can present as FUO; usually there is enlargement of lymph nodes or spleen. Some lymphomas present with intra-abdominal disease only. CT scan is helpful in detecting these tumors. Leukemia also may present as FUO, sometimes with a normal peripheral blood smear. Bone marrow examination reveals an increased number of blast forms. Hypernephroma, atrial myxoma, primary hepatocellular carcinoma, and tumor metastatic to the liver also may present as FUO. Liver function abnormalities (predominantly alkaline phosphatase) are common in all these tumors except atrial myxoma. Myxoma can be suspected in the presence of heart murmur and multisystem embolization (mimicking endocarditis) and is readily diagnosed by echocardiogram. Radiographic studies of the abdomen and retroperitoneum (CT scan or ultrasound) generally detect the other tumors. Colon carcinoma also must be considered in the differential diagnosis, since as many as a third or more of patients with this diagnosis may present with low-grade fever, and in some this is the only sign of disease.

Other Causes of FUO

Collagen vascular diseases account for approximately 10 per cent of cases of FUO. Systemic lupus erythematosus is readily diagnosed serologically and thus accounts for a small proportion of cases of FUO. Vasculitis remains an important etiology of FUO and should be suspected in febrile patients with "embolization/infarctions" or with "multisystem disease." Giant cell arteritis should be considered in older patients with FUO, particularly in the presence of polymyalgia rheumatica symptoms (see Chapter 107). Juvenile rheumatoid arthritis, or Still's disease, can present as FUO with joint symptoms. An evanescent rash, sore throat, and leukocytosis occur in this disorder, which is diagnosed on clinical criteria in the absence of other potential causes of fever.

Granulomatous diseases without a defined etiology have been associated with FUO. Sarcoidosis is a multisystem granulomatous disorder often involving the lungs, skin, and lymph nodes. The majority of patients are anergic to skin test antigens. Diagnosis is based upon the demonstration of discrete noncaseating granulomas. Granulomatous hepatitis can present with prolonged fevers, occasionally lasting for years. Serum alkaline phosphatase levels are generally elevated; liver biopsy reveals granulomas, and no underlying etiology can be demonstrated.

A number of miscellaneous disorders make up the remainder of FUO cases, including Crohn's disease, familial Mediterranean fever, and hypertriglyceridemia. Drug-related fevers and recurrent pulmonary emboli always demand consideration in the differential diagnosis. A significant minority of FUO's (approximately 10 per cent) remain undiagnosed after careful evaluation. The majority of these patients have experienced an undefinable but self-limited illness, with fewer than 10 per cent of these patients developing an underlying serious disorder when followed up years later.

Factitious or Self-Induced Fever. Patients with factitious or self-induced illness present unique ethical and therapeutic problems. Once the possibility of factitious or self-induced illness is considered, the doctor-patient relationship is changed. Typically, the physician can rely on the good faith of the patient's history. In the case of factitious or self-induced illness, the physician must assume a more detached role in order to establish the diagnosis. Patients with factitious fever are typically young, often female. Many have been or are employed in health-related professions. Usually articulate and well-educated, these patients are adept at manipulating their family, friends, and physicians. In these instances, a consultant new to the patient may provide a detached and helpful perspective on the problem.

Clues to factitious fever include the absence of a toxic appearance despite high temperature readings, lack of an appropriate rise in pulse rate with fever, and absence of the physiological diurnal variation in temperature. Suspected factitious readings can be evaluated by immediately repeating the reading with the nurse or physician in attendance. Use of electronic thermometers allow rapid and accurate recording of a patient's temperature.

Self-injection of pyrogen-containing substances, usually bacteria-laden culture medium, urine, or feces, can produce bacteremia and high fever; usually these bacteremic episodes are polymicrobial and intermittent, often suggesting a diagnosis of intra-abdominal abscess. However, patients with self-induced bacteremia may appear remarkably well between episodes of fever, in contrast to most patients with abscesses. Illicit ingestion of medications known by the patient to produce fever can also present a very difficult diagnostic problem. Clues to the presence of self-induced illness are subtle. The patients are often emotionally immature; some exaggerate their importance and fabricate unrelated aspects of their history. Some are surprisingly stoic about the apparent seriousness of their illness and the procedures employed

to diagnose or treat them. In some instances, interview of family members can elicit clues to the possibility of factitious or self-induced illness. Confirming the diagnosis is crucial and, in many instances, requires search of the patient's hospital room. Although most will deny their role in inducing or feigning illness, the diagnosis must be explained, and psychiatric care is essential. These complicated patients are at risk for inducing life-threatening disease; some respond to psychiatric counseling.

REFERENCES

Aduan RP, Fauci AS, Dale DC, et al: Factitious fever and self-induced infection. A report of 32 cases and review of the literature. Ann Intern Med 90:230–242, 1979.
Dinarello CA, Cannon JG, Wolff S: New concepts of the pathogenesis of fever. Rev Infect Dis 10:168–169, 1988.
Larson EB, Featherstone HJ, Petersdorf RG: Fever of undetermined origin: Diagnosis and follow-up of 105 cases, 1970–1980. Medicine 61:269–292, 1982.

85

BACTEREMIA AND SEPTICEMIA

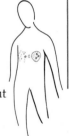

At the outset, several terms must be distinguished. Sepsis refers to the presence of pathogenic microorganisms or their toxins in tissue or blood. Bacteremia, therefore, is a special form of sepsis and is quite variable in terms of its clinical manifestations. Septicemia, in contrast, is systemic disease associated with the presence and persistence of pathogenic organisms or toxins in the blood. Septicemia therefore usually is an expression of bacteremia. Septicemia, in turn, may lead to septic shock—a blood pressure less than 80 mm Hg systolic and unresponsive to appropriate volume replacement.

The presence of bacteria in the blood indicates that the rate of entrance of organisms from a local infection into the circulation exceeds the capacity of the clearance mechanisms of the reticuloendothelial system and the capillary beds. The bacteremia may be low-grade, intermittent, and of little consequence. As the intensity of the local infection increases, however, high-grade bacteremia itself causes symptoms and signs, justifying the designation septicemia. In pneumococcal bacteremia, for example, mortality increases only when over 1000 colony-forming units of pneumococci are present per milliliter of blood. Quantitative blood cultures rarely are performed, however, so that the intensity and significance of bacteremia must be judged on clinical grounds.

The clinical syndromes of septicemia and septic shock are due to local or circulating microbial prod-

ucts. These syndromes, therefore, may occur without demonstrable bacteremia (Table 85–1).

EPIDEMIOLOGY

Septicemia due to gram-negative enteric organisms is the most serious infectious disease of medical progress. Only 100 cases of gram-negative bacteremia were reported before 1920. Bacteremias among the Enterobacteriaceae were virtually restricted to *Escherichia coli* and *Salmonella* species. Antibiotic usage has been associated with a dramatic increase in incidence of gram-negative rod bacteremia, a broadening of the spectrum of causative agents to include *Klebsiella*, *Pseudomonas*, *Serratia*, *Enterobacter*, and *Proteus*, and an increase in the fraction of bacteremic episodes resulting from hospital-acquired infections.

TABLE 85–1. SEPTICEMIA WITH NEGATIVE BLOOD CULTURES

Prior administration of antibiotics
Severe local infection (often intra-abdominal, mixtures of aerobic and anaerobic bacteria)
Fastidious, slow-growing organism in blood
Infections due to organisms not routinely cultured (e.g., tuberculosis, fungal, severe viral)
Toxemia—toxic shock syndrome

TABLE 85–2. RISK FACTORS FOR SEPSIS

Underlying Disease or Condition
  Immunodeficiency—hypogammaglobulinemic states,
    neutropenia
  Immunosuppression—corticosteroid and cytotoxic drug
    treatment, e.g., renal allograft recipients
  Leukemia and lymphoma
  Advanced solid tumors
  Metabolic diseases—uremia, chronic liver disease, diabetes
    mellitus
  Neurologic diseases—paraplegia
  Intravenous drug abuse
Invasive Medical Devices/Instrumentation
  Indwelling urinary catheter
  Plastic intravenous cannula
  Monitoring devices (arterial line, Swan-Ganz catheter)
  Genitourinary instrumentation
Therapeutic Procedures
  Hemodialysis
  Genitourinary or abdominal surgery
  Splenectomy

Other factors that contribute to the upsurge in frequency of gram-negative sepsis are use of invasive monitoring devices, indwelling catheters, extensive surgical procedures, and the growing number of immunosuppressed patients. Patient groups at particular risk of sepsis are shown in Table 85–2. Overall, an estimated 100,000 to 300,000 cases of gram-negative bacteremia occur in the United States each year.

Gram-negative septicemia may occur without a recognized tissue site of origin; however, more commonly it is secondary to infection in the urinary tract, lungs, peritoneal cavity, biliary tract, soft tissue, or wounds.

Gram-positive bacteremia, particularly that caused by *Staphylococcus aureus*, also has become an increasing problem owing to the abuse of intravenous drugs and the therapeutic placement of chronic venous access sites.

PATHOGENESIS

Toxic bacterial products account for the cardiovascular and ventilatory derangements characterizing septic shock, as depicted in Figure 85–1. The main toxic product in gram-negative organisms is endotoxin; in gram-positive organisms the peptidoglycan/teichoic acid complex; and, in yeast, polysaccharide substances. These microbial products are responsible for intravascular activation of the complement, clotting, and fibrinolytic pathways and may directly activate neutrophils. Bacterial products induce release of interleukin-1 (IL-1) and cachetin/tumor necrosis factor (TNF) by mononuclear phagocytes. IL-1 and TNF are key mediators of the clinical syndrome of septicemia. IL-1 and TNF both cause fever and appear to act in synergy in the pathogenesis of shock. IL-1 in addition promotes release of neutrophils from the bone marrow, and both IL-1 and TNF induce hepatic synthesis of acute-phase reactants associated with inflammation (haptoglobin, C-reactive protein).

CLINICAL FINDINGS

The history and physical examination usually indicate the site of origin of the bacteremia. The findings attributable to septic shock depend on whether the patient is evaluated early or late. Shaking chills, often accompanied by nausea, vomiting, and diarrhea, mark the early toxic state characteristic of "warm shock." Patients appear hot, dry, flushed, and animated. Hyperventilation, confusion, apprehension or lethargy, and obtundation are apparent. In "cold shock," patients are cold, clammy, hypotensive, and lethargic. At this stage, findings of end-organ dysfunction due to hypoperfusion may predominate. These include a bleeding diathesis, jaundice, cyanosis, congestive heart failure, oliguria, and acidosis.

Skin lesions when present are particularly helpful, since they not only suggest sepsis but may provide a clue to the specific etiology. Ecthyma gangrenosum is a round or oval lesion 1 to 15 cm in diameter, with a central vesicle that evolves into a necrotic ulcer, set on an erythematous, indurated base (Fig. 85–2). The typical lesion is caused by *Pseudomonas* species septicemia in neutropenic hosts and results from direct infection of blood vessel walls by bacteria. Other Enterobacteriaceae, particularly *Aeromonas* and *Serratia* species, cause similar lesions on occasion. *Candida tropicalis* may cause hyperpigmented macular lesions in the neutropenic patient. *Vesiculobullous* and petechial skin lesions, cellulitis, and diffuse erythema also may appear in the septic patient. A sunburn-like rash also is characteristic of the toxic shock syndrome (see Chapter 84). Biopsy and aspiration of skin lesions sometimes allow rapid etiological diagnosis. For example, smears of material expressed from purpuric lesions have a high diagnostic yield (>80 per cent) in meningococcemia.

LABORATORY FINDINGS

The white blood cell count is increased or decreased with an increased proportion of circulating immature neutrophils (band forms). Vacuolization of circulating neutrophils is a useful finding, since it suggests bacterial infection with a high probability of bacteremia. Such changes as toxic granulations and Döhle bodies (pale intracytoplasmic inclusions), on the other hand, merely are indicative of neutrophil immaturity. The platelet count may be decreased in sepsis, the prothrombin and partial thromboplastin times prolonged, and the bilirubin and blood urea nitrogen increased. Sometimes laboratory abnormalities relating to specific end-organ damage are so striking that misdiagnosis or faulty localization of the site of infection may result. An example is the disseminated intravascular coagulation of sepsis that may be suggestive of a primary hematological disease. Most patients with fever and confusion should have a lumbar puncture. If meningitis is present, the selection of antibiotics must assure good penetration into cerebrospinal fluid.

Bacteriological diagnosis is, of course, essential.

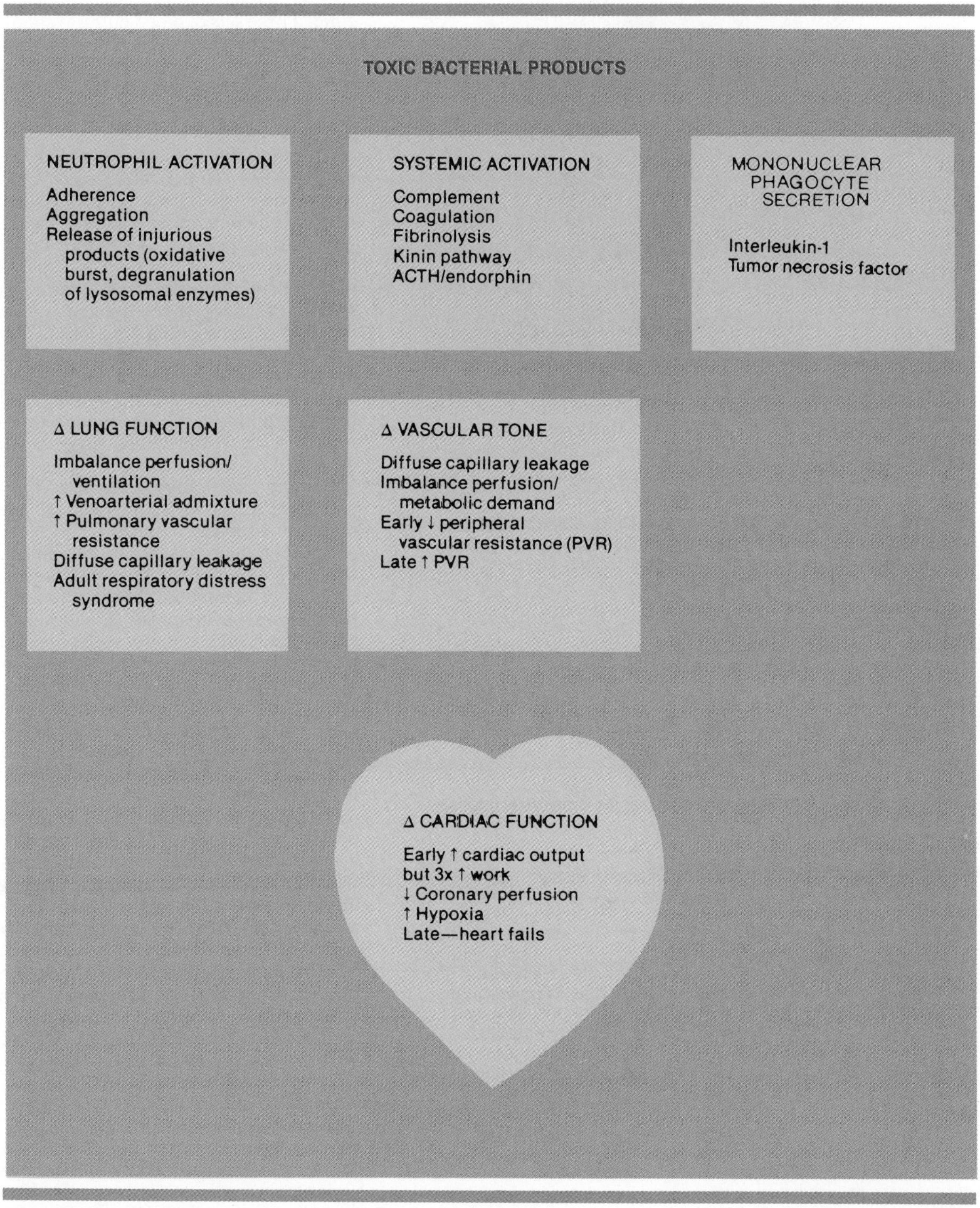

FIGURE 85–1. Pathogenesis and pathophysiology of septic shock.

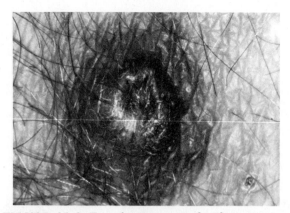

FIGURE 85–2. Typical appearance of ecthyma gangrenosum.

Gram's stained preparations should be prepared from urine, sputum, and pus. The Gram's stain not only allows rapid diagnosis but also may indicate organisms that are not easily cultured (fastidious, slow-growing bacteria or anaerobes, for example). Gram's and Wright's stains of a buffy coat smear also may be ex-

TABLE 85–3. FACTORS AFFECTING SELECTION OF ANTIBIOTICS IN THE PATIENT WITH PRESUMED SEPSIS

Community or hospital acquisition of infection
Underlying disease of the host, particularly the presence of neutropenia
Likely source of bacteremia
Organisms suspected on clinical grounds
Results of previous cultures from the patient
Meningitis present
Prevailing sensitivities of bacteria in the hospital, particularly patterns of aminoglycoside resistance and prevalence of methicillin-resistant staphylococci

TABLE 85–4. ANTIBIOTIC REGIMENS FOR THE SEPTIC PATIENT

CLINICAL SETTING	LIKELY BACTERIA	ANTIBIOTICS
Uncertain source	Enterobacteriaceae Staphylococcus	Gentamicin[a] or tobramycin + nafcillin
Abdominal or pelvic source likely	Enterobacteriaceae Enterococcus Bacteroides fragilis	Gentamicin or tobramycin + ampicillin + clindamycin[b] or metronidazole
Neutropenic patient	Pseudomonas species Enterobacteriaceae Staphylococcus species	Tobramycin + ticarcillin + nafcillin[a]

[a]Selection of an aminoglycoside and an antistaphylococcal drug depends on patterns of bacterial sensitivity in the individual hospital. For example, in many areas the frequency of resistant staphylococci is high enough to require initial use of vancomycin rather than nafcillin.
[b]Avoid clindamycin if potential gastrointestinal side effects would be difficult to recognize (e.g., patient with abdominal pain or ileus).

tremely helpful, as intracellular organisms, particularly gram-positive cocci and meningococci, are present in over one third of cases of sustained bacteremia. Three sets of blood cultures should be obtained, each from a different venipuncture site.

TREATMENT AND OUTCOME

The mortality of bacteremic shock remains in the range of 40 to 60 per cent despite rapid institution of what should be effective antibiotics. In large part, the adverse outcome reflects a lethal bacterial load at the time of diagnosis and/or a serious underlying disease.

Management of the infection dictates removal of such potential infective foci as intravenous catheters, surgical drainage of accessible abscesses, and administration of appropriate antibiotics. The possibility of infected intravenous catheters or intravenous infusates should be considered at the first suggestion of sepsis. However, stabilization and survival may depend on interrupting the vicious circle that culminates in septic shock. If the setting suggests toxic shock syndrome (e.g., a menstruating woman with a rash and tampon in place), the foreign body should be removed and local niches of staphylococcal infection incised and drained if appropriate.

Appropriate antibiotics should be administered immediately. The selection of antibiotics depends on a number of factors indicated in Table 85–3. Two antibiotics with overlapping activities clearly are necessary to treat *Pseudomonas* species infection in neutropenic patients and probably in patients with severe burns. In general, the administration of synergistic combinations of antibiotics also appears to be associated with improved outcome in patients with severe underlying disease. An additional rationale for two-drug regimens stems from problems incurred by the use of aminoglycosides in most septic patients. Treatment with a second effective agent is particularly important while aminoglycoside pharmacokinetics are being assessed and dosage schedules optimized in the individual patient. In addition, aminoglycosides are ineffective when the pH is low, as may occur in pulmonary infection. Initial antibiotic regimens suggested for patients with sepsis are presented in Table 85–4. If blood cultures are negative at 48 hours and there is no evidence of serious local infection, consideration should be given to stopping the antibiotics. If toxic shock syndrome is suspected, the patient should be treated with an antistaphylococcal drug despite negative blood culture.

Hemodynamic stabilization of the patient with septic shock requires assessment of cardiac function. This usually necessitates monitoring with a central venous or a Swan-Ganz catheter. In the warm stage of shock, peripheral vascular resistance and left ventricular end-diastolic pressure (LVEDP) are decreased; isotonic intravenous fluids are needed, sometimes in large amounts. Pressors may be necessary as well. Dopamine is the inotropic agent of choice, since it increases cerebral, coronary, renal, and mesenteric perfusion when used at low doses. Some patients require intubation and mechanical ventilation, including positive end-expiratory pressure, to maintain acceptable oxygenation. In the cold state of shock, congestive heart failure with increased LVEDP limits the use of fluids. Afterload reduction with agents such as nitroprusside is a rational form of therapy but usually requires concomitant administration of pressor agents.

Recent studies do not support the use of corticosteroids in septic shock. A promising new approach to the management of septic shock is to detoxify bacterial products. Antibody to the lipopolysaccharide core improves the survival of patients in profound septic shock but has thus far been used only on an experimental basis in humans. The use of monoclonal antibodies directed against bacterial toxins or host proteins mediating sepsis (IL-1 and TNF) ultimately may revolutionize management.

The optimal use of preventive measures would have the greatest impact on the morbidity and mortality of septic shock. The pneumococcal polysaccharide vaccine, for example, is effective and available but tre-

mendously underutilized. Antibiotics should be used only when indicated and then in narrow spectrum and for appropriately short intervals. Intravenous catheters and indwelling urinary catheters should be used only when unavoidable; when necessary, they should be inserted, changed at regular intervals, and maintained by experienced personnel, preferably organized in special teams.

REFERENCES

Sheagren JN: Shock syndromes related to sepsis. In Wyngaarden JB, Smith LH Jr (eds): Cecil Textbook of Medicine. 18th ed. Philadelphia, WB Saunders Co, 1988, pp 1538–1541.

Tracey KJ, Beutler B, Lowry SF, et al: Shock and tissue injury induced by recombinant human cachetin. Science 234:470, 1986.

Young LS, Martin WJ, Meyer RD, et al: Gram-negative rod bacteremia: Microbiologic, immunologic and therapeutic considerations. Ann Intern Med 86:456, 1977.

86

INFECTIONS OF THE NERVOUS SYSTEM

Infections of the central nervous system (CNS) range from fulminating, readily diagnosed septic processes to indolent illnesses requiring exhaustive searches to identify their presence and define their cause. Neurological outcome and survival depend largely on the extent of CNS damage present before effective treatment begins. Accordingly, it is essential that the physician move quickly to achieve a specific diagnosis and institute appropriate therapy. The initial evaluation, however, must take into account both the urgency of beginning antibiotic treatment in bacterial meningitis and the potential hazard of performing a lumbar puncture in the presence of focal neurological infection or mass lesions.

Patients with CNS infection present with some combination of fever, headache, altered mental status, depressed sensorium, focal neurological signs, and stiff neck. The history and physical examination, results of lumbar puncture, and neuroradiographic procedures provide the mainstays of diagnosis. The order in which the latter two procedures are performed is critical. A subacute history, evolving over seven days to two months, of unilateral headache with focal neurologi-

cal signs implies a mass lesion that may or may not be infectious. A brain-imaging procedure should be performed first; lumbar puncture is potentially dangerous, as it may precipitate cerebral herniation, even in the absence of overt papilledema. By contrast, patients admitted with fulminating symptoms of fever, headache, lethargy, confusion, and stiff neck should have an immediate lumbar puncture and, if abnormal, the institution of antibiotics for presumed bacterial meningitis. If the distinction between focal and diffuse CNS infection is unclear or not adequately evaluable, as in the comatose patient, cultures of blood, throat, and nasopharynx should be obtained, antibiotic therapy started, and an emergency scanning procedure performed. If the latter is unavailable, lumbar puncture should be delayed pending evidence that no danger of herniation exists. Inevitably, this approach means that some patients will receive parenteral antibiotics several hours before a lumbar puncture is performed. In acute bacterial meningitis, 50 per cent of CSF cultures will be negative by 4 to 12 hours after institution of antibiotics; negative CSF cultures are even more likely if the causative organism is a sensitive pneumococcus. Should the CNS infection actually represent acute bacterial meningitis, however, the characteristics of the CSF still would suggest the diagnosis, since neutrophilic pleocytosis and hypoglycorrhachia (low CSF sugar) usually persist for at least 12 to 24 hours after antibiotics are instituted. Furthermore, Gram's stained preparation (or assay for microbial antigen by CIE or latex agglutination) should indicate the causative organism even after antibiotics have rendered the CSF culture-negative. Blood and nasopharyngeal cultures obtained before therapy also are likely to be positive in view of the high frequency of isolation of causative organisms from these fluids. The approach of treating suspected CNS infections promptly, therefore, does not significantly compromise management, although it may lead to prolonged broad-spectrum treatment in some patients because of the inability to obtain antibiotic sensitivity tests. This approach to the use of scanning procedures is germane only for adults with community-acquired CNS infection. In children, technically adequate CT scans require heavy sedation; therefore, scanning procedures must be reserved for more stringent indications.

MENINGITIS

Definition. Meningitis is an inflammation of the leptomeninges caused by infectious or noninfectious processes. The most common types of infectious meningitis are bacterial, viral, tuberculous, and fungal. The most common noninfectious causes are subarachnoid hemorrhage, sarcoidosis, and cancer. Infectious meningitis will be considered in three categories: acute bacterial meningitis, aseptic meningitis, and subacute to chronic meningitis.

BACTERIAL MENINGITIS

Epidemiology. Three fourths of cases of acute bacterial meningitis occur before the age of 15 years. *Neisseria meningitidis* causes sporadic disease or epidemics in closed populations. Most cases occur in winter and spring and involve children or adults less than 50 years of age. *Haemophilus influenzae* men-

TABLE 86–1. MENINGITIS AND MENINGOENCEPHALITIS IN THE IMMUNOCOMPROMISED HOST

ABNORMALITY	INFECTIOUS AGENT
Complement deficiencies (C6-C8)	*Neisseria meningitidis*
Splenectomy	*Haemophilus influenzae* *Streptococcus pneumoniae* *Neisseria meningitidis*
Sickle cell disease	*Streptococcus pneumoniae* *Haemophilus influenzae*
Impaired cellular immunity	*Listeria monocytogenes* *Cryptococcus neoformans* *Toxoplasma gondii* Cytomegalovirus

ingitis is even more selectively a disease of childhood, most cases developing by the age of 10 years. Infections are sporadic, although secondary cases may occur in close contacts. In contrast, pneumococcal meningitis is a disease seen in all age groups. Extensive clinical series of adults hospitalized 20 years ago showed a relative frequency of 68 per cent pneumococcal, 18 per cent meningococcal, and 10 per cent *Haemophilus influenzae* meningitis. At University Hospitals of Cleveland in the period from 1972 to 1981 the relative frequencies were 40 per cent, 30 per cent, and 20 per cent, respectively, in keeping with the general experience that serious *Haemophilus influenzae* infections are increasingly common in adults.

Close contact with a patient with meningococcal or *Haemophilus influenzae* disease is particularly important in the development of secondary cases of meningitis and other severe disease manifestations (sepsis, epiglottitis) as well. For example, the risk of meningococcal disease is 500 to 800 times greater in a close contact of a patient with meningococcal meningitis than in a noncontact. Asymptomatic pharyngeal carriers of *Haemophilus* species also can spread infection to their contacts.

Pathogenesis and Pathophysiology. The bacteria that cause most community-acquired meningitis transiently colonize the oropharynx and nasopharynx of healthy individuals. Meningitis may occur in nonimmune hosts following bacteremia from an upper respiratory site (meningococcus or *Haemophilus* species) or pneumonia and by direct spread from contiguous foci of infection (nasal sinuses, mastoids).

The pathogenesis of acute bacterial meningitis is best understood for meningococcal disease. The carrier state occurs when meningococci adhere to pharyngeal epithelial cells via specialized filamentous structures termed pili. The production of IgA protease by pathogenic *Neisseria* species favors adherence by inactivating a major host barrier to colonization. Organisms enter and pass through epithelial cells to subepithelial tissues, where they multiply in the nonimmune individual and produce bacteremia. The localization of organisms to the CSF is not well-understood but presumably depends on invasive properties of the capsular polysaccharide which permit penetration of the blood-brain barrier. Immunity is conferred by bactericidal antibody and presumably is acquired by earlier colonization of the pharynx with nonpathogenic meningococci and cross-reacting bacteria. The presence of blocking IgA antibody may increase susceptibility transiently in some individuals.

Table 86–1 summarizes host factors conferring a particular risk of bacterial meningitis. Bacterial meningitis remains confined to the leptomeninges and does not spread to adjacent parenchymal tissue. Focal and global neurological deficits develop because of involvement of blood vessels coursing in the meninges and through the subarachnoid space; in addition, cranial nerves and cerebral tissue can be affected by the attendant inflammation, edema, and scarring as well as by the development of obstructive hydrocephalus.

Gram-negative enteric meningitis occurs mainly in

severely debilitated persons or individuals whose meninges have been breached or damaged by head trauma, a neurosurgical procedure, or a parameningeal infection.

Clinical Presentation. Patients with bacterial meningitis may present with fever, headache, lethargy, confusion, irritability, and stiff neck. Three syndromes predominate. About 25 per cent of cases begin abruptly with fulminant illness; mortality is high in this setting. More often, meningeal symptoms progress over one to seven days. Finally, meningitis may superimpose itself on one to three weeks of an upper respiratory–type illness; diagnosis is difficult in this group. Occasionally, no more than a single additional neurological symptom or sign hints at disease more serious than a routine upper respiratory infection. Stiff neck is absent in about one fifth of all patients with meningitis, notably in the very young, the old, and the comatose. A petechial or purpuric rash is found in one half of patients with meningococcemia; while not pathognomonic, palpable purpura is very suggestive of *Neisseria meningitidis* infection. About 20 per cent of patients with acute bacterial meningitis have seizures, and a similar fraction have focal neurological findings.

Laboratory Diagnosis. The CSF in acute bacterial meningitis usually contains 1,000 to 10,000 cells per microliter, mostly neutrophils (Table 86–2). Glucose content falls below 40 mg/dl and protein rises above 150 mg/dl in most patients. The Gram's stained preparation of CSF is positive in 80 to 88 per cent of cases. However, certain cautionary notes are appropriate. Cell counts can be lower (occasionally zero) early in the course of meningococcal and pneumococcal meningitis. Also, predominantly mononuclear cell pleocytosis may occur in patients who have received antibiotics before the lumbar puncture. A similar mononuclear pleocytosis may be seen in *Listeria monocytogenes* meningitis, a disease often associated with impaired cellular immunity. For several reasons, Gram's stained preparations of CSF may be negative or misinterpreted when meningitis is caused by *Haemophilus influenzae*, *Neisseria meningitidis*, or *Listeria monocytogenes*; the presence of gram-negative diplococci and coccobacilli may be difficult to appreciate, particularly when the background consists of amorphous pink material. Also, bacteria tend to be pleomorphic in CSF and may assume atypical forms. In the case of *Listeria*, CSF colony counts are low (10^3/μl). If interpretation of the Gram's stained CSF is not clear-cut, broad-spectrum antibiotics should be instituted while awaiting the results of cultures. If the initial Gram's stained preparation does not contain organisms, examining the stained sediment prepared by concentrating up to 5 ml of CSF with a cytocentrifuge may reveal the causative organism.

Cultures of CSF, blood, fluid expressed from purpuric lesions, and nasopharyngeal swabs have a high yield. The last mentioned is particularly valuable in the patients who have received antibiotic therapy before hospitalization, since most such drugs do not achieve substantial levels in nasopharyngeal secretions.

Recognition of meningitis may be difficult following head trauma or neurosurgery, since the symptoms, signs, and laboratory findings of infection can be difficult to separate from those of trauma. A low CSF glucose usually indicates infection. The causative organism, characteristically an enteric rod, may already have been cultured from an extraneural site, such as a wound or urine. The known antibiotic sensitivities of such isolates, therefore, may provide a valuable guide to initial treatment of meningitis.

All patients with meningitis caused by *S. pneumoniae*, *H. influenzae*, and unusual agents or mixed infections should have radiographs of nasal sinuses and mastoids to exclude a parameningeal focus of infection.

Differential Diagnosis. Classic acute bacterial meningitis resembles few other diseases. Ruptured brain abscess should be considered, particularly if the CSF white blood cell count is unusually high and focal neurological signs are present. Parameningeal foci of infection usually cause fever, headache, and local signs, but stiff neck occurs only if the meninges are penetrated. In the absence of that catastrophe, a modest pleocytosis may be present. CSF glucose, however, is usually normal. In patients with bacterial meningitis already given antibiotic treatment, the CSF may be sterile, but neutrophils commonly are present in CSF and the glucose level is depressed. Early in the evolution of viral or tuberculous meningitis, the pleocytosis may be predominantly neutrophilic. Serial examinations, however, will show a progressive shift to a mononuclear cell predominance. Acute viral meningoencephalitis may be difficult to distinguish clinically from bacterial meningitis; the evolution of CSF findings and the clinical course usually decide the matter.

Treatment and Outcome. Bacterial meningitis requires the prompt institution of appropriate antibiotics. If the Gram's stained smear of CSF indicates pneu-

TABLE 86–2. TYPICAL CSF FINDINGS IN CNS INFECTION

	CELLS	PER CENT NEUTROPHILS	GLUCOSE	PROTEIN
Bacterial meningitis	1,000–10,000/μl	>50%	<40 mg/dl	>150 mg/dl
Aseptic meningitis	10–2,000/μl	early 2/3 >50%	normal	<100 mg/dl
Herpes simplex virus encephalitis	0–1,100/μl	<50%	normal	<100 mg/dl
TBC meningitis	100–500/μl	early >50% late <50%	<40 mg/dl	>150 mg/dl

mococcal or meningococcal disease, penicillin G should be administered intravenously in a dose of 25,000 units/kg q2h (up to 24 million units per day). The alternative drug for patients with severe penicillin allergy is chloramphenicol (25 mg/kg intravenously q6h). Suspected cases of *Haemophilus influenzae* meningitis should be treated with cefotaxime 2g q4h intravenously, or ceftriaxone 2g q12h intravenously. In a case of suspected community-acquired meningitis, if the Gram's stained preparation of CSF is negative, but clinical and laboratory findings suggest bacterial meningitis, penicillin and cefotaxime therapy should be started. Third-generation cephalosporins are the indicated choice for treating sensitive gram-negative enteric organisms causing meningitis. Agents such as ceftazidine 2g q12h intravenously, may be effective against *Pseudomonas aeruginosa*. If the organism is resistant to cephalosporins, the patient should be treated with a combination of intraventricular plus parenteral aminoglycoside and a beta-lactam antibiotic selected on the basis of the sensitivity of the isolate (e.g., ticarcillin or piperacillin). The placement of an intraventricular reservoir facilitates treatment of such patients. Regardless of the results of in vitro sensitivity testing, chloramphenicol is not an adequate drug for treatment of gram-negative bacillary meningitis; its use has been associated with unacceptably high mortality rates.

The management of bacterial meningitis extends beyond the patient. Contacts must be protected, as they are at substantial risk of developing meningococcal meningitis or serious *H. influenzae* disease. At the time one first suspects bacterial meningitis, respiratory isolation procedures should be initiated. One should begin antibiotic prophylaxis of contacts when the clinical course or Gram's stained preparation of CSF suggests meningococcal or *H. influenzae* meningitis. Recommended doses for household and other intimate contacts of patients with meningococcal meningitis are rifampin, 10 mg/kg (up to 600 mg) twice daily for two days. The goal of prophylaxis of contacts of *H. influenzae* type B meningitis is to protect children less than four years of age. Since the organism may be passed from patient to asymptomatic adults to at-risk child, rifampin, 20 mg/kg (up to 600 mg) daily for four days, should be given to all members of the household and day care center of the index case who have contact with children less than four years old. Despite par-

enteral antibiotic therapy, patients with *N. meningitidis* or *H. influenzae* meningitis may have persistent nasopharyngeal carriage and should receive rifampin treatment before discharge from the hospital.

Although hospital contacts of patients with meningococcal meningitis are at low risk of acquiring the carrier state and disease, occasional secondary cases do occur. Accordingly, personnel with close contact with the patient's respiratory secretions should receive prophylactic antibiotics. All individuals receiving rifampin prophylaxis should be warned that their urine and tears will turn orange and that oral contraceptives will be inactivated temporarily by the antiestrogen effects of the drug.

About 30 per cent of patients with bacterial meningitis die of the infection. Of the survivors, deafness (6 to 10 per cent) and other serious neurological sequelae (1 to 18 per cent) are common. The prognosis in individual cases depends largely on the level of consciousness and extent of CNS damage at the time of first treatment. Misdiagnosis (40 per cent of patients) and attendant delays in starting antibiotics are factors in morbidity which the physician must try to offset. Patients with fulminant meningitis should be treated with antibiotics within 30 minutes of reaching medical care. Even after antibiotic therapy and presumed cure, bacterial meningitis may recur. The pattern of recurrence usually suggests a parameningeal infective focus or dural defect (Table 86–3).

The most common types of bacterial meningitis can be prevented by vaccinating susceptible individuals. Effective polysaccharide vaccines are available for some strains of *N. meningitidis* and *S. pneumoniae* and for *H. influenzae* type B.

ASEPTIC MENINGITIS

Leptomeningitis associated with negative Gram's stains of CSF and negative cultures for bacteria has been designated aseptic meningitis, a somewhat unfortunate designation which implies a benign illness that resolves spontaneously. It is important, however, to assume a high level of vigilance in this group of patients, as they may have a potentially treatable but progressive illness.

Epidemiology. Viral infections are the most frequent cause of aseptic meningitis. Of those cases in which a specific causal agent can be established, 97 per cent are due to enteroviruses (particularly Coxsackie virus B and ECHO viruses), mumps, lymphocytic choriomeningitis virus (LCM), herpes simplex virus, and leptospirosis. Viral meningitis is a disease mainly of children and young adults (70 per cent of patients are less than 20 years of age). Seasonal variation reflects the predominance of enteroviral infection, so that most cases occur in summer or early fall. Mumps usually occurs in winter and LCM in fall or winter.

Pathogenesis/Pathophysiology. Localization to the meninges occurs during systemic viremia. The

TABLE 86–3. 3 R's OF CNS INFECTION

R	DETERIORATION	POSSIBILITIES
Recrudescence	During Rx, same bacteria	Wrong Rx
Relapse	3–14 days after stopping treatment, same bacteria	Parameningeal focus
Recurrence	Delayed, same or other bacteria	Congenital or acquired dural defects

basis for the meningotropism of those viruses that cause aseptic meningitis is not understood. Herpes simplex virus type 2 may cause meningitis during the course of primary genital herpes.

Clinical Presentation. The syndrome of aseptic meningitis of viral origin begins with the acute onset of headache, fever, and meningismus associated with CSF pleocytosis. The headache often is described as the worst ever experienced and is exacerbated by sitting, standing, or coughing. In typical cases, the course is benign. The development of changes in sensorium, seizures, or focal neurological signs shifts the diagnosis to encephalitis or meningoencephalitis. Additional clinical features may suggest a particular infectious agent. Patients with mumps may have or may develop parotitis or orchitis and usually give a history of appropriate contact. LCM infection often follows exposure to mice, guinea pigs, or hamsters and causes severe myalgias; an infectious mononucleosis-like illness can ensue with rash and orchitis. Leptospirosis often follows exposure to rats or mice or swimming in water contaminated by their urine; aseptic meningitis occurs in the second phase of the illness. Aseptic meningitis also can be seen in persons with HIV infection, either as a manifestation of primary infection by the virus or as a later complication. The pleocytosis generally is modest, the protein only slightly elevated, and glucose normal or slighted depressed. HIV can be detected in CSF by culture or antigen detection.

Laboratory Diagnosis. In viral meningitis, the CSF shows a pleocytosis of 10 to 2000 WBC/μl. Two thirds have mainly neutrophils in the initial CSF specimen. However, serial lumbar punctures reveal a rapid shift (within six to eight hours) in the CSF differential count toward a mononuclear cell predominance. CSF protein is normal in one third of cases and almost always less than 100 mg/dl. CSF glucose characteristically is normal, although minimal depression occurs in mumps (30 per cent), LCM (60 per cent), and less frequently in ECHO virus and HSV meningitis. Serial lumbar punctures show a 95 per cent reduction in cell count by two weeks. Stool cultures have the highest yield for viral isolation (40 to 50 per cent); CSF and throat cultures each are positive in about 15 per cent of cases. Serologies also may indicate a specific causative agent; a fourfold rise in antibody titer is helpful in confirming the significance of a virus isolated from the throat or stool.

Differential Diagnosis. Partially treated bacterial meningitis and a parameningeal focus of infection may be particularly difficult to distinguish from aseptic meningitis. Serial lumbar punctures may be helpful in establishing the former and x-ray films of paranasal sinuses and mastoids the latter. Also in the differential diagnosis are infectious agents that are not cultured on routine bacterial meningitis and are considered below as causing subacute meningitis.

Treatment and Course. Viral meningitis is generally benign and self-limited. HSV meningitis associated with primary genital herpes occasionally causes sufficient symptoms to warrant treatment with acyclovir.

SUBACUTE MENINGITIS

Certain infectious and noninfectious diseases can present as a subacute or chronic meningitis. Chronic meningitis refers to a clinical syndrome of at least four weeks' duration and will be discussed in Chapter 122. More germane to the differential diagnosis of aseptic meningitis is a neurological disease that develops over a course of several days to weeks, clinically takes the form of meningitis or meningoencephalitis, and is associated with a predominantly mononuclear pleocytosis in the CSF. The infectious causes of this syndrome may cause a subacute to chronic meningitis (Table 86–4).

At the outset it is important to consider the possible role of human immunodeficiency virus (HIV) as directly causing this syndrome or predisposing to specific opportunistic infections, such as cryptococcosis or toxoplasmosis, which frequently present as subacute meningitis. The patient in a high-risk category for AIDS requires special consideration in this regard (see Chapter 97).

Tuberculous meningitis results from the rupture of a parameningeal focus into the subarachnoid space. The presentation is generally one of semiacute or subacute meningitis, with a neurological syndrome being present for less than two weeks in over half of patients. Headache, fever, meningismus, and altered mental status are characteristic, with papilledema, cranial nerve palsies (II, III, IV, VI, or VII), and extensor plantar reflexes each occurring in roughly one fourth of cases. Initial CSF may show predominance of neutrophils, but the differential shifts to mononuclear cells within the next seven to ten days. Acid-fast bacilli are identified in the CSF of 10 to 20 per cent of patients; the intermediate strength tuberculin skin test is positive in 65 per cent. Since delay in institution of treatment is associated with increased mortality, therapy is initiated before confirmation of the diagnosis in most cases. The clinical suspicion of tuberculosis is heightened by a history of remote tuberculosis in one half of patients; concurrent pulmonary disease occurs in about one third, so that the diagnosis may be supported by smears or culture of pulmonary secretions. Appropriate therapy consists of isoniazid, rifampin,

TABLE 86–4. SUBACUTE TO CHRONIC MENINGITIS

CAUSATIVE AGENT	ASSOCIATION
Human immunodeficiency virus	Direct involvement or opportunistic infection
Mycobacterium tuberculosis	May have extraneural tuberculosis
Cryptococcus neoformans	Compromised host
Coccidioides immitis	Southwestern United States
Histoplasma capsulatum	Ohio and Mississippi River valleys
Treponema pallidum	Acute syphilitic meningitis, secondary meningovascular syphilis
Lyme disease	Tick bite, rash, seasonal occurrence

and ethambutol. "Vasculitis" related to entrapment of cerebral vessels in inflammatory exudate may lead to stroke syndromes. This has been offered as a rationale for the use of corticosteroids as adjunctive therapy. Although evidence of their advantage remains unproved, some authorities believe that corticosteroids should be given, in tapering doses, for four weeks when the diagnosis of tuberculosis is established, particularly if cranial palsies appear or stupor or coma supervenes.

Cryptococcal meningitis is the most common fungal meningitis and can occur in apparently normal as well as immunocompromised hosts. The presentation is of insidious onset followed by weeks to months of progressive meningoencephalitis, sometimes clinically indistinguishable from the course of tuberculosis. Certain associations are useful in this differential diagnosis. The presence of immunosuppression suggests cryptococcosis, whereas chronic debilitating disease, miliary infiltrates on chest radiograph, or the syndrome of inappropriate antidiuretic hormone suggests tuberculosis. An India ink preparation of CSF reveals encapsulated yeast in 50 per cent of cases. More than 90 per cent have cryptococcal polysaccharide antigen in CSF or serum. Fungal cultures should be obtained of urine, stool, sputum, and blood; they may be positive in the absence of clinically apparent extraneural disease. Treatment of cryptococcal meningitis requires amphotericin B. Addition of flucytosine allows use of less amphotericin B. Preliminary data suggest that a new imidazole, fluconazole, may be effective in the treatment of cryptococcal meningitis.

Coccidioides immitis is a major cause of granulomatous meningitis in semiarid areas of the southwestern United States; *Histoplasma capsulatum* may cause a similar syndrome in endemic areas (Ohio and Mississippi River valleys).

Acute syphilitic meningitis is a manifestation of secondary syphilis and may be accompanied by a characteristic rash (Chapter 96). Hydrocephalus and cranial nerve (VII and VIII) abnormalities may develop. CSF and serum serologies are strongly positive, and the disease is responsive to penicillin. Meningovascular syphilis occurs two to ten years after the primary lesion and is characterized by meningoencephalitis, with associated vasculitis producing multiple infarcts of the cerebrum or spinal cord. Again, CSF serologies reveal the diagnosis. Although the meningeal signs respond to penicillin therapy, recovery from the focal abnormalities may be incomplete. Late neurosyphilis is discussed in Chapter 122.

Lyme disease, a tick-borne spirochetosis (Chapter 84), is associated in 15 per cent of clinically affected individuals with meningitis, encephalitis, or cranial or radicular neuropathies. Characteristically, the neurological disease begins several weeks after the typical skin rash, erythema chronicum migrans. Furthermore, the skin rash may have been so mild as to go unnoticed and usually has faded by the time neurological manifestations appear. The diagnosis should be suspected when a patient develops subacute or chronic meningitis during late summer or early fall, with CSF changes consisting of a modest mononuclear pleocytosis, protein values below 100 mg/dl, and normal glucose levels. The diagnosis is established serologically. Patients usually respond to therapy with antibiotics.

ENCEPHALITIS

Definition. Acute viral and other infectious causes of encephalitis usually produce fever, headache, and stiff neck, and additionally alterations in consciousness, focal neurological signs, and seizures.

Epidemiology. A large number of viral and nonviral agents can cause encephalitis (Table 86–5). Seasonal occurrence may help to limit the differential diagnosis. Arthropod-borne viruses peak in the summer (California encephalitis and western equine encephalitis in August, St. Louis encephalitis slightly later). The tick-borne infections (Rocky Mountain spotted fever) occur in early summer, enterovirus infections in later summer and fall, and mumps in the winter and spring. Geographic distribution is also helpful. Eastern equine encephalitis is confined to the coastal states. Serological surveys indicate that infections by encephalitis viruses are most often subclinical. It is not clear why a few among infected subjects develop encephalitis.

Herpes simplex virus (HSV) is the most frequent and devastating cause of sporadic, severe focal encephalitis; overall it is implicated in 10 per cent of all cases of encephalitis. There is no age, sex, seasonal, or geographic preference.

Pathogenesis. Viruses reach the CNS by the blood stream or peripheral nerves. HSV presumably reaches the brain by cell-to-cell spread along recurrent branches of the trigeminal nerve which innervate the meninges of the anterior and middle fossae. Although this would explain the characteristic localization of necrotic lesions to the inferomedial portions of the temporal and frontal lobes, it is not clear why such spread is so rare, one case of HSV encephalitis occurring per million in the population per annum.

Clinical Features. The course of HSV encephalitis will be considered here in detail because of the

TABLE 86–5. INFECTIOUS AGENTS CAUSING ENCEPHALITIS AND MENINGOENCEPHALITIS

VIRUSES	NONVIRAL
Herpes simplex	*Rickettsia rickettsii*
Epstein-Barr	*Rickettsia typhi*
Varicella-zoster	*Mycoplasma pneumoniae*
Cytomegalovirus	*Leptospira* species
Mumps	*Brucella* species
Measles	*Mycobacterium tuberculosis*
California encephalitis	*Histoplasma capsulatum*
St. Louis encephalitis	*Cryptococcus neoformans*
Eastern Equine encephalitis	*Naegleria* species
Western Equine encephalitis	*Acanthamoeba* species
Coxsackie	*Toxoplasma gondii*
ECHO	*Trypanosoma* species
Rabies	*Plasmodium falciparum*
Human immunodeficiency virus	*Borrelia burgdorferi*

importance of establishing the diagnosis of this now treatable entity. Patients affected by HSV commonly describe a prodrome of one to seven days of upper respiratory tract symptoms followed by the sudden onset of headache, fever, behavioral abnormalities, delirium, difficulty with speech, and seizures, often focal.

Laboratory Diagnosis. The CSF shows a predominantly lymphocytic pleocytosis. In HSV encephalitis, the cell count is 0 to 1100 WBC/μl (median 130). Protein is moderately high (median 80 mg/dl). CSF glucose is reduced in only 5 per cent of individuals within three days of onset but becomes abnormal in additional patients later in the course. In about 5 per cent the CSF is normal. Other laboratory findings at onset are of little help, although focal abnormalities may be present in the EEG and develop in CT or MRI brain images by the third day in most patients. Acyclovir offers such high likelihood of therapeutic benefit in HSV encephalitis, with so little risk in this highly fatal and neurologically damaging disease, that we rarely perform brain biopsy unless an alternative, treatable diagnosis seems very likely. A low CSF glucose should increase suspicion that a granulomatous infection is present (tuberculosis, cryptococcosis). If brain imaging remains inconclusive in such circumstances, biopsy may be appropriate.

Viral cultures of stool, throat, buffy coat, and brain biopsy specimens and indirect immunofluorescence or immunoperoxidase staining of tissues may provide a specific diagnosis, but both viral isolation and serological evidence of a rise in antibody titer usually come too late to guide initial treatment. In the case of HSV encephalitis, serologies are particularly helpful in the 30 per cent of individuals with a primary infection. Also, CSF titers of antibody to HSV, which reflect local production of antibody, may show a diagnostic fourfold rise.

Differential Diagnosis. Acute (demyelinating) encephalomyelitis, infective endocarditis producing diffuse brain embolization, meningoencephalitis caused by *Cryptococcus neoformans* or *M. tuberculosis*, acute bacterial cerebritis, acute thrombotic thrombocytopenic purpura, cerebral venous thrombosis, vascular disease, and primary and metastatic tumors may all simulate HSV encephalitis.

Treatment and Outcome. The course of viral encephalitis depends on the etiologic agent. Untreated HSV encephalitis has a high mortality (70 per cent), and survival is associated with severe neurological residua. Acyclovir therapy improves survival and greatly lessens morbidity in patients if initiated early, before deterioration to coma. Prognosis is particularly favorable in patients less than 30 years old.

RABIES

Rabies encephalitis is always fatal, requiring one to place major attention on prevention. Currently, zero to six cases of rabies occur each year in the United States, and approximately 20,000 people receive postexposure prophylaxis.

The incubation period for rabies is generally 20 to 90 days, during which the rabies virus replicates locally and then migrates along nerves to the spinal cord and brain. Rabies begins with fever, headache, fatigue, and pain or paresthesias at the site of inoculation; confusion, seizures, paralysis, and stiff neck follow. Periods of violent agitation are characteristic of rabies encephalitis. Attempts at drinking produce laryngospasm, gagging, and apprehension. Paralysis, coma, and death supervene. When rabies is suspected, protective isolation procedures should be instituted to avoid additional exposure of the hospital staff to saliva and other infected secretions. Confirmation of the diagnosis is possible by assaying rabies-neutralizing antibody or isolating virus from saliva, CSF, and urine sediment. Immunofluorescent rabies antibody staining of a skin biopsy taken from the posterior neck is a rapid means of establishing the diagnosis.

Indications for prophylaxis are based on the following principles: (1) The patient must have been exposed. Nonbite exposure is possible if mucous membranes or open wounds are contaminated with animal saliva; exposure to bat urine in heavily contaminated caves has been followed by rabies. (2) Small rodents (rats, mice, chipmunks, squirrels) and rabbits rarely are infected with rabies and have not been associated with human disease. Consultation with local or state health authorities is essential, since certain areas of the United States are considered rabies-free. In other areas, if rabies is present in wild animals, dogs and cats have the potential to transmit rabies. Domestic dogs and cats should be quarantined for 10 days after biting someone; if no signs of illness develop, there is no risk of transmission by their earlier bite. Other animals should be destroyed and their brains examined for rabies virus by direct fluorescent antibody testing. If the biting animal escapes, postexposure prophylaxis is usually indicated. Bites of a bat, skunk, and racoon require treatment unless the animal is caught. Unusual behavior of animals and truly unprovoked attacks (as opposed to those incurred during handling or feeding) increase the likelihood of rabies.

Currently, postexposure management consists of (1) thorough wound cleansing, (2) human rabies immune globulin 20 IU/kg, one half infiltrated locally in the area of the bite and one half intramuscularly, and (3) human diploid cell rabies vaccine, 1.0 ml intramuscularly five times during a one-month period. Individuals at high risk of exposure to rabies should be vaccinated. Veterinarians, laboratory workers, and those who frequent caves belong in this category.

MYELITIS

Several viruses are associated with disease of the spinal cord (myelitis); all except varicella-zoster are uncommon in the United States. Dermatomal varicella-zoster infection is discussed in Chapter 84. In some instances, the infection spreads from the dorsal root sensory ganglia into the spinal cord. If anterior horn cells are affected, paralysis may develop in muscles supplied by the same dermatomal segment involved by the rash. More widespread infection of the spinal cord causes transverse or diffuse myelopathy. Varicella-zoster also can lead to trigeminal neuralgia, or facial nerve palsy (Ramsay Hunt syndrome, see Chapter 122) or arteritis of the internal carotid artery followed by hemiplegia.

Poliomyelitis was at one time a major public health problem in the United States and remains so in developing countries. Small epidemics still are reported, however, when patients refuse vaccination for religious reasons; occasional sporadic cases result from vaccination with attenuated poliovirus. The disease is characterized by symptoms of acute viral meningitis, including headache, fever, and stiff neck, followed in about 10 per cent by paralysis of voluntary muscles supplied by anterior horn cells of either spinal cord or brain stem. Muscle paralysis is asymmetrical and often patchy and may be profound; sensory systems remain unaffected. The spinal fluid contains an increased number of lymphocytes with an elevated protein and normal glucose concentration. Illness indistinguishable from poliomyelitis also can be caused by other enteroviruses. The disorder should not be mistaken for Guillain-Barré syndrome (Chapter 116), which is a nonfebrile, essentially symmetrical paralytic illness, often accompanied by sensory abnormalities. Both poliomyelitis and Guillain-Barré syndrome produce their most serious symptoms by paralyzing respiratory muscles so as to require respiratory support.

Brain abscess and focal CNS infection are discussed in Chapter 122.

REFERENCES

Bacterial Meningitis

Spagnuolo PJ, Ellner JJ, Lerner PI, et al: *Hemophilus influenzae* meningitis: The spectrum of disease in adults. Medicine 61:74, 1982.
Swartz MN: Bacterial meningitis. *In* Wyngaarden JB, Smith LH Jr (eds): Cecil Textbook of Medicine. 18th ed. Philadelphia, WB Saunders Co, 1988, pp 1604–1611.

Aseptic Meningitis

Lepow ML, Carver DH, Wright HT, et al: A clinical, laboratory and epidemiologic investigation of aseptic meningitis during the 4-year period 1955–1958. N Engl J Med 266:1181, 1962.

Encephalitis

Johnson R: Viral Infections of the Nervous System. New York, Raven Press, 1982.
Nahmias AJ, Whitley RJ, Visintine AN, et al: HSV encephalitis; Laboratory evaluations and their diagnostic significance. J Infect Dis 145:829–836, 1982.
Price RW: Herpes virus infections of the nervous system. *In* Wyngaarden JB, Smith LH Jr (eds): Cecil Textbook of Medicine. 18th ed. Philadelphia, WB Saunders Co, 1988, pp 2195–2198.
Sawyer J, Ellner JJ, Ransahoff DF: To biopsy or not to biopsy in suspected herpes simplex encephalitis. Medical Decision Making 8:95–101, 1988.

87

INFECTIONS OF THE HEAD AND NECK

INFECTIONS OF THE EAR

Otitis externa is an infection of the external auditory canal. The process may begin as a folliculitis or pustule within the canal. Staphylococci, streptococci, and other skin flora are the most common pathogens. Some cases of otitis externa have been associated with swimming in hot tubs. This infection (swimmer's ear) is usually due to *Pseudomonas aeruginosa*.

Patients with otitis externa complain of ear pain that is often quite severe, and they may also complain of itching. Examination reveals an inflamed external canal; the tympanic membrane may be uninvolved. (Patients with otitis media, in contrast, will not have involvement of the external canal unless the tympanic membrane is perforated.) Otitis externa with cellulitis can be treated with systemic antibiotics such as dicloxacillin or erythromycin and local heat. In the ab-

sence of cellulitis, irrigation and administration of topical antibiotics such as neomycin and polymyxin are sufficient. Patients with diabetes mellitus are at risk for an invasive external otitis (malignant otitis) due to *P. aeruginosa*. In malignant otitis externa, pain is a presenting complaint and infection rapidly invades the bones of the skull and may result in cranial nerve palsies, invasion of the brain, and death. Treatment must include debridement of as much necrotic tissue as is feasible and at least four to six weeks of treatment with an aminoglycoside plus a penicillin derivative active against *Pseudomonas* (e.g., carbenicillin). Ceftazidime and imipenem may also be especially effective for this infection.

Otitis media is an infection of the middle ear seen primarily among preschool children but occasionally in adults as well. Infection caused by upper respiratory tract pathogens is facilitated by obstruction to drainage through edematous, congested eustachian tubes. *Streptococcus pneumoniae, Haemophilus influenzae,* and *Branhamella catarrhalis* are the most common pathogens, and virus infection may predispose to acute otitis media. Fever, ear pain, diminished hearing, vertigo, or tinnitus may be seen. In young children, however, localizing symptoms may not be appreciated. The tympanic membrane may appear inflamed, but to diagnose otitis media with certainty, either fluid must be seen behind the membrane or diminished mobility of the membrane must be demonstrated by tympanometry or after air insufflation into the external canal.

Treatment with ampicillin, trimethoprim-sulfamethoxazole, or cefaclor is generally effective; addition of decongestants is of no proven value. Complications of otitis media are uncommon but include infection of the mastoid air cells (mastoiditis), bacterial meningitis, brain abscess, or subdural empyema.

INFECTIONS OF THE NOSE AND SINUSES

Rhinitis is a common manifestation of numerous respiratory virus infections. It is characterized by mucopurulent or watery nasal discharge that may be profuse. When due to respiratory virus infection, there may be associated pharyngitis, conjunctival suffusion, and fever. Rhinitis can also be caused by hypersensitivity responses to airborne allergens. Patients with allergic rhinitis often have a transverse skin crease on the bridge of the nose a few millimeters from the tip. The demonstration of eosinophils in a wet preparation of nasal secretions readily distinguishes allergic rhinitis from rhinitis of infectious origin. (Eosinophils can be identified in wet preparations by the presence of large refractile cytoplasmic granules.) Occasionally, following head trauma or neurosurgery, cerebrospinal fluid (CSF) may leak through the nose. "CSF rhinorrhea" places patients at risk for bacterial meningitis. CSF is readily distinguished from nasal secretions by its low protein and relatively high glucose concentrations.

Sinusitis is an infection of the air-filled paranasal sinuses that may complicate viral upper respiratory infections. Allergic rhinitis and structural abnormalities of the nose that interfere with sinus drainage also predispose to sinusitis. Acute sinusitis is primarily caused by upper respiratory tract bacterial pathogens, *Streptococcus pneumoniae* and *Haemophilus influenzae,* and less often by anaerobes and staphylococci.

Sinusitis may be difficult to distinguish from a viral upper respiratory illness that, in many instances, precedes sinus infection. Patients may complain of headache, "stuffiness," and purulent nasal discharge. Headache may be exacerbated by bending over. There may be tenderness over the involved sinus, and pus may be seen in the turbinates of the nose. Failure of a sinus to light up on transillumination may suggest the diagnosis; sinus radiographs revealing opacification, mucosal thickening, or air-fluid levels establish the diagnosis of sinusitis. Most patients with sinusitis can be treated with a 10-day course of ampicillin, amoxicillin, or trimethoprim-sulfamethoxazole, and nasal decongestants. Patients who appear toxic or otherwise are severely ill should undergo sinus puncture for drainage, Gram's stain, and culture. Sinusitis may be complicated by bacterial meningitis, brain abscess, or subdural empyema. Therefore, patients with sinusitis and neurologic abnormalities must be evaluated carefully for these complications by CT scan if a space-occupying lesion is suspected or by CSF examination if meningitis is suspected (see Chapter 86).

Rhinocerebral mucormycosis is an invasive infection arising from the nose or sinuses caused by fungi of the order Mucorales. This infection can result in progressive bony destruction and invasion of the brain. Rhinocerebral mucormycosis is seen primarily among poorly contolled diabetics, recipients of organ transplants, and patients with hematological malignancy.

Black necrotic lesions of the palate or nasal mucosa are characteristic. Most patients have a depressed sensorium at presentation. Vascular thrombosis and cranial nerve palsies are common. Diagnosis is made by demonstration of the broad ribbon-shaped nonseptate hyphae on histological examination of a scraping or biopsy specimen. Differential diagnosis includes infection due to *Pseudomonas aeruginosa* or to other fungi such as *Aspergillus* species, and cavernous sinus thrombosis. Rhinocerebral mucormycosis is a surgical emergency. Treatment involves correction of the underlying process if possible, broad surgical debridement, and administration of amphotericin B.

INFECTIONS OF THE MOUTH AND PHARYNX

Stomatitis

Stomatitis or inflammation of the mouth can be caused by a wide variety of processes. Patients with stomatitis may complain of diffuse or localized pain in the mouth, difficulty swallowing, and difficulty managing oral secretions. Various nutritional deficiencies (vitamins B_{12} and C, folic acid, and niacin) can also produce stomatitis and soreness of the mouth.

Thrush is an infection of the oral mucosa by *Candida* species. Thrush may be seen among infants and also in patients receiving broad-spectrum antibiotics or corticosteroids (systemic or inhaled), among patients with leukopenia (e.g., acute leukemia), and among patients with impairments in cell-mediated immunity (e.g., AIDS). In its milder form, thrush is manifested by an asymptomatic white, "cheesy" exudate on the buccal mucosa and pharynx, which when scraped leaves a raw, bleeding surface. In more severe cases, there may be pain and also erythema surrounding the exudate. The diagnosis is suggested by the characteristic appearance of the lesions and is confirmed by microscopic examination of a KOH preparation of the exudate, which reveals yeast and the pseudohyphae characteristic of *Candida.* Thrush related to administration of antibiotics and corticosteroids should resolve after the drugs are withdrawn.

Otherwise, thrush can be managed with clotrimazole troches. Refractory thrush or *Candida* involving the esophagus should be treated with ketoconazole or intravenous amphotericin B.

Oral Ulcers and Vesicles
(Table 87–1)

Aphthous Stomatitis. Aphthae are discrete shallow painful ulcers on erythematous bases which may be single or multiple and are usually present on the labial or buccal mucosa. Attacks of aphthous stomatitis may be recurrent and quite debilitating. Symptoms may last for several days to two weeks. The cause of these ulcerations is unknown, and treatment is symptomatic with saline mouth wash or topical anesthetics.

Herpes Simplex Virus Infection. Although most recurrences of oral herpes simplex infections occur on or near the vermillion border of the lips, the primary attack usually involves the mouth and pharynx. Generalized symptoms of fever, headache, and malaise often precede the appearance of oral lesions by as much as 24 to 48 hours. The involved regions are swollen and erythematous. Small vesicles soon appear which rupture, leaving shallow, discrete ulcers that may coalesce. The diagnosis can be made by scraping the base of an ulcer. Wright's or Giemsa stain of this material may reveal the multinucleated giant cells characteristic of herpes simplex infection. Viral cultures are more sensitive but also expensive. Treatment of primary infection with acyclovir will decrease the duration of symptoms but has no effect on the frequency of recurrence.

Vincent's Stomatitis. This is an ulcerative infection of the gingival mucosa due to anaerobic fusobacteria and spirochetes. Breath is often foul, and the ulcerations are covered with a purulent, dirty-appearing, gray exudate. Gram's stain of the exudate reveals the characteristic gram-negative fusobacteria and spirochetes. Treatment with penicillin is curative. Untreated, the infection may extend to the peritonsillar space (quinsy) and even involve vascular structures in the lateral neck (see below).

Syphilis. Syphilis may produce a painless primary chancre in the mouth or a painful mucous patch that is a manifestation of secondary disease. The diagnosis should be considered in the sexually active patient

TABLE 87–1. ORAL VESICLES AND ULCERS

Aphthous stomatitis
Primary herpes simplex infection
Vincent's stomatitis
Syphilis
Coxsackievirus A (herpangina)
Fungi (histoplasmosis)
Behçet's syndrome
Systemic lupus erythematosus
Reiter's syndrome
Crohn's disease
Erythema multiforme
Pemphigus
Pemphigoid

with a large (>1 cm) oral ulceration and should be confirmed serologically, since darkfield examination may be confounded by the presence of nonsyphilitic oral spirochetes.

Herpangina. This is a childhood disease that causes tiny discrete ulcerations of the soft palate and is due to infection with coxsackievirus A.

Fungal Disease. Occasionally, an oral ulcer or nodule may be a manifestation of disseminated infection due to histoplasmosis. These ulcers are generally mildly or minimally symptomatic and are overshadowed by the constitutional symptoms of disseminated fungal illness.

Systemic Illnesses Causing Ulcerative or Vesicular Lesions of the Mouth. Recurrent aphthous oral ulcerations may be part of Behçet's syndrome. Oral ulcerations have been associated with connective tissue diseases, such as systemic lupus erythematosus and Reiter's syndrome and with Crohn's disease. Although isolated oral bullae and ulcerations may be seen in patients with erythema multiforme, pemphigus, and pemphigoid, almost all patients will have an associated skin rash. The "iris" or "target" lesion of erythema multiforme is diagnostic. Otherwise, biopsy will establish the diagnosis. Corticosteroids may be life-saving for pemphigus. Corticosteroids are also used in the treatment of erythema multiforme majorum (Stevens-Johnson syndrome), although proof of their efficacy is not available.

APPROACH TO THE PATIENT WITH "SORE THROAT"

This section will discuss the clinical approach to patients with sore throat and will also discuss several less common but serious illnesses that can present as a "sore throat." When evaluating a patient with a sore throat, it is first important to distinguish between the relatively common and benign sore throat syndromes (viral or streptococcal pharyngitis) and the less common but more dangerous causes of sore throat. Patients with viral or streptococcal pharyngitis often give a history of exposure to individuals with upper respiratory tract infections. Symptoms of cough, rhinitis, and hoarseness (indicating involvement of the larynx) suggest a viral upper respiratory tract infection, although it is important to remember that hoarseness may also be seen with more serious infections such as epiglottitis.

Examination of the Throat. Two points regarding examination of the throat need emphasis. The first is that complete examination of the oral cavity is important. Not only will a thorough examination give clues as to the etiology of the complaint, but it may also provide early diagnosis of an asymptomatic malignancy at a time when cure is feasible. The second point is that the normal tonsils and mucosal rim of the anterior fauces are generally a deeper red than the rest of the pharynx in healthy subjects. This should not be mistaken for inflammation. Patients with pharyngitis often have a red, inflamed posterior pharynx. The tonsils are often enlarged and red and may be covered with a punctate or diffuse white exudate. Lymph nodes of the anterior neck are often enlarged.

If any of the seven *danger signs* listed in Table 87–2 is present, the clinician must suspect an illness other than viral or streptococcal pharyngitis. Symptoms persisting longer than one week are rarely due to streptococci or viruses and should prompt consideration of other processes (see "Persistent or Penicillin-unresponsive Pharyngitis" below). Respiratory difficulty, particularly stridor, difficulty handling oral secretions, or difficulty swallowing should suggest the possibility of epiglottitis or soft tissue space infection. Severe pain in the absence of erythema of the pharynx may be seen with some of the "extrarespiratory" causes of sore throat, as well as in some cases of epiglottitis or retropharyngeal abscess. A *palpable mass* in the pharynx or neck suggests a soft tissue space infection, and *blood in the ear or pharynx* may be an early indication of a lateral pharyngeal space abscess eroding into the carotid artery.

A good history and careful examination will distinguish between the common and benign causes of a sore throat, and the unusual but often more serious causes.

Pharyngitis

A list of agents that have been associated with pharyngitis is shown on Table 87–3. Almost half of all cases are due to respiratory viruses or group A streptococci. Most of the remainder of the cases are without defined etiology. Most cases occur during the winter months. In practice, once a diagnosis of pharyngitis is established clinically, it is most important to distinguish between group A streptococcal infections, which should be treated with penicillin, and viral infections, which should be treated symptomatically (e.g., salicylates, saline gargles). Since clinical criteria do not reliably distinguish streptococcal from nonstreptococcal pharyngitis, all patients with pharyngitis should have a throat swab cultured for streptococci. Recently test kits have become available that rapidly detect group A streptococcal antigen on throat swabs with high levels of accuracy. These tests may be substituted for culture and provide more rapid diagnosis of group A streptococcal infection.

Pharyngitis and Respiratory Virus Infections. Many patients with common colds due to rhinovirus or coronavirus or with influenza will have an associated pharyngitis. Other cold symptoms—rhinorrhea, conjunctival suffusion, and mild cough—suggest a cold virus; fevers and myalgias suggest influenza. Symptoms generally resolve in a few days without treatment.

Infectious mononucleosis due to Epstein-Barr virus is often associated with pharyngitis. Patients will often also complain of malaise and fever. On examination, the pharynx may be inflamed and the tonsils hypertrophied and covered by a white exudate. Cervical lymph node enlargement is often prominent, and generalized lymph node enlargement and splenomegaly are common. Examination of a peripheral blood smear reveals atypical lymphocytes, and the presence of heterophile antibodies (e.g., Monospot) or a rise in antibodies to EBV viral capsid antigen will confirm the diagnosis.

Streptococcal Pharyngitis. Streptococcal pharyngitis may produce mild or severe symptoms. The pharynx is generally inflamed, and exudative tonsillitis is common but not universal. Fever may be present and cervical lymph nodes may be enlarged and tender. Clinical distinction between streptococcal and nonstreptococcal pharyngitis is inaccurate, and patients with pharyngitis should therefore have a swab of the posterior pharynx cultured on sheep blood agar plates or tested for streptococcal antigen. The growth of group A beta-hemolytic streptococci or detection of group A streptococcal antigen is an indication for treatment with penicillin (or erythromycin if the patient is penicillin-allergic). Antibiotics may shorten the duration of symptoms due to this infection but are given primarily to decrease the frequency of rheumatic fever, which may follow untreated streptococcal pharyngitis.

Corynebacterial Disease. Diphtheria, caused by *Corynebacterium diphtheriae*, is a rare disease in the United States, with only three cases reported to the CDC in 1980. The grey pseudomembrane bleeds when removed and rarely may cause death via airway obstruction. Most morbidity and mortality in diphtheria are related to the elaboration of a toxin with neurologic and cardiac effects. Treatment consists of antitoxin plus erythromycin. A self-limited pharyngitis, often associated with a diffuse scarlatiniform rash, may be caused by *Corynebacterium hemolyticum*. This infection can be treated with penicillin or erythromycin.

TABLE 87–2. SEVEN DANGER SIGNS IN PATIENTS WITH "SORE THROAT"

1. Persistence of symptoms longer than one week without improvement
2. Respiratory difficulty, particularly stridor
3. Difficulty handling secretions
4. Difficulty in swallowing
5. Severe pain in the absence of erythema
6. A palpable mass
7. Blood, even in small amounts, in the pharynx or ear

TABLE 87–3. CAUSES OF PHARYNGITIS

Viral
    Respiratory viruses*
    Herpes simplex
    Epstein-Barr virus
    Coxsackievirus A (herpangina)
Mycoplasma pneumoniae
Bacterial
    Group A streptococcus*
    Vincent's fusospirochetes
    Corynebacterium diphtheriae
    Corynebacterium hemolyticum
    Neisseria gonorrhoeae
Fungal
    Candida species (thrush)

* Most frequent identifiable causes of pharyngitis

Epiglottitis

Epiglottitis, usually an aggressive disease of young children, occurs in adults as well. Early recognition of this entity is critical, because delay in diagnosis or treatment frequently results in death, which may occur abruptly, within hours after the onset of symptoms. This diagnosis must be considered in any patient with a sore throat and any of the following key symptoms or signs: (1) difficulty in swallowing, (2) copious oral secretions, (3) severe pain in the absence of pharyngeal erythema (the pharynx of patients with epiglottitis may be normal or inflamed), and (4) respiratory difficulty, particularly stridor. Patients with epiglottitis often display a characteristic posture; they lean forward in order to prevent the swollen epiglottis from completely obstructing the airway and resist any attempt at placement in the supine position. The diagnosis can be confirmed by lateral x-rays of the neck or by indirect laryngoscopy with visualization of the swollen erythematous epiglottis. This should be performed with the patient in the sitting position to minimize the risk of laryngeal spasm. Furthermore, the physician must be prepared to perform emergency tracheostomy should spasm occur. Therapy has two major objectives: protecting the airway and providing appropriate antimicrobial coverage. Prophylactic tracheotomy is often indicated if respiratory distress increases under observation. As the most likely pathogen is *Haemophilus influenzae*, which may be beta-lactamase producing, good antibiotic choices are chloramphenicol, trimethoprim-sulfamethoxazole, or a second or third-generation cephalosporin. Corticosteroids may relieve some inflammatory edema; however, their role in this disease remains unproven. Patients with respiratory difficulty should have their airway protected by endotracheal intubation or tracheostomy. Patients without respiratory complaints may be monitored continuously in an intensive care setting and intubated at the first sign of respiratory difficulty. Young children who are close contacts of patients with invasive disease due to *H. influenzae* are themselves at particular risk of serious infection. Children less than four years of age who are close contacts of the index patient and all family members in a household with children less than four years of age should receive prophylaxis with rifampin (20 mg/kg orally up to 600 mg twice daily for eight doses).

Soft Tissue Space Infections

Quinsy. Quinsy is a unilateral peritonsillar abscess or phlegmon that is an unusual complication of tonsillitis. The patient has pain and difficulty swallowing and often trouble handling oral secretions. Trismus (inability to open the mouth due to muscle spasm) may be present. Examination reveals swelling of the peritonsillar tissues and lateral displacement of the uvula. Digital examination may reveal a mass. In the phlegmon stage, penicillin therapy may be adequate; abscess requires surgical drainage. Untreated, quinsy may result in glottal edema and respiratory embarrassment or lateral pharyngeal space abscess.

Lateral Pharyngeal Space Abscess. This rare infection is associated with serious morbidity because of its proximity to vascular structures. Extension to the jugular vein may result in thrombophlebitis with septic pulmonary emboli and bacteremia (syndrome of "postanginal sepsis"). Erosion of the carotid artery may also complicate this infection with resultant exsanguination. This is often preceded by small amounts of blood in the ear or pharynx. This infection is generally associated with tenderness and a mass at the angle of the jaw. Prompt surgical intervention may be life-saving.

Retropharyngeal Space Abscess. This complication of tonsillitis is rare in adults, since by adulthood the lymph nodes that give rise to this infection are generally atrophied. Most cases in adults are secondary to trauma (e.g., endoscopic) or extension of a cervical osteomyelitis. The patient often has difficulty swallowing and may complain of dyspnea, particularly when sitting upright. Diagnosis may be suspected by the presence of a posterior pharyngeal mass and confirmed by lateral neck films.

Ludwig's Angina. This cellulitis/phlegmon of the floor of the mouth generally is secondary to an odontogenic infection. The tongue is pushed upward, and there is often firm induration of the submandibular space and neck. Laryngeal edema and respiratory compromise may also occur and necessitate protection of the airway. Penicillin is the antibiotic of choice; some patients may require a broad guillotine incision across the submandibular space to provide decompression and adequate drainage, although incision may be unnecessary if the airway can be protected.

Extrarespiratory Causes of Sore Throat

Several extrarespiratory causes of sore throat should be kept in mind. The older patient who complains of soreness in his throat when he climbs stairs or when he is upset may be suffering from angina pectoris with an unusual radiation. The hypertensive patient who presents with an abrupt onset of a "tearing pain" in his throat may have a dissecting aortic aneurysm. In these patients, swallowing is generally unaffected. Patients with DeQuervain's subacute thyroiditis may present with fever and pain in the neck radiating to the ears. In patients with thyroiditis, the thyroid is generally tender and the sedimentation rate is increased. Patients with vitamin deficiencies may complain of soreness in the mouth and throat (see Table 87–1). Examination may reveal a red "beefy" tongue with flattened papillae, resulting in a smooth appearance.

Persistent or Penicillin-unresponsive Pharyngitis

Most cases of viral or streptococcal pharyngitis are self-limited, and symptoms generally resolve within three to four days. Persistent sore throat should prompt consideration of the following possibilities:

Soft Tissue Abscess or Phlegmon. Rarely, an untreated tonsillitis extends to the soft tissues of the pharynx, producing a potentially life-threatening infection (see above).

Pharyngeal Gonorrhea. Although most cases of pharyngeal gonorrhea are asymptomatic, mild pharyngitis may be seen occasionally. This infection will not respond to doses of penicillin used for pharyngitis; moreover, the gonococcus is relatively resistant to phenoxymethyl penicillin (PenV). The gonococcus will not likely be identified on routine culture medium; isolation generally requires culture of a fresh throat swab on a selective medium such as Thayer-Martin (see Chapter 96).

Infectious Mononucleosis. One virus that can produce a more protracted exudative pharyngitis is the Epstein-Barr virus, causative agent of infectious mononucleosis. Adenopathy, splenomegaly, generalized malaise, and rash may accompany this illness. Peripheral blood smear usually reveals numerous atypical lymphocytes. The patient should be advised to abstain from contact sports, as traumatic rupture of the enlarged spleen may be fatal.

Acute Lymphoblastic Leukemia. Persistent exudative tonsillitis may be a presentation of acute lymphoblastic leukemia (ALL). Diagnosis can be suspected by examination of the peripheral blood smear; however, some experience may be required to distinguish between the blasts of ALL and the atypical lymphocytes of infectious mononucleosis.

Other Leukopenic States. Stomatitis/pharyngitis may be the presenting complaint of patients with *aplastic anemia* or with *agranulocytosis.* As some of these cases are drug-induced (e.g., propylthiouracil, phenytoin, etc.), a complete medication history on initial presentation may suggest this possibility. Prompt discontinuation of the offending drug may be life-saving.

Although sore throat is a common complaint of patients with relatively benign illness, rarely it is the presenting complaint of a patient with a serious or life-threatening disease. Any of the key signs or symptoms shown in Table 84–2 should alert the clinician to the possibility of an extraordinary process.

REFERENCES

Evans FO, Sydnar JB, Moore WEC, et al: Sinusitis of the maxillary antrum. N Engl J Med 293:735–739, 1975.

Krause RM: Streptococcal diseases. *In* Wyngaarden JB, Smith LH Jr (eds): Cecil Textbook of Medicine. 18th ed. Philadelphia, WB Saunders Co, 1988, pp 1572–1580.

Mayo Smith MF, Hirsch PJ, Wodzinski SF, Schiffman FJ: Acute epiglottitis in adults: An eight year experience in the State of Rhode Island. N Engl J Med 314:1133, 1986.

88

INFECTIONS OF THE LOWER RESPIRATORY TRACT

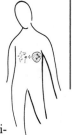

Pneumonia currently accounts for about 10 per cent of admissions to adult medical services in North America and is one of the leading causes of death during the productive years of life. Although pneumonia ranks sixth among the causes of death in the United States today, it is first among the potentially lethal illnesses that are readily reversible by the alert physician. Every physician must therefore be adept at the *rapid* diagnosis and management of the patient with pneumonia. Viruses, chlamydia, rickettsia, mycoplasma, bacteria, protozoans, and parasites can all produce serious infection of the lower respiratory tract. Careful history and physical examination can provide clues to the likely etiology of infection. The clinical spectra of pneumonias caused by different pathogens overlap considerably, however. Microscopic examination of respiratory secretions provides a rapid and essential step in the differential diagnosis of pneumonia.

PATHOGENESIS OF PNEUMONIA

Microbes can enter the lung to produce infection by hematogenous spread, by spread from a contiguous focus of infection, by inhalation of aerosolized particles, or, most commonly, by aspiration of oropharyngeal secretions. In the latter instance, the organisms colonizing the oropharynx will determine the flora of the aspirated secretions and presumably the nature of the resultant pneumonia. Some organisms like *Streptococcus pneumoniae* may transiently colonize the oropharynx in healthy individuals. Others such as gram-negative bacilli are more prevalent in the upper respiratory tract of debilitated and hospitalized patients. Aspiration of normal oropharyngeal flora may lead to necrotizing pneumonia caused by mixtures of oral anaerobic bacteria.

Inoculum size (the number of bacteria aspirated) may be an important factor in the development of pneumonia. Studies using radioisotopes have demonstrated that up to 45 per cent of healthy men aspirate some oropharyngeal contents during sleep. In most instances the bacteria aspirated are relatively avirulent and back-up defenses, including cough and mucociliary clearance, are adequate to prevent the development of pneumonia. Individuals with structural disease of the oropharynx or patients with impaired cough reflexes due to drugs, alcohol, or neuromuscular disease are at particular risk for the development of pneumonia due to aspiration. The specialized ciliated cells of the bronchial mucosa are covered by a layer of mucus that traps foreign particles, which are propelled upward by rhythmic beating of the cilia to a point where a cough can expel the particles. Impaired mucociliary transport as may be seen in persons with chronic obstructive pulmonary disease may predispose to bacterial infection. Denuding of the respiratory epithelium by infection with the influenza virus may be one mechanism whereby influenza predisposes to bacterial pneumonia.

Infection by *Mycobacterium tuberculosis* is usually acquired through inhalation of aerosolized contaminated droplet nuclei. A primary infection is established in the parenchyma of the lungs and in the draining lymph nodes which may result in a progressive primary infection, but in most instances it resolves after producing a mild respiratory illness. The organism remains alive, sequestered within host macrophages,

and contained by host cell-mediated defenses. Reactivation of infection may never occur or may occur without apparent precipitating events or at times when host cell-mediated immune responses are impaired. Examples of these impairments include starvation, intercurrent viral infections, administration of corticosteroids or cytotoxic drugs, and illnesses associated with immunosuppression such as Hodgkin's disease and AIDS.

EPIDEMIOLOGY

Common pathogens of community-acquired and nosocomial pneumonia are shown in Table 88–1. As a general rule, the pneumococcus is an important pathogen in all age groups, and influenza and tuberculosis become more frequent with increasing age. Although *Mycoplasma* occasionally produces pneumonia in the elderly, it is primarily a pathogen of the young. Certain systemic disorders appear to be associated with pneumonias due to particular organisms (Table 88–2). The exposure history may be helpful in suggesting specific causative agents (Table 88–3). Pneumonias associated with bone marrow suppression and malignant disorders are discussed in Chapter 98.

DIAGNOSTIC APPROACH TO THE PATIENT

A critical historical point in the differential diagnosis of pneumonia is the duration of symptoms. Pneumonia due to the pneumococcus, *Mycoplasma*, or virus is usually an acute illness. Symptoms are measured in hours to a few days, although there may occasionally be a longer viral prodrome before bacterial superinfection. In contrast, symptoms of pneumonia lasting 10 days or more are rarely due to the common aerobic pulmonary pathogens and should raise suspicion of mycobacterial, fungal, or anaerobic pneumonia (anaerobes can produce acute or chronic infection) or the presence of an anatomic defect such as an endobronchial mass.

Occupational, exposure, and travel history often provide clues to the etiology of some less common pneumonias (Table 88–3). Although these pneumonias are uncommon, they should be considered in the appropriate setting because, if improperly treated, some may be fatal.

A history of rhinitis or pharyngitis suggests respiratory virus or *Mycoplasma* pneumonia, although infection with the influenza virus may predispose to bacterial pneumonia. Diarrhea has been associated with *Legionella* species pneumonia in some but not all outbreaks. A persistent hacking, nonproductive cough characterizes some *Mycoplasma* infections; symptoms of grippe—malaise and myalgias— are common in influenza and may also be seen with *Mycoplasma* pneumonia. A true rigor is very suggestive of a bacterial (often pneumococcal) pneumonia. Whereas small pleural effusions may be seen in nonbacterial pneumonias, severe pleuritic pain in a patient with pneu-

TABLE 88–1. IMPORTANT PATHOGENS CAUSING PNEUMONIA

Young healthy adult	*Streptococcus pneumoniae*, *Mycoplasma pneumoniae*, virus
Elderly	*Streptococcus pneumoniae*, influenza, *M. tuberculosis*
Debilitated	*Streptococcus pneumoniae*, influenza, oral flora, *M. tuberculosis*, gram-negative bacilli
Hospitalized	Oral flora, *Staphylococcus aureus*, gram-negative bacilli

TABLE 88–2. SPECIFIC DISORDERS AND ASSOCIATED PNEUMONIAS

Seizures	Aspiration (mixed anaerobes)
Alcoholism	Aspiration, *Streptococcus pneumoniae*, gram-negative bacilli
Diabetes mellitus	Gram-negative bacilli, *Mycobacterium tuberculosis*
Hemoglobinopathy	*Streptococcus pneumoniae*, *Mycoplasma pneumoniae*
Chronic lung disease	*Streptococcus pneumoniae*, *Haemophilus influenza*, *Pasteurella multocida*, gram-negative bacilli
Chronic renal failure	*Streptococcus pneumoniae*, *M. tuberculosis*

TABLE 88–3. EXPOSURES ASSOCIATED WITH PNEUMONIA

Cattle, goats, sheep	Q fever, brucellosis
Rabbits	Tularemia
Birds	Psittacosis, histoplasmosis*
Southwestern United States	Coccidioidomycosis
Mississippi and Ohio River valleys	Histoplasmosis, blastomycosis
Southeast Asia	Tuberculosis, melioidosis

*Exposure to bird and bat droppings.

monia is suggestive of bacterial infection. Night sweats are seen in chronic pneumonias and suggest tuberculous or fungal disease.

Most patients with pneumonia have fever and tachycardia. Fever without a concomitant rise in pulse rate may be seen in legionellosis, *Mycoplasma* infections, and other "nonbacterial" pneumonias. Patients with pulmonary tuberculosis often maintain high fevers in relative comfort when compared to patients with acute bacterial pneumonia. Respirations may be shallow in the presence of pleurisy. Tachypnea, cyanosis, and the use of accessory muscles for respiration suggest serious illness. Foul breath suggests anaerobic infection. Mental confusion in a patient with pneumonia should immediately raise the suspicion of meningeal involvement, which occurs most commonly in patients with pneumococcal pneumonia. Any infection may cause confusion in an elderly patient. Nonetheless, patients with pneumonia who are confused must be evaluated by examination of cerebrospinal fluid.

Physical evidence of consolidation—dullness to percussion, bronchial breath sounds, rales, increased fremitus, and whispered pectoriloquy—suggest bacterial pneumonia. Early in the course of pneumonia, however, physical examination may be normal.

RADIOGRAPHIC PATTERNS IN PATIENTS WITH PNEUMONIA

Clinical/radiographic dissociation is seen often in patients with *Mycoplasma pneumoniae* pneumonia. Chest radiographs of patients with *Mycoplasma* infection often suggest a more serious infection than does the appearance of the patient or the physical examination. The converse is true in patients with *Pneumocystis carinii* infection, who may appear quite ill despite normal or nearly normal chest radiographs. This may also be true early in the course of acute bacterial pneumonias, when pleuritic chest pain, cough, purulent sputum, and inspiratory rales may precede specific x-ray findings by many hours. A "negative" x-ray can never "rule out" the possibility of acute bacterial pneumonia when the patient's symptoms and signs point to this diagnosis. A lobar consolidation suggests a bacterial pneumonia; however, patients with chronic lung disease often fail to manifest clinical or radiographic evidence of consolidation during the course of bacterial pneumonia. Interstitial infiltrates suggest a nonbacterial process but may also be seen in early staphylococcal pneumonia. Enlarged hilar lymph nodes suggest a concomitant lung tumor but may also be seen in primary tuberculous, viral, or fungal pneumonias. Large pleural effusions should suggest streptococcal pneumonia or tuberculosis. Pneumatoceles are seen in patients after respirator-mediated barotrauma but occur frequently in the evolution of staphylococcal pneumonia, particularly among children. The presence of cavitation identifies the pneumonia as necrotizing. This virtually excludes viruses and *Mycoplasma* and makes pneumococcal infection unlikely (Table 88–4).

TABLE 88–4. NECROTIZING PNEUMONIAS

COMMON	RARE	? NEVER
Tuberculosis	*Streptococcus pneumoniae*	*Mycoplasma pneumoniae*
Staphylococcus	*Legionella*	
Gram-negative bacilli	*Pneumocystis carinii*	Virus
Anaerobes		
Fungi		

OTHER LABORATORY FINDINGS

In patients with bacterial pneumonia, the white blood cell count is often (but not invariably) elevated. Among patients with pneumococcal infection, WBC counts of 20,000 to 30,000 per μl or more may be seen. A left shift with immature forms is common. Patients with nonbacterial pneumonias tend to have lower WBC counts. Modest elevations of serum bilirubin (conjugated) may be seen in many bacterial infections but are particularly common in patients with pneumococcal pneumonia.

DIAGNOSIS AND MANAGEMENT OF THE PATIENT WITH PNEUMONIA

When the patient presents with abrupt onset of shaking chills, followed by cough, pleuritic chest pain, fever, rusty or yellow sputum, and shortness of breath, and the physical examination reveals tachypnea and even minimal signs of alveolar inflammation (e.g., harsh breath sounds at one lung base), the presumptive diagnosis of bacterial pneumonia should be made, sputum should be examined, and appropriate therapy should be begun regardless of radiographic findings. The radiographic abnormalities may lag for several hours after the clinical onset of pneumonia.

EXAMINATION OF RESPIRATORY SECRETIONS

Examination of respiratory secretions is essential for accurate diagnosis and proper treatment of pneumonia. When history and physical examination suggest pneumonia, a specimen of sputum must be Gram-stained and examined immediately. The adequacy of the specimen can be ascertained by (1) the absence of squamous epithelial cells and (2) the presence of polymorphonuclear leukocytes (10 to 15 per high-power field). The presence of alveolar macrophages and bronchial epithelial cells confirms the lower respiratory tract source of the specimen. A specimen with many (more than five per high-power field) squamous epithelial cells is of no value for either culture or Gram's stain, since it is contaminated with upper respiratory tract secretions.

In some cases, the patient cannot produce an adequate sputum sample. Unless the patient appears quite well and by all clinical criteria has a mild viral or *Mycoplasma* pneumonia, a nasotracheal aspiration should be performed. This is done by placing the patient supine, hyperextending the neck, and passing a well-lubricated red rubber suction catheter from the nose to the posterior pharynx. During inspiration, the tube is then passed swiftly past the glottis into the trachea, suction is applied, and secretions are collected in a Lugen's trap. The vigorous coughing stimulated by this procedure often produces an additional excellent expectorated specimen.

If nasotracheal aspiration still fails to provide a good specimen for analysis, transtracheal aspiration should be considered. The sicker the patient and the greater the likelihood of a penicillin-resistant pathogen, the more important it is to get an adequate sample of sputum for examination and culture. Severe hypoxia or hypercarbia, bleeding diathesis, or inability of the patient to remain motionless during the needle insertion is a contraindication to transtracheal aspiration. With the patient supine and with his/her neck hyperextended, local anesthetic is injected over the cricothyroid membrane. A small gauge blade is used to make a tiny nick in the skin. A 14-gauge needle containing a large-bore plastic catheter is then inserted through the incision and directed toward the coccyx with the bevel of the needle facing upward. The catheter is then threaded down the trachea and the needle is withdrawn. With the catheter in place, a 20-ml syringe is used to aspirate tracheal contents. If this is not successful, 2 ml of sterile saline (without preservatives) is injected through the catheter and aspirated. This specimen should be Gram's stained and cultured aerobically and anaerobically. (Note: Expectorated sputum and sputum obtained through nasotracheal aspiration cannot be cultured anaerobically because of universal contamination with oral flora.)

The Gram's stained specimen should be examined using an oil immersion lens. The presence of a predominant organism, particularly if found within white blood cells, suggests that this is the pathogen. In cases of aspiration of mouth flora, there is a mixture of oral streptococci, gram-positive rods, and gram-negative organisms. In some cases, there may be inflammatory cells and no organisms seen on Gram's stain. This finding suggests a number of possibilities, many of which are nonbacterial pneumonias (Table 88–5). Unless the diagnosis of acute bacterial pneumonia is clear, an acid-fast stain or fluorescent auramine-rhodamine stain of sputum for mycobacteria should be performed. If legionellosis is suspected, immunofluorescence stains for *Legionella* can be performed, although the yield on expectorated sputum is low. The demonstration of elastin fibers in a KOH preparation of sputum establishes a diagnosis of necrotizing pneumonia (see Table 88–4). Importantly, this test can be positive in the absence of radiographic evidence of cavitation. Blood cultures should be obtained and may be positive in approximately 20 to 30 per cent of patients with bacterial pneumonia.

Results of sputum cultures must be interpreted with caution, since pathogens causing pneumonia may fail to grow and sputum isolates may not be the pathogens responsible for infection. Careful screening of sputum specimens using Gram's stain (see above) will increase the accuracy of culture results. A tuberculin skin test and control skin tests such as mumps, *Candida*, and *Trichophyton* should be applied in all cases of pneumonia of uncertain etiology. If the tuberculin is negative but tuberculosis remains a diagnostic possibility, a second strength tuberculin (250 TU) should be placed. In the absence of anergy (no response to control skin tests), a negative 250 TU tuberculin makes reactivation tuberculosis unlikely but does not exclude the diagnosis.

SPECIFIC PATHOGENIC ORGANISMS

Viral Agents. Viral infection is usually limited to the upper respiratory tract, and only a small proportion of infected patients develop pneumonia. In children, viruses are the most common cause of pneumonia, and respiratory syncytial virus is the most frequent organism. In adults, viruses are estimated to account for less than 10 per cent of pneumonias, and

TABLE 88–5. SPUTUM GRAM'S STAIN REVEALING INFLAMMATORY CELLS AND NO ORGANISMS

POSSIBILITIES	CLINICAL SETTING	CONFIRMATION OF DIAGNOSIS	TREATMENT
Prior antibiotic treatment			
Viral pneumonia	Winter months—influenza, may be mild or life-threatening	Serologies, virus culture	Amantadine for influenza
Mycoplasma pneumonia	Hacking, nonproductive cough	Cold agglutinins, serologies	Erythromycin
Legionella	Chronic lung disease—hospital-acquired, summer prevalence	DFA* of sputum, bronchial brush biopsy, or pleural fluid, culture, serologies	Erythromycin
Psittacosis	Exposure to birds, e.g., parrots, turkeys	Serologies	Tetracycline
Q fever	Exposure to cattle, South Africa	Serologies	Tetracycline or chloramphenicol

*Direct immunofluorescence assay

influenza is the most common organism. Patients at increased risk of influenzal pneumonia include the aged, patients with chronic disease of the heart, lung, or kidney, and women in the last trimester of pregnancy. Cytomegalovirus has developed prominence as a cause of pneumonia in immunosuppressed patients, particularly in AIDS and the post-transplantation state, in which it has a mortality rate of about 50 per cent. When varicella occurs in adults, some 10 to 20 per cent develop pneumonia, which commonly leaves a pattern of diffuse punctate calcification on chest radiograph. Measles is occasionally complicated by a typical viral pneumonia. Viral pneumonias typically occur in community epidemics and usually develop one to two days after the onset of "flu-like" symptoms. Major features include a dry cough, dyspnea, generalized discomfort, unremarkable physical examination, and an interstitial pattern on chest radiograph. A presumptive diagnosis may be made on the basis of the clinical presentation and the epidemiologic setting. Viral isolation or serology is required for confirmation but is rarely of clinical value.

Streptococcus pneumoniae. The pneumococcus is still the most common bacterial cause of pneumonia in the community and in hospital. The organism colonizes the oropharynx in up to 25 per cent of healthy adults. An increased predisposition to pneumococcal pneumonia is observed in persons with sickle cell disease, prior splenectomy, chronic lung disease, hematologic malignancy, alcoholism, and renal failure. Clinical features include fever, rigors, chills, cough, respiratory distress, signs of pulmonary consolidation, confusion, and herpes labialis. By the second or third day of illness, the chest radiograph typically shows lobar consolidation with air bronchograms, but a patchy bronchopneumonic pattern may also be found. Abscess or cavitation rarely occurs. Sterile pleural effusions occur in up to 25 per cent of cases and empyema in 1 per cent. Typically, a leukocytosis of 15,000 to 30,000 cells/μl with neutrophilia is found, but leukopenia may be observed with fulminant infection and among alcoholics. Demonstration of gram-positive diplococci on Gram's stain of sputum is helpful in the rapid diagnosis of pneumonia but may fail to demonstrate organisms in some cases of pneumococcal pneumonia. Positive blood cultures are found in 20 to 25 per cent of patients. Penicillin G remains the treatment of choice, although recently resistant forms have emerged, sensitive only to vancomycin.

Staphylococcus aureus. This accounts for 2 to 5 per cent of community-acquired pneumonia, 11 per cent of hospital-acquired pneumonia, and up to 26 per cent of pneumonia following a viral infection. Persistent nasal colonization is observed in 15 to 30 per cent of adults, and 90 per cent of adults display intermittent colonization. Presentation is similar to that of pneumococcal pneumonia, but contrasting features include the development of parenchymal necrosis and abscess formation in up to 25 per cent and empyema in 10 per cent. A hematogenous source of infection, such as septic thrombophlebitis, infective endocarditis, or an infected intravascular device should be sus-

pected in cases of staphylococcal pneumonia, particularly if the chest radiograph reveals multiple or expanding nodular or wedge-shaped infiltrates. If the pneumonia is hematogenous in origin, blood cultures are usually positive and associated skin lesions occur in 40 per cent. Sputum Gram's stain may reveal grape-like clusters of gram-positive cocci. S. aureus is recovered very easily from mixed culture samples so that its absence in a purulent specimen usually excludes it as a cause of the pneumonia. Treatment requires a penicillinase-resistant agent such as nafcillin or vancomycin.

Streptococcus pyogenes. This is now a rare cause of pneumonia, probably accounting for less than 1 per cent of all cases. Carriage rate in the pharynx, about 3 per cent in adults, is less than with the other gram-positive cocci. Presentation is similar to that observed with S. pneumoniae and S. aureus, except that empyema, often massive, is found in 30 to 40 per cent of cases. Gram's stain reveals gram-positive cocci in pairs or chains. Penicillin G is the treatment of choice.

Gram-Negative Bacilli. GNB have emerged as pathogens of major importance with the introduction of potent antibiotics and the proliferation of intensive care units. They are frequently encountered in patients with debilitating diseases such as chronic alcoholism, cystic fibrosis, neutropenia, diabetes mellitus, malignancy, and chronic diseases of the lungs, heart, or kidney. They are ubiquitous throughout the hospital, contaminating equipment and instruments, and are the major source of nosocomial pneumonia.

Specific organisms are associated with certain situations; e.g., *Klebsiella pneumoniae* is particularly common in chronic alcoholics, *Escherichia coli* pneumonia is associated with bacteremias arising from the intestinal or urinary tracts, and *Pseudomonas aeruginosa* is almost universal in cystic fibrosis. Precise etiological diagnosis is confounded by the frequency with which these organisms colonize the upper airways in predisposed patients. Treatment in this situation generally includes the use of a penicillinase-resistant penicillin or a cephalosporin and an aminoglycoside. *Haemophilus influenzae* is a gram-negative coccobacillus often present in the upper respiratory tract, particularly among patients with chronic obstructive pulmonary disease. Its isolation from sputum in these patients is to be expected. Confirmation of its role in the pathogenesis of pneumonia depends on isolating the organism in the blood, pleural fluid, or lung tissue. Nevertheless, many cases of pneumonia due to this organism will not be confirmed using these rigid criteria, and in a patient with pneumonia the demonstration of gram-negative coccobacilli on Gram's stain of sputum should prompt institution of treatment with ampicillin plus a beta-lactamase inhibitor, a second or third-generation cephalosporin, or trimethoprim/sulfamethoxazole, since 20 per cent of these organisms may show resistance due to beta-lactamase production.

Mycoplasma pneumoniae. Not only is this a common cause of pneumonia in young adults, but it also produces a wide range of extrapulmonary features that may be the only findings. Less than 10 per cent of infected patients develop symptoms of lower respiratory tract infection. Respiratory findings resemble those of viral pneumonia. Hacking, nonproductive cough is characteristic. Nonpulmonary features include myalgias, arthralgias, skin lesions (rashes, erythema nodosum and multiforme, Stevens-Johnson syndrome), and neurological complications (meningitis, encephalitis, transverse myelitis, neuropathy). Cold agglutinins can be demonstrated at the bedside by observing red blood cell clumping on the walls of a glass tube containing anticoagulated blood that had been incubated on ice for at least 10 minutes; they are also occasionally positive in other respiratory infections. A specific complement fixation test allows confirmation of the diagnosis. Tetracycline or erythromycin decreases the duration of symptoms and hastens radiographic resolution but does not eradicate the organism from the respiratory tract.

Legionella Species. These are fastidious GNB that were responsible for respiratory infections long before the outbreak of Legionnaires' disease in 1976. They are distributed widely in water, and outbreaks have been related to their presence in cooling towers, condensers, potable water, and even hospital shower heads. Infection may occur sporadically or in outbreaks. Although healthy subjects are affected, there is an increased risk in patients with chronic diseases of the heart, lungs, or kidneys, malignancy, and impairment of cell-mediated immunity. After an incubation period of two to ten days the illness usually gradually begins with a dry cough, respiratory distress, fever, rigors, malaise, weakness, headache, confusion, and gastrointestinal disturbance. The chest radiograph shows alveolar shadowing that may have a lobar or patchy distribution, with or without pleural effusions. The diagnosis is clinically suggested by the combination of a rapidly progressive pneumonia, dry cough, and multiorgan involvement. Gram's stain of sputum shows neutrophils and no organisms.

Diagnosis can be made by four methods. (1) Indirect fluorescent antibody testing of serum is positive in 75 per cent of patients, but up to eight weeks is required for seroconversion. (2) Direct fluorescent antibody testing of respiratory secretions is the most rapid method of establishing the diagnosis and has a specificity of 95 per cent. Sensitivity of this method is greater in specimens obtained from bronchoscopy or transtracheal aspirate than expectorated sputum. (3) Fresh fluids and tissues should be evaluated by the direct fluorescent antibody technique. (4) The organism can be cultured on charcoal yeast extract medium, but up to ten days are required for growth.

Erythromycin is the treatment of choice and appears to result in a fourfold reduction in mortality. Patients usually respond within 12 to 48 hours, and it is very unusual for fever, leukocytosis, and confusion to persist beyond four days of therapy.

Tuberculosis. Approximately 25,000 new cases of tuberculosis occur in the United States each year, with a worldwide incidence of 7 to 10 million. These figures will increase because tuberculosis is the major communicable complication of AIDS. *Mycobacterium tu-*

berculosis is transmitted by the respiratory route from an infected patient with cavitary pulmonary tuberculosis to a susceptible host not previously infected with the organism. Primary infection usually is manifest only by development of a positive tuberculin skin test. Occasionally the patient develops sufficient symptoms of fever and nonproductive cough to visit a physician and a chest radiograph is taken; patchy or lobular infiltrates are noted in the anterior segment of the upper lobes or in the middle or lower lobes, often with associated hilar adenopathy. Pleurisy with effusion is a less common manifestation of primary tuberculosis. Primary infection usually is self-limited, but hematogenous dissemination seeds multiple organs and latent foci are established which become the nidus for delayed reactivation. Overall, 5 to 15 per cent of infected individuals develop disease. Factors associated with progression to clinical disease are age (the periods of greatest biological vulnerability to tuberculosis being infancy, childhood, adolescence, and old age); underlying diseases that depress the cellular immune response (see Chapter 98); diabetes mellitus, gastrectomy, silicosis, and sarcoidosis; and interval since primary infection, with disease progression most likely in the first few years after infection.

Early progression of infection to disease is known as progressive primary tuberculosis and may be manifest as miliary tuberculosis, sometimes with meningitis, or as pulmonary disease of the apical and posterior segments of the upper lobes or lower lobe disease.

Most commonly, tuberculosis represents delayed reactivation. Factors influencing reactivation are not well understood. Symptoms begin insidiously with night sweats or chills and fatigue; fever is noted by less than 50 per cent of patients, and hemoptysis by less than 25 per cent. Physical examination may be unremarkable or may show dullness and rales in the upper lung fields, occasionally with amphoric breath sounds. Chest radiograph may show cavitary disease with infiltrates in the posterior segment of the upper lobes or apical segments of the lower lobes.

Extrapulmonary tuberculosis also reflects reactivation of latent foci and accounts for approximately 15 per cent of cases. Miliary tuberculosis is discussed in Chapter 84, meningeal tuberculosis in Chapter 86, and tuberculosis of bones and joints in Chapter 93.

Because of the growing proportion of elderly individuals in our society and the growing prevalence of HIV infection, "atypical" presentations of tuberculosis are increasingly common. The elderly and patients with diabetes mellitus are more likely to have lower lobe tuberculosis. In HIV-infected patients, extrapulmonary tuberculosis is almost as common as pulmonary involvement, and tuberculin skin tests are likely to be negative. The index of suspicion must be high in these settings.

Before starting antituberculosis drug treatment, two or three sputum samples should be obtained for cultures; bronchoscopy and bronchial washing are indicated only if sputum smears are negative for acid-fast bacilli. It is important to obtain baseline evaluation of liver function for individuals to receive potentially hepatotoxic drugs (isoniazid, rifampin, pyrazinamide);

color vision, visual fields, and acuity when ethambutol will be used; and audiometry for patients who are to receive streptomycin.

The main principle of chemotherapy of tuberculosis is to avoid resistance by treating with at least two drugs to which the organism is likely to be sensitive. Pulmonary tuberculosis assumed to be caused by sensitive organisms should be treated with daily isoniazid (5 mg/kg up to 300 mg) plus rifampin (10 mg/kg up to 600 mg) daily for nine months. Additional or alternative drugs are necessary if the patient has life-threatening disease as assurance against unsuspected drug resistance, or when the likelihood of resistance is deemed high (Asians, Hispanics, individuals acquiring infection in an area with high levels of resistance, or persons exposed to a patient known to harbor drug-resistant bacilli). In such instances, ethambutol (15 to 25 mg/kg), pyrazinamide (15 to 30 mg/kg), or streptomycin (15 mg/kg IM) should be added to the regimen until drug sensitivities are known. At that point the regimen can be tailored to consist of two drugs to which the organism is sensitive. Close monitoring during treatment is mandatory to maximize compliance and minimize side effects.

Contact tracing is critical, as recent infection or additional cases of tuberculosis are likely in some household contacts. Preventive therapy with isoniazid is discussed below.

TREATMENT AND OUTCOME

Bacterial Pneumonia

As soon as the causative organism is identified on Gram's stain, antibiotics must be administered without delay. If the pathogen is readily identified, the antibiotic choices are straightforward (Table 88–6). Patients with *Mycoplasma* and viral pneumonia can generally be treated on an ambulatory basis. An occasional young patient with no underlying disease can also be managed at home, provided that the patient is reliably attended by friends or family and has ready access to a physician or hospital. Otherwise, patients with bacterial pneumonia should be hospitalized.

Supplemental oxygen should be provided if the patient is tachypneic or hypoxemic. Patients at risk for the development of respiratory insufficiency should be monitored in a critical care setting. Patients who are not capable of adequately coughing up respiratory secretions should have frequent clapping and drainage; meticulous attention must be paid to suctioning of oral secretions. Patients with suspected pulmonary tuberculosis should be isolated from other patients.

Patients treated for pneumococcal pneumonia should begin to improve within 48 hours after institution of antibiotics; patients with pneumonia caused by gram-negative bacilli, staphylococci, and oral anaerobes may remain ill for longer periods after initiation of treatment. Several possibilities should be considered among patients who fail to improve or who deteriorate while on treatment:

Endobronchial Obstruction. Physical examination may fail to reveal sounds of consolidation, and radiographs may show evidence of lobar collapse. Bronchoscopy can establish the diagnosis.

Undrained Empyema. Radiographs may not always distinguish between fluid and consolidation; ultrasonography and computerized tomographic scans can identify the fluid and provide direction for its drainage.

Purulent Pericarditis. This should be suspected in a very ill patient with pneumonia involving a lobe adjacent to the pericardium. Chest pain and electrocardiographic evidence of pericarditis are usually absent. Distended neck veins and pericardial friction rubs are present in a minority of cases. Echocardiogram or chest ultrasonography reveals fluid in the pericardium. If purulent pericarditis is suspected, emergency pericardiocentesis can be life-saving (see Chapter 10).

Incorrect Diagnosis or Treatment. In cases in which clinical response is poor, the patient's hospital course and admission sputum stains should be reviewed by a clinician with expertise in diagnosis and treatment of pneumonia. Misinterpretation of sputum Gram's stained preparations—either failure to recognize an important pathogen or a treatment decision based upon examination of an inadequate specimen—are avoidable pitfalls of medical practice.

Approach to the Patient with Pleural Effusion and Fever

The approach to such patients is quite straightforward; the fluid must be examined. If a bacterium other than *Streptococcus pneumoniae* is seen on Gram's

TABLE 88–6. INITIAL ANTIBIOTICS FOR TREATMENT OF PNEUMONIA

PATHOGEN	TREATMENT
Streptococcus pneumoniae	Penicillin G, 1.2 million units/day[1]
Mycoplasma pneumoniae	Erythromycin, 500 mg P.O. q.i.d.
Haemophilus influenzae[2]	Trimethoprim-sulfamethoxazole, 80 mg/400 mg q6h, or cefuroxime, 1g q8h I.V.
Staphylococcus aureus	Nafcillin, 3 gm I.V. q6h
Legionella pneumophila	Erythromycin, 750 mg q6h
Mixed oral flora (anaerobes)	Penicillin, 2–10 million units/day[3]
Gram-negative rods	Aminoglycoside (e.g., gentamicin, 1.7 mg/kg I.V. q8h) plus third-generation cephalosporin, 8–12 gm/day[4]
Tuberculosis	Isoniazid, 300 mg/day, plus rifampin 600 mg/day

[1]Erythromycin, 500 mg q6h for penicillin-allergic patients
[2]Beta-lactamase–producing *H. influenzae* has caused disease in adults. If patient is very ill, avoid ampicillin and use instead trimethoprim-sulfamethoxazole or a third-generation cephalosporin.
[3]Clindamycin, 600 mg q6h, if patient fails to respond to penicillin.
[4]Add beta lactam antibiotic active against *Pseudomonas aeruginosa* (e.g., carbenicillin 30 gm/day) if *Pseudomonas* is a possibility. Antibiotics can be adjusted when sensitivity data are available.

TABLE 88–7. PREVENTION OF PNEUMONIA: CANDIDATES FOR PNEUMOCOCCAL AND INFLUENZA VACCINES

	PNEUMOCOCCAL VACCINE (ONE TIME ONLY)	INFLUENZA VACCINE (YEARLY)
Patients ≥ 65 years	Yes	Yes
Chronic lung or heart disease	Yes	Yes
Sickle cell disease	Yes	Consider
Asplenic patients	Yes	No
Hodgkin's disease	Yes	Consider
Multiple myeloma	Yes	Consider
Cirrhosis	Yes	Consider
Chronic alcoholism	Yes	Consider
Chronic renal failure	Yes	Consider
Cerebrospinal fluid leaks	Yes	No
Residents of chronic care facilities	Consider	Yes
Diabetes mellitus	Yes	Yes

TABLE 88–8. INDICATIONS FOR PROPHYLAXIS WITH INH

Documented new skin test conversion to tuberculin over past two years
Tuberculin-positive contacts of patients with active TB
Tuberculin-negative contacts of patients with active TB[1]
Positive tuberculin skin test of unknown duration
    Patients under 35 years of age
    Patients with radiographic evidence of inactive tuberculosis who have
        never received an adequate course of antituberculous drugs
Consider INH prophylaxis for patients with positive tuberculin skin tests
    and:
    gastrectomy
    diabetes mellitus
    prolonged (> one month) administration of corticosteroids or
        immunosuppressive drugs
    renal transplantation
    silicosis
    infection with human immunodeficiency virus

[1]These individuals should have repeat skin tests three months after INH is begun. If the repeat test is negative, INH may be discontinued.

stain of pleural fluid or grown in culture, chest tube drainage is required. A pleural effusion infected with the pneumococcus can often be treated with simple needle aspiration and antibiotics. Among patients with pneumonia, even fluids that do not reveal organisms on Gram's stain but that have a pH of less than 7.00 and/or a glucose concentration below 40 mg/dl may require chest tube drainage for satisfactory resolution.

Pleurisy caused by *Mycobacterium tuberculosis* is often an acute illness. In most cases, a pneumonia is not present or readily appreciated. Inflammatory cells—polymorphonuclear leukocytes, mononuclear leukocytes, or both—are present in the pleural fluid. Notably absent are mesothelial cells, whose presence in numbers exceeding 0.5 per cent of the total cell count makes a tuberculosis effusion unlikely. Pleural fluid glucose levels are often depressed but may be normal. Mycobacteria are rarely seen on stains of pleural fluid. As many as one third of patients do not have positive tuberculin skin tests. Other possible causes of pleural effusion in this setting include pulmonary infarction (less than half of the cases produce a hemorrhagic exudate), malignancy (most do not have fever), and connective tissue disorders such as SLE and rheumatoid arthritis. If the etiology of the effusion is not apparent, a biopsy of the pleura is required.

PREVENTION

Pneumococcal pneumonia may be preventable by immunizing patients at high risk with polyvalent pneumococcal polysaccharide vaccine. The current polyvalent vaccine is 60 to 80 per cent effective in individuals with normal immune responses. Booster immunizations should not be given because of the possibility of serious reactions. Yearly immunization with influenza vaccine is also recommended for many of these patients; by decreasing the attack rate of influenza, immunization also decreases morbidity and mortality due to secondary bacterial pneumonia (Table 88–7).

Patients without active tuberculosis but with skin test reactivity to tuberculosis are at risk for reactivating their infection. The development of active tuberculosis can be prevented in most instances by treatment for one year with isoniazid, 300 mg/day. Indications for prophylaxis are shown in Table 88–8.

REFERENCES

Johanson WG Jr: Introduction to pneumonia. *In* Wyngaarden JB, Smith LH Jr (eds): Cecil Textbook of Medicine. 18th ed. Philadelphia, WB Saunders Co, 1988, pp 1551–1554.

Karnad A, Alvarez S, Berk SL: Pneumonia caused by gram-negative bacilli. Am J Med 79 (Suppl 1A):61, 1985.

89

INFECTIONS
OF THE HEART AND VESSELS

INFECTIVE ENDOCARDITIS (IE)

Infective endocarditis ranges from an indolent illness with few systemic manifestations, readily responsive to antibiotic therapy, to a fulminant septicemic disease with malignant destruction of the heart valves and life-threatening systemic embolization. The varied features of endocarditis relate in large measure to the different infecting organisms. Viridans streptococci are the prototype of bacteria that originate in the oral flora, infect previously abnormal heart valves, and may cause minimal symptomatology despite progressive valvular damage. *Staphylococcus aureus*, in contrast, can invade previously normal valves and destroy them rapidly.

EPIDEMIOLOGY

The average age of patients with endocarditis has increased in the antibiotic era owing to the greater frequency of underlying degenerative heart disease and nosocomial endocarditis. Rheumatic heart disease remains a predisposing factor in 20 to 30 per cent of patients with IE. About 15 per cent of patients have congenital heart disease (exclusive of mitral valve prolapse). The propensity to develop endocarditis varies with the congenital lesion. For example, infection of a bicuspid aortic valve accounts for one fifth of cases of IE occurring over the age of 60; a secundum atrial septal defect, however, rarely becomes infected. Mitral valve prolapse is the predisposing condition in over one third of cases of endocarditis restricted to the mitral valve. Intravenous drug users have a unique propensity to develop IE of the tricuspid valve, although infection of the mitral or aortic valve also is common.

PATHOGENESIS

Endocarditis ensues when bacteria entering the blood stream from an oral or other source lodge on heart valves that may already bear platelet-fibrin thrombi. The frequency of bacteremia is quite high after dental extraction (18 to 85 per cent) or peridontal surgery (32 to 88 per cent) but also is significant following everyday activities such as tooth brushing (0 to 26 per cent) and chewing candy (17 to 51 per cent). The production of extracellular dextran by some strains of *Streptococcus* is responsible for their adherence to dental enamel and also is a factor in the entrapment of circulating organisms on damaged valves and platelet-fibrin thrombi. The localization of infection is partly determined by the production of turbulent flow. The mitral valve is the most frequent site

of infection. Vegetations usually are found on the valve surface facing the lower pressure chamber (e.g., atrial surface of the mitral valve), a relative haven for deposition of bacteria from the swift blood stream. Occasionally "jet lesions" develop where the regurgitant stream strikes the heart wall or the chorda tendineae. Once infection begins, bacteria proliferate freely within the interstices of the enlarging vegetation; in this relatively avascular site they are protected from serum bactericidal factors and leukocytes.

The infection may cause rupture of the valve tissue itself or of its chordal structures, leading to either gradual or acute valvular regurgitation. Some virulent bacteria (for example, *Staphylococcus aureus*) or fungal vegetations may become large enough to obstruct the valve orifice or create a large embolus. Aneurysms of the sinus of Valsalva may occur and can rupture into the pericardial space. The infection may invade the interventricular septum, causing intramyocardial abscesses or septal rupture that can involve the conduction system of the heart. Peripheral septic emboli may occur with left-sided endocarditis and septic pulmonary emboli with right-sided endocarditis.

CLINICAL FEATURES

Some cases of streptococcal endocarditis become manifest clinically within two weeks of initiating events such as dental extraction. Diagnosis usually is delayed an additional four to five weeks or more, however, because of the paucity of symptoms. If the causative organism is slow-growing and produces an indolent syndrome, symptoms may be extremely protracted (six months or longer) before definitive diagnosis. The symptoms and signs of IE relate to systemic infection, emboli (bland or septic), metastatic infective foci, congestive heart failure, or immune complex–associated lesions. The most common complaints in patients with IE are fever, chills, weakness, shortness of breath, drenching night sweats, loss of appetite, and weight loss. Musculoskeletal symptoms develop in nearly one half of patients and may dominate the presentation. Proximal arthralgias are typical and are frequently accompanied by oligoarticular arthritis of the lower extremities. Fever is present in 90 per cent of patients. Fever is more often absent in elderly or debilitated patients or in the setting of underlying congestive heart failure, renal dysfunction, or previous antibiotic treatment. Heart murmurs are frequent (85 per cent); changing murmurs (5 to 10 per cent) and new cardiac murmurs (5 per cent) are unusual but highly suggestive of the diagnosis of IE. With endocarditis involving the aortic or the mitral valve, congestive heart failure occurs in two thirds of patients

TABLE 89–1. PERIPHERAL MANIFESTATIONS OF INFECTIVE ENDOCARDITIS

PHYSICAL FINDING (frequency)	PATHOGENESIS	MOST COMMON ORGANISMS
Petechiae (20–40%) (red, nonblanching lesions in crops on conjunctivae, buccal mucosa, palate, extremities)	Vasculitis or emboli	*Streptococcus, Staphylococcus*
Splinter hemorrhages (15%) (linear, red-brown streaks most suggestive of IE when proximal in nailbeds)	Vasculitis or emboli	*Staphylococcus, Streptococcus*
Osler's nodes (10–25%) (2–5 mm painful nodules on pads of fingers or toes)	Vasculitis	*Streptococcus*
Janeway lesions (<10%) (macular, red or hemorrhagic, painless patches on palms or soles)	Emboli	*Staphylococcus*
Roth's spots (<5%) (oval, pale retinal lesions surrounded by hemorrhage)	Vasculitis	*Streptococcus*

and may begin precipitously, for example, with perforation of a valve or rupture of chorda tendineae. At least one of the peripheral manifestations of endocarditis occurs in one half of patients (Table 89–1). Splenomegaly (25 to 60 per cent) is more likely when symptoms have been prolonged. Clubbing occurs in 10 to 15 per cent of patients.

The clinical syndrome of IE differs in users of intravenous drugs. Tricuspid valve infection is most common. Patients most often present with fever and chills, but may present with pleuritic chest pain caused by septic pulmonary emboli. Round, cavitating infiltrates may be found on chest radiograph. The infective foci are initially centered in blood vessels; only after they erode into the bronchial system does cough develop, productive of bloody or purulent sputum.

Serious systemic emboli may cause dramatic findings, at times masking the systemic nature of IE. Embolism to the splenic artery may lead to left upper quadrant pain, sometimes radiating to the left shoulder, a friction rub, and/or left pleural effusion. Renal, coronary, and mesenteric arteries are frequent alternative sites of clinically important emboli. CNS embolization is one of the most serious complications of IE, since it may produce irreversible and disabling neurological deficits.

Overall, neurological manifestations occur in one third of patients with IE. In addition to stroke due to vascular occlusion by an embolus, toxic encephalopathy, which may mimic psychosis, and meningoencephalitis also occur. The consequences of embolization depend on the site of lodging and the bacterial pathogen. Organisms such as viridans streptococci initially produce a syndrome entirely attributable to the vascular occlusion; however, damage to the blood vessel can result in formation of a mycotic aneurysm that may leak or burst at a later date. *S. aureus*, in contrast, produces progressive infection extending from the site of embolization; brain abscess and purulent meningitis are common sequelae.

The kidney can be the site of abscess formation, multiple infarcts, or immune complex glomerulonephritis. When renal dysfunction develops during antibiotic therapy, drug toxicity is an additional possibility.

LABORATORY FINDINGS

Nonspecific laboratory abnormalities occur in IE and reflect chronic infection. These include anemia, reticulocytopenia, increased erythrocyte sedimentation rate, hypergammaglobulinemia, and circulating immune complexes and rheumatoid factor. The presence of rheumatoid factor may be a helpful clue to diagnosis in patients with culture-negative endocarditis. Urinalysis frequently shows proteinuria (50 to 60 per cent) and microscopic hematuria (30 to 50 per cent). The presence of red blood cell casts is indicative of immune complex–mediated glomerulonephritis.

The bacteremia of IE is continuous and low-grade (often 1 to 100 bacteria/ml in subacute cases). Three sets of blood cultures should be obtained in the first 24 hours of hospitalization. Two or three additional blood cultures are important if the patient has received antibiotic therapy in the preceding one to two weeks and if initial blood cultures are negative at 48 to 72 hours. In most series, 15 to 20 per cent of patients with the clinical diagnosis of IE have negative blood cultures, usually because of previous antibiotic therapy.

Echocardiography is a useful technique for identifying vegetations in endocarditis. The finding of vegetations is helpful diagnostically and also indicates an increased risk of valvular destruction with congestive heart failure, systemic embolization, and death. Echocardiographic findings may be misleading, however, and the absence of vegetations on echocardiogram does not exclude the diagnosis of IE.

DIFFERENTIAL DIAGNOSIS

The diagnosis of IE usually is firmly established on the basis of the clinical findings and results of blood cultures. In fact, in streptococcal infection, the speciation of the blood culture isolate may provide circumstantial evidence for or against infection of the heart valves (Table 89–2). The identity of the causative organism may be helpful for other bacteria as well; the ratio of IE to non-IE bacteremias is approximately 1:1 for *Staphylococcus aureus*, 1:7 for group B streptococci, and 1:200 for *Escherichia coli*. *Streptococcus*

TABLE 89–2. RELATIVE FREQUENCY OF IE AND NON-IE BACTEREMIAS FOR VARIOUS STREPTOCOCCI*

SPECIES	IE/NON-IE
Streptococcus mutans	14:1
Streptococcus bovis	6:1
Streptococcus faecalis	1:1
Group B streptococci	1:7
Group A streptococci	1:32

* Modified from Parker MT, Ball LC: Streptococci and aerococci associated with systemic infection in man. J Med Microbiol 9:275, 1976.

bovis bacteremia and endocarditis are often (>50 per cent) associated with colonic carcinomas and polyps, so that isolation of this organism warrants thorough evaluation of the lower gastrointestinal tract.

The initial presentation of IE can be misleading: The young adult may present with a stroke, pneumonia, or meningitis, or the elderly patient may present simply with confusion. The index of suspicion of IE, therefore, must be high, and blood cultures should be obtained in these varied settings, particularly if antibiotic usage is contemplated.

Major problems in diagnosis arise if antibiotics have been administered before blood is cultured or if blood cultures are negative. Attempts to culture slow-growing organisms, including those with particular nutritional requirements, should be planned by discussion with a clinical microbiologist. The differential diagnosis of culture-negative endocarditis includes acute rheumatic fever, multiple pulmonary emboli, atrial myxoma, and nonbacterial thrombotic endocarditis (NBTE). NBTE (sometimes called marantic endocarditis) occurs in patients with severe wasting, whether due to malignancy or other conditions. Also, patients with systemic lupus erythematosus may develop sterile valvular vegetations, termed Libman-Sacks lesions, on the undersurfaces of the valve leaflets. These diagnoses should be considered and excluded, if possible, before beginning therapy for presumed culture-negative IE.

MANAGEMENT AND OUTCOME

The outcome of endocarditis is determined by the extent of valvular destruction, the size and friability of vegetations, and the choice of antibiotics. These, in turn, are influenced by the nature of the causative organism and delays in diagnosis. The goal of antibiotics is to halt further valvular damage and to cure the infection. Surgery may be necessary for hemodynamic stabilization, prevention of embolization, or control of drug-resistant infection.

Antibiotics should be selected on the basis of the clinical setting (Table 89–3) and started as soon as blood cultures are obtained if the diagnosis of IE appears highly likely and the course is suggestive of active valvular destruction or systemic embolization. The an-

tibiotics can be adjusted later on the basis of culture and sensitivity data.

Antibiotics

Several general considerations are important in choosing a regimen of antibiotics. A number of different regimens have been advocated for the treatment of IE due to each of the causative organisms. Since few have been subjected to valid comparative trials, the selection of drugs, dosages, and duration is somewhat empirical. Similarly, although sophisticated laboratory tests such as serum bactericidal activity are used to monitor and adjust drug regimens, they have not been standardized or validated adequately.

Most viridans streptococci and nonenterococcal group D streptococci, such as S. bovis, are exquisitely sensitive to penicillin. The penicillin concentration inhibiting growth of such organisms is less than 0.1 μg/ml, and they are killed by similar concentrations of penicillin. A variety of antibiotic regimens has been advocated to treat this form of IE and several appear to be equally effective. Aqueous penicillin G, 12 million units intravenously per day for four weeks, is curative in almost all patients. In the stable patient at low risk of complications, some or most of the antibiotic course can be administered on an outpatient basis.

Treatment of enterococcal endocarditis and IE caused by other penicillin-resistant streptococci is much less satisfactory because of frequent relapses and high mortality. The recommended regimen is aqueous penicillin G, 20 million units IV per day, plus gentamicin or tobramycin, 3 to 5 mg/kg IV per day. The lower dose of aminoglycoside is associated with less nephrotoxicity. Tobramycin is the preferred aminoglycoside because of its slightly lower risk of nephrotoxicity, unless sensitivity testing reveals greater potency of gentamicin. The aminoglycoside dose should be adjusted according to measured serum levels and

TABLE 89–3. SYNDROMES SUGGESTING SPECIFIC BACTERIA CAUSING INFECTIVE ENDOCARDITIS

Indolent Course
  Viridans streptococci
  Streptococcus bovis
  Streptococcus faecalis
  Fastidious gram-negative rods
Aggressive Course
  Staphylococcus aureus
  Streptococcus pneumoniae
  Streptococcus pyogenes
  Neisseria gonorrhoeae
Drug Users
  Staphylococcus aureus
  Pseudomonas aeruginosa
  Streptococcus faecalis
  Candida sp.
  Bacillus sp.
Frequent Major Emboli
  Haemophilus sp.
  Bacteroides sp.
  Candida sp.

the bactericidal activity of serum. Streptomycin, 0.5 gm IM q12h, can be substituted as the aminoglycoside if the organism is sensitive; however, streptomycin is associated with irreversible vestibular and auditory toxicity in some patients.

Although the value of serum bactericidal determinations has not been established rigorously, most experts rely on them as a general guide to the adequacy of antibiotic regimens for enterococcal endocarditis. A drug regimen is considered adequate for treatment of IE if trough serum bactericidal activity is present at dilutions of 1:8 or greater. In view of the high frequency of relapses, regimens to treat enterococcal infection should be continued for four to six weeks. Culture-negative endocarditis should be treated similarly.

Staphylococcus aureus endocarditis should be treated with nafcillin, 12 gm IV/day. Infection with a methicillin-resistant species of *Staphylococcus* necessitates the use of vancomycin. The addition of an aminoglycoside hastens clearance of bacteremia and is indicated in the patient with a fulminant septic presentation and in the initial treatment of left-sided endocarditis. Once sepsis is controlled, the aminoglycoside should be discontinued. Minimal bactericidal concentrations of antibiotic should be determined. If the bactericidal concentration is over 32 times the bacteriostatic concentration, the organism can be considered drug-tolerant. Patients with IE caused by tolerant staphylococci may have a more complicated clinical course. If the organism fulfills the criteria for tolerance, determination of serum bactericidal activity is appropriate; if this proves inadequate (i.e., bactericidal activity <1:8 dilution of serum), addition of a drug (aminoglycoside or rifampin) or substitution of vancomycin for nafcillin should be considered. The duration of antibiotic therapy for staphylococcal endocarditis of the mitral or aortic valve is a minimum of six weeks.

In the patient with streptococcal or staphylococcal IE and history of serious penicillin allergy, vancomycin can be substituted for penicillin. Outcome generally is comparable, although auditory or renal toxicity may occur with vancomycin.

Pseudomonas endocarditis is a particular problem in intravenous drug users. Therapy should be initiated with tobramycin, 8 mg/kg/day IV, and ticarcillin, 250 mg/kg/day IV. The unusually high doses of aminoglycosides have improved the outcome of medical therapy of *Pseudomonas* infection of the tricuspid valve with surprisingly few side effects such as nephrotoxicity. Left-sided *Pseudomonas aeruginosa* infections, however, generally require surgery for cure. Although third-generation cephalosporins have attractive in vitro efficacy against *Pseudomonas* species, in vivo development of resistance and clinical failure have limited their usefulness in this setting. Some young adults have rapid clearance of aminoglycosides, so it is particularly critical to evaluate pharmacokinetics and adjust dosages as appropriate when these agents are employed.

Fungal endocarditis is refractory to antibiotics and requires surgery for management. Amphotericin B generally is administered to such patients but is not in itself curative.

Surgery

The indications for early surgery in IE need to be individualized and forged by discussions with the cardiac surgeon. Refractory infection is a clear indication for surgery; as noted, the requirement for surgery is predictable in IE caused by certain organisms. Persistence of bacteremia for longer than seven to ten days, despite the administration of appropriate antibiotics, frequently reflects paravalvular extension of infection with development of valve ring abscess or myocardial abscesses. Medical cure is not possible in this setting. A prolonged febrile course is not unusual, however (10 per cent of patients remain febrile for more than two weeks) and is not an independent indication for surgery, particularly when tricuspid endocarditis is complicated by multiple septic pulmonary emboli with necrotizing pneumonia. Delayed defervescence also is common, despite appropriate antimicrobial therapy, with endocarditis due to *Staphylococcus aureus* and enteric bacteria.

Congestive heart failure is the most frequent indication for early cardiac surgery. The extent of valvular dysfunction may be difficult to gauge clinically, particularly in patients with acute aortic regurgitation (AR); in the absence of compensatory ventricular dilatation, classic physical signs associated with AR such as wide pulse pressure may not be present. Echocardiography, fluoroscopy, and cardiac catheterization may be necessary to evaluate the extent of aortic regurgitation in some instances. However, when congestive heart failure develops in the patient with *S. aureus* IE, aortic valvular destruction usually is extensive, necessitating early surgery. Delaying surgery to prolong the course of antibiotic therapy is never appropriate if the patient is hemodynamically unstable. Prosthetic valve endocarditis seldom occurs following cardiac valve replacement for IE, and its incidence is not influenced by duration of preoperative antibiotics.

Recurrent major systemic embolization is another indication for surgery. If valvular function is preserved, vegetations sometimes can be removed without valve replacement. Septal abscess, although often difficult to recognize clinically, and aneurysms of the sinus of valsalva are absolute indications for surgery.

PROSTHETIC VALVE ENDOCARDITIS (PVE)

PVE complicates approximately 3 per cent of cardiac valve replacements. Two separable clinical syndromes have been identified. Early PVE occurs within 60 days of surgery and most often is caused by *S. epidermidis*, gram-negative enteric bacilli, *S. aureus*, or diphtheroids. The prosthesis may be contaminated at the time of surgery or seeded by bacteremia from extracardiac sites (intravenous cannula, indwelling urinary bladder catheter, wound infection, pneumonia).

In addition to forming vegetations, which may be quite bulky and cause obstruction, particularly of mitral valve prostheses, circumferential spread of infection often causes dehiscence and paravalvular leak at the site of an aortic prosthesis. The combination of vancomycin, 2 gm/day IV, and tobramycin, 3 to 5 mg/kg/day IV, plus rifampin, 600 mg/day orally, is indicated to treat *S. epidermidis* infection. Other infections should be treated with synergistic combinations of antibiotics based on in vitro sensitivity testing. Surgery is mandatory in the presence of moderate to severe CHF. The mortality of early PVE is approximately 75 per cent.

Late PVE usually is caused by viridans streptococcal bacteremia from an oral site that seeds a re-endothelialized valve surface. Treatment with aqueous penicillin G, 20 million units IV daily, plus tobramycin, 3 to 5 mg/kg/day IV, is appropriate. Prognosis for cure with antibiotic therapy alone is better in patients infected with penicillin-sensitive streptococci. Moderate to severe CHF is the main indication for surgery. The mortality of late PVE is approximately 40 per cent.

PROPHYLAXIS OF INFECTIVE ENDOCARDITIS

Patients with prosthetic heart valves or mitral or aortic valvular heart disease are at relatively high risk of developing IE. Mitral valve prolapse associated with a systolic murmur is another significant risk factor. Neither the value of antibiotic prophylaxis nor the optimal regimens have been established definitively. Recommended regimens are presented in Table 89–4.

Devices that are associated with high rates of infection and bacteremia (intravenous cannulas, indwelling urinary bladder catheters) should be avoided in hospitalized patients at risk for IE if at all possible; established local infections should be treated promptly and vigorously.

BACTERIAL ENDARTERITIS AND SUPPURATIVE PHLEBITIS

Bacterial endarteritis usually develops by one of three mechanisms: (1) Arteries, particularly those with intimal abnormalities, may become infected as a consequence of transient bacteremia. (2) During the course of IE, septic emboli to vasa vasorum may lead to mycotic aneurysms. (3) Blood vessels also may be infected by direct extension from contiguous foci and trauma.

A septic presentation is characteristic of endarteritis due to organisms such as *S. aureus*. Besides sepsis, the major problem caused by endarteritis is hemorrhage. About 3 to 4 per cent of patients with IE develop intracranial mycotic aneurysms. Mycotic aneurysms in IE typically are situated peripherally and in the distribution of the middle cerebral artery. Focal seizures, focal signs, or aseptic meningitis may herald cata-

TABLE 89–4. PROPHYLAXIS OF INFECTIVE ENDOCARDITIS

INDICATIONS	REGIMEN*
Oral	
Aortic or mitral valve disease in patients undergoing dental procedure with bleeding gums	1. Penicillin V 2.0 gm orally 1 hr before and 1.0 gm 6 hr after procedure
As above for penicillin-allergic patient or when chronic penicillin prophylaxis has been used to prevent rheumatic fever	2. Erythromycin 1.0 gm orally 1 hr before and 0.5 gm orally 6 hr after procedure
Parenteral	
Patient with prosthetic heart valve undergoing dental, gastrointestinal, or genitourinary procedure. Patient with aortic or mitral valve disease undergoing gastrointestinal surgery or genitourinary instrumentation or surgery	1. Ampicillin 2.0 gm IM or IV plus gentamicin 1.5 mg/kg IM or IV 30 min before procedure Repeat parenteral antibodies 8 hours after procedure.
Penicillin-allergic patient with prosthetic heart valve undergoing dental procedure	2. Vancomycin 1.0 gm IV over a 1-hr period beginning 1 hr before procedure
Penicillin-allergic patient with aortic or mitral valve disease undergoing gastrointestinal surgery or genitourinary instrumentation or surgery. Penicillin-allergic patient with prosthetic valve undergoing gastrointestinal or genitourinary procedure	3. Vancomycin 1.0 gm IV plus gentamicin 1.5 mg/kg IV beginning 1 hr before procedure

*These are empiric suggestions. Additional doses of antibiotic may be given if there is risk of prolonged bacteremia.

strophic rupture of such aneurysms. These premonitory findings, therefore, indicate the need for evaluation with arteriography; neurosurgical intervention should be contemplated if accessible lesions are demonstrated. Other forms of bacterial endarteritis also require combined medical and surgical management; antibiotic selection should be based on the results of in vitro sensitivity testing.

Suppurative thrombophlebitis usually is a complication of the use of intravenous plastic cannulas. Burn patients, especially those with lower extremity catheterization, are at particular risk. Typically, intravenous cannulas have been left in place five days or more. Symptoms may be delayed until several days after removal of the catheter and reflect septicemia, septic pulmonary emboli, or metastatic abscess formation. Local findings at the site of infection are present in only one third of burn patients with this complication. Therefore, surgical exploration is imperative when the diagnosis of suppurative phlebitis is first suspected. Involved segments of vein must be excised. Antibiotics should be selected so as to assure coverage of the most common pathogens, *Staphylococcus aureus* (nafcillin, 12 gm/day IV) and Enterobacteriaceae (gentamicin, 5 mg/kg/day IV). When infection of an intravenous cannula is suspected, the catheter should be removed and two-inch segments rolled across a blood agar plate. The growth of more than 15 colonies suggests infection. The infusate also should be cultured.

Suppurative phlebitis is preventable. Steel "scalp vein" needles are associated with 40-fold less risk of infection than plastic cannulas and should be used preferentially for intravenous therapy. When plastic peripheral intravenous cannulas are necessary, they should be inserted aseptically and replaced at least every 48 hours.

REFERENCES

Durack DT: Infective endocarditis. *In* Wyngaarden JB, Smith LH Jr (eds): Cecil Textbook of Medicine. 18th ed. Philadelphia, WB Saunders Co, 1988, pp 1586–1596.
Reller LB: The serum bactericidal test. Rev Infect Dis 8:803, 1986.

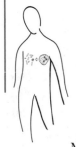

90

SKIN AND SOFT TISSUE INFECTIONS

Normal skin is remarkably resistant to infection. Most common infections of the skin are initiated by breaks in the epithelium. Hematogenous seeding of the skin by pathogens is less frequent.

Some superficial infections, such as folliculitis and furuncles, may be treated with local measures. Other superficial infections (e.g., impetigo and cellulitis) require systemic antibiotics. Deeper soft-tissue infections such as fasciitis and myonecrosis require surgical debridement. As a general rule, infections of the face and hand should be treated particularly aggressively because of the risks of intracranial spread in the former, and the potential loss of function due to closed-space infection in the latter.

SUPERFICIAL INFECTIONS OF THE SKIN

CIRCUMSCRIBED INFECTIONS OF THE SKIN

Vesicles, pustules, nodules, and ulcerations are the lesions in this category (Table 90–1).

Folliculitis is a superficial infection of hair follicles. The lesions are crops of red papules or pustules; careful examination using a hand lens reveals hair in the center of most papules. Staphylococci, yeast, and, occasionally, *Pseudomonas* species are the responsible pathogens. Local treatment with cleansing and hot compresses is usually sufficient. The skin lesions of disseminated candidiasis seen in neutropenic patients may resemble folliculitis. In this setting, skin biopsy readily distinguishes these two processes; in disseminated disease, yeast are found within blood vessels and not simply surrounding the hair follicle.

Furuncles and carbuncles are subcutaneous abscesses due to *Staphylococcus aureus*. The lesions are red, tender nodules that may have a surrounding cellulitis and occur most prominently on the face and back of the neck. They often drain spontaneously. Furuncles may be treated with local compresses. The larger carbuncles require incision and drainage if fluctuant. Antistaphylococcal antibiotics should be given if the patient has systemic symptoms such as fever or malaise, if there is accompanying cellulitis, or if the lesions are on the face.

Impetigo is a superficial infection of the skin due to group A streptococci, although occasionally *Staphy-*

TABLE 90–1. CIRCUMSCRIBED CUTANEOUS INFECTIONS

DESCRIPTION	PREDOMINANT ORGANISM
Folliculitis	*Staphylococcus aureus*
Furuncles, carbuncles	*Staphylococcus aureus*
Impetigo	Group A streptococci
Ecthyma gangrenosum	Gram-negative bacilli (systemic infection)

VESICULAR OR VESICULO-PUSTULAR LESIONS OF THE SKIN

Impetigo
Folliculitis
Herpes simplex virus infection
Varicella-zoster virus infection
Rickettsialpox

ULCERATIVE LESIONS OF THE SKIN

Pressure sores
Stasis ulcerations
Diabetic ulcerations
Mycobacterial infection
Fungal infection
Ecthyma gangrenosum

lococcus aureus may also be found in the lesions. The disease is seen primarily among children who initially develop a vesicle on the skin surface; this rapidly becomes pustular and breaks down, leaving the characteristic dry golden crust. This infection is highly contagious—usually spread by the child's hands to other sites on the child's body or to other children. Gram's stain reveals gram-positive cocci in chains (streptococci); occasionally, clusters of staphylococci are also seen. Certain strains of streptococci causing impetigo have been associated with the later development of post-streptococcal acute glomerulonephritis. The differential diagnosis of impetigo includes herpes simplex infection and varicella. These viral lesions may become pustular; Gram's stain of an unruptured viral vesicle or pustule should not, however, contain bacteria. Tzanck prep (see Chapter 82) can establish the diagnosis of herpes simplex or varicella if the differential diagnosis is uncertain. Penicillin is the treatment of choice for impetigo, since staphylococci represent secondary infection and will disappear when the streptococci are eradicated. Antibiotics do not appear to affect the development of post-streptococcal glomerulonephritis but will prevent the spread of infection to others.

Ecthyma gangrenosum (see Fig. 85–2) is a cutaneous manifestation of disseminated gram-negative rod infection, usually due to *Pseudomonas aeruginosa* in neutropenic patients. The initial lesion is a vesicle or papule with an erythematous halo. Although generally small (<2 cm), the initial lesion may exceed 20 cm in diameter. In a short time the vesicle ulcerates, leaving a necrotic ulcer with surrounding erythema or a violaceous rim. Gram's stain of an aspirate may reveal gram-negative rods; cultures of the aspirate are generally positive. Biopsy of the lesion shows venous thrombosis, often with bacteria demonstrable within the blood vessels. Since these lesions are manifestations of gram-negative rod bacteremia, treatment should be instituted immediately with an aminoglycoside plus a third-generation cephalosporin with good activity against *Pseudomonas aeruginosa* (e.g., ceftazidime) until the results of culture and sensitivity studies are known. (See also Chapter 85.)

Herpes Simplex Virus. Oral infections due to this virus are discussed in Chapter 87, and genital infection in Chapter 96. On occasion, infection with this virus occurs on extraoral or extragenital sites, usually on the hands. This is most often the case in health care workers, but also may result from sexual contact or from autoinoculation. The virus may produce a painful erythema, usually at the junction of the nail bed and skin (whitlow). This progresses to a vesiculopustular lesion. At both stages of infection, herpetic whitlow can resemble a bacterial infection—paronychia. When more than one digit is involved, herpes is much more likely. It is important to distinguish between herpetic and bacterial infections, since incision and drainage of a herpetic whitlow is contraindicated. Puncture of the purulent center of a paronychia and Gram's stain of the exudate allow prompt and accurate diagnosis. In the case of herpetic whitlow, bacteria are not present unless the lesion has already drained and become superinfected. In the case of a bacterial paronychia, bacteria are readily seen. Recurrences of herpetic whitlow may be seen but are generally less severe than the primary infection. Treatment with oral acyclovir may shorten the duration of symptoms.

Varicella-zoster Virus (see also Chapter 84). Primary infection with varicella-zoster virus (chickenpox) is thought to occur via the respiratory route but may also occur through contact with infected skin lesions. Viremia results in crops of papules that progress to vesicles, then pustules followed by crusting. The lesions are most prominent on the trunk. This is almost always a disease of childhood. Systemic symptoms may precede development of the characteristic rash by one or two days but are mild except in the case of an immunocompromised patient or primary infection in the adult. In the immunocompromised, chickenpox can produce a fatal systemic illness. In otherwise healthy adults, chickenpox can be a serious illness with life-threatening pneumonia. Clinical diagnosis is based on the characteristic appearance of the rash. Impetigo and folliculitis are readily distinguished clinically or by Gram's stain of the pustule contents. Disseminated herpes simplex virus infection is seen only in the immunocompromised host or in patients with eczema. Only viral culture will distinguish herpes simplex from herpes zoster in these settings. Most patients with rickettsialpox, which is confused with chickenpox rarely, also have an ulcer or eschar that precedes the generalized rash by three to seven days and represents the bite of the infected mouse mite, which transmits the disease.

Immunocompromised children exposed to varicella should receive prophylaxis with zoster immune globulin. Immunocompromised patients with varicella should be treated with acyclovir.

After primary infection, the varicella-zoster virus persists in a latent state within sensory neurons of the dorsal root ganglia. The infection may reactivate, producing the syndrome of zoster (shingles). Pain in the distribution of the affected nerve root precedes the rash by a few days. Depending upon the dermatome, the pain may mimic pleurisy, myocardial infarction, or gallbladder disease. A clue to the presence of early zoster infection is the presence of dysesthesia—an unpleasant sensation when the involved dermatome is gently stroked by the examiner's hand. The appearance of papules and vesicles in a dermatomal distribution confirms the diagnosis. Herpes zoster infections of certain dermatomes merit special attention. The Ramsay Hunt syndrome can be caused by infection involving the geniculate ganglia and presents with painful eruption of the ear canal and tympanic membrane, often associated with an ipsilateral seventh cranial nerve (facial nerve) palsy. Infection involving the second branch of the fifth cranial nerve (trigeminal nerve) often produces lesions of the cornea. This infection should be treated promptly with systemic acyclovir to prevent loss of visual acuity. A clue to possible ophthalmic involvement is the presence of vesicles on the tip of the nose. (See also Chapter 116).

In most instances, dermatomal zoster is a disease of the otherwise healthy adult. However, immunocompromised patients are at greater risk for reactivation of this virus. Patients with zoster should receive a careful history and physical evaluation; in the absence of specific suggestive findings, these patients do not require an exhaustive evaluation for a malignancy or immune deficiency.

Cutaneous Mycobacterial and Fungal Diseases. Mycobacteria and fungi can produce cutaneous infection, manifesting generally as papules, nodules, ulcers, crusting lesions, or lesions with a combination of these features. *Mycobacterium marinum*, for example, can produce inflammatory nodules that ascend via lymphatic channels of the arm among individuals who keep or are exposed to fish; similar lesions due to *Sporothrix schenckii* may be seen among gardeners. *Blastomyces dermatitidis* and *Coccidioides immitis* are other fungi that produce skin nodules or ulcerations.

As a general rule, a chronic inflammatory nodule, crusted lesion, or nonhealing ulceration that is not readily attributable to pressure, vascular insufficiency, or venous stasis should be biopsied. Mycobacteria and fungi should be carefully sought, using acid-fast and silver stains and appropriate cultures.

Ulcerative Lesions of the Skin. A common factor in the pathogenesis of many skin ulcers is the presence of vascular insufficiency. Microbial infection of these lesions is secondary but often extends into soft tissue and bone.

Pressure sores occur at weight-bearing sites among individuals incapable of moving. Patients with strokes, quadriplegia, or paraplegia or patients in coma who remain supine rapidly develop skin necrosis at the sacrum, spine, and heels, since pressures at these weight-bearing sites can exceed local perfusion pressure. Patients kept immobile on their sides will ulcerate over the greater trochanter of the femur. As the skin sloughs, bacteria colonize the necrotic tissues; abetted by further pressure-induced necrosis, the infection extends to deeper structures. Infected pressure sores are common causes of fever and occasional

causes of bacteremia in debilitated patients. Not infrequently, a necrotic membrane hides a deep infection. The physician should probe the extent of a pressure sore using a sterile glove; potential sites of deeper infection should be probed with a sterile needle. Necrotic material must be debrided and the ulceration may be treated with topical antiseptics and relief of pressure. Systemic antibiotics are indicated when bacteremia, osteomyelitis, or significant cellulitis is present. Anaerobes and gram-negative rods are the most frequent isolates. Skin grafting can be used to repair extensive ulceration in patients who can eventually be mobilized. Prevention of pressure sores by frequent turning and by inspection of pressure sites among immobilized patients is far more effective than treatment. The use of specialized beds that distribute pressure more evenly may be of particular value among these patients.

Stasis Ulceration. Patients with lower extremity edema are at risk for skin breakdown and formation of stasis ulcers. These may become secondarily infected; but unless cellulitis is present, systemic antibiotics are not necessary and treatment is aimed at reducing the edema.

Diabetic Ulcers. Patients with diabetes mellitus often develop foot ulcers. Peripheral neuropathy may result in distribution of stress to sites on the foot not suited to weight-bearing and may also result in failure to sense foreign objects stepped on or caught within the shoe. The resulting ulceration heals poorly. This may be related to vascular disease, poor metabolic control, or both. Secondary infection with anaerobes and gram-negative bacilli progresses rapidly to involve bone and soft tissue. Prevention of these events requires meticulous foot care, avoidance of walking barefoot, the use of properly fitting shoes, and checking the inside of the shoe before use. Once an ulcer develops, the physician should evaluate the patient promptly. Bed rest and topical antiseptics are always indicated. Systemic antibiotics active against anaerobes and gram-negative bacilli should be employed for all but the most superficial and clean wounds. In most instances, this requires admission to the hospital. Aggressive management is indicated, since, if left untreated or improperly treated, the proximate bones and soft tissues of the entire foot may become involved. Once this occurs, eradication of infection without amputation may be difficult.

More Diffuse Lesions of Skin (Table 90–2)

Erysipelas. Erysipelas is an infection of the superficial layers of the skin; it is almost always caused by group A streptococci. This infection, seen primarily among children and the elderly, most commonly occurs on the face. Erysipelas is a bright red to violaceous raised lesion with sharply demarcated edges. This sharp demarcation distinguishes erysipelas from the deeper tissue infection—cellulitis—the margins of which are not raised and merge more smoothly with uninvolved areas of skin. Fever is generally present, and bacteremia is uncommon; rarely, the pathogen can be isolated by aspiration of the leading edge of the

TABLE 90–2. DIFFUSE CUTANEOUS AND SUBCUTANEOUS BACTERIAL INFECTIONS

DESCRIPTION	PREDOMINANT ORGANISMS
Erysipelas	Group A streptococci
Cellulitis	Group A streptococci, *Staphylococcus aureus*, *Haemophilus influenzae*, *Clostridium perfringens*, other anaerobic organisms, gram-negative bacilli
Fasciitis	Group A streptococci, *Clostridium perfringens*, other anaerobic organisms, Enterobacteriaceae
Myonecrosis	*Clostridium perfringens*, other anaerobic organisms

erythema (clysis culture). Penicillin, 2 to 6 million units/day, is curative, but defervescence is gradual.

Cellulitis. Cellulitis is an infection of the deeper layers of the skin. Cellulitis has a particular predilection for the lower extremities, where venous stasis predisposes to infection. Cellulitis predisposes to recurrent infection, perhaps by impairing lymphatic drainage. A breakdown in normal skin barriers almost always precedes this infection. Lacerations, small abscesses, or even tiny fissures between the toes due to minor fungal infection antedate the onset of pain, swelling, and fever. Although shaking chills often occur, bacteremia is infrequently documented. Linear streaks of erythema and tenderness indicate lymphatic spread. Regional lymph node enlargement and tenderness are common. Patches of erythema and tenderness may occur a few centimeters proximal to the near edge of infection; this is probably due to spread through subcutaneous lymphatics. Cellulitis of the calf is often difficult to distinguish from thrombophlebitis. Rupture of a Baker's cyst or inflammatory arthritis may also mimic cellulitis. Pain within the joint on passive motion suggests arthritis, but after Baker's cyst rupture, examination of the joint may be relatively benign. Lymph node enlargement and lymphatic streaking virtually confirm the diagnosis of cellulitis. Most cases of lower extremity cellulitis are due to group A beta-hemolytic streptococci, but on occasion, *Staphylococcus aureus* is responsible. Gram-negative bacilli often cause cellulitis in neutropenic and other immunosuppressed patients. Cellulitis of the face or upper extremities, particularly among children, may be due to *Haemophilus influenzae.* Among patients with diabetes mellitus, streptococci and staphylococci are the predominant pathogens of cellulitis. However, if the cellulitis is associated with an infected ulceration of the skin, there is a good chance that anaerobic bacteria and gram-negative rods are also involved.

As in the case of erysipelas, cultures of blood and clysis cultures of the leading edge of infection rarely yield the pathogen. Almost all patients with cellulitis should be hospitalized and treated with a semisynthetic penicillin active against staphylococci and streptococci, such as nafcillin 6 to 12 gm/day. If *Haemophilus* is suspected, trimethoprim-sulfamethoxazole, a third-generation cephalosporin, or chloramphenicol is an effective agent. Diabetics with foot ulcers complicated by cellulitis should be treated with agents active against anaerobes (e.g., clindamycin) plus agents active against enteric gram-negative rods (e.g., an aminoglycoside). Radiologic studies should be performed on patients with ulcers to determine if osteomyelitis is present (see Chapter 93). Prevention of cellulitis can be achieved by institution of measures aimed at reducing venous stasis and edema. Patients with recurrent cellulitis may benefit from eradication of fungal infection of toes or interdigital regions if present. Repeated attacks of cellulitis may be prevented by monthly one-week courses of an oral antibiotic such as erythromycin.

Soft Tissue Gas. Crepitus on palpation of the skin indicates the presence of gas in the soft tissues.

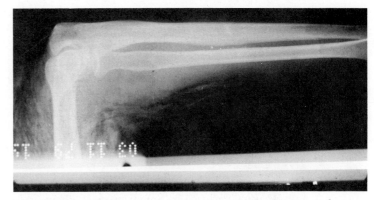

FIGURE 90–1. Radiograph in a case of clostridial myonecrosis showing gas within tissues. (Courtesy of Dr. J. W. Tomford.)

Although this often reflects anaerobic bacterial metabolism, subcutaneous gas can also be found after respirator-induced barotrauma or after application of hydrogen peroxide to open wounds.

In the setting of soft tissue infection, crepitus suggests the presence of gas-forming anaerobes. Roentgenograms will occasionally demonstrate gas before crepitus is appreciated (Fig. 90–1). The presence of gas requires emergent surgical incision to determine the extent of necrosis and requirements for debridement. Involvement of the muscle establishes the diagnosis of myonecrosis (see below) and mandates extensive debridement. Despite the often extensive crepitus seen in clostridial cellulitis, exploration reveals the muscles to be uninvolved, and proper treatment is limited to debridement of necrotic tissue, open drainage, and antibiotics, usually penicillin G, 10 to 20 million units/day, and chloramphenicol, 4 gm/day. Thus the principles of treatment for anaerobic soft tissue infections are (1) removal of necrotic tissue, (2) drainage, and (3) appropriate antibiotics. These apply to superficial anaerobic infections (clostridial cellulitis), deeper anaerobic infections (anaerobic fasciitis—see below), and deepest infections (anaerobic myonecrosis—see below).

DEEPER INFECTIONS OF THE SKIN AND SOFT TISSUE

Fasciitis is a deep infection of the subcutaneous tissues that generally occurs following trauma, sometimes minor, or surgery. Most cases are caused by beta-hemolytic streptococci with or without staphylococci; some are due to mixtures of anaerobic organisms and gram-negative bacilli. Because fasciitis involves subcutaneous tissues, the skin may appear normal or may have a red or dusky hue. The clue to this diagnosis is the presence of subcutaneous swelling. In some instances, crepitus is present. The patient appears more toxic than one would expect from judging only the superficial appearance of the skin. Radiographs may reveal gas within tissues: its absence does not exclude the diagnosis. Men with diabetes mellitus, urethral trauma, or obstruction may develop an aggressive fasciitis of the perineum called Fournier's gangrene. Perineal pain and swelling may antedate the characteristic discoloration of the scrotum and perineum. Prompt debridement of all necrotic tissue is critical to cure of these infections. Once the diagnosis is suspected, the patient must be taken to the operating room, where incision and exploration will determine if fasciitis is present. Gram's stain of necrotic material will guide antibiotic choice.

INFECTIONS OF MUSCLE

Pyomyositis. Pyomyositis is a deep infection of muscle usually caused by *Staphylococcus aureus* and occasionally by group A beta-hemolytic streptococci or enteric bacilli. Most cases occur in warm or tropical regions, and most occur among children. Nonpenetrating trauma may antedate the onset of symptoms, suggesting that infection of a minor hematoma during incidental bacteremia may be causative. Patients present with fever and tender swelling of the muscle; the skin is uninvolved or minimally involved. In older patients, myositis may mimic phlebitis. Diagnosis can be readily made, if suspected, by needle aspiration or ultrasonography. Drainage and appropriate antibiotics are usually curative.

Clostridial Myonecrosis (Gas Gangrene). This anaerobic infection generally occurs following a contaminated injury to muscle. Within a day or two of injury, the involved extremity becomes painful and begins to swell. The patient becomes toxic appearing, often delirious. The skin may appear uninvolved at first, but eventually may develop a bronzed-blue discoloration. Crepitus may be present but is not as prominent as in patients with clostridial cellulitis (a more benign lesion). Rarely clostridial myonecrosis occurs spontaneously in the absence of trauma; most of these patients have an underlying malignancy, usually involving the bowel. Regardless of etiology, this illness progresses rapidly, producing extensive necrosis of muscle. Hypotension, hemolytic anemia caused by bacterial lecithinase, and renal failure can complicate this illness. Gram's stain of the thin and watery wound exudate reveals large gram-positive rods and very few inflammatory cells. Emergency surgery with wide debridement is essential if the patient is to survive. Large doses of penicillin (10 to 20 million units/day) may prevent further spread of the bacilli. Chloramphenicol may be used in patients with hypersensitivity to penicillin. Hyperbaric oxygen therapy is of uncertain value.

REFERENCES

Finegold DS: The diagnosis and treatment of gangrenous and crepitant cellulitis. *In* Remington JS, Swartz MN: Current Clinical Topics in Infectious Diseases. Vol 2. New York, McGraw-Hill Book Co, 1981.

Swartz MN: Cellulitis and superficial infections. *In* Mandell GL, Douglas RG, Bennett JE (eds): Principles and Practice of Infectious Diseases. 2nd ed. New York, John Wiley and Sons, 1984.

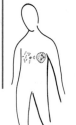

91

HEPATIC ABSCESS

Abscesses of the liver are generally due to infection by bacteria or, less commonly in the United States, by amebae. The diagnosis is often missed, since many patients have only subtle clinical indications of liver disease or none at all.

Pathogenesis

Pyogenic liver abscess is a disease seen predominantly among individuals with other underlying disorders. Structural and neoplastic diseases involving the biliary tract predominate. Obstruction to biliary drainage allows infected bile to produce ascending infection of the liver. Inflammatory diseases of the bowel such as appendicitis and diverticulitis also predispose to hepatic abscess via spread through portal veins. On occasion, penetrating or blunt trauma predisposes to hepatic abscess; tissue injury may allow bacterial infection by seeding during transient episodes of portal bacteremia.

Hepatic abscess complicates fewer than 2 per cent of cases of colitis due to *Entamoeba histolytica*, presumably occurring via portal spread.

Clinical and Laboratory Features

Clinical findings in patients with hepatic abscess are often nonspecific. Most are febrile, but only about half have abdominal pain and tenderness; two thirds have palpable hepatomegaly; less than one in four is jaundiced, although half have elevated serum bilirubin levels. About half of patients with pyogenic liver abscess have positive blood cultures. In patients with liver abscess the alkaline phosphatase is generally elevated and disproportionate to the modest elevation in bilirubin. In contrast, patients with the nonspecific jaundice that occasionally accompanies bacterial infection at other sites generally have elevated bilirubin levels (as much as 5 to 10 mg/dl or more) and only slightly elevated alkaline phosphatase levels.

In liver abscess, chest roentgenogram may reveal an elevated right hemidiaphragm and atelectasis or effusion at the right lung base. The diagnosis is best achieved by contrast-enhanced computerized tomography of the abdomen. Pyogenic abscesses may be single or multiple; multiple abscesses often arise from a biliary source of infection. Amebic abscesses are generally single and are usually located in the right lobe of the liver. Only a minority of patients with amebic liver abscess have concurrent intestinal amebiasis; a positive stool examination for amebae, however, may suggest the diagnosis. Antibody titers against E. histolytica are almost always positive in patients with amebic liver abscess.

Microbiology

Anaerobes, microaerophilic streptococci, and gram-negative bacilli are the predominant agents of pyogenic liver abscess. Occasionally Staphylococcus aureus causes multiple hepatic abscesses during the course of bacteremic seeding of multiple organs. Of the protozoa, only Entamoeba histolytica is known to cause hepatic abscess.

Differential Diagnosis

In patients with bacteremia and abnormal liver function studies, the jaundice of sepsis may be distinguished from the mild jaundice of liver abscess by a relatively high bilirubin/alkaline phosphatase ratio and clinical indications of a primary extrahepatic source of bacteremia. Patients with cholecystitis and cholangitis are at risk, albeit low, for the development of hepatic abscess. In both cholecystitis and cholangitis the onset of illness is more abrupt than in patients with hepatic abscess. Tenderness among patients with cholecystitis is generally quite localized over the gallbladder. Patients with cholangitis are often very ill and jaundiced.

The Fitz-Hugh–Curtis syndrome or gonococcal perihepatitis may share some clinical manifestations of hepatic abscess and should be suspected in the young sexually active woman with fever and right upper quadrant tenderness. Tumors involving the liver may produce fever and a clinical and radiologic picture mimicking hepatic abscess. This is complicated by the occasional concurrence of malignancy with hepatic abscess. Patients with echinococcal cysts may present with a slowly expanding mass in the liver. Fever in the absence of cyst rupture is rare.

Diagnosis and Treatment

If pyogenic abscess is suspected, needle aspiration is indicated. Using ultrasound or CT guidance, a percutaneous catheter can be inserted into the abscess cavity for both diagnostic and therapeutic purposes. The pus should be Gram's stained and cultured aerobically and anaerobically. Unless the Gram's stain indicates otherwise, initial therapy for pyogenic liver abscess should include a drug active against anaerobes (clindamycin or chloramphenicol) plus an aminoglycoside. Antibiotics should be continued for at least four to six weeks. Duration of therapy may be guided by serial CT scans. Surgery is required to relieve biliary tract obstruction and to drain loculated abscesses or abscesses that do not respond to percutaneous drainage and antibiotics. Patients with pyogenic liver abscess should be evaluated for an intra-abdominal source of infection.

If epidemiological features strongly suggest an amebic abscess, metronidazole is the drug of choice. Needle aspiration is necessary only to exclude pyogenic infection or if the abscess is large or close to other viscera into which it may rupture. In the case of amebic abscess, the anchovy paste material obtained by needle drainage is not pus but necrotic liver tissue. Large numbers of white cells suggest pyogenic abscess or bacterial superinfection. Trophozoites of Entamoeba histolytica are infrequently seen on aspiration of abscesses. They are often seen on biopsy of the abscess capsule and may be cultured on certain enriched media.

REFERENCE

Scharschmidt BF: Parasitic, bacterial, fungal, and granulomatous liver disease. In Wyngaarden JB, Smith LH Jr (eds): Cecil Textbook of Medicine. 18th ed. Philadelphia, WB Saunders Co, 1988, p 834.

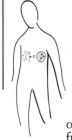

92

ACUTE INFECTIOUS DIARRHEA

Acute diarrheal illnesses caused by bacterial, viral, or protozoal pathogens vary from mild bowel dysfunction to fulminant, life-threatening diseases. Using the best techniques available, a specific causative agent can be identified in 70 to 80 per cent of cases (Table 92–1).

PATHOGENESIS AND PATHOPHYSIOLOGY: GENERAL CONCEPTS

All pathogens that produce acute diarrhea must be ingested. Normally, the low pH of the stomach, the rapid transit time of the small bowel, and antibody produced by cells in the lamina propria of the small bowel are adequate to keep the jejunum and proximal ileum relatively free of microorganisms (although not sterile). Furthermore, the ileocecal valve inhibits proximal migration of the huge numbers of bacteria that reside in the large bowel.

Pathogenic microorganisms are able to pass through the hostile environment of the stomach if (1) they are acid-resistant (e.g., *Shigella*), (2) they are ingested in huge numbers that allow for a few survivors (e.g., *Vibrio cholerae* or *Escherichia coli*), or (3) they are ingested with food and therefore partially protected in the neutralized environment. People with decreased gastric acidity, either natural or surgically induced, are at an increased risk to develop acute diarrheal disease.

Once in the small bowel, the organisms must either colonize (e.g., V. *cholerae*, E. *coli*) and/or invade (e.g., rotavirus, Norwalk agent) the local mucosa, or pass through into the terminal ileum (*Salmonella*) or colon (*Shigella*) to colonize and invade the mucosa in those sites. The active peristalsis of the small bowel is an effective deterrent to the successful colonization of most organisms. The organisms (e.g., V. *cholerae*, E. *coli*) that are able to colonize this area have developed special colonization factors such as fimbria (hairlike projections from the cell wall) or lectins (special proteins that attach to specific carbohydrate-binding sites) that allow them to adhere tightly to the mucosal cell surface.

Organisms that do not have special colonization properties pass into the terminal ileum and colon, where they compete with the established flora. The normal fecal flora produce substances that serve to prevent most newly introduced bacterial species from proliferating. (*Bacteroides*, for example, produces fatty acids; certain other enteric bacteria produce specific colicins). The ability of the colonic enteropathogens to invade intestinal mucosa allows these microorganisms (e.g., *Shigella*) to multiply preferentially.

Diarrheas Caused by Enterotoxigenic Pathogens

In the enterotoxin-induced or secretory diarrheas the patient seldom has fever or other major systemic symptoms, and there is little or no inflammatory response. The diarrhea is watery, often voluminous, with a low protein concentration and an electrolyte content that reflects its source. Rapid loss of this diarrheal fluid results in predictable saline depletion, base-deficit acidosis, and potassium deficiency. The amount and rate of fluid loss determine the severity of the illness. Certain of the secretory diarrheas, such as those caused by V. *cholerae* or E. *coli* enterotoxins, can result in massive intestinal fluid losses, exceeding 1 liter per hour in adults.

Characteristically, large numbers of bacteria (10^5 to 10^8) must be ingested with grossly contaminated food or water (although a small inoculum may produce disease in individuals with achlorhydria). The enterotoxin-producing bacteria then colonize, but do not invade, the small bowel mucosal cells. After multiplying to large numbers (10^8 to 10^9 organisms per milliliter of fluid), the bacteria produce enterotoxins that bind to mucosal cells, causing hypersecretion of isotonic fluid at a rate that overwhelms the reabsorptive capacity of the colon. The V. *cholerae* enterotoxin rapidly binds to monosialogangliosides of the gut mucosa and causes sustained stimulation of cell-bound adenylate cyclase. This results, via both an increased secretion and decreased absorption of electrolytes, in net secretion of large quantities of isotonic fluid into the gut lumen. The disease runs its course in two to seven days, during which time continued fluid and electrolyte repletion are of critical importance. E. *coli* produces two other major bacterial enterotoxins. The labile toxin (LT) of E. *coli* is similar in structure and nearly identical in mode of action to cholera enterotoxin. The E. *coli* heat-stable toxins (ST) are much smaller than LT and

TABLE 92–1. MAJOR ETIOLOGIC AGENTS IN ACUTE DIARRHEAL ILLNESSES

INVASIVE/ DESTRUCTIVE PATHOGENS	NONINVASIVE PATHOGENS	BACTERIAL TOXINS (FOOD POISONING)
Shigella	*Escherichia coli*	*Staphylococcus aureus*
Salmonella	*Vibrio cholerae*	*Clostridium*
Campylobacter jejuni		*perfringens*
Vibrio parahaemolyticus		*Bacillus cereus*
Yersinia enterocolitica		
Clostridium difficile		
Rotavirus		
Other viruses		
Entamoeba histolytica		

act via a different biochemical pathway (stimulation of cellular guanylate cyclase), but also stimulate secretion of isotonic fluid into the gut lumen.

Three conditions provide well-recognized exceptions to the above schema of enterotoxigenic diarrheas. In each of these exceptions, the culpable enterotoxin exerts its effect by some means other than stimulation of one of the known secretory mechanisms of the small bowel mucosa, and the resulting fluid losses are seldom voluminous.

1. Enterotoxins may be ingested directly in food, as with staphylococcal and *Bacillus cereus* food poisoning. These organisms grow to high concentration in the food rather than the small intestine and often cannot be recovered from the stool. Distinctive features of staphylococcal food poisoning include a short incubation period (two to six hours), high attack rates (up to 75 per cent of population at risk), and prominent vomiting (probably due to direct effect of absorbed toxin on the CNS). *Bacillus cereus* produces two distinct enterotoxins, one of which is similar to the *E. coli* LT, and the other to the staphylococcal enterotoxin; therefore two different clinical syndromes may be produced, one indistinguishable from staphylococcal food poisoning, and the other similar to the diarrhea caused by enterotoxigenic *E. coli*. The former syndrome is usually associated with ingestion of contaminated rice.

2. *Clostridium perfringens*, usually contracted by eating contaminated meat or poultry, produces an enterotoxin in the small bowel. Like staphylococcal food poisoning, *C. perfringens* toxicity has a short incubation period, a high attack rate, and generally causes a relatively brief diarrhea (<36 hours) with a small volume of liquid lost. However, unlike staphylococcal enterotoxin, *C. perfringens* enterotoxin damages gut mucosa.

3. *Clostridium difficile*, unlike the previously described organisms, colonizes the large bowel. This organism produces enterotoxins that cause severe mucosal damage, yielding colonic lesions that may be indistinguishable from those caused by *Shigella*. *C.*

difficile diarrhea is usually associated with or follows antibiotic usage. Diagnosis is reliably made by assaying stool for toxins. Inflammatory cells may be present on methylene blue–stained stool samples.

Diarrheas Caused by Invasive Pathogens

Diarrheas caused by mucosal invasion by microorganisms are often accompanied by fever and myalgias. Cramping abdominal pain may be prominent, and small amounts of stool are passed at frequent intervals, often associated with tenesmus. These organisms often induce a marked inflammatory response, so that the stool contains pus cells, large amounts of protein, and often gross blood. Significant dehydration rarely results from this kind of diarrhea, since the diarrheal fluid volume is small relative to that caused by the secretory enterotoxins, seldom exceeding 750 ml per day in adults. Although certain clinical features are statistically more frequent in invasive diarrheas caused by specific enteropathogens (i.e., more severe myalgias with shigellosis, higher temperature spikes with salmonellosis), epidemiologic characteristics are more helpful than signs or symptoms in determining the etiologic agent in invasive diarrheal illnesses (Table 92–2).

Acute shigellosis occurs when susceptible individuals ingest fecally contaminated water or food. Unlike *Salmonella* infections, which require a large inoculum, shigellosis can occur after ingestion of only 10 to 100 microorganisms. Largely for this reason, direct person-to-person transmission (e.g., in day-care centers) is more common with shigellosis than with other bacterial enteric infections. The organism multiplies in the small intestine, during which time a watery noninflammatory diarrhea may occur. Later, the organisms invade the colonic epithelium, causing the characteristic bloody stool. Unlike *Salmonella*, *Shigella* rarely causes bacteremia. The disease usually resolves spontaneously after three to six days, but the clinical course can be shortened by antimicrobials (Table 92–2).

Acute salmonellosis usually results from ingestion

TABLE 92–2. EPIDEMIOLOGIC CHARACTERISTICS OF COMMON INVASIVE ENTERIC PATHOGENS

MICROORGANISMS	EPIDEMIOLOGIC FEATURES	ANTIBIOTICS
Shigella	Outbreaks in child-care centers or custodial institutions. Person-to-person transmission	Yes
Salmonella	Zoonosis. Survives dessication in processed dairy, poultry, and meat products	No
Campylobacter jejuni	Zoonosis. Worldwide distribution. Transmitted in dairy products	Maybe
Yersinia enterocolitica	Zoonosis. Occasionally transmitted in dairy products	Maybe
Vibrio parahaemolyticus	Coastal salt waters. Transmitted by inadequately cooked shrimp and shellfish	No
Clostridium difficile	Almost always follows antimicrobial therapy	Yes
Rotavirus	Outbreaks among children. Worldwide distribution. Unusual and mild in adults	No
Norwalk virus	Microepidemic pattern. No specific age predilection	No
Entamoeba histolytica	Person-to-person transmission. Very rare in United States, Canada, and Western Europe	Yes

of contaminated meat, dairy, or poultry products. In the industrialized world, *Salmonella* is often transmitted via commercially prepared dried, processed foodstuffs. Unlike *Shigella*, *Salmonella* is remarkably resistant to dessication. The nontyphoidal salmonellae invade primarily the distal ileum. The organism characteristically causes a short-lived (two to three days) illness characterized by fever, nausea, vomiting, and diarrhea. (This is in marked contrast to the three- to four-week febrile illness, usually not associated with diarrhea, that is caused by *Salmonella typhi*.)

Campylobacter jejuni may be responsible for up to 10 per cent of acute diarrheal illnesses worldwide. This organism may invade both the small intestine, most commonly the terminal ileum, and the colon, which may account for the broad spectrum of symptoms, ranging from an acute shigella-type syndrome to a milder, but more protracted, diarrheal illness. Since the organism is enzootic in domestic animals, epidemiologic features are helpful only in occasional point-source outbreaks.

In addition to *Shigella*, *Salmonella*, and *Campylobacter*, three other organisms—*Yersinia enterocolitica*, *Vibrio parahaemolyticus*, and *enteroinvasive E. coli* (EIEC—distinct from the enterotoxigenic *E. coli*)—also cause tissue invasion and acute diarrheal illnesses that may be clinically indistinguishable from those caused by the more commonly recognized invasive bacterial enteropathogens (Table 92–2). Another distinct *E. coli* strain, enterohemorrhagic *E. coli*, produces bloody diarrhea without evidence of mucosal inflammation (i.e., grossly bloody stool with few or no leukocytes).

Viruses must grow in host cells; by definition, therefore, both the rotavirus and the Norwalk agent produce invasive diarrheal disease. Both these organisms damage the villous epithelial cells, with the degree of injury ranging from modest distortion of epithelial cells to sloughing of villi. Presumably both the rotavirus and the Norwalk agent cause diarrhea by interfering with the absorption of normal intestinal secretions. Affected patients may have low-grade fever and mild to moderate cramping abdominal pain. The stool is usually watery and its contents resemble those of a noninvasive process, with few inflammatory cells, probably because of lack of damage to the colon.

While few protozoa cause acute diarrheal illness, *Giardia lamblia* is an important pathogen. In North America, Rocky Mountain water sources are frequent origins of microepidemics. As is the case in shigellosis, ingestion of only a few organisms is required to establish infection. The organisms multiply in the small bowel, attach to and occasionally invade the mucosa, but do not cause gross damage to the mucosal cells. Clinical manifestations span the spectrum from an acute, febrile diarrheal illness to chronic diarrhea with associated malabsorption and weight loss. Diagnosis may be made by identification of the organism in either the stool or duodenal mucus or by small bowel biopsy. *Entamoeba histolytica* may cause intestinal syndromes ranging from mild diarrhea to fulminant amebic colitis with multiple bloody stools, fever, and severe abdominal pain. Although *E. histolytica* has a worldwide distribution, it is an uncommon cause of diarrhea in the United States. Two other protozoa, *Cryptosporidium* and *Isospora belli*, occasionally cause self-limited acute diarrheal illness in normal individuals and may cause voluminous, life-threatening diarrheal disease in patients with AIDS. Stool examination is critical to distinguish between the cysts of *Giardia*, *Entamoeba*, and *Isospora*, which respond to appropriate antimicrobials, and *Cryptosporidium*, for which no treatment is known to be effective.

Although most diarrheagenic pathogens produce either invasive (cytopathic) or enterotoxic (secretory) diarrhea, both processes contribute to the illness in some situations. Certain strains of *Shigella*, nontyphoidal *Salmonella*, *Y. enterocolitica*, and *C. jejuni* both invade and possess the capacity to produce enterotoxins in vitro. Such enterotoxins may play a contributory role in the acute disease process. The invasive capacity of these organisms is, however, of paramount importance in their ability to produce disease.

GENERAL EPIDEMIOLOGIC CONSIDERATIONS

In developing countries, where sanitation is generally inadequate, young children (up to two years of age) contract multiple episodes of diarrhea (often four to eight per year), a process that engenders intestinal immunity to the majority of enteropathogens in their immediate environment. Most of these diarrheal episodes are mild, but some are life-threatening. In these areas, enterotoxigenic *E. coli* and rotavirus together cause the large majority of diarrheal illnesses. *Shigella* infections are far less common during this period.

In the industrialized world, infants and small children have fewer episodes of diarrhea, and the most common etiologic agent is the rotavirus. Most episodes are mild. Enterotoxigenic *E. coli* and *Shigella* infections infrequently occur except in a few defined population groups (e.g., individuals in custodial institutions). On the other hand, throughout the world, clinically significant diarrhea in adults is relatively unusual except in specific defined epidemics or common-source outbreaks due to contaminated food or water. The same etiologic agents are largely responsible for the acute diarrheas of both adults and children. This is made apparent by immunologically inexperienced adults from the developed world who visit developing countries. Such tourists have an extremely high incidence of diarrheal disease (traveler's diarrhea), and the organisms responsible are the same ones as those causing most childhood diarrhea in the country visited.

Gender preference is an important epidemiological consideration in the patient with acute diarrheal disease, as the pathogens most frequently responsible for "gay bowel syndrome" (see Table 96–4) differ from those that most commonly occur in the general population.

DIAGNOSIS

In managing acute diarrheal illnesses, determining the specific etiologic agent is much less important than promptly repleting lost electrolytes. All pathogens that cause serious diarrheal disease produce similar electrolyte losses. The fluid losses represent the chief cause of serious morbidity and mortality. Determination of the specific cause is less important, since antimicrobial therapy has proven value in only a minority of cases (Table 92–2). Discerning the epidemiology of the illness is often more helpful than laboratory techniques in identifying cases in which antimicrobial therapy is likely to be helpful. Figure 92–1 provides a useful schematic approach to diagnosis and management.

The examination of a methylene blue-stained stool preparation for erythrocytes and pus cells may be helpful in distinguishing between acute diarrheal illnesses caused by invasive and noninvasive pathogens. This is easily accomplished by adding one drop of methylene blue dye to one drop of liquid stool or mucus, allowing the preparation to air dry, and examining under the high dry microscope lens. Few, if any, leukocytes or red cells are seen in the stools of patients with diarrhea caused by noninvasive organisms (e.g.,

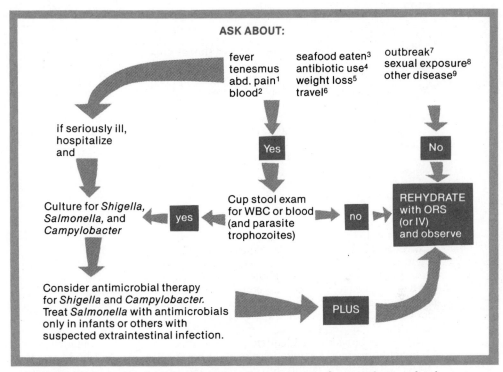

FIGURE 92–1. Approach to the diagnosis and management of acute infectious diarrhea.

1. If unexplained abdominal pain and fever suggest an appendicitis-like syndrome, culture for *Yersinia enterocolitica*.
2. Bloody diarrhea, in the absence of fecal leukocytes, suggests enterohemorrhagic *E. coli* or amebiasis (where leukocytes are destroyed by the parasite).
3. Ingestion of inadequately cooked seafood prompts consideration of *Vibrio* infections or Norwalk-like viruses.
4. Associated antibiotics should be stopped and *C. difficile* considered.
5. Persistence (>10 days) with weight loss prompts consideration of giardiasis or cryptosporidiosis.
6. Travel to tropical areas increases the chance of enterotoxigenic *E. coli* as well as viral, protozoal (*Giardia, Entamoeba, Cryptosporidium*), and, if fecal leukocytes are present, invasive bacterial pathogens.
7. Outbreaks should prompt consideration of *S. aureus, B. cereus, C. perfringens*, ETEC, *Vibrio, Salmonella, Campylobacter*, or *Shigella* infection.
8. Sigmoidoscopy in symptomatic homosexual males should distinguish proctitis in the distal 15 cm (caused by herpesvirus, gonococcal, chlamydial, or syphilitic infection) from colitis (*Campylobacter, Shigella* or *C. difficile* infections).
9. Immunocompromised hosts should have a wide range of viral (e.g., CMV, HSV, rotavirus), bacterial (e.g., *Salmonella, Mycobacterium avium-intracellulare*), and protozoal (e.g., *Cryptosporidium, Entamoeba*, and *Giardia*) agents considered. (Adapted from Guerrant RL, Shields DS, Thorson SM, et al: Evaluation and diagnosis of acute infectious diarrhea. Am J Med 78:91–98, 1985.)

enterotoxigenic *E. coli* and *V. cholerae*). Variable numbers of leukocytes and red cells are present in diarrheas secondary to invasive bacteria (e.g., *Shigella*) or cytopathic toxins (*C. difficile* toxin).

The precise diagnosis of any diarrheal illness lasting longer than four to five days is important, as specific antimicrobial therapy may be helpful, e.g., with giardiasis. Additionally, Crohn's disease or ulcerative colitis may be present.

MANAGEMENT: GENERAL PRINCIPLES OF ELECTROLYTE REPLETION THERAPY

Intravenous Fluids

All acute diarrheal diseases respond to a similar fluid repletion regimen. Voluminous infectious diarrhea in adults consistently produces the same pattern of fecal electrolyte loss. The electrolyte characteristics differ somewhat in diarrhea in young children in that the mean sodium and chloride concentrations are 15 to 20 mEq/L less than in adults. Sodium and chloride concentrations in stool may be even less with diarrheal diseases of viral etiology, in which massive fluid loss seldom occurs.

The fluid losses of massive diarrhea can rapidly be corrected by infusing fluids intravenously that approximate those that have been lost. Lactated Ringer's solution is readily available and provides uniformly good results. With patients who are hypotensive, the intravenous fluids should initially be infused rapidly, at a rate of up to 100 ml/min, until a strong radial pulse is restored. The rate can then be slowed until skin turgor has returned to normal. Subsequent maintenance fluid administration can be guided by the patient's clinical appearance, including his vital signs, the appearance of neck veins, and skin turgor. Clinical evaluation *alone* provides an adequate guide to fluid replacement in most acute diarrheal illnesses. If intravenous fluids are administered in adequate quantities throughout the diarrheal illness, virtually every patient with diarrhea caused by toxigenic bacteria should be restored to health. Complications (e.g., acute renal failure secondary to hypotension) are exceedingly rare if these principles are followed.

Oral Fluids

In most patients with acute diarrheal illness, fluid repletion can also be achieved via the oral route, using isotonic glucose-containing electrolyte solutions. Oral therapy is based upon the fact that glucose facilitates sodium absorption by the small bowel and that glucose-facilitated sodium absorption remains intact during enterotoxigenic diarrheal illnesses. A uniformly effective solution can be prepared by the addition of 20 gm glucose, 3.5 gm sodium chloride, 2.5 gm sodium bicarbonate, and 1.5 gm potassium chloride to a liter of drinking water (Table 92–3). Such fluids should be administered initially in large quantities, 250 ml every 15 minutes in adults, until clinical observations indicate that fluid balance has been restored. Thereafter, one administers fluids in quantities sufficient to maintain normal balance; if stool output is measured, roughly 1.5 liters of glucose-electrolyte solution should be given orally for each liter of stool. The oral fluid regimen does *not* decrease the volume of fluid lost via the intestinal tract, but rather facilitates absorption of adequate fluid to counterbalance the toxin-induced fluid secretion.

Since a similar pattern of fluid loss occurs in diarrheal illnesses caused by other intestinal pathogens, patients with fluid depletion caused by invasive microbial agents (e.g., rotavirus, *Salmonella*) also respond well to oral glucose-electrolyte therapy. Although the pathogenesis of diarrheal disease caused by the rotavirus is quite different from that caused by enterotoxigenic bacteria, patients with rotavirus illness consistently respond well to oral glucose-electrolyte replacement.

Antimicrobial Therapy

Most acute infectious diarrheas do not require antibiotic therapy (Table 92–2). Of the noninvasive bacterial diarrheas, only in cholera do antibiotics dramatically decrease the volume of diarrhea. Oral tetracycline, 40 mg/kg in four divided doses daily for 48 hours, is the drug of choice.

Of the invasive bacterial diarrheas, short-term antimicrobial treatment significantly decreases the duration and severity of shigellosis. In North America, ampicillin, 40 mg/kg in four divided doses daily for 48 hours, is the drug of choice. Because of the increasing frequency of plasmid-mediated antimicrobial resistance, sensitivity testing is necessary to determine the appropriate antibiotic in many other areas of the world.

Antimicrobial therapy *may* be helpful in decreasing the duration and severity of enteritis caused by *Yersinia* and *Campylobacter*. Oral erythromycin appears to be the drug of choice for *Campylobacter jejuni*, and trimethoprim-sulfamethoxazole is the preferred treatment for *Yersinia enterocolitica*. Antimicrobials are of no known value in *V. parahaemolyticus* infections and are contraindicated in uncomplicated nontyphoidal *Salmonella* enteritis, as they may prolong the fecal shedding of salmonella.

Antimicrobial therapy is, paradoxically, indicated for treatment of antibiotic-associated diarrhea (AAC). AAC develops in 1 to 15 per cent of patients who receive broad-spectrum antimicrobials and is caused by cytotoxins produced by *Clostridium difficile*, which

TABLE 92–3. ORAL REHYDRATION FLUID

CONSTITUENTS (gm/L)	ELECTROLYTE CONTENT (mmol/L)
NaCl—3.5 gm	Na—90
NaHCO₃—2.5 gm	Cl—80
KCl—1.5 gm	K—20
Glucose—20 gm	HCO₃—30
	glucose—110

proliferate in the colonic mucosa when the normal flora is disturbed. Although generally characterized by mild diarrhea, AAC may result in a potentially lethal pseudomembranous colitis. In all moderate to severe cases (fever, mucosal ulceration, and/or pseudomembranes), vancomycin (250 mg q6h orally for seven days) should be initiated on the basis of strong clinical suspicion, before the diagnosis is confirmed by stool assay for *C. difficile* toxins.

Antimicrobials decrease the duration and severity of giardiasis. In adults, metronidazole, given 750 mg every eight hours for three days, and quinacrine, 300 mg/day for seven days, appear to be equally effective in adults. Acute intestinal amebiasis demands antimicrobial therapy. Metronidazole, 750 mg every eight hours for five days, is the drug of choice in adults. The duration of diarrhea caused by *Isopora belli* is significantly shortened by administration of trimethaprim/sulfamethoxazole (TMP/SMX) twice daily for five days.

Antimicrobial Prophylaxis

Prophylactic antimicrobials are effective in preventing traveler's diarrhea, a generally self-limited illness caused most often by enterotoxigenic *E. coli*. Doxycycline, TMP/SMX and norflaxacin are also effective. However, because of the rapid response of most patients to early treatment with any of these three agents, the advantages of prophylactic drugs are, in most instances, outweighed by their potential risks (adverse reactions).

Symptomatic Therapy

Adjuvant symptomatic therapy is not essential but may provide modest symptomatic relief in acute infectious diarrheas associated with cramping abdominal pain. Bismuth subsalicylate, 0.6 gm every six hours, may ameliorate symptoms of traveler's diarrhea. Agents that decrease intestinal motility (e.g., codeine, diphenoxylate, loperamide) also relieve the cramping abdominal pain associated with many acute diarrheal illnesses, but are potentially hazardous because they may enhance severity of illness in shigellosis, the prototype of invasive bacterial diarrheas.

REFERENCES

Guerrant RE: Enteric *Escherichia coli* infections. *In* Wyngaarden JB, Smith LH Jr (eds): Cecil Textbook of Medicine. 18th ed. Philadelphia, WB Saunders Co, 1988, pp 1653–1656.

Guerrant RE, Shields DS, Thorson SM, et al: Evaluation and diagnosis of acute infectious diarrhea. Am J Med 78:91–98, 1985.

Pierce N: Cholera. *In* Wyngaarden JB, Smith LH Jr (eds): Cecil Textbook of Medicine. 18th ed. Philadelphia, WB Saunders Co, 1988, pp 1651–1653.

Stevens DP: Giardiasis: Host-pathogen biology. Rev Infect Dis 4:851–856, 1982.

93

INFECTIONS INVOLVING BONES AND JOINTS

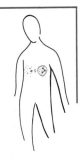

ARTHRITIS

In adults, almost all cases of infectious arthritis occur via hematogenous seeding of the joint. Rarely, intra-articular trauma results in septic arthritis. Bacteria, viruses, mycobacteria, and fungi can all produce an arthritis by infection of the joint. Additionally, certain viruses such as hepatitis B virus can produce a polyarthritis via immune complex deposition. Immune mechanisms may also underlie arthritis syndromes seen in Lyme disease and after diarrhea due to *Salmonella*, *Shigella*, and *Yersinia* infections; the majority of individuals with post-dysentery arthritis syndrome share the HLA B27 antigen (see Chapter 110).

ACUTE ARTHRITIS

Underlying joint disease, particularly rheumatoid arthritis, predisposes to septic arthritis. Many patients with septic arthritis give a history of joint trauma antedating symptoms of infection. Conceivably, disruption of capillaries during an unrecognized and transient bacteremia allows bacteria to spill into hemorrhagic and traumatized synovium or joint fluid, resulting in the initiation of infection.

Microbiology of Acute Infectious Arthritis (Table 93–1)

Staphylococcus aureus is the most common cause of septic arthritis. Patients with underlying joint disease

TABLE 93–1. INFECTIOUS ARTHRITIS—ACUTE

	ETIOLOGIC AGENT	CHARACTERISTICS
Bacterial	Staphylococcus aureus	Most common overall. Usually monoarticular, large joint involvement.
	Neisseria gonorrhoeae	Most common in young, sexually active adults. Commonly polyarticular in onset. Often associated with skin lesions.
	Pseudomonas aeruginosa	Largely restricted to intravenous drug users. Often involves sternoclavicular joint.
Viral	Hepatitis B, rubella, mumps	Usually polyarticular, with minimal joint effusions, normal peripheral WBC count.

and intravenous drug abusers are at particular risk for infection with this organism. *Pseudomonas aeruginosa* is another important cause of septic arthritis among intravenous drug abusers.

Other gram-negative bacilli are infrequent causes of septic arthritis and are seen primarily among elderly debilitated patients with chronic arthritis. In adults under 30, *Neisseria gonorrhoeae* is the most likely pathogen. Isolates causing disseminated gonococcal infection (DGI) with arthritis are generally resistant to killing by normal serum.

Clinical Presentation

Symptoms of septic arthritis are generally present for only a few days before the patient seeks medical attention. Fever is usual; shaking chills may occur. The knee is the most commonly affected joint and is generally painful and swollen. Fluid can be demonstrated in most infected joints, and there is marked limitation of motion. In some cases, however, particularly among patients with underlying rheumatoid arthritis who are receiving corticosteroids, physical findings indicating infection may be subtle. In these individuals, who are at particular risk for septic arthritis, superimposed infection may be difficult to distinguish from a flare-up of underlying disease. Symmetrical symptoms in multiple joints are more indicative of a rheumatoid flare-up. Approximately 10 per cent of cases of septic arthritis, however, involve more than one joint.

Differential Diagnosis of Acute Monoarticular or Oligoarticular Arthritis

Crystal deposition (uric acid—gout, calcium pyrophosphate—pseudogout), rheumatoid arthritis, systemic lupus erythematosus, and degenerative joint disease can also produce an acute monoarticular arthritis. All red, warm, tender joints must be aspirated. The synovial fluid should be cultured anaerobically and aerobically. A Gram's stained preparation should be examined; a wet mount of fluid should be examined using a polarized microscope to look for

crystals. Synovial fluid leukocyte counts and chemistries are of limited value in the differential diagnosis of a suspected septic joint. As a general rule, however, synovial fluid WBC counts in excess of 100,000/μl suggest either infection or crystal-induced disease (see Table 100-4). Blood cultures should be obtained in all cases of suspected septic arthritis.

Treatment of Acute Infectious Arthritis

The two major modalities for treatment of acute septic arthritis are drainage and antibiotics. During the first needle aspiration of a septic joint, one should remove as much fluid as possible. Initial antibiotic choice should be based upon the clinical presentation and results of Gram's stain. Staphylococcal infection can be treated with penicillinase-resistant penicillin or vancomycin. Gonococcal infections respond to high doses of penicillin (10 to 20 million units/day). Arthritis due to gram-negative rods should be treated with an aminoglycoside plus another drug active against gram-negative bacilli, such as a cephalosporin. In IV drug users, the second drug should be active against *Pseudomonas*; therefore, an extended-spectrum penicillin such as carbenicillin, or a third-generation cephalosporin such as ceftazidime, is indicated. Arthritis due to *Staphylococcus aureus* or gram-negative bacilli should be treated with antibiotics for four to six weeks. Otherwise, two to three weeks of antibiotics are sufficient to eradicate infection.

Septic joints (with the notable exception of joints infected with the gonococcus) generally reaccumulate fluid after treatment is initiated. These reaccumulations must be removed by repeated needle aspirations as often as necessary. Indications for open surgical drainage of the joint include failure of the synovial fluid white blood cell count to fall after five days of antibiotic treatment and repeated needle aspirations, and presence of loculated fluid within the joint. Septic arthritis of the hip is generally drained surgically because of the difficulty and potential hazard of repeated needle aspirations of this joint. Early surgical drainage also should be considered for joint infections due to gram-negative rods, and *Staphylococcus aureus*. Osteomyelitis is an uncommon complication of untreated or inadequately treated septic arthritis. In instances in which the diagnosis and treatment have been delayed, radiographs of the involved joint should be obtained at the beginning and termination of treatment.

POLYARTICULAR ARTHRITIS

Arthritis involving multiple joints is infrequently attributable to direct microbial invasion. In many instances, a polyarticular arthritis represents an immunologically mediated process. *Acute rheumatic fever*, a delayed immune-mediated response to group A streptococcal infection, may present with a migratory, asymmetric, arthritis of the knees, ankles, elbows, and wrists. Heart involvement, subcutaneous nodules, or erythema marginatum is present in a minority of cases. Most have serologic evidence of recent streptococcal infection. Antistreptolysin O, anti–DNA-ase, and antihyaluronidase antibodies are usually present. The importance of making this diagnosis lies primarily in the requirement for long-term prophylaxis against streptococcal infection and the clinical response of this process to salicylates.

Viral infections such as *hepatitis B*, *rubella*, and *mumps* may be associated with polyarthritis. These processes are self-limited. Serum sickness, polyarticular gout, sarcoidosis, rheumatoid arthritis, and other connective tissue disorders must be considered in the differential diagnosis. Since 10 per cent of cases of septic arthritis involve more than one joint, all acutely inflamed joints containing fluid should be tapped to exclude bacterial infection.

Disseminated gonococcal infection (see Chapter 96) may present with fever, tenosynovitis, or arthritis involving several joints and a characteristic rash. The rash may be petechial but usually consists of a few to a few dozen pustules on an erythematous base. Cultures of the joint fluid are usually negative at this stage, but blood cultures are often positive; Gram's stain of a pustule may reveal the pathogen. High-dose penicillin is curative.

CHRONIC ARTHRITIS (Table 93–2)

Mycobacteria and fungi may produce an indolent, slowly progressive arthritis, usually involving only one joint or contiguous joints such as those of the wrist and hand. Fever may be low-grade. Cultures of joint fluid may be negative. Some patients with tuberculous arthritis have no evidence of active disease in the lungs. As a general rule, patients with inflammatory chronic monoarticular arthritis should have a synovial biopsy for culture and histology. Granulomas indicate the likelihood of fungal or mycobacterial infection. Cultures should confirm the diagnosis. Serologic studies may be helpful when coccidioidomycosis is suspected, as synovial cultures are often negative.

Fungal arthritis is treated with amphotericin B. Mycobacterial arthritis must be treated for 18 months with at least two drugs active against the isolate. Since some mycobacterial isolates causing joint disease are nontuberculous, extensive susceptibility testing may be needed to guide antimicrobial therapy.

A spirochete is the pathogen responsible for Lyme disease. Several months to two years after the bite of the ixodid tick and the characteristic rash of erythema chronicum migrans, some patients develop an intermittent arthritis involving one or more joints—usually including the knees. This chronic arthritis may result in joint destruction, but fever is unusual. Treatment

TABLE 93–2. INFECTIOUS ARTHRITIS— CHRONIC

Tuberculosis
Nontuberculous mycobacteria
Fungi
Lyme disease (oligoarticular)

TABLE 93–3. FACTORS PREDISPOSING TO HEMATOGENOUS OSTEOMYELITIS

SETTING	LIKELY PATHOGENS
Intravenous drug abuse	*Staphylococcus aureus*
	Pseudomonas aeruginosa
Intravenous catheters	*Staphylococcus aureus*
	Staphylococcus epidermidis

with high doses of penicillin (20 million units/day) for 10 days will halt the progression of disease in the majority of cases (see Chapter 84).

SEPTIC BURSITIS

Septic bursitis is almost always due to *Staphylococcus aureus* and involves either the olecranon or prepatellar bursa. In most instances, there is a history of antecedent infection or irritation of the skin overlying the bursa. On examination, the skin over the bursa is red and often peeling. The bursa has a doughy consistency and may reveal fluid on careful examination. Needle aspiration and antistaphylococcal antibiotics are generally curative.

OSTEOMYELITIS

Infections of the bone occur either as a result of hematogenous spread or via extension of local infection.

Hematogenous Osteomyelitis (Table 93–3)

This infection occurs most commonly in the long bones or vertebral bodies. The peak age distributions are in childhood and old age. Individuals predisposed to hematogenous osteomyelitis include IV drug abusers who are at risk for infections with *Staphylococcus aureus* and *Pseudomonas aeruginosa* and patients with hemoglobinopathy in whom nontyphoidal *Salmonella* often infect infarcted regions of bone. Recently *Staphylococcus epidermidis* has emerged as an important nosocomial pathogen among patients with infected intravenous catheters. Like patients with septic arthritis, patients with hematogenous osteomyelitis often give a history of trauma antedating symptoms of infection, suggesting that transient, unrecognized bacteremia might allow initiation of infection in traumatized tissue.

Patients with acute hematogenous osteomyelitis generally present with acute onset of pain, tenderness, and fever; there may also be soft tissue swelling over the affected bone. In most instances, physical examination distinguishes acute osteomyelitis from septic arthritis, since range of joint motion is preserved in osteomyelitis. In the first two weeks of illness, roentgenograms may be negative or show only soft-tissue swelling; technetium scans or gallium scans are almost always positive, but technetium scans may also be positive in the setting of increased vascularity or increased bone formation of any etiology. After two weeks of infection, radiographs generally show some abnormality, and untreated osteomyelitis may produce areas of periosteal elevation or erosion followed by increased bone formation (sclerosis). The erythrocyte sedimentation rate is generally elevated, as is the white blood cell count.

A patient with back pain and fever must be considered to have a serious infection until proven otherwise. Spasm of the paravertebral muscles is common in patients with vertebral osteomyelitis, but nonspecific. Point tenderness over bone suggests the presence of local infection. A good history should be obtained and a careful neurological examination performed. Abnormalities of bowel or bladder or of strength or sensation in the lower extremities suggest the possibility of spinal cord involvement via spinal epidural abscess with or without osteomyelitis. Acute spinal epidural abscess is a *surgical emergency*. The challenge is to make the diagnosis before neurological signs appear (see Chapter 122). Emergency myelogram will confirm the diagnosis and mandates prompt surgical decompression to avoid disastrous neurological sequelae. Magnetic resonance imaging (MRI) provides excellent definition of epidural or paravertebral abscess and is the diagnostic procedure of choice when available.

Although most cases of hematogenous osteomyelitis have an acute presentation, some cases, particularly those involving the vertebral bodies among IV drug abusers, may have an indolent course. These patients may have an illness of over one year's duration characterized by pain and low-grade fever. Radiograms are abnormal but may reveal only collapse of a vertebral body. This most often occurs in infections due to *Pseudomonas aeruginosa*, but *Candida* species and *Staphylococcus aureus* may also occasionally present in this manner.

Blood cultures are positive in about half of acute cases of osteomyelitis. Patients with acute osteomyelitis should have a needle biopsy and culture of the involved bone unless blood culture results are known beforehand. Antibiotic treatment should be continued for four to six weeks using agents active against the pathogen.

OSTEOMYELITIS SECONDARY TO EXTENSION OF LOCAL INFECTION

There are several major settings in which local infection predisposes to osteomyelitis (Table 93–4). The first is after penetrating trauma or surgery where local infection gains access to traumatized bone. In postsurgical infections, staphylococci and gram-negative bacilli predominate. Generally, there is evidence of wound infection with erythema, swelling, increased postoperative tenderness, and drainage. A traumatic incident often associated with osteomyelitis is a bite—either human or animal. Human bites, if deep enough, may result in osteomyelitis due to anaerobic mouth flora. Cat bites notoriously result in the development of osteomyelitis because thin, sharp, long cat's teeth often penetrate the periosteum. *Pasteurella multocida* is a frequent pathogen in this setting. A four- to six-week course of penicillin G, 10 million units/day, is indicated.

The intimate relationship of the teeth and periodontal tissues to the bones of the maxilla and mandible may predispose to osteomyelitis following local infection. Debridement of necrotic tissue and penicillin comprise the treatment of choice, since penicillin-sensitive anaerobes are the usual agents of these infections.

The third setting in which local infection predisposes to osteomyelitis is that of an infected sore or ulcer. Pressure sores of the sacrum or femoral region may erode into contiguous bone and produce an osteomyelitis (see Chapter 90) due to a mixed flora containing anaerobic organisms. Patients with diabetes mellitus often develop ulcerations of their toes and feet, with eventual development of osteomyelitis. Anaerobes, streptococci, staphylococci, and gram-negative bacilli are often involved in these infections (see Chapter 90). Treatment involves debridement (often amputation in the case of diabetics) and antibiotics active against the pathogens involved.

CHRONIC OSTEOMYELITIS

Untreated or inadequately treated osteomyelitis results in avascular necrosis of bone and the formation of islands of nonvascularized and infected bone called sequestra. Patients with chronic osteomyelitis may tolerate their infection reasonably well, with intermittent episodes of disease activity manifested by increased local pain and the development of drainage of infected material through a sinus tract. Some patients have tolerated chronic osteomyelitis for decades. A normochromic normocytic anemia of chronic disease is common in this setting, and occasionally amyloidosis and rarely osteogenic sarcoma complicate this disorder.

Staphylococcus aureus is responsible for the great majority of cases of chronic osteomyelitis; the major exception is among patients with sickle cell anemia, in which nontyphoidal Salmonellae may cause chronic infection of the long bones.

Cultures of sinus tract drainage do not reliably reflect the pathogens involved in the infection. Diagnosis and cure are best effected by surgical debridement of necrotic material followed by long-term administration of antibiotics active against the organism found in the surgical specimens.

Mycobacteria, especially *Mycobacterium tuberculosis*, can produce a chronic osteomyelitis. The an-

TABLE 93–4. OSTEOMYELITIS SECONDARY TO CONTIGUOUS SPREAD

SETTING	LIKELY MICRO-ORGANISMS
Surgery, trauma	*Staphylococcus aureus*, aerobic gram-negative bacilli
Cat or dog bites	*Pasteurella multocida*
Human bites	Penicillin-sensitive anaerobes
Periodontal infections	Penicillin-sensitive anaerobes
Cutaneous ulcers	Mixed aerobic and anaerobic organisms

terior portions of vertebral bodies are the most common sites of infection. Hematogenous dissemination and lymphatic spread are the most likely routes of infection. Paravertebral abscess may complicate this infection. Diagnosis is usually confirmed by histologic examination and culture of biopsy material. Long-term (two years) treatment with antituberculous drugs is usually curative.

REFERENCES

Goldenberg DL, Reed JI: Bacterial arthritis. N Engl J Med 312:764–770, 1985.
Waldvogel FA: Osteomyelitis. *In* Wyngaarden JB, Smith LH Jr (eds): Cecil Textbook of Medicine. 18th ed. Philadelphia, WB Saunders Co, 1988, p 1622.

94

INFECTIONS OF THE URINARY TRACT

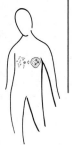

The urethra, bladder, kidneys, and prostate are all susceptible to infection. Most urinary tract infections cause local symptoms, yet clinical manifestations do not always pinpoint the site of infection. In addition, the criteria used by different clinical laboratories to define infection of the urinary tract are also variable. This chapter will attempt to simplify the clinical and laboratory approach to diagnosis and treatment of urinary tract infections. Infections associated with indwelling urinary catheters are discussed in Chapter 98.

Urethritis

Urethritis is predominantly an infection of sexually active individuals, usually observed in males. The symptoms are pain and burning of the urethra during urination, and there is generally some discharge at the urethral meatus. Urethritis may be gonococcal in origin. However, nongonococcal urethritis (NGU) is now more frequent in North America. NGU may be due to *Chlamydia trachomatis* or *Ureaplasma urealyticum* and less commonly to *Trichomonas vaginalis* or *Herpesvirus hominis*. Diagnosis and management of urethritis are considered in Chapter 96.

Cystitis and Pyelonephritis

Epidemiology. Bacterial infection of the bladder (cystitis) and kidney (pyelonephritis) is more frequent in females, and the incidence of infection increases with age. Factors that predispose to urinary tract infection include instrumentation (e.g., catheterization, cytoscopy), pregnancy, and possibly diabetes mellitus.

Pathogenesis. Although some infections of the kidney may arise as the result of hematogenous dissemination, most urinary tract infections "ascend" via a portal of entry in the urethra. Most pathogens responsible for community-acquired urinary tract infections are part of the subject's normal bowel flora. *Escherichia coli* is the most common isolate and, in the female, colonization of the vaginal and periurethral mucosa may antedate infection of the urinary tract. The longer and protected male urethra may account for the lower incidence of urinary tract infection in men. Motile bacteria may swim "upstream," and reflux of urine from the bladder into the ureters may predispose to the development of kidney infection. Congenital anomalies or obstruction of urine flow at any level also predispose to infection.

Clinical Features. Pain, discomfort, or burning sensation on urination and frequency of urination are common symptoms of infection of the urinary tract. Back or flank pain or the occurrence of fever suggests that infection is not limited to the bladder (cystitis), but involves the kidney (pyelonephritis) or prostate as well. However, clinical presentation often fails to distinguish between simple cystitis and pyelonephritis. Approximately one half of infections that appear clinically to involve the bladder only can be shown by instrumentation and other specialized techniques to actually affect the kidneys. Elderly or debilitated patients with infection of the urinary tract may have no symptoms referable to the urinary tract and may present only with fever, altered mental status, or hypotension.

Laboratory Diagnosis of Urinary Tract Infection. Analysis of a midstream urine sample obtained from patients with infection of the bladder or kidney should reveal white blood cells and may also have red cells and slightly increased amounts of protein. The presence of an increased number (see below) of white cells (pyuria) in a midstream urine sample indicates the likelihood of a urinary tract infection. However, since most laboratories count white blood cells by examining the sediment of a centrifuged urine sample, and since urinary white blood cell count may vary according to the degree of urine concentration, quantitation of pyuria is imprecise. As a general rule, more than 5 to 10 white blood cells per high-power field on a centrifuged specimen of urine is abnormal. Resuspending a sedimented urine should be done gently using a Pasteur pipette; in this way casts are not disrupted; the presence of white blood cell casts in an infected urine sample indicates the presence of pyelonephritis. Bacteria may be seen in sedimented urine and can be readily identified using Gram's stain.

At present, most clinical laboratories consider bacterial growth of greater than 10^5 colony-forming units/ml to be indicative of infection. Recent studies indicate that smaller numbers of bacteria can produce lower urinary tract infections (see below). A hazard in interpreting results of urine culture is that if the sample is allowed to stand at room temperature for a few hours before planting on culture plates, bacteria can multiply. This results in spuriously high bacterial counts. For this reason, urine for culture should not be obtained from a catheter bag. Specimens that are not plated immediately should be refrigerated. Biochemical tests to detect bacteriuria are not reliable. Detection of antibody on the surface of bacteria freshly voided in urine is an indication that the kidney (or occasionally the prostate) is infected.

Treatment and Outcome. Patients with cystitis may be treated with a 7-day course of antibiotics such as sulfisoxazole, ampicillin, or trimethoprim-sulfamethoxazole. Recent studies suggest that most patients with cystitis are cured by a single high dose of antibiotic (e.g., 3 gm amoxicillin or 2 gm sulfisoxazole). Culture and sensitivity confirm the diagnosis and ascertain if the antibiotic is active against the pathogen. Because of the difficulty in clinical distinction between cystitis and upper tract disease, some patients treated for cystitis with a single dose of an antibiotic may relapse because of unrecognized upper tract disease.

Occasionally, urine cultures obtained from a patient with symptoms of urinary tract infection and pyuria are reported as "no growth" or "insignificant growth." This has been labeled the "urethral syndrome." Low numbers of bacteria (as few as 100/ml urine) may produce such infections of the urinary tract. In other instances, the urethral syndrome may be caused by *Chlamydia* or *Ureaplasma*, which will not grow on routine culture media. Thus, if a patient with the urethral syndrome has responded to antibiotics, the course should be completed; otherwise, if symptoms and pyuria persist, the patient should receive a 7- to 10-day course of tetracycline, which is active against *Chlamydia* and *Ureaplasma*. Other considerations for patients with lower urinary tract symptoms and no or "insignificant" growth on cultures of urine include vaginitis, herpes simplex infection, and gonococcal infection. (*Neisseria gonorrhoeae* will not grow on routine media used for urine culture.) Thus, a pelvic examination and culture for gonococci may be indicated in this setting if the patient is sexually active.

The presence of fever suggests that infection involves more than just the bladder. Young, febrile patients with UTI may be treated on an ambulatory basis with trimethoprim-sulfamethoxazole for two weeks, provided that (1) they do not appear toxic, (2) they have friends or family at home, (3) they have good provisions for follow-up, and (4) they have no poten-

tially complicating features such as diabetes mellitus, history of renal stones, history of obstructive disease of the urinary tract, or sickle cell disease. Gram's stain of urine in patients hospitalized for pyelonephritis will guide initial therapy. Gram-negative rod infection may be treated initially with an aminoglycoside plus ampicillin or a cephalosporin. The finding of gram-positive cocci in chains suggests that enterococci are the pathogens. This infection should be treated, at least initially, with ampicillin plus an aminoglycoside. Gram-positive cocci in clusters may be staphylococci. *Staphylococcus saprophyticus* is a likely agent in otherwise healthy women and is sensitive to most antibiotics used in the treatment of UTI. In the older patient, *Staphylococcus aureus* should be considered, and this infection may be treated with a penicillinase-resistant penicillin such as nafcillin. Gram-positive cocci in the urine may represent a case of endocarditis with septic embolization to the kidney.

Therapy should be simplified when reports of antimicrobial susceptibility are available. Repeat urine culture after two days of effective treatment should show sterilization or marked decrease in urinary bacterial count. If the patient fails to demonstrate some clinical improvement after two to three days of treatment or if the patient presents with the clinical picture of sepsis or has been febrile for more than one week, a complicating feature should be suspected. Intra- or perinephric abscess or obstruction due to a stone or an enlarged prostate may underlie this presentation. Plain films of the abdomen may occasionally reveal a radiopaque stone, but ultrasonography is a good first diagnostic procedure in this setting. This will generally detect obstruction and collections of pus and may also detect stones greater than 3 mm in diameter. Obstruction must be relieved and abscesses drained to result in cure.

All patients with UTI should have repeat urine cultures one to two weeks after treatment is completed to check for relapse. If relapse occurs, the patient may have pyelonephritis, prostatitis, or neuropathic or structural disease of the urinary tract. If a six-week course of antibiotics active against the bacterial isolate is not effective in eradicating infection, the possibility of structural abnormalities or prostatic infection should be investigated. Urologic evaluation should be performed for all males with urinary tract infection (excepting urethritis) because of the high frequency of correctable anatomic lesions in this population.

Some women have frequent episodes of urinary tract infection due to different bacterial isolates. In some instances, these reinfections are related to sexual activity. A single dose of an active antibiotic such as cephalexin just after sexual contact and voiding after sexual contact can decrease reinfection rate in these women. In other cases, in which no precipitating factor can be found and infections are frequent, prophylaxis with one half a tablet of trimethoprim-sulfamethoxazole nightly has been effective.

On occasion, urine cultures reveal bacterial growth in the absence of symptoms. If the sample has been obtained properly and repeat culture reveals the same organism, this is termed *asymptomatic bacteriuria*. This is generally observed in elderly or middle-aged individuals and, in the absence of structural disease of the urinary tract or diabetes mellitus, may not require treatment. Asymptomatic bacteriuria occurring during pregnancy should be treated because of the high risk of pyelonephritis in this setting.

The occurrence of pyuria in the absence of bacterial growth on culture of urine ($<10^2$ colonies/ml) may be termed *sterile pyuria*. If this occurs in the patient with lower urinary tract symptoms, chlamydial or gonococcal infection, vaginitis, or herpes simplex infection should be considered. In the absence of lower urinary tract symptoms, sterile pyuria may be seen among patients with interstitial nephritis of numerous causes, or tuberculosis of the urinary tract. Patients with renal tuberculosis often have nocturia and polyuria. More than half of male patients also have involvement of the genital tract, most commonly the epididymis. Diagnosis can be made by biopsy of genital masses, when present, and by three morning cultures of urine for mycobacteria.

Prostatitis

Although prostatic fluid has antibacterial properties, the prostate can become infected, usually by direct invasion through the urethra. Symptoms of urinary tract infection, back or perineal pain, and fever are common. Some patients experience pain with ejaculation. Rectal examination usually reveals a tender prostate. Patients with acute prostatitis generally have an abnormal urinary sediment and pathogenic bacteria (usually gram-negative enteric rods) in cultures of urine.

Acute prostatitis may be due to the gonococcus but is most often due to gram-negative bacilli. Treatment is directed against the pathogen observed on Gram's stain of urine and is generally effective. Chronic prostatitis should be suspected in males with recurrent urinary tract infection. The urine sediment may be relatively benign in patients with chronic prostatitis. In this instance, comparison of the first part of the urine sample, midstream urine, excretions expressed by massage of the prostate, and postmassage urine should reveal bacterial counts more than 10-fold greater in the prostatic secretions and postmassage urines than in first-void and midstream samples. Treatment of chronic prostatitis is hampered by poor penetration of most antimicrobials into the prostate. Long-term treatment with trimethoprim-sulfamethoxazole has cured approximately one third of patients and prevented symptomatic relapse in another third. Ciprofloxacin also appears to be effective in this setting.

REFERENCES

Andriole VT: Urinary tract infections and pyelonephritis. In Wyngaarden JB, Smith LH Jr (eds): Cecil Textbook of Medicine. 18th ed. Philadelphia, WB Saunders Co, 1988, p 628.
Komaroff AL: Acute dysuria in women. N Engl J Med 310:368–374, 1984.

95

NOSOCOMIAL INFECTIONS

A nosocomial or hospital-acquired infection is an infection, not present on admission to the hospital, that first appears 72 hours or more after hospitalization. A patient admitted to a hospital in the United States has an approximately 5 to 10 per cent chance of developing a nosocomial infection. These infections result in significant morbidity and mortality (approximately 1 per cent of these infections are fatal and an additional 4 per cent contribute to death) and greatly increased medical costs (over 1 billion dollars per year).

Numerous factors are associated with a greater risk of acquiring a nosocomial infection. These include factors that are not avoidable by optimal medical practice such as age and severity of underlying illness. Contributing factors that can be minimized by thoughtful patient management include prolonged duration of hospitalization, the inappropriate use of broad-spectrum antibiotics, the use of indwelling catheters, and the failure of health care personnel to wash their hands.

APPROACH TO THE HOSPITALIZED PATIENT WITH SUSPECTED NOSOCOMIAL INFECTION

The first clue to the presence of a nosocomial infection is often a rise in temperature. The only sign of infection, particularly in the elderly or demented patient, may be a change in mental status (Table 95–1). Some patients with serious infection do not initially develop fever but instead become tachypneic or con-

TABLE 95–1. SIGNS OF INFECTION IN THE HOSPITALIZED PATIENT

Fever
Change in mental status
Tachypnea
Hypotension
Leukocytosis

fused for no apparent reason. Analysis of arterial blood gases may reveal at first a respiratory alkalosis, followed by a metabolic acidosis due to increased levels of lactate. Arterial oxygen content may be normal or depressed.

When evaluating a hospitalized patient for a new fever (Table 95–2) or suspected nosocomial infection, the physician should first assess the stability of the patient. Hypotension, tachypnea, or new obtundation mandate rapid evaluation and treatment. Review the patient's problem list; ascertain if the patient was subjected to a potentially hazardous intervention recently (e.g., genitourinary tract instrumentation or administration of blood products). If the patient can cooperate, elicit a history directed at possible causes of the fever. Often the patient has a specific complaint that helps identify the source of the fever. Examine the skin carefully. Maculopapular rashes often accompany drug fevers; ecthyma gangrenosum can be a sign of gram-negative sepsis (see Chapter 85). Surgical wounds should be examined for the presence of infection. Among debilitated patients, pressure sores located near the sacrum or over the greater trochanters may become infected and produce fever. Abscesses at these sites may be covered by a necrotic membrane so that exploration with a gloved finger or sterile needle may be required to demonstrate a focus of pus. Patients receiving multiple intramuscular injections may develop fever due to the development of sterile abscesses at the injection sites. Headache or sinus tenderness may be present in patients with sinusitis—this may be a problem among patients after nasogastric or nasotracheal intubation. Nuchal rigidity may be a sign of nosocomial meningitis, although it may be absent in some cases, and generalized rigidity is often seen in elderly demented patients without CNS infection. Examine the nose and oropharynx and attempt to elicit symptoms of viral upper respiratory tract infections. These do occur in hospitals. A pleural friction rub may indicate a recent pulmonary thromboembolism as a cause of fever; rales or other evidence of consolidation

TABLE 95–2. COMMON CAUSES OF FEVER IN THE HOSPITALIZED PATIENT

Pneumonia
Catheter-related infection
Surgical wound infection
Urinary tract infection
Drugs
Pulmonary emboli
Infected pressure sores

may indicate a nosocomial pneumonia; basilar rales and even egophony and bronchial breath sounds may also be due to atelectasis in debilitated patients. A new S_4 gallop or pericardial friction rub may be the only clinical manifestation of a myocardial infarction.

The abdomen may also be a source of fever in the hospitalized patient. The patient with antibiotic-induced colitis generally has fever, diarrhea, and abdominal pain. Patients with indwelling urinary catheters are at particular risk of infection. These patients should have a careful examination of the prostate—looking for abscess or tenderness—and of the urine—looking for white blood cells and bacteria.

The extremities must be examined carefully, particularly the sites of current and old intravenous catheter placements, for evidence of phlebitis. If no other source of fever is found and an intravenous catheter has been in place, it should be replaced and a segment of the catheter should be rolled on an agar plate for culture.

Deep vein thrombophlebitis and pulmonary thromboemboli are life-threatening complications of hospitalization whose only clinical manifestations may be fever. The lower extremities should be examined and measured carefully. An asymmetry in leg or calf circumference, which may not be obvious without a measurement, may be an important clue to an underlying thrombosis. A crystal induced arthritis is another potential source of fever in a hospitalized patient (see Chapter 113). Gout and pseudogout may be precipitated by acute infections.

The patient's medication list should be reviewed for drugs likely to produce fever. In this regard antimicrobial agents (particularly penicillins, sulfa drugs, and cephalosporins) are among the most common causes of drug-induced fevers. A drug fever can occur at any time but usually occurs during the second week of drug administration. A review of the peripheral blood smear can give important clues as to the cause of the fever. Eosinophilia may suggest drug-reaction and lymphocytosis a viral process. A left shift and vacuolization within neutrophils suggest a bacterial infection. Unless the etiology of the fever is apparent and bacteremia is unlikely, cultures of blood should be obtained.

NOSOCOMIAL PNEUMONIA

Although some hospital-acquired pneumonias occur as a result of bacteremic spread, the vast majority occur via aspiration of oropharyngeal contents. The oropharynx of the patient admitted to the hospital rapidly becomes colonized with aerobic gram-negative bacilli and often staphylococci. The administration of broad-spectrum antibiotics, severe underlying illness, respiratory intubation, and prolonged duration of hospitalization predispose to colonization.

Sedation, loss of consciousness, and other factors that depress the gag and cough reflexes place the colonized patient at greater risk for aspiration and the development of nosocomial pneumonia. The development of a new pulmonary infiltrate in a hospitalized patient may represent pneumonia, atelectasis, aspiration of gastric contents, drug reaction, or pulmonary infarction. If pneumonia is suspected, prompt definition of the pathogen and appropriate treatment are critical, since nosocomial pneumonia carries a 20 to 50 per cent mortality. If the patient cannot produce good quality sputum, nasotracheal or transtracheal aspiration should be performed (see Chapter 88). Antibiotic therapy is guided by the results of Gram's stain of the sputum or of the tracheal aspirate. Gram-negative rods are the predominant pathogens in this setting; these infections should be treated with an aminoglycoside plus an extended-spectrum penicillin or cephalosporin until results of culture and sensitivity are known. In certain hospitals, nosocomial pneumonia due to *Legionella* species is frequent, and erythromycin should be included in the initial treatment regimen. Patients with nosocomial pneumonia should also receive respiratory therapy consisting of clapping, postural drainage, and promotion of coughing to assist in bringing up secretions.

The patient in the intensive care unit with an endotracheal tube in place is at particular risk for nosocomial pneumonia. This patient has an ineffective gag reflex and often a depressed cough as well. He is therefore entirely dependent upon suctioning by the staff to clear secretions from his airways. The airways of these patients become rapidly colonized with bacteria. Epidemics of nosocomial pneumonia have sometimes been associated with contamination of tubing and machinery used for ventilation or respiratory therapy, but more often infection is due to transmission of pathogens on the hands of medical personnel. Large-volume nebulizers, when contaminated, are also capable of delivering droplets containing bacteria to the lower respiratory tract. Patients whose airways are simply colonized but whose lower respiratory tracts are not infected should not be treated with antibiotics, despite positive sputum cultures. Premature treatment of colonization results in replacement of the initial colonists by more resistant organisms, whereas delay in treatment of nosocomial pneumonia can result in death due to overwhelming infection. The physician must therefore be able to distinguish accurately between colonization and infection. The development of new fever, leukocytosis, pulmonary infiltrate, and/or deterioration of respiratory status as ascertained by blood gas determinations indicate infection (pneumonia) rather than colonization. A Gram's stain of sputum should be performed to identify the predominant organism(s). The appearance of elastin fibers in KOH preps of sputum is a very specific indicator of bacterial infection in this setting (see Chapter 82). The appearance of these fibers may actually precede the development of infiltrates on chest radiograph. This test, however, detects only about one half of nosocomial pneumonias in the ICU.

Nosocomial pneumonias are best prevented by (1) avoiding excessive sedation; (2) providing frequent suctioning and respiratory therapy—drainage and clapping—to patients who have difficulty managing secretions; (3) avoiding the use of large-volume reservoir nebulizers; (4) avoiding the injudicious use of broad-spectrum and/or high-dose antibiotic therapy; (5) frequent handwashing by medical and nursing personnel.

INTRAVASCULAR CATHETER–RELATED INFECTIONS

Infections related to intravascular catheters may occur via bacteremic seeding or through infusion of contaminated material, but the vast majority of these infections occur via bacterial invasion at the site of catheter insertion.

Intravenous catheters may produce a sterile phlebitis. Certain drugs such as tetracycline or erythromycin, when administered intravenously, are particularly likely to produce phlebitis. Bacteria migrating through the catheter insertion site may colonize the catheter and then produce a septic phlebitis or bacteremia without evidence of local infection. Factors associated with a greater risk of IV catheter–related infection are shown in Table 95–3. *Staphylococcus epidermidis* and *Staphylococcus aureus* are the predominant pathogens in this setting, followed by the enteric gram-negative rods. A peripheral catheter (and all readily removable foreign bodies) should be replaced if bacteremia occurs and no other primary site of infection is found. The catheter should also be removed if fever without an obvious source occurs or if local phlebitis develops. The value of culturing a peripheral catheter tip is uncertain unless semiquantitative techniques are used (i.e., rolling the catheter across an agar plate). During the evaluation of a hospital-acquired fever, an inflamed vein should be examined carefully, and after the catheter is removed the inflamed portion of the vein should be compressed in an attempt to express pus through the catheter entry site. If pus can be expressed or the patient remains febrile or bacteremic while on appropriate antibiotics, the vein should be surgically explored and excised if septic phlebitis is found.

Central venous catheters remain in place longer than peripheral catheters and are therefore associated with a greater overall infection rate. This is particularly true if total parenteral nutrition is provided by this route. Patients receiving parenteral nutrition are at particular risk for systemic infection with *Candida* spe-

TABLE 95–3. FACTORS ASSOCIATED WITH GREATER RISKS OF INTRAVENOUS CATHETER–RELATED INFECTION

Duration of catheterization > 72 hours
Plastic catheter > steel needle
Lower extremities and groin > upper extremity
Cutdown > percutaneous insertion
Emergency > elective insertion
Breakdown in skin integrity, e.g., burns
Inserted by physician > IV therapy teams

TABLE 95–4. FACTORS PREDISPOSING TO NOSOCOMIAL URINARY TRACT INFECTION

Indwelling catheters
Duration of catheterization
Open drainage (versus closed-bag drainage)
Interruption of closed drainage system
Use of broad-spectrum antibiotics (*Candida*)

cies and gram-negative bacilli as well as with staphylococci. Pus at the catheter insertion site or positive blood cultures without another source are indications for catheter removal. In an attempt to decrease percutaneous spread of bacteria to intravascular sites, most centers are now placing long Silastic catheters into the subclavian vein after subcutaneous tunneling. These catheters may be kept in place for prolonged periods with a lower infection risk. As a general rule, persistent bacteremia while on appropriate antibiotics, recurrent bacteremia, and fungemia with *Candida* or related yeasts explanation are indications for catheter removal.

PRESSURE SORES

See Chapter 90.

NOSOCOMIAL URINARY TRACT INFECTION

Placement of an indwelling catheter into the urethra of a hospitalized patient facilitates access of pathogens to an ordinarily sterile site. Factors that predispose to infection are shown in Table 95–4. The most common pathogens are enteric gram-negative rods; however, among immunocompromised patients and patients receiving broad-spectrum antibiotics, *Candida* species are also important causes of infection. Prophylactic antibiotics, irrigation, urinary acidification, and use of antiseptics are of no value in prevention of infection in this setting. Nosocomial urinary tract infections can be best prevented by instituting the following:

1. Catheterize only when necessary. (Monitoring of intake and output or urinary incontinence are generally not appropriate indications for catheterization.)

2. Remember that repeated straight ("in-and-out") catheterizations are less likely to produce infection than indwelling catheters. Many patients with dysfunctional bladders (e.g., with multiple sclerosis) have used this technique for years without developing significant urinary tract infections.

3. If an indwelling catheter is unavoidable, observe the following guidelines:

   a. Remove the catheter as soon as possible.

   b. Emphasize handwashing.

   c. Maintain a closed and unobstructed drainage system. (Urine specimens for culture and analysis may be obtained by inserting a 22-guage needle aseptically through the distal end of the catheter wall.) Do not disconnect the catheter from the drainage bag.

   d. Secure the catheter in place.

   e. Keep the catheter bag below the level of the bladder.

   f. Irrigate the catheter only if it is obstructed.

Asymptomatic bacterial colonization of the catheterized bladder need not be treated. If the patient has fever or local symptoms, antibiotic treatment is indicated. *Candida* infection of the bladder often resolves once broad-spectrum antibiotics are discontinued. If *Candida* infection persists, the catheter may be changed; if infection still persists, twice-daily irrigation of the catheter with amphotericin B can eradicate the organism.

The best way to prevent catheter-related infections of the urinary tract is to avoid catheterization unless absolutely necessary.

REFERENCES

Kunin CM: Detection, Prevention and Management of Urinary Tract Infections. 4th ed. Philadelphia, Lea & Febiger, 1986.

Salata RA, Lederman MM, Shlaes DM, et al: Diagnosis of nosocomial pneumonia in intubated, intensive-care unit patients. Am Rev Resp Dis 135:426–432, 1987.

Wenzel RP: Prevention and treatment of hospital-acquired infections. *In* Wyngaarden JB, Smith LH Jr (eds): Cecil Textbook of Medicine. 18th ed. Philadelphia, WB Saunders Co, 1988, pp 1541–1549.

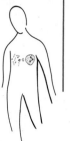

96

SEXUALLY TRANSMITTED INFECTIONS

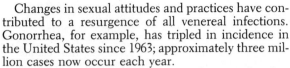

Changes in sexual attitudes and practices have contributed to a resurgence of all venereal infections. Gonorrhea, for example, has tripled in incidence in the United States since 1963; approximately three million cases now occur each year.

Sexually transmitted diseases can be considered in broad groups according to whether major initial manifestations are (a) genital sores, (b) urethritis, cervicitis, and pelvic inflammatory disease, or (c) vaginitis. Human immunodeficiency virus infections are discussed in Chapter 97.

GENITAL SORES

Six infectious agents cause most genital lesions (Table 96–1). The appearance of the lesions, natural history, and laboratory findings allow a clear-cut distinction among the possible causes in most instances. The two most common and significant infections are herpes simplex virus infection and syphilis.

HERPES SIMPLEX VIRUS INFECTION (*HSV*)

Genital herpes infection has reached epidemic proportions, causing a corresponding increase in public awareness and concern. Genital herpes differs from the other sexually transmitted disease in its tendency for spontaneous recurrence. Its importance stems from the morbidity, both physical and psychic, of the recurrent genital lesions, the danger of transmission of a fulminant, often fatal disease to newborn infants, and the observed association with cervical carcinoma.

Epidemiology

HSV has a worldwide distribution. Humans are the only known reservoir of infection, which is spread by direct contact with infected secretions. Of the two types of HSV, HSV-2 is the more frequent cause of genital infection. The major risk of infection is in the 14- to 29-year-old cohort and varies with sexual activity. The prevalence of HSV-2 antibody is 3 per cent in nuns and 70 per cent in prostitutes.

After exposure, HSV replicates within epithelial cells and lyses them, producing a thin-walled vesicle. Multinucleated cells are formed with characteristic intranuclear inclusions. Regional lymph nodes become enlarged and tender. HSV also migrates along sensory neurons to sensory ganglia, where it assumes a latent state. Inside the sacral ganglia, HSV DNA can be demonstrated, but the virus does not replicate and is inactive metabolically. Just how viral reactivation occurs is uncertain. During reactivation, the virus, however, appears to migrate back to skin along sensory nerves.

Clinical Presentation

Primary genital lesions develop two to seven days after contact with infected secretions. In males, painful vesicles appear on the glans or penile shaft; in females, on the vulva, perineum, buttocks, cervix, or vagina. A vaginal discharge frequently is present, usually accompanied by inguinal adenopathy, fever, and malaise. Sacroradiculomyelitis or aseptic meningitis can complicate the primary infection. Perianal and anal HSV infections are common, particularly in male homosexuals; tenesmus and rectal discharge often are the main complaints.

The precipitating events associated with genital relapse of HSV infection are poorly understood. In individual cases, stress or menstruation may be implicated. Overall, genital recurrences develop in about 60 per cent of HSV-infected patients. Clinically apparent recurrences are more frequent in males with HSV-2 infection. The frequency of asymptomatic cervical recurrence in women is not known. Many patients describe a characteristic prodrome of tingling or burning for 18 to 36 hours before the appearance of lesions. Recurrent HSV genital lesions are fewer in number, usually stereotyped in location, often restricted to the external genitalia, and associated with few systemic complaints.

Laboratory Diagnosis

The appearance of the characteristic vesicles is strongly suggestive of HSV infection. However, diagnosis should be confirmed by Tzanck smear (see Chapter 82), Pap smear, or viral isolation. Serologies for HSV may be useful in the diagnosis of primary infection.

Treatment

Acyclovir shortens the course of primary genital HSV infection. Intravenous or oral administration is recommended for severe cases with fever, systemic symptoms, and extensive local disease. Antiviral agents do not purge the latent stage of virus, however, and cannot prevent recurrent infections. Prophylactic oral acyclovir decreases the frequency of recurrences by 60 to 80 per cent when used over a four- to six-month period; oral acyclovir also hastens recovery from severe recurrent episodes. Cervical shedding of HSV from active lesions late in pregnancy, near the time of parturition, is an indication for Caesarean section. The risk to the neonates exposed to asymptomatic shedding of HSV during parturition is uncertain.

SYPHILIS

Syphilis is of unique importance among the venereal diseases because early lesions heal without specific

TABLE 96–1. DIFFERENTIATION OF DISEASES CAUSING GENITAL SORES

DISEASE	PRIMARY LESION	ADENOPATHY	SYSTEMIC FEATURES	DIAGNOSIS/Rx
Herpes genitalis, 5–10% sexually active adults, due to *Herpesvirus hominis* (II) Primary	Incubation 2–7 days. Multiple painful vesicles on erythematous base. Persist 7–10 days.	Tender, soft adenopathy.	Fever	Tzanck smears pos. Tissue culture isolation, over four-fold rise in antibodies to HSV. Rx: acyclovir.
Recurrent	Grouped vesicles on erythematous base, painful. Last 3–21 days.	None	None	Tzanck, tissue culture pos. Titers not helpful.
Syphilis, 75,000 cases U.S./yr caused by *Treponema pallidum*	Incubation 10–90 days (m. 21). Chancre: papule that ulcerates. Painless, border raised, firm, ulcer is indurated, base smooth. Usually single. May be genital or almost anywhere. Persists 3–6 wk, leaving thin atrophic scar.	1 wk after chancre appears. Bilateral or unilateral. Firm, discrete, moveable, no overlying skin changes, painless, nonsuppurative. May persist for months.	Later	Cannot be cultured. Pos. darkfield. VDRL pos. 77%; FTA-ABS, 86% (see Table 96–3).
Chancroid, 1,000 cases U.S./yr caused by *Haemophilus ducreyi*	Incubation 3–5 days. Vesicle or papule to pustule to ulcer. Soft, not indurated. Very painful.	1 wk after primary in 50%. Painful, unilateral (2/3), unilocular, suppurative.	None	Organism in Gram's stains of pus. Can be cultured (75%) but direct yields highest from lymph node. Erythromycin 2 gm/day or trimethoprim-sulfamethoxazole 160/800 mg b.i.d. × 10–14 days.
Lymphogranuloma venereum, 600–1,000 cases U.S./yr due to *Chlamydia trachomatis*	Incubation 5–21 days; painless papule, vesicle, ulcer, evanescent (2–3 days), noted in only 10–40%.	5–21-day post primary, 1/3 bilateral, tender, matted iliac/femoral "groove sign," multiple abscesses, coalescent, caseating, suppurative, sinus tracts, thick yellow pus, fistulas, strictures, genital ulcerations.	Fever, arthritis, pericarditis, proctitis, meningoencephalitis, keratoconjunctivitis, preauricular adenopathy, edema of eyelids, erythema nodosum.	LGV C.F. pos. 85–90% (1–3 wk); must have high titer (>1:16) as crossreacts with other *Chlamydia*. Also pos. STS, rheumatoid factor, cryoglobulins. Rx tetracycline 2 gm/day × 2–4 wk.
Granuloma inguinale, 50 cases U.S./yr caused by *Calymmatobacterium granulomatis*	Incubation 9–50 days. At least one painless papule that gradually ulcerates. Ulcers are large (1–4 cm), irregular, nontender, with thickened, rolled margins and beefy red, friable, exuberant cobblestone granulation tissue at base. Older portions of ulcer show characteristic depigmented scarring, while advancing edge contains new papules.	No true adenopathy. In 1/5, subcutaneous spread via lymphatics leads to indurated swelling or abscesses of groin—"pseudobuboes."	Metastatic infection of bones, joints, liver.	Scraping or deep curetting at actively extending border—Wright's/Giemsa stain reveals short, plump, bipolar staining "Donovan bodies" in macrophage vacuoles. Rx tetracycline 2 gm/day × 10 days or trimethoprim-sulfamethoxazole.
Condyloma acuminatum (genital warts). Frequent, due to papillomavirus	Characteristic large, soft, fleshy, cauliflower-like excrescences around vulva, glans, urethral orifice, anus, perineum.	None	None per se. Association with HIV infection	Chief importance is in distinction from others. Topical podophyllin ± cryosurgery, laser resection.

therapy; however, serious systemic sequelae pose a major risk to the patient, and transplacental infections to the offspring.

Epidemiology

Primary syphilis occurs mostly in sexually active 15- to 30-year olds. At least one third of new cases in the United States are in homosexual males. Approximately 50 per cent of the sexual contacts of a patient with primary syphilis become infected. The long incubation period of syphilis becomes a key factor in designing strategies for contact tracing and management. Unless successful follow-up seems certain, contacts of proven cases must be treated with penicillin.

Pathogenesis

Treponema pallidum penetrates intact mucous membranes or abraded skin, reaches the bloodstream via the lymphatics, and disseminates. The incubation period for the primary lesion depends on inoculum size, with a range of 3 to 90 days.

Natural History and Clinical Presentation

Primary syphilis is considered in Table 96–1.

Secondary syphilis develops six to eight weeks after the chancre. Skin, mucous membranes, and lymph nodes are involved. Skin lesions may be macular, papular, papulosquamous, pustular, follicular, or nodular. Most commonly they are generalized, symmetrical, and of like size and appear as discrete erythematous, macular lesions of the thorax or red-brown hyperpigmented macules on the palms and soles. In moist intertriginous areas, large, pale, flat-topped papules coalesce to form highly infectious plaques or "condylomata"; they are teeming with spirochetes as assessed by darkfield microscopy. Mucous patches are painless, dull erythematous patches or grayish-white erosions. They too are infectious and darkfield-positive. Systemic manifestations of secondary syphilis include malaise, anorexia, weight loss, fever, sore throat, arthralgias, and generalized, nontender, discrete adenopathy. Specific organ involvement also may develop: gastritis (superficial, erosive), nephritis or nephrosis (immune complex–mediated, remits spontaneously or with treatment of syphilis), and symptomatic or asymptomatic meningitis (see Chapter 122). One fourth of patients have relapses of the mucocutaneous syndrome within two years of onset. Thereafter, infected patients become asymptomatic and noninfectious except via blood transfusions or transplacental spread.

Late syphilis develops after 1 to 10 years in 15 per cent of untreated patients. The skin gumma is a superficial nodule or deep granulomatous lesion that may develop punched-out ulcers. Superficial gummas respond dramatically to therapy. Gummas also may involve bone, liver, and the cardiovascular or central nervous system. Deep-seated gummas may have serious pathophysiological consequences; treatment of the infection often does not reverse organ dysfunction.

Gradually progressive cardiovascular syphilis begins within 10 years in over 10 per cent of untreated patients, most frequently males. Patients develop aortitis with medial necrosis secondary to an obliterative end-arteritis of the vasa vasorum. There may be asymptomatic linear calcifications of the ascending aorta or (in decreasing frequency) aortic regurgitation, aortic aneurysms (saccular or fusiform, most commonly thoracic), or obstruction of coronary ostia.

Central nervous system syphilis develops in 8 per cent of untreated patients 5 to 35 years following primary infection and includes meningovascular syphilis, tabes dorsalis, and general paresis (see Chapter 122). Although general paresis and tabes are classified as separate neurological syndromes, many patients show elements of both. Late CNS syphilis also may be asymptomatic despite cerebrospinal fluid abnormalities indicating active inflammation.

Diagnosis and Treatment

The clinical diagnosis of syphilis must be confirmed by darkfield examination and/or serologies. Spirochetes are seen in darkfield preparations of chancres or moist lesions of secondary syphilis. Saprophytic treponemes confuse darkfield diagnosis of oral lesions. Serologic diagnosis is considered in Table 96–2. The differential diagnosis of primary syphilis consists of herpes simplex and three conditions that are relatively

TABLE 96–2. SEROLOGIES IN SYPHILIS

	VDRL	FTA-ABS
Technique	Standard nontreponemal test. Antibody to cardiolipin-lecithin.	Standard treponemal test. Antibody to Nichol's strain *Treponema pallidum* after absorption on nontreponemal spirochetes.
Indications	Screening and assessing response to therapy. Should be quantified by diluting serum.	Confirmation of specificity of positive VDRL. Remains reactive longer than VDRL. Useful for late syphilis, particularly neurosyphilis.
Per Cent Positive in Syphilis		
Primary	77%	86%
Secondary	98%	100%
Early latent	95%	99%
Late latent and late	73%	96%
False Positives	Weakly reactive is nonspecific (positive treponemal serologies in 30%). Positive VDRL should be repeated and, if positive, FTA-ABS performed. Relative frequency of false positives determined by prevalence of syphilis in the population.	Borderline positive is frequent (80%) in pregnancy. Should be repeated.

rare in the United States: chancroid, lymphogranuloma venereum, and granuloma inguinale. The characteristics of these diseases are presented in Table 96–1.

The presence of neurosyphilis requires modifying the standard antibiotic treatment of syphilis. For this reason, a lumbar puncture should be performed in all patients with late latent syphilis (at least one year after primary syphilis) or syphilis of unknown duration. An elevated CSF white blood cell count, elevated protein, and positive VDRL on diluted samples of CSF establish the diagnosis of neurosyphilis. A patient with persistent positive blood VDRL and a positive CSF VDRL or FTA-ABS should be considered and treated as a case of neurosyphilis. Because the VDRL may be negative in late syphilis, the presence of a positive serum FTA-ABS in a patient with a neurologic syndrome consistent with syphilis is a sufficient indication for treatment. A small proportion (2 to 3 per cent) of patients with neurosyphilis may undergo abrupt deterioration following treatment with penicillin; this Jarisch-Herxheimer reaction, of uncertain cause, may be ameliorated by concomitant treatment with corticosteroids. Lumbar puncture should be repeated at six-month intervals for three years to assure adequacy of treatment as reflected by normalization of CSF and progressive decline in CSF VDRL titer. Retreatment may be necessary if CSF abnormalities persist or recur. Treatment protocols are shown in Table 96–3.

Syphilis serologies must be followed after treatment. Using the recommended treatment schedules, 1 to 5 per cent of patients with primary syphilis will develop recurrence (? relapse, ? reinfection). Serologies in adequately treated primary syphilis should be negative by two years after therapy (usually by 6 to 12 months). Seventy-five per cent of patients with secondary syphilis will be seronegative by two years. If the VDRL does not become negative or achieve a low fixed titer in patients with primary, secondary, or early latent syphilis, lumbar puncture should be performed to evaluate the possibility of asymptomatic neurosyphilis, and the patient should be retreated with penicillin. Patients

with late or late latent syphilis should show a decline in antibody titer or low fixed titers by two years. Two to 10 per cent of patients with CNS syphilis will relapse following treatment. However, it is rare for asymptomatic patients to develop symptomatic disease after penicillin therapy. Every patient should be seronegative or "serofast" with a low fixed titer before termination of follow-up. If not, therapy should be repeated.

URETHRITIS, CERVICITIS, AND PELVIC INFLAMMATORY DISEASE

These syndromes can be considered broadly as gonococcal and nongonococcal in etiology.

GONORRHEA

Gonorrhea is among the most common of venereal diseases. The morbidity of gonococcal infections now exceeds that of syphilis. *N. gonorrheae* is second only to *Chlamydia trachomatis* as a cause of sexually transmitted diseases in the United States.

Epidemiology

The incidence of gonorrhea reached a plateau in the United States between 1975 and 1980, possibly reflective of a decrease in the size of the at-risk cohort. Reinfection is the norm, and it is not unusual for one sexually active patient to have 20 or more discrete infections. Particular risk factors are urban habitat, low socioeconomic status, unmarried status, number of different sexual contacts, and male homosexuality. Fifty per cent of females having intercourse with a male with gonococcal urethritis will develop symptomatic infection. The risk for males is 20 per cent after a single sexual contact with an infected female. Orogenital contact and anal intercourse also transmit disease. Asymptomatic infection of males is an important factor in transmission. Forty per cent of male contacts of symptomatic women have asymptomatic urethritis. About one quarter of them develop symptomatic infection within seven days; a like number spontaneously become culture-negative within this period. The remaining 50 per cent remain culture-positive and asymptomatic but capable of transmitting infection for periods of up to six months.

Pathogenesis

Neisseria gonorrhoeae is a gram-negative, kidney bean–shaped diplococcus. Specialized projections from the organism, the pili, aid in attachment to mucosal surfaces, contribute to resistance to killing by neutrophils, and constitute an important virulence factor. Production of an IgA protease by the organism is another factor in pathogenicity. In females, several factors alter susceptibility to infection. Group B blood type increases susceptibility, while diverse factors such as vaginal colonization with normal flora, iron and IgA content of vaginal secretions, and high progesterone levels may be protective. Spread from the cervix to the upper genital tract is associated with menstruation be-

TABLE 96–3. TREATMENT FOR SYPHILIS

CLINICAL CATEGORY	REGIMEN OF CHOICE	HISTORY OF PENICILLIN ALLERGY
Primary Secondary Early latent Healthy contact*	Benzathine penicillin 2.4 MU I.M. once	Tetracycline or erythromycin 2 gm/ day × 15 days
Late latent or late	Benzathine penicillin 2.4 MU I.M. q week × 3	No regimen adequately evaluated ? Tetracycline or erythromycin 2 gm/ day × 30 days
Neurosyphilis	Aqueous penicillin G 20 MU IV q.d. × 10 days	Same as for late latent or late

* Contact of patient with active skin or mucous membrane lesions.

cause changes in the pH and biochemical constituents of cervical mucous lead to increased shedding of gonococci; cervical dilatation, reflux of menses, and binding of the gonococcus to spermatozoa may be additional factors in ascending genital infection and dissemination. Intrauterine contraceptive devices increase the risk of endometrial spread of infection two- to nine-fold (oral contraceptives are associated with a two-fold decrease).

Clinical Presentation

In males who develop symptomatic urethritis, disturbing symptoms of spontaneous purulent discharge and severe dysuria usually develop 2 to 7 days after sexual contact. Prompt treatment usually follows so that more extensive genital involvement is uncommon.

In females, cervicitis is the most frequent manifestation and results in a copious yellow vaginal discharge. Overall, 20 per cent of females with gonococcal cervicitis develop pelvic inflammatory disease (PID), usually beginning at a time close to the onset of menstruation. PID is manifest as endometritis (abnormal menses, midline abdominal pain), salpingitis (bilateral lower abdominal pain and tenderness), or pelvic peritonitis. Salpingitis can cause tubal occlusion and sterility. Gonococcal perihepatitis (Fitz-Hugh-Curtis syndrome) also may complicate pelvic inflammatory disease and present as right upper quadrant pain.

Females also may develop urethritis with dysuria and frequency. One fourth of women complaining of urinary tract symptoms and 60 per cent of those with symptoms but no bacteriuria have urethral cultures positive for N. gonorrhoeae.

Anorectal gonorrhea occurs in homosexual males and heterosexual females. In males, the resultant rectal pain, tenesmus, mucopurulent discharge, and bleeding may represent the only site of infection. Anorectal disease also may be asymptomatic and recognized only by cultures of asymptomatic contacts of patients with gonorrhea. In females, asymptomatic anorectal involvement is a frequent complication of symptomatic genitourinary disease (44 per cent); isolated anorectal infection (4 per cent) as well as acute or chronic proctitis (2 to 5 per cent) are rare. Treatment failures are frequent in anorectal gonorrhea (7 to 35 per cent).

Pharyngeal gonorrhea occurs in homosexual males or heterosexual females following fellatio and less frequently in heterosexual males. Symptoms of pharyngitis occurring in this setting may be due to associated trauma or to gonococcal pharyngitis. Pharyngeal gonorrhea rarely is the sole site of gonococcal infection (5 to 8 per cent). Infection of the pharynx is important, however, as a source of dissemination, particularly in males.

Extragenital dissemination occurs in approximately 1 per cent of males and 3 per cent of females with gonorrhea. Strains of N. gonorrhoeae causing dissemination differ from other gonococci in several respects. They are more penicillin-sensitive and resist the nor-

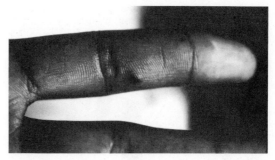

FIGURE 96–1. Typical skin lesion of disseminated gonococcal infection.

mal bactericidal activity of antibody and complement. The latter finding may be due to their binding of a naturally occurring blocking antibody. Dissemination of gonococcal infection may take the form of the "arthritis-dermatitis syndrome" with 3 to 20 papular, petechial, pustular, necrotic, or hemorrhagic skin lesions, usually found on the extensor surfaces of the distal extremities (Fig. 96–1). Associated findings are an asymmetric polytenosynovitis, with or without arthritis, which predominantly involves wrists, fingers, knees, and ankles. Joint fluid cultures usually are negative in the arthritis-dermatitis syndrome, leading to speculation that circulating immune complexes, demonstrable in most patients, are important in its pathogenesis. Biopsy of skin lesions reveals gonococcal antigens (by immunofluorescent antibody staining) in two thirds of cases. Blood cultures are positive in 50 per cent. Septic arthritis is another manifestation of dissemination; N. gonorrhoeae is the most frequent cause of septic arthritis in 16- to 50-year-olds. Sometimes the history indicates an antecedent syndrome suggestive of bacteremia. The joint fluid cultures usually are positive (particularly when the leukocyte count in joint fluid exceeds 80,000/μl), and blood cultures are usually negative. Gonococcemia rarely may lead to endocarditis, meningitis, myopericarditis, or toxic hepatitis.

Laboratory Diagnosis and Management

Gram's stain of the urethral discharge will determine the cause of urethritis in most males with gonorrhea, typical intracellular diplococci being diagnostic (Fig. 96–2). The finding of only extracellular gram-negative diplococci is equivocal. The absence of gonococci on smear of a urethral discharge from a male virtually excludes the diagnosis. Diagnosis by Gram's staining of cervical exudates is relatively specific but insensitive (<60 per cent). Modified Thayer-Martin medium contains antibiotics that inhibit the growth of other organisms and increases the yield of gonococci from samples likely to be contaminated; it is not necessary for culture of normally sterile fluids such as joint fluid, blood, and cerebrospinal fluid. Specimens from these sites should be cultured on chocolate agar. The addition of 3 per cent trimethoprim to Thayer-Martin medium inhibits fecal Proteus and is useful for anorectal cultures. Other important considerations for the

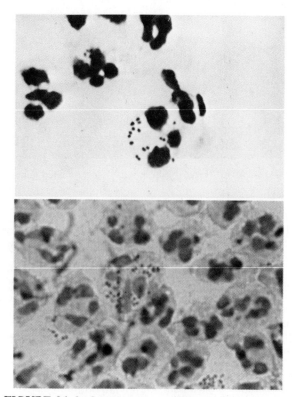

FIGURE 96–2. Gram stain of urethral discharge showing typical intracellular diplococci associated with neutrophils.

isolation of gonococci include the use of synthetic swabs (unsaturated fatty acids in cotton may be inhibitory), the introduction of a very thin swab or loop 2 cm into the male urethra, and the avoidance of vaginal douching (12 hr), urination (2 hr), and vaginal speculum lubricants before culture. In all suspected cases of gonorrhea, the urethra, anus, and pharynx should be cultured. In females, 20 per cent of cases in which initial cultures were negative yield N. *gonorrhoeae* when cultures are repeated. Current recommendations for the treatment of uncomplicated gonorrhea are 4.8 million units procaine penicillin intramuscularly or 3.0 gm amoxicillin orally, plus 1.0 gm probenecid. The addition of a course of tetracycline (2 gm/day orally for seven days) is appropriate to treat concurrent chlamydial infection. In fact, tetracycline alone appears to be adequate for treatment of male urethritis. Spectinomycin, 2.0 gm intramuscularly as a single injection, is an effective alternative except in pharyngeal infections. Acute pelvic inflammatory disease should be treated with procaine penicillin followed by tetracycline, 2 gm/day orally for 10 days. Seriously ill females with PID should be hospitalized. If they appear toxic, the initial antibiotic regimens should be broad-spectrum. The combination of cefoxitin and doxycycline is usually effective. Evaluation by ultrasonography for the presence of a pelvic abscess or peritonitis usually is warranted in this setting. Surgery in indicated to drain a tubo-ovarian or pelvic abscess. Disseminated gonococcal infection should be treated with aqueous penicillin G, 20 million units per day for three to five days, followed by oral ampicillin (2 gm/day) to complete a 10-day course. In the penicillin-allergic patient, tetracycline is an acceptable alternative for the treatment of PID and ceftriazone for disseminated infection. Cephalosporins should not be used, however, if the history suggests an IgE-mediated allergy to penicillin (anaphylactoid reaction, angioedema, urticaria). In such a case, tetracycline is indicated.

If a patient fails to respond to treatment, the isolates should be tested for penicillinase production. Penicillinase-producing gonococci are common in southeast Asia but are rare in most regions of the United States. Depending on the clinical manifestations, spectinomycin, ceftriazone, or tetracycline can be substituted as therapy.

A VDRL should be obtained in all patients with gonorrhea. If negative, no further follow-up is necessary, since procaine penicillin in the dosage used is effective in treating incubating syphilis. This is not true of therapy with alternate drugs; if they are used, the VDRL should be repeated after 4 weeks. Because of both intrinsic and beta-lactamase–mediated penicillin resistance of gonococci, cultures should be repeated after treatment. In males, these should be obtained at 7 to 14 days; in females at 7 to 14 days and again at six weeks. Anal cultures should be part of the routine follow-up of females, since persistent anorectal carriage may be the source of delayed relapse. Postgonococcal urethritis occurs in 30 to 50 per cent of males two to three weeks after penicillin therapy. It usually is caused by C. *trachomatis* or U. *urealyticum*.

NONGONOCOCCAL URETHRITIS, CERVICITIS, AND PID

The diagnosis of nongonococcal urethritis (NGU) requires the exclusion of gonorrhea, since considerable overlap exists in the clinical syndromes.

Epidemiology

At least as many cases of urethritis are nongonococcal as gonococcal. Typically, NGU predominates in higher socioeconomic groups. *Chlamydia trachomatis* causes 30 to 50 per cent of NGU and can be isolated from 0 to 11 per cent of asymptomatic, sexually active males. *C. trachomatis* also can be isolated from 20 per cent of males with gonorrhea and presumably represents a concurrent infection. Some cases of *Chlamydia*-negative NGU are due to *Ureaplasma urealyticum* or *Trichomonas vaginalis*.

Clinical Syndromes

NGU is less contagious than gonococcal disease. The incubation period is 7 to 14 days. Characteristically, patients complain of urethral discharge, itching, and dysuria. Importantly, the discharge is not spontaneous but becomes apparent after stripping the urethra in the morning. The mucopurulent discharge consists of thin, cloudy fluid with purulent specks; these characteristics do not always allow clear distinction from gonococcal disease. *Trichomonas vaginalis* causes a typically scanty discharge.

C. *trachomatis* also is a common cause of epididymitis in males under 35 years of age and can produce proctitis in homosexual males, as well as in women.

Chlamydial infections are more common than gonococcal infections in females but frequently escape detection. Two thirds of females with mucopurulent cervicitis have chlamydial infection. Similarly, many females with the acute onset of dysuria, frequency, and pyuria, but sterile bladder urine, have C. *trachomatis* infection. C. *trachomatis* is at least as common a cause of salpingitis as is the gonococcus.

Laboratory Diagnosis

Ordinarily the distinction between gonococcal and nongonococcal infections relies mainly on Gram's stained preparations of exudate and cultures. In a male with urethritis and typical gram-negative diplococci associated with neutrophils, the diagnosis of gonococcal urethritis is clear-cut and culture unnecessary. Coincident NGU cannot be excluded, however. If interpretation of the Gram's stain is not straightforward in males and in all females, culture on Thayer-Martin medium is appropriate. Again, however, the presence of *N. gonorrhoeae* does not preclude concurrent NGU. Techniques for isolation and detection of chlamydia are widely available and should be a routine means of evaluating genital infections.

Treatment

The patient and all sexual contacts should be treated with a seven-day course of tetracycline, 2 gm per day orally. Recurrence may occur and requires longer periods (2 to 3 weeks) of treatment.

TABLE 96–4. ORGANISMS CAUSING THE GAY BOWEL SYNDROME

Neisseria gonorrhoeae
Chlamydia trachomatis
Herpesvirus hominis
Treponema pallidum
Shigella species
Salmonella species
Campylobacter species
Entamoeba histolytica
Giardia lamblia
Cryptosporidium species
Strongyloides stercoralis

GAY BOWEL SYNDROME

Male homosexuals may present with proctitis/proctocolitis causing anorectal pain, mucoid or bloody discharge, tenesmus, or abdominal pain. Constipation or diarrhea can occur, too. Sigmoidoscopy should be performed with culture and Gram's stain of discharge. Potential causative organisms are shown in Table 96–4. The diarrheal syndromes are considered in Chapter 92. Ten per cent of patients harbor two or more pathogens. Proctitis also may occur in male homosexuals without a definable pathogen (42 per cent). Diarrhea in the patient infected with human immunodeficiency virus has an entirely different set of implications, as will be discussed in Chapter 97.

VAGINITIS

Table 96–5 considers salient features in the diagnosis and management of patients with vaginitis.

TABLE 96–5. VAGINITIS

DISEASE	EPIDEMIOLOGY/ PATHOGENESIS	CLINICAL FINDINGS	LABORATORY DIAGNOSIS	TREATMENT
Candidiasis	Yeast are part of normal flora. Overgrowth and disease favored by broad-spectrum antibiotics, high estrogen levels (pregnancy, before menses, oral contraceptives), diabetes mellitus, tight clothing.	Itching, little or no urethal discharge, occasional dysuria. Labia pale or erythematous with satellite lesions. Vaginal discharge thick, adherent with white curds. Balanitis in 10% of male contacts.	Vaginal pH = 4.5 (normal), negative whiff test, yeast seen on wet mount in 50%, culture positive.	Miconazole or clotrimazole cream or suppositories for 7 days.
Trichomonas vaginalis	STD. Incubation 5–28 days. Symptoms begin or exacerbate with menses.	Discharge, soreness, irritation, mild dysuria, dyspareunia. Copious loose discharge, 1/5 yellow/green, 1/3 bubbly.	Elevated pH. Wet mount shows large numbers of WBC, trichomonads. Positive whiff test (10% KOH causes fishy odor).	Metronidazole, 2 gm as single dose. Treat sexual contacts.
Nonspecific	Synergistic infection, *Gardnerella vaginalis* and anaerobes, (*Mobiluncus* sp.).	Vaginal odor, mild discharge, little inflammation. Greyish, thin, homogeneous discharge with small bubbles.	Elevated pH; positive whiff test. Wet prep contains clue cells (vaginal epithelial cells with intracellular coccobacilli), few WBC.	Metronidazole, 500 mg b.i.d. × 7 days. Do not treat contacts unless recurrent vaginitis.

REFERENCES

Holmes KK, Mardh P-A, Sparling PF, Weisner PJ (eds): Sexually Transmitted Diseases. New York, McGraw-Hill Book Co, 1984.

Sparling PF: Sexually transmitted diseases. In Wyngaarden JB, Smith LH Jr (eds): Cecil Textbook of Medicine. 18th ed. Philadelphia, WB Saunders Co, 1988, pp 1701–1723.

Stamm WE, Guinan ME, Johnson C, et al: Effect of treatment regimens for Neisseria gonorrhoeae on simultaneous infection with Chlamydia trachomatis. N Engl J Med 310:545, 1984.

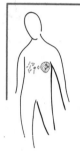

97

THE ACQUIRED IMMMUNODEFICIENCY SYNDROME AND OTHER HIV-RELATED DISORDERS

The acquired immunodeficiency syndrome (AIDS) is the most serious expression of a series of related disorders due to infection by the human immunodeficiency virus (HIV-1). The recognition of an epidemic of immunodeficiency has led to a case definition, originally designed for surveillance purposes, that defines AIDS as an illness that occurs in previously healthy individuals, with no underlying or iatrogenic cause of immunosuppression, who develop one of the infections listed in Table 97–1 or one of the other conditions specified in Table 97–2.

EPIDEMIOLOGY

The first cases of AIDS were described in 1981 among sexually active homosexual men residing in New York, Los Angeles, and San Francisco. Subsequent analyses revealed that AIDS-like illnesses had occurred in Central Africa for several years prior to 1981. Since that time, the disease has spread throughout the nation and the world. As of July, 1989, over 100,000 cases fulfilling strict diagnostic criteria for AIDS were reported to the United States Centers for Disease Control. Over half of these persons have died. The World Health Organization recorded more than 200,000 cases of AIDS in 144 countries by the middle of 1989. (This represents serious underreporting from several regions.) The best current estimates are that, by mid-1989, over 5 million persons worldwide will be infected with HIV. By 1993, unless more effective antiviral agents are developed, there will have been nearly half a million persons in the United States with CDC-defined AIDS (Fig. 97–1).

The pattern of spread of HIV-1 involves exposure to infected blood via shared needles, transfusions of contaminated blood and blood products, vertical spread from mother to infant, or transmission via heterosexual or homosexual relations. Almost three fourths of the United States cases have occurred among homosexual or bisexual males. Intravenous drug users are the next largest group of North American AIDS patients (Table 97–3). Other groups at increased risk of HIV-1 infection include recent immigrants to the United States from Central Africa and

TABLE 97–1. OPPORTUNISTIC INFECTIONS INDICATIVE OF A DEFECT IN CELLULAR IMMUNE FUNCTION ASSOCIATED WITH AIDS

Protozoan Infection
Pneumocystis carinii pneumonia
Disseminated toxoplasmosis, or Toxoplasma encephalitis, excluding congenital infection
Chronic Cryptosporidium enteritis (>1 mo)
Chronic Isospora belli enteritis (>1 mo)

Fungal Infection
Candida esophagitis, bronchopulmonary candidiasis*
Cryptococcal meningitis or disseminated infection
Disseminated histoplasmosis*†
Disseminated coccidioidomycosis*†

Bacterial Infection
Disseminated Mycobacterium avium-intracellulare or Mycobacterium kansasii
Extrapulmonary Mycobacterium tuberculosis*†
Recurrent Salmonella septicemia†

Noncongenital Viral Infection
Chronic (>1 mo) mucocutaneous herpes simplex or bronchial or esophageal herpes simplex
Histologically evident cytomegalovirus infection of any organ except liver, spleen, or lymph nodes
Progressive multifocal leukoencephalopathy secondary to JC virus

Helminthic Infection
Strongyloidiasis (disseminated beyond the gastrointestinal tract)*

---

* Not listed in original CDC definition of AIDS, but subsequently added
† Requires laboratory evidence of HIV infection

the Caribbean, hemophiliac recipients of pooled antihemophilic factor concentrates, and recipients of contaminated blood transfusions. In many of the latter instances, units of transfused blood have been traced back to asymptomatic donors who were subsequently found to have been infected with HIV-1. Transmission by contaminated blood and blood products has now been largely eliminated in North America by appropriate screening of donors and testing of donated blood.

AIDS is now occurring with increasing frequency among heterosexual contacts of men and women belonging to groups at risk for AIDS and among newborn children of infected mothers. By the early 1990's, over 8 per cent of North Americans with AIDS will have been infected by heterosexual intercourse.

HIV-1 has been cultured from lymphocytes, monocytes, and macrophages obtained from blood, semen, and vaginal and cervical secretions of infected individuals. The virus also exists in a cell-free form in these fluids. It is not clear whether cell-to-cell contact or the exposure of uninfected cells to free virus is the more common or efficient way that new infections occur. The virus has also been obtained, less consistently, from the cerebrospinal fluid, and rarely in very low concentration from the saliva of patients infected by HIV-1. No clearly documented cases of HIV transmission via body fluids other than blood or genital secretions are known.

HIV-1 infection can be heterosexually transmitted bidirectionally through vaginal intercourse. In Africa, heterosexual activity is the major route of acquisition

TABLE 97–2. OTHER CONDITIONS FULFILLING CRITERIA FOR AIDS

CONDITION	COMMENTS
Neoplasm	
Kaposi's sarcoma (in a person <60 years old)	Most commonly present in homosexual males in U.S. Uncommon elsewhere and among other risk groups
High grade, B-cell non-Hodgkin's lymphoma*† (e.g., Burkitt's lymphoma)	Unusual in U.S. except in AIDS
Undifferentiated non-Hodgkin's lymphoma†	
Immunoblastic sarcoma†	
Primary brain lymphoma†	Limited to brain. Hard to diagnose. May be multicentric
Systemic Illness	
HIV wasting syndrome*†	Unintentional loss of >15 per cent of body weight
Neurological Impairment	
HIV encephalopathy*†	Variety of symptoms, dementia most common (see text)

* Not listed in original CDC definition of AIDS, but subsequently added
† Requires laboratory evidence of HIV infection

TABLE 97–3. GROUPS AT HIGHEST RISK FOR AIDS

Homosexual or bisexual men
Intravenous drug abusers
Recent immigrants from Central Africa or the Caribbean with a history of multiple sexual partners
Hemophiliacs
Recipients of blood transfusions before 1985
Sexual contacts of persons belonging to above groups at risk
Newborn offspring of individuals at risk for AIDS

of HIV-1 infection. Among gay and bisexual males, receptive anal intercourse is the major means of transmission of infection, although rare cases of infection are thought to have occurred after receptive oral exposure to ejaculation. Multiple studies indicate that nonsexual, nonparenteral contact with infected persons does *not* transmit HIV-1 infection. A few hospital and laboratory workers have become infected with HIV-1 after needlesticks, following exposure of mucous membranes or traumatized skin to blood, or after exposure to very high concentrations of virus particles grown in tissue cultures. Needlestick exposure of health care workers to blood from HIV-1–infected individuals has resulted in seroconversion of less than 0.6 per cent of exposed persons. Rigorous adherence to infection control measures is clearly essential for maximal protection of health care workers.

A second human immunodeficiency virus (HIV-2) was identified in Western Africa in the mid-1980's. While HIV-2 has been associated with AIDS-like syndromes, the vast majority of HIV-2 seropositive persons are asymptomatic. Whether these seropositive individuals are infected with a less virulent strain, or simply represent more recent exposure to an equally virulent virus, is not yet known. Although HIV-2

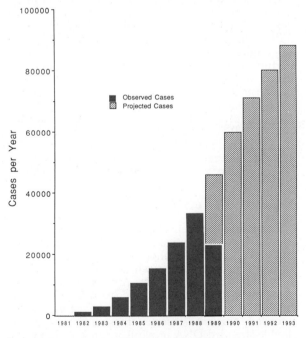

FIGURE 97–1. Observed and projected annual incidence of AIDS in the United States from 1981 through 1993. Current estimates indicate a continued annual increase in the incidence of AIDS through the mid-1990's.

shares many biologic and genetic characteristics with HIV-1, each of the two viruses also has genes that are unique. HIV-2 is more closely related to the simian immunodeficiency virus (SIV). Sporadic HIV-2 infections in the United States have occurred in persons of West African origin.

HTLV-I (human T-cell lymphotropic virus-I), the first pathogenic human retrovirus, was identified several years prior to the recognition of HIV-1 as the cause of AIDS. HTLV-I is endemic in southern Japan and the Caribbean and in certain parts of Africa. It is also present among IV drug users in Europe and the United States and thus has the potential for further spread. Its modes of transmission are similar to those of HIV-1 and 2, but the perinatal routes (breast milk as well as transplacental) appear to account for a far greater proportion of the known cases of HTLV-I infection. Two distinct clinical illnesses, an aggressive adult T-cell leukemia and a relatively indolent spastic paraparesis (originally designated tropical spastic paraparesis), may be associated with HTLV-I infection. However, as compared to HIV-1, individuals infected with HTLV-I are much less likely to develop clinical illness. Fewer than 1 per cent of HTLV-I–infected persons develop either T-cell malignancies or spastic paraparesis; both of the clinical syndromes most frequently develop in the fourth through the sixth decades of life, 30 to 50 years after the presumed acquisition of the HTLV-I infection. The extent of sub-

clinical neurological and/or immunological impairment in populations infected with this virus is not known. Persons infected with both HTLV-I and HIV-1 appear to become immunocompromised more rapidly than those infected with HIV-1 alone.

NATURAL HISTORY OF HIV-1 INFECTION

The great majority of individuals infected with HIV-1 develop, within three months of their initial exposure, readily detectable antibodies against specific components of HIV-1. Some individuals are asymptomatic during this seroconversion period but many—perhaps the majority—experience a generally mild, short-lived "retroviral syndrome" manifested by transient maculopapular or urticarial skin eruptions, aseptic meningitis, and/or a mononucleosis-like syndrome with fever, malaise, and generalized lymphadenopathy. After these initial symptoms, individuals generally remain asymptomatic for several years, although slowly progressive immunological impairment is proceeding all the while (Fig. 97–2). The mean T4 helper lymphocyte count decreases inexorably following HIV-1 infection, but the rate of decrease shows considerable variation from individual to individual. Exposure to other immunosuppressive viruses, such as HTLV-I, hepatitis B, herpes simplex, cytomegalovirus, Epstein-Barr virus, and human herpesvirus type 6 (HH6), may accelerate the impairment of immune function, but there are no conclusive data in this regard. The first clinical manifestations of HIV-1 infection may be reflected solely by persistent generalized lymphadenopathy, weakness, hematologic abnormalities, or intellectual impairment. On the other hand, the sudden appearance of symptoms of a serious opportunistic infection or tumor may be the first evidence of disease. Thus, there is a wide spectrum of manifestations of HIV-1 infection. In the San Francisco experience, more than 50 per cent of men with HIV-1 infections documented for 10 years have developed AIDS. Less than 25 per cent of the men in this cohort remained completely asymptomatic after 10 years. The rate of development of opportunistic illnesses appears to increase with time after infection.

PATHOPHYSIOLOGY

The HIV-1 outer-envelope glycoprotein has high affinity for the CD4 antigen—a molecule found on the surface of T helper lymphocytes, monocytes and macrophages, microglia of the central nervous system, and Langerhans cells of the skin. A virus bound to CD4 gains entry to the cell and uncoats (Fig. 97–3). The RNA viral genome is reverse transcribed by a virus-encoded enzyme—reverse transcriptase—and the double-stranded DNA provirus is integrated into the host chromosome, where it may remain in a latent state. Various factors may activate transcription of proviral DNA in vitro. Lymphocyte-activating signals such as antigens or mitogens induce host transactivating factors to activate transcription of latent virus.

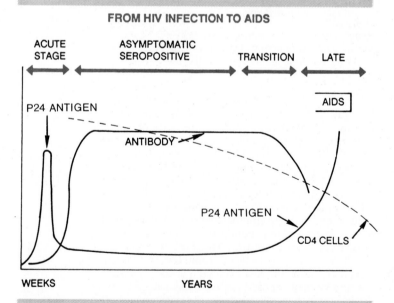

FROM HIV INFECTION TO AIDS

ACUTE STAGE | ASYMPTOMATIC SEROPOSITIVE | TRANSITION | LATE

AIDS

P24 ANTIGEN

ANTIBODY

P24 ANTIGEN

CD4 CELLS

WEEKS | YEARS

FIGURE 97–2. This diagram indicates schematically the course of events following infection by HIV. Following infection, many patients experience a mild "retroviral syndrome." This is usually followed by an asymptomatic period of several years before clinically significant immunodeficiency and opportunistic infections and/or neoplasms occur. The viral core P24 antigen, thought to be a marker of increased viral replication, is transiently detectable in serum during the acute stage of infection, and then reappears years later as immune competence becomes severely impaired. (From Baltimore D: Confronting AIDS: Update 1988. Washington, National Academy Press, 1988.)

Other viruses such as herpes simplex and cytomegalovirus also contain proteins capable of activating latent HIV-1. Viral messenger RNA codes for the synthesis of core proteins, reverse transcriptase, and envelope; whole virus containing two copies of the RNA genome is then assembled, and virus buds from the infected cell.

Patients with AIDS have a profound deficiency in T helper lymphocytes. Cytopathic effects of the virus may contribute to the striking depletion of CD4+ T helper cells in persons with AIDS. Yet among seropositive individuals, the frequency of latently infected T helper cells is estimated to be not more than 10^{-3}, and even fewer cells (an estimated 10^{-4} to 10^{-5}) can be shown to be synthesizing viral messenger RNA at any one time. Thus, the mechanisms contributing to cell loss in this disease are not yet completely understood. Anergy—the failure to demonstrate delayed-type hypersensitivity to recall antigens—occurs in more than 90 per cent of AIDS patients.

Laboratory evidence of immunodeficiency and immunological regulatory impairment (dysregulation) is striking. In vitro infection of T helper lymphocytes results in cytopathic effects, cell lysis, and multiple cell fusion into giant syncytia. T lymphocytes proliferate less readily in response to various stimuli and show impaired production of the lymphokines, interleukin-2 and interferon-γ. Cytotoxic lymphocytes kill virus-infected cells and tumor cells less effectively in vitro. B lymphocyte function is also abnormal; polyclonal hyperglobulinemia is common, but B lymphocyte function as measured by in vitro tests. Impaired B cell function appears to be a greater problem in young children with AIDS, in whom repeated infections by encapsulated bacteria may dominate the clinical course. The most critical underlying problem, however, is the progressive cell-mediated immunodeficiency.

Among asymptomatic HIV-1–infected individuals subclinical immunodeficiency is frequent, with immunological abnormalities that are similar to but less severe than those in patients with AIDS. In these asymptomatic individuals, generalized lymph node enlargement is common.

CLINICAL MANIFESTATIONS

Some individuals with HIV-1 infection have a prodrome including generalized lymph node enlargement, episodes of fever, night sweats, weight loss, and diarrhea, which may last for weeks to months before the development of opportunistic infections or neoplasms. In other individuals, the abrupt onset of an opportunistic infection (e.g., *Pneumocystis carinii* pneumonia) may be the first clinical manifestation of illness.

Mucosal Disease
Candida stomatitis (thrush), herpes zoster (commonly polydermatomal), and refractory candidal vaginitis are often forerunners of AIDS. Hairy leukoplakia, a fimbriated, plaque-like lesion of the tongue

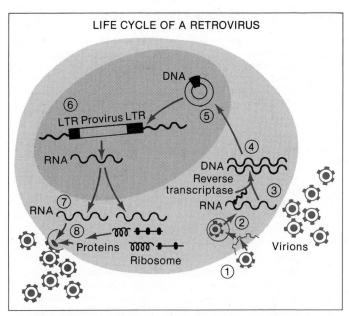

FIGURE 97–3. Viral life cycle: (1) Retrovirus enters the cell by a specific receptor; (2) virus is uncoated in an endosome; and (3) viral RNA is transcribed to double-stranded viral DNA (4) and is transported to the nucleus (5) and integrates into the cellular genome (6). Viral DNA is transcribed as genomic RNA and viral messenger RNA (7), which is translated into new viral protein and assembled at the cell membrane to complete the viral life cycle by budding (8).

or buccal mucosa, often occurs in HIV-infected patients before the development of AIDS.

Thrush often can be suppressed successfully by oral antifungal agents (e.g., clotrimazole troches). The occurrence of esophageal candidiasis, manifesting clinically as pain or difficulty in swallowing, fulfills criteria for the diagnosis of AIDS. Esophageal involvement necessitates treatment with ketoconazole or amphotericin B. Chronic ulcerative perioral or perianal herpes simplex infection, seen frequently in patients with HIV-1 infection, establishes an AIDS diagnosis if lesions persist for four weeks or more. Diagnosis can be confirmed by demonstrating multinucleated giant cells in a Wright's stain of a scraping obtained from the base of the ulcer. Acyclovir is the treatment of choice and may require chronic administration after the acute ulcers have healed.

Kaposi's sarcoma, a malignancy of endothelial cell origin primarily infecting homosexual men, is histologically similar to Mediterranean Kaposi's sarcoma but follows a more aggressive course. The lesions of Kaposi's sarcoma can arise anywhere on the skin or in the mucosa of the mouth or gastrointestinal tract; occasionally they first appear in enlarged lymph nodes. The lesions are vascular, can be raised or flat, may be pink, brown, or blue in color, and often resemble insect bites, bruises, or nevi. The diagnosis is established by biopsy, especially of an older lesion. Some lesions may regress or stabilize after administration of interferon-α or cytotoxic drugs (e.g., vinblastine, vincristine), but no treatment has been consistently effective.

TABLE 97—4. NERVOUS SYSTEM COMPLICATIONS OF HIV INFECTION

Direct HIV-1 Infection
Acute meningoencephalitis
Aseptic meningitis
AIDS dementia complex
HIV-1 encephalitis
Vacuolar myelopathy
Peripheral neuropathy (axonal)
Opportunistic Neoplasms
Primary brain lymphoma
Metastatic lymphoma

Opportunistic Infections
Cerebral toxoplasmosis
Cryptococcal meningitis
Cytomegalovirus encephalitis
Progressive multifocal
leukoencephalitis
Varicella-zoster virus
encephalitis/myelitis
Other or Unknown Etiologies
Acute or chronic
demyelinating
polyneuropathy
Metabolic encephalopathies
(e.g., hypoxia from
pneumonia)
Vasculitis

The relative frequency of Kaposi's sarcoma as an AIDS-defining lesion in North American males has decreased from greater than 24 per cent in 1984 to less than 12 per cent in 1989; the reason for the relative decrease is not known.

Systemic Infection

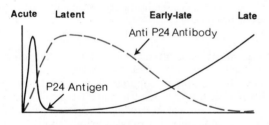

Central nervous system events

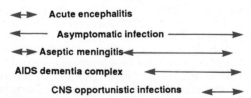

FIGURE 97–4. As with other manifestations of HIV-1 infection, neurological disease may be divided into four phases. (1) In the "acute retroviral syndrome," either acute aseptic meningitis or acute encephalitis may occur, followed by full recovery. (2) This is followed by a latent phase, usually of several years duration, during which no neurological abnormalities are apparent. (3) In the third phase, concomitant with increasing CNS damage by HIV-1, AIDS dementia may begin. (4) In the final phase, concomitant with severe immunosuppression, CNS dementia may progress rapidly and major opportunistic CNS infections and/or tumors may develop. Although only a minority of patients have clinically apparent aseptic meningitis, the majority exhibit moderate to severe intellectual dysfunction in the final phase of the illness. (Adapted from Price RW, Bruce B, Sidtis J, et al: The brain in AIDS: Central nervous system HIV-1 infection and AIDS dementia complex. Science 239:586, 1988, with permission.)

Nervous System Diseases

Neurologic manifestations of AIDS are common and may be fatal (Table 97–4). HIV-1 itself may cause aseptic meningitis either early or late in the course of the infection, and may also cause an acute encephalitis or a chronic progressive AIDS dementia complex (Fig. 97–4). The virus may also result in neuropathy, myelopathy, or focal CNS lesions. Lumbar puncture may reveal elevated CSF protein, sometimes with a reactive lymphocytosis, and the virus will often grow from the spinal fluid.

Although intellectual impairment is rarely seen early in the course of HIV infection, progressive AIDS dementia may precede the development of opportunistic infections. AIDS dementia complex, the most common CNS manifestation of HIV infection, results from direct invasion of the brain by the virus. It usually begins insidiously and progresses over months or years (see Chapter 122). Occasionally the disorder may be acute or subacute in onset. AIDS dementia complex is characterized by poor concentration and memory, slowing of thought processes, and behavioral abnormalities, usually social withdrawal and apathy. A few patients become agitated, confused, or paranoid or develop hallucinations. Motor abnormalities are common, including impaired rapidly alternating movements, impaired ocular motility, and mild gait ataxia. As the disease progresses, patients become more and more demented and may develop a myelopathy characterized by spastic weakness of the lower extremities and incontinence. Sometimes the myelopathy precedes signs of intellectual impairment. The patients eventually become completely withdrawn and bedridden before death from an opportunistic infection.

The AIDS dementia must be distinguished from the potentially treatable opportunistic infections that may also affect the brain (Table 97–4). Computed tomography (CT) and magnetic resonance imaging (MRI) scans in the AIDS dementia complex usually demonstrate cerebral atrophy. On MRI, patchy white matter abnormalities are frequently seen. The CSF may show mild mononuclear pleocytosis with an elevated protein count. Treatment with zidovudine (AZT) may retard progression of the dementia in some patients.

Opportunistic CNS infections and tumors characteristically occur late in the course of HIV infection, at a time of advanced immunosuppression. Patients with cryptococcal meningitis may complain of persistent headache, difficulty in concentrating, and lethargy. Prior to the appearance of AIDS, approximately half of the cases of cryptococcal meningitis occurred among individuals without underlying immunosuppressive conditions. Thus, the occurrence of cryptococcal meningitis in a previously healthy individual is suggestive but not diagnostic of AIDS. AIDS patients with cryptococcal meningitis often have cryptococcal fungemia. Virtually all have a positive test for cryptococcal antigen in the CSF, which establishes the diagnosis. The infection can be suppressed with amphotericin B, but relapses are the rule. Thus, AIDS patients with cryptococcal infection must receive maintenance therapy for life, with either amphotericin or fluconazole.

Toxoplasmosis of the central nervous system, presenting as single or multiple brain lesions, occurs frequently in AIDS patients. Serological tests are usually not diagnostic, but the characteristic ring-enhancing lesions on CT scan in an HIV-infected patient with focal neurological signs provide adequate criteria to initiate treatment for toxoplasmosis (see Fig. 122–3). Pyrimethamine and sulfadiazine, combined with folinic acid, is the treatment of choice; therapy must be continued indefinitely. Progressive multifocal leukoencephalopathy, a demyelinating disease due to papovavirus, can produce progressive dementia, visual impairment, and hemiparesis in AIDS patients. MRI reveals characteristic lesions of white matter. There is no known treatment. Varicella-zoster rarely also causes a focal leukoencephalitis in persons with AIDS. Cytomegalovirus-induced chorioretinitis often affects patients with advanced AIDS and may lead to blindness. Progression of the retinal disease may be retarded by gancyclovir, a derivative of acyclovir, or foscarnet (phosphonoformate), both investigational in the United States. Primary lymphoma of the central nervous system also occurs with increased frequency among patients with AIDS; response to systemic or intrathecal therapy is generally poor.

Pulmonary Disease

Pneumocystis carinii pneumonia (PCP) is the most common life-threatening opportunistic infection complicating AIDS. In North America, over 60 per cent of the initial AIDS-defining infections are due to PCP. Affected patients complain of shortness of breath, nonproductive cough, and fever. In contrast to the often acute onset of PCP in other immunocompromised patients, AIDS patients with PCP may have pulmonary symptoms for weeks before presentation. Arterial hypoxemia is common; the chest radiograph generally reveals a mixed, often subtle interstitial and alveolar pattern. The diagnosis may be made by cytological examination of induced sputum or, if necessary, bronchoalveolar lavage.

Treatment with high doses of intravenous trimethoprim-sulfamethoxazole for three weeks is generally effective, but the drug combination produces an unusually high frequency of side effects in AIDS patients, including marrow depression, rash, and fever, which limit its effectiveness. Intravenous pentamidine is comparably effective. Side effects of pentamidine include azotemia, occasional marrow depression, and chemical hepatitis, as well as hypoglycemia, which may occur or persist for days after the drug is stopped. Other drugs that appear useful include combinations of oral trimethroprim with dapsone, and trimetrexate. The use of aerosolized pentamidine for milder cases has shown encouraging results and has minimized toxic side effects. Organisms persist in repeat biopsy specimens and relapse is frequent. Following an initial episode of PCP pneumonia, prophylaxis with either oral trimethoprim-sulfamethoxazole twice daily or aerosolized pentamidine greatly decreases the likelihood of recurrent episodes of PCP pneumonia. Prophylaxis is also effective in preventing the initial episode of PCP pneumonia in patients with CDC-defined AIDS (e.g., individuals with Kaposi's sarcoma).

Gastrointestinal Disease

The sexual practices of some homosexual men (e.g., oral-anal contact) predispose them to infection by a variety of gastrointestinal pathogens (see Table 96–4). Homosexual men with AIDS often have intermittent or persistent severe watery diarrhea. In some instances, diarrhea results from common treatable sexually transmitted pathogens such as Shigella or Campylobacter; in others, unusual protozoa such as *Cryptosporidium* or *Isospora belli* are the causative microorganisms. If stool cultures and examinations for parasites are negative, the responsible microorganism may sometimes be found by mucosal biopsy (e.g., cytomegalovirus). In approximately half the patients, an etiological microorganism is not identified.

Other Infections

Disseminated CMV infection is common among AIDS patients. The virus is often present in the urine and in biopsy or postmortem examinations of lung, liver, gut, and brain. Invasive disease (e.g., chorioretinitis, colitis) may respond to treatment with gancyclovir. Both pulmonary and extrapulmonary disease caused by *M. tuberculosis* is especially common in HIV-infected individuals; it may appear early in the course of HIV-1 infection and usually responds well to appropriate therapy (see Chapters 84 and 88). *Mycobacterium avium-intracellulare* (MAI) is a saprophytic mycobacterium that, on rare occasion, produces an indolent pneumonia in otherwise healthy individuals. In patients with AIDS, MAI frequently produces disseminated infection. The organism can be cultured from blood but may require several weeks to grow. Acid-fast smears of stool sometimes reveal MAI. Culture and histological examination of bone marrow may be more sensitive in diagnosis.

MAI resists the action of most antibiotics. Combinations of antimycobacterial drugs can eradicate bacteremia in some patients but they almost never provide a cure. MAI bacteremia was distinctly unusual before the AIDS epidemic, even in patients with severe immunodeficiency. Salmonellosis, often associated with persistent bacteremia, may be difficult to eradicate in AIDS patients. Infections caused by certain encapsulated bacteria (e.g., S. *pneumoniae*, H. *influenzae*) are more frequent among patients with HIV-1 infection but usually respond to prompt administration of appropriate antibiotics. By contrast, infections such as listeriosis, aspergillosis, and nocardiosis, common among other groups of patients with impaired cell-mediated immunity, are relatively uncommon in patients with AIDS. These observations suggest that "cell-mediated host defenses" are heterogeneous and can be selectively impaired.

DIAGNOSIS AND LABORATORY FINDINGS

At present, the physician makes a clinical diagnosis of AIDS based upon criteria indicated in Tables 97–1 and 97–2. An abnormal distribution of lymphocyte phenotypes, with decreases in both the absolute number and percentage of T helper cells, is almost invariably present. In the patient with HIV-1 infection, it is unusual for a major AIDS-defining opportunistic infection to occur until the absolute T4 helper lymphocyte count has fallen below 200 cells/µl in the peripheral blood.

Anemia and leukopenia are common. Some patients with HIV-1 infection have a syndrome resembling immune thrombocytopenic purpura (ITP), probably due to binding of immune complexes to platelets, resulting in rapid clearance of platelets from the circulation by reticuloendothelial cells. Thrombocytopenic purpura may occur months or years before other clinical manifestations of HIV-1 infection and often disappears spontaneously or after short-term steroid therapy. Splenectomy is rarely necessary.

Abnormal tests of liver function are common and may be related to infection with cytomegalovirus, hepatitis A or B, non-A non-B hepatitis, or *Mycobacterium avium-intracellulare*. Serum albumin is often low, and total immunoglobulins are usually elevated, reflecting a polyclonal increase. Increased serum beta-2 microglobulin levels are also present. Virtually all AIDS patients have serum antibody against HIV antigens. The p24 (core) antigen is characteristically present early in the course of infection; it disappears entirely as serum antibody develops but reappears years later as immunocompromise becomes more severe (Fig. 97–2).

APPROACH TO THE PATIENT AT RISK FOR AIDS

The long latency period (median of 10 years in adults) following HIV-1 infection and the absence of definitive predictive tests produce great uncertainty among individuals with asymptomatic HIV-1 infection and related syndromes such as generalized lymph node enlargement. Persons who think they are at risk for HIV-1 infection should have access to confidential serological screening. Noninfected individuals in high-risk behavior groups should be informed of means of minimizing their exposures to the causative agent. Homosexual men should be advised to limit the number of sexual partners and either to avoid anal intercourse altogether or always to use a condom. Intravenous drug users should understand that sharing needles is dangerous. They require counseling and encouragement to undergo detoxification in therapeutic communities or with methadone. Persons whose behavior places them at high risk of HIV-1 infection should not donate blood, regardless of their serological status. The screening of blood donors for antibody to HIV is an additional safeguard. There is no evidence that either asymptomatic HIV-1–positive individuals or AIDS patients pose any risk to schoolmates, co-workers, or household members who are not their sexual partners.

TREATMENT OF HIV-1 INFECTION

The identification of the structure and life cycle of HIV has led to broadened insights as to potential therapeutic approaches (Fig. 97–3). The virus utilizes an enzyme unique to retroviruses, reverse transcriptase, which converts its RNA form into a DNA provirus that integrates into the host cell genome. Zidovudine (AZT), an inhibitor of reverse transcriptase, is effective in postponing death in persons with AIDS and in delaying the onset of opportunistic illnesses in persons with symptomatic HIV-1 infection. Persons with oral thrush, unexplained fevers, weight loss, night sweats, and low numbers of T helper lymphocytes (below 200 cells/ml) are at high risk for the development of opportunistic infections, and generally receive prophylaxis against PCP as well as treatment with zidovudine. Asymptomatic HIV-1 seropositive persons are now participating in studies to assess the benefits of zidovudine over longer periods of time. Zidovudine also inhibits erythropoiesis, and over 20 per cent of patients taking zidovudine for more than one year require periodic transfusions. Patients who are least immunocompromised, as gauged by T4 lymphocyte counts, are least likely to become anemic. Other inhibitors of reverse transcriptase (e.g., phosphonoformate, dideoxyadenosine) are undergoing clinical trials.

In preclinical and early clinical trials the efficacy of agents that block binding of HIV-1 to cellular receptors is being evaluated. Research efforts are also directed toward inhibiting viral transcription by interfering with the activity of viral regulatory gene products. Agents potentially capable of inhibiting viral assembly are also being evaluated for their usefulness in the management of HIV-1 infections. Substances under investigation include intravenously administered CD-4 molecules that may act as "decoys" to prevent HIV from binding to cellular CD-4 receptors, the use of granulocyte-monocyte–colony-stimulating factor (GM-CSF) to correct leukopenia in zidovudine-treated patients, and the use of erythropoietin to prevent anemia in patients treated with antiviral drugs. Early attempts at reconstituting the immune system of AIDS patients by the use of immunostimulatory drugs such as interferon, interleukin-2, and other cytokines were not successful. It may be possible in the future to add immunostimulatory agents to antiretroviral drugs to help reconstitute the immune system.

The future holds promise, but carefully executed clinical trials will take time. At present, prevention is the most critical element in slowing the spread of this devastating epidemic as it is not likely that an effective vaccine will be developed, evaluated, and made available for widespread application in the near future.

REFERENCES

Carpenter CCJ, Mayer KH: Advances in AIDS and HIV infection. Adv Intern Med 33:45–80, 1988.

Fischl MA, Richman DD, Grieco MH, et al: The efficacy of AZT in the treatment of patients with AIDS and AIDS-related complex. N Engl J Med 317:185–191, 1987.

Gallo RC, Groopman JE: The acquired immunodeficiency syndrome. *In* Wyngaarden JB, Smith LH Jr (eds): Cecil Textbook of Medicine. 18th ed. Philadelphia, WB Saunders Co., 1988, pp 1794–1808.

Institute of Medicine: Confronting AIDS: Update 1988. Washington, DC, National Academy Press, 1988.

Price RW, Bruce B, Sidtis J, et al: The brain in AIDS: Central nervous system HIV-1 infection and AIDS dementia complex. Science 239:586, 1988.

98

INFECTIONS IN THE IMMUNOCOMPROMISED HOST

Immunosuppression is an increasing by-product of diseases and modern approaches to their treatment. The immunocompromised host suffers from increased susceptibility to opportunistic infection, defined as infection caused by organisms of low virulence that comprise normal mucosal and skin flora or by resident microbial agents usually maintained in a latent state.

Immunocompromise is not an all-or-none phenomenon. The extent of immunosuppression varies with the underlying cause and must exceed a threshold to predispose to opportunistic infections. Importantly, the type of immunosuppression predicts the spectrum of agents likely to cause infections. Accordingly, opportunistic infections can best be considered in categories that reflect the nature of immunocompromise.

DISORDERS OF CELL-MEDIATED IMMUNITY

Cell-mediated immunity is the major host defense against facultative intracellular parasites, as discussed in Chapter 81. The list of diseases and situations that produce impaired cell-mediated immunity is presented in Table 98–1. However, only certain of these result in increased susceptibility to infection with intracellular parasites. Foremost among acquired immunodeficiencies are HIV infection (see Chapter 97), Hodgkin's disease and other lymphomas, hairy-cell leukemia, and advanced solid tumors. Severe malnutrition, as well as treatment with high-dose corticosteroids, cytotoxic drugs, or radiotherapy, can produce a similar predilection to infections. Congenital immunodeficiencies are associated with severe infections early in childhood and will not be considered here. Patients with impaired cell-mediated immunity are especially susceptible to organisms shown in Table 98–2.

Thus, with depression of cell-mediated immunity, organisms ordinarily constituting the normal flora such as *Candida* species act as virulent opportunistic pathogens capable of causing deep-seated infections. Latent viruses, fungi, mycobacteria, and protozoa reactivate to cause locally progressive and/or disseminated disease. Often the signs, symptoms, and laboratory abnormalities suggesting the diagnosis are subtle.

The association between defective cell-mediated immunity and disease produced by the infectious agents listed in Table 98–2 is clear-cut. Sometimes, treatment of the underlying disease causing immunodeficiency or progression of this disease produces a more severe and generalized compromised state, which predisposes to infection by additional microorganisms. For example, during chemotherapy for lymphoma, bacterial infections predominate. Disease progression also results in local factors favoring bacterial infections such as mucosal breakdown and tumor masses obstructing bronchi, ureters, or the biliary tract. The result is a marked increase in severe bacterial infection and septicemia late in the course of many diseases associated with impaired cell-mediated immunity.

DISORDERS OF HUMORAL IMMUNITY

The acquired disorders of antibody production associated with increased frequency of infection are common variable immunodeficiency, chronic lymphocytic leukemia, lymphosarcoma, and multiple myeloma. The paraproteinemic states belong in this category because of secondary decreases in levels of functioning antibody. Therapy with cytotoxic drugs may produce similar immunocompromise.

Infections due to the pneumococcus, *Haemophilus influenzae*, streptococci, and staphylococci predominate early in the course of the humoral immunodeficiency. As the underlying disease itself progresses, infections due to gram-negative bacilli become more frequent. Treatment of the underlying condition with corticosteroids and cytotoxic drugs causes additional defects in cell-mediated immunity, providing susceptibility to infections with the group of pathogens presented in Table 98–2.

TABLE 98–1. CONDITIONS CAUSING IMPAIRED CELL-MEDIATED IMMUNITY

Infectious diseases—measles, chickenpox, typhoid fever, tuberculosis, leprosy, histoplasmosis, HIV infection
Vaccinations—measles, mumps, rubella
Malignancies—Hodgkin's disease, lymphomas, advanced solid tumors
Drugs—corticosteroids, cytotoxic drugs
Miscellaneous—sarcoidosis, uremia, diabetes mellitus, malnutrition, old age

TABLE 98–2. INFECTIONS IN PATIENTS WITH IMPAIRED CELL-MEDIATED IMMUNITY

Viruses—varicella-zoster, herpes simplex, cytomegalovirus, JC virus
Fungi—Pathogenic: *Histoplasma*, *Coccidioides*; Saprophytic: *Cryptococcus*, *Candida*, *Aspergillus*, *Zygomycetes*
Bacteria—*Listeria*, *Nocardia*, *Mycobacterium tuberculosis*, *Legionella pneumophila*, non-tuberculous mycobacteria
Protozoa—*Pneumocystis carinii*, *Toxoplasma gondii*, *Cryptosporidium* species
Helminths—*Strongyloides stercoralis*

In sickle cell anemia, heat-labile opsonic activity is abnormal. Complement depletion by erythrocyte stroma causes impairment of opsonization of pneumococci and *Salmonella* species, leading to frequent infections with these organisms. Impaired reticulo-endothelial system function due to erythrophagocytosis and functional asplenia also may predispose patients with sickle cell disease to serious bacterial infections. The predisposition to infection is age-related; once children with SS disease develop antibodies to pneumococcal capsular polysaccharide, they lose their thousand-fold increased susceptibility to severe pneumococcal infection.

IMPAIRED NEUTROPHIL FUNCTION

Many inherited and acquired diseases impair neutrophil function. The defect may be extrinsic or intrinsic to the neutrophil. Impaired chemotaxis is a significant factor predisposing patients with inherited C3 and C5 deficiencies to frequent bacterial infections (see Chapter 81). Corticosteroid therapy also interferes with chemotaxis. Whereas circulating neutrophil counts may be normal or increased in patients treated with corticosteroids, these cells are dysfunctional, since they do not localize normally to the site of infection. Defective cell-mediated immunity also contributes to the spectrum of infections promoted by corticosteroids.

Intrinsic defects in neutrophils are rare but provide insights into the microbicidal mechanisms of these cells. Neutrophils from patients with chronic granulomatous disease (CGD) cannot develop an oxidative burst. Catalase-negative organisms produce sufficient hydrogen peroxide to facilitate their own killing by CGD neutrophils through the myeloperoxidase pathway. Catalase-producing organisms such as staphylococci, *Serratia*, *Nocardia*, and *Aspergillus* scavenge the hydrogen peroxide that they produce; these infectious agents, therefore, cannot be killed by CGD neutrophils and produce serious, deep-seated infections.

The most severe intrinsic neutrophil defects occur in the Chédiak-Higashi syndrome. Patients have giant granules in their leukocytes and defective microtubule assembly. The result is impaired chemotaxis, abnormal phagolysosomal fusion, delayed bacterial killing, and recurrent infections. Diagnosis of this rare syndrome is aided by phenotypic abnormalities: partial albinism, depigmentation of the iris, peripheral neuropathies, and nystagmus.

TABLE 98–3. INFECTIOUS AGENTS THAT FREQUENTLY CAUSE INFECTIONS IN NEUTROPENIC PATIENTS

Bacteria—*Pseudomonas, Klebsiella, Serratia, Escherichia coli, Staphylococcus aureus, Staphylococcus epidermidis, Corynebacterium J-K*
Fungi—*Candida, Aspergillus, Zygomycetes*
Viruses—Cytomegalovirus, *Herpesvirus hominis*
Protozoa—*Pneumocystis carinii*

NEUTROPENIA

As the neutrophil count falls below 500/µl, an exponential increase occurs in the frequency and severity of infections. Most reliable data originate from patients with acute leukemia. For example, in one study, neutrophil counts of 100 to 500 µl were associated with infections during 35 per cent of hospitalized days, whereas at counts below 100/µl this increased to 55 per cent. However, granulocytopenia of other etiologies produces a comparable risk of infection. In patients with chronic and cyclical neutropenias, the susceptibility to infection varies inversely with the monocyte count; the mononuclear phagocytes provide some of the antibacterial capacity of the missing neutrophils. Following chemotherapy of acute leukemia, neutropenia usually is sustained and associated with damage to mucosal barriers to infection. Patients become susceptible to organisms that are ubiquitous in the environment and ordinarily compose the normal flora (Table 98–3).

DIAGNOSTIC PROBLEMS IN THE COMPROMISED HOST

PULMONARY INFILTRATES

The immunocompromised patient with pulmonary infiltrates presents a particularly vexing diagnostic problem. The pulmonary infiltrates could represent infection, extension of underlying tumor, complication of chemotherapy, or some combination of these. Specific diagnosis is necessary. Unfortunately, noninvasive serodiagnostic tests rarely are helpful in this setting, yet concomitant thrombocytopenia too often increases the risk of lung biopsy.

The clinical setting and radiographic appearance of the pulmonary infiltrate influence the probable yield of lung biopsy and the decision as to whether to proceed. For example, in patients with leukemia, parenchymal infiltrates occurring before or within three days of initiating chemotherapy usually are bacterial, as are focal infiltrates developing later in the course. Major efforts should be directed at obtaining adequate sputum samples for Gram's stain and culture (see Chapter 88); the evolution of the pneumonitis during antibiotic therapy becomes a useful factor in deciding whether to proceed with lung biopsy.

In contrast, diffuse infiltrates occurring *after* treatment of leukemia are more suggestive of opportunistic infection. *Pneumocystis carinii* is an important treatable cause of diffuse infiltrates and occurs most often after treatment for acute lymphocytic leukemia or in patients with an acquired deficiency of cell-mediated immunity (see also Chapter 97). In these settings, the diagnosis should be established by examination of induced sputum, by bronchoalveolar lavage, or, less commonly, by transbronchial biopsy. If these diagnostic approaches are not helpful, empirical therapy with trimethoprim-sulfamethoxazole may be initiated.

The indications and timing of lung biopsy, when needed, must be individualized. Delay in proceeding

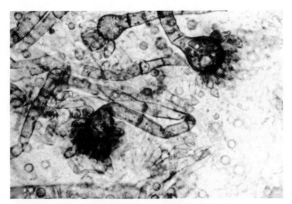

FIGURE 98–1. Fruiting head of *Aspergillus fumigatus* on lung biopsy. Aspergillosis usually causes an expanding perihilar pulmonary infiltrate. Prompt institution of amphotericin B therapy may lead to a good clinical response.

with biopsy, to a point at which the patient is severely hypoxic, nullifies the chances of affecting the outcome with therapy, even if the biopsy shows a potentially treatable disease.

Once the decision has been made to perform a biopsy, the next question is which procedure to use. Fiberoptic transbronchial biopsy has provided a good diagnostic yield, particularly in the evaluation of diffuse pulmonary lesions. This technique should not be performed in the thrombocytopenic patient. It is imperative that the tissue obtained be processed and examined quickly. Open lung biopsy has an additional yield of 50 to 75 per cent in the patient with a nondiagnostic transbronchial biopsy and should be performed without delay if the tempo of progression of the patient's illness mandates immediate diagnosis. Open lung biopsy can generally be performed in thrombocytopenic patients if prophylactic transfusions can achieve an increment in the platelet count and diminish the bleeding time.

Early treatment of most pulmonary infections in immunocompromised hosts, even aspergillosis (Fig. 98–1), is associated with an initially favorable outcome. The long-term result, however, is dependent on the natural history of the underlying disease process.

DISSEMINATED MYCOSES

Disseminated mycoses represent another major diagnostic problem in the immunocompromised host. Fungal infections are found postmortem in over one half of patients with leukemia and lymphoma; usually the nature of the infection has not been established antemortem. Culture of a saprophytic organism such as *Candida* from superficial sites does not establish pathogenicity. Even in patients with widespread infection, however, fungemia is a late event.

How, then, can the diagnosis of fungal infection be established early, at a time when the infection is potentially curable? It is important to search for superficial lesions accessible to scraping, aspiration, or biopsy (Fig. 98–2). Dissemination of *Candida tropicalis*

frequently causes hyperpigmented macular or pustular skin lesions that show the organism on biopsy. Cryptococcal polysaccharide antigen may be present in serum or CSF of the patient with disseminated cryptococcosis. Serodiagnosis for other fungi has, in general, been disappointing. In the absence of adequate diagnostic procedures, empirical use of antifungal drugs is often indicated in the immunocompromised host when there is appropriate clinical suspicion of disseminated mycoses (for example, in the neutropenic patient with fever for more than seven days despite broad-spectrum antibiotic therapy).

PREVENTION AND TREATMENT OF INFECTIONS IN THE NEUTROPENIC PATIENT

PREVENTION

Acute bacterial infections and septicemia arising from organisms comprising the gut flora occur frequently in granulocytopenic patients and may have fever as their sole manifestation. Prophylactic nonabsorbable antibiotics and protective isolation have generally failed to prevent such infection. Recently, trimethoprim-sulfamethoxazole has been given prophylactically and has been shown to decrease the number of infections and bacteremic episodes in some neutropenic patients. Trimethoprim-sulfamethoxazole prophylaxis is not effective in patients with acute nonlymphocytic leukemia, however, and enthusiasm for its use in other settings has waned because of its bone marrow toxicity and selection of resistant organisms. Quinolones, such as ciprofloxacin, may be at least as effective in preventing bacterial infections and less toxic; quinolones lack activity, however, against *Pneumocystis carinii*.

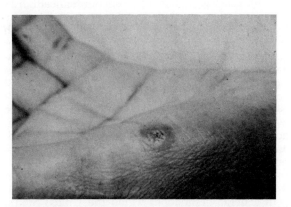

FIGURE 98–2. Skin lesion in a 76-year-old woman treated with corticosteroids and cytotoxic drugs for chronic lymphocytic leukemia and presenting with nodular pulmonary infiltrates and lymphocytic meningitis. Fluid expressed from the lesion contained encapsulated yeast seen on India ink preparation and yielded *Cryptococcus neoformans* on culture.

Prophylactic granulocyte transfusions decrease the occurrence of bacterial sepsis in patients with acute myelogenous leukemia but are costly, and do not affect overall remission rate and duration of survival.

TREATMENT

Empirical antibiotic therapy is indicated in febrile granulocytopenic patients, since up to two thirds have an underlying infection. Selection of two drugs with activity against *Pseudomonas aeruginosa*, such as tobramycin and ticarcillin, is essential. This two-drug regimen also provides adequate initial antibiotic coverage of staphylococcal infections, although clinical experience favors the use of other drugs for their definitive therapy. Despite the early empirical use of antibiotics, the outcome of bacterial infections is poor unless the initial neutrophil count exceeds 500/μl, the count rises during treatment, or the pathogen is a gram-positive organism.

The appropriate duration of antibiotic therapy of febrile neutropenic patients is uncertain. Many physicians continue antibiotics until neutropenia resolves. Empirical addition of amphotericin B therapy is indicated in the neutropenic patient who remains febrile for at least one week despite broad-spectrum antibiotics. In this setting, it often is best to continue broad-spectrum antibiotics for the duration of the neutropenia unless the cause of the fever can be clearly defined.

REFERENCES

Pizzo PA, Young LS: Limitations of current antimicrobial therapy in the immunosuppressed host: Looking at both sides of the coin. Am J Med 76:78, 1984.
Root RK: The compromised host. *In* Wyngaarden JB, Smith LH Jr (eds): Cecil Textbook of Medicine. 18th ed. Philadelphia, WB Saunders Co, 1988, pp 1529–1538.

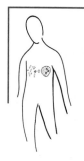

99

INFECTIOUS DISEASES OF TRAVELERS

Over 10 million Americans travel to developing countries each year. They often encounter health risks with which they and their doctors are unfamiliar. The Centers for Disease Control (CDC) publish "Health Information for International Travel," which provides general guidelines for travelers. Specific recommendations must be adjusted to specific locations within a country, as well as to the duration and type of travel anticipated.

Some confusion exists in advice to travelers, since legal requirements and medically indicated precautions are generally separate issues. Both must be addressed and are subject to sudden change. Thus, current information should always be obtained from travelers' clinics, from local health departments, or from the Centers for Disease Control.

In general, destinations within the United States, Canada, Western Europe, Australia, and New Zealand require no specific health precautions. In contrast, a six-week backpacking trip through East Africa may require six or seven different vaccinations given over six to eight weeks, several prescription medications, and patient education.

IMMUNIZATIONS

Only yellow fever and cholera vaccinations are required by law for international travel. Although not generally considered "travel" immunizations, routine immunizations are not up to date in many Americans because immunity was allowed to lapse (e.g., diphtheria-tetanus) or proper immunization was not done in their youth (e.g., measles and polio). Other immunizations are strongly recommended for travel to specific areas.

Yellow Fever. This live attenuated virus vaccine is recommended for travel to areas in South America and Africa where yellow fever is endemic. It is required by law for travel out of a yellow fever endemic area into most other countries (not the United States).

Cholera. This vaccine is of limited effectiveness, and cholera is not a disease of North American tourists. Vaccination is given only to meet the legal requirement for travel between some Third World countries that have endemic cholera. Because of vicissitudes of international travel (unexpected transit into a neighboring country) and uncertainty of obtaining sterile, disposable needles overseas, cholera vaccine is given primarily to protect against unwanted needle sticks in foreign quarantine stations.

Measles and Mumps. Up to 20 per cent of college freshman have no serological evidence of prior measles/mumps infection or immunization and must be presumed to be susceptible. Individuals born after 1956 (measles) and 1970 (mumps), with no documented record of immunization, should receive live attenuated virus vaccination.

Diphtheria-Tetanus. A booster within the last five years eliminates the need for a tetanus booster if the traveler sustains an injury overseas.

Polio. Most young adults have been immunized with at least four doses of trivalent oral polio vaccine (OPV). Many adults (>18 years of age) cannot remember, however, whether they received all serotypes of OPV (mass campaigns used monovalent vaccines) and should be given inactivated polio vaccine (IPV). IPV should be boosted every five years for international travel.

Gamma Globulin. Most travelers from industrialized nations are susceptible to hepatitis A. Hepatitis is the most common serious infectious disease contracted abroad. Published attack rates vary from 1/150 to 1/500 for a routine two-week trip to most developing countries. Immune serum globulin (ISG) is effective in reducing the risk of hepatitis A. For adults, 2 cc is given intramuscularly for trips of less than two months' duration, while 5 cc is of benefit for up to four to six months. ISG should ideally not be given with or prior to immunizations with live attenuated virus vaccines.

Meningococcal Meningitis. Vaccination with the quadrivalent polysaccharide vaccine (A, C, Y, + W-135) is recommended for travel to northern India, Nepal, certain parts of sub-Saharan Africa, and Saudi Arabia.

Typhoid. Typhoid vaccination is clearly indicated for travelers with achlorhydria, immunosuppression, or sickle cell anemia. Vaccination is often recommended for prolonged travel (more than three weeks) to areas with poor sanitation.

Other Vaccines. Some travelers need special consideration, including missionaries, physicians, and anthropologists, who live for prolonged periods in developing countries or are at special risk for contracting certain highly contagious diseases. Consideration should be given to immunization with hepatitis B, Japanese-B encephalitis, plague, rabies, and BCG vaccines.

MALARIA PROPHYLAXIS

Malaria prophylaxis is a major problem for international travelers because of the increase in drug resistance and the toxicities of existing antimalarial drugs (e.g., Fansidar). The need for, and the type of, prophylaxis is usually dependent upon the exact itinerary within a given country. For example, malaria does not occur in most urban centers in Southeast Asia such as Bangkok, but highly drug-resistant strains of

Plasmodium falciparum may be encountered just a few miles into the countryside. Recommended chemoprophylactic regimens change frequently and are often out of date in textbooks. Detailed information on malaria risk is contained in the annual "Health Information for International Travel," which is updated frequently.

Travelers to areas where chloroquine-sensitive *P. falciparum* strains are common (Central America, most parts of India and Southeast Asia, the Middle East, and most parts of West Africa) should take chloroquine phosphate (300 mg base or 500 mg salt) weekly starting two weeks before, during, and for six weeks after leaving malaria endemic areas. No completely safe and effective chemoprophylaxis is available for chloroquine-resistant *P. falciparum* malaria. Therefore, travelers, in addition to taking weekly chloroquine, should carry antibiotics for presumptive treatment for acute malaria (three tablets of pyrimethamine/sulfadoxine sold under the trade name Fansidar), which are self-administered for a temperature over 102°F when appropriate medical care is unavailable.

In sulfa-allergic patients, daily doxycycline (100 mg) is given alone. Neither regimen is very effective in Burma or Thailand, where combined chloroquine and Fansidar resistance is common. Combined resistance is a growing problem in East Africa. The preferred chemoprophylaxis in these areas as well as chemoprophylaxis for prolonged travel in any area endemic for chloroquine-resistant malaria is controversial. Recommendations include weekly Fansidar (associated with 1/11,000 to 1/25,000 risk of fatal reactions in users) and the use of other drugs in addition to chloroquine (including proquanil and amodiaquine). Some authorities recommend no prophylaxis with instructions to seek medical advice immediately when a fever develops. Emphasis should be given to the use of netting, screens, and insect repellants as well as prompt diagnosis and treatment of any febrile episodes overseas.

TRAVELER'S DIARRHEA

Between 20 and 50 per cent of persons traveling to a Third World country develop diarrhea during or shortly after their trip. Traveler's diarrhea is usually caused by toxigenic *E. coli*. The average duration of an episode of traveler's diarrhea is four days. About 10 per cent of episodes last longer than one week. The diarrhea may be accompanied by abdominal cramping, nausea, headache, low-grade fever, vomiting, or bloating. Less than 5 per cent of persons have fever (>101°F), bloody stools, or both. Travelers with these symptoms do not have simple traveler's diarrhea and should see a physician at once.

Both this problem and more serious medical illness can be avoided through care with food and water. All water should be presumed to be unsafe, and dairy products should generally be avoided.

Pepto-Bismol (bismuth subsalicylate) can be used as a prophylactic measure (two tablespoons four times a day) or used to treat acute bouts of diarrhea (one ounce every 30 minutes for eight doses). Lomotil (diphenoxylate) and Imodium (loperamide) may give some symptomatic relief of diarrhea but should be avoided if the diarrhea is severe, fever exists, or blood is present in the stool. Bactrim (TMP-SMZ), doxycycline, or one of the quinalones can be taken orally for three to five days to treat episodes of diarrhea. These regimens dramatically reduce the duration of symptoms and treat a wide variety of bacterial pathogens, including *Shigella* and *Salmonella* species as well as enterotoxigenic *E. coli*. Prophylactic antibiotics are not generally recommended except for very short trips because the risk of adverse drug reactions outweighs the potential benefits (see Chapter 92).

GENERAL HEALTH INFORMATION

Other potentially dangerous activities overseas including petting dogs and cats (rabies), swimming in fresh water (schistosomiasis), walking barefoot (hookworm or strongyloidiasis), and insect bites (e.g., dengue, sleeping sickness, malaria).

SPECIAL PROBLEMS

Pregnant Women. Most vaccines are contraindicated in pregnant women and greatly complicate pretravel preparations. Chloroquine probably can be used safely, but travel to chloroquine-resistant malaria areas is risky and should be strongly discouraged. No drug regimen to prevent or treat chloroquine-resistant malaria is safe in pregnancy, and malaria in a pregnant woman is a medical emergency for both the mother and the fetus.

AIDS. Both travelers and host countries are concerned with AIDS. The People's Republic of China has recently required HIV serologic testing for all travelers applying for more than a three-month visa, and this practice may soon extend to other countries.

Most international travelers are concerned about the risk of acquiring AIDS. Prostitutes pose a particular risk in certain developing countries. The most important concerns, however, are contaminated blood or nonsterile needles that might be used in an emergency. The greatest risk is for travel to Central and East Africa, where HIV infection is at least as common as in the United States. Only a few hospitals in these countries now have sterile, disposable needles and adequate blood screening.

THE RETURNING TRAVELER

Three clinical problems often arise in travelers soon after return. Fever is most important, since delay in the diagnosis of *P. falciparum* malaria can be fatal. Fever should always be considered malaria until proven otherwise in travelers returning from malaria-endemic countries. Tuberculosis, hepatitis, amebic liver abscess, and typhoid fever should then be considered. Traveler's diarrhea that is unresponsive to antibiotics and persists until the traveler returns home is often caused by *Giardia*. Antibiotic-resistant bacteria, amebiasis, temporary lactose intolerance, and bacterial overgrowth should then be considered. Eosinophilia in a returning traveler is less common but is usually caused by helminth infections. A stool examination for ova and parasites may be negative during the tissue-migrating phase of many parasites or in tissue nematode infections such as filariasis or onchocerciasis.

Finally, some diseases acquired abroad can take several years to manifest symptoms. All travelers should be advised to remind their doctor of past international travel when presenting with an unknown illness.

REFERENCES

Centers for Disease Control: Health Information for International Travel. U.S. Public Health Service, Department of Health and Human Services. Publication No [CDC] 87-8280, 1987 (updated weekly by CDC).

Jong EC (ed): The Travel and Tropical Medicine Manual. Philadelphia, WB Saunders Co, 1987.

Steffan R, Rickenbach M, Wilhelms U, et al: Health problems after travel to developing countries. J Infect Dis 156:84–91, 1987.

MUSCULOSKELETAL AND CONNECTIVE TISSUE DISEASES

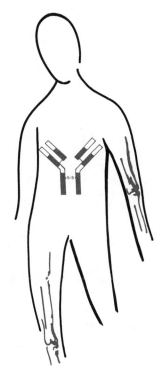

100

RHEUMATIC DISEASES

The rheumatic diseases are a diverse group of disorders that affect the supporting tissue and parenchyma of different organ systems. Although these disorders are often referred to as collagen vascular diseases, the preferred designation is connective tissue disease or systemic rheumatic disease.

It is convenient to think of rheumatic disorders as inflammatory or noninflammatory processes. Rheumatoid arthritis is a prototypical inflammatory disease, whereas fibromyalgia is a noninflammatory ailment. The inflammatory processes are generally classified as either autoimmune or nonautoimmune. An autoimmune disease is a process in which an immune response is mounted against self tissue antigens. Systemic lupus erythematosus (SLE) is an autoimmune syndrome; gout is a nonautoimmune, inflammatory process. The symptoms and signs that characterize the rheumatic disorders tend to be variable and overlapping. Because their etiologies remain unknown, several rheumatic diseases are syndromes, or collections of symptoms and signs, that are recognized as specific entities when grouped together. Both mixed connective tissue disease and fibromyalgia are well-recognized syndromes.

The natural history of the rheumatic diseases is often variable and unpredictable. A prolonged *latent interval* during which symptoms and signs wax and wane before diagnosis is a characteristic feature of disorders such as Sjögren's syndrome or rheumatoid arthritis. This may make identification of the onset and duration of the process difficult to estimate accurately. The physician often makes the diagnosis of SLE retrospectively. Alternatively, the onset can often be precipitous, a feature common to subacromial bursitis and pseudogout. After the diagnosis has been established, many rheumatic diseases continue to exhibit a wide spectrum of symptoms and signs over time. Both inflammatory and noninflammatory rheumatic disorders characteristically manifest constitutional symptoms of fatigability, malaise, anorexia, and a loss of sense of well-being. Fluctuating symptoms or episodic exacerbations and remissions are common and reflect a *periodicity* that is observed in both inflammatory and noninflammatory processes.

EVALUATION OF THE PATIENT

A detailed history and physical examination are indispensable in the evaluation and treatment of the rheumatic diseases. A diagnosis can often be made by these means alone. Routine laboratory and radiographic studies often play an ancillary role in the diagnosis and management of these disorders, but diagnosis of complicated or subtle problems may require more extensive testing to assist in diagnosis and to de-termine therapeutic choices. The use of tests or procedures to "rule out" a variety of diagnoses provides little useful information. Instead, the necessity to obtain accurate and useful information requires that sufficient time be spent in obtaining a detailed history and in performing a comprehensive examination. Such information provides an invaluable perspective on the individual's current illness and directs the clinician's subsequent evaluation.

Patients with rheumatic disorders most frequently seek medical assistance because they have pain or do not feel well. The characteristics, the duration, the pattern, and the origin of the pain should be established by detailed questioning. Activities that worsen or improve the pain should be noted. Neck and shoulder girdle pain are common complaints. The origin of neck pain is likely to be different in the middle-aged or elderly person from that in an adolescent. Aching posterolateral neck pain with radiation into the lateral aspect of the arm in the absence or presence of paresthesias in a middle-aged person is likely to represent nerve root, or radicular, pain. In contrast, generalized aching pain involving multiple muscle groups, marked fatigability, malaise, headaches, and abdominal distress may represent fibromyalgia in a young woman.

A detailed family history should determine whether parents, grandparents, sibs, or other second- or third-degree family members have similar disorders. Although rheumatoid arthritis is usually an isolated disorder, roughly 10 per cent of cases are familial. Similar familial patterns occur in other connective tissue disorders, including osteoarthritis, spondyloarthritides, and systemic lupus erythematosus. Moreover, a familial history of other rheumatic disorders is also commonly obtained. The recognition that a proband with systemic lupus erythematosus has a maternal cousin with progressive systemic sclerosis and a maternal aunt with Sjögren's syndrome suggests penetrance of an autoimmune gene(s) on the maternal side.

The Physical Examination

A comprehensive physical examination is necessary in the evaluation of connective tissue disorders. Because many apparent local musculoskeletal complaints have their origin distant from the region of pain, the identification of the underlying process may be delayed if only a limited examination is performed. Moreover, the comprehensive examination often provides unanticipated clues. The apparent subacromial bursitis may actually reflect referred pain from an unsuspected neoplasm metastatic to the cervical spine. The recognition of weight loss by history and of an abdominal mass on examination may lead to earlier detection of the primary neoplasm. Thus, shortcuts in the examination can lead to erroneous diagnoses and prolonged delay in further evaluation and treatment. The examination of the locomotor system must include a simultaneous evaluation of the nervous system. The evaluation of muscle weakness of the legs and an associated gait disturbance requires integration of both systems. In the performance of a neuromuscular evaluation, a systemic approach is essential. The neurological examination is reviewed in Chapter 113. To begin, the *tonus* and *bulk* of the major muscle groups should be assessed. While palpating the muscle groups, the clinician should look for generalized tenderness of a muscle group or localized areas of tenderness (tender zones). In addition, note should be made whether any changes are symmetrical or asymmetrical. The evaluation of a suspected myopathy requires that the observer take the time to look for fasciculations or myokymia. Analysis of muscle strength includes manual testing, having the patient sit up from a supine position and stand from a sitting position, and observing stance and gait. The joint examination includes the temporomandibular joints; the small joints of the hands and feet; the non–weight-bearing wrists, elbows, and shoulders; and the weight-bearing hips, knees, and ankles. The architecture of these joints and their function should be initially noted and tested. Abnormal architecture of a joint may be due to active synovitis, effusion, or deformity. A joint may be acutely deformed owing to synovitis, effusion, or subluxation. Subluxation connotes malalignment of a joint and includes varus and valgus defects. Chronic deformity often stems from subluxation and/or contracture. A joint contracture refers to a fixed and limited degree of extension. Because edema around the ankles is sometimes confused with synovitis, a careful analysis is necessary. Next, the joint should be palpated to ascertain squeeze tenderness, synovitis, effusions, synovial cysts, and para-articular tenderness. The function of a joint can be tested by analyzing its range of motion. Each joint has a well-defined, physiological angle through which it moves. Depending upon the specific joint, this range of motion may include not only flexion and extension, but internal and external rotation, forward flexion, abduction, adduction, plantar flexion, and dorsiflexion. The extent of a joint's abnormal architecture and mobility should be carefully recorded in the medical record in order to gauge the effect of therapy or a change in disease activity in the future. Because pain or dysfunction in the area of a joint is not necessarily articular in origin, attention should be directed to the para-articular region. Para-articular pain has multiple etiologies, including enthesopathy (pain at the attachment of the tendon or ligament to bone), bursitis, and tendinitis (Fig. 100–1).

The cervical, thoracic, and lumbar vertebral regions exhibit varying architecture depending upon age and sex. In general, the cervical and lumbar regions exhibit lordosis, whereas the thoracic spine shows a kyphosis. The range of motion of the cervical spine can be estimated by testing flexion, lateral mobility, and extension. The movement of the thoracic cage can be gauged by measurement of the difference in chest circumference between inspiration and expiration. Lumbar mobility can be estimated by testing flexion, lateral

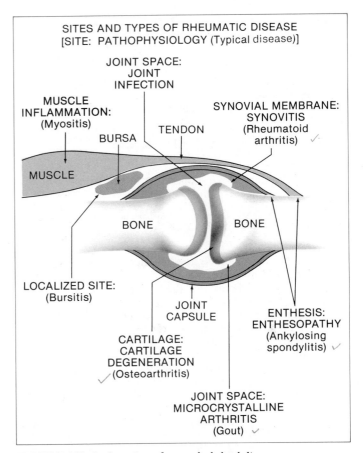

FIGURE 100–1. Location of musculoskeletal disease processes.

bending, and extension. During this examination, evidence of tender zones along the paravertebral muscles and buttocks, as well as sacroiliac joint tenderness, should be sought.

UNDERSTANDING LABORATORY TESTS USED IN EVALUATION OF RHEUMATIC DISEASES

The Erythrocyte Sedimentation Rate (ESR)

In the absence of a laboratory test to identify a specific etiologic agent, other tests are performed to provide an index of the inflammatory response. The ESR, the most commonly employed test of the acute phase response, strongly suggests a systemic inflammatory response.

Of the methods for measuring the ESR, the Westergren method is the simplest and most reproducible. Some of the factors that contribute to an accelerated rate of sedimentation of red cells in disease are listed in Table 100–1. Of these factors, an elevated fibrinogen correlates most closely with an accelerated sedimentation rate. Similarly, certain factors are known

TABLE 100–1. SOME FACTORS THAT CAN ALTER THE ERYTHROCYTE SEDIMENTATION RATE*

ACCELERATION	DECREASE
Hyperfibrinogenemia	Increased serum viscosity
Inflammatory disorders	Sickle cell disease
Rouleaux formation	Spherocytosis
Hyperglobulinemia	Acanthocytosis
Hypochromasia	Polycythemia
Microcytosis	Leukemoid reaction
Hyperlipidemia	Hypofibrinogenemia
Pregnancy	Cachexia
	Congestive heart failure
	High doses of corticosteroids

* After Sox HC, Liang MH: The erythrocyte sedimentation rate. Guidelines for rational use. Ann Intern Med 104:515, 1986.

to produce a falsely low sedimentation rate, as summarized in Table 100–1.

In most laboratories, the normal ESR for men under the age of 50 is between 0 and 15 mm/hr, and for women under the age of 50 between 0 and 20 mm/hr. With increasing age, the range of normal increases. Thus, in healthy persons in the sixth decade or older, the ESR may be elevated in the absence of illness.

The clinical indication for the use of the ESR is the suspicion of an inflammatory disorder. The ESR is often utilized to follow the progress of treatment with anti-inflammatory or disease-remittive agents. The ESR can be unexpectedly normal or only slightly accelerated in certain viral illnesses, including infectious mononucleosis and hepatitis. The ESR should be interpreted as only a crude index of disease activity.

C-Reactive Protein

A second test of the acute phase response that reflects a systemic inflammatory response is the C-reactive protein (CRP). CRP is produced in the liver in small amounts in healthy individuals. During tissue injury, the protein behaves as an acute phase reactant, and its concentration in plasma can exceed 1000-fold normal levels. In contrast to the ESR, serum CRP concentrations rise and subsequently fall rapidly. Thus, the test may be helpful during the early phase of an inflammatory disease.

Serum Immunoglobulins

Serum immunoglobulins are described in Chapter 81 (see Table 81–1 and Figure 81–2). Two techniques are routinely utilized in the clinical laboratory for the characterization and quantitation of serum immunoglobulins. Serum protein electrophoresis separates the serum proteins into characteristic zones; then, scanning of the profile by a densitometer provides a useful technique to identify alterations in the proportions of these proteins. Thus, serum protein electrophoresis is often employed as a screening technique to identify the absence of components, monoclonal immunoglobulin spikes, or beta-gamma bridging. A detailed classification of the alterations of normal serum protein electrophoresis during disease has been developed. In the evaluation of rheumatic diseases, the most common pattern encountered on serum protein electrophoresis is nonspecific, polyclonal increases in IgG, IgM, and/or IgA that occur in response to either acute or chronic inflammation. Quantitation of the serum immunoglobulins is useful in certain rheumatic diseases. Both systemic lupus erythematosus and rheumatoid arthritis can be associated with partial or complete deficiencies of IgA. Similarly, a seronegative inflammatory arthritis resembling rheumatoid arthritis occasionally complicates hypogammaglobulinemia.

Autoantibodies Directed Against Nuclear and Cytoplasmic Antigens

Autoantibodies are composed of IgG, IgA, and/or IgM isotypes directed against self tissue antigens. The antigens include molecules localized to the cell surface, nucleus and/or cytoplasm, and circulating molecules. Such autoantibodies are found predominantly in the sera of individuals with autoimmune diseases. Serological tests to detect autoantibodies are routine in the evaluation of rheumatic disorders and monitoring of treatment.

When the clinical symptoms and signs point to a specific connective tissue disease, an antinuclear antibody (ANA) test may be indicated to delineate the disorder further. Because the ANA can be positive in other, unrelated diseases, this test should not be indiscriminately used to "rule out" a connective tissue disorder. The ANA is detected by indirect immunofluorescence. If immunofluorescence is present, the highest dilution giving a visual fluorescent pattern is reported as the titer of ANA. Depending upon the tissue substrate used, a titer greater than 1:10 or 1:20 is considered significant. A homogeneous pattern of fluorescence indicates antideoxyribonucleoprotein; a rim pattern indicates anti-DNA antibody; and a speckled pattern indicates extractable nuclear antigens.

Autoantibodies have been divided into four major groups: those directed against antigenic determinants within the nucleus; those against cytoplasmic antigens; those against cell surface molecules; and those against autologous immunoglobulins. Anti-native DNA (nDNA) antibodies are routinely used to assess disease activity in SLE, are often indicative of active renal disease, and are employed to monitor the progress of therapy. The titer of ANA is not a reliable indicator of active disease; the circulating anti-nDNA correlates more closely with disease activity. Furthermore, the occurrence of anti-nDNA strongly suggests SLE, although it is occasionally present in low concentrations in other disorders. Although anti–single-strand DNA is present in SLE and may be operative in the pathogenesis of the disease, the antibody is not specific for SLE; it is also found in other rheumatic and nonrheumatic disorders.

Table 100–2 summarizes the commonly observed autoantibodies to histones, DNA nonhistone nuclear proteins, and RNA-protein complexes, and their frequencies in the rheumatic diseases. Antihistone antibodies occur in drug-induced LE, SLE, and rheu-

matoid arthritis. Of the ANAs present in drug-induced
LE, the majority are directed against histones. The
anti-Sm antibody is directed against an RNase-resist-
ant nonhistone nuclear antigen. The antibody, when
present, is specific for SLE but is present in only 20
to 30 per cent of lupus sera. Anti-nRNP antibody is
commonly found in mixed connective tissue disease
(an overlap syndrome). Autoantibodies to nuclear SS-
A and SS-B antigens exhibit a speckled immunofluorescence pattern. Anti-Scl-70 and anti-centromere/ki-
netochore are serological markers for scleroderma and
CREST* syndrome, respectively. Anti–PM-1, anti–
Jo-1, anti–Mi-2, and anti-Ku are autoantibodies detectable in the sera of individuals with polymyositis,
dermatomyositis, or a polymyositis/scleroderma overlap disorder.

Rheumatoid Factors

Rheumatoid factors are antibodies directed against
antigenic determinants on the Fc fragment of IgG.
Although IgG and IgM rheumatoid factors are the
most common, rheumatoid factors can be of the IgM,
IgG, and IgA classes.

The role of rheumatoid factors in homeostasis is not
known. Yet the presence of such factors in 5 to 10 per
cent of normal persons and their increased incidence
during chronic infections suggest that rheumatoid factors operate in concert with other immune mechanisms. Rheumatoid factors are known to activate complement, to convert soluble immune complexes into
insoluble complexes, and to enhance phagocytosis,
chemotaxis, and kinin generation. The observation
that rheumatoid factor exhibits a wide range of functions underscores the concept that these antiglobulins
can mediate physiological responses as well as form
antigen-antibody complexes that can contribute to inflammation in rheumatoid arthritis.

Rheumatoid arthritis patients with positive tests for
rheumatoid factors (i.e., "seropositive" patients) develop more severe disease, in general, than those individuals without rheumatoid factors, termed "seronegative" patients. Also, IgM rheumatoid factors are
associated with more severe and more progressively
disabling disease than IgG rheumatoid factors. Thus,
the measurement of IgM rheumatoid factors is the
most helpful determination.

The presence of a rheumatoid factor is not tanta-
mount to the diagnosis of rheumatoid arthritis. IgM
rheumatoid factors are present in approximately 30 per
cent of other rheumatic diseases. Moreover, there is
a variable incidence of these antiglobulins in the elderly well population, in certain acute and chronic
infections, and in hepatic and pulmonary disorders.

The Classic and Alternative Complement Pathways

The complement cascade contains at least 25 individual serum proteins that interact with and modify

---

* CREST = Calcinosis, Raynaud's phenomenon, Eso-
phagal dysmotility, Sclerodactyly, and Telangiectasia.

TABLE 100–2. ANTINUCLEAR ANTIBODIES IN SYSTEMIC RHEUMATIC DISEASES

ANA	DISEASE ASSOCIATION (FREQUENCY, %)
Autoantibodies to DNA	
Native DNA (nDNA)	SLE (50–70%)
Single-strand DNA (ssDNA)	SLE, other rheumatic and nonrheumatic diseases
Autoantibodies to Histones	
H1, H2A, H2B, H3, H4	Drug-induced LE (95–100%)
	Rheumatoid arthritis (15–20%)
	SLE (30–80%)
Autoantibodies to Nonhistone Nuclear Antigens	
Sm	SLE (20–30%)
U1-RNP (nRNP)	Overlap syndrome (95–100%)
	SLE (30–40%)
SS-A (Ro)	Sjögren's syndrome (60–70%)
	SLE (30–40%)
	Neonatal lupus syndrome
SS-B (La)	Sjögren's syndrome (50–60%)
	SLE (15%)
Scl-70	Scleroderma (15–20%)
Centromere	CREST* (70–90%)
PM-1	Polymyositis (50%)
	Polymyositis/scleroderma overlap (87%)
	Dermatomyositis (17%)
Jo-1	Polymyositis (31%)
	Dermatomyositis (5%)
Mi-2	Dermatomyositis (30%)

Modified from Tan EM: Autoantibodies to nuclear antigens (ANA): Their immunobiology and medicine. Adv Immunol 33:173, 1982.
* CREST = Calcinosis, Raynaud's, Esophageal dysmotility, Sclerodactyly, Telangiectasia.

the function of the immune system (see Chapter 81).
The cascade is divided into three portions: (1) the classic arm, (2) the alternative or properdin arm, and (3)
the terminal attack sequence.

The classic pathway can be activated by immune
complexes. Although not all antigen-antibody complexes bind complement equally, larger immune complexes attach to C1q, resulting in the sequential activation of C1r, C1s, C4, C2, and the fragments C3a
and C3b.

The alternative or properdin arm of the complement system can be activated by IgA, bacterial polysaccharides and endotoxins, and perhaps IgE. The activated intermediate products factor B, factor D, and
properdin (P) finally interact with C3, resulting in the
cleavage fragments C3a and C3b.

The terminal attack sequence is activated upon
cleavage of C3. This results in the sequential activation of C5, C6, C7, C8, and C9. Adherence to the
target of the C5-C9 complex results in lysis and destruction.

Complement measurements are helpful in gauging
the activity of certain rheumatic diseases. The CH50,
or total hemolytic complement, depends upon intact
and functional classic and terminal pathways, resulting in effective target (red blood cell) lysis. In general,

normal CH50 levels imply that there is no enhanced activation of the pathway leading to "consumption" of individual complement components and that there are normal levels of these components. In contrast, decreased CH50 levels suggest either depletion of complement proteins by an immune-mediated process or an inherited deficiency of an individual protein. In the presence of decreased CH50 levels due to an immune mechanism, low levels of C1q, C4, C2, and C3 are ordinarily observed.

Assessment of the complement system in a patient with a suspected or documented rheumatic disorder is best provided by determining the CH50, C3, and C4 levels. Under certain clinical circumstances, as when monitoring the results of therapy of lupus glomerulonephritis, the clinician may serially follow C4 and C3 levels as well as CH50. Whatever complement levels are measured, it is important to monitor them at regular intervals over time to establish a response to therapy.

In the evaluation of individuals with symptoms of an obscure connective tissue disorder, it is often useful to consider an inherited complement component deficiency disorder. Isolated deficiencies of nearly all components have been recognized. This can be assessed by the CH50, which is usually low or absent. Subsequently, the presence of a heterozygous or homozygous deficiency of an isolated complement protein can be established by family studies.

Deficiencies of components of the classic complement pathway are associated with an increased frequency of rheumatic disorders, including systemic lupus erythematosus and hereditary angioneurotic edema. Deficiencies of C1, C4, and C2 are associated with systemic lupus erythematosus. In this circumstance, the SLE is milder, exhibits less renal involvement, has more extensive cutaneous involvement, and exhibits only low titers of ANA. A deficiency of functionally active C1 inhibitor (C1-INH) can result in angioedema. Two major forms of the deficiency are recognized: the congenital type, designated hereditary angioneurotic edema, and the acquired form, which is associated with systemic lupus erythematosus and lymphoid malignancies. The C1 inhibitor is a protease inhibitor present in normal human plasma that regulates enzymes of the coagulation, complement, and fibrinolytic or kinin-producing pathways. The more common type of hereditary angioneurotic edema is observed in 85 per cent of patients and is characterized by low levels of functional C1 inhibitor and C1 inhibitor antigen. The second form of hereditary angioneurotic edema occurs in 15 per cent of patients who manifest low levels of functional C1 inhibitor but normal or increased levels of a dysfunctional C1 inhibitor protein (i.e., normal or increased C1 inhibitor antigen). Table 100–3 summarizes the complement deficiencies associated with rheumatic or infectious diseases and malignancies.

The Synovial Fluid Analysis

A small amount of synovial fluid is present in the normal diarthrodial (synovium-lined) joint. This fluid provides both nutrients to the avascular cartilage and lubrication during joint movement. Characteristics of normal and pathological synovial fluids are presented in Table 100–4.

Analysis of the synovial fluid is integral to the evaluation of an arthritic disorder. Examination of the fluid makes it possible to categorize a synovitis as noninflammatory or inflammatory based upon the total leukocyte count and the per cent neutrophils. Table 100–4 provides such a classification of effusions. Synovial fluid analysis includes a description of the appearance, viscosity, and mucin clot formation. Gram's stain can identify the presence of extracellular or intracellular bacteria. A Wright stain is done to perform a leukocyte differential count. Inspection of the fluid for crystals is performed under both white light and polarizing microscopy. Examination of the synovial fluid expedites diagnosis because one can often identify the presence of infection or the type of crystals. All inflammatory synovial fluids should be cultured regardless of whether bacteria are identified by Gram's stain. Additional pertinent studies include a total protein and glucose (with simultaneous blood total protein and glucose). Special studies may include cytology for malignant cells; levels of complement (with simultaneous blood complement); antigammaglobulins; and specific antigens by countercurrent immunoelectrophoresis.

Association Between Rheumatic Diseases and HLA Specificities

The human leukocyte antigens (HLA) are cell-surface molecules controlled by genes located at the major histocompatibility complex on the short arm of the sixth chromosome of man. These gene products are divided into two classes. The class I molecules, which comprise the HLA-A, B, and C loci of the major

TABLE 100–3. COMPLEMENT COMPONENT DEFICIENCIES IN RHEUMATIC AND INFECTIOUS DISEASES AND MALIGNANCIES*

COMPLEMENT COMPONENT	DISEASE
C1q	Glomerulonephritis
C1r	Glomerulonephritis; SLE-like disorder
C1s	SLE-like disorder
C1-INH	Hereditary angioedema; discoid lupus; SLE; SLE-like disorder
C4	SLE; Sjögren's syndrome
C2	SLE; discoid lupus; polymyositis; Henoch-Schönlein purpura; Hodgkin's disease; vasculitis; glomerulonephritis; common variable hypogammaglobulinemia
C3	Vasculitis; SLE-like disorder; glomerulonephritis
C5	SLE; Neisseria infections
C6, C9	Neisseria infections
C7	SLE; rheumatoid arthritis; Raynaud's phenomenon and sclerodactyly; vasculitis; Neisseria infections
C8	SLE; Neisseria infections

* After Ruddy S: Complement. In Cohen AS (ed): Laboratory Diagnostic Procedures in the Rheumatic Diseases. 3rd ed. Orlando, FL, Grune & Stratton, 1985, p 152.

TABLE 100–4. SYNOVIAL FLUID ANALYSIS*

DIAGNOSIS	APPEAR-ANCE	TOTAL WHITE CELL COUNT PER CUBIC MILLIME-TER†	POLYMORPHO-NUCLEAR CELLS	MUCIN CLOT TEST	SYNOVIAL FLUID–BLOOD GLUCOSE DIFFER-ENCE (MEAN MILLI-GRAMS PER DEC-ILITER)	MISCELLA-NEOUS (CRYSTALS, ORGANISMS)
Normal	Clear, pale yellow	0–200 (200)	<10%	Good	No significant difference‡	—
Group I (noninflammatory effusions)						
Degenerative joint disease; traumatic arthritis	Clear to slightly turbid	50–4000 (600)	<30%	Good	No significant difference	—
Group II (noninfectious, mildly inflammatory)						
Systemic lupus erythematosus; scleroderma	Clear to slightly turbid	0–9000 (3000)	<20%	Good (occasionally fair)	No significant difference	Occasional LE cell; decreased complement
Group III (noninfectious severe inflammatory effusions)						
Gout	Turbid	100–160,000 (21,000)	~70%	Poor	10	Monosodium urate crystals
Pseudogout	Turbid	50–75,000 (14,000)	~70%	Fair-poor	Not enough data	Calcium pyrophosphate dihydrate crystals
Rheumatoid arthritis	Turbid	250–80,000 (19,000)	~70%	Poor	30	Decreased complement
Group IV (infectious inflammatory effusions)						
Acute bacterial	Very turbid	150–250,000 (80,000)	~90%	Poor	90	Culture positive for gram-positive or gram-negative bacteria
Tuberculosis	Turbid	2500–100,000 (20,000)	~60%	Poor	70	Culture positive for *M. tuberculosis*

* From Cohen AS: Specialized diagnostic procedures in the rheumatic diseases. *In* Wyngaarden JB, Smith LH Jr (eds): Cecil Textbook of Medicine. 18th ed. Philadelphia, WB Saunders Co, 1988, p 1994.
† Averages in parentheses.
‡ Less than 10 mg/dl difference.

histocompatibility complex, are found on all nucleated cells but not on sperm and mature erythrocytes. The class I molecules act as recognition structures for the discrimination between self and nonself during immunological interactions. The HLA class II molecules, composed of the HLA-DR, DP, and DQ loci, are expressed primarily on antigen-presenting accessory cells (e.g., macrophages) and on B lymphocytes. These molecules bind polypeptides derived from antigens degraded within accessory cells and initiate a cellular immune response by presenting the polypeptide fragments of antigen to the antigen receptor on helper T lymphocytes. The interaction between accessory cells and T lymphocytes is restricted to autologous cells by these class II molecules because the T cell must recognize the class II molecule before an effective interaction between T cell and accessory cell can take place.

TABLE 100–5. SELECTED HLA AND DISEASE ASSOCIATIONS IN CAUCASIAN PATIENTS*

DISEASE	ANTIGEN	APPROXIMATE RELATIVE RISK
Ankylosing spondylitis	B27	81.8
Reiter's syndrome	B27	40.4
Acute anterior uveitis	B27	8.0
Reactive arthritis (*Yersinia*)	B27	17.6
Rheumatoid arthritis	DR4	6.4
Juvenile rheumatoid arthritis		
Seropositive	DR4	7.2
	DW4	25.8
	DW14	47
	DW4/DW14	116
Pauciarticular	DR5	2.9
Systemic lupus erythematosus	DR3	2.7
Behçet's disease	B5	3.3
Sjögren's syndrome	DR3	5.6

Adapted from Schwartz BD: The major histocompatibility complex and disease susceptibility. *In* Wyngaarden JB, Smith LH Jr (eds): Cecil Textbook of Medicine. 18th ed. Philadelphia, WB Saunders Co, 1988, p 1967.

A highly significant relationship exists between ankylosing spondylitis and the expression of HLA-B27 on leukocytes. Similar but less striking HLA-disease associations are present in other rheumatic diseases (Table 100–5). HLA typing is not useful at this time as an adjunct in the diagnosis of rheumatic diseases. However, the recognition that certain HLA specificities can predispose to disease has prompted further analysis of the mechanisms by which alterations in the genome lead to disease.

REFERENCES

Cohen AS (ed): Laboratory Diagnostic Procedures in the Rheumatic Diseases. 3rd ed. Orlando, FL, Grune & Stratton, 1985.

Fritzler M: Antinuclear antibodies in the investigation of rheumatic diseases. Bull Rheum Dis 35:1, 1985.

Tan EM: Autoantibodies to nuclear antigens: Their immunobiology and medicine. Adv Immunol 33:167, 1982.

101

RHEUMATOID ARTHRITIS

Rheumatoid arthritis (RA) is an inflammatory synovitis of unknown etiology. While the predominant symptoms and signs may involve virtually all synovial joints, RA is often associated with extra-articular involvement of other organ systems. The organs frequently affected include the skin, eye, cardiovascular system, bronchopulmonary system, spleen, and nervous system. Thus, RA is a systemic inflammatory disorder.

IMMUNOPATHOLOGY

The initial event inciting the synovitis is not known. The earliest synovial response to the inciting event is inflammation. In the initial phase, there is hypertrophy of the synovium characterized principally by synoviocyte hyperplasia and increased numbers of blood vessels. Polymorphonuclear leukocytes, B and T lymphocytes, and occasional plasma cells infiltrate the synovium. Upon phagocytosis of immune complexes, polymorphonuclear leukocytes release proinflammatory prostenoids, oxygen radicals, and leukotrienes, which interact synergistically with other mediators to produce vasodilation, edema, heat, and loss of function. Simultaneously, the lining synoviocytes augment the production of synovial fluid, resulting in the accumulation of an effusion. Moreover, the monokine interleukin-1 (IL-1) is found in increased concentrations in RA synovial fluid and contributes to inflammation. IL-1 interacts with substance P, a neurotransmitter of pain impulses in the nervous system, that is released into the inflamed joint. In the joint, substance P activates macrophages to secrete oxygen radicals, prostenoids, and increased amounts of IL-1. The effusions of RA are described in Table 100–4. Rheumatoid factor is also frequently present.

If untreated, the synovitis of rheumatoid arthritis becomes self-perpetuating and chronic. The synovium becomes thickened and boggy, and the predominantly neutrophilic infiltrate is replaced by macrophages, fibroblasts, lymphocytes (approximately 70 to 75 per cent T lymphocytes), and plasma cells. On pathologic section, the synovium takes on a villous appearance. Inward overgrowth of the hypertrophic synovium across the surface of the articular cartilage results in the formation of *pannus*. The inflammatory reaction at the cartilage-pannus junction may eventually result in articular cartilage degradation, paraarticular osteopenia, and ultimately the characteristic marginal erosions observed on x-ray. The degradation of cartilage leaves large, gaping surface ulcers, and with articulation, the rubbing of bone against bone produces crepitus and pain.

Rheumatoid nodules are granulomatous lesions that occur in approximately 20 per cent of individuals with RA and characteristically form at surface sites of friction, such as the extensor surfaces of the arms and tendon sheaths. Moreover, rheumatoid nodules also form in various organ systems, including the heart, lung, and brain. The origin of rheumatoid nodules is controversial. Pathologic studies indicate that these lesions develop about capillaries. Histopathologically, there is a central area of necrosis, an intermediate layer of palisading histiocytes, and a superficial layer comprising lymphocytes and plasma cells. Thus, the rheumatoid nodule could reflect a local response to vasculitis.

CLINICAL MANIFESTATIONS OF RA

RA affects 2 to 3 per cent of the general population. The disease afflicts women in the childbearing years three times more frequently than men. In the older age groups ($\geq$ seventh decade), there is a trend toward more equal involvement of men and women.

RA is an idiopathic, symmetric synovitis affecting similar joints bilaterally. The criteria for the diagnosis of RA are presented in Table 101–1. Occasionally, however, the disease presents as a monoarthritis or asymmetrical oligoarthritis. Over time, the arthritis is additive and assumes a symmetrical distribution. Very early in its course, the predominant symptoms may be vague: variable aching, polyarthralgias, and fatigability with little, if any, definitive clinical evidence of synovitis. It is during this early phase that alternative diagnoses such as fibrositis and polymyalgia rheumatica are considered. Over months, synovitis insidiously evolves, usually in the feet and hands. A second, commonly observed onset is frank synovitis in an otherwise healthy individual. The synovitis most commonly affects the metatarsophalangeal joints of the feet and the metacarpophalangeal and proximal interphalangeal joints of the hands, although other joints can be simultaneously involved. A third but uncommon mode of presentation is that of a rapidly progressive and debilitating polyarticular synovitis, often associated with extra-articular organ system involvement. The fourth and least common onset is the occurrence of extra-articular disease in the absence of clinical evidence of synovitis. An example of the latter is the histopathological diagnosis of a rheumatoid nodule prior to the occurrence of synovitis. While these modes of onset may or may not be associated with the early presence of IgM rheumatoid factors, the aggressive form of RA is often characterized by high titers of rheumatoid factor.

The clinical course of RA is highly variable but usually pursues one of three patterns. The most common is a sporadic course punctuated by variable intervals

TABLE 101–1. CRITERIA FOR RHEUMATOID ARTHRITIS

CRITERIA	CLASSIFICATION
Morning stiffness	Classic rheumatoid arthritis: 7 criteria
Pain on motion or tenderness in at least one joint	Definite rheumatoid arthritis: 5 criteria; joint signs or symptoms continuous for at least six weeks
Swelling (soft tissue or fluid) of at least one joint	Probable rheumatoid arthritis: 3 criteria; joint signs or symptoms continuous for at least six weeks
Swelling of at least one other joint	Possible rheumatoid arthritis: 2 criteria; joint signs or symptoms continuous for at least three weeks
Symmetric joint swelling, same joint on both sides of body (excluding terminal phalangeal joint)	
Subcutaneous nodules	
Roentgenographic changes (at least bony decalcification)	
"Rheumatoid factor" (any method)	
"Poor" mucin precipitate	
Characteristic histological changes—synovium	
Characteristic histological changes—nodules	

After Kellgren et al (eds): The Epidemiology of Chronic Rheumatism, Vol 1, 1963. Courtesy of Blackwell Scientific.

of disease inactivity. The periods of spontaneous remission extend for months to years. This course holds the most favorable prognosis. A second commonly observed pattern is the insidious and relentless progression of synovitis and periodic, debilitating flares. Such flares are accompanied by severe polyarticular pain, flagrant synovitis, joint effusions, marked stiffness, low-grade fevers, and prostration. Because the synovitis involves the joints and tendon sheaths alike, joint subluxations can occur. Pannus formation leads to erosive articular disease and progressive loss of joint function and integrity with eventual fibrosis of tendon sheaths creating joint contractures. The prognosis depends upon the severity and is directly related to treatment intervention. The third, least common clinical course is rapid and aggressive and has been termed "malignant." There is severe polyarticular synovitis, rheumatoid nodules, weight loss, very high titers of rheumatoid factor, and hypocomplementemia. Extra-articular organ involvement of the skin (vasculitis), eyes (scleritis, corneal ulcers), lungs (nodules, interstitial fibrosis), heart (myopericarditis), blood (Felty's syndrome), and nervous system (neuropathy) frequently complicate this aggressive disease (Table 101–2). In the absence of effective treatment, the disease is debilitating and disabling owing to joint contractures, deformities, and the complications of the extra-articular involvement.

The small joints of the hands and feet are the earliest and most common diarthrodial articulations affected. Initially, the synovitis of the proximal interphalangeal (PIP) joints results in fusiform swelling associated with warmth, erythema, pain, and limitation of motion. Independent of PIP involvement, the metacarpophalangeal (MCP) joints develop soft-tissue swelling, squeeze tenderness, and limitation of motion due to synovitis.

TABLE 101–2. EXTRA-ARTICULAR ORGAN SYSTEM INVOLVEMENT IN RHEUMATOID ARTHRITIS

ORGAN SYSTEM	EXTRA-ARTICULAR MANIFESTATIONS
Skin	Cutaneous vasculitis
	Rheumatoid nodules
Eye	Episcleritis
	Scleritis
	Scleromalacia perforans
	Corneal ulcers/perforation
	Uveitis
	Retinitis
	Glaucoma
	Cataract
Lung	Pleuritis
	Diffuse interstitial fibrosis
	Vasculitis
	Rheumatoid nodules
	Caplan's syndrome
	Pulmonary hypertension
Heart and blood vessels	Pericarditis
	Myocarditis
	Coronary arteritis
	Valvular insufficiency
	Conduction defects
	Vasculitis
	Felty's syndrome
Nervous system	Mononeuritis multiplex
	Distal sensory neuropathy

With the exception of severe RA, the distal interphalangeal (DIP) joints are rarely affected.

Chronic synovitis of joints and tendon sheaths often leads to permanent deformities. Because the metatarsophalangeal (MTP) joints of the feet are commonly affected, subluxations of the heads of the MTP's and foreshortening of the extensor tendons give rise to "hammer toe" or "cock-up" deformities. A similar process in the hands results in volar subluxation of the MCP joints and ulnar deviation of the fingers. An exaggerated inflammatory response of an extensor tendon can result in a spontaneous, often asymptomatic rupture. Hyperextension of a PIP joint and flexion of the DIP joint produces a *swan-neck deformity*. The *boutonniere deformity* is a fixed flexion contracture of a PIP joint and extension of a DIP joint.

The radiocarpal, intercarpal, and carpometacarpal joints of the wrists are frequently affected in RA. There is variable tenosynovitis of the dorsa of the wrists, and ultimately, interosseous muscle atrophy and diminished movement due to articular destruction and/or bony ankylosis. Volar synovitis can lead to a compression neuropathy termed carpal tunnel syndrome (see Chapter 117).

Chronic synovitis of the elbows, shoulders, hips, knees, and/or ankles each creates special secondary disorders. Destruction of the elbow articulations can lead to flexion contractures, loss of supination and pronation, and/or subluxations. When the shoulder is involved, limitation of shoulder mobility, dislocation, and spontaneous tears of the rotator cuff resulting in

chronic pain can occur. A result of long-term synovitis of the knee is hypertrophy of the gastrocnemius-semi-membranous bursa (Baker's cyst) of the popliteal fossa. Dissection of the cyst distally into the leg and rupture can mimic acute thrombophlebitis.

Involvement of the cervical spine by RA tends to be a late occurrence in more advanced disease. Pain localized to the lateral neck just inferior to the mastoid bone may be the first indication of inflammation of the C1-C2 articulation. Chronic inflammation of the supporting ligaments of C1-C2 eventually produces laxity, sometimes giving rise to atlantoaxial subluxation. There is posterior displacement of the odontoid process, with a consequent increase in the preodontoid space of greater than the normal range of 2 to 3 mm. Spinal cord compression can result from anterior dislocation of C1 or by vertical subluxation of the odontoid process of C2 into the foramen magnum.

TREATMENT

RA is an eminently treatable disorder, especially if the medical regimen is initiated early in the course of the disease. The objectives of treatment are (a) pain relief, (b) reduction or suppression of inflammation, (c) avoidance or early recognition of side effects, (d) preservation or restoration of function, and (e) maintenance of life style. The response to therapy can be gauged by the physician's global assessment of the patient's well being and by the criteria listed in Table 101–1.

The conservative therapy of RA requires a multi-faceted approach. The importance of an ongoing educational program in RA cannot be overstated. Education should emphasize the benefits of a balanced daily program of rest and exercise. Physical and occupational therapy instruction in the appropriate exercises, along with the judicious application of splinting, can prevent and treat deformities, enhance muscle tone and strength, and preserve or improve function.

The pharmacological therapy of RA often necessitates a combination of agents. It has been useful to approach therapy logically utilizing a "treatment pyramid." Treatment is initiated with either aspirin or a nonsteroidal anti-inflammatory agent. The use of aspirin should result in a therapeutic serum salicylate level of 20 to 30 mg/dl. Because of the potential side effects of acetylated salicylates such as gastrointestinal hemorrhage secondary to peptic ulcer or gastritis, or a bleeding diathesis resulting from aspirin-induced inhibition of platelet aggregation, the use of a nonacetylated derivative, choline magnesium salicylate, should be considered. A second group of agents includes the antimalarials and gold salts. Hydroxychloroquine is the most common antimalarial in use in the United States. Although the specific mechanism(s) by which these agents reduce synovitis in RA remains unknown, antimalarials do produce anti-inflammatory activity by stabilizing lysosomal membranes, reducing phagocytic and chemotactic functions of polymorphonuclear leukocytes, and inhibiting prostaglandin formation. If an efficacious response is not obtained within six months, the agent is discontinued. The major toxicity of the antimalarials is their potential to deposit on the cornea, to produce macular pigmentation, or to result in field defects. Although emphasis has been placed upon these potential adverse reactions, the occurrence of visual impairment due to hydroxychloroquine is rare and can be prevented by routine ophthalmologic exams.

Gold salts are the standard disease-modifying therapeutic agents used in RA. They are regarded as remitting agents. Although the precise mode(s) of action in RA is unknown, these agents appear to alter macrophage function and complement metabolism. Two intramuscular forms of the agent are currently available: gold thioglucose and gold sodium thiomalate. The indication for initiating treatment with gold salts remains controversial. In general, the agents are more efficacious when begun early in the course of seropositive disease. In the absence of significant side effects, a total of 1 gm is given and the response to therapy is then assessed. If there is improvement in disease activity (Tables 101–1 and 101–2), therapy is maintained with an increasing time interval between injections. Since there are multiple potential adverse reactions to the gold salts, these agents should be carefully monitored for hematologic, dermatologic, and renal side effects at regular intervals.

Other chemotherapeutic remitting agents are also utilized in the therapy of RA. These include penicillamine, methotrexate and azathioprine. Since these agents produce untoward side effects, it is necessary to monitor the blood count, differential, platelet count, and urinalysis at regular intervals.

Corticosteroids are routinely used in both the acute and chronic management of RA. Although these agents are clearly beneficial in the therapy of an acute flare, their long-term use is not warranted, since steroids neither cure nor alter the natural course of the disease. In fact, the prolonged use of corticosteroids, even in small or "maintenance" doses, is fraught with numerous unwanted complications, including cataracts, osteopenia, myopathy, and accelerated atherosclerosis. Nevertheless, corticosteroids are indicated in the immediate therapy of rapidly progressive RA complicated by anorexia, weight loss, fever, anemia, leukopenia, vasculitis, pleuropericarditis, Felty's syndrome, and/or hypocomplementemia. Moreover, intra-articular corticosteroids are useful following arthrocentesis to quell the synovitis, reduce pain, and improve function.

REFERENCES

Cohen AS (ed): Laboratory Diagnostic Procedures in the Rheumatic Diseases. 3rd ed. Orlando, FL, Grune & Stratton, 1985.

Fassbender HG: Normal and pathological synovial tissue with emphasis on rheumatoid arthritis. *In* Cohen AS, Bennett JC (eds): Rheumatology and Immunology. 2nd ed. Orlando, FL, Grune & Stratton, 1986.

Greenberg PD, Zvaifler NJ: Rheumatoid arthritis. *In* Cohen S, McCluskey R, Ward P (eds): Mechanisms of Immunopathology. New York, John Wiley & Sons, 1979.

102

SYSTEMIC LUPUS ERYTHEMATOSUS

Systemic lupus erythematosus (SLE) is an acute and chronic inflammatory process of unknown etiology which involves multiple organ systems. It is the prototype autoimmune disorder. This disorder, which afflicts women eight times more frequently than men, predominantly strikes women during their childbearing years. While the general prevalence is approximately 1 in 2100, the disease is observed three times more often in black than white women.

There is a strikingly wide spectrum of disease activity in SLE. When the lesions are confined to the skin, the disorder has been previously termed discoid lupus erythematosus. Although this terminology is still in use, discoid LE is now regarded as a part of the broad spectrum of SLE. In contrast to this benign form of the disease, SLE can be a fulminant, debilitating, and life-threatening disease. Acute proliferative glomerulonephritis can be associated with severe hypertension and the rapid onset of end-stage renal failure, a cause of death. Other common causes of death include hemorrhage secondary to thrombocytopenia, nervous system involvement, and infection. With improved management during the past two decades, the 10-year survival rate is now greater than 85 per cent, and the quality of life has been vastly improved.

CLINICAL MANIFESTATIONS

Both the clinical presentation and course of SLE are highly variable. Since SLE is a syndrome, not a specific disease entity, the disorder can present as symptoms and signs involving one or more major organ systems. Moreover, SLE can manifest as a single symptom that resolves spontaneously, not to be followed by another symptom for months or years, long after the initial ailment is forgotten. Such an insidious onset is common in SLE. By contrast, SLE can present precipitously de novo as a rapidly progressive, multisystem illness. The ARA Diagnostic and Therapeutic Criteria Committee has published revised criteria for the classification of SLE, which can be used by the clinician as a guide in establishing the diagnosis.

Nonspecific constitutional symptoms often accompany disease activity in SLE. The most common symptoms include fatigue, anorexia, weight loss, and fever (Table 102–1).

Skin lesions of SLE are among the most common signs of the disease, occurring in 85 per cent of individuals (Table 102–1). They include alopecia, painless oral ulcers, a discoid rash, photosensitive skin eruptions, urticaria, bullae, and the classic butterfly rash.

Several distinct skin lesions have been observed in SLE. Among these, discoid lesions and vasculitis are commonly observed. In discoid lesions there is a characteristic vacuolar appearance to the dermoepidermal junction where immunoglobulin and complement can be deposited. Using immunofluorescence techniques, a band of granular deposits comprising IgG, IgA, IgM, and/or complement is found. This skin biopsy staining technique, the lupus band test, signifies the deposition of immune complexes in tissue, and the presence of IgG and C3 correlates with active systemic disease, particularly glomerulonephritis.

Vasculitis affects several organ systems in SLE. The presence of inflammation of the capillaries, arterioles, or venules of the skin is called leukocytoclastic vasculitis. Depending upon the age of the lesions, there is either a polymorphonuclear leukocytic or lymphocytic infiltrate of the vessel wall, fibrinoid necrosis, red blood cell extravasation, endothelial cell hypertrophy, interruption of the vessel wall, and deposition of immunoglobulins, complement, and fibrin.

Raynaud's phenomenon of varying severity is observed in about one third of SLE patients. Only a small proportion of patients exhibit fixed Raynaud's phenomenon in warm surroundings or develop digital ulcers.

Polyarthralgias and polyarthritis are the most common manifestations of SLE (Table 102–1). A symmetrical, nondeforming arthritis affecting the small joints of the hands, wrists, knees, and metatarsophalangeal joints occurs and, during early disease, is often confused with rheumatoid arthritis. The presence of prolonged morning stiffness in one half of patients, rheumatoid nodules (7 per cent), and rheumatoid factors (15 to 20 per cent) in persons with active disease often makes the distinction of SLE from RA difficult, especially in the absence of other distinguishing features of SLE.

Other musculoskeletal disorders also complicate SLE (Table 102–1). Myalgias occur in up to one third of patients and tend to be unrelated to the degree of disease activity. In contrast to muscle aching, a true inflammation of muscles occasionally is observed in SLE. It is characterized by painless proximal muscle weakness and is clinically similar to idiopathic polymyositis. When SLE coexists with scleroderma and polymyositis, it is termed an overlap syndrome.

Renal disease occurs in approximately one half of patients with SLE (Table 102–1). Usually presenting within the first 24 months of disease, the findings on urinalysis include proteinuria, microscopic hematuria, and cylindruria. The presence of red and white cell casts, proteinuria, and hematuria in the urine reflects active glomerular disease (See Chapter 31 and Table 31–7).

Polyserositis refers to inflammation of the serosal surfaces of the pericardium, thorax, and abdomen and is characterized by pain (Table 102–1). Involvement of the pericardium can often be documented by the presence of a pericardial friction rub and echocardiographic and electrocardiographic findings characteristic of pericarditis. Pericarditis is commonly associated with myocarditis, and this can lead to a transient or persistent tachyarrhythmia and electrocardiographic evidence of myocardial ischemia. Pleurisy and pleural effusion can result from inflammation of the pleura. Pleuritic pain can also be secondary to acute lupus pneumonitis, which occurs in fewer than 10 per cent of SLE patients. Diffuse abdominal pain and ascites reflect inflammation of the abdominal serosa. However, the pain of serositis must be differentiated from other causes of abdominal pain, especially mesenteric arteritis, acute pancreatitis due to pancreatic vasculitis, or occult perforation of a viscus due to corticosteroid therapy.

Hepatosplenomegaly and systemic adenopathy are commonly observed in SLE (Table 102–1). Clinically significant liver disease has been regarded as unusual in SLE. However, there is a relationship between the symptoms of SLE and chronic active hepatitis. Chronic active hepatitis should be considered in SLE patients with abnormal liver function studies.

The neuropsychiatric manifestations of SLE vary greatly (Table 102–1). Psychosis and seizures can start at any time in the course of SLE. Vascular headaches tend to be associated with active disease, although milder forms are seen during periods of remission as well. Other neurologic disorders that may complicate SLE include CVA, chorea, cranial nerve palsies, peripheral neuropathies, transverse myelopathy, and aseptic meningitis. Although the intracranial arteries can exhibit a perivascular cellular infiltrate producing a vasculopathy, cerebral vasculitis is uncommon.

Hematologic disorders are commonly identified by laboratory testing (Table 102–1). These include anemias of different types, leukopenias (neutropenia, lymphopenia), and thrombocytopenia.

The relationship between SLE and pregnancy continues to be an important issue. Women with active SLE, especially glomerulonephritis, who become pregnant have an increased frequency of exacerbation of their disease as well as missed abortions, stillbirths, and fetal wastage. In addition, they more often have premature labor and delivery. Children born to mothers with SLE have an increased risk of congenital heart block, and this appears to be associated with the transplacental transfer of anti–SS-A. However, women with SLE in remission can have normal pregnancies and do not appear to have an increased rate of exacerbations of their disease nor of fetal wastage or stillbirths.

Drug-induced lupus is a disorder in which a pharmacologic agent induces the symptoms and signs of SLE over time. A list of the agents reported to be associated with an SLE-like syndrome is presented in Table 102–2. Although there is convincing evidence that certain drugs induce a lupus syndrome, the data for the remainder are speculative. Review of some cases diagnosed as drug-induced lupus suggests that a number of these patients had premorbid signs of SLE.

Hydralazine and procainamide are the prototype agents associated with a drug-induced lupus syndrome. The incidence of hydralazine-induced lupus in an unselected group of hypertensive patients was approximately 10 per cent and in patients taking procainamide long term 5 to 30 per cent. Hydralazine causes a syndrome characterized by fever, arthritis, erythematous skin rashes, pleurisy, leukopenia, hypergammaglobulinemia, a positive LE cell test, ANA, and a biological false-positive VDRL. Procainamide, considered the most potent inducer of the drug-induced lupus syndrome, is characterized by arthralgias or arthritis, pleuropericarditis (with or without effusions), rashes, pulmonary infiltrates, and ANA. In both types of drug-induced lupus syndrome, neurologic and renal disease are uncommon, and anti-nDNA and anti-Sm antibodies are absent. In general, withdrawal of the offending agents leads to resolution of the symptoms within days to weeks. However, the ANA can persist for months to years.

IMMUNOPATHOGENESIS

The mechanism by which the immune system is regulated by the presence of genetically determined cell surface molecules encoded by the major histocompatibility loci has been an area of intense interest and research. Since the prevalence of SLE in first-degree relatives of SLE probands is approximately 1.5 per cent and the concordance of SLE in monozygotic twins is about 70 per cent, there appears to be a genetic basis for SLE. The relationship between genetically determined complement component deficiencies and SLE also supports this hypothesis. An association clearly exists between SLE and the major histocompatibility complex (see Table 100–5).

Both the cellular and humoral effector arms of the immune system are impaired in SLE. Several exper-

TABLE 102–1. COMMON CLINICAL ABNORMALITIES IN PATIENTS WITH SLE*

ABNORMALITY	APPROXIMATE FREQUENCY (%)
Constitutional	
Fatigue	90
Fever	80
Weight loss, anorexia	60
Musculoskeletal	
Arthritis, arthralgia	90
Myalgia, myositis	30
Skin and mucous membranes	
Butterfly rash	60
Alopecia	50
Photosensitivity	40
Raynaud's phenomenon	30
Mucosal ulcers	30
Discoid lupus	20
Urticaria	10
Edema or bullae	10
Eye (conjunctivitis/episcleritis/sicca syndrome	20
Gastrointestinal	30
Serosal (pleurisy, pericarditis, peritonitis)	50
Lymphoreticular	
Lymphadenopathy	50
Splenomegaly	30
Hepatomegaly	30
Hypertension	30
Bacterial infections	40
Pneumonitis (all)	30
"lupus"	10
Renal (all)	50
severe	20
Central nervous system	
Personality disorders	50
Seizures	20
Psychoses	20
Stroke or long tract signs	10
Migraine headaches	10
Cardiac	
Myocarditis	30
Murmurs and valvular disease	30
Coronary artery disease	20
Hematologic	
Anemia (all)	70
Hemolytic	10
Purpura (all)	50
Thrombocytopenia	10
Peripheral neuropathy	10

* From Steinberg AD: Systemic lupus erythematosus. *In* Wyngaarden JB, Smith LH Jr (eds): Cecil Textbook of Medicine. 18th ed. Philadelphia, WB Saunders Co, 1988, p 2015.

TABLE 102–2. DRUGS ASSOCIATED WITH A LUPUS-LIKE SYNDROME*

DEFINITE	POSSIBLE	UNLIKELY
Hydralazine	Anticonvulsants	Griseofulvin
Procainamide	Chlorpromazine	Phenylbutazone
Isoniazid	Methyldopa	Oral contraceptives
	Penicillamine	Gold salts
	Quinidine	Sulfonamides
	Propylthiouracil	Penicillin
	Practolol	
	Lithium carbonate	
	Nitrofurantoin	

* After Weinstein A: Drug-induced SLE. Prog Clin Immunol 4:1, 1980.

imental approaches have identified a defect of suppressor T lymphocyte function during active SLE. Although the suppressor dysfunction improves with disease remission, a residual defect appears to persist even during remission. A disorder of helper T lymphocyte function has also been demonstrated. By contrast, there is exaggerated B cell activity in SLE characterized by the production of antibodies directed against numerous immunogens. One hypothesis to explain the hypergammaglobulinemia resulting from B cell hyperactivity holds that impaired suppressor cells cannot regulate B cell function, and, in particular, fail to suppress autoantibody production by forbidden B cell clones.

Immune complexes play a central role in the inflammatory response in SLE. Upon deposition or in situ formation, antigen-antibody complexes induce the activation of the classic complement cascade, the release of various vasoactive peptides and anaphylatoxins, the ingress of polymorphonuclear leukocytes, and the aggregation of platelets. This inflammatory response may ultimately result in destruction of the vessel wall, thrombosis, ischemia, and end-organ destruction.

TREATMENT

When the diagnosis of SLE is made, it is necessary to make a decision as to whether therapy is indicated. This decision rests largely on the degree of disease activity. The SLE patient who is asymptomatic, has no physical stigmata of active disease, but manifests certain abnormal laboratory studies may present a perplexing problem. Under these circumstances, the decision to treat depends upon the type of abnormal studies. Persistently low complement levels by themselves do not require therapy, whereas hemolytic anemia or thrombocytopenia does. In contrast, falling complement levels, rising titers of anti-nDNA, and a change in the urinary sediment suggesting active renal disease signify activation of the disease and demand a prompt therapeutic decision.

Several different drugs are utilized in the management of SLE. Aspirin and the nonsteroidal anti-inflammatory agents are indicated for the treatment of arthralgias or mild synovitis, pleurisy, headache, myalgia, and low-grade fever. Side effects include a modest rise in hepatic transaminases or deterioration in renal function studies, which are reversible with alteration of dosage.

Hydroxychloroquine, an antimalarial agent, has long been recognized to be effective in the treatment of arthralgias, arthritis, and skin disease in SLE. The major drawbacks to this agent are its slow onset of action (about three months) and potential ocular toxicity (see Chapter 101).

The use of adrenal corticosteroids in SLE has gained prominence because of their potent anti-inflammatory effect. Although the indications for initiating corticosteroids are imprecise, clinical, serological, and biochemical evidence for enhanced disease activity constitutes a general guideline. The principal objective of corticosteroid therapy is control of the inflammatory response in order to prevent end-organ damage and deterioration. High-dose intravenous bolus therapy with methylprednisolone (1 gm/day for three consecutive days) has been efficacious in the therapy of poorly responsive glomerulonephritis.

The decision about when to taper the dosage of corticosteroids depends upon the patient's response to therapy. Improvement or resolution of symptoms and signs, a reduction of the anti-nDNA titer, and an increase of the complement levels toward normal concentrations constitute evidence of lessening disease activity. In general, corticosteroids are tapered slowly to prevent a flare of SLE. At a dosage of approximately 10 to 12.5 mg/day of prednisone, disease activity may break through. Such an occurrence, far from uncommon, may require readjustment of the dosage upward, a time interval to re-establish control, and an even slower decrement in dosage. In fact, at a level of 10 mg/day, tapering by 1 mg weekly or more slowly may be necessary.

Lupus nephritis may progress, and there can be continuous deterioration of kidney function despite appropriate corticosteroid therapy. Under these circumstances immunosuppressive agents should be considered. Evidence now indicates that these agents, which principally include azathioprine and cyclophosphamide, when combined with steroids, significantly improve outcome of therapy by preventing further end-organ destruction.

REFERENCES

Schur PH: The Clinical Management of Systemic Lupus Erythematosus. New York, Grune & Stratton, 1983.

Tan EM, Cohen AS, Fries JF, et al: The 1982 revised criteria for the classification of systemic lupus erythematosus. Arthritis Rheum 25:1271, 1982.

103
SJÖGREN'S SYNDROME

Sjögren's syndrome is a chronic connective tissue disorder characterized by inflammation and dysfunction of the exocrine glands, particularly the salivary and lacrimal glands. The disease is categorized as (a) the primary form, or (b) the secondary form, which is commonly associated with RA, SLE, or, less commonly, other connective tissue disorders. The combination of xerophthalmia and xerostomia is referred to as the sicca complex. Keratoconjunctivitis sicca refers to loss of integrity of the corneal epithelium due to desiccation.

CLINICAL FEATURES

Round cell infiltration of the lacrimal and salivary glands produces insidious destruction of glandular tissue, resulting in the sicca complex. There is dryness of the eyes due to decreased and altered tear production, giving the sensation of grittiness or of the presence of a foreign body. With time, there is variable conjunctival injection, reduced visual acuity, and photosensitivity. Prolonged desiccation leads to the development of erosions and sloughing of the corneal epithelium (filamentary keratitis), as demonstrated by rose bengal staining and slit lamp examination. The extent of xerostomia appears to be more variable, even in the presence of striking xerophthalmia. The frequency of dental caries is increased due to diminution of the volume of saliva, which possesses antibacterial factors.

Dryness of other mucosal surfaces as a result of the same inflammatory response is common. In the respiratory tract there may be epistaxis, dysphonia, bronchitis, or pneumonia. Inspissation of secretions in the eustachian tubes leads to obstruction, chronic otitis media, and hearing impairment. Mucosal gland involvement of the gastrointestinal tract produces dysphagia, reduced gastric acid output, constipation, and pancreatic insufficiency. Dyspareunia may occur due to vaginal dryness.

Several prominent extraglandular features can complicate the course of Sjögren's syndrome. Renal tubular acidosis results from infiltrative interstitial nephropathy. Both peripheral and cranial neuropathy have been attributed to vasculitis of the vasa nervorum. Other associated neuromuscular disorders include myopathy, polymyositis, and cranial vasculitis. Dyspnea may be the presenting symptom of underlying diffuse interstitial pneumonitis due to lymphocytic infiltration. An obstructive ventilatory defect has been attributed to peribronchial lymphocytic infiltration. Nonthrombocytopenic purpura of the dependent regions is associated with a polyclonal hypergammaglobulinemia. Raynaud's phenomenon occurs in about one fifth of patients. Chronic Hashimoto's thyroiditis is present in a small proportion of patients with Sjögren's syndrome. Also, hepatomegaly, chronic active hepatitis, biliary cirrhosis, and adult celiac disease have been occasionally observed with Sjögren's syndrome. Table 103–1 lists disorders associated with Sjögren's syndrome.

Systemic lymphadenopathy may reflect benign lymphatic hyperplasia, a pseudolymphoma, or frank lymphoma. Although these can occur early in the course of Sjögren's syndrome, death due to lymphoma often ensues after years of illness. Although the histologic type of the lymphoma is variable, the lymphoma is of B cell origin. Other lymphoproliferative disorders observed with Sjögren's syndrome include Waldenström's macroglobulinemia and myeloma. Markers of increased risk of malignancy include persistent parotid swelling, systemic lymphadenopathy, splenomegaly, and a progressive decrement of a previously elevated class of immunoglobulin and/or rheumatoid factor.

DIAGNOSIS

The diagnosis of Sjögren's syndrome is based upon the results of Schirmer's filter paper test, ophthalmologic exam, and minor salivary gland biopsy. Xerophthalmia is confirmed by the wetting of 5 mm or less of filter paper in 5 minutes in an unanesthetized eye. The demonstration of superficial corneal erosions by rose bengal staining and filamentory keratitis by slit lamp examination indicates more advanced keratoconjunctivitis sicca.

Biopsy of the minor salivary glands of the lower lip in Sjögren's syndrome demonstrates lymphocytic infiltration of the acinar glands and progressive destruction of glandular tissue. The extent of inflammation

TABLE 103–1. DISORDERS ASSOCIATED WITH SJÖGREN'S SYNDROME

Rheumatoid arthritis
Systemic lupus erythematosus
Progressive systemic sclerosis
Overlap syndrome
Polymyositis/dermatomyositis
Graft-versus-host disease
Malignant lymphoma
Chronic Hashimoto's thyroiditis
Chronic active hepatitis
Biliary cirrhosis
Graves' disease
Premature ovarian failure
Celiac disease
Dermatitis herpetiformis
Myasthenia gravis
Pemphigus
Lipodystrophy

can be quantitatively scored using the "focus score." Each aggregate of 50 or more lymphocytes equals a focus, and the number of foci per 4 sq mm of tissue represents the focus score. A score of greater than 1 is compatible with Sjögren's syndrome.

Sjögren's syndrome appears to exhibit a genetic basis. Immunogenetic studies have identified an excess of the HLA antigens B8, DR3, and MT2 (DRw52). The relationship between these B cell alloantigens and DR3 and Sjögren's syndrome suggests that the development and expression of disease is regulated, in part, by immune response genes.

Autoantibodies are commonly found in both primary and secondary Sjögren's syndrome. Antinuclear antibodies are present in up to 80 per cent of persons. IgM rheumatoid factor is found in 60 to 70 per cent. Antibodies to SS-A occur in 50 to 75 per cent in primary Sjögren's syndrome, in 70 to 85 per cent of SLE with Sjögren's syndrome, and in 30 to 40 per cent of patients with SLE overall. Antibodies to SS-B occur in 50 to 60 per cent of Sjögren's syndrome patients, and in only 15 per cent of SLE patients without Sjögren's syndrome (Table 100–2).

THERAPY

The treatment of Sjögren's syndrome is directed at the alleviation of symptoms and complications of xerophthalmia and xerostomia. Xerophthalmia can be treated with artificial tears or with surgical punctal occlusion. Staphylococcal blepharitis should be immediately treated with topical or, if necessary, systemic antibiotics. Xerostomia is managed by maintaining oral hydration and the liberal use of sialogogues. Bronchopulmonary infections require both supportive regimens and antibiotics. Dyspareunia is treatable with commercial water-soluble vaginal lubricants. The use of corticosteroids or immunosuppressive agents is confined to more severe disease of the kidneys or bronchopulmonary tract and systemic vasculitis.

REFERENCES

Lass J, Kammer GM: Complications and management of ocular complications associated with the rheumatic diseases. Seminars Ophthalmol 2:292–305, 1987.
Talal N: Sjögren's syndrome. In Rose N, Mackay I (eds): The Autoimmune Diseases. New York, Academic Press, 1985, pp 145–159.

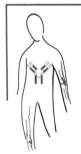

104

POLYMYOSITIS AND DERMATOMYOSITIS

Polymyositis (PM) and dermatomyositis (DM) are inflammatory myopathies of striated muscle of unknown etiology. Although the onset of disease can occur in any age group, the clinical course of these disorders in childhood differs from that in adulthood. Women are afflicted twice as often as men. The incidence in the general population has been estimated to be between 1:200,000 and 1:280,000 per year.

CLASSIFICATION

A classification for PM and DM is based upon their association with other diseases (Table 104–1).

TABLE 104–1. CLASSIFICATION OF POLYMYOSITIS AND DERMATOMYOSITIS*

GROUP	DESCRIPTION
1	Primary idiopathic polymyositis
2	Primary idiopathic dermatomyositis
3	Dermatomyositis or polymyositis associated with neoplasia
4	Childhood dermatomyositis or polymyositis associated with vasculitis
5	Polymyositis or dermatomyositis associated with connective tissue disorder (overlap group)

* After Bohan A, Peter J, Bowman R, Pearson C: A computer-assisted analysis of 153 patients with polymyositis and dermatomyositis. Medicine 56:255, 1977.

CLINICAL COURSE

There is no single presentation or course that typifies either PM or DM. The majority of persons with PM manifest proximal muscle weakness. In dermatomyositis, both the skin rash and proximal muscle weakness occur early in the course. The skin rash consists of a scaly, erythematous eruption over the PIP and MCP joints (Gottron's sign), elbows, knees, medial maleoli, face, and elsewhere. Involvement of the upper eyelids, appearing as a dusky lilac suffusion, is termed a heliotrope rash. Both disorders may be punctuated by spontaneous exacerbations and remissions. Moreover, either disorder can present precipitously with rapid loss of muscle strength leading to acute respiratory distress and death.

When these inflammatory myopathies are associated with another connective tissue disorder, it is designated an overlap syndrome. Interestingly, the ratio of females to males affected increases to 9:1. In addition, PM occurs three times more often than DM. The associated disorders include, in descending order of frequency, scleroderma, SLE, and RA. Although relatively uncommon in PM or DM alone, arthralgias, Raynaud's phenomenon, and myalgias are actually more common than proximal muscle weakness in the overlap syndrome.

The occurrence of malignancy with inflammatory myopathy is relatively uncommon (8.5 per cent) but increases with age. When present, about two thirds of malignancies coexist with dermatomyositis. Carcinomas of the breast, lung, ovaries, colon, endometrium, prostate, and stomach are the leading tumors. In 70 per cent the myositis precedes the diagnosis of malignancy by nearly two years. It is currently recommended that a search for malignancy be conducted in persons with PM or DM over age 50 years.

Cardiopulmonary manifestations include nonspecific ST-T wave changes (23 per cent), arrhythmias (6 per cent), altered Q waves (6 per cent), bundle branch block (5 per cent), congestive heart failure (3.3 per cent), heart block (2.2 per cent), and restrictive lung disease (20 per cent).

When considered as a group of disorders (Table 104–1), the leading cause of death is metastatic malignant disease followed by sepsis. Other causes include profound muscle weakness and cardiovascular failure.

LABORATORY FINDINGS

The CPK is the most reliable serum enzyme and correlates with the activity of disease. The occurrence of a normal CPK in the presence of active myositis is exceedingly uncommon (< 2 per cent). A normal enzyme level may be accounted for by advanced muscle atrophy and loss of muscle mass. ANA is present in 25 per cent and the rheumatoid factor in up to 40 per cent. The sedimentation rate correlates poorly with disease activity and the clinical course. The triad of EMG findings includes (a) small-amplitude, short-duration polyphasic motor unit potentials; (b) fibrillations, positive sharp waves, and insertional irritability; and (c) bizarre, high-frequency discharges. A normal EMG in the presence of active disease is uncommon (10.7 per cent).

The muscle biopsy is an essential component in confirming the clinical diagnosis of PM or DM. The most common histopathological abnormality is degeneration of muscle fibers. Other pathologic findings include an inflammatory infiltrate, centralization of nuclei, regeneration, and interstitial fibrosis.

THERAPY

Treatment of PM or DM includes physical therapy, corticosteroids, and, if indicated, immunosuppressive agents. An intensive course of physical and occupational therapy improves muscle strength and tonus and assists in activities of daily living once muscle inflammation is suppressed.

The initial dosage of corticosteroids depends upon the severity of disease but often is the equivalent of 60 mg of prednisone. Approximately three quarters of patients normalize the CPK within 57 to 102 days. Muscle strength progressively improves with this regimen. The dosage of corticosteroids is tapered on the basis of clinical and biochemical evidence of resolution of disease activity.

An indication for the addition of immunosuppressive therapy is failure of therapy with corticosteroids alone within a four- to six-week interval. The addition of an immunosuppressive agent often provides a "steroid-sparing effect," allowing the daily corticosteroid dosage to be reduced to lower levels. The agents of choice include methotrexate and azathioprine. It is often necessary to maintain long-term therapy with corticosteroids and/or immunosuppressive agents to control disease activity.

PROGNOSIS

The prognosis of PM and DM has improved substantially with the introduction of corticosteroid and immunosuppressive agents. A recent study demonstrated a survival rate of 87 to 91 per cent over a 15-year interval, in those cases not associated with malignancy.

REFERENCES

Hochberg MC, Feldman D, Stevens MB: Adult onset polymyositis/dermatomyositis: An analysis of clinical and laboratory features and survival in 76 patients with a review of the literature. Semin Arthritis Rheum. 15:168, 1986.

Messner RP: Polymyositis. In Wyngaarden JB, Smith LH Jr (eds): Cecil Textbook of Medicine. 18th ed. Philadelphia, WB Saunders Co, 1988, pp 2034–2037.

105

PROGRESSIVE SYSTEMIC SCLEROSIS (SCLERODERMA)

Progressive systemic sclerosis (PSS) is characterized by (a) inflammation, (b) fibrosis, and (c) degeneration of the integument. These pathologic alterations are associated with similar changes and prominent vascular lesions in the gastrointestinal tract, synovium, heart, lung, and kidneys. As a result of progression of these lesions, there is thickening (collagenous), tightening and induration (sclerosis) of the skin, and destruction of the normal architecture of visceral organs, culminating in death due to hypertensive renal disease, malabsorption and cachexia, heart failure, or pulmonary disease.

CLINICAL FEATURES

PSS is a disorder of indeterminate etiology which affects women three times more frequently than men. The onset of disease ranges between the third and fifth decades.

Several sequential phases of the disorder occur in the integument over time. The initial phase, characterized by bilateral, painless pitting edema of the hands, forearms, legs and feet, generally extends over a few weeks to several months. The swollen fingers appear tight and demonstrate variable but limited function. During the second phase, the edema is gradually absorbed, leaving indurated skin. The integument is thickened, tight, and inelastic. This represents the well-known sclerodermatous stage. The third phase is characterized by a taut and shiny appearance. A melanotic hyperpigmentation often develops in a patchy distribution in the affected areas. There is loss of the skin folds, creases, and hair of the fingers. The face takes on the classic appearance of the Mauskof (mouse-head), in which there are pursed lips, bitemporal muscle atrophy, loss of subcutaneous tissue and muscle of the face and neck, and a taut and shiny skin of the malar region and forehead. Other prominent changes in the skin include calcinosis circumscripta (subcutaneous calcifications) and telangiectasias of the fingers, face, lips, and forearms. Raynaud's phenomenon is present in virtually all persons with PSS. This phenomenon is discussed in Chapter 108.

Rheumatic symptoms occur commonly in PSS. Although polyarthralgias are a frequent accompaniment of PSS, active synovitis leading to joint effusions, limitation of range of motion, and severe flexion contractures can present a difficult management problem. Radiographs demonstrate bony resorption of the tufts of the terminal phalanges and subcutaneous calcinosis. Severe, relentless disease often leads to autoamputation of digit(s).

Loss of subcutaneous tissue and muscle bulk steadily progresses over time with consequent weight loss. The myopathy of PSS is the result of an inflammatory myositis indistinguishable from polymyositis and is often referred to as sclerodermatomyositis.

Cardiovascular disorders may complicate the course of PSS. Progressive fibrosis of the myocardium eventually results in the development of a cardiomyopathy. In addition, fibrosis of the conducting pathways can lead to arrhythmias and conduction disturbances. Other disorders include pulmonary arterial hypertension, pericarditis, and pericardial effusions.

Several pulmonary complications of PSS can lead to pulmonary insufficiency and death. Chest radiographs demonstrate a reticular or reticulonodular pattern of interstitial fibrosis. The earliest and most sensitive indicator of pulmonary involvement is a reduced diffusing capacity of carbon monoxide. Progressive diminution of the diffusing capacity with time often predicts gradual progression of the restrictive ventilatory defect.

The gastrointestinal tract is a major target organ in PSS. Esophageal dysfunction may be asymptomatic or be manifested by dysphagia, esophagitis, and/or esophageal reflux (see Chapter 36). Radiographic visualization by barium contrast and esophageal motility studies often demonstrates disordered or absent motility. There may be marked dilatation of the inferior two thirds of the esophagus and strictures may result from chronic reflux esophagitis, ulceration, and healing by fibrosis. Histopathology of the esophagus reveals loss of smooth muscle and increased collagen deposition in the lamina propria and submucosa. Similar histopathologic alterations elsewhere in the gastrointestinal tract result in reduced motility, causing bacterial overgrowth that leads to malabsorption, weight loss, and inanition. Classic radiographic findings on barium contrast studies include the loop sign (dilatation of the second and third segments of the duodenum due to atony) and wide-mouth diverticula of the large bowel (due to atrophy of the muscularis).

Progressive involvement of the kidneys, leading to severe hypertension, renal failure, and death, is a common sequence of events in PSS. Often precipitous and unheralded by prior clinical renal disease, the hypertension can result in encephalopathy and rapid, irreversible renal failure associated with markedly elevated renin levels. Histopathology of the kidney demonstrates arteriolar lesions characterized by intimal hyperplasia, fibrinoid necrosis of the arcuate and interlobular vessels, and infarction. Overall, the outlook for patients developing scleroderma hypertensive crises is poor, despite occasional encouraging responses to angiotensin-converting enzyme inhibitors.

LABORATORY FINDINGS

Although no laboratory tests are specific for PSS, several abnormalities can be observed. Anemias occur owing to autoimmune hemolytic mechanisms, a microangiopathic process, or chronic disease. Hypertensive renal disease results in proteinuria, cylindruria, and microscopic hematuria.

Antinuclear antibodies exhibiting speckled or nucleolar patterns occur in more than 65 per cent of PSS patients. In particular, autoantibodies directed against the Scl-70 nonhistone nuclear protein occur in 15 to 20 per cent of patients and are regarded as a marker for PSS.

VARIANTS OF PSS

Disorders that manifest certain clinical stigmata of PSS are now well recognized and can be properly termed PSS variants. CREST syndrome refers to calcinosis, Raynaud's phenomenon, esophageal dysfunction, sclerodactyly, and telangiectasia. It is distinguished by cutaneous thickening confined to the fingers, slow evolution over decades, lack of visceral involvement, and autoantibodies to centromere in 70 to 90 per cent of patients. In contrast to PSS, the early edematous phase characterized by swollen fingers can persist for prolonged intervals in CREST. The calcium deposits may be more diffuse and larger, and the telangiectasia may appear on the face and trunk as well as the extremities. Raynaud's phenomenon is a prominent sign of CREST. Bony erosions leading to dissolution of the tufts or, in more severe cases, the phalanges can complicate the course of CREST. Moreover, the pulmonary hypertension observed in long-standing CREST can be more severe than that of PSS, owing to marked sclerosis of small pulmonary arteries often unassociated with interstitial fibrosis. Although hepatic parenchymal disease is rare in CREST, biliary cirrhosis is found in some women. Cranial neuropathies and sensory neuropathies, especially involving the trigeminal nerve, are more commonly observed in CREST than PSS. When compared with PSS, CREST patients enjoy a relatively benign prognosis.

Linear scleroderma is a localized form of the disease that usually develops during childhood and is characterized by a band of sclerosis of one or more extremities or in the frontoparietal region of the forehead and scalp (scleroderma en coup de sabre). Involvement of the face and scalp can result in ipsilateral hemiatrophy of the face. Linear scleroderma can also coexist with morphea and may induce an unusual form of hyperostosis (melorheostosis). A nonerosive arthritis of the fingers is occasionally observed. However, visceral involvement does not occur, nor is there a transition to PSS.

Finally, a newly recognized scleroderma-like disorder characterized by induration and inflammation of the fascia has been designated diffuse fasciitis with eosinophilia. The hands, forearms, legs, and feet are predominantly affected; however, over time, the face and trunk can also become involved. During the formative stage of eosinophilic fasciitis, peripheral eosinophilia and a polyclonal hypergammaglobulinemia are often observed. Corticosteroids reduce the symptoms, eliminate the eosinophilia, and reverse the fascial thickening, in striking contrast to their ineffectiveness in PSS.

TREATMENT

Although no therapy is available that can induce remission of the skin and visceral manifestations of PSS, several different measures are available that provide partial relief of symptoms and control end-organ damage. D-Penicillamine induces skin softening; however, its long-term effects on the course and prognosis of scleroderma remain uncertain. The more recent availability of effective antihypertensive agents has resulted in improved control of hypertensive crises and stabilization of renal function. Hypertension should be aggressively and promptly treated. Moreover, there is evidence that control of blood pressure in some patients has resulted in reduction of skin thickening, lending support to the hypothesis that a defective microcirculation plays a role in the pathogenesis of PSS. Because of their inhibition of angiotensin-converting enzyme and the reduction of renin, captopril or enalapril is the agent of choice in the hypertensive crises due to scleroderma kidney.

The use of corticosteroids in PSS has yielded disappointing results. In general, corticosteroids are reserved for use in controlling the myopathy or signs associated with the overlap syndrome.

REFERENCES

LeRoy EC: Scleroderma (systemic sclerosis). In Kelly WN, Harris ED Jr, Ruddy S, et al (eds): Textbook of Rheumatology. 2nd ed. Philadelphia, WB Saunders Co, 1985, pp 1183–1205.
Medsger TA Jr: Systemic sclerosis (scleroderma), eosinophilic fasciitis, and calcinosis. In McCarty DJ (ed): Arthritis and Allied Conditions. 10th ed. Philadelphia, Lea and Febiger, 1985, p 994.

106

OVERLAP SYNDROME

The overlap syndrome, also designated mixed connective tissue disease, refers to the concurrent expression of selected symptoms and signs of polymyositis (PM), SLE, and PSS in a single individual. Although the overlap syndrome has been observed in virtually all age ranges, it occurs most commonly in women during the fourth decade.

CLINICAL FEATURES

Like SLE and RA, the overlap syndrome often develops insidiously over a prolonged period. Therefore, it is not until a group of findings is recognized by the physician that the diagnosis is entertained. The most common features of the syndrome are listed in Table 106–1. In general, any of the features described in SLE, PSS, and polymyositis may be found in such patients.

Clinically significant renal disease is uncommon in the overlap syndrome (Table 106–1). Proteinuria and microscopic hematuria have led to kidney biopsies, which usually demonstrate minimal change disease of the mesangium. Diffuse membranous or membranoproliferative glomerulonephritis similar to that observed in SLE is rare.

TABLE 106–1. CLINICAL FEATURES OF OVERLAP SYNDROME*

SIGN	FREQUENCY (%)
Polyarthralgia/polyarthritis	95
Raynaud's phenomenon	85
Esophageal dysmotility	67
Decreased pulmonary diffusing capacity	67
Swollen hands	66
Myositis	63
Lymphadenopathy	39
Skin rash	38
Sclerodermatous change	33
Fever	33
Serositis	27
Splenomegaly	19
Hepatomegaly	15
Neurologic abnormalities	10
Sicca complex	7
Hashimoto's thyroiditis	6
Renal disease, definite or possible	5

* After Sharp GC: Mixed connective tissue disease. Bull Rheum Dis 25:828, 1975.

LABORATORY FEATURES

Laboratory abnormalities found in SLE, PSS, and polymyositis are variably found in patients with the overlap syndrome. Antinuclear antibodies exhibiting a speckled immunofluorescent pattern directed against nuclear ribonucleoprotein (RNP) are often present. The titers of antibody are characteristically high and persist during periods when disease is quiescent.

TREATMENT

The therapy of the overlap syndrome combines supportive and medical regimens. Considering the wide range of potential stigmata that can occur in each patient, it is apparent that the therapeutic regimen should be tailored to the individual and that it should be flexible should new manifestations develop.

REFERENCE

Sharp GC, Singsen BH: Mixed connective tissue disease. *In* McCarty DJ (ed): Arthritis and Allied Conditions. 10th ed. Philadelphia, Lea and Febiger, 1985, p 962.

107

THE VASCULITIDES

The term vasculitis refers to inflammation of a blood vessel. When the inflammation specifically involves only arterial vessels, it is designated arteritis. Similarly, an inflammatory response of a dermal venule is a venulitis. Often, vasculitis is described as necrotizing when there is obliteration of the vessel by the byproducts of inflammation, resulting in local thrombosis, hemorrhage, and infarction.

CLASSIFICATION OF THE VASCULITIDES

The vasculitides are classified anatomically based upon the predominant size and distribution of the affected vessel. Although the concept of the clinical syndromes developed from the detailed elucidation of the histopathology, the size of the involved vessel does not

TABLE 107–1. CLASSIFICATION OF VASCULITIS*

Hypersensitivity angiitis
Allergic granulomatosis
Wegener's granulomatosis
Polyarteritis nodosa
Giant cell (cranial, temporal) arteritis

* After Zeek PM: Periarteritis nodosa: A critical review. Am J Clin Pathol 22:777, 1952.

necessarily dictate the clinical syndrome. For example, medium muscular arteries are involved in polyarteritis nodosa, allergic granulomatosis, and Wegener's granulomatosis. Despite this overlap, the classification of the vasculitides presented in Table 107–1 is clinically useful.

IMMUNOPATHOGENESIS

Although the precise immunopathogenesis of the vasculitides remains incompletely understood, the fundamental event that triggers an inflammatory response of vessels appears to be the deposition or in situ formation of antigen-antibody complexes. In humans, circulating immune complexes of varying size and capability of binding complement have been isolated from individuals with different clinical vasculitic disorders. Moreover, immunofluorescent studies of biopsied tissue have conclusively demonstrated the presence of immunoglobulins and complement in the vessel wall. The finding of the hepatitis B surface antigen and antibody in the serum as well as the hepatitis B surface antigen, immunoglobulin, and complement in the vessel walls of individuals with polyarteritis nodosa suggests that the hepatitis B virion may be directly involved in the pathogenesis of this disorder. Yet, despite the presence of the hepatitis B surface antigen in polyarteritis nodosa and native DNA in systemic lupus erythematosus as two putative antigens, the identification of the antigens comprising the vast array of circulating immune complexes is yet to be elucidated.

HYPERSENSITIVITY ANGIITIS

Hypersensitivity angiitis is the most common form of vasculitis and is usually localized to the integument. It is characterized by infiltration of the dermal arterioles, capillaries, and/or venules with either polymorphonuclear or mononuclear leukocytes. Pathologically, there is infiltration of the vessel wall, leukocytoclasis, red blood cell extravasation, thrombosis of the vessel lumen, and fibrinoid necrosis. Thus, this process is often referred to as a necrotizing leukocytoclastic vasculitis.

The distinctive dermal lesions of hypersensitivity angiitis are purpuric papules and urticaria. Other types of cutaneous lesions associated with this form of vasculitis include infarcts, hemorrhagic or nonhemorrhagic bullae, and superficial erosions. The lesions of cutaneous vasculitis usually appear first on the lower extremities as erythematous macules that evolve into *palpable purpura*. Although the lesions preferentially concentrate in the dependent regions inferior to the knees, a similar process can be observed less often on the upper extremities, particularly on the fingers.

There are no specific laboratory tests that identify cutaneous vasculitis. The ESR can be either normal or elevated. Similarly, the total hemolytic complement can be normal or depressed. Circulating immune complexes can be detected, usually in low concentrations. The hepatitis B surface antigen and antibody are absent. Skin biopsy can confirm the diagnosis of cutaneous vasculitis.

Certain discrete disorders exhibit a cutaneous necrotizing vasculitis. *Henoch-Schönlein purpura*, also referred to as anaphylactoid purpura, is a hypersensitivity vasculitis characterized by fever, abdominal pain, nonthrombocytopenic purpura, arthralgia, and renal disease. The classic triad of purpura, arthritis, and abdominal pain occurs in about 80 per cent of patients. Although the disorder can afflict persons of any age, children and young adults are most commonly affected, the peak age being four to eight years. The disease occurs most often in the spring, and may be preceded by an upper respiratory tract infection. Although the average duration of disease is 6 to 16 weeks, 5 to 10 per cent of persons who recover will relapse with renal disease characterized by glomerulonephritis.

Mural vasculitis of the gastrointestinal tract can result in colicky abdominal pain, intestinal bleeding, obstruction, infarction, intussusception, or perforation. The glomerulonephritis of Henoch-Schönlein purpura is usually self-limited but can progress to fatal renal failure or nephrotic syndrome. Immunofluorescence studies have demonstrated the deposition of immunoglobulin and complement in both the kidneys and cutaneous vessels. Serum complement levels are ordinarily normal in Henoch-Schönlein purpura. However, the serum IgA level may be elevated, and IgA is often deposited in the skin and kidney.

A second disorder characterized by hypersensitivity vasculitis is a syndrome of arthralgia, purpura, weakness, and mixed cryoglobulinemia termed *essential mixed cryoglobulinemia*. There are recurrent bouts of palpable purpura of the lower extremities, hepatosplenomegaly, lymphadenopathy, and polyarthralgias. A diffuse proliferative glomerulonephritis may lead to terminal renal failure. The laboratory findings include a moderate anemia, IgM rheumatoid factors, ANA, hypocomplementemia, and cryoglobulins containing IgG and IgM. Certain autoimmune and neoplastic disorders have been associated with this syndrome: lymphoma, renal tubular acidosis, Sjögren's syndrome, rheumatoid arthritis, thyroiditis, and primary biliary cirrhosis.

Hypersensitivity vasculitis, characterized pathologically as either an arteriolitis or venulitis, can also be associated with drug reactions, bacterial infections (i.e., streptococcal), serum sickness, subacute bacterial endocarditis, chronic active hepatitis, ulcerative colitis, Sjögren's syndrome, retroperitoneal fibrosis, and Goodpasture's syndrome.

Treatment of hypersensitivity angiitis includes management of the associated entities (i.e., drug reactions, bacterial infections) and drug therapy. Because there is no specific, curative therapy, several pharmacological agents are used individually or in combinations to suppress the inflammatory response and to promote healing: colchicine, nonsteroidal anti-inflammatory agents, dapsone, corticosteroids, methotrexate, azathioprine, and/or cyclophosphamide. Management of cutaneous ulcers requires fastidious local care and debridement to prevent infection.

POLYARTERITIS NODOSA

Polyarteritis nodosa is a vasculitis involving primarily the medium muscular arteries, and to a lesser extent, small muscular arteries. Although the disease principally affects males of middle age, it can occur in any age group of both sexes.

The kidneys are the most commonly involved organ system. Inflammation of the arcuate arteries as well as other medium-size vessels may or may not result in segmental aneurysmal dilatations. A rapidly progressive, necrotizing glomerulonephritis can lead to the sudden onset of severe hypertension, nephrotic syndrome, and renal failure. Spontaneous rupture of aneurysms can result in retroperitoneal hemorrhage or a perinephric hematoma.

The heart becomes involved during polyarteritis nodosa in approximately 70 per cent of patients. Coronary arteritis can produce angina pectoris or frank myocardial infarction. Pericarditis, often diagnosed post mortem, is another source of retrosternal chest pain.

Polyarteritis nodosa also involves the gastrointestinal tract in about 65 per cent of patients, causing abdominal pain, intestinal bleeding, obstruction, or perforation. Rupture of mesenteric aneurysms can lead to intraperitoneal hemorrhage, hypovolemic shock, and death.

Neurological involvement contributes significantly to the morbidity of the disease in about 60 per cent of patients. Disorders of the peripheral nervous system are attributable to arteritis of the vasa nervorum and ultimate occlusion. The peripheral neuropathies include mononeuritis multiplex, distal sensorimotor polyneuropathy, cutaneous neuropathy, and extensive mononeuritis. Mononeuritis multiplex is characterized by paresthesias, pain, weakness, and sensory loss of the affected limb due to infarction of several peripheral nerves.

Vasculitis of the central nervous system (CNS) in polyarteritis nodosa is estimated to occur in 20 to 40 per cent of cases. Encephalopathy secondary to severe hypertension and/or primary neuronal dysfunction produces a global cognitive disorder. Vasculitis affecting different anatomical structures of the CNS presents as focal or multifocal defects of function of the brain or spinal cord. Such defects can lead to seizures and hemorrhagic or ischemic strokes.

Polyarteritis nodosa affects the integument in only 5 to 15 per cent of patients. The most common sign of skin involvement is nodules of the legs or, less commonly, the arms. These nodules, which measure 0.5 to 1.0 cm, pulsate and are painful. Livedo reticularis and peripheral gangrene also occur.

The laboratory findings of polyarteritis nodosa often reflect the presence of a severe systemic inflammation. The erythrocyte sedimentation rate, serum immunoglobulin levels, C-reactive protein, white blood cell count, and platelet count are all frequently elevated. The presence of anemia may be due to blood loss or renal failure. Microscopic hematuria, cylindruria, and proteinuria result from glomerulonephritis. Hypocomplementemia may be present, but the ANA and rheumatoid factor are absent. Thirty per cent exhibit hepatitis B surface antigenemia. The cerebrospinal fluid is normal unless there has been a subarachnoid hemorrhage.

The definitive diagnosis necessitates biopsy of an affected organ, such as the skin, muscle, testis, sural nerve, or kidney. Angiography of the renal, hepatic, and mesenteric arteries is often performed to seek evidence of aneurysmal formation and/or tapering and "cut-offs" of vessels due to vasculitis. However, the absence of aneurysms does not exclude the diagnosis of polyarteritis. If CNS vasculitis is suspected, angiography will also be necessary, since neither the MRI nor CT scan provides sufficient evidence to confirm the diagnosis.

Effective treatment necessitates a combination of a corticosteroid and immunosuppressive agents. The current recommended initial therapy is prednisone, 1 to 2 mg/kg/day, and cyclophosphamide, 2 mg/kg/day. Prednisone is tapered gradually as the clinical response allows, and cyclophosphamide may be necessary to maintain remission.

ALLERGIC GRANULOMATOUS VASCULITIS OF CHURG AND STRAUSS

The Churg-Strauss syndrome is characterized by (a) hypereosinophilia, (b) allergic rhinitis and/or asthma, and (c) a systemic vasculitis of the medium and small muscular arteries involving two or more extrapulmonary sites.

Three phases of the disease have been identified. A prodromal period may exist over many years during which the predominant clinical findings are atopic. Allergic rhinitis usually precedes the onset of extrinsic asthma. During the second phase, hypereosinophilia and eosinophilic tissue infiltration occur. The final phase is characterized by the development of a systemic necrotizing vasculitis.

Asthma occurs in all cases of Churg-Strauss syndrome and is a criterion for the diagnosis. At the onset of vasculitis, asthma may remit or exacerbate. Hypereosinophilia and tissue infiltration with eosinophils is a second criterion of the Churg-Strauss syndrome. Treatment with corticosteroids usually abolishes the eosinophilia.

The vasculitis of Churg-Strauss syndrome involves both the medium and smaller muscular arteries, and, in this way, can be similar to Wegener's granulomatosis and PAN with involvement of cardiac, renal, gastrointestinal, or nervous systems. The onset of vasculitis may be preceded by constitutional symptoms, weight loss, and fever.

The treatment of Churg-Strauss syndrome is similar to that of the other systemic necrotizing vasculitides. The Churg-Strauss vasculitis generally responds readily to high-dose corticosteroids (i.e., prednisone, 60 mg per day). A dramatic drop in the eosinophil count, the white blood cell count, and ESR documents this response. Less often the disease responds only partially, and it becomes necessary to add cyclophosphamide.

WEGENER'S GRANULOMATOSIS

Wegener's granulomatosis is a systemic necrotizing vasculitis primarily involving the medium and small muscular arteries. It is characterized by (a) granulomatous vasculitis of the upper and lower respiratory tract, and (b) a necrotizing glomerulonephritis.

The disease occurs in equal proportions of males and females. Although the peak incidence is in the fourth and fifth decades with an average age of 40, the range varies between the ages of 15 and 75 years.

The majority of individuals in whom the diagnosis of Wegener's granulomatosis is eventually made present with symptoms of upper respiratory tract disease (Table 107–2). The most common complaints include nasal ulcers, rhinorrhea, and sinus pain. Sinusitis and otitis media can both occur. Biopsy of sinus mucosa often demonstrates the necrotizing granulomata.

Ocular inflammation also develops in more than half of all patients. The findings include conjunctivitis, episcleritis, scleromalacia, corneal ulcers, and retinal artery thrombosis.

The lungs become involved in the majority of patients. Common symptoms of pulmonary disease include hemoptysis, cough, and pleurisy. Although variable and often nonspecific, the radiographic findings of solitary or multiple infiltrates or nodules and multilocular, irregular cavities reflect the presence of a necrotizing granulomatous process in the absence or presence of vasculitis. Biopsy of the lung usually provides documentation of the process.

Kidney disease, which occurs in about 85 per cent of cases, is a later manifestation of Wegener's granulomatosis. The pathologic lesions are a focal or diffuse proliferative glomerulonephritis and interstitial nephritis. The glomerulonephritis often results in an active urinary sediment characterized by proteinuria, hematuria, and cylindruria. If left untreated, a rapidly progressive and terminal renal failure results.

Dermal vasculitic lesions have been observed in more than one third of persons with Wegener's granulomatosis. Both nodular lesions and purpuric papules suggest a granulomatous vasculitis.

Joint pains in the absence of active synovitis are a complaint in about one half of patients. Although synovitis occurs, it is very uncommon.

There is no laboratory test that is specific for the diagnosis of Wegener's granulomatosis. Because of the presence of widespread inflammation, the ESR is elevated and a normochromic, normocytic anemia is often observed. A polyclonal hypergammaglobulinemia is characterized by elevated IgG and IgA levels. Abnormalities of urinalysis, BUN, and creatinine reflect renal disease.

The diagnosis of Wegener's granulomatosis is made on the basis of the clinical signs of upper and lower respiratory tract disease (i.e., sinusitis, rhinitis, otitis, pulmonary nodules or infiltrates) associated with glomerulonephritis and a biopsy demonstrating necrotizing vasculitis with granuloma formation. In addition, other organ systems can be simultaneously involved.

The current therapy for Wegener's granulomatosis utilizes cytotoxic chemotherapy. Cyclophosphamide is the agent of choice, and critically ill patients should be treated with intravenous cyclophosphamide until the course of the disease is stabilized and it is deemed advisable to switch to oral therapy.

Although treatment with corticosteroids alone is insufficient to control disease activity and induce remission, short term administration of these agents is useful in relieving the sequelae of inflammation, particularly that of the eye.

TABLE 107–2. FREQUENCY OF ORGAN SYSTEM INVOLVEMENT IN WEGENER'S GRANULOMATOSIS*

ORGAN	PER CENT
Respiratory tract	100
Kidneys	85
Eyes	55
Joints	48
Skin/muscle	40
Ear	36
Heart	17
Nervous system	15

* After Kornblut AD, Wolff S, Defries HO, Fauci A: Wegener's granulomatosis. Laryngoscope 90:1453, 1980.

POLYMYALGIA RHEUMATICA AND GIANT CELL ARTERITIS

Polymyalgia rheumatica (PMR) is an idiopathic disorder characterized by aching and myalgias of the shoulder and pelvic girdle musculature, neck, and proximal extremities. Usually having its onset in women (2:1) in the sixth decade or older, the yearly incidence is approximately 54 per 100,000 population. Occasional cases occur in younger persons.

Symptoms of aching, stiffness after rest, and myalgias often begin precipitously, although the disease may progress relatively slowly over time. Polyarthralgias or a true synovitis can be present. Other commonly observed constitutional features include fever, weight loss, malaise, and anorexia.

The physical examination reveals tender muscles but no weakness or atrophy. Synovitis of the knees with or without small effusions occur. In contrast, synovitis of the small joints of the hands and feet is rare.

There are no specific laboratory tests to identify PMR. However, the Westergren sedimentation rate is elevated above 35 mm/hr in nearly all patients. A normochromic, normocytic anemia is present in one half of patients. There is no increase in the incidence of rheumatoid factor, ANA, or other autoantibodies. Complement levels are normal or elevated. The muscle enzymes (CPK, aldolase, SGOT) are normal. Neither electromyographic evaluation nor muscle biopsy has provided diagnostic benefit. Synovial fluid analysis usually reveals a noninflammatory or mildly inflammatory picture (WBC = 0–9000/cu mm, predominantly lymphocytes) with normal glucose and complement levels. Synovial biopsy may show a nonspecific, mild synovial hyperplasia.

The differential diagnosis includes infections, neoplasia (i.e., plasma cell dyscrasia), fibromyalgia, and painful myopathies. Giant cell arteritis can present or be associated with PMR in 20 to 40 per cent of patients.

Giant cell arteritis is a granulomatous vasculitis that usually affects individuals over the age of 50. The approximate annual incidence of the disease is 12 cases per 100,000 individuals over age 50. The mean age of onset is 69 years, with a range of 48 to 90 years. Sixty-four per cent of patients are women.

The onset of giant cell arteritis may be precipitous or insidious. When the disorder co-exists with PMR, proximal extremity aching, stiffness, fatigue, and headache are the presenting symptoms in 20 to 40 per cent of patients. Other constitutional symptoms include recurrent and unexplained fevers, anorexia, weight loss, and malaise. The low-grade fever is present as an early sign of disease activity in one half of patients. Neuropsychiatric signs include confusion, depressive reactions, psychosis and, rarely, dementia. The synovitis observed with giant cell arteritis is a manifestation of PMR.

The symptoms of claudication, headache, visual changes, and scalp tenderness are the result of arteritis. Claudication can occur in muscle groups in which the blood flow is compromised by vasculitis. The most common sites include the muscles of mastication, deglutition, the extremities, and the tongue. Jaw claudication, a symptom in one third to one half of patients, is a consequence of impaired blood flow of the temporal or maxillary arteries.

The visual alterations of giant cell arteritis include transient blurring, ptosis, diplopia, and transient, permanent partial, or complete blindness. These symptoms are the result of arteritis affecting the posterior ciliary or ophthalmic vessels or, less commonly, the central retinal artery. Although blindness is usually preceded by other visual changes for weeks or months, it can occur precipitously without warning.

Headache and scalp tenderness, very common symptoms, are due to arteritis of the temporal or occipital vessels. Headache may be one of the earliest symptoms, since it is reported as an initial complaint in 30 to 45 per cent of patients. The new onset of an ill-defined headache of variable severity in an older person should raise the suspicion of giant cell arteritis.

Although several laboratory abnormalities can be observed, none is specific for the disorder. Hematologic abnormalities often present are a normochromic, normocytic anemia, leukocytosis of less than 20,000/cu mm, and a thrombocytosis of less than 1,000,000/cu mm. Alterations in plasma proteins result from the response to inflammation and include elevated fibrinogen, α-2-globulin, IgG, total hemolytic complement, C4, and C3. The erythrocyte sedimentation rate is often greater than 60 mm/hr and remains a sine qua non for the diagnosis of giant cell arteritis.

When the diagnosis is suspected, a biopsy of a clinically involved or symptomatic portion of the temporal artery should be obtained. If the temporal artery appears clinically uninvolved, biopsy of a 5-cm segment should be taken to obtain sufficient tissue to identify the commonly observed "skip" lesions of temporal arteritis. Temporal arteriography has demonstrated low sensitivity, gives frequent false-positive results, and does not enhance the value of the temporal artery biopsy. However, a history of claudication of an extremity and the presence on examination of a bruit implicates large vessel arteritis and should be confirmed by angiography.

The treatment of choice is corticosteroids. The usual initial daily dosage is the equivalent of prednisone, 60 mg. If there is a moderate to high likelihood of giant cell arteritis, corticosteroid therapy should be instituted immediately, *prior to biopsy*, to avert the dreaded potential of blindness. Although prior steroid therapy can alter the histopathologic changes after one week of treatment, the characteristic histologic findings are present if biopsy is performed within one week. The response to therapy is monitored clinically by resolution of symptoms as well as by the ESR. Upon remission and return of the ESR to normal levels, the corticosteroid dosage can be tapered as the ESR is periodically monitored. Whether the corticosteroid therapy can be discontinued in giant cell arteritis depends upon the clinical course.

REFERENCES

Cupps T, Fauci A: The Vasculitides. Philadelphia, WB Saunders Co, 1981.

Fauci A, Haynes B, Katz P, Wolff S: Wegener's granulomatosis: Prospective clinical and therapeutic experience with 85 patients for 21 years. Ann Intern Med 98:76, 1983.

Haynes BF, Allen NB, Fauci AS: Diagnostic and therapeutic approach to the patient with vasculitis. Med Clin North Am 70:355, 1986.

Lanham J, Elkan K, Pusey C, Hughes G: Systemic vasculitis with asthma and eosinophilia: A clinical approach to the Churg-Strauss syndrome. Medicine 63:65, 1984.

108

RAYNAUD'S PHENOMENON

Raynaud's phenomenon is a disorder characterized by a triphasic color change of the affected anatomical region due to local arterial vasospasm. When unassociated with another disorder, this phenomenon is commonly designated Raynaud's disease.

Raynaud's phenomenon is a relatively common malady, affecting 5 to 10 per cent of the normal population. Approximately 1000 new cases are identified yearly per million adults. When compared with the annual incidence rates of rheumatoid arthritis (750), systemic lupus erythematosus (75), progressive systemic sclerosis (10), and dermatomyositis/polymyositis (10), Raynaud's phenomenon is a relatively common connective tissue disorder. Three out of four affected persons are female, and the median age of onset is 39.5 years.

CLINICAL FEATURES

Raynaud's phenomenon is usually triggered by a stimulus such as exposure to cold or emotional stress. Occasionally, the reaction occurs de novo. Raynaud's phenomenon primarily affects the acral regions, including the hands and feet. Other less commonly involved structures include the ears, nose, nipples, and tongue. The process is classically divided into three phases: initial pallor of the skin resulting from vasoconstriction and subsequent reduced cutaneous blood flow. Following arterial constriction, the second phase of cyanosis results from limited blood flow through the dermal vessels. Upon rewarming, the third stage of hyperemia can be appreciated as the dermal arterial vessels dilate and blood flow returns to baseline. The duration of the reaction is quite variable, from minutes to hours. Indeed, severe Raynaud's phenomenon can exhibit a predominant phase of cyanosis, even in the absence of an ongoing stimulus, and this has been termed "fixed" Raynaud's phenomenon. Thus, neither the duration of each phase nor the extent of dermal changes of each phase need be equivalent. Moreover, pain may or may not accompany an episode of Raynaud's phenomenon.

The severity and frequency of attacks of Raynaud's phenomenon are often dependent on the presence of an associated disorder. In its primary form, Raynaud's disease can be unilateral or bilateral, long-standing, and uncommonly complicated by cutaneous gangrene. However, the occurrence of vasospastic signs well in advance of a connective tissue disorder is common. Thus, more severe vasospastic disease may be premonitory to an insidiously evolving disorder such as scleroderma. Advanced Raynaud's phenomenon can result in gangrene and/or autoamputation of the affected structure.

PATHOPHYSIOLOGY

The precise etiopathogenesis of Raynaud's phenomenon remains unknown. Segmental, often widely distributed local defects of small arterial vessels have been postulated. Histopathology demonstrates variable degrees of intimal thickening with luminal narrowing, endothelial swelling, increased numbers of intracellular cytoplasmic filaments that may be contractile elements, and adventitial fibrosis.

The roles of the various vasoactive mediators in the pathogenesis of Raynaud's phenomenon are currently under investigation. Since this disorder is characterized by vasospasm, vasodilation, and thrombosis, prostaglandins may mediate, in part, these exaggerated local responses. Thromboxane A2, synthesized by the endothelium and platelets, promotes vasoconstriction and platelet aggregation. By contrast, prostacyclin, also synthesized by endothelium, produces vasodilation and inhibits platelet aggregation. An inhibitor of thromboxane, dazoxiben,* produces temporary improvement of the vasospasm. Similarly, prostacyclin* promotes vasodilation, providing temporary resolution of the process.

DISORDERS ASSOCIATED WITH RAYNAUD'S PHENOMENON

The individual presenting for diagnosis of Raynaud's phenomenon should be comprehensively evaluated for a disorder associated with this process. The most common rheumatic diseases associated with Raynaud's phenomenon include scleroderma (> 90 per cent), overlap syndrome (80 per cent), SLE (30 per cent), dermatomyositis/polymyositis (20 per cent), and rheumatoid arthritis (10 per cent).

The initial evaluation must include a comprehensive history and physical examination aimed at identifying remote or recent symptoms and signs of other disorders that can be related to Raynaud's phenomenon. The use of particular drugs or the exposure to certain toxins should be sought. A knowledge of the patient's occupational exposures is critical, since workers in certain trades, such as vinylchloride workers, have an increased incidence of Raynaud's phenomenon. The examination may reveal evidence of an evolving connective tissue disorder or neurovascular compression. Widefield nailfold capillaroscopy is a simple, rapid, reliable, and inexpensive technique to identify gross anatomical alterations in the capillaries which may herald a systemic rheumatic disease.

The use of particular laboratory tests in the initial and subsequent evaluation of Raynaud's phenomenon

---

* Investigational drug for this purpose.

is warranted. A complete blood count, Westergren sedimentation rate, urinalysis, ANA, anti–SS-A and anti–SS-B, serum protein electrophoresis, and cryoglobulins can provide evidence of a connective tissue disorder or paraproteinemia. A chest x-ray and cervical spine films assist in excluding the diagnosis of a thoracic outlet syndrome due to an aberrant first cervical rib, but do not rule out compression due to a hypertrophied scalenus anticus muscle. Arteriography is rarely efficacious in diagnosis.

Since Raynaud's phenomenon may precede the onset of an associated disorder, the patient with apparent Raynaud's disease should be monitored yearly for an indefinite period. Surveillance of such persons often permits the early recognition and treatment of complicating diseases such as rheumatoid arthritis or monoclonal gammopathy.

THERAPY

The management of Raynaud's phenomenon usually requires the use of simple general measures. Only a minority of patients require pharmacological agents. The direct exposure to cold should be avoided. Multiple layers of warm clothing, especially gloves, should be recommended. The continued use of tobacco should be discouraged owing to the relationship between thromboangiitis obliterans and Raynaud's phenomenon. The use of beta-adrenergic blocking drugs in the treatment of hypertension should be discontinued owing to their capacity to promote vasoconstriction.

If these measures still fail to control Raynaud's phenomenon, medical therapy should be considered. The application of a quarter inch of a nitroglycerin-containing ointment to the skin prior to cold exposure can reduce or eliminate the vasospasm without producing untoward side effects. More advanced disease may necessitate agents that promote vasodilation. The calcium channel blocking agents appear to inhibit smooth muscle contraction by regulating the slow calcium channel influx. Although the numbers of patients rigorously studied have been small, preliminary results with nifedipine* indicate efficacy. Alternatively, the postganglionic alpha blocker prazosin* often lessens the symptoms of Raynaud's phenomenon but may be associated with untoward effects of palpitations and orthostatic hypotension.

Another mode of management has been sympathectomy. The results of sympathectomy have been complicated by a high recurrence rate. The efficacy of the newly developed superselective digital sympathectomy awaits further analysis.

REFERENCES

Campbell PM, LeRoy EC: Raynaud's phenomenon. Sem Arthritis Rheum 16:92, 1986.
Lafferty K, Roberts V, DeTrafford J, Cotton L: On the nature of Raynaud's phenomenon. Lancet 2:313, 1983.

* Investigational drug for this purpose.

109

NONARTICULAR RHEUMATISM

Nonarticular rheumatism is the currently preferred designation for a group of disorders that affect the soft or supporting tissues: fascia, tendons, ligaments, bursae, and intervertebral disks. These disorders are very common in the general population and often produce acute and chronic pain syndromes. While certain types of nonarticular rheumatism are readily recognizable and easily treatable, others often remain undiagnosed for prolonged periods and/or are very difficult to manage effectively. The prototype disorder of nonarticular rheumatism is the myofascial pain syndrome, also referred to as fibromyalgia.

THE FIBROMYALGIA SYNDROME

The fibromyalgia syndrome is a disorder, or group of disorders, of unknown etiology characterized by chronic and generalized muscular aching, stiffness, joint pains, variable fatigability, paresthesias, poor sleep habits, headaches, anxiety, and irritable bowel syndrome. This disorder occurs in women of childbearing age (20 to 50 years) six times more frequently than in men. Until recently, the disorder was regarded as psychosomatic in origin; however, carefully conducted clinical studies have further defined and characterized fibromyalgia, and suggested that, although the disorder lacks precise pathologic definition, an organic etiology appears likely.

The person with fibromyalgia describes fatigue upon arising in the morning and prolonged morning stiffness lasting several hours. Some individuals experience both morning and evening stiffness. Certain forms of exercise or manual labor tend to aggravate the muscular soreness and stiffness. There is a sensation of swelling of the joint, especially the small joints of the hands. The nonrheumatic symptoms of headache, sleep disorder, paresthesias, anxiety, and irritable bowel syndrome occur independently. Factors that augment fibromyalgia include changing weather conditions, humid or cold weather, stress, fatigue or overactivity. Symptoms tend to be relieved by rest, warm weather, amelioration of stress, hot showers, massage, and, in some persons, stretching exercises.

The physical examination of persons with fibromyalgia unassociated with other disorders (primary fibromyalgia) usually reveals a healthy-appearing adult. The locomotor examination characteristically demonstrates (a) tenderness with palpation of joints with no evidence of synovitis, deformity, or limitation of range of motion; (b) tender zones over distinct muscle groups; (c) tenderness of certain costochondral junctions; and (d) marked cutaneous erythema following palpation of tender zones. Persons with fibromyalgia often exhibit 12 or more tender zones.

The laboratory evaluation in fibromyalgia is unrevealing. Tests for the identification of inflammation are negative. Biopsies of skin, fascia, and muscle demonstrate either nonspecific findings or no pathologic changes. Similarly, the electromyographic examination may demonstrate some insertional activity but is generally unrevealing.

The management of fibromyalgia should begin with an explanation of the disorder to the patient. It should be emphasized that fibromyalgia characteristically runs a course punctuated by exacerbations and remissions; that it is not a psychosomatic disorder, but that anxiety and stress can exacerbate symptoms; and that the disorder does not produce crippling or disability. Patients should be encouraged to continue gainful employment, but the type of job may have to be changed if it requires activities that are recognized to exacerbate symptoms. The importance of regular periods of rest, vacation, and relaxation, which are known to ameliorate symptoms, should be explained. The participation in a regular program of nonstressful stretching exercises can be tried, since this has proven effective in partially relieving symptoms in a subset of patients.

Medical and psychiatric treatment may be useful in the long-term management of fibromyalgia. Brief psychotherapy is being evaluated for its effectiveness in coping with the disorder. The use of amitriptyline, 10 to 25 mg, in the early evening may improve the sleep disorder and reduce aching. Other modalities that have been utilized to reduce pain include salicylates and nonsteroidal anti-inflammatory agents. The disorder does not respond to corticosteroids. Additional adjunctive treatments that have provided relief include transcutaneous electric stimulation (TENS), and biofeedback (see also Myofascial Pain, Chapter 116).

REFERENCES

Bole GG: Nonarticular rheumatism. *In* Wyngaarden JB, Smith LH Jr (eds): Cecil Textbook of Medicine. 18th ed. Philadelphia, WB Saunders Co, 1988, pp 2047–2048.

Yunus M, Masi A, Calabro J, et al: Primary fibromyalgia (fibrositis): Clinical study of 50 patients with matched normal controls. Sem Arthritis Rheum 11:151, 1981.

110

THE SPONDYLOARTHROPATHIES

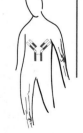

The spondyloarthropathies are a group of interrelated disorders that share certain epidemiologic, pathogenetic, clinical, and pathologic features. The entities that compose this group include (a) ankylosing spondylitis, (b) Reiter's syndrome, (c) psoriatic arthritis, (d) arthritis associated with chronic inflammatory disease of the intestine, (e) Whipple's disease, and (f) postinfectious "reactive" arthropathies.

ANKYLOSING SPONDYLITIS

Ankylosing spondylitis (AS) is the prototype of the spondyloarthropathies. It is characterized by *enthesopathy*, the presence of inflammation at the site of ligamentous insertion into bone; sacroiliitis; spondylitis; inflammatory ocular disease; an asymmetrical oligoarthritis predominantly of the large joints of the lower limbs; and an association with HLA-B27 (see Table 100–5).

Prevalence

The prevalence of AS in Caucasians is 1 per cent of the general population. Among American blacks, the prevalence of AS is approximately one quarter that of Caucasians. Although the ratio of affected males to females is equal in sacroiliitis, the ratio is 3:1 in the presence of spondylitis. The disease usually has its onset in the second and third decades. There is a prominent familial incidence of AS and of other spondyloarthropathies among first-degree family members of affected persons.

Clinical Features

AS usually presents during young adulthood with vague symptoms of mid- and low-back stiffness and pain. There is often a history of long-standing soreness and stiffness of the back after prolonged rest, which is partially alleviated with mobility and exercise. Radiation of the pain into the buttocks and down the posterior aspect of the leg may occur. The prominent stiffness after rest may prompt the patient to arise from bed at night to walk about.

Thoracic cage pain also occurs in AS. Owing to involvement of the central cartilaginous joints of the anterior thoracic cage, the pain can have a pleuritic quality. In particular, pain from the manubriosternal and sternoclavicular joints is very common.

Enthesopathic pain is also common in AS and is frequently a presenting complaint. The pain is due to dactylitis, Achilles tendinitis, plantar fasciitis, and iliac crest involvement.

Polyarthralgias and/or polyarthritis is another frequent complaint during the course of AS. The proximal synovial joints, including the shoulders, hips and knees, are more often involved than the smaller distal joints. As in RA, there is prolonged early morning stiffness and swelling of joints; however, the synovitis can be asymmetrical and only uncommonly results in severe, erosive articular disease.

Acute anterior uveitis occurs in approximately one quarter of patients with AS. There is pain, redness, and photophobia that is usually episodic and may be unilateral or bilateral.

Examination of the patient with early AS can demonstrate reduced spinal mobility, partial or complete loss of the physiologic lumbar lordosis, and increased thoracic kyphosis. Later findings include restriction of chest wall expansion during deep inspiration (<2.5 cm), the gradual development of a stooped posture, fixation of the spine with head held in flexion, and a shuffling gait. The presence of peripheral joint synovitis is variable.

Pathology

AS is a chronic inflammatory arthritis predominantly affecting the axial skeleton. The target joints are both synovial and nonsynovial. The inflammatory arthritis of the axial skeleton induces an exuberant fibrotic response. Over time, the fibrotic scar calcifies,

leading to ossification of ligaments, bony bridging between vertebral bodies (syndesmophytes), and irreversible skeletal immobility.

Radiologic Features

The long-standing pathologic changes produce characteristic radiographic features in AS. Inflammation of the sacroiliac joints leads to gradual destruction of cartilage and subchondral erosions, giving the radiographic appearance of "pseudo-widening." An osteoblastic response of the affected bone then results in sclerosis of the joint margins. Subsequent fusion of the joint results from the ingrowth of osteoid tissue, calcification, and bony bridging of the joint margins. The final radiographic feature is juxta-articular osteopenia.

Osteitis of subchondral vertebral bone and periostitis of the anterior face of the vertebral body can destroy the superior and inferior margins, flattening the normal concave surface and giving the radiographic picture of squaring of the bodies. This finding, most common in thoracic vertebrae, can be the earliest radiographic change of AS.

Healing of the chondritis and osteitis is associated with fibrosis, calcification, new bone formation with replacement of the annulus fibrosus, and development of syndesmophytes that bridge the margins of adjacent vertebral bodies. The gradual ossification of the annulus fibrosus, formation of syndesmophytes, and ossification of the perispinal ligaments eventually immobilize the spine and give the radiographic appearance of the "bamboo" spine.

Laboratory Studies

There is no laboratory test that is specific for AS. Early in the disease process the elevated sedimentation rate reflects the inflammatory process; in the presence of chronic disease, the sedimentation rate may or may not be raised. A mild or moderate rise in the alkaline phosphatase indicates the presence of bony resorption during osteitis.

There is an excellent correlation between AS and the presence of HLA-B27. Approximately 90 per cent of Caucasian patients with AS possess B27, compared with 8 per cent of the general population. In black Americans with AS the incidence of B27 approximates 50 per cent, in contrast to a 4 per cent incidence in the black population at large. Thus, in patients in whom the diagnosis is uncertain, determining the presence of B27 may assist in making the early diagnosis of AS; in contrast, testing for the presence of B27 in persons with clinically evident AS is unnecessary, since it does not alter management.

Treatment

The management of AS is predicated upon a vigorous approach to physical therapy and the judicious use of certain nonsteroidal anti-inflammatory agents. Although nonsteroidal anti-inflammatory drugs do not alter the course of AS, by providing analgesia they promote function. The long-term objective of the exercise regimen is to halt the insidious development of disabling axial immobility and to preserve maximal motion and function. At times, the use of a custom-designed "spondylitic" jacket to maintain maximal upright posture and to relieve distressing paravertebral muscular pain is beneficial.

REITER'S SYNDROME

Reiter's syndrome is a seronegative spondyloarthritis characterized by (a) urethritis, (b) conjunctivitis, and (c) arthritis. The disease most commonly affects young males (male to female ratio approximates 10–15:1) during the third and fourth decades but can rarely be observed in women, adolescents, and elderly persons.

Epidemiology and Immunogenetics

The onset of Reiter's syndrome often occurs following venereal infections or dysentery. The venereal relationship appears more frequently in the United States. *Chlamydia* can be cultured from the urethra of untreated patients in 33 to 47 per cent of cases. Moreover, anti-chlamydial antibodies can eventually be detected in about one half of patients. However, there is no evidence to confirm that *Chlamydia* is an etiologic agent of Reiter's syndrome. The postdysenteric form of Reiter's syndrome, which is found more frequently in Africa, Europe, and the Far and Middle East, usually results from a gastrointestinal infection with *Shigella flexneri*, but may also follow enteric infections with *Salmonella* spp., *Y. enterocolitica*, or *C. jejuni*. Because the joint fluids of Reiter's syndrome usually yield no bacterial growth, postdysenteric Reiter's syndrome has been regarded as a reactive arthritis.

The observation that Reiter's syndrome can, in some cases, be familial and is associated with sacroiliitis or ankylosing spondylitis led to immunogenetic analysis of the disorder. The genotype HLA-B27 is found by serotyping in 75 per cent of Caucasian and 37 per cent of black patients. Although the precise significance of the B27 allotype remains uncertain, this cellular surface antigen may predispose individuals with certain bacterial infections (i.e., *Shigella, Salmonella, Yersinia enterocolitica*) to the eventual development of a reactive arthritis such as Reiter's syndrome.

Clinical Features

Characteristically, Reiter's syndrome develops one to four weeks following venereal exposure or diarrhea. Urethritis, often the earliest symptom, is characterized by burning and frequency. A concurrent cystitis can be found in both females and males. Since the penile discharge is clear and mucoid, it resembles nonspecific urethritis. A notable association with the urethritis is a perimeatal erosion of the glans penis.

A profuse and watery diarrhea can precede the onset of urethritis in Reiter's syndrome. Following an epidemic of *Shigella* dysentery, approximately 2 out of every 1000 affected persons can be expected to develop Reiter's syndrome.

The conjunctivitis of Reiter's syndrome is a mild, noncatarrhal, bilateral inflammation of the bulbar and palpebral conjunctiva. It is characterized by an eva-

nescent irritation with burning usually lasting one to two days, or, less commonly, as long as several weeks. The process is ordinarily self-limiting. In contrast, the development of an acute anterior iridocyclitis, which occurs in less than one third of persons, can be complicated by pain and potential visual loss if not treated.

Mucocutaneous lesions are commonly observed during Reiter's syndrome. Lesions of the oropharynx can be identified on the buccal mucosa, tongue, palate, and pharyngeal mucosa. Such lesions can take the form of *painless* vesicles, elevated erythematous papules, or superficial ulcers. The lesions of the penis, termed *circinate balanitis*, begin as small, painless vesicles that can coalesce to form larger, painless lesions. Once present, balanitis generally resolves within a few weeks but can last several months. The third cutaneous lesion of Reiter's syndrome is *keratoderma blennorrhagicum*. This painless rash, which occurs in 20 per cent of patients and is found most often on the plantar surfaces of the feet, has the appearance of a brown or yellow cone-shaped papule. Coalescence of the papules leads to large desquamating lesions.

The arthritis of Reiter's syndrome often presents precipitously and frequently affects the knees and ankles. The distribution of the arthritis is asymmetrical and can be monarticular or pauciarticular. The synovitis can also involve any other joint, including the small digital articulations and the sacroiliac joints. When involved, the joints become hot, swollen, and painful and can develop effusions.

A particularly notable feature of Reiter's syndrome is the enthesopathy. Although enthesopathic signs are present in other forms of spondyloarthritides, these symptoms are present so often, especially during the early phase of the disorder, as to suggest the diagnosis of Reiter's syndrome. Enthesopathic signs include tendinitis of the extensor hallucis longus; tendinitis at the insertion of the Achilles tendon on the calcaneus; pain on the anterior surface of the patella; periostitis of the digital bones of the feet; and pain over the surfaces of the distal tibias.

The onset of Reiter's syndrome can be abrupt, occurring over several days or more gradually over several weeks. Patients sustaining the precipitous onset can appear quite toxic and exhibit hectic fevers, weight loss, malaise, and debilitation. The recognition of Reiter's syndrome in a young male presenting in this manner can be difficult in the absence of the complete clinical picture. Yet the presence of urethritis and diarrhea, especially if a history of enthesopathy can be elicited, should suggest the diagnosis of Reiter's syndrome.

The long-term outcome of Reiter's syndrome is variable. Approximately two thirds of patients experience no further acute episodes, while the remaining one third experience recurrent or sustained disease activity. Ankylosing spondylitis complicates the course of Reiter's syndrome in 15 per cent of cases.

Laboratory Findings

There are no laboratory tests that specifically identify Reiter's syndrome. During active disease a normocytic, normochromic anemia, leukocytosis (<30,000/cu mm), and elevation of the ESR are often observed. IgM rheumatoid factors are absent. The urinalysis can show microscopic hematuria and pyuria, but cultures are sterile. Serum and synovial fluid complement levels can be elevated on the basis of an acute phase response but are of no diagnostic significance.

Radiographic Findings

Radiographic changes are notably absent early in the disease course. Later, after the appearance of peripheral synovitis, juxta-articular osteoporosis can be observed about affected joints. Periostitis of the os calcis is common but not diagnostic. The sacroiliitis associated with Reiter's syndrome tends to be asymmetrical, later becoming symmetrical. The ankylosing spondylitis is notable radiographically for nonmarginal syndesmophytes bridging the vertebrae.

Treatment

The management of Reiter's syndrome requires both supportive and preventive measures. In general, the mucocutaneous lesions do not necessitate treatment unless there are ulcerations or extensive spread of the skin lesions. In this situation, the use of a topical corticosteroid preparation is often beneficial. The eyes should be carefully examined by an ophthalmologist and treatment initiated if there is iridocyclitis. Failure to diagnose iridocyclitis or to effectively manage this complication can lead to progressive visual impairment. A regimen of bed rest, physical therapy, and nonsteroidal anti-inflammatory agents is often very effective in the symptomatic management of the arthritis. The use of corticosteroids in the treatment of synovitis is of limited benefit and therefore should be avoided. However, the local injection of corticosteroids and an anesthetic in regions of tendinitis temporarily ameliorates the pain. In the absence of a response of the synovitis to this regimen, low-dose oral methotrexate can be used.

PSORIATIC ARTHRITIS

Psoriatic arthritis (PsA) is an inflammatory arthritis that occurs in approximately 5 to 7 per cent of patients with psoriasis. Based on clinical, epidemiological, and immunogenetic findings, PsA is a distinct rheumatic disease and not a variant of RA or other inflammatory spondyloarthritides. Yet patients with PsA often share clinical, radiographic, pathological, and immunogenetic features with Reiter's syndrome and other spondyloarthritides.

Clinical Presentation

The diagnosis of PsA remains a clinical one, dependent on symptoms and findings on examination.

Because PsA is a systemic disorder, patients often describe multiple constitutional complaints. The severity and extent of psoriasis and onychodystrophy do not necessarily parallel the activity of the arthritis. The symptoms of fatigability, morning stiffness, and articular pain and swelling are similar to those found in RA. Thus, the frequent family or personal history of psoriasis or both help provide the initial clue to the diagnosis of PsA.

Because ankylosing spondylitis (including sacroiliitis) occurs in one fifth to one third of individuals with PsA, the symptoms of back pain should be thoroughly investigated. Such complaints as low back pain and stiffness after resting, improvement of soreness and stiffness with exercise, and chest wall pain suggest an inflammatory rather than a structural etiology of the back pain (Table 110–1).

Three different distributions of synovitis at the onset of disease typify PsA. Patients with PsA classified as group I have an asymmetrical oligo- or polyarticular synovitis involving any joint, especially the DIP joints, PIP joints, or both, of the hands and feet. About one half of all individuals with PsA exhibit an asymmetrical arthritis at disease onset. Although PsA was classically described as affecting the DIP joints of the hands, distal involvement alone occurs in only a small minority of patients. Some patients who initially present with an asymmetrical oligo- or polyarticular synovitis develop a symmetrical pattern over time. Other common findings on physical examination include "sausage digits" and onychodystrophy. Sausage digits of the fingers or toes, or both, result from interphalangeal involvement and attendant flexor tendon sheath effusion. Onychodystrophy, a manifestation of psoriasis, occurs in about two thirds of patients with an asymmetrical arthritis.

In general, the course of disease in asymmetrical synovitis is less aggressive and disabling than in other forms of PsA.

PsA presents as a symmetrical arthritis (group II) affecting any pairs of joints, including the DIP joints, PIP joints, or both, of the hands and feet, in about 25 per cent of affected individuals. In contrast to individuals with an asymmetrical distribution of arthritis, one half may experience an erratic, destructive, deforming, and progressively disabling disease course.

Psoriatic spondyloarthritis (Group III) is the coexistence of either sacroiliitis or ankylosing spondylitis with psoriasis. With the exception of their psoriasis, persons with psoriatic spondyloarthritis have physical stigmata similar to those with idiopathic ankylosing spondylitis or sacroiliitis.

TABLE 110–1. SYMPTOMS AND SIGNS IN PSORIATIC SPONDYLOARTHRITIS*

Symptoms
  Back stiffness and pain >3 months
  Improvement of back pain and stiffness with exercise
  Thoracic pain
  Radiation of pain to buttocks
  Dyspnea with effort
Signs
  Chest expansion <2.5 cm, resulting in restrictive pulmonary defect
  Limitation of motion of spine
  Inflammatory ocular disease

* After Kammer GM: Clinical significance of subgroups in psoriatic arthritis. IM—Int Med Spec 2:40, 1981.

A major complication of PsA is arthritis mutilans. This is a severe, deforming, and destructive arthritis that has a relentless course and principally affects the small joints of the hands and feet; it occurs with approximately equal frequency in the three groups. Radiographically, it is characterized by osteolysis and bone resorption of the metacarpals, metatarsals, phalanges, and tufts and by ankylosis and osteoporosis. Unfortunately, history or physical examination gives no clues that can predict the eventual occurrence of arthritis mutilans.

Laboratory and Radiographic Findings

No laboratory studies are specific for PsA. Because of the presence of widespread inflammation, the Westergren erythrocyte sedimentation rate, the C-reactive protein, and other acute phase reactants (i.e., complement) are elevated during disease activity. The occurrence of rheumatoid factors in a patient with otherwise definite PsA should not dissuade the clinician from that diagnosis. Other commonly observed but nonspecific abnormal laboratory findings include the anemia of chronic disease, polyclonal hypergammaglobulinemia, hyperuricemia, low titer ANA, and circulating immune complexes.

The radiographic features of the peripheral joints include soft-tissue swelling, demineralization, loss of cartilage space, erosions, bony ankylosis, subluxation, and subchondral cysts. Several radiographic findings are classically observed in arthritis mutilans. These findings include "whittling," "pencil-in-cup," *"la main en lorgnette"* (opera-glass hand), and *"doigt en lorgnette"* (telescope finger). Of particular interest is the usual simultaneous occurrence of osteoporosis, osteolysis, and bony ankylosis.

Immunogenetic Findings

The frequency of B27 in all individuals with PsA is about one in three. More recent genetic studies have also shown that the HLA antigens B17, Bw38, Bw39, and DRw4 are significantly increased in persons with PsA. It remains to be demonstrated, however, what the role of these tissue antigens is in the inheritance, susceptibility, and severity of the disease.

Treatment of PsA

Optimal management of acute PsA or a flare of the disease currently combines several modalities: bed rest, a program of physical therapy, orthotics, and drug therapy. The agents used for short-term treatment provide anti-inflammatory action to reduce synovitis and control pain. Such agents include aspirin and nonsteroidal anti-inflammatory drugs.

A minority of patients fail to respond to the conservative regimen outlined above. To control the inflammatory process, corticosteroids are often used on a short-term basis.

For long-term management, nonsteroidal anti-inflammatory agents alone can be employed in mild, nonerosive PsA. In the presence of more severe disease with attendant erosive arthritis, a remittive agent should be used. Several agents, including gold salts, 6-mercaptopurine, and methotrexate, have been successful. Methotrexate has been used extensively in the treatment of both severe psoriasis and PsA. The use of remittive agents may be complicated by dermatoses, bone marrow toxicity, and hepatotoxicity. Care must be taken to follow the clinical course at regular intervals and to obtain appropriate laboratory studies to exclude toxicity.

ARTHRITIS ASSOCIATED WITH INFLAMMATORY BOWEL DISEASE

Inflammatory bowel disease (IBD) is an idiopathic chronic inflammatory process involving the gastrointestinal tract. Both ulcerative colitis and regional enteritis can be associated with an inflammatory arthritis. Two distinct types of arthritis are observed in these disorders: a peripheral arthritis and ankylosing spondylitis. These entities are discussed in Chapter 38.

REFERENCES

Calin A: The spondyloarthropathies. *In* Wyngaarden JB, Smith LH Jr (eds): Cecil Textbook of Medicine. 18th ed. Philadelphia, WB Saunders Co, 1988, p 2004.

Fox R, Calin A, Gerber R, et al: The chronicity of symptoms and disability in Reiter's syndrome: An analysis of 181 consecutive patients. Ann Intern Med 91:190–193, 1979.

Kammer G, Soter N, Gibson B, et al: Psoriatic arthritis: a clinical, immunologic and HLA study of 100 patients. Sem Arth Rheum 9:75–97, 1979.

Ziff M, Cohen SB: The spondyloarthropathies. *In* Advances in Inflammation Research, Vol 9. New York, Raven Press, 1985.

111

OSTEOARTHRITIS

Osteoarthritis is the most frequently encountered disorder of connective tissue affecting the joints in human beings. Although the disease has been described as a "wear and tear" process leading to the degeneration of articular cartilage in the elderly age range, this characterization is an imprecise oversimplification. Instead, osteoarthritis should be viewed as an insidious, slowly evolving disorder of the articular cartilage occurring over decades, which becomes *symptomatic* during the sixth through ninth decades. More specifically, osteoarthritis is a disease of both articular cartilage and subchondral bone. There is structural disorganization and deterioration of cartilage leading to focal and, later, diffuse erosions of the surface cartilage. The erosions are a result of pitting and fissuring of the cartilage. Contiguous erosions become larger ulcerations, finally resulting in large areas of destroyed cartilage over the articular surface. The progressive loss of cartilage is often associated with proliferation of new bone and cartilage at the joint margins, the result of which is osteochondrophyte spur formation. In general, there is little, if any, primary synovitis associated with the destruction of cartilage and osteophyte formation, and, therefore, osteoarthritis is not regarded as an inflammatory arthritis but as a structural arthritis. The underlying subchondral bone, when directly exposed following cartilage loss, shows drop-out of osteocytes, osteoblastic and osteoclastic activity, and regions of osteolysis adjacent to subarticular osteosclerosis. Thus, osteoarthritis is an insidious, slowly advancing disease resulting in progressive destruction of articular cartilage, osteophyte formation, subchondral bone collapse, and sclerosis, which produces variable clinical disability of an affected joint.

Osteoarthritis is a worldwide disorder found in approximately the same frequency in all geographic regions. Pathologic studies have demonstrated that by age 40 many persons exhibit some asymptomatic degenerative changes in the cartilage of weight-bearing joints. However, by age 75 virtually all persons have developed osteoarthritis in one or more joints. Thus, the prevalence of symptomatic osteoarthritis does increase with age. When all ages are considered, the prevalence of the disease is equal among males and females. However, certain stresses applied repetitively over long periods of time, as occur in certain occupations, appear to predispose to the development of osteoarthritis.

Osteoarthritis is classified as primary (Table 111–1) or secondary. The disorder is considered primary when it occurs in the absence of any identifiable underlying process. In contrast, it is termed secondary when it complicates a previously established pathologic process such as congenital hip dysplasia or slipped femoral epiphysis.

More recently, primary osteoarthritis has been recognized to exist in clinically different forms, or subsets. On the basis of clinical, histopathologic, and radiographic findings, four types have been identified: primary generalized osteoarthritis, erosive osteoarthritis, diffuse idiopathic skeletal hyperostosis, and chondromalacia patellae (Table 111–1).

The most common distribution of joint involvement in osteoarthritis is the distal interphalangeals, proximal interphalangeals, the first carpometacarpals, hips, knees, first metatarsophalangeals, and the cervical and lumbar apophyseal joints. Although most individuals with osteoarthritis have only a few affected joints, primary generalized osteoarthritis often involves the majority of joints listed above sequentially over time. Unlike inflammatory arthritides such as rheumatoid arthritis, there are no systemic signs of early morning stiffness and profound fatigability. Instead, there is a gradual increase in the degree of a deep, poorly localized pain. Pain is worse following use of the affected joint and better with rest. With progression of the disease, every little motion of the affected joint induces pain, and there is often nocturnal pain. The pain is the result of several co-existent factors, including direct pressure upon exposed subchondral bone; trabecular microinfarcts; periosteal elevation; distortion of the joint capsule; and, when present, a secondary inflammatory synovitis.

Examination of the affected joint reveals several notable clinical findings suggestive of osteoarthritis. Tenderness upon palpation often affects widely separated areas of the joint. There may be joint enlargement due to proliferative changes in the cartilage and bone with osteophyte formation. Although large effusions are uncommon, the joint, especially the knee, can exhibit a mild synovitis with a small effusion. Palpation of the para-articular structures may demonstrate medial or lateral joint line tenderness and anserine bursitis. Passive range of motion can elicit variable crepitus and limitation of motion. Varus or valgus deformities are observed during the more advanced stages of osteoarthritis of the knees due to cartilage loss and collapse of subchondral bone. Thus, gait disturbances of variable severity can be observed. Similarly, advanced joint disease, with attendant splinting, often results in muscle atrophy, enhancing the characteristic limp.

TABLE 111–1. CLASSIFICATION OF PRIMARY OSTEOARTHRITIS*

Peripheral joints: first CMC, first MTP, DIP, PIP, hip, knee
Spine: intervertebral and apophyseal joints
Variant subsets
  Erosive inflammatory osteoarthritis
  Generalized osteoarthritis
  Diffuse idiopathic skeletal hyperostosis
  Chondromalacia patellae

* After Moskowitz RW, Howell DS, Goldberg VM, Mankin HJ (eds): Osteoarthritis: Diagnosis and Management. Philadelphia, WB Saunders Co, 1984, p 3.

Specific joints are commonly affected in osteoarthritis. Osteophyte formation and loss of the joint space of the distal interphalangeal joint are termed a Heberden's node, and involvement of the proximal interphalangeal joint is called a Bouchard's node.

There are no specific identifying laboratory features of osteoarthritis. Because there is no substantial inflammatory response, there are no acute phase reactants such as an accelerated sedimentation rate or elevated serum complement levels. The blood count is also within normal limits. Synovial fluid analysis generally shows a clear yellow fluid and a good mucin clot formation. The leukocyte count is usually less than 500 to 750/cu mm, with fewer than 25 per cent granulocytes. The total protein is often less than 3.0 gm/dl. The synovial fluid glucose is normal. Fibrosis and fragments of cartilage embedded in the synovium are often present.

Optimal management of the osteoarthritic joint requires the sequential or simultaneous use of several treatment modalities. These include physical and occupational therapy, drug therapy, and reconstructive surgery. The application of such modalities as exercise, the use of orthoses and adaptive devices, and education in conjunction with a capable therapist will prevent the devastating loss of joint and muscle function which leads to disability. A program of exercises will be more effectively carried out if the patient has sufficient symptomatic relief of pain with appropriate drug therapy. At present, there are no known pharmacological agents that can reverse or block the natural course of osteoarthritis. Therefore, agents are selected which provide analgesic and/or anti-inflammatory properties. If assessment indicates primarily a mechanical joint dysfunction, but little inflammation, then use of a non-narcotic analgesic agent is sufficient. The presence of more advanced disease with evidence of synovitis as well as pain is an indication for a nonsteroidal anti-inflammatory agent.

Although the majority of patients with osteoarthritis can be successfully managed conservatively, an increasing proportion of individuals is requiring reconstructive joint surgery. In general, three indications for considering a surgical procedure include (a) progressive and irreversible loss of joint function; (b) pain, especially nocturnal pain; and (c) diminishing capacity to carry out activities of daily living independently.

The surgical management of osteoarthritis can be divided into four basic approaches: (a) osteotomy, (b) debridement, (c) arthrodesis, and (d) arthroplasty.

REFERENCES

Howell DS: Osteoarthritis (degenerative joint disease). *In* Wyngaarden JB, Smith LH Jr (eds): Cecil Textbook of Medicine. 18th ed. Philadelphia, WB Saunders Co, 1988, pp 2039–2041.

Moskowitz RW, Howell DS, Goldberg VM, Mankin HJ (eds): Osteoarthritis. Diagnosis and Management. Philadelphia, WB Saunders Co, 1984.

112

THE CRYSTAL-INDUCED ARTHRITIDES

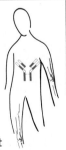

CHONDROCALCINOSIS AND ASSOCIATED DISORDERS

Crystal-induced arthritides include gout, discussed in Chapter 61, chondrocalcinosis, and apatite-induced diseases, which will be considered here. Chondrocalcinosis results from the deposition of calcium pyrophosphate dihydrate (CPPD) crystals in cartilage. The clinical disorder, pseudogout, is polyarticular, most often idiopathic, but is also associated with aging and certain metabolic disorders (Table 112–1). It affects about 5 per cent of the adult population and may resemble clinically gout, rheumatoid arthritis, neurotrophic arthritis, or osteoarthritis.

Pseudogout is an acute inflammatory arthritis that results from the phagocytosis of IgG-coated CPPD crystals by synovial fluid neutrophils and the subsequent release of inflammatory mediators. Pseudogout accounts for approximately one quarter of all cases of CPPD deposition disease and predominantly affects men. Initially monarticular, the attack soon becomes oligo- or polyarticular. Although the acute arthritis can be self-limiting, lasting for one to several days, more severe attacks involving both the peripheral and axial joints can more slowly resolve over several weeks. The precipitating factors are often similar to those inducing an acute gouty arthritis. The large joints of the lower extremities are more likely to be affected as op-

TABLE 112–1. RELATIONSHIP OF CPPD DEPOSITION TO METABOLIC DISORDERS

Hemochromatosis
Hyperparathyroidism
Hypothyroidism
Gout
Hypomagnesemia
Hypophosphatasia
Wilson's disease
Ochronosis

posed to the small joints in acute gout. The knee joint is involved in over one half of all cases of pseudogout. The diagnosis of pseudogout should not depend upon the radiographic findings alone, since chondrocalcinosis is observed in only 75 per cent of pseudogout. The presence of chondrocalcinosis can be identified radiographically by the characteristic punctate or linear radiodensities in the joint fibrocartilaginous lateral menisci of the knees or hyaline articular cartilage. Other areas frequently exhibiting these findings include the wrists and pelvis.

The diagnosis of pseudogout and its differentiation from other acute inflammatory arthritides make arthrocentesis a necessary procedure in its evaluation. Acute infectious arthritis and gout can clinically resemble pseudogout. Moreover, both monosodium urate and CPPD crystals can coexist within the same joint. CPPD crystals are rhomboid in shape and produce weakly positive birefringence under compensated polarizing microscopy. The crystals can be observed within neutrophils or are free-floating. The synovial fluid exhibits a leukocytosis with a predominance of neutrophils and has a low viscosity (see Table 100–4).

CPPD crystal disease can also exhibit a symmetrical polyarticular distribution and can clinically resemble rheumatoid arthritis in about 5 per cent of cases. Patients having this form of the disease describe prolonged morning stiffness, fatigability, and malaise. The course of the disease is punctuated by mild attacks of many months in duration. Examination reveals polyarticular synovitis and, less often, flexion contractures. Although there can be elevation of the sedimentation rate and IgM rheumatoid factors (10 per cent), radiographs show secondary osteoarthritic changes of affected joints, and the synovial fluid has a normal glucose and complement in the presence of CPPD crystals.

Progressive osteoarthritis complicated by flexion contractures occurs in about one half of all cases of CPPD crystal disease. This form, known as pseudo-osteoarthritis, usually affects women and involves the knees, wrists, MCPs, hips, shoulders, elbows, and ankles. The process can be symmetrical or asymmetrical. Although radiographs may or may not demonstrate the punctate or linear calcifications of the cartilage, CPPD crystals are found in synovial fluid even in radiographically negative joints.

Asymptomatic persons found inadvertently to have CPPD crystal deposits by radiographs are said to have lanthantic CPPD deposition disease. In contrast, the combination of tabes dorsalis, Charcot knee joint deformities, and CPPD crystal deposits produces a painful, disabled joint. The finding of CPPD crystals in these destructive joint processes is referred to as pseudoneurotrophic.

The management of CPPD deposition disease is similar to that of gout. Clinically symptomatic disease responds to rest, joint protection, and the initiation of a nonsteroidal anti-inflammatory agent. Colchicine has been found to be efficacious in pseudogout as well as gout. Following aspiration of a joint with marked synovitis, the instillation of a corticosteroid preparation may hasten resolution of the inflammatory process. Maintenance therapy, when necessary, consists of a nonsteroidal anti-inflammatory agent and colchicine.

The third crystal-induced rheumatic syndrome is associated with apatite crystals, $Ca_5(PO_4)_3OH$. The spectrum of clinical manifestations ranges from calcific tendinitis to frank arthritis that is typically episodic and monarticular. "Milwaukee shoulder" is an inflammatory and destructive arthritis associated with rotator cuff tear in which apatite crystals play an etiologic role.

The differentiation of apatite-induced inflammation from acute septic arthritis, gout, or pseudogout is made by synovial fluid examination. Apatite crystals are non-birefringent globules or clumps under polarized light and stain with alizarin red under light microscopy.

Systemic diseases, including chronic renal failure, scleroderma, and dermatomyositis, can be associated with apatite deposition. CPPD and apatite disease can also coexist with osteoarthritis, with chronic gout, and with rheumatoid arthritis.

REFERENCES

Gibilisco PA, Schumacher HR, Hollander JL, et al: Synovial fluid crystals in osteoarthritis. Arthritis Rheum 28:511, 1985.

McCarty DJ: Diagnostic mimicry in arthritis—patterns of joint involvement associated with calcium pyrophosphate dihydrate crystal deposits. Bull Rheum Dis 25:804, 1974–75.

Schumacher HR, Somlyo AP, Rose RL, et al: Arthritis associated with apatite crystals. Ann Intern Med 87:411, 1977.

SECTION
XIII
NEUROLOGIC DISEASES

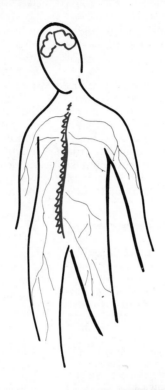

113

EVALUATION OF THE PATIENT

Disorders of the nervous system are not easy to define precisely. In the broadest sense, all symptoms of disease are neurological, since the ability of the patient to recognize that he is ill requires that (1) sensory pathways carry information from the diseased organ to the brain and (2) the brain interpret that information as a symptom of something wrong. Furthermore, the brain can generate within itself symptoms (see p. 693) identical to those it receives from the body's peripheral organs and interprets as signs of bodily dysfuction. For example, both emotionally generated anxiety and a catecholamine-secreting pheochromocytoma can cause headache, shortness of breath, and feelings of panic.

By convention, neurological diseases are defined as those in which there is either a structural or a physiological abnormality in the central or peripheral nervous system. Exceptions exist: Most headache is caused by extracranial non-neural dysfunction but is considered a neurological disease; the same holds true for much back pain, a condition caused most often by abnormal muscle or joint function. About 10 per cent of patients who visit the office of their primary care physician complain of symptoms suggesting a neurological disorder. The figure for hospital admissions is 25 per cent. Table 113–1 lists the most common complaints leading to neurological referral and some possible disorders causing those complaints.

As the above paragraph implies, disorders of the nervous system place special requirements upon the physician's clinical skills. Symptoms of nervous system disease can be mimicked by those of systemic or psychiatric illness (e.g., somewhat similar headaches may be caused by brain tumor, giant cell arteritis, or involutional depression). The physician must systematically approach patients whose complaints are potentially neurological and answer four fundamental questions, as outlined in Table 113–2.

While the physician is considering the possibility or the nature of a primary neurological disorder, he must pay close attention to the patient's psychological state. Few illnesses frighten patients as much as those of the nervous system, with its threat of dementia, paralysis, and loss of control of bodily functions. Kindness, reassurance, and control of symptoms such as pain mark the humane approach to the diagnosis of a patient with neurological disease. A final requirement is to recognize that the nervous system regenerates poorly and that once neurological function is lost, it is rarely regained. Therefore, an appropriate combination of care and speed are necessary to make the correct diagnosis and institute appropriate treatment. At times, in the presence of severe and potentially irreversible crises, one must attempt to stabilize the nervous system even before beginning the diagnostic exercise.

TABLE 113–1. COMMON COMPLAINTS IN NEUROLOGICAL PRACTICE

| COMPLAINTS | EXAMPLES | |
	STRUCTURAL	PHYSIOLOGICAL OR PSYCHOPHYSIOLOGICAL
Headache	Brain tumor	Migraine or tension
Backache	Herniated disc	Myofascial pain syndromes
Dizziness	Meniere's disease	Hyperventilation attacks, perceptual imbalance
Weakness and/or fatigue	Myasthenia gravis	"Neurasthenia"
Memory loss	Alzheimer's dementia	Depression, preoccupation
Episodic alterations of consciousness	Seizures, syncope	Anxiety, hyperventilation

TABLE 113–2. CRUCIAL STEPS IN NEUROLOGICAL DIAGNOSIS

Does the patient have a nervous system disorder?
  Do psychological mechanisms play a role in the genesis of symptoms?
Where in the nervous system is the disorder?
  Central or peripheral, brain or spinal cord, left or right, single or multiple?
What are the mechanisms (pathophysiology)?
  Structural or physiological, vascular, neoplastic, inflammatory, etc.
What is the cause (etiology)?
  Specific tests

THE NEUROLOGICAL HISTORY

In most respects, the neurological history is similar to the general medical history. The purpose (to supply diagnostic information that will direct the physical and laboratory examinations and lead to an appropriate diagnosis) and the format (e.g., chief complaint, present illness, past history, social history, review of systems) are the same (Table 113–3). However, because many neurological diseases are not accompanied by either abnormal physical or laboratory findings, the neurological history often supplies a greater proportion of the diagnostically relevant information than does a medical history. Furthermore, because neurological abnormalities affect such important functions as thinking, moving, and feeling, most important abnormal physical signs will already have created symptoms perceived by the patient. (Exceptions occur in demented patients and those with lesions of the nondominant parietal lobe, characterized by denial of disability.) Findings on examination not previously recognized by the patient or his family are likely to be irrelevant or even misleading. By contrast, recent symptoms, such as mild weakness or alterations of sensation, often reflect disease even if the process is still too subtle to be detected by the most meticulous neurological examination. Because neurological symptoms are so keenly sensed, a careful history often allows the examiner to localize the disease anatomically and to understand its pathophysiology even before he begins the physical examination.

Taking the neurological history ordinarily occupies the majority of the time initially spent in evaluating a patient suffering from a neurological disorder. At the completion of the history, the physician should be able either to make a definitive diagnosis or to formulate three or four diagnostic hypotheses that can be tested by physical and laboratory examinations. Because an almost infinite number of potential questions can be asked of a patient with a neurological disorder, one must develop a strategy to achieve maximal useful information in a reasonable period of time. Specific questions should be tailored to the patient's complaints and to the physician's knowledge of neurological illness. Certain guidelines aid in taking complete and accurate histories:

Require Precision. Do not accept jargon or diagnoses from the patient. For example, a patient who complains of dizziness may mean vertigo (a vestibular symptom), lightheadedness (potentially caused by cardiovascular disease), syncope, ataxia, diplopia, or psychogenic dissociation—all of which have very different implications. "Sinus headache" is a diagnostic term often given to describe headaches that are rarely caused by sinusitis but are usually migraine or tension headache.

Both Listen and Ask. Elicit the history in the patient's own words and, whenever possible, without interruption. Excessive interruptions can imply that one is hurried or disinterested and may lead patients to exclude vital information. When the patient is allowed to tell his story, important information often emerges about fears and anxieties. However, the physician must ask direct questions to encourage relevance, achieve precision, and place each symptom in its correct context. If the information is not volunteered, ask about the temporal profile of the complaint: was the onset abrupt or gradual? Is it static, progressive, waxing and waning, or improving? Inquire into the intensity and frequency of the symptoms and the events and factors that precipitate or relieve them, and determine how the symptoms affect the patient's daily life and any other symptoms associated with the major complaint. For example, although a patient may complain of headache, careful questioning may yield a clinical description of trigeminal neuralgia (p. 712) or cluster headaches (p. 709) so characteristic as to allow no other diagnosis.

Form Hypotheses. Do not be a passive recipient of the patient's story. Most patients supply excessive information, much not diagnostically pertinent. One must sift and distill the information in order to retain what is relevant and weed out the irrelevant. Concurrently, one must form anatomical and/or pathophysiological hypotheses about the nature of the

TABLE 113–3. IMPORTANT ELEMENTS OF THE NEUROLOGICAL HISTORY

Chief complaint and present illness
  Require the patient to describe symptoms precisely.
  Onset sudden or gradual?
  Course progressive, remitting, improving, stable?
  Aggravating and relieving factors?
  Associated symptoms?
Other history (past and present)
  Previous neurological symptoms?
  Previous or present medical illnesses, allergies, exposure to toxins?
Social and psychological history
  How does illness affect daily life and vice versa?
Review of systems
  Mood
  Sexual function
  Nutrition, weight
  Drugs and medicinals
  Sleep habits

symptoms and gradually refine them into etiologic terms as the history develops. For example, in a patient complaining of weakness of the right arm and leg, the hypotheses might include a lesion of the left hemisphere, the brain stem, or the cervical spinal cord. As the history discloses weakness in the face and difficulty with language, the latter two hypotheses can be discarded and the left hemispheral lesion accepted. An additional history of slowly progressive weakness accompanied by headaches and lethargy suggests an intracranial mass, possibly hematoma, tumor, or abscess, and a history of heavy smoking with recent cough could imply a metastatic lung tumor. Hypotheses should favor illnesses that are *probable* (i.e., common diseases are more likely than rare diseases), *serious* (e.g., brain tumors should be excluded before diagnosing tension headache), *treatable* (e.g., combined systems disease and spinal cord meningioma should be ruled out before making a diagnosis of multiple sclerosis), and *novel* (some patients do have rare diseases, and these should not be forgotten in taking the history).

Always Take a Complete History. Even if the diagnosis seems clear from the chief complaint and the present illness, check other aspects of the history to ensure that other physical or psychological disabilities are not playing a role. In particular, inquire about the patient's mood (e.g., is he depressed or suicidal?), his usually daily activities and whether the illness interferes with them, his sexual function, the nature of psychological and physical support at home, and his own view of his illness and how it affects him.

End by Summarizing. Summarize for the patient the history, asking if the summary is correct and if anything has been missed. Such a summary offers a chance to supply information and to correct misunderstandings. It also tends to reassure patients and allows them an additional opportunity to present sensitive or embarrassing material.

Obtain Further History from the Family and Friends. If the history appears incomplete, and particularly if part of the illness involves changes in mental state or consciousness, the family, friends, and colleagues should be asked to corroborate the story and to supply missing elements, giving their views on how the signs and symptoms affect the patient's daily life.

Gear the Neurological Examination to Hypotheses Generated by the History. It is neither possible nor desirable to perform all elements of the neurological examination on every patient. Thus, the hypotheses generated during the course of the history determine which of the nonroutine neurological maneuvers the physician will carry out during his examination. For example, a complaint of intermittent numbness in an upper extremity should lead to tests for thoracic outlet compromise, even though that is not part of the routine neurological examination. Hypotheses generated during the history also direct subsequent laboratory testing, even in the presence of a normal neurological examination. For example, if the history strongly suggests dysfunction of the left cerebral hemisphere (e.g., focal seizures), failure to find a hemiparesis on examination does not rule out a brain tumor and a magnetic resonance image (MR) or a computed tomographic scan (CT) should be performed. Even if such tests are initially uninformative, a strongly suggestive history requires that the doctor follow the patient closely, repeating the test if necessary.

THE NEUROLOGICAL EXAMINATION

All major aspects of the nervous system must be examined systematically (Table 113–4). A screening neurological examination, as outlined here, takes only a few minutes. More time may be required to evaluate areas that the history suggests may be disordered. Details of those examinations are given in the chapters that follow. The *level of arousal* must be noted: is the patient awake and alert, drowsy and lethargic, responsive only when externally stimulated (stuporous),

TABLE 113–4. IMPORTANT ELEMENTS OF THE NEUROLOGICAL EXAMINATION

Level of arousal
Mental status
 Orientation, mood, language, memory, intellect, thought
Station and gait
Cranial nerves
Motor system
 Strength, tone, muscle bulk, adventitious movements
Sensory system
 Pin, temperature, vibration, object identification, proprioception
Reflexes
 Deep tendon
 Abdominals
 Plantar
 Anal wink
Autonomic system
 Blood pressure
 Sphincter
Vascular system
 Carotid pulse and bruits; distal arteries

or psychologically unarousable, even to vigorous external stimulation (comatose). The *mental state* can be examined during the history. A person who gives an articulate and comprehensive history with accurate attention to both detail and dating of the complaints almost always has retained normal cognitive functions. Still, one may occasionally be fooled and it is useful to check (1) orientation, particularly for place and date, (2) short-term memory (the most vulnerable memory function) by asking the patient to repeat three unrelated words five minutes after he has heard them, and (3) capacity to abstract, by interpreting proverbs and by recognizing similarities and differences (boy-dwarf, apple-pear). Because anxiety can interfere with cognitive functions, one must be patient and reassuring. Patients usually do not object to cognitive tests if one begins gently by indicating that he is going to test the patient's memory. Many patients who do object are hiding cognitive abnormalities. A formal quantitative screening examination such as the "mini mental status" examination (see Table 114–19) is useful for following a patient suspected of suffering cognitive dysfunction.

Observe the patient's *stance and walk.* If possible this should be done with the patient at least partially undressed so that the alignment of the spine can be observed. A patient who can turn briskly, walk on heels and toes, do a deep-knee bend, and tandem walk has no substantial disability of motor or coordinative functions of the lower extremities. In the absence of specific complaints, these functions need not be tested further.

Examine the *cranial nerves*; visual acuity and visual fields should be tested in all patients and the optic fundi scrutinized for abnormalities of the blood vessels, retina, or optic discs. Pupillary activity, ocular movements, corneal reflexes, jaw movement, facial movement, hearing, swallowing, speaking, and breathing should be tested quickly as well. On the other hand, postural tests of labyrinthine function need not be assessed in the absence of a history of dizziness or vertigo.

Abnormalities of *upper extremity* form, strength, and proprioception can be assessed by having the patient extend his arms forward in a supinated position and spread his fingers. If, with the eyes closed, neither arm drifts and there are no tremors or adventitious movements of the fingers, and if the patient can accurately touch his index finger in rapid succession to his nose and the examiner's outstretched finger, it is likely that, in the absence of complaints, no neurological abnormalities affect the upper extremities. If, however, he complains of weakness or sensory loss, one must test these functions individually.

Sensation can further be assessed by testing in succession the ability of the patient to identify objects placed in his hand when his eyes are closed, to perceive position and vibration in the hands and feet (for vibration, the examiner can use his own perception as the norm, recognizing that in older persons vibration perception normally declines somewhat), and to recognize anywhere on his body the sharp from the dull end of a pin. Any significant sensory loss of the extremities will almost certainly have been described by the sentient patient during the history and demands careful sensory testing of each dermatome and peripheral nerve in the area of complaint. *Deep tendon reflexes* from biceps, triceps, brachioradialis, knees, and ankles are a sufficient screening test. Test the plantar responses, recalling that an equivocal Babinski sign is more likely to be misleading than helpful. *Autonomic activity* and *sphincter functions* are usually examined as part of the general medical examination, but one seeks a history of sphincter disturbance, and careful assessment of sphincter tone, voluntary sphincter contraction, and the anal wink reflex is essential. Always test for postural hypotension when evaluating autonomic impairment or dizziness. The carotid arteries, the aorta, and peripheral pulses should be palpated and auscultated for evidence of vascular disease, but be aware of transmitted cardiac bruits.

The physician should be careful not to be misled by equivocal neurological signs. In office practice the neurological examination can mislead almost as often as it helps, particularly when subtle sensory or reflex asymmetries are found. Patients, in their anxiety to be helpful, often hyperdiscriminate, so that they interpret mild changes in the pressure of the examining pin as differences in sensation and falsely interpret as vibration the pressure of the unstruck tuning fork. When persons complain of sensory disturbance, it is often wise to let them map its distribution before the examiner attempts to do so.

DIAGNOSTIC TESTS: SCOPE AND LIMITATIONS

New technology has remarkably increased the accuracy of diagnosis and physiological evaluations. However, if used inappropriately, high technology tests needlessly raise the cost of medical care; furthermore, their results threaten to become the goals of care rather than a means to diagnosis. Since the doctor's practice influences this aspect of health care costs, a judicious physician must consider, before ordering, the precise advantages that each positive or negative test can confer on a patient's evaluation and treatment (Table 113–5).

Tissue Analysis

Lumbar Puncture (LP). LP, a safe and simple technique for analyzing cerebrospinal fluid (CSF), indirectly assesses biochemical abnormalities in the extracellular fluid of the central nervous system. Because headache and backache can follow lumbar puncture, the procedure is not routine but is done for a specific indication (Table 113–6). The test is mandatory and usually diagnostic when the leptomeninges or surface of the brain are infiltrated by infectious agents or tumor. The test also establishes the diagnosis (in the presence of a normal CT scan) of pseudotumor cerebri (p. 804) or idiopathic intracranial hypotension (p. 805). The total protein concentration gives nonspecific in-

TABLE 113–5. COMMON NEUROLOGICAL LABORATORY TESTS: APPROXIMATE COSTS*

Lumbar puncture (spinal tap)	$ 175.00
Myelogram	1100.00
Computed tomography (CT)	
Brain	420.00
Vertebral-paravertebral area	420.00
Magnetic resonance (MR) imaging	850.00
Brain	
Spinal cord	
Angiography	
Arteriograms	1100.00
Cerebral, spinal	
Digital intravenous angiogram (DIVA)	1100.00
Vessels of neck	
Cerebral venous sinuses	
Electrodiagnostic tests	
EEG	174.00
EMG and nerve conduction velocity	396.00
Neuromuscular transmission	210.00
Evoked potentials	
Visual	207.00
Auditory	207.00
Sensory	207.00
Muscle biopsy	$87.00 for processing plus surgeon's fee

* Cost includes mean laboratory and professional fees at major New York City hospitals, 1988.

formation about the presence of nervous system disease and assists in the diagnosis of polyneuropathies. Protein electrophoresis may assist in the diagnosis of multiple sclerosis and other inflammatory diseases of the nervous system. No patient should be anticoagulated for a presumed stroke unless an LP (or a CT scan) have ruled out intracranial hemorrhage. The diagnosis of subarachnoid hemorrage is usually made by identifying blood in the subarachnoid space on CT scan, eliminating the need for an LP. There are only a few contraindications. Lumbar puncture should not be performed in patients with known or suspected intracranial mass lesions until after a brain image has been obtained to assure the safety of the procedure. In every patient who undergoes LP, sufficient fluid should be obtained and sampled to procure maximal information. The tests in Table 113–6 are those most commonly ordered. The most common complication of LP is headache resulting from intracranial hypotension (see p. 805). Post-LP headache, usually mild, follows about 20 per cent of LP's and cannot be prevented by a period of post-LP bed rest. The smaller the LP needle, the lower the incidence of headache.

Tissue Biopsy. Diagnostic biopsies of muscle, less often of peripheral nerve or brain, can give information achievable in no other way (Table 113–7). Select for biopsy only those patients in whom the test is likely to yield information that is not only diagnostic and prognostic but also of therapeutic benefit.

Imaging Techniques (Fig. 113–1)

Computed Tomography. Modern techniques of imaging (MR and CT) identify most structural diseases of the brain and spinal cord. A negative test often re-

TABLE 113–6. CONSIDERATIONS FOR PERFORMING A LUMBAR PUNCTURE (LP)

Indications for Test

Absolute
  Suspicion of central nervous system infection
  Before anticoagulant therapy for cerebrovascular disease (if no CT)
Relative
  Suspicion of nervous system disease
  Intrathecal therapy for meningeal leukemia or fungal meningitis
  Symptomatic treatment of severe headache from subarachnoid
    hemorrhage or pseudotumor cerebri

Contraindications

Absolute
  Tissue infection in region of puncture site
Relative
  Spinal cord tumor, known or probable brain tumor
  Bleeding tendency (anticoagulant or thrombocytopenia)
  Increased intracranial pressure due to mass lesions

Diagnostic Evaluation of Cerebrospinal Fluid

Sediment
  Cell count and differential
  Cytological examination for neoplastic cells
  Stains for bacteria and fungi
  Culture for organisms
Supernatant Fluid
  Protein concentration
  Protein electrophoresis (gamma globulin, oligoclonal bands)
  Glucose concentration
  Serological tests for syphilis
  Viral antibodies and cultures
  Spectrophotometric test for bilirubin, oxyhemoglobin, or
    methemoglobin

Complications of Test

Common
  Headache
  Backache
Rare
  Transtentorial or foramen magnum herniation
  Worsening of spinal tumor symptoms
  Spinal epidural hematoma (patients with bleeding tendency)
  Herniated or infected disc
  Reaction to anesthetic agent
  Meningitis (contaminated needle)

TABLE 113–7. TISSUE ANALYSIS FOR NEUROLOGICAL DIAGNOSIS

TISSUE	INDICATION(S)	COMMENT
Muscle	Weakness suggesting myopathy (helps distinguish specific myopathies and myopathy from neuropathy)	Histochemical and enzyme analyses require special laboratory processing
Peripheral nerve (usually sural)	Polyneuropathy (helps distinguish demyelination from axonal neuropathy)	Should be performed only at specialized centers. Has low diagnostic yield for specific diseases.
Brain	Tumors (for specific diagnosis). Occasionally for puzzling infections, some dementias	Not indicated for suspected herpes simplex unless antiviral therapy fails

assures the patient (and his physician) that no serious structural disease is present. However, the tests are expensive, often cannot diagnose metabolic or inflammatory disorders, and should not substitute for clinical judgement (Table 113–8). Depending on their density and the quality of the instrument, lesions as small as 5 mm can be seen, and abnormal permeability of the blood-brain barrier can be identified by intravenous injection of iodinated contrast material into a vein (contrast enhancement). The CT scan is the diagnostic test of choice for assessing the presence of structural disease of the brain or spine associated with acute trauma, suspected intracranial or subarachnoid hemorrhage, bony lesions of the cranium or skull, cervical or lumbar root lesions, and brachial or lumbosacral plexus lesions. CT also is used instead of MR when the patient is agitated, is severely claustrophobic, or harbors metal implantations. CT can identify mass lesions and ventricular size, distinguish hemorrhage from infarct, identify most subdural hematomas and brain tumors, and assess the degree of cerebral atrophy. Subarachnoid blood is usually detected, and lesions of the pituitary gland and orbits can be identified readily. The CT scan often does not detect lesions less than 5 mm in diameter or infiltrating brain tumors that do not alter the blood-brain barrier. Very recent infarcts and isodense hematomas also show up poorly. For those disorders MR is preferred.

Magnetic Resonance Imaging (MR). MR is available in many centers and promises to replace CT scanning as the imaging technique of the future. MR is unaffected by bone and usually does not require the injection of contrast material. An intravenous paramagnetic contrast material (gadolinium DPTA) will soon be available to mark areas of blood-brain barrier breakdown. The material is safer than iodine and promises to add another dimension to MR diagnosis of tumors. Furthermore, images can be procured in any plane, whereas CT images are limited to horizontal and coronal planes. MR also has better resolution than CT and frequently reveals lesions, including tumors, arteriovenous anomalies, and areas of demyelination that CT scanning fails to detect. A complete MR scan requires 30 to 45 minutes of immobility on the part of the patient. Because of the high magnetic field, the test is contraindicated in patients harboring cardiac pacemakers or metal aneurysm clips. It also is difficult to apply in critically ill patients who may be intubated or require close attention to airway. There are no other known risks and no irradiation is involved.

Myelography. Suspected abnormalities of the spinal cord should first be assessed by a plain x-ray. Substantial lesions of bone can thus be identified. In order to identify compression of the spinal cord, nerve roots, or cauda equina, myelography is performed by injection of iodinated contrast material, usually water-soluble, into the spinal canal. The contrast material is run up and down the canal and visualized fluoroscopically, and roentgenograms are taken. The test is particularly valuable for identifying herniated discs; compression of the spinal cord, cauda equina, or nerve roots; and intrinsic or extrinsic tumors and vascular

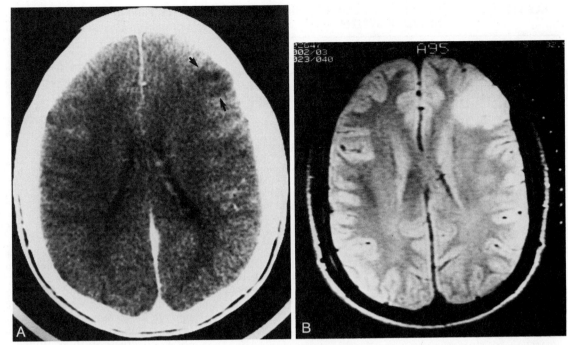

FIGURE 113–1. Comparison of imaging techniques in a patient suffering from a low-grade glioma of the left frontal lobe. The CT scan (A) was taken after an injection of double the standard dose of contrast material. It shows only a vague area of hypodensity in the frontal lobe (arrows). MR scan (B) taken at the same level within a few days of the CT scan reveals a large area of hyperdensity caused by the altered proton density of the low-grade tumor. A biopsy revealed a low-grade glioma. The patient had suffered from a single generalized convulsion and had no other neurological signs or symptoms.

malformation of the spinal cord. MR is rapidly replacing myelograms for diagnosing many diseases, particularly spinal cord compression, tumors, and herniated discs.

Angiography. The blood vessels of the brain and spinal cord can be visualized either by injection of contrast material directly into an artery or by the injection of a larger amount of contrast material intravenously and enhancement of the image by computerized subtraction techniques. The latter approach, digital intravenous angiography (DIVA), is less accurate but can be used as an outpatient test in the search for surgically treatable causes of cerebrovascular disease and is the technique of choice for identifying cerebral venous sinuses. Arterial angiography is required for

the identification of most small intracranial aneurysms and for definitive outlining of spinal arteriovenous anomalies.

Electrodiagnostic Studies (Table 113–9)

Electroencephalography (EEG). EEG records the electrical activity of the cerebral cortex. It is particularly helpful in the differential diagnosis of seizures, especially if an attack occurs spontaneously or can be evoked during the recording process. EEG often identifies the presence and type of epilepsy. It also helps differentiate seizures from metabolic encephalopathy, and it aids in distinguishing between organic and psychogenic causes of unresponsiveness. The absence of EEG activity, properly recorded, supports the diagnosis of brain death. A new, still experimental technique, *magnetoencephalography*, records the magnetic field produced by the brain's electrical activity and promises to localize epileptic activity better than does EEG.

Nerve Conduction Studies (Table 113–10). Percutaneous electrical stimulation of a peripheral nerve generates an action potential. For motor nerves, electrodes are placed over a muscle to record the evoked muscle action potential. One stimulates the nerve innervating that muscle at various points along its length and determines the conduction velocity from the time required to travel from each site of stimulation to the

TABLE 113–8. INDICATIONS FOR CT RATHER THAN MR OF BRAIN OR SPINE

Acute trauma
Suspected intracranial or subarachnoid hemorrhage
Cervical or lumbar root disease
Brachial or lumbosacral plexus lesions
Bony lesions of cranium or skull base
MR contraindicated
  Metallic attachments to patient
  Agitated or severely claustrophobic patient
  Cardiac pacemaker or cerebral aneurysm clips

TABLE 113–9. NONINVASIVE ELECTRICAL STUDIES OF THE NERVOUS SYSTEM

TEST	SOME INDICATIONS	COMMENT
Electroencephalogram (EEG)	Any brain dysfunction, especially epilepsy	Sensitive but not specific; inexpensive
Visual evoked potentials (VER)	Tests integrity of optic nerve and cerebral visual pathway	Sensitive for asymptomatic optic neuritis, e.g., from multiple sclerosis
Brain stem auditory evoked potentials (BAER)	Tests integrity of auditory pathways	Sensitive for acoustic nerve tumors and brain stem disease
Somatosensory evoked potentials (SEP)	Tests integrity of central sensory pathways	Sensitive for spinal cord and lower brain stem disease
Nerve conduction velocity (see Table 113–10)	Tests rate of conduction in peripheral nerve	Distinguishes demyelination from axonal disease; sometimes establishes site of nerve compression
Neuromuscular transmission studies	Myasthenia gravis, Lambert-Eaton syndrome, botulism	Noninvasive but unpleasant
Electromyogram (EMG)	Identifies denervated areas of muscle, detects reduced muscle action, identifies myopathic changes	Helps identify lower motor neuron disorders, nerve root compression, etc.; helps distinguish neurogenic from myopathic disorders

onset of the evoked muscle response. For sensory nerves, one stimulates cutaneous nerve branches distally and places recording electrodes over the nerve at various proximal sites. The *F-response* provides a measure of conduction in the proximal portions of a motor nerve and ventral root. The *H-reflex* provides the electrical equivalent of the stretch reflex by stimulating sensory fibers of the posterior tibial nerve in the popliteal fossa and recording the efferent evoked action potential from the soleus muscle. These peripheral nerve and muscle electrophysiological studies assist in determining whether disease involves nerve, muscle, or both and in determining the distribution of the abnormality. They facilitate the differentiation of demyelinating neuropathy from axonal neuropathy, neuropathy from radiculopathy, and primary muscle disease from disease of the motor unit. Demyelinating neuropathies affect mainly large fibers and slow the conduction velocity. When disease damages axons in addition to myelin, there is a decrease in the number of axons that can be electrically activated, resulting in a diminution in the size of the compound action potential.

Electromyography (EMG). EMG is performed by inserting a needle electrode into a muscle to record the structure's electrical activity (Fig. 113–2). Normal muscle is silent at rest, but denervated or diseased muscle membranes become spontaneously excitable, generating *fibrillation potentials* of small amplitude. When the nerve itself is diseased, entire motor units may become spontaneously active. The resulting *fasciculations* are often visible percutaneously and can be detected by the electrode. Furthermore, when damaged axons cease to innervate muscle fibers, the remaining axons gradually sprout collaterals that reinnervate the denervated fibers; as a result, during voluntary contraction the few remaining muscle units show a decrease in their number and an increase in the size of their electrical potentials. When the patient voluntarily contracts the muscle being examined, action potentials appear and with full voluntary contraction cannot be distinguished one from the other (interference pattern). With neurogenic weakness, the interference pattern is reduced or disappears because of the paucity of voluntary reaction potentials. By contrast, as muscle fibers degenerate in primary disease of muscle, the size of motor units decreases, since each nerve now innervates fewer fibers. During voluntary contraction the number of activated units is normal, but their amplitude is smaller; the interference pattern remains normal. In primary myopathies, the distribution of abnormality helps in characterizing the myopathy itself. Table 113–10 provides guides to the usefulness and pertinent changes in electrophysiological tests in various neuromuscular disorders. The EMG must be interpreted in light of the clinical findings, since occasional fibrillation potentials may be

TABLE 113–10. DIFFERENTIATION AMONG MYOPATHY, AXONOPATHY, MYELINOPATHY, AND RADICULOPATHY USING ELECTROPHYSIOLOGIC STUDIES

	MYOPATHY	AXONOPATHY	MYELINOPATHY	RADICULOPATHY
Nerve conduction velocity	Normal	Normal	Slow	Normal
F-response	Normal	Normal	Delayed-absent	Delayed-absent
H-reflex*	Normal	Normal	Delayed-absent	Delayed-absent
EMG				
Voluntary contraction	Predominance of small motor units	Predominance of large motor units	Normal	Normal, some large motor units
Spontaneous activity	Fibrillations	Fibrillations, fasciculations	Normal	Fibrillations, fasciculations

* Usually studied with posterior tibial nerve stimulation, recording the soleus contraction, thus providing an index of S1 root function only.

FIGURE 113–2. Electromyogram from normal and abnormal muscle. *A*, The trace shows two normally innervated motor units (left) and the needle electromyogram shows those units at rest, with minimal activity (only one unit is active) and during maximal contraction. When all units are active the normal baseline cannot be seen (complete interference pattern). *B*, Denervated muscle after damage to the motor neuron or peripheral nerve supplying motor unit B. The surviving motor unit has taken over two of the fibers supplied by B; other fibers have become atrophied. The resting tracing shows fibrillation potentials (spontaneous discharge of denervated fibers). Minimal voluntary activity fires a giant motor unit, indicating that there has been sprouting of motor neuron A. With maximal contraction, loss of motor units leads to an incomplete interference pattern. *C*, Myopathic muscle. There is random loss of muscle fibers in all motor units, although the nerve remains normal. Fibrillation potentials are rarely seen unless there is involvement of nerve terminals as well. Minimum voluntary activity fires a small motor unit of short duration. With maximal contraction there is a complete interference pattern of smaller than normal amplitude. (Modified from Patten J: Neurological Differential Diagnosis. New York, Springer-Verlag, 1977.)

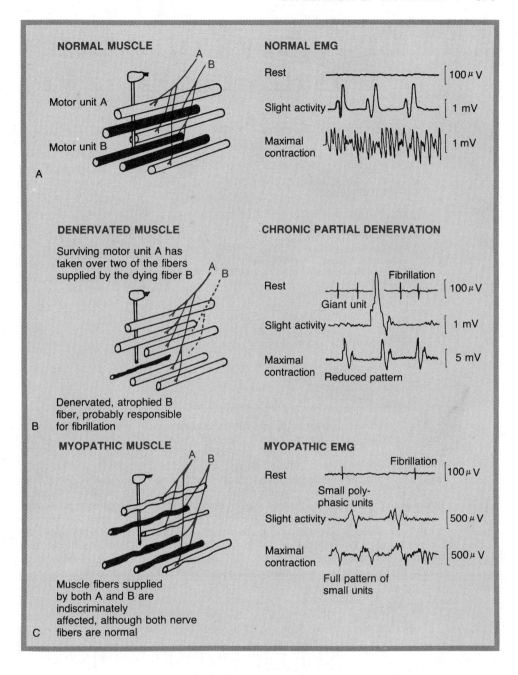

found in normals and confusingly similar changes sometimes are found in myopathies and neuropathies. Table 113–10 indicates how the above electrical tests are used to differentiate nerve from muscle disease.

Neuromuscular Transmission Studies. Diseases of the neuromuscular junction (p. 761) are characterized by normal nerve conduction velocity and usually a normal EMG. Repetitive electrical activation of the neuromuscular junction, however, will produce either an abnormal diminution (myasthenia gravis) or an abnormal facilitation (Lambert-Eaton pseudomyasthenia, botulism) of the successively evoked muscle action potential.

REFERENCES

Bannister R: Brain's Clinical Neurology. 6th ed. London, Oxford Press, 1985.

Mumenthaler M (trans. by O Appenzeller): Neurologic Differential Diagnosis. New York, Thieme-Stratton, 1985.

Ross RT: How to Examine the Nervous System. 2nd ed. New York, Medical Examination Publishing Co, 1985.

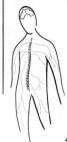

114

DISORDERS OF CONSCIOUSNESS AND HIGHER BRAIN FUNCTION

The conscious state expresses the interaction of two major neurological functions: one, the level of arousal, and the other, the mental content and expressed behavior of the awakened state. Arousal, i.e., the recurrent cycling of wakefulness from sleep, expresses a normal, phylogenetically primitive activity critically regulated in the human brain by the reticular core of the brain stem that extends from the level of the rostral pons forward to the ventromedian thalamus. Mental content and learned behavior, by contrast, are manifestations of much more complicated brain mechanisms that require arousal for their full expression but represent the product of the interactive workings of many millions of nerve and supporting cells located in the extensive gray matter of the cerebral hemispheres and their related subcortical nuclei.

This chapter discusses alterations in consciousness from several aspects. It first addresses problems related to normal sleep and the frequent but seldom incapacitating disorders that affect that state. The chapter then proceeds to discuss a variety of pathological alterations of the conscious state that represent more serious threats to the brain and the integrity of the individual.

A. SLEEP AND ITS DISORDERS

Sleep represents the active physiological interruption of arousal, regulated by brain stem autonomic mechanisms. Both the pattern and the necessary amount of sleep vary widely from person to person. Some healthy persons sleep as little as four to five hours per day, while others seem unable to function with less than nine or ten. Moderate exercise reduces the latent period required to fall asleep and generally increases the depth and somewhat the length of sleep as well. Anxiety, preoccupation, depression, drugs such as caffeine, and somatic conditions such as fever, pain, and cardiopulmonary disease all contribute to subjective difficulties in sleeping. Distressing insomnia or hyposomnia can have several aspects. Older persons generally sleep with less satisfaction than do younger ones. Some insomniacs complain of an increased latent period before sleep occurs, while others report middle-of-the-night or early-morning awakenings. Although subjectively distressing, such common variations produce little or no physiological harm. Scientific observations of hyposomnia indicate that periods of sleep almost always last longer than the subject believes; what is recalled are the awakenings. Forced severe insomnia, however, whether induced by anxiety, pain, disease, or work requirements, does appear to reduce mental efficiency.

Insomnia of recent origin is best handled by reassurance with efforts directed toward correcting underlying medical or psychological problems and, if necessary, the parsimonious prescribing of mild sedatives. Such cautious approaches may fail to please all patients, but the realities are that most chronic insomnia is extremely difficult to treat effectively because almost all soporifics sooner or later induce tolerance. Acute insomnia due to intercurrent illness, acute physical or emotional pain, jet lag, and the like is best treated in otherwise healthy persons with small doses (e.g., 0.25 mg or less) of the short-acting benzodiazepine triazolam at bedtime. Milder agents such as benadryl, chloral hydrate, or flurazepam may be preferable for elderly patients or those with fever or systemic illness. Tricyclic antidepressants, with the entire dose taken at bedtime, help in the management of the insomnia of depression. Alcohol, although widely employed, is a poor choice of sedative; it shortens the sleep latency interval but tends to shorten the duration of sleep and to produce unpleasant hangovers. Tolerance often occurs, resulting in increasing doses to achieve effect.

Hypersomnia of recent origin can be a symptom of overwhelming fatigue or psychological depression. In all other instances it deserves consideration as possibly reflecting serious neurological disease. Chronic or recurrent hypersomnia is a symptom most often of narcolepsy or of one of the sleep apnea syndromes described on page 167.

Narcolepsy is a chronic disorder of unknown cause characterized by a recurrent uncontrollable drowsiness, usually starting in the late teens or early 20's, and associated with one or more of the following experiences: (1) sleep attacks consisting of sudden, uncontrollable, and inappropriately timed episodes of rapid eye movement sleep that interrupt normal schedules of wakefulness; (2) cataplexy, a phenomenon of abrupt muscular hypotonia precipitated by surprise or emotion; (3) hypnagogic hallucinations, intense dreamlike experiences occurring during the penumbra between sleep and wakefulness; (4) sleep paralysis, an overwhelming sense that one cannot move, occurring during the moments of awakening from sleep. All these features may be experienced to some degree by normal persons, but in narcolepsy the symptoms intensify to the point of disrupting social and vocational occupations or producing dangerous situations such as drowsy driving. The predisposition to narcolepsy appears to be inherited as an autosomal dominant trait, with most narcoleptics possessing the HLA-DR2 antigen. The clinical expression, however, varies considerably. Its cause is unknown, although a defect in central pharmacological neurotransmission has been postulated. Medications are of limited value, although therapy with methylphenidate helps some sufferers. In intractable cases, symptomatic treatment with monoamine oxidase inhibitors or other amphetamine congeners occasionally brings relief.

The *Klein-Levin syndrome* is a rare disease of adolescent boys and young men marked by episodic periods of hypersomnia and hyperphagia lasting days to weeks. The condition usually subsides in adulthood.

Sleep disturbances that can occur in otherwise normal persons include enuresis (bedwetting), night terrors, nightmares, sleep walking, and sleep talking. All of these conditions affect children more than adults. Efforts to establish consistent psychiatric correlations have been unsuccessful. Although tension, anxiety, or other psychological problems may accentuate the tendencies, they are probably not the cause. Imipramine, 25 to 50 mg at bedtime, helps some cases of enuresis, while several of the other disorders improve with the taking of short-acting benzodiazepines at bedtime. Most of the conditions subside during late adolescence or adulthood.

REFERENCE

Kales A, et al: Sleep disorders. Sleep apnea and narcolepsy. Ann Intern Med 106:434–443, 582–592, 1987.

B. PATHOLOGICAL ALTERATIONS OF CONSCIOUSNESS

The recognition, accurate etiologic diagnosis, and prompt treatment of impaired or abnormal conscious states constitutes an important challenge to physicians in every branch of medicine. Aside from brief intoxication or fainting, the appearance of almost any acute or subacute global disorder of higher brain function implies the possibility of a serious threat to a patient's immediate personality or future well being.

It sometimes can require careful examination and considerable judgment to estimate a patient's level of consciousness. This is because the physiologically normal level extends widely along a continuum that ranges from fully awake, intelligent attention at one extreme to states of almost totally uncommunicative psychological withdrawal at the other. Furthermore, a number of variations in behavior that can be either normal or abnormal depending on individual circumstances can lie along this functionally declining scale. Examples include distractability, agitation, inattention, partial disorientation, seeming confusion, preoccupied misperception, hypersomnolence, and even, following prolonged sleep deprivation, a degree of

TABLE 114–1. CONSCIOUSNESS AND ITS ALTERATIONS: DEFINITIONS

Consciousness. The awake state of awareness of self and environment, judged externally by evidence of the individual's capacity to express learned and anticipatory behavior.

Coma. An eyes-closed state of unarousable behavior in which patients lack any recognizable evidence of learned responses to internal or external stimulation.

Stupor. A state of psychological unresponsiveness that can be interrupted only by vigorous and sustained external stimulation.

Hypersomnia. Sleep behavior that consistently exceeds the subject's norm by 25 to 30 per cent or more. Most pathological hypersomnia is accompanied by a degree of delirium or reduced intellectual capacity.

Delirium. An acute or subacute state characterized by a confused reduction in the clarity of awareness of the environment. Symptoms include partial disorientation coupled with misperceptions, poor judgment, delusions, and the erroneous recollection of events. Prolonged confusional states may be difficult to distinguish from the early stages of chronic dementia. A more agitated or severe form of delirium can accompany toxic or infectious illnesses. Affected patients become boisterous and restless and suffer hallucinations, usually of a visual nature. A dreamlike state characterized by a loss of self-recognition can occur, as can reversals of sleep-wake cycles, accompanied by episodic insomnia or hypersomnia.

Vegetative state. A condition of severe brain damage in which sleep-wake cycles remain or recover but the body has become mindless, that is, has lost all evidence of awareness of self or environment. Relatively normal thermal control, chewing, swallowing, breathing, and circulatory regulation remain, but such patients express no cognitive reactions and their behavioral responses consist of no more than primitive motor reflexes or instinctive emotional patterns.

Locked-in state. An uncommon condition in which severe damage to efferent (motor) neural pathways temporarily or permanently prevents communication. Sufficient oculomotor activity may be spared to permit coded signalling in response to questions or inner needs. Affected patients possess self-aware consciousness but cannot express it satisfactorily because of paralysis of communication. Either bilateral interruption of the corticospinal tracts in the brain stem or severe motor polyneuropathy can cause the condition. An equivalent, but more transient, helpless experience affects conscious patients who are intubated for life-support ventilation.

Brain death. The permanent loss of all essential brain functions, despite the continued activity of artificially supported heart, lungs, and other viscera. The state has been accepted as representing death of the person in most of the United States as well as Western Europe. Table 114–2 provides diagnostic criteria.

---

physiological unarousability that can at least transiently imitate pathological unconsciousness. To provide a frame of diagnostic reference, Table 114–1 defines the most common, sustained alterations of consciousness encountered in the medical setting. States of brief loss of consciousness are listed later in Table 114–13.

SUSTAINED IMPAIRMENTS OF NORMAL CONSCIOUSNESS

Sustained impairments of consciousness are defined as lasting for a matter of hours to indefinitely. In medical terms, sustained disturbances of consciousness are caused by either (1) pathological interruptions of the upper brain stem arousal mechanisms or (2) global-diffuse organic impairments of cerebral regions regulating mental and behavioral function. These two an-

atomical patterns often coincide. Restricted, focal psychological impairments such as aphasia, selective perceptual loss, or specific learning deficits are customarily identified by the deficit in question and not designated as altered states of consciousness. They are described in a later section.

MECHANISMS OF COMA AND APPROACH TO DIAGNOSIS

Mechanisms

Disorders that can damage the brain so extensively or strategically as to interrupt consciousnes fall into three general categories (Table 114–3): (1) Supratentorial mass lesions that either (a) directly invade or destroy the posterior ventromedial diencephalon or (b) enlarge sufficiently to compress these basal diencephalic areas severely or herniate them through the tentorial notch. (2) Subtentorial lesions that bilaterally damage or destroy the midbrain–upper pontine reticular activating system. (3) Diffuse metabolic or multifocal structural abnormalities that simultaneously or in close succession cause widespread, severe cerebral hemispheric dysfunction. These latter conditions can depress reticular arousal mechanisms either directly or by abruptly removing their normal cerebral feedback stimulation from the cerebrum. Many of these diffuse or multifocal conditions have chemical rather than structural causes. They produce no abnormalities on brain imaging and often create an intellectual challenge in diagnosis and management.

Approach to the Patient

Once consciousness is impaired and the history is obtained, physical and laboratory tests provide crucial clues. Physically, an evaluation of motor and neuroophthalmological signs plus an appraisal of the breathing pattern often yields the most useful information in reaching an initial localizing diagnosis and estimating cause and prognosis. Brain imaging abets clinical localization and, in the case of mass or destructive lesions, often points to specific etiologies. Systematic studies of blood, urine, CSF, and other tissues offer specific answers to the causes of many of the metabolic encephalopathies. The following paragraphs amplify these principles.

Supratentorial Lesions. The most frequent supratentorial causes of acutely or subacutely altered consciousness consist of expanding hemispheric masses that squeeze the surrounding cerebrum, either shifting it downward to displace the diencephalon against the midbrain or down and laterally to compress the temporal lobe against the thalamus and midbrain. (The anatomy is illustrated in Figure 121–1.)

Characteristically, supratentorial mass lesions cause signs of focal cerebral dysfunction before they produce discernible changes in consciousness (Table 114–4). The initial clinical signs may be behavioral-psychological or, if they affect sensorimotor systems, can cause abnormalities in these functions on the opposite side of the body. Because of the functional anatomy, even when deep forebrain compression or displacement begins to impair arousal and cause abnormal bilateral motor signs, the brain stem–controlled pupillary reflexes, conjugate eye movements, and oculovestibular responses remain largely or completely spared in early supratentorial coma. Unless diencephalic compression is halted, however, the process proceeds to transtentorial herniation, described below.

Primary destructive or invasive lesions of the posterior paramedian thalamus are a well-established but unusual supratentorial cause of stupor and coma. The area can be selectively damaged by stroke caused by basilar artery occlusion; from neoplasms, particularly primary lymphomas; by granulomas such as those of sarcoid, or in the course of acute encephalitis. With any of these conditions the chief clinical manifestation usually consists of gradually or acutely progressing hypersomnia, sometimes with nearly unarousable sleep lasting most of the 24-hour day. Specific diagnosis depends on other signs of thalamic or brain stem dysfunction plus information gained from imaging studies and cerebrospinal fluid analysis.

Herniation Syndromes. Transtentorial herniation can occur in two patterns (Table 114–5). *Central compression-herniation* consists of displacement and compression of the midline diencephalon caudally toward and through the tentorial notch so that it eventually herniates against the midbrain. As this occurs, the level of arousal declines, bilateral upper motor neuron signs tend to replace early focal cerebral motor changes, and signs of hypothalamic dysfunction, including small, light-reactive, equal pupils, ensue. Evidence of brain stem dysfunction, (e.g., eye movement changes) appears only as the midbrain becomes severely compressed by the downward shift. *Uncal (lateral) herniation* occurs when a lesion occupying the temporal fossa expands, pushing the uncus over the edge of the ipsilateral tentorium so as to compress the third nerve and midbrain (see Fig. 121–1). Reduced consciousness and bilateral motor signs appear relatively late, the earliest evidence of serious trouble usually being incipient parasympathetic paralysis of the pupil. Either form of herniation, however, warns of impending upper brain stem compression and calls for quick and effective action to prevent irreversible neurological damage.

Subtentorial Lesions. As noted above, in order for subtentorial lesions to cause coma they necessarily must damage or depress the function of the reticular activating system located in the dorsal medial brain stem tegmentum of the upper pons and midbrain. Since the reticular formation surrounds or lies adjacent to oculomotor pathways and upper brain stem cranial nerve nuclei, signs of damage to these latter structures always accompany the onset of stupor or coma caused by subtentorial lesions. Furthermore, subtentorial lesions causing coma almost always have a structural nature that MR or, less reliably, CT brain images will identify. Table 114–3 lists their most common causes and Table 114–6 gives their characteristic signs and symptoms.

Metabolic, Diffuse, and Multifocal Disorders Producing Altered Consciousness. Table 114–3 lists the major examples of these conditions. They tend to af-

TABLE 114–2. CRITERIA FOR DIAGNOSIS OF BRAIN DEATH

1. Nature and duration of coma is known
   a. Known structural disease or irreversible systemic metabolic cause
   b. No chance of drug intoxication or hypothermia; no paralyzing or sedative drugs recently given for treatment
   c. Six-hour observation of no brain function is sufficient in cases of known structural cause when no drug or alcohol is involved in cause or treatment; otherwise, 12 to 24 hours plus a negative drug screen is required
2. Absence of cerebral and brain stem function
   a. No behavioral or reflex response to noxious stimuli above foramen magnum level
   b. Fixed pupils
   c. No oculovestibular responses to 50 ml ice water calorics
   d. Apneic off ventilator with oxygenation for 10 minutes
   e. Systemic circulation may be intact
   f. Purely spinal reflexes may be retained
3. Supplementary (optional) criteria* (any one acceptable)
   a. EEG isoelectric for 30 minutes at maximal gain
   b. Auditory-evoked responses reflect absent function in vital brain stem structures
   c. No circulation present on cerebral blood flow examination

* May be useful if medicolegal issues are in question or when taking organs for transplantation, especially at six-hour intervals.

TABLE 114–3. COMMON CAUSES OF STUPOR AND COMA

I. Supratentorial lesions
   A. Compressing or herniating diencephalon against the upper brain stem (common)
      1. Cerebral hemorrhage
      2. Large cerebral infarction
      3. Subdural hematoma
      4. Epidural hematoma
      5. Brain tumor
      6. Brain abscess (rare)
   B. Directly invading or destroying the posterior ventromedial diencephalon (less common)
      1. Neoplasms
      2. Infarcts
      3. Encephalitis
II. Subtentorial lesions (compressing or damaging the midbrain–upper pontine reticular formation)
   A. Pontine or cerebellar hemorrhage
   B. Midbrain–upper pontine infarction
   C. Tumor
   D. Cerebellar abscess
   E. Acute demyelination
III. Metabolic and diffuse lesions
   A. Exogenous psychoactive drugs or poisons
   B. Anoxia or ischemia
   C. Mixed encephalopathies: pathologic aging, postoperative state, systemic infection, therapeutic drugs in various combinations
   D. Hepatic, renal, pulmonary, pancreatic insufficiency
   E. Hypoglycemia
   F. Infections
         Meningitis
         Encephalitis
   G.. Multifocal small structural lesions, e.g., metastases, emboli, thrombi
   H. Concussion and postictal states
   I. Ionic and electrolyte disorders
   J. Nutritional deficiency
IV. Psychogenic unresponsiveness

TABLE 114—4. CHARACTERISTICS OF SUPRATENTORIAL LESIONS LEADING TO COMA

Initiating symptoms usually cerebral-focal: Aphasia; focal seizures; contralateral hemiparesis, sensory change, or neglect; frontal lobe behavioral changes; headache.

Dysfunction moves rostral to caudal: e.g., focal motor → bilateral motor → altered level of arousal.

Abnormal signs usually confined to a single or adjacent anatomic level (not diffuse).

Brain stem functions spared unless herniation develops.

TABLE 114—5. SIGNS OF CENTRAL AND UNCAL HERNIATION

	CENTRAL	UNCAL
Arousal	Declines early	Declines late
Pupils	Small, equal, reactive	Ipsilateral dilation
Oculocephalics	Full, conjugate	Unilateral third nerve palsy
Motor	Decerebrate early	Decerebrate late
Breathing	Sighs, yawns, periodic (Cheyne-Stokes)	Central hyperventilation, late

TABLE 114—6. CHARACTERISTICS OF SUBTENTORIAL LESIONS CAUSING COMA

Onset of coma often sudden

Symptoms of brain stem dysfunction may precede coma

Localizing brain stem signs always present

Caloric responses disconjugate or absent

Pupil(s) abnormal: pinpoint (pons), fixed (midbrain), irregular and/or unequal (midbrain-pontine)

Often "bizarre" signs: ocular bobbing, ataxic breathing, etc.

Often signs of cerebellar or bilateral motor dysfunction

TABLE 114—7. CHARACTERISTICS OF METABOLIC ENCEPHALOPATHY

Confusion, lethargy, delirium often precede or replace coma

Motor signs, if present, usually symmetrical

Bilateral asterixis, myoclonus appear

Pupillary reactions usually preserved; tonic calorics often present

Sensory abnormalities usually absent

Hypothermia common

Abnormal signs reflect incomplete brain dysfunction at multiple anatomical levels simultaneously

fect the brain diffusely and, characteristically, produce symptoms and signs of both widespread cerebral and concurrent brain stem dysfunction. Depending on the particular illness, its severity, and its rate of appearance, initiating symptoms in metabolic-multifocal encephalopathy can include either changes in the forebrain's cognitive capacities or a reduction in arousal.

Acute, self-induced drug overdose, or sudden, severe hypoglycemia, for example, each can precipitate acute coma with few prodromal symptoms. By contrast, mild drug intoxication or a moderate reduction in blood sugar is more likely to be reflected by confused or bizarre behavior. If the history is lacking or indefinite, an important clue to diagnosis in all the recoverable metabolic encephalopathies is that except for poisoning with drugs that contain anticholinergic agents, almost no reversible examples paralyze the pupillary light reflex. Also, except for certain drug poisonings, most metabolic comas fail to block reflex oculovestibular responses.

SIGNS AND SYMPTOMS. Table 114–7 lists the most common signs and symptoms. Characteristic in the early stages is an acute or subacute delirium accompanied by restlessness and reduced alertness. The presence of confusion often makes a clear history difficult to obtain. Bedside evaluation of mental status (see Table 114–19) shows impaired recall, poor concentration, and often disorientation. Confabulation, obtundation, and stupor follow in varying degrees and combinations depending on the intensity of the disorder and how rapidly it progresses. Fluctuations in behavior are common; some patients may alternate widely between stupor and agitation. Nearly always, symptoms of confusion or delirium tend to be accentuated by nightfall and unfamiliar surroundings.

Characteristic motor changes include tremor, asterixis, and multifocal myoclonus (defined on page 736). The tremor of delirium tends to be coarse, irregular, rapid at 8 to 10 Hz, and intensified by movement. Bilateral asterixis or multifocal myoclonus arising acutely or subacutely and accompanying a recent impairment of consciousness is pathognomonic of metabolic encephalopathy. Seizures, hyperactive stretch reflexes, and even focal signs sometimes accompany several of the metabolic encephalopathies (e.g., drug withdrawal, global cerebral anoxia, hypoglycemia, hyperosmolar coma, fulminating hepatic encephalopathy). Such focal signs usually are transient and always are accompanied by other neurological changes that reflect diffuse or multifocal brain disease.

Pupillary light reflexes are nearly always preserved in metabolic coma, exceptions including poisoning with hyoscine, strong narcotics, or glutethimide; the deliberate or accidental contact with mydriatics; or exposure to irreversible anoxia-asphyxia. Except in cases of severe sedative overdose, spontaneous conjugate eye movements or conjugate oculovestibular reflexes are preserved until the terminal phases of most metabolic comas.

Breathing alterations are common with metabolic encephalopathy; vigorous hyperpnea (Kussmaul breathing) accompanies the metabolic acidosis of diabetes, uremia, lactacidosis and organic alcohol ingestion, whereas less prominent overbreathing reflects the alkaloses of hepatic disease, septic shock, and early salicylism. Hypoventilation is prominent in CO_2 encephalopathy, whether due to pulmonary disease or medullary respiratory depression such as caused by drugs or hypoglycemia.

PSYCHOGENIC UNRESPONSIVENESS

Psychogenic unresponsiveness can accompany several disorders, including catatonic withdrawal due to schizophrenia or severe depression as well as in hysteria or malingering. All these conditions can produce clinical pictures that superficially resemble metabolic coma. Certain signs will differentiate, however (Table 114–8). Careful examination of such cases reveals a normal general physical and somatic neurological examination. Psychogenically unresponsive patients may resist answers during attempts to appraise mental status, but, unless they are hysterical or malingering, they do not give wrong ones. Those with closed eyes resist passive opening of the lids, and when they are passively raised, they shut abruptly when released; neither is true in organic coma. Pupils are briskly reactive unless mydriatics have been self-instilled, ice water calorics give normal responses, and the EEG is normal. One must always remember, however, that fear, anxiety, or other emotions commonly superimpose psychological symptoms on the signs of acute illness and must be taken into account diagnostically and treated sympathetically.

DIAGNOSIS OF COMA AND EMERGENCY MANAGEMENT

A careful history discloses most causes of coma. When that is unavailable or misleading (some families, for example, hide evidence of drug ingestion) one proceeds as in Table 114–9. Once ventilation and the circulation are protected, brain images usually indicate whether or not a surgically treatable condition exists. If not, some of the clues given in Table 114–10 may suggest which tests to do first. Lumbar puncture is best withheld if an MR or CT scan shows an acute intracranial mass, including cerebral hemorrhage. If meningitis is suspected, however, one must proceed with lumbar puncture immediately, since to delay diagnosis and hold back appropriate antimicrobial therapy invites serious complications or death. An EEG is helpful only in the unusual case in which serial seizures (status epilepticus) due to petit mal or partial complex seizures (p. 793) produce a severe confusional state.

Most coma of unknown cause that begins rapidly or abruptly in previously healthy persons outside the hospital results from self-induced drug poisoning, and patients lacking definite alternate diagnoses must be managed for this possibility until another cause is definitively established (see Section F and Table 114–21). Among older persons, especially those with chronic illness or receiving multiple medications, other puzzling metabolic encephalopathies also are common. This especially occurs in the hospital setting where confusion, obtundation, or delirium due to a mixture of adverse causes can complicate the course of many acute medical or surgical illnesses. The laboratory profile given in Table 114–11 plus a search for offending medications in doubtful instances frequently gives the answer to such conditions. Table 114–12 outlines the major emergency steps that will protect the patient acutely in almost all of the major conditions producing sustained loss of consciousness.

TABLE 114–8. SIGNS OF PSYCHOGENIC PSEUDOCOMA

Lids close actively and often resist examiner's attempt to open them
Breathing: eupnea or acute hyperventilation
Pupils responsive or dilated (self-administered cycloplegia)
Oculocephalic responses unpredictable; calorics produce quick nystagmus
Motor responses unpredictable and often asymmetrical or bizarre
No pathological reflexes. EEG normal awake

TABLE 114–9. KEY TO CLINICAL DIAGNOSIS OF COMA

Pursue history diligently and provide immediate life-support (see Table 114–12).
How do signs of dysfunction evolve?
 Rostral-caudal? (Supratentorial)
 Focal brain stem from onset? (Subtentorial)
 Multifocal diffuse? (Metabolic-diffuse)
 Do they represent nonphysiological abnormalities? (Psychogenic)
Obtain emergency brain image.
Move to specific tests or treatment.

TABLE 114–10. HELPFUL CLUES IN EARLY DIAGNOSIS OF COMA

Fever	Meningitis, encephalitis, postictal state, acute bacterial endocarditis, scopolamine poisoning
Hypothermia	Myxedema, hypoglycemia, drug poisoning, brain stem infarct
Signs of trauma	Cerebral contusion; extradural, subdural, or parenchymal hematoma
Severe hypertension	Cerebral or subarachnoid hemorrhage; hypertensive encephalopathy
Hypotension	Occult (usually gastrointestinal) bleeding, septic shock, hypovolemia, poor cardiac output, depressant drug poisoning
	Tachycardia > 180 per min, bradycardia < 40 min: poor cardiac output
Arrhythmias	Tricyclic overdose, myocardial infarction
Hyperventilation	Diabetic ketosis; uremia; organic alcohol poisoning; lactic acidosis, hepatic coma; salicylate poisoning
Hypoventilation	Pulmonary insufficiency, depressant drug or opiate poisoning, low brain stem infarct or hemorrhage
Petechiae	Meningococcemia; thrombocytopenic and nonthrombocytopenic purpura; bacterial endocarditis
Pink skin	Carbon monoxide
Stiff neck	Acute meningitis, subarachnoid hemorrhage

TABLE 114–11. LABORATORY TESTS IN METABOLIC ENCEPHALOPATHY

IMMEDIATE	LATER IF INDICATED
Glucose	Liver function tests including arterial ammonia
Na^+	Sedative drug screen
Ca^{++}	Blood and CSF culture
BUN	Full electrolytes, including Mg^{++}
Arterial blood pH, P_{CO_2}, P_{O_2}	Coagulation profile
Lumbar puncture	EEG

Hb, Hct, WBC, smear. Electrolyte and chemistry screen

TABLE 114–12. EMERGENCY MANAGEMENT OF COMA

1. Assure airway and oxygenation
2. Maintain adequate systemic circulation
3. Give thiamine, 50 to 100 mg intravenously
4. Give glucose after first obtaining blood for analysis
5. Stop generalized seizures
6. Restore blood acid-base and osmolar balance but do not change serum sodium by more than 15 mOsm per day
7. Treat infection specifically
8. Ameliorate extreme body temperature (>41 or <35°C)
9. Consider naloxone
10. Control agitation-tremulousness with diazepam

REFERENCE

Plum F, Posner JB: Diagnosis of Stupor and Coma. 3rd ed. rev. Philadelphia, FA Davis Co, 1982.

BRIEF AND EPISODIC ALTERATIONS OF CONSCIOUSNESS

All of the disorders listed in Table 114–13 can produce recurrent, short-lived, relatively stereotyped alterations in perceptions, psychological feeling states, somatic functions, or global consciousness. Although each of these conditions produces fairly characteristic symptoms and signs, only hypoglycemia, seizure disorders, or certain forms of syncope (e.g., with cardiac arrhythmia) produce diagnostic laboratory findings. Indeed, even these latter usually must be obtained during the episodes. Accordingly, the cause of most episodes of brief loss of consciousness must be inferred from retrospective evidence. In such instances, the patient's age, his medical history, and, especially, an accurate recounting of symptoms or reports of direct observers provide the greatest help in diagnosis.

Syncope describes brief loss of consciousness due to a global reduction in cerebral blood flow. The disorder almost always is due to an abrupt or semiabrupt loss of cardiac output, most frequently secondary to

TABLE 114–13. BRIEF, OFTEN RECURRENT DISORDERS OF NEUROLOGICAL FUNCTION

Brief loss of consciousness
Syncope (Table 8–9)
Hypoglycemia (Ch. 74)
Seizures (Chapter 120)
Recurrent psychological disturbances
Hyperventilation attacks
Panic attacks
Fugue states (p. 694)
Episodic neurological dysfunction without impaired arousal
Transient global amnesia (p. 686)
Cerebral transient ischemic attacks (p. 769)
Drop spells
Migraine (p. 708)

acutely impaired right heart output (cardiac rhythm maintained) or severe left heart output (asystole or severe arrhythmia) (see Table 9–9).

Syncope due to reduced right heart filling usually results from pooling of blood in capacitance veins of the lower extremities or trunk. Most often, this comes from the triggering of vasodepressor reflex mechanisms. Orthostatic hypotension secondary to depleted blood volume, hypotensive drugs, and neurological disease, as well as mechanical increases in pulmonary resistance such as can accompany severe coughing or acute pulmonary infarction, are less frequent mechanisms. Cardiac tamponade interferes with both right and left heart filling and output.

Vasodepressor syncope (simple fainting) exceeds in frequency all other causes of acute brief unconsciousness combined. Simple fainting tends to be a recurrent problem in some individuals; a few give a family history of the disorder. No associated neurological or cardiologic abnormality can be found in most cases. Attacks are engendered by emotional crises, acute painful visceral stimuli, hyperventilation after micturition, and, in susceptible persons, various combinations of alcohol, hunger, and drugs. Often, one can identify no precipitating cause. Attacks begin in some persons with a brief prodrome of anxiety, giddiness, diaphoresis, and nausea before collapse. Others precipitously sink to the floor as heart rate and blood pressure fall and cardiac output declines. Except with prolonged asystole, syncope always occurs in the erect or sitting position, never when supine. Patients are pale and sweaty and may have one or two generalized clonic twitches as a result of a profound faint (convulsive syncope). Incontinence is unusual, but vomiting, micturition, and diarrhea commonly follow the attack. In young persons with a negative physical examination and characteristic history, physiological or structural disease almost never is present and laboratory studies need not be extensive. Hysteria and drug-alcohol intoxication are the chief resemblers. Table 120–5 outlines the differences from minor seizures. Simple fainting can affect persons older than 50 years, but a first episode in that age group deserves careful evaluation to rule out serious cardiac disorders. Cerebral transient ischemic attacks rarely simulate syncope. Occasionally, vasodepressor syncope accompanies attacks of severe migraine in adolescents and young adults.

Syncope recovers too quickly to treat except posturally by placing the subject supine and elevating the lower extremities; there are no effective preventive measures except when severe cardiac disorders are found and corrected. Avoiding offending foods as well as eliminating bouts of alcoholic ingestion without accompanying food helps when the history incriminates such associations.

Other causes of briefly altered unconsciousness are uncommon or discussed elsewhere (Table 114–13). Hyperventilation attacks more closely resemble the syndrome of panic than syncope. Affected patients may complain of feeling unreal, floating, or dizzy, but they do not lose contact with the environment. Perioral paresthesias, a sense of suffocating dyspnea, and carpopedal spasm are diagnostic. Treatment consists of attempting to provide the sufferer with insight and emphasizing the benign nature of the condition. Propranolol, up to 40 mg three times daily, may help to reduce the frequency of panic attacks. The drug is especially helpful in warding off stage fright.

REFERENCES

Day SC, Cook ET, Funkenstein H, et al: Evaluation and outcome of emergency room patients with transient loss of consciousness. Am J Med 73:15, 1982.

Kapoor WN, Peterson J, Wieand H, Karpf M: Diagnostic and prognostic implications of recurrences in patients with syncope. Am J Med 83:700, 1987.

C. FOCAL DISTURBANCES OF HIGHER BRAIN FUNCTION

REGIONAL SYNDROMES

The human cerebral cortex contains the final receiving areas for somatic and special sensory information as well as the primary motor cortex that executes all voluntary movement. Lying between these main sensorimotor regions are the very large areas of the association cortex, which converts sensation into perception and integrates instinctive and acquired memory into symbolic communication as well as planned, emotionally influenced behavior (Fig. 114–1). Increasing neurobiological evidence indicates that certain areas of the association cortex preferentially serve relatively specific aspects of higher brain function. Accordingly, damage to such regions often produces specifically recognizable psychological symptoms. This principle especially applies to functions such as language and orientation to extracorporeal space that are strongly lateralized in one hemisphere or the other.

Injury to a *frontal lobe* often produces one or more of the syndromes indicated in Table 114–14. The frontal lobes are large structures, however, and the nature and degree of symptoms depend on the locus, specific nature, and size of any damage that occurs, as well as its rate of enlargement. Relatively small abnormalities involving the posterior frontal areas of either hemisphere can cause seizures, motor deficits, or, on the dominant side, aphasia. By contrast, behavioral abnormalities with more anterior frontal lobe disturbances usually become apparent only when they grow to a large size or spread bilaterally.

Small lesions of the parietal lobe that lie outside the immediate postcentral gyrus often produce no clinically detectable symptoms. Large lesions such as can accompany stroke or malignant neoplasms produce abnormalities of the kind that are briefly summarized in Table 114–15.

Temporal lobe functions contribute to language, memory, and emotional capacities, and aspects of their damage are discussed below as well as in Chapter 120, describing complex partial seizures.

LANGUAGE AND APHASIA

Verbal language is a complex function to which many parts of the brain contribute. The critical areas

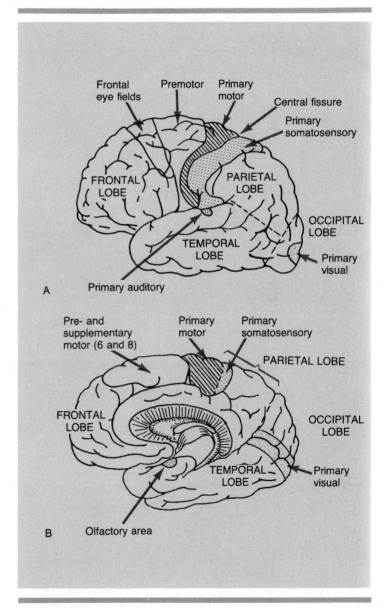

FIGURE 114–1. Major anatomic and functional areas of the cerebral hemispheres. *A,* Lateral surface. *B,* Medial surface.

TABLE 114–14. SYNDROMES OF FRONTAL LOBE DAMAGE

Contralateral upper motor neuron spastic weakness, more distal than proximal

Contralateral seizures: focal hand, face, foot (rare); adversive body or eyes

Aphasia (dominant hemisphere)

Social hyposensitivity

Impaired conceptualization and planning

TABLE 114–15. SYNDROMES OF PARIETAL LOBE DAMAGE

Postcentral cortex: Homunculus-patterned contralateral impairment of somesthetic abstraction: stereoanesthesia-astereognosis

Inferior parietal lobe

  Dominant: Aphasia, apraxia, acalculia, right-left disorientation

  Nondominant: Spatial disorientation; perceptual neglect, especially contralaterally; inappropriate affect, sometimes delirium

for language processing consist of Wernicke's area, which extends posteriorly along the superior temporal gyrus from the primary auditory cortex; the adjacent posterolateral temporal cortex and inferior parietal lobe cortex; and the inferior, posterolateral part of the frontal lobe cortex, called Broca's area (Fig. 114–2).

Language is a strongly lateralized function, arising entirely or predominantly from the above-described areas of the left hemisphere in roughly 95 per cent of the population. Dominance for handedness is less exclusive: about 15 per cent of persons are left-handed

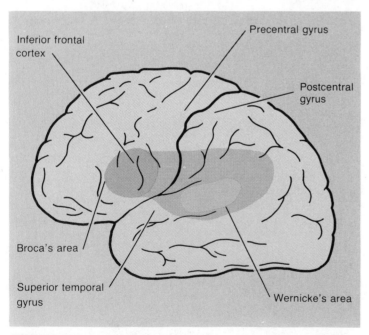

FIGURE 114–2. Primary language areas in the dominant cerebral hemisphere. Damage to Broca's area or Wernicke's area produces characteristic language abnormalities, as described in the text. Injury to the surrounding stippled areas causes less classic language impairments, including conduction aphasia.

Labels on figure:
Inferior frontal cortex
Precentral gyrus
Postcentral gyrus
Broca's area
Superior temporal gyrus
Wernicke's area

or ambidextrous, but only a third of left-handers possess a right hemisphere that is dominant for language. However, even though verbal language in many or most right-handed persons is an exclusive property of the left hemisphere, most left-handers tend to have some language function in both hemispheres. Accordingly, almost no left-handers become completely and permanently aphasic after an injury or even surgical removal of either the right or left hemisphere.

Aphasia or *dysphasia* consists of a loss or impairment of language function as a result of damage to or dysfunction in the specific language areas of the dominant hemisphere. The condition must be distinguished from *dysarthria*, a disturbance in the articulation of speech, from the nonsensical *word salad* of schizophrenia, and from the *jargon* phrases emitted during severe delirious reactions. The following paragraphs describe the major types of aphasia as well as certain other speech disorders with which they may be confused.

Wernicke's aphasia, sometimes called receptive aphasia, consists of an incapacity to recognize the nature or meaning of symbolic sensory stimuli, including language, or to connect learned words with either inner thoughts or stored memories. Affected patients cannot recognize any message, whether spoken, written, or symbolized, the only occasional exceptions being abrupt commands, e.g., "stop." Despite their severe loss of comprehension, however, they speak a fluent nonsense with a natural, meaningless rhythm. Insight is minimal and prognosis for total recovery is poor. Causative lesions damage the dominant posterior superior temporal lobe and, usually, adjacent parietal lobe structures as well.

Broca's aphasia is characterized by severe disturbances in expressing either spontaneous or commanded speech and writing. Comprehension is relatively better but incompletely preserved, with things spoken being better understood than things read. The vulnerable region includes Broca's area, described above. Largely because of vascular distributions, many patients with Broca's aphasia also have an associated right hemiparesis or hemiplegia, the result of a concurrent internal capsular lesion.

Both Broca's expressive aphasia and Wernicke's receptive language defect can occur in incomplete or mixed forms, but the general rule holds true that predominantly expressive language defects correlate with frontal lesions whereas receptive and word-finding difficulties correlate with temporoparietal abnormalities. An example of this principle occurs in conduction aphasia, characterized by a fluent, Wernicke-like aphasia coupled with the ability of the patient to repeat after the examiner phrases and often long sentences. The latter ability implies that Wernicke's and Broca's areas as well as the major connections between them must be relatively intact, so that the responsible lesions must lie near to but not within the primary speech areas.

Global aphasia describes the combined severe loss of all major aspects of language function due to frontotemporal damage in the dominant hemisphere. Affected patients can neither comprehend nor express language except, perhaps, in the form of brief expletives or phrases. Most have a right hemiplegia. Insight is poor, as is prognosis for full recovery.

Mutism, the inability to speak or make sounds, can occur with several disorders, as indicated in Table 114–16. All but hysterical mutism produce associated signs of organic brain disease.

Anarthria consists of the inability to speak because of abnormal innervation or mechanical disease of the vocal apparatus. Affected patients make sounds and express their frustration over being unable to speak. Neurogenic causes of anarthria include severe bulbar or pseudobulbar palsy, conditions readily diagnosed by the presence of other signs and symptoms of nuclear or supranuclear paralysis.

Apraxia refers to a disturbance of or an inability to perform learned motor acts despite the retention of sufficient sensory and language function to understand the command and enough crude motor capacity to carry it out (praxis). The condition most commonly accompanies deep lesions of the frontal or, especially, parietal lobes. Lesions are often multifocal, such as occur with the degenerative dementias or after multiple strokes.

Agnosia is the inability to recognize a complex sensory stimulus despite the preservation of elemental perceptions and the absence of a defect in language. The phenomenon accompainies certain post-Rolandic lesions, including postcentral gyrus (astereognosis) or parts of the parieto-occipital association cortex (inability to identify or grasp the significance of faces, body parts, colors, or observed objects). It occurs most often with multiple strokes or one of the degenerative dementias.

MEMORY

The establishment of memory and learning is identical. Disturbances of memory include defects in past memory, called *retrograde amnesia*, and the inability to form new memories from ongoing events, called *anterograde amnesia*.

Patterns of Memory Failure. Memory can be divided into immediate, intermediate, and remote epochs. *Immediate memory* consists of holding in the mind material just heard or read with no necessary intervening storage process. *Intermediate memory* covers the time span beginning within a few seconds past and extending backward for 24 to 48 hours or more. *Long-term memory* extends beyond that epoch, but this too has its gradations, for many childhood memories tend to be well recalled even as more recent ones begin to fade. Illustrating this principle, standard I.Q. tests that include definitions of words and functions learned before the age of 14 years often give normal scores in adults suffering from diseases that severely impair or destroy recent and anterograde memory.

Memory Mechanisms. The brain possesses substantial *instinctive memory*, reflected in many aspects of automatic human behavior and motor skills.

TABLE 114–16. FREQUENT CAUSES OF MUTISM (No Voluntary Sounds)

Acute lesions of left frontal or pre-Broca area (transient)
Acute epileptic attacks (paroxysmal)
Deep bilateral frontal lesions (sustained)
Bilateral midbrain–upper pons corticospinal damage (locked-in)
Hysteria or malingering (situational)

Learned memories are generated from perceptions of the external world and inner thoughts and have at least three distinct components: perception-registration of the experience, storage, and retrieval. Storage of both perceived events and motor skills is distributed widely in the brain, especially in the areas of the association cortex that lie adjacent to primary sensory perceptual regions or, for motor skills, in the prefrontal regions. The agnosias described above provide examples of damage to such distributed areas. Memory formation and retrieval, by contrast, appear to require the integrity of the hippocampal areas of the temporal lobe, as well as certain subcortical nuclei. Considerable redundancy of function characterizes the memory-transacting areas. Reflecting this, purely unilateral damage to, for example, the left hippocampus may produce modest impairments in verbal memory, but severe memory impairment requires much more extensive and usually bilateral injury.

Bilateral damage or surgical removal of the hippocampus in the adult results in profound and usually permanent deficits in intermediate memory affecting especially the verbal-visual-spatial spheres. Proportional defects in anterograde learning accompany the retrograde loss. At the subcortical level, bilateral damage to several paramedian areas of the thalamus and, probably, the mammillary bodies, results in a profound multidimensional disturbance of memory. The prominent memory loss that often accompanies Huntington's disease suggests that striatal mechanisms may contribute to the normal memory process.

Cerebral memory mechanisms depend in an incompletely understood way on cholinergic and other autonomic projections that link the subcortical basal forebrain with the hippocampus and the association cortex of the temporal, parietal, and frontal lobes. Degeneration of these projections is a prominent accompaniment of the dementia of Alzheimer's and certain other dementias.

Clinical Memory Disorders. Many middle-aged and elderly persons report an increasing, relatively isolated difficulty in recalling proper names and recent events of minor importance. This "benign forgetfulness" bears no consistent relationship to the progressive dementias and is best treated with prompt and vigorous reassurance.

More serious amnesias accompany or follow severe thiamine deficiency (e.g., Korsakoff's syndrome), the organic dementias discussed in the next section, severe head trauma, brain anoxia or ischemia, encephalitis, and, less frequently, intracranial mass lesions.

Korsakoff's syndrome is a profound recent memory

TABLE 114–17. ORGANIC AND PSYCHOGENIC AMNESIA COMPARED

	ORGANIC	PSYCHOGENIC
Time frame	Recent worse than remote	Unpredictable mixture of recent and remote, often for circumscribed events
Pattern	Anterograde amnesia as bad as retrograde	No anterograde amnesia except in total fugues ("who am I?")
	Emotionally important events recalled better	Such events often "forgotten"
Self-recognition	Intact except with severe delirium or seizures	May be denied
Behavior	Same questions asked repeatedly	Often no questions asked

loss, usually accompanied by lack of insight, disorientation to time and place, and confabulation. Nutritional Korsakoff's syndrome most frequently affects alcoholics and often accompanies or follows the florid signs and symptoms of acute Wernicke's encephalopathy or delirium tremens. Other causes include global cerebral anoxia-ischemia, status epilepticus, and subarachnoid hemorrhage, all of which can selectively and bilaterally damage vulnerable neurons in the hippocampus and medial diencephalon.

Even modest head trauma temporarily interrupts memory-mediating neural connections. Concussive injuries frequently produce an initially severe degree of retrograde and a lesser degree of anterograde amnesia; in most instances the memory loss almost disappears with time. A less fortunate prognosis accompanies prolonged post-traumatic coma. When this lasts more than two to three weeks, most patients over 25 years old never fully recover from memory impairment.

Permanent or prolonged amnesia occasionally can follow bilateral cerebral infarction, large brain tumors, or surgical operations affecting the hippocampus. Herpes simplex encephalitis has a predilection to produce necrotic-inflammatory lesions in the limbic system lying along the medial surfaces of the temporal lobes and characteristically leaves severe amnesia in its wake.

Transient global amnesia (TGA) is a condition marked by periods lasting from several minutes to as long as 12 hours or so of abruptly beginning, acute alert confusion. A severe deficit in retrograde memory accompanies the beginning of the attack and gradually disappears as it wears off. Affected persons can identify themselves but are severely disoriented for time and place and distressed about the experience. Most TGA attacks affect middle-aged or elderly persons and appear to reflect temporary vascular insufficiency affecting the hippocampal memory areas or their immediate neural connections. Temporal lobe seizures or hysterical fugue states represent the principal conditions to be distinguished. Most attacks neither leave residual limitations nor carry a strong risk of recurrence.

Psychogenic memory impairment can affect either recent or remote recall, usually in clinically recognizable patterns (Table 114–17). Anxiety, forced inattention, or reduced arousal may result in inconsistent responses to testing, with persons accurately recounting some current events but claiming to forget others. In general, organic disturbances in memory are marked by variability in what is remembered, emotionally reinforced material being recalled better than neutral events. With organic memory loss, disorientation is worst for time, less for place and persons, and never for self. In most instances, events of the recent past are forgotten more than remote ones, and the providing of cues often improves recall. By contrast, psychogenic amnesia tends to be greatest for emotionally important events, may elide from the patient's memory well-defined blocks of past events while leaving intact the recall of preceding or following material, and may affect remote memories equally with recent ones.

Treatment. Patients with acute post-traumatic amnesia show a high rate of spontaneous recovery. Improvement of memory loss from other organic disorders is less predictable except when the amnesia can be traced to an excess use of medication or a temporary systemic disorder such as hepatic, renal, or pulmonary insufficiency. Neither medications nor diets have proved useful in treating the organic amnesias.

REFERENCES

Mesulam MM: Principles of Behavioral Neurology. Philadelphia, FA Davis Co, 1985.
Squire LR: Memory: Neural organization and behavior. *In* Plum F (ed): Handbook of Physiology. Section 1: The Nervous System. Vol 5: Higher Functions of the Brain. Bethesda, American Physiological Society, 1987, pp 295–373.

D. DEMENTIA

GENERAL CONSIDERATIONS

Dementia describes a sustained or permanent, multidimensional decline of intellectual function that interferes seriously with the individual's normal social or economic adjustment.

Static dementia is a state that occurs abruptly or acutely and remains either fixed or improves very little thereafter. The condition can follow any process that structurally damages large portions of the association areas of the cerebral hemispheres. Severe head injury, global brain ischemia from cardiac arrest, large intracranial neoplasms or hemorrhages with their surgical removal, or infections such as severe encephalitis or meningitis are typical examples. *Progressive dementias* may begin either suddenly or insidiously but, by definition, worsen with the passage of time, often ending in hopeless incapacity or death.

Table 114–18 indicates the most common causes of the progressive dementias and provides rough estimates of their frequencies. The figures emphasize the relatively greater problem of the progressive "primary" dementias, especially of the Alzheimer type. AIDS-related dementia is an increasing problem among young homosexual males and intravenous drug abusers in metropolitan areas.

Early Clinical Manifestations. Acute, static dementia seldom provides a problem in diagnosis. Most often the diagnostic problem following a sudden brain injury becomes not whether a mental decline has occurred but to what degree and how the patient can restructure his world to his new, possibly permanent limitations.

Early diagnosis in the progressive dementias is often difficult. Initial symptoms involve deterioration in mood, personality, recent memory, judgment, and the capacity to form abstractions. Families or work associates usually notice a change before the patient does, and persons who live by intellectual efforts show their limitations earlier than do those with routine or manual jobs. Some patients become so apathetic as to seem depressed; in others great anxiety or increased irritability disrupts a once pleasant personality. Some persons with early dementia become paranoid or depressed. Loss of recent memory is a universal feature. Appointments are missed, plans forgotten, and stories of recent events become narrated repeatedly with no insight. Eventually orientation fails, first for days, then years, then months, and finally for place. Interest lags. Debts may be accumulated silently, property unwisely sold, accounts lost, and meals cooked twice over or served half-cold. Mental capacities can fluctuate suddenly without apparent relationship to external events. In Alzheimer's disease and some of the other progressive primary dementias, social amenities tend to be retained until late in the course. By contrast, incontinence, soup on the shirt, and a disheveled appearance characterize the mental deterioration that accompanies frontal lobe disease, intracranial mass lesions, or chronic drug-alcohol abuse.

Diagnosis. The principal questions are: (1) Does a true decline in intellect exist? (2) If so, what is its probable cause?

The clinical examination of all patients with subacute or chronic central nervous system disease should include at least a brief evaluation of mental function such as represented by the Mini Mental Status (Table 114–19). For further quantitation the Wechsler Adult Intelligence Scale (WAIS) provides useful information but requires the assistance of a trained psychologist. In mild to moderate dementia the verbal score of the WAIS provides an index of learning capacity, whereas the performance part reflects current mental abilities. A discrepancy of more than 15 points between the two reflects acquired brain dysfunction.

TABLE 114–18. MAJOR CAUSES OF PROGRESSIVE DEMENTIA

1.	Senile dementia, Alzheimer type	50%
2.	Multi-infarct (arteriosclerotic)	10%
3.	Combination of 1 and 2	15%
4.	Communicating hydrocephalus	
5.	Alcoholic or post-traumatic	15%
6.	Huntington's chorea	
7.	Intracranial mass lesions	
8.	Uncommon or mixed with above:	10%

Chronic drug use; Creutzfeldt-Jakob; metabolic (thyroid, liver, nutritional); degenerative (spinocerebellar, amyotrophic lateral sclerosis, parkinsonism, multiple sclerosis, Pick's, Wilson's, epilepsy); AIDS dementia; static post-anoxic dementia

The laboratory evaluation of dementia depends on the combined results of the history, general physical and neurological examination, and preliminary laboratory results. Potentially treatable forms of chronic confusion or potential dementia include intracranial mass lesions, thamine deficiency, pellagra, myxedema, hypercalcemia, cyanocobalamin (vitamin B_{12}) deficiency, drugs and toxins, hepatic encephalopathy, Wilson's disease, syphilis, granulomatous meningitis, and hydrocephalus. In the absence of leads from the history or examination, the tests listed in Table 114–20 will detect most of these treatable disorders.

Pseudodementia is a term applied to reversible states in which reduced cognitive functions are caused by

TABLE 114–19. MINI MENTAL STATUS EXAMINATION*

TEST	SCORE
What is the year, season, date, day, month?	5
Where are you: state, county, town, place, floor	5
Name three objects: State slowly and have patient repeat (repeat until patient learns all three)	3
Do reverse serial 7's (five steps) or spell "WORLD" backwards	5
Ask for three unrelated objects above	3
Name from inspection a pencil, a watch	2
Have patient repeat No if's, and's, or but's	1
Follow a three-stage command (1 pt each) (Take a paper in your hand, fold it, and put it on the floor)	3
Read and obey, Close your eyes	1
Write a simple sentence	1
Copy intersecting pentagons	1

* Out of a possible total score of 30, most patients with true dementia score below 15, whereas those with uncomplicated depression score above 25. Mixed or transient cognitive impairments produce scores in between normals and those with irreversible dementia.

TABLE 114–20. LABORATORY SCREENING TESTS TO IDENTIFY A TREATABLE DEMENTIA

All cases: CBC; full chemistry screen; serum B_{12}; VDRL; serum free T_4 index and TSH. Brain CT or MR image

If clinical indices suggest: Erythrocyte sedimentation rate, lumbar puncture (cells [including examination of sediment for cytology], protein, glucose, VDRL, culture); EEG chronic drug intoxication or depressive illness. Aging persons are especially susceptible to both conditions. Among drugs, the barbiturates, benzodiazepines, butyrophenones, tricyclic antidepressants, MAO inhibitors, anticholinergics, corticosteroids, and digitalis are frequently responsible (see Table 114–26).

The apathy, semimutism, akinesia, anxiety, and indifference of psychological depression sometimes can simulate dementia (see Table 114–23). In contrast to demented patients, however, those with depression complain repeatedly of their poor memory. They commonly eat little, often are severely constipated, sleep

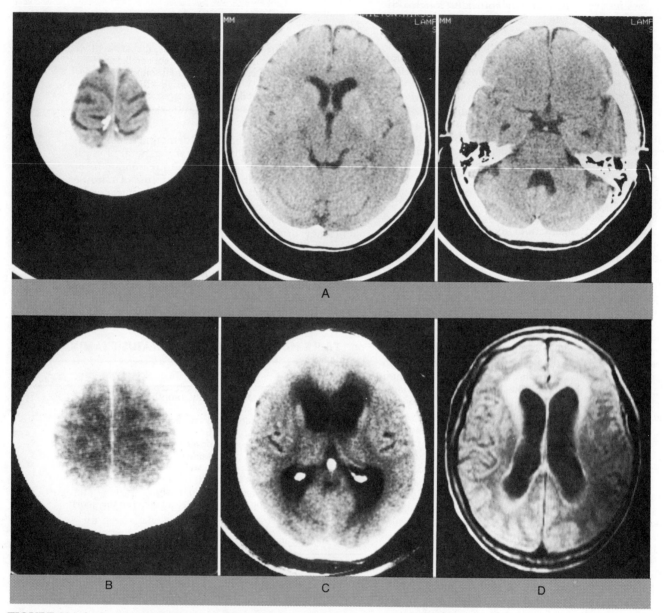

FIGURE 114–3. Communicating hydrocephalus. A 61-year-old woman seven years following uncomplicated removal of carcinoma of the lung developed symptoms of headache and depression of mood in the setting of her husband's catastrophic stroke. Neurological examination and CT evaluation (A) were unremarkable, although in retrospect the fourth ventricle was slightly dilated. Over the next four months she became increasingly withdrawn, occasionally incontinent, and finally disoriented. She developed a broad-based ataxic gait and CT scan showed (B) absent sulcal markings at the vertex with (C) ventricular dilatation. NMR confirmed the ventricular enlargement (D) and showed periventricular increased signals typical of edema. Spinal fluid contained increased protein, hypoglycorrhachia (glucose 25 mg/dl) and malignant cells. CSF pressure was 180 mm in the lateral recumbent positions. Her alertness and gait temporarily improved following spinal drainage.

less than normal, and tend to behave best at night. They make errors because of indifference or obstinant refusal rather than poor comprehension. Such depressed patients may stumble over tests requiring attention, but they rarely forget major recent events or political figures, and when they do cooperate they perform adequately on mental status examinations. By contrast, patients with incapacitating dementia are disoriented, their nights are more agitated and confused than their days, they have difficulty following commands, attention and recent memory are severely impaired, and they often suffer difficulties in language and specific learned motor functions. Brain imaging procedures show anatomic abnormalities in many of the dementias, and the EEG is nonspecifically slow in most of the dementias but not in depression.

THE MOST FREQUENT DEMENTIAS

Alzheimer's Presenile and Senile Dementia (ASD). This devastating, increasingly frequent disorder occasionally affects persons younger than 50 years but is uncommon up to age 65. Subsequently, the prevalence increases to more than 20 per cent of those who live beyond age 80 years. The etiology of ASD is unknown, but recent attention has focused on a possible hereditary factor associated with a gene abnormality on chromosome 21. Pathologically, the condition includes neuronal degeneration in the deeper levels of the cerebral cortex and hippocampus as well as in basal forebrain nuclei that project cholinergic fibers to the cortex and other areas of the cerebrum. Noradrenergic and serotonergic projections can be impaired as well. The neuropeptide, somatostatin, is reduced in the cortex. Brain images usually show only moderate cerebral atrophy. Histological examination discloses in the cortex characteristic fibrillary degeneration in neurons, together with amyloid-cored plaques containing cellular debris. A major current hypothesis regards an abnormality in the larger precursor protein of this amyloid as important in causing the disease. Clinically, the onset of ASD usually is insidious, with memory impairment, personality alterations, and affective shallowness giving way at varying rates to severe event and spatial amnesia, as well as language errors. Social amenities are preserved until late. Focal neurological abnormalities or convulsions are not a feature. Specific diagnostic laboratory markers are lacking. The duration of ASD varies widely between extremes of 3 to 20 years, with patients declining slowly toward a terminal vegetative state. Death comes from pneumonia or intercurrent illness. Variants have been described in association with parkinsonism and motor neuron disease. No effective treatment has been established.

Multi-infarct Dementia. This occurs as a result of successive large and small strokes, affecting the cerebral hemispheres and their deep subcortical nuclei. Hypertension, diabetes mellitus, or hyperlipidemia causes the most common vascular changes, although similar results can follow several other disorders capable of causing multiple cerebral arterial occlusions. The usual clinical picture is of successive, cumulative episodes of focal neurologic worsening, resulting in a disheveled appearance, accompanied commonly by aphasia, focal neurologic deficits and CT or MRI scans that show multiple lucencies reflecting past infarctions. Many patients develop pseudobulbar palsy and some, incontinence. Occasionally, successive small strokes in hypertensive patients result in a less obviously episodic decline, but in any event evidence of severe heart and vascular disease is present.

Progressive Hydrocephalic Dementia. This condition is caused by chronic communicating hydrocephalus resulting from interference with CSF absorption pathways over the surface of the hemispheres. The ultimate cause in some cases is inflammatory or neoplastic meningitis with subarachnoid hemorrhage being responsible in others; in many instances the initiating mechanism escapes detection. The condition affects mostly persons older than 55 years and is marked by nonspecific changes in memory and intellect, apathetic fatigability and, usually, the development of a broad-based, moderately spastic ataxic gait, accompanied by extensor plantar responses. Urinary incontinence is common. Diagnosis depends on the clinical findings. Brain images show abnormal cerebral ventricular dilatation and reduction in vertex sulcal markings, usually coupled with evidence of periventricular edema (Fig. 114–3). Some patients improve following surgical ventricular shunting, but no laboratory test reliably predicts the postoperative outcome.

Other Dementias. Huntington's disease is an autosomal, dominantly transmitted disorder producing chorea and dementia, discussed on page 738. *Creutzfeldt-Jakob disease*, a rare, progressive dementia, affects persons of either sex, mainly between the ages of 40 and 65 years. Usually within 6 months, prominent intellectual deterioration occurs, accompanied by signs of corticospinal tract dysfunction, myoclonus, and, sometimes, muscle atrophy. In the late stages characteristic EEG changes develop. The illness is caused by a "slow virus" (p. 811). It has been inadvertently transmitted to healthy recipients by corneal transplants and deep brain electrodes taken from unrecognized cases as well as by injections of growth hormone prepared from human pituitary glands taken at autopsy.

REFERENCES

Cummings JL, Benson DF: Dementia, A Clinical Approach. Boston, Butterworths, 1983.
Friedland RP, et al: Alzheimer Disease: Clinical and biological heterogeneity. Ann Intern Med 109:298, 1988

E. DISORDERS OF MOOD AND BEHAVIOR

Many patients confront the physician with an abnormality of mood (anxiety, depression, indifference, anger) or behavior (inappropriateness, obsessiveness) that appears to play a major role in their illness. All such moods and behaviors must arise from the brain and therefore ultimately are neurogenic. However, for pragmatic reasons, medicine distinguishes "organic" from "psychogenic" disorders of mood and behavior, the former caused by clearly identifiable structural or metabolic abnormalities of the brain, the latter by more or less identifiable environmental stresses or by endogenous predisposition. The distinction is potentially useful because behavioral symptoms of an organic nature usually require treatment different from those of a psychological nature. There are, however, two major problems with the organic-psychogenic distinction: (1) Often the distinction is clinically difficult. The appearance of psychological depression can be mimicked by frontal lobe brain tumors, and occasional patients with temporal lobe epilepsy develop illnesses indistinguishable from schizophrenia. On the other hand, some patients with conversion reactions develop neurological signs (i.e., hemiparesis, sensory loss) that closely resemble those of structural brain disease or can even be superimposed on organic signs. (2) The two categories of illness at times overlap so much that the distinction is useless. For example, a patient with structural disease of the brain (e.g., Alzheimer's or post-traumatic) may become anxious or depressed because the brain disease has rendered him unable to cope with environmental stresses that he formerly could handle. These psychological abnormalities may be prominent at a time when structural abnormalities are so subtle as to be undetectable by the physician, but sedative drugs used to treat the anxiety may exacerbate the dementia. On the other hand, patients suffering from anxiety or depression related to life stresses may complain only of face, neck, or back pain engendered by muscle tension and postural abnormalities associated with the anxiety (p. 692). A diagnostic work-up may in fact reveal structural disease of the temporomandibular joint, neck, or back which could be responsible for much of the pain. Nevertheless, the physician discovers that only when he appropriately treats the anxiety and depression is he able to ameliorate the somatic symptoms.

Since all mood and behavior *must* be associated with alterations of electrical or biochemical (or both) activity in the brain, it is likely that the future will bring greater knowledge of the physiology of brain function and lead to a clearer understanding of the interface between so-called organic and psychogenic illnesses. In the meantime, however, one must sift out for each patient the relative degrees of psychological as well as physical distress and give due weight to each in devising treatment. This chapter deals with illnesses that are thought to have primarily a psychological origin (organic disorders are described in other chapters) and follows in its classification the Diagnostic and Statistical Manual of Mental Disorders (American Psychiatric Association, DSM-III) (Table 114–21). This manual provides objective diagnostic criteria for psychiatric disorders which, if rigorously applied, will prevent most diagnostic errors.

SCHIZOPHRENIC DISORDERS

These are a group of symptomatic disorders, possibly of different etiologies, characterized by disturbances of mind and personality, including hallucinations, delusions, and altered behavior toward others. The common thread consists of a disturbance in the form and content of thought and a deterioration in psychosocial functioning which often causes downward social mobility. The disorder, which affects about 1 per cent of the population, can be mimicked by structural or physiological-pharmacological disease of the brain, particularly that involving the limbic system, and thus the diagnosis requires that such structural disease be absent. The symptoms of schizophrenia begin before the age of 45, usually during adolescence or early adulthood. Most patients suffer from auditory hallucinations in which they either hear their own thoughts aloud or hear voices commenting on their action, often in a derogatory fashion. At times, several voices discuss the patient, usually in the third person. In addition to the hallucinations, affected patients suffer from delusions, such as, for example, that their actions or thoughts are controlled by outside forces and they are forced to carry out unwanted acts. To the examiner, schizophrenic patients often appear vague, unresponsive, and unemotional, with awkward and slowed thinking and ideas poorly related one to another. The affect is often flat or inappropriate, the patient laughing as he discusses serious problems. In addition, schizophrenic patients may show facial grimaces or tics that at times can resemble chorea or other extrapyramidal disorders. Occasional patients become immobile (catatonia), resembling the apathy and indifference of frontal lobe disturbances.

The cause of the schizophrenic disorders is unknown. Studies of identical twins have shown a strong genetic basis for the disorder, but no structural or biochemical abnormality of the brain has been identified. An abnormality of chromosome 5, identified in one

TABLE 114–21. PSYCHOGENIC DISORDERS OF MOOD AND BEHAVIOR

1. Schizophrenic disorders
2. Affective disorders
3. Anxiety disorders
4. Somatoform disorders
5. Dissociative disorders
6. Factitious disorders
7. Not attributable to a mental disorder, e.g., malingering

large pedigree, has not been confirmed in another. Some recent studies employing CT scans suggest that schizophrenics have atrophic brains, but the finding is far from universal.

The diagnosis rests first on the recognition of the constellation of distinctive symptoms and second on the ruling out of other potential causes for the emotional and personality disorders. Schizophrenic patients, if their cooperation can be assured, are oriented and have no abnormality of cognitive functions; by contrast, careful testing reveals that patients suffering from structural or metabolic disease of the brain manifested by selective symptoms suggesting schizophrenia demonstrate disorientation or other cognitive abnormalities. The clinical problem is that often cooperation cannot be assured in either group. Sometimes it is difficult to distinguish schizophrenia from an affective psychosis (see below). The distinction is important, since the treatment is different and the prognosis is considerably better in the affective psychoses than it is in schizophrenia.

The treatment of schizophrenia requires considerable expertise. Neuroleptic drugs including phenothiazine, butyrophenones, and thioxanthenes are the mainstay and have been in large measure responsible for allowing most schizophrenic patients to be treated outside mental institutions. However, the drugs are difficult to use, in part because of problems with patient compliance. Furthermore, they are fraught with side effects. With the doses required to control the psychotic symptoms, some patients may develop akathisia and/or dystonic reactions or extrapyramidal disorders of the *Parkinson* type. The latter sometimes requires anticholinergic drugs to be added to the phenothiazines. In addition, long-term use of phenothiazines leads in more than 10 per cent of patients to *tardive dyskinesias* in the form of either continuous orolingual facial movements or less commonly dystonic movements of the trunk or extremities. Tardive dyskinesia may persist even when the neuroleptics are discontinued, and it responds poorly to therapy. Thus, one should attempt to control psychotic symptoms with the smallest possible dose. In addition to drug therapy, it is often useful to try to establish a milieu in which patients can be comfortable and supported without being stressed. The recognition that such therapy is efficacious has led to the founding of halfway houses for chronically ill patients. If appropriate treatment is begun early, one third to one half of patients remit and another 30 per cent are able to live in the community.

AFFECTIVE DISORDERS

This category includes a group of disorders characterized by an excessive disturbance of mood, either elation or depression, the mood abnormality not being due to any other physical or mental disorder. The major affective disorders include recurrent episodes of either manic or depressive behavior or both (bipolar disorders), with attacks of either or both kinds repeating on several occasions during a lifetime but usually clearing after weeks or months even without treat-

ment. The pathogenesis is unknown, although monozygotic twin studies indicate a major genetic component. In one study a gene on chromosome 11 appears to predispose to the autosomal dominant inherited bipolar disease of Amish families. Other investigators find that some cases may be associated with a gene on the X chromosome. Unlike the schizophrenic disorders, between episodes most patients appear entirely normal.

Depression. The most common affective disorder is depression. Depression is a feeling of sadness and misery, usually accompanied by lowered self-esteem and ranging from feelings of inadequacy and incompetence to a full-blown delusion that the patient is evil and responsible for many of the world's ills. The delusions (usually of a bizarre nature) distinguish "psychotic" from situational depressions (i.e., excessive sadness related to a true environmental event). Both groups of patients, however, suffer from physical symptoms as well as depression of mood. Depressed patients usually have either insomnia, usually falling asleep reasonably promptly but waking early in the morning and being unable to return to sleep, or hypersomnia, sleeping 12 to 16 hours a day. There may be loss of appetite, constipation, and frequently weight loss. A few patients eat excessively and gain weight. Severely depressed patients are slow in their responses and appear apathetic and indifferent. They frequently complain of aches, pains, and other somatic symptoms (headache is particularly common) that may be either psychophysiological or delusional. Some patients complain only of the somatic symptoms and deny depression (masked depression). Psychomotor retardation may lead the physician to suspect either that the patient has serious organic disease or that he is suffering from dementia (pseudodementia of depression). However, tests of cognitive functions, if the patient cooperates, are normal.

The diagnosis of depression may be difficult, but it is important. Depression, no matter what its underlying cause, can be treated, but if untreated may lead to prolonged illness, lengthy and unnecessary medical testing, and even suicide. There are several diagnostic problems. The first is to distinguish depression from physical illness. Many patients complaining of somatic symptoms have lost weight and may look so ill that the physician searches for a disease such as cancer without considering depression as the primary process. Early morning awakening, loss of appetite, and, particularly, unexplained headache, however, should suggest depression; direct questioning about mood is essential and often rewarding. Patients should be asked if they feel blue or hopeless. If so, patients should be asked gently and supportively if they have considered suicide as an option. An affirmative answer greatly strengthens the diagnosis and increases the gravity. Exploring the nature of the patient's plans for suicide helps determine the level of risk.

The second diagnostic task is to identify depression in the setting of established physical illness or environmental stress. Depression arising in a patient with a chronic illness (e.g., multiple sclerosis or cancer) can too easily be disregarded because it is believed to be appropriate to the situation. However, profound depression, even in terminal patients, is not the rule but adds great misery when it occurs. If it is discovered, the physician should consider it an added illness meriting specific treatment.

The third problem is to distinguish depression from dementia (Table 114–22). Many depressed patients are so inattentive to their environment that they appear to have lost cognitive functions. One particularly important clue is that the pseudodemented depressive patient generally answers a question of cognition with "I don't know," whereas a truly demented patient often gives an answer even though it is incorrect. Pseudodemented patients also much more frequently ask if they are losing their minds.

Finally, the physician must distinguish structural disease of the brain from psychogenic depression. Patients with large frontal lobe brain tumors, some with hydrocephalus or subdural hematomas and many with myxedema, can give the apathetic appearance of being withdrawn and depressed. Unless accompanied by other neurological signs, the signs and symptoms of neurogenic pseudodepression may be indistinguishable from those of psychological illness, and some such patients may even respond to antidepressant drugs. Generally, however, one finds other clinical signs of neurological dysfunction that suggest structural disease of the brain (e.g., abnormalities of motor function and language with frontal tumors or infarcts, and with hydrocephalus, abnormalities of gait, and sometimes urgency incontinence). In doubtful instances a CT or MR scan provides accurate differentiation.

Depression usually responds to appropriate treatment with antidepressant drugs. This is true not only of "pure" psychogenic depression but also of situational or reactive depression and, to a lesser degree, even that associated with structural disease of the nervous system. The tricyclic antidepressant drugs such as amitriptyline, given in appropriate doses (from 75 to 300 mg/day), often relieve symptoms promptly. These drugs should be started in low doses (e.g., 10 to 20 mg at bedtime) and gradually increased, particularly in elderly patients, to avoid excessive sedation and sometimes hallucinations. If the drug is given as a single dose at night, it promotes sleep, frequently relieving almost immediately one of the most disturbing symptoms in the depressed patient. The full psychological benefit usually takes two to four weeks. Other antidepressant drugs include monoamine oxidase inhibitors, tetracyclic antidepressants, and trazadone, a new drug unrelated to any of the others. Benzodiazepines such as diazepam (Valium) and flurazepam (Dalmane) are *not* useful. Furthermore, if used to treat anxiety or insomnia, they may exacerbate an unrecognized depression. If antidepressant drug therapy fails, electroshock therapy is often efficacious, particularly in patients with psychotic depression. Usually four to eight treatments terminate an episode.

Mania. Manic symptoms are the antithesis of depression, producing elation, grandiosity, and constant restless activity. In the earliest stages of mania, patients may in fact become more productive. As the disease progresses, however, they deteriorate. They are easily distracted, show flight of ideas, and become so grandiose and implausible as to be recognized by all around them as "crazy." Such patients have a decreased need for sleep and with intense mania may go for days without sleep and yet deny fatigue.

The elated mood can suddenly change to anger, and the patient may become violent with little or no provocation. The diagnosis is usually easy because the symptoms are so characteristic and are rarely imitated by other disorders. Occasionally structural disease of the limbic system can mimic mania, and the ingestion of corticosteroid drugs may cause an indistinguishable clinical picture. Sometimes one has difficulty distinguishing a manic episode from schizophrenic illness with agitated behavior, but the extreme self-confidence that accompanies the former usually establishes the diagnosis.

The treatment of mania is difficult, in part because patients feel well and see no need for medicine. Phenothiazines or butyrophenones often control agitated behavior. Lithium is the mainstay. The drug is given in a dose of 900 to 2400 mg/day, with careful monitoring of plasma lithium levels to keep the concentration below 2 mEq/L. Excessive lithium levels lead to confusion, disorientation, tremor, anorexia, and, sometimes, seizures with permanent neurologic damage. Maintenance lithium in patients with a history of manic psychosis often prevents further episodes.

Anxiety Disorders (Table 114–23). Anxiety is an unpleasant mood of tension and apprehension related to fear but not focused on an object of immediate danger. The symptom is common and frequently is appropriate for a particular life situation or illness and if not excessive or sustained may focus the mind and improve performance. Anxiety is generally accompanied by autonomic symptoms including tachycardia, perspiration, dry mouth, and sometimes hyperventilation. The autonomic symptoms may create a vicious circle in which perception of the autonomic changes, particularly palpitations (tachycardia) and lightheadedness (hyperventilation), increase the anxiety, thus in turn increasing the autonomic symptoms.

The cause of the primary anxiety disorders (those

TABLE 114–22. SOME FEATURES DIFFERENTIATING PSEUDODEMENTIA FROM DEMENTIA

PSEUDODEMENTIA	DEMENTIA
Symptoms of short duration suggest pseudodementia.	Symptoms of long duration suggest dementia.
Patients frequently complain of cognitive loss.	Patients rarely complain of cognitive loss.
Patients' complaints of cognitive dysfunction are usually detailed.	Patients' complaints of cognitive dysfunction are usually imprecise.
"Don't know" answers are typical.	Patient usually gives an incorrect answer.

Modified from Wells CE, Duncan GW: Neurology for Psychiatrists. Philadelphia, FA Davis Co, 1977, pp 92–95.

TABLE 114–23. THE PRIMARY ANXIETY DISORDERS

Phobic disorders
    Agoraphobia with panic attacks
    Agoraphobia without panic attacks
    Social phobia
    Simple phobia
Anxiety states
    Panic disorder
    Generalized anxiety disorder
    Obsessive-compulsive disorder
Post-traumatic stress disorder
    Acute
    Chronic or delayed
Atypical anxiety disorder

Modified from Brown JT, Mulrow CD, Stoudemire CA: The anxiety disorders. Ann Intern Med 100:558–564, 1984.

that occur in the absence of identifiable physical or environmental cause) is unknown. The disorder is common, with a prevalence rate of about 1 per cent with increased incidence particularly of agoraphobia in women. In susceptible patients the disorder can often be produced by infusions of sodium lactate or isoproteranol and by benzodiazepine receptor antagonists. In a recent study, positron emission tomography in patients with a panic disorder revealed a pathological asymmetry in the parahippocampal region. There is also a genetic factor, since anxiety disorders have a higher concordance in monozygotic than in diazygotic twins, generally run in families, and are often associated with alcoholism. A disproportionate number of patients also have mitral valve prolapse.

Clinically, anxiety states can be characterized by (1) *phobias*, which can vary from simple phobic fears of particular objects, to agoraphobia, fear of either being alone or being in public places, (2) panic attacks that occur in spontaneous sudden episodes marked by fear, apprehension, and feelings of impending doom without underlying cause (Table 114–24), and (3) a generalized and constant feeling of fear and apprehension.

The diagnosis is usually not difficult, but sometimes patients focus on the physical and autonomic aspects of anxiety or the panic attack, complaining of palpitations and dizziness (sometimes misinterpreted as vertigo) rather than the feelings of anxiety, leading the physician to suspect an organic disorder. Frequently, having such patients hyperventilate will reproduce their symptoms and distinguish the disorder from a primary cardiac or neurological abnormality. By contrast, structural disease occasionally may be responsible for attacks of autonomic dysfunction that appear to be panic in origin. Some temporal lobe seizures produce an aura of intense fear or anxiety associated with abnormalities of pulse and respiration, in early stages indistinguishable from panic attacks. In most patients with temporal lobe structural disease, however, the attack culminates in a psychomotor or generalized convulsion, thus establishing the diagnosis. Sudden changes in cardiovascular function, such as arrhythmias or acute hypertension (as from a pheochromocytoma), can mimic panic or anxiety attacks. This is particularly true with pheochromocytomas, which release substances that cause the sensation of anxiety.

Behavioral therapy and pharmacological agents are reported to be efficacious for some panic attacks. Behavioral modification in which the patient is desensitized by exposure to the fear-producing object has been particularly useful in the treatment of phobias. Generalized anxiety disorders and panic attacks respond less well. However, pharmacological agents are often effective. Useful drugs include monoamine oxidase inhibitors, tricyclic antidepressants, and the anxiolytic agents such as the benzodiazepines. Beta blockers such as propranolol appear to be useful in patients with major autonomic symptoms, especially in those suffering from the combination of mitral valve prolapse and panic attacks.

Somatoform Disorders. The essential features of this group of conditions are physical symptoms unexplained by either demonstrable organic findings or known physiological mechanisms, accompanied by evidence of severe psychological conflicts. These disorders differ from factitious disorders or malingering in that the symptom production is believed not to be under conscious control, although this distinction may be difficult to make. Somatoform disorders are often grouped together under the rubric "hysteria," conversion reaction (in which the patient relieves his anxiety by converting psychological to physical symptoms), or Briquet's syndrome.

The pathogenesis of somatoform disorders is not known. Although psychological mechanisms undoubtedly play an important role, a substantial pro-

TABLE 114–24. DIAGNOSTIC CRITERIA FOR PANIC DISORDER*

I.   At least three panic attacks within a three-week period in circumstances other than marked physical exertion or a life-threatening situation. The attacks are not specifically precipitated by exposure to a particular phobic stimulus.

II.   Panic attacks are manifested by discrete periods of apprehension or fear, and at least four of the following symptoms appear during each attack:
    A. Dyspnea
    B. Palpitations
    C. Chest pain or discomfort
    D. Choking or smothering sensations
    E. Dizziness, vertigo, or unsteady feelings
    F. Feelings of unreality
    G. Paresthesias (tingling in hands or feet)
    H. Hot and cold flashes
    I. Sweating
    J. Faintness
    K. Trembling or shaking
    L. Fear of dying, of "going crazy," or of doing something uncontrolled during an attack

III.   The disorder is not due to a physical disorder or another mental disorder, such as major depression, somatization disorder, or schizophrenia.

IV.   The disorder is not associated with agoraphobia.

* Source: Diagnostic and Statistical Manual III. American Psychiatric Association.

portion of patients with conversion symptoms suffer a physical, often a neurological, illness as well. The conversion reaction may be either an embellishment of the underlying disorder or a different and more florid sign, both of which serve to call attention to the patient's distress over the physical illness. For example, a patient with weakness of the extensors of the wrist and fingers from a radial nerve palsy may demonstrate paralysis of the entire arm, all but that of the radial nerve distribution being psychogenic in origin.

Somatoform disorders can produce almost any of the symptoms of physical illness (Table 114–25). Most conversion reactions produce symptoms that involve the nervous system and consist of sensory loss, paralysis, blindness, hearing loss, speech loss, or seizures. (Many patients with "pseudoseizures" also have true epilepsy.) Abnormalities of consciousness or gait may also be symptoms of a conversion reaction. Even more difficult to diagnose are non-neurological somatic complaints such as nausea, multiple aches and pains, excessive fatigue, and weakness.

The diagnosis of conversion reactions often is far from easy. When the symptoms are neurological, the diagnosis must be based on an examination that indicates that the findings are inexplicable on a physiological basis. Thus, for example, a patient who complains of complete sensory loss on one side of the body, including absence of vibration and position sense, but who is able to use the arm normally for fine movements with eyes both open and closed, cannot have his symptoms explained by a physiological disease of the nervous system. In addition to demonstrating the absence of somatic disease and the nonphysiological nature of the symptoms and signs, every effort should be made to discover a reason for the development of the somatoform disorder at that particular time. For example, the symptoms may have extricated the patient from a difficult environmental situation (secondary gain) or a patient complaining of paralysis may have recently lost a loved one to a stroke. In all instances, however, one must be very careful, even when the evidence suggests conversion symptoms, to be certain that the situation is not caused by an overreaction to or extension of an underlying physical or neurological illness. At times only careful follow-up will ultimately establish the diagnosis. The physician's diagnosis of hysteria will be correct most of the time in patients who give a dramatic or complicated medical history beginning before age 35, have symptoms as indicated in Table 114–25 and show no evidence for another diagnosis that explains the symptoms.

Conversion reactions are hard to treat. Physical, particularly neurological, symptoms in their early stages can often be relieved by a matter-of-fact approach in which the physician reassures the patient that he is going to get well but avoids initiating a long discussion of the symptom's pathogenesis. He then demonstrates to the patient his or her ability to do things that were thought to be impossible. Firmness and support often restore strength to a hemiplegic hysteric and sight to a blind one. At the same time, psychological support should be given to relieve anxiety and to ameliorate the environmental stresses that produced the symptoms in the first place. Many such patients, however, are intractable to treatment. Even those in whom one eradicates one set of symptoms may return with new and different ones.

DISSOCIATIVE DISORDERS

A dissociative disorder is a sudden, temporary alteration in the normal integration of consciousness or self-identity that is not caused by known structural or physiological disease of the nervous system. Such disturbances can take the following forms: (1) *Amnesia,* either for a circumscribed period of time (localized amnesia) or for all of life's events (generalized amnesia). (2) *Fugue states,* episodes in which individuals disappear from home, travel to another place, assume a new identity, and fail to recall their previous identity. Following recovery there is no recollection of the events that took place during the fugue state. (3) *Multiple personalities* (the Three Faces of Eve syndrome), two or more distinct personalities, one of which is dominant at a particular time, controlling the behavior of the individual. (4) *Depersonalization disorders,* in which patients suffer a change in their perception of themselves so that the usual sense of one's reality is temporarily lost or changed ("I feel as if I am outside my body, watching myself"). There is usually a feeling of unreality ("The world does not seem real").

Depersonalization reactions may be difficult to distinguish from structural or physiological disease of the brain, particularly that arising from temporal lobe and other limbic system disorders (multiple personalities is an exception, almost never being mimicked by neu-

TABLE 114–25. SOMATIZATION DISORDER*

A. Onset of symptoms before age 30; symptoms present for several years
B. Complaints of at least 14 of the following symptoms for women and 12 for men:

Sickly: has been sickly much of his or her life

Conversion or pseudoneurological symptoms: difficulty swallowing, loss of voice, deafness, diplopia, blurred vision, blindness, fainting or loss of consciousness, memory loss, seizures or convulsions, trouble walking, paralysis or muscle weakness, urinary retention, or difficulty urinating

Gastrointestinal symptoms: abdominal pain, nausea, vomiting, bloating, intolerance of several foods, diarrhea

Female reproductive symptoms: excessively painful menstruation, menstrual irregularity, excessive bleeding, severe vomiting throughout pregnancy or causing hospitalization during pregnancy

Psychosexual symptoms: for the major part of the individual's life after opportunities for sexual activity: sexual indifference, lack of pleasure during intercourse, pain during intercourse

Pain: pain in back, joints, extremities, genital area (other than during intercourse); pain on urination; other pain (other than headaches)

Cardiopulmonary symptoms: Shortness of breath, palpitations, chest pain, dizziness

* Modified from American Psychiatric Association: Diagnostic and Statistical Manual of Mental Disorders. 3rd ed. Washington, DC, American Psychiatric Association. 1980.

rogenic disease). The differential diagnosis of psychogenic amnesia is discussed on page 686 (see also Table 114–17).

A psychogenic fugue state may be confused with temporal lobe or petit mal status epilepticus, in which individuals may also wander long distances with an imperfect knowledge of their environment. During a psychogenic fugue state, the patient is alert, oriented, and purposeful, even when committing violent acts. On the other hand, patients with prolonged epileptic attacks are usually confused and perplexed and not able to carry out complex acts, merely performing the same automatic activity over and over again and requiring help even to carry out the simplest act. Such patients are rarely violent, although they may strike out if attempts are made to restrain them. Furthermore, in psychogenic fugue states there is usually an identifiable emotional or environmental stress that precipitates the episode. In psychomotor or petit mal status epilepticus, the interictal EEG is often abnormal and other forms of epilepsy including generalized seizures may coexist.

Depersonalization reactions may be described by the patient as dizziness and thus be mistaken for vertigo (p. 723) or may be confused with an aura of temporal lobe epilepsy. A clear description from the patient establishes the difference between depersonalization and vertigo or syncope. The differentiation between a depersonalization reaction and the aura of temporal lobe epilepsy is more difficult. Generally, patients with depersonalization episodes have fewer episodes that last longer and never culminate in automatic activity. Patients with temporal lobe epilepsy are likely to have multiple episodes that are stereotypical and short-lived and often culminate in a psychomotor seizure. The interictal EEG may be abnormal in temporal lobe epilepsy but not in a depersonalization reaction.

In all of the dissociative disorders a meticulous history usually distinguishes neurogenic from psychogenic dissociation. In rare patients, the differentiation from temporal lobe dysfunction may be difficult or impossible. In those rare patients, EEG and MR scan may be indicated. Generally the diagnosis should be made by the examination and the patient treated by psychiatric methods.

FACTITIOUS DISORDERS AND MALINGERING

Factitious disorders are characterized by physical or psychological symptoms under voluntary control of the patient. Factitious disorders are distinguished from malingering because in the former the illness is feigned for no discernible reason, whereas in the latter there is a clear gain to the individual (such as avoiding standing trial, getting out of jail, procuring compensation for an alleged injury). Patients with factitious disorders may feign either psychological (Ganser's syndrome) or physical symptoms (Munchausen's syndrome), with an intensity and self-destructive effect that suggest psychotic thinking. Psychological symptoms include psychosis and/or dementia. Patients may report hallucinations, amnesia, or suicidal ideation. A particularly characteristic symptom of Ganser's syndrome is the tendency to give an approximate but incorrect answer to a question (question: how many legs has a horse? answer: 5; question: what is 8×6? answer: 49).

Patients with Munchausen's syndrome may report a symptom (common ones are nausea, dizziness, abdominal pain) or may actually produce abnormal findings. In the days before electronic thermometers, patients caused "fever" by rubbing the thermometer or holding it close to a light bulb. In one series describing patients with fever of unknown cause, over 1 per cent turned out to be factitious. In a particularly malignant form of the syndrome, some patients have been known to take anticoagulants to cause bleeding or bruising, to take diuretics to cause potassium loss and muscle weakness, to bleed themselves to cause anemia, or to inject talc into their joints to cause arthritis. Such patients produce these abnormalities in order to be hospitalized and often submit to extensive diagnostic and sometimes surgical procedures. They may travel from hospital to hospital in different parts of the country, and many have had 30 or 40 hospitalizations with multiple surgical procedures. Many such patients have a knowledge of medicine from prior work in a hospital. When they are confronted with the correct diagnosis, they usually deny the allegation and sign out of the hospital, only to appear subsequently in another institution with similar complaints. The fixation is often delusional and may be shared by a relative (folie a deux). Even more bizarre are occasional parents who produce symptomatic illness in their children (Munchausen's syndrome by proxy) and submit them to extensive diagnostic and therapeutic work-ups. Reported examples have included the giving of sedative drugs to children to produce episodic coma or the addition of blood or fecal material to urine to cause apparent hematuria or urinary tract infection.

The pathogenesis of Munchausen's syndrome is not known, but the patients, by definition, have underlying major mental illness or personality disorders. The individual's goal is simply to become a patient. Although the diagnosis can be difficult, diagnostic clues usually are available from the beginning to help avoid prolonged work-up. In most such patients, symptoms are vague and out of proportion to the physical findings. There is usually an extensive past history of physical illness and multiple diagnostic and therapeutic procedures. Despite the dreadful background, these patients usually look healthy. Finally, the symptoms and signs are almost always more prominent when medical attention is present. For example, patients writhing in pain from abdominal distress cease to do so once the nurse leaves the room.

The diagnosis is usually made readily once considered. A surreptitious search of the patient's room may disclose the drugs or instruments that lie behind the abnormal laboratory values, or skin lesions may be located only at sites where the medical actor can reach to scratch.

Munchausen's syndrome appears to be relatively intractable to treatment, since patients usually refuse psychiatric assistance. Therapeutic endeavors should be directed toward identifying the illness and attempting to prevent repetitive entry to hospitals. A few victims can be sustained by close contact with a knowledgeable physician.

Malingering is the voluntary production of false or grossly exaggerated physical or psychological symptoms in the pursuit of a goal that is better recognized by understanding the individual's circumstances than unraveling his or her psychology. Examples abound in the military (where physical symptoms can be used to avoid or limit onerous duty), in the last year before retirement from a variety of jobs (particularly persons in uniform, to whom additional compensation is given for physical illness), in patients who have suffered an injury such as an automobile accident (where lawsuits are pending), and in patients who are trying to evade criminal prosecution or to obtain drugs from a physician.

The diagnosis of malingering can be made with cer-

tainty only if the patient confesses that he is "faking." Otherwise, even when the physician can determine that the physical sign is not physiological, it may be difficult to distinguish malingering from factitious disorders, conversion reactions, or psychophysiological musculoskeletal syndromes. The diagnosis depends solely on the judgment as to whether the symptom production is in pursuit of a goal that is recognizable and understandable under the circumstances. When the situation is unclear, the patient must be given the benefit of the doubt.

REFERENCES

Cowley DS, Roy-Byrne PP: Hyperventilation and panic disorder. Am J Med 83:929–937, 1987.
Pincus JH, Tucker GJ: Behavioral Neurology. 3rd. ed. New York, Oxford Press, 1985.
Spitzler R (ed): Diagnostic and Statistical Manual of Mental Disorders. 3rd. ed. Washington, DC, American Psychiatric Association, 1980.

F. DRUG AND ALCOHOL ABUSE

Almost any drug as well as many household substances, including some common plants, can produce toxic changes if taken in large amounts. Most abused drugs, as well as those ingested for suicidal purposes, exert their primary effects on the brain.

THERAPEUTIC DRUG OVERDOSE

This condition is frequent, especially among the elderly, whose susceptibility is enhanced both by poor memories for what they have taken and their involutionally weakened neurological and metabolic reserves. The chief offenders are listed in Table 114–26. Several of these agents, such as digitalis or corticosteroids, can cause confusion and hallucinations in "standard" therapeutic doses, especially in patients over age 70.

TABLE 114–26. THERAPEUTIC DRUGS THAT POTENTIALLY CAUSE DELIRIUM

Digitalis	Yellowed vision; paranoid complex hallucinations
Sedatives Anxiolytics Antidepressants Antipsychotics	Dull confusion, occasionally agitation, withdrawal, irritability, and insomnia. Some have anticholinergic effects
Corticosteroids, salicylates levodopa, theophylline, cimetidine, amantadine, etc.	Occasionally confusion, hallucination, or organic psychosis

RECREATIONAL-SEDATIVE DRUG ABUSE AND POISONING (Table 114–27)

Almost all drugs that affect higher brain function possess in varying combinations and severity the addiction-promoting potentials of *psychological dependence* leading to craving, *tolerance-habituation* leading to the ingestion of increasing amounts of drugs to achieve a constant effect, and *physical dependence* leading to neurogenic *withdrawal phenomena* unless the drug is taken continuously. Individual susceptibility to these changes varies widely and is influenced by both environmental and inherited qualities.

Marijuana

This widely used, predominantly inhaled agent depends primarily on metabolites of delta-9-tetrahydro cannabis for its pharmacological action. Autonomic effects include conjunctival congestion, tachycardia, flushing, orthostatic hypotension, dry mouth, and, sometimes, vomiting. Psychic reactions depend considerably on the user and on the setting in which the drug is inhaled. Users report perceptual enhancement, euphoria, a sense of timelessness, infectious joviality, and drowsiness. Coordination and reaction time are impaired. Mild tolerance and physical dependence usually develop, but most persons suffer only moderately adverse effects. Physiological effects include respiratory tract irritation, tachycardia, decreased sperm formation, and, possibly, reduced fertility. Enduring psychic changes are uncertain. Acutely, depression, panic, paranoia, and toxic psy-

TABLE 114–27. COMMON DRUG POISONINGS AFFECTING BEHAVIOR

DRUG	SIGNS AND SYMPTOMS		DIAGNOSTIC TEST	TREATMENT: INTENSIVE CARE PLUS
	MILD	SEVERE		
Opiates Heroin Morphine Meperidine (Demerol) Methadone Hydromorphone Oxycodone Levorphanol	"Nodding" drowsiness, small pupils, urinary retention, slow and shallow breathing; skin scars and subcutaneous abscesses; duration 4–6 hours; with methadone, duration to 24 hours	Coma, pinpoint pupils, low irregular breathing or apnea, hypotension, hypothermia, pulmonary edema	Response to naloxone Urine	Naloxone, 0.4 mg IV; repeat at 15-min intervals if responds and gradually increase intervals; repeat in 3 hours if necessary; if no response by second dose, suspect another cause; find and treat infection.
Depressants Alcohol Barbiturates Chloral hydrate Glutethimide (Doriden) Meprobamate (Equanil) Methaqualone (Quaalude, Sopor, Mandrax) Benzodiazepines, (Librium, Valium, Tranxene, Ativan, Dalmane, etc.) Ethchlorvynol (Placidyl)	Confusion, rousable drowsiness, delirium, ataxia, nystagmus, dysarthria, analgesia to stimuli Hallucinations, agitation, motor hyperactivity, myoclonus, tonic spasms Often taken with another sedative or alcohol if poisoning is attempted	Stupor to coma, pupils reactive, usually constricted, rarely fixed, oculovestibular response absent, motor tonus usually flaccid, respiration and blood pressure depressed; hypothermia. With methaqualone: coma, occasional convulsions, tachycardia, cardiac failure, bleeding tendency	Blood, urine, breath Blood Blood Blood Blood Blood	Intubate, ventilate, lavage; drainage position; antimicrobials; keep mean blood pressure above 90 mm Hg and urine output above 300 ml per hour; avoid analeptics; hemodialyze severe phenobarbital poisoning; otherwise, diuresis of little help.
Stimulants Amphetamines Methylphenidate	Hyperactive, aggressive, sometimes paranoid, repetitive behavior; dilated pupils, tremor, hyperactive reflexes; hyperthermia, tachycardia, arrhythmia Acute torsion dystonia	Agitated, assaultive paranoid; occasionally convulsions; hypothermia; circulatory collapse	Blood	Chlorpromazine
Cocaine	Similar to but less prominent than above; less paranoid, often euphoric	Twitching, irregular breathing, tachycardia, arrhythmia, occasionally convulsions	Blood, urine	Diazepam, plus symptomatic
Psychedelics: LSD, psilocybin, phencyclidine, PCP (angel dust)	Confused, perceptual distortions, distractable, withdrawn or eruptive, leading to accidents or violence; dilated pupils; restless, hyperreflexic; less often, hypertension or tachycardia	Panic		Reassure; diazepam satisfactory; avoid phenothiazines
Scopolamine-atropine (knockout drops, Transderm delirium)	Agitated or confused, visual hallucinations, dilated pupils, flushed and dry skin	Florid delirium, hallucinations, amnesia, fever, tachyarrhythmia, dilated pupils, urinary retention		Reassure; sedate lightly, avoid phenothiazines; if severe, do not leave alone.
Antidepressants Tricyclics (Tofranil, Elavil, Desipramine, etc.)	Restlessness, drowsiness, tachycardia, ataxia, sweating	Agitation, vomiting, hyperpyrexia, sweating, muscle dystonia, convulsions, tachyarrhythmia, QT prolongation	Blood	Symptomatic; gastric lavage. If severe, anticonvulsants and antiarrhythmics

Table continues on following page

TABLE 114–27. COMMON DRUG POISONINGS AFFECTING BEHAVIOR (*Continued*)

DRUG	SIGNS AND SYMPTOMS		DIAGNOSTIC TEST	TREATMENT: INTENSIVE CARE PLUS
	MILD	SEVERE		
MAO inhibitors (Parnate, Nardil, Eutonyl, etc.)	Hypertensive crises, agitation, drowsiness, ataxia	Hypotension, headache, chest pain, agitation, coma, seizures, and shock	Clinical	Symptomatic; gastric lavage; avoid meperidine.
Neuroleptics (phenothiazines, butyrophenones, etc.)	Acute dystonia, somnolence, hypotension	Coma, convulsions (rare), arrhythmias, hypotension	Blood	Anticholinergics; diphenhydramine; symtomatic; gastric lavage
Lithium	Mild lethargy	Intention tremor, distracted lethargy, muteness, coma, multifocal seizures, slow or fluctuating course	Blood	Hydrate if mild; hemodialyze for delirium, coma, or convulsions.
Acid-forming Intoxicants Methanol (formic); ethylene glycol (oxalic and hippuric); other organic alcohols	Inebriation with hyperpnea	All produce progressive hyperventilation, drunkeness, stupor, eventually convulsions and death. Early blindness with methanol	Blood: increasing anion-gap acidosis	Inhibit hepatic alcohol dehydrogenase by giving alcohol until acidosis is controlled; treat acidosis vigorously.
Salicylate Aspirin	Tinitus, dyspnea	Older persons: confusion or toxic delirium leading to stupor, convulsions, coma	Blood salicylate >55 mg/dl	Alkaline diuresis

Adapted from Plum F, Posner JB: Disturbances of consciousness and arousal. *In* Wyngaarden JB, Smith LH Jr (eds): Cecil Textbook of Medicine. 18th ed. Philadelphia, WB Saunders Co, 1988, pp 2069–2070.

chosis have been reported. Some chronic heavy users become unable to undertake goal-directed efforts, but whether the traits precede or follow cannabis use is uncertain.

CNS Depressants

The drugs most frequently abused under this heading include benzodiazepines (diazepam [Valium], chlordiazepoxide [Librium]), short-acting barbiturates (pentobarbital [Nembutal], secobarbital [Seconal], amylbarbital [Amytal]), and other sedatives, especially methaqualone (Quaalude), glutethimide (Doriden), and methyprylon (Noludar). The agents are mostly ingested orally and are widely used to counteract insomnia and anxiety. Most self-medicators develop only mild habituation, but severe addiction can develop among secret sedative users, much as it does among closet alcoholics. Street use of all the drugs is usually combined with marijuana, alcohol, or cocaine.

Withdrawal symptoms commonly follow the removal of any of these drugs after heavy usage, usually beginning two to six days after cessation. Symptoms consist of heightened insomnia, anxiety, and apprehension, together with tremulousness and mild autonomic changes. Withdrawal from chronic heavy barbiturate use is particularly distressing and causes symptoms and signs similar to those of the alcohol abstinence syndrome (p. 700). Treatment is similar to

that of alcohol withdrawal syndromes and consists of reintroducing the drug, then tapering it gradually to avoid symptoms. Overprescribing by physicians commonly underlies addiction to these drugs; accordingly, benzodiazepines are best given to patients in limited amounts to curb severe anxiety or insomnia. They should not be prescribed chronically. Barbiturates probably should be avoided except for the treatment of epilepsy. All CNS depressant drugs tend to intensify pre-existing feelings of psychological depression, contraindicating their use for treating such symptoms.

Cocaine

This powerfully addicting agent is predominantly insufflated but also can be taken by mouth, vein, or mucous membrane absorption. Its use has increasingly and rapidly spread among adolescents and young adults, especially in the free-based form termed "crack." Mortality is climbing apace. Physiological effects include local anesthesia, fever, tachycardia, hypertension, pupillary dilatation, peripheral vasoconstriction, tachypnea, and anorexia. Psychologically, users report feelings of increased energy, alertness, and self-confident psychic power, often coupled with irritability and some anxiety. The last-mentioned symptoms often lead to combining cocaine use with sedatives. Reportedly, intravenous use or the smoking of crack induces an intense, euphoric "rush" followed by a craving to repeat the experience. Complications include social dissolution associated with craving, ulceration of the nasal septum, intracranial stroke-causing angiitis, occasionally convulsions and, with high doses, coma and death. Amphetamine abuse can cause many of the same experiences and complications. Treatment of cocaine abuse consists of withdrawal in a protective, supportive environment plus the giving of benzodiazepines or phenothiazines as necessary to control severe agitation. Psychological dependence is strong, leading to repetitive or continuous use, with a "crash" of debilitated disorganization and deep sleep at the end. Postwithdrawal craving reportedly is intense and protracted, leading to frequent recidivism even after weeks or months of abstinence.

Opiates

Heroin, morphine, methadone, and meperidine are the chief offenders, in that order. Two principal medical problems arise with their usage: accidental or intentional overdose and the development of complications resulting from idiosyncratic reactions, infections, and immunological abnormalities. Efforts by amateur chemists to produce psychedelic congeners have sometimes generated molecular variants with disastrous results, as exemplified by a recent mini-epidemic of chemically induced severe parkinsonism.

Acute overdose with opiates produces stupor or coma, pupillary miosis, and slow, irregular, shallow breathing. Body temperature and blood pressure fall, seizures can occur, and some patients develop acute pulmonary edema. Treatment of acute overdose consists of immediately giving naloxone, a powerful opiate antagonist, intravenously or, if no veins can be found, intramuscularly. If no immediate response occurs, the injection should be repeated immediately. Since the effects of naloxone wear off within two to three hours and the depressant effects of the opiates can last much longer, the antagonist should be repeated at two- to three-hour intervals until all evidence of a response disappears. Stuporous or hypoventilating patients who do not respond immediately should be treated according to the general program for care of the patient in coma (Table 114–12).

Chronic opiate addicts can develop severe withdrawal symptoms consisting of yawning, anxiety, restlessness, rhinorrhea, lacrimation, and influenzal symptoms within minutes after receiving naloxone. In an emergency, the symptoms can be reduced by clonidine or ameliorated by small doses of narcotics. The use of naloxone should be confined to overdose situations and not employed in a nonemergency setting either as a diagnostic measure or to induce withdrawal.

Complications of illicit narcotic use include arrhythmias, pulmonary edema, and convulsions due to adulterants. Opiate users suffers a high incidence of bacteriological infections of skin, veins, blood, heart, and lung. Many develop viral hepatitis and AIDS (Ch. 98). Serious neurological complications consist of neuropathy, myelopathy, optic neuritis, and a myriad of infections, including tetanus and brain abscess.

Tricyclic Antidepressants

These agents possess potentially serious cardiovascular effects, oral doses of more than 2 gm often being lethal. Since behavioral changes can take some hours to develop and blood levels may not be easily available, patients reporting acute self-overdose should have an immediate ECG. The presence of a widened QRS to greater than 100 msec indicates serious toxicity and a need for intensive supervision and cardiac monitoring. A more common presentation consists of a state of stupor or coma, combined with anticholinergic signs reminiscent of atropine poisoning and the presence of cardiac arrhythmias on the ECG. Treatment in alert patients consists of ipecac-induced vomiting or in stuporous ones of gastric lavage followed by activated charcoal instillation. Convulsions and arrhythmias are treated by appropriate standard measures, including ventricular pacing in the event of serious arrhythmia. Physostigmine given intravenously sometimes produces transient awakening but its use is inadvisable, since it risks producing arrhythmias and seizures. Otherwise, management follows that outlined in Table 114–12. Most tricyclics have half-lives of many days, so that monitoring and intensive treatment can be required for as long as a week in severe cases.

Salicylate Poisoning

Salicylate intoxication can occur in older adults as an accident of overzealous attempts to relieve pain and in adolescents and young adults due to intentional overdose. Salicylates in high doses uncouple oxidative phosphorylation and aspirin itself adds acid radicals. The resulting acid-base disturbance in adults is almost diagnostic: tissue glycolysis produces intracellular lactacidosis, which produces an acid urine and stimulates the brain stem respiratory centers. The result is a mixed respiratory alkalosis–metabolic acidosis with an elevated pH, a low Pa_{CO_2} and low serum bicarbonate. Early symptoms include tinnitus, deafness, disequilibrium, drowsiness, and a moderate delirium. With blood levels greater than 60 mg/dl, stupor, coma, and potentially fatal convulsions can ensue. Treatment consists of gastric lavage and the giving of bicarbonate solutions using alkaline diuresis as an end point.

Phencyclidine (PCP)

PCP is currently the most widely abused of the psychedelic-hallucinogenic group of drugs that include, among numerous others, LSD, amphetamines, and scopolamine. Users describe various experiences, most prevalent of which is a state of altered perception in which dreams and heightened reality become indistinguishable. Excess inhalation or ingestion of PCP can induce ataxia, confusion, aggressive violence, prolonged psychotic states, coma, or convulsions. Treatment is symptomatic, but the bad trip may be shortened by acidifying the urine with ammonium chloride and applying continuous gastric suction to accelerate excretion of the drug.

Nonethyl Alcohols

Most poisoning from these agents occurs by alcoholics or drug abusers unaware of the toxic nature of the substance. Methanol, isopropyl alcohol, and ethylene glycol all produce potentially fatal metabolic acidosis through their metabolic products. Paraldehyde acidosis may have a similar mechanism. The hepatic enzyme alcohol dehydrogenase acts on all three substrates to produce acid products. The alcohol dehydrogenase inhibitor, 4-methylpyrazol, effectively halts this highly toxic step and is the current drug of choice. If it is unavailable, the next potentially life-saving step is to slow metabolism of the poison by administering ethyl alcohol by mouth or vein in intoxicating amounts. Severe poisoning requires that ethanol blood levels of 100 to 150 mg/dl be maintained for at least 48 to 72 hours while stabilizing blood acid-base levels with the bicarbonate buffer. Ethylene glycol may cause subsequent renal damage from oxylate and hippurate crystalluria.

ALCOHOL AND ITS COMPLICATIONS

Ethyl alcohol is the oldest and still most widely taken addicting psychotropic drug. Used by nearly half of all Americans and abused by 1 in 20, the agent creates a huge medical and sociological problem. Alcohol generates a direct and associated death rate that lags behind only vascular disease and cancer and a total life-year work-loss rate that probably exceeds all other illnesses.

Pharmacology

Ethanol is usually ingested as a fraction of some vehicle of distinctive taste such as beer (5 per cent), wine (12 per cent), or various stronger agents containing 20 to 50 per cent alcohol (40 to 100 proof). Ethanol enters the blood within minutes from the stomach and intestine and, being lipid-soluble, quickly penetrates all aqueous body compartments, including the brain and alveolar air. Ethanol is excreted by physical diffusion through the lungs and detoxified by hepatic dehydrogenase at a rate that approximates 8 ml/hour, clearing about 15 mg/dl/hour from the blood.

Blood levels of alcohol correlate directly with clinical signs and symptoms, chronic alcoholics showing great tolerance compared to novice drinkers (Table

TABLE 114–28. BLOOD-ALCOHOL LEVELS AND SYMPTOMS

LEVEL (mg/dl)	SPORADIC DRINKERS	CHRONIC DRINKERS
50 (party level)	Congenial euphoria	No observable effect
75	Gregarious or garrulous	Often no effect
100	Incoordinated. Legally intoxicated	Minimal signs
125–150	Unrestrained behavior Episodic dyscontrol	Pleasurable euphoria or beginning incoordination
200–250	Alertness lost → lethargic	Effort required to maintain emotional and motor control
300–350	Stupor or coma	Drowsy and slow
>500	Some will die	Coma

114–28). Acutely, in less than near-fatal amounts, aside from producing vasodilatation and gastric irritation, alcohol exerts almost all its ill affects on the central nervous system. The molecular action is unknown, but alcohol acts entirely as a depressant, although not simultaneously on all CNS structures. Thus the earlier euphoriant-excitatory stage reflects a removal of higher inhibitory effects from limbic impulses, while larger doses increasingly depress first forebrain and then brain stem functions, including those that regulate pain sensation and arousal. Death from acute intoxication usually results from central respiratory depression followed by circulatory failure.

Clinical Features

Acute Intoxication. The behavioral effects of acute intoxication vary with the user, ranging among social drinkers from pleasant conviviality to angry argumentativeness. A small number of younger male drinkers develop pathologically severe, aggressive, violent behavior ("dyscontrol") for which they later claim no memory. The syndrome has potentially dangerous consequences and calls for total abstinence and immediate psychiatric referral. *Alcoholic blackouts*, periods of amnesia lasting for several hours or more during or at the end of a heavy drinking bout, are a sign of serious intoxication bordering on anesthesia. When recurrent, they signify impending or already existing alcoholic addiction.

Treatment of acute alcoholic attacks depends upon the degree of intoxication and the associated blood levels. Mild drunkenness requires no treatment. More severe intoxication producing heavy drowsiness or stupor deserves attention, especially if one does not know whether or not additional drugs have been ingested. The level of CNS depression can increase rapidly as alcohol is absorbed, and stuporous drunks need close attention to vital functions. Alcoholic deep stupor or coma requires hospital monitoring until symptoms subside. Patients with associated severe trauma or fever need especially close evaluation for masked neurological injury, blood loss, or infection.

Withdrawal Syndromes. Headache, giddiness, difficulty in concentrating, nausea, and mild tremulousness characterize the well-known *hangover*. Classic but unproved remedies or preventives include forcing nonalcoholic fluids while still intoxicated, avoiding the ingestion of agents such as red wines or brandies, and taking antacids. When hangover appears, another alcoholic drink aborts most of the symptoms but represents an early step toward the development of chronic alcoholism.

The serious withdrawal states of chronic alcoholism consist of, respectively, prominent tremulousness, rum fits, and delirium tremens (DTs). They usually are preceded by years of problem drinking and are precipitated by a continuous alcoholic ingestion lasting many days or weeks.

Tremulousness, insomnia, and agitation, although much more common, symptomatically blend into delirium tremens and are discussed below. Each reflects a state of central adrenergic hyperexcitation that emerges as alcohol's inhibitory influence dissipates.

Withdrawal convulsions (rum fits) consist of single or short runs of generalized seizures, usually with no focal features. Their necessary stimulus consists of no more than a falling blood alcohol level and, in contrast to the more delayed appearance of DTs, they can occur during the course of a prolonged spree within hours of the last drink. About one third are followed by the DTs if abstinence continues. Treatment is symptomatic, using diazepam to stop the seizures and dampen the often associated tremulousness. Interictal laboratory tests, including CT scans and EEGs, show no specific abnormality, although if focal seizures occur a CT scan should be obtained to rule out a localized brain lesion such as subdural hematoma. Prophylactic anticonvulsants confer no protection.

Delirium tremens represents the most serious and occasionally fatal withdrawal complication of alcohol, usually appearing only after a decade or more of fairly continuous, heavy drinking. The course is worsened when complicated by systemic infection, hepatic insufficiency, or head trauma. A somewhat similar although less florid condition affects patients withdrawing from chronic heavy barbiturate use, and the treatment described below applies equally well to that syndrome and alcoholic DTs. Either alcoholic or *barbiturate withdrawal* DTs can arise unexpectedly in patients abruptly withdrawn from these drugs because of admission to hospital for other conditions such as trauma, emergency surgery, etc.

In contrast to the immediate appearance of less severe tremulousness or rum fits, DTs most often emerge only three to five days after complete alcohol or drug withdrawal. First symptoms consist of severe tremulousness, disorientation, visual hallucinations, and agitation. Signs of beta-adrenergic autonomic hyperactivity are prominent, including fear, sweating, tachycardia, hypertension, tachypnea, and incontinence. Many patients are malnourished and display associated signs of hepatic insufficiency, gastritis, dehydration, infection, polyneuropathy, myopathy, or Wernicke's syndrome (see below). Treatment consists of sedation with a drug cross-tolerant for alcohol, the benzodiazepine diazepam being most useful (Table 114–29). Huge amounts may be required: authorities report as much as 15 to 215 mg may be necessary to control agitation initially, and some patients may need as much as 1200 mg given intravenously during the first 60 hours in order to remain calm.

Acute alcoholic hallucinosis is less common than the DTs but arises in a similar setting. The disorder is characterized by days or weeks of auditory hallucinations accompanied by comparatively less agitation or mental confusion. Although the auditory hallucinations, which are sometimes paranoid, can resemble an acute schizophrenic reaction, the history of chronic heavy drinking followed by withdrawal is diagnostic.

Chronic Alcoholism. This condition is widespread and requires the physician's constant vigilance to detect it sufficiently early to modify its course. Psychological dependence, closet drinking, increasing social lapses, more than an occasional mild hangover or, among spouses, an increasing number of nights out with the boys (or girls) are danger signals. Blackouts,

TABLE 114–29. TREATMENT OF SEVERE TREMULOUSNESS OR DELIRIUM TREMENS

1. Attempt control by reassurance and observation.

2. Treat systemic problems promptly.

3. Treat uncontrollable agitation: Control with diazepam 10 mg IV given slowly followed by 5–10 mg IV slowly every 5 minutes to induce calmness. Once calm, maintain with diazepam 5–10 mg IV or more every 1-4 hours.

4. Continuously supply and balance electrolytes and vitamins, especially thiamine.

absenteeism, drunken driving, occupational downgrading, or any medical complications including poorly explained, repeated physical injury imply serious trouble.

Even to get a potential alcoholic to consider that he or she has a psychological-medical problem commonly is a thankless and unsuccessful task. To accomplish this usually requires sustained and effective treatment by an experienced psychotherapist plus the patient's participation in a vigorous reinforcement group, such as Alcoholics Anonymous. Several industries and large universities recently have established such groups, reportedly with success running as high as 70 per cent or higher when persons can be persuaded that their

TABLE 114–30. MAJOR NON-NEUROLOGICAL COMPLICATIONS OF ALCOHOLISM

Heart
　Cardiomyopathy
　Arrhythmia
　Hyperlipidemia

Gastrointestinal
　Gastritis
　Hepatitis-cirrhosis
　Pancreatitis
　Head, neck, and esophageal cancer
　Malabsorption

Blood
　Iron or folate deficiency
　Anemia
　Thrombocytopenia
　Prothrombin deficiency

Endocrine
　Male sexual impairment
　Increased fetal risk

Immune System
　Increased susceptibility to infection and impaired healing

Electrolyte Disturbances
　Hypocalcemia
　Hypomagnesemia
　Hypophosphatemia
　Acute water intoxication
　Alcoholic hyperosmolality
　Alcoholic ketosis

jobs are on the line and that the employer is genuinely interested. Recovery or improvement rate is less once severe social disruption begins. Disulfiram (*Antabuse*) produces conditioned avoidance to alcohol by introducing a violently adverse reaction to its ingestion. It is reserved for treating the severe alcoholic and is best supervised by experienced therapists.

Complications of Alcohol

Drunkenness contributes to a large fraction of death and severe injury from traffic accidents, trauma, murder, suicide, and the inadvertent overdose of other drugs. Chronic complications as indicated in Table 114–30 can affect many body organs. Some of these may be due to a direct, but tenuously established, toxic effect. Nutritional deprivation, however, causes the majority. Alcohol contains 7 calories per gram, but most of its vehicles include negligible amounts of vitamins, trace metals, or other nutrients, including protein. Alcoholics, supplying their immediate energy needs by carbohydrates, can wear the mask of nutritional good health for years while their brains, nerves, livers, and hearts degenerate in a pattern which, sooner or later, allows no turning back.

TOXIC AND DEFICIENCY NEUROLOGICAL DISORDERS RELATED TO ALCOHOLISM AND NUTRITIONAL DEPRIVATION (Table 114–31)

In addition to chronic alcoholism, severe nutritional insufficiencies can accompany any debilitating, energy-consuming illnesses, such as metastatic cancer, disseminated infection, thyrotoxicosis, advanced connective tissue disease, impaired intestinal absorption, and chronic behavioral disorders. Nutritional insufficiency with these illnesses only occasionally is confined to a single vitamin or nutrient fraction, although thiamine lack is perhaps most prevalent. Signs that suggest nutritional failure include apathetic listlessness, darkening of the skin, a sore red tongue, fissuring at the corners of the mouth, burning feet, progressive unexplained weight loss, and unexplained anemia. This section focuses on the most common neurological disorders, all of which, in the United States, occur more with alcoholism than any other single disorder.

Chronic severe alcoholics suffer an increased incidence of middle-life onset *optic neuropathy*, a con-

TABLE 114–31. MAJOR NEUROLOGICAL COMPLICATIONS OF SEVERE ALCOHOLISM

Amblyopia and optic atrophy
Progressive cerebral degeneration and dementia
Peripheral neuropathy
Myopathy
Wernicke-Korsakoff disease
Parenchymatous cerebellar degeneration
Cerebral leukodystrophy (Marchiafava-Bignami disease)

dition marked by reduced visual acuity, central or paracentral scotomas, and normal optic fundi. Dietary and vitamin therapies sometimes bring improvement. Advanced problem drinkers as young as the fourth decade also can develop CT-imaged *cerebral atrophy* and signs of early dementia. Abstinence sometimes reverses the severity of these changes.

Alcoholic-Nutritional Peripheral Neuropathy. This disorder in the United States usually occurs only in company with advanced, mixed nutritional deprivation and usually improves only with total replacement and weight gain. The disorder produces axonal degeneration affecting predominantly the small pain- and temperature-mediating fibers in the distal lower extremities. Since the larger, touch-mediating peripheral fibers determine sensory nerve conduction velocities, that function can remain normal in the early stages of the neuropathy. Distal motor loss occurs relatively early. Spontaneous, often burning, pain and autonomic neuropathy commonly affect advanced cases. Deep tendon reflexes disappear in a distal-to-proximal pattern. Recovery, often incomplete, requires months or years of renourishment.

Alcoholic myopathy is confined to chronic, severe alcoholics and can have either an acute or a chronic onset. The acute form consists of sudden transient rhabdomyolysis, often following a cluster of rum fits or, possibly, other trauma. It includes muscle pain, tenderness, cramping, weakness, and an elevated serum creatine kinase. Severe cases can develop myoglobinuria with associated renal complications. Chronic myopathy, a less blatant and distinctive disorder, consists of diffuse proximal muscle wasting and weakness disproportional to any existing neuritic impairment. It improves gradually with nutritional replacement.

Wernicke-Korsakoff Disease. This condition reflects the acute and chronic central nervous system effects of severe, sustained thiamine depletion in the face of a continued caloric intake. In the United States, severe alcoholism most often causes the disorder, but other vitamin-impoverished diets, including nonsupplemented hospital glucose infusions, hemodialysis, various restrictive food faddisms, and polished rice alone can lead to the same condition. The pathological process consists of axonal demyelination, neuronal loss, glial proliferation, endothelial thickening, and petechial pericapillary hemorrhages affecting the brain. The oculomotor nuclei, the vestibular nuclei, the medullary autonomic nuclei, and the brain stem reticular formation suffer the greatest damage. At higher levels the mammillary bodies, the mediodorsal thalamic nuclei, and scattered cortical regions including the hippocampus suffer most.

The clinical manifestations of Wernicke's disease reflect the major neuropathological alterations. Acutely such patients are confused, often drowsy or semistuporous, ataxic, and dysarthric. Partial or complete external ophthalmoplegia and nystagmus are cardinal features. Further examination often discloses tachycardia, orthostatic hypotension, hypothermia, and a diffuse analgesia. The pupils seldom are affected, but almost any motor cranial nerve can be partially paralyzed. Most patients have at least mild signs of peripheral neuropathy, but these can be altogether absent. Treatment consists of giving thiamine 50 mg parenterally, upon suspicion of the diagnosis, followed by replenishment of blood volume and electrolytes. Glucose administration should not precede thiamine treatment, as its metabolic processing can precipitate acute worsening. Evidence of severe anemia, hepatic insufficiency, or infection should be corrected and the patient watched closely for evidence of impending seizures or DTs. General good nourishment and efforts to halt the destructive slide of chronic alcoholism necessarily follow.

Differential diagnosis of Wernicke's disease is readily made on clinical grounds, provided one has enough history to suspect thiamine deficiency. The eye signs provide a critical clue: only acute idiopathic polyneuropathy, myasthenia gravis, botulism, and intoxication with phenytoin are likely to cause a similarly acute symmetrical or asymmetrical bilateral external ophthalmoplegia. Of these, only Wernicke's disease and, rarely, phenytoin intoxication produce mental changes. Furthermore, the response to thiamine injection is usually diagnostic: the ophthalmoplegia usually begins to improve within a matter of hours to a day or so, a response produced with no other disorder.

Korsakoff's amnestic syndrome usually emerges as the acute confusional delirium of Wernicke's disease subsides. Affected patients show a profound, relatively isolated loss of recent memory for events. This, coupled with a placid lack of insight, often leads to absurd conversations or answers to questions (confabulation). Arousal, language functions, and remote memories are spared. Korsakoff's arises only after either several preceding attacks of Wernicke's encephalopathy or an unusually severe one. Treatment is as for Wernicke's. About half the patients treated for the first time improve to the point of regaining independence.

Acute Cerebellar Degeneration. This arises most often in male alcoholics as a complication of an acute superimposed severe alcoholic spree rather than following the prolonged drinking periods that usually precede the Wernicke-Korsakoff syndrome. The disease is caused by an unknown mechanism of neuronal degeneration in the anterior and superior cerebellar vermis, leading to a gradually or suddenly appearing broad-based, stiff-legged ataxia unaccompanied by incoordination in the upper extremities or nystagmus. Many patients have an associated nutritional peripheral neuropathy whose treatment sometimes improves their functional difficulties.

Central Pontine Myelinolysis (CPM). This disorder occurs as a complication of severe hyponatremia or its treatment, usually following the correction of serum sodium levels at or below 110 mEq/L. Such severe hyponatremia can be a complication of prolonged alcoholism but more often represents a complication of severe medical illness. The disorder consists of the development of a symmetrical zone of demyelination affecting the basis pontis of the brain stem, leading to lethargy or stupor, a quiet confused delirium, and more or less severe quadriparesis. Evidence is strong that the disorder especially follows the overly rapid correction of severe hyponatremia: Most authorities currently recommend raising the serum sodium by no more than about 0.5 mEq per hour. Most examples of CPM become visible on MR or CT brain images within a week or so after onset. Many patients treated symptomatically recover in a matter of weeks.

REFERENCES

Dreisbach RH, Robertson WO: Handbook of Poisoning. 12th ed. Norwalk, CO, Appleton and Lange, 1987.

Kissin B: Alcohol abuse and alcohol-related illness. *In* Wyngaarden JB, Smith LH Jr (eds): Cecil Textbook of Medicine. 18th ed. Philadelphia, WB Saunders Co, 1988, pp 48–52.

115

DISORDERS OF AUTONOMIC FUNCTION

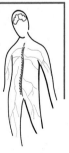

The autonomic nervous system contains three major components. One operates principally via the hypothalamus and links the brain to the pituitary gland and thence to the peripherally located endocrine organs. Its functions and disorders are discussed in this text with the endocrine system. The second component diffusely projects cholinergic, noradrenergic, and serotonergic pathways that travel rostrally from, respectively, ventral basal forebrain nuclei, the locus ceruleus of the pontine tegmentum, and the raphe nuclei of the midbrain and pons. These ascending projections appear to modulate arousal as well as the activities of higher levels of brain function, but their precise activities currently are poorly understood and will not be discussed further at this time. The third, classically known system consists of the descending autonomic sympathetic and parasympathetic pathways that connect the hypothalamus and other brain stem centers to the viscera so as to help regulate internal homeostasis. This section describes some of the more common examples of its disorders.

HYPOTHALAMUS (HT)

Direct damage to the HT can impair normal arousal mechanisms, interfere with trophic regulation of the pituitary gland, blunt normal learning memory and emotion, and disrupt the mechanisms that regulate normal water balance, heat regulation, and caloric appetite.

Disorders of Water Balance. Disease of the HT can produce three principal disorders of water balance: (1) Hypoplasia of or direct damage to the supraoptic or paraventricular nuclei or their major connections to the posterior pituitary gland leads to antidiuretic hormone (ADH) deficiency and the disorder *diabetes insipidus.* (2) Neurogenic imbalance or biologically erroneous signals from peripheral receptors or their CNS connections can lead to *inappropriately increased ADH* secretion, producing excessive hemodilution and hyponatremia. (3) HT-engendered failure of thirst coupled with reduced ADH secretion causes the rare condition of *essential hypernatremia,* in which appetite for water (thirst) is lacking despite pathologically elevated serum sodium levels. The condition usually is associated with partial insufficiency of central ADH regulation.

Disturbances of Temperature Regulation. Sustained relative *hypothermia* or *poikilothermia,* with body temperatures varying with the environment and falling below 35°C, follows destructive lesions of the posterior hypothalamus or adjacent midbrain. Hypothermia also can accompany several metabolic comas as well as depressant drug poisoning. In addition, deficiencies in appropriate autonomic responses to both dehydration and ambient cooling frequently affect alcoholics and elderly persons, increasing their suscep-

tibility to exposure and intensifying fluid loss and hypothermia. Several small epidemics of exposure-induced hypothermia have been reported among residents of insufficiently heated nursing homes.

Special low recording thermometers usually are required to quantify the diagnosis of severe hypothermia, although stupor or coma, a reduction in amplitude of vital signs, and the patient's coldness to touch are qualitatively obvious. When core temperature lies between 31° and 35°C, treatment consists of gradual rewarming by blankets in an ambiently warm room. Heating blankets set at 38°C, tub immersions at 40° to 42°C, or warmed peritoneal dialysis can be employed for persons with colder core temperatures. Fluids and auxiliary treatment are guided by specific cardiac or infectious complications.

Paroxysmal hypothermia is an uncommon disorder, probably a form of diencephalic epilepsy, in which body temperature episodically drops to 32°C or less, associated with reduced alertness, mental slowness or confusion, and, usually, cardiorespiratory irregularities. Some affected patients respond to antiepileptic therapy.

Hyperthermia appears in several forms, including that from hypothalamic damage as well as with heat exhaustion, heat stroke, and malignant hyperthermia. *Neurogenic hyperthermia* occurs as an acute phenomenon in association with acute head injury, surgical trauma, hemorrhages into the hypothalamic region, or encephalitis affecting this area. Fever can rise to potentially fatal levels of 42°C or higher. If standard antipyretic measures fail, adding small doses of opiates sometimes ameliorates the elevated temperature. Subacute or chronic fever almost never results from primary noninflammatory central nervous system disease.

Heat exhaustion and heat stroke (Table 115–1) result from combinations of high environmental temperature, increased generation of body heat, and decreased bodily adaptive functions. Muscular heat cramps are common following exhausting exercise in hot weather. They respond quickly to fluid and salt ingestion. More extensive heat exhaustion and heat stroke represent potentially more serious problems. *Heat exhaustion* results from a gradual net loss of water or salt and water. Its least serious form consists of muscle cramps progressing to eventual impairment of cardiovascular mechanisms manifested by feelings of giddiness, dizziness, syncope, and, in a more protracted and severe stage, fever and delirium. The presence of sweating continues until the late stages. Treatment consists of cool spongings or tubs plus generous salt and water replacement.

Heat stroke, a potentially fatal disorder, characteristically affects its victims during the first severe heat wave of the new season or upon the sudden movement of vigorously active young persons from a cool to a hot climate, such as occurs with active troops during war. As is true with heat exhaustion, risk factors include a lack of acclimatization, old age and infirmity, alcoholic excess and, especially, the ingestion of anticholinergic or antipsychotic drugs. The disorder re-

TABLE 115–1. HEAT EXHAUSTION AND HEAT STROKE COMPARED

	HEAT EXHAUSTION	HEAT STROKE
Time of occurrence	Any hot weather	First sustained heat wave
Principally affected	Elderly hypodipsics, young heavy laborers, strenuous athletes, etc.	Elderly; infirm; obese; alcoholics; psychotics
Principal pathogenesis	Salt or water loss	Failure of heat loss
Contributing factors	Prolonged exercise	Antiperspirants; anticholinergics, phenothiazines, diuretics, neuroleptics; age; dehydration
Body temperature	37–38.5°C	39–43°C
Sweating	Usually present	Absent
Treatment	Fluids and adjusted electrolytes	Prompt body cooling (ice immersion)

sults when high ambient temperatures and humidity impair or prevent adequate heat loss. Tissue damage ensues when core temperatures rise above 43°C. Clinical signs include hyperpyrexia greater than 41°C; hot, dry skin; and increasing prostration, confusion, stupor and, finally, coma accompanied by signs of brain stem dysfunction. Associated abnormalities can include tachycardia, ST and T wave abnormalities on the EKG, hypotension, consumption coagulopathy, signs of dehydration, and both potassium and sodium depletion as well as hepatic damage. Treatment is aimed at bringing core temperature below 39°C in an ice tub bath and meeting systemic problems, including high-output heart failure, as they arise. Mortality and the development of permanent neurological disability relate directly to the duration of hyperthermia and whether or not pressor agents are required to support the circulation.

Malignant hyperthermia is a rare disorder that occurs in two drug-related settings, one with anesthetics, the other with neuroleptics. The anesthesia-related disorder results from a genetically determined, autosomal dominant defect in muscle that leads to excessive calcium release from sarcoplasm during anesthetic induction. Immediately following the preoperative giving of succinylcholine followed by an inhalation anesthetic, diffuse, severe skeletal muscle contraction takes place, producing generalized rigidity, increased heat production, and potentially fatal fevers of 39 to 42°C or greater. Treatment consists of quick interruption of anesthesia and surgery, with vigorous measures taken to counteract fever and systemic lactacidosis. Blood relatives of those who show the disorder should be pretested by anesthesiologists for potential susceptibility before receiving general anesthesia. The *neuroleptic malignant syndrome*, a less frequent idiosyncratic response, follows a similar clinical pattern, with hyperthermia, muscle rigidity, autonomic instability, and reduced consciousness following upon the administration of one or more of the drugs cited in Table 115–2. The pathogenesis in this disorder is less clearly known, but the approach to treatment is similar, consisting of neuroleptic withdrawal plus symptomatic attention to hyperthermia and serum lactacidosis. Dantrolene and, less often, procainamide have been reported to counter the muscle rigidity in some but not all examples of both hyperthermic syndromes.

AUTONOMIC INSUFFICIENCIES

Generalized systemic autonomic insufficiency can occur on either a central or a peripheral basis. Diffuse, moderate sympathetic-parasympathetic dysfunction accompanies occasional cases of parkinsonism and several of the late-life cerebellar degenerations. *Shy-Drager disease* is an uncommon midlife, degenerative disorder that affects central autonomic pathways, accompanied by variable abnormalities in extrapyramidal and, occasionally, other motor systems. Cardinal symptoms and signs include male impotence, anhid-

TABLE 115–2. CHIEF DRUG GROUPS ASSOCIATED WITH THE NEUROLEPTIC MALIGNANT SYNDROME

Phenothiazines	Sudden discontinuation of anti-
Butyrophenones	Parkinson drugs
Thioxanthines	Dopamine-depleting agents
Other antipsychotic agents	

rosis, orthostatic hypotension, absent autonomic cardiovascular reflexes, impaired pupillary control, gastrointestinal hypomotility, urinary retention or incontinence, hoarseness, and signs of parkinsonism or cerebellar dysfunction. Late in the disease the capacitance veins of the abdomen and lower extremities completely lose their constrictor reflexes. As a result, patients develop refractory bradycardia, orthostatic hypotension, and symptoms of lightheadedness or syncope when assuming the erect or even the sitting position. Treatment is symptomatic and consists of counteracting the hypotension with elastic stockings, increasing fluid intake, and giving mineralocorticoids to assist in blood volume expansion.

Autonomic abnormalities including severe hypotension also can accompany a number of peripheral neuropathies, especially those of diabetic neuropathy, syphilitic tabes dorsalis, and inherited amyloid disease. Moderate autonomic dysfunction consisting of persistent tachycardia, impaired volume reflexes, and mild orthostatic insufficiency also accompanies most examples of acute inflammatory neuropathy. A few patients with inflammatory neuropathy can experience major defects in peripheral sympathetic and parasympathetic control due to a predominant or selective involvement of these fibers.

Neurogenic Bladder Dysfunction. Micturition represents a parasympathetically regulated reflex act, normally subordinated to higher cerebral control. The afferent and efferent components of the reflex travel between the bladder and the lower sacral spinal cord, and the cord contains all the necessary components for completion of the reflex. Centrally, several levels of the spinal cord and brain stem enhance the reflex and facilitate complete bladder emptying. The cerebrum acts primarily to inhibit the micturition reflex, thereby normally governing its appropriate time and place of action.

Cerebral disorders disinhibit the micturition reflex threshold. Medial frontal lobe lesions can cause urgency incontinence (brief warning, full emptying), while diffuse cerebral disorders causing dementia lead to the incontinence of indifference. Subcortical and incomplete spinal disorders causing spasticity lower the micturition reflex threshold, resulting in urinary urgency, usually with small volumes and complete emptying. (Urinary tract infections produce similar symptoms.) Spinal transection at first inhibits reflex micturition due to spinal shock, then facilitates it as reflex hyperactivity returns in the distal spinal stump. Lacking influences from higher centers, spinal reflex micturition seldom completely empties the bladder unless specific rehabilitation retraining is carried out.

Peripheral bladder denervation occurs with lesions of the sacral cord, cauda equina, or afferent or efferent nerves. Reflex micturition is lost, and the bladder dilates until the intrinsic intravesical pressure overcomes urethral resistance to produce overflow incontinence. Within weeks to months multifocal autonomous contractions involve the bladder wall, reflecting parasympathetic denervation hypersensitivity. Urine is ejected as either a semicontinuous dribble or in repeated small, ineffective volumes. The bladder increasingly distends and generally requires recurrent catheterization to avoid chronic infections.

Three forms of treatment exist for urinary bladder difficulties. Patients with intermittent or small volume incontinence often can be helped by wearing soft, dry perineal padding. Anticholinergic drugs such as oxybutynin chloride in small amounts can overcome moderate degrees or urgency incontinence. With more severe degrees of the problem, the drugs can be adjusted to create urinary retention, which the patient can then learn to manage safely by self-catheterization.

Male sexual dysfunction has several potential causes, as listed in Table 72–3 and discussed in the associated text. Neurological abnormalities account for as many as 15 to 20 per cent, especially among older persons. Organic symptoms are limited to loss of libido, failure to sustain an effective erection (impo-

tence), and failure to attain normal ejaculation-emission. The absence of nocturnal penile tumescence is more characteristic of organic than psychogenic causes. Temporal lobe–limbic system damage is often associated with reduced male libido, while lesions affecting descending or peripheral parasympathetic fibers commonly interfere with the capacity to gain and maintain an erection. For such men, corporeal self-injection of papaverine has been reported to be more than 90 per cent succcessful. Some paraplegics can be taught relatively normal reflex erection and ejaculation. Most persons, however, with severely or completely impaired spinal or peripheral parasympathetic pathways will require prosthetic assistance if they are to satisfy a partner in sexual intercourse.

REFERENCES

Guzé BH, Baxter LR: Neuroleptic malignant syndrome. N Engl J Med 313:163, 1985.

Hart GR, Anderson RJ, Crumpler CP, et al: Epidemic classical heat stroke: Clinical characteristics and course of 28 patients. Medicine 61:189, 1982.

Williams ME, Pannill FC: Urinary incontinence in the elderly. Physiology, pathophysiology, diagnosis and treatment. Ann Intern Med 97:895, 1982.

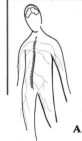

116

DISORDERS OF SENSORY FUNCTION

A. PAIN AND PAINFUL SYNDROMES

PAIN AS A SIGNAL OF DAMAGE

Pain (Table 116–1) is the most common symptom for which patients seek medical assistance, and chronic pain is among the most vexing problems that physicians face. Pain has two aspects: the first is an emotionally neutral perception of a stimulus that is usually sufficiently strong to produce tissue damage; the second is an affective response to the perception of that stimulus. Pain implies damage to the organism, either physical or psychological, and chronic pain if untreated will itself damage the organism.

DIAGNOSIS OF PAINFUL DISORDERS

Pain can be either acute or chronic; pain of more than six months duration is usually considered chronic. Several clinical features differentiate acute from chronic pain. Patients suffering from *severe* acute pain usually give a clear description of its location, character, and timing. Signs of autonomic nervous system hyperactivity with tachycardia, hypertension, diaphoresis, mydriasis, and pallor are often present. Acute pain usually responds well to analgesic agents, and psychological factors often play only a minor role in pathogenesis. By contrast, patients suffering from chronic pain describe less precisely the localization, character, and timing of the pain, and, because the autonomic nervous system adapts, signs of autonomic hyperactivity disappear. Furthermore, chronic pain usually responds less well to analgesic agents, and psychological colorings are usually more pertinent than in acute pain. All of these factors may lead the physician to believe that the patient exaggerates his complaints. Since there are no reliable objective tests to assess chronic pain, the physician is advised to accept his patient's report, taking into consideration his age, cultural background, environment, and other psychological background known to alter reaction to pain.

Chronic pain can be divided into three somewhat overlapping categories in decreasing order of frequency: (1) *Psychophysiological disorders*. Structural disease, such as a herniated disc or torn ligaments, may once have been present, but whether or not structural disease was ever present, psychological factors have engendered chronic physiological alterations, such as muscle spasm, which produce pain long after the underlying deficit has healed. Such patients tend to respond poorly to analgesic drugs, but often respond well to combination therapy directed at the end-organ (i.e., injection of trigger points in muscles) and at correcting or at least discussing disturbing psychological factors. (2) Chronic pain associated with *structural disease*, such as occurs with rheumatoid arthritis, metastatic cancer, or sickle cell anemia, may be characterized by episodes of pain alternating with pain-free intervals or by unremitting pain waxing and waning in severity. Psychological factors may play an important role in exacerbating or relieving pain, but treatment of the pain by analgesics or correcting the underlying disease is usually more helpful. (3) *Somatic delusions*. Pain caused by neither structural nor physiological disorders occurs in patients with profound psychiatric disturbances such as psychotic depression or schizophrenia. The history of the pain is so vague and bizarre and its distribution so unanatomical as to suggest the diagnosis. These patients respond *only* to psychiatric therapy. History, examinations, laboratory studies, and management must be pursued with these principles in mind.

Pain associated with either structural or psychophysiological disorders can arise from somatic, visceral, or neural structures. *Somatic pain* results from activation of peripheral receptors and somatic efferent

TABLE 116–1. ASPECTS OF PAIN

Definition: An unpleasant sensory and emotional experience associated with either actual or potential tissue damage, or described in terms of such damage (International Association for Study of Pain)

Temporal Characteristics
Acute (less than 6 months)
Chronic (more than 6 months)

Physiology
Somatic
Visceral
Neural (deafferentation)

Pathogenesis
Structural
Psychophysiological
Delusional

nerves, without injury to the nerves themselves. The pain can be either sharp or dull but is typically well-localized and intermittent. *Visceral pain* results from activation of visceral nociceptive receptors and visceral efferent nerves and is characterized as a deep aching, cramping sensation, often referred to cutaneous sites. *Deafferentation* or *causalgic pain* results from injury to peripheral receptors, nerves, or central nervous system. It is typically burning and dysesthetic and often affects an area of sensory loss (e.g., postherpetic neuralgia). The autonomic nervous system plays a significant modulatory role in all three types of pain, most prominently in visceral and deafferentation pain. Somatic and visceral pain are readily managed with a wide variety of nonopioid and opioid analgesics, anesthetic blocks, and neurosurgical approaches. In contrast, deafferentation pain responds minimally to nonopioid and opioid analgesics and anesthetic and neurosurgical procedures.

Referred pain is perceived at a site remote from the source of the noxious disturbance. It is usually cutaneous and evoked by disease of deep structures innervated by the same dermatome. Referred pain may be associated with cutaneous hyperalgesia and even relieved by procaine injection into the area of referral. When pain is referred to the same dermatome or myotome that includes the diseased structure [e.g., pain down the medial aspect of the arm (T1-T2) produced by myocardial infarction or angina pectoris, or diaphragmatic irritation causing shoulder pain (C4)], it is often helpful in diagnosis. However, pain is sometimes referred at a great distance from the primary site to segments not similarly innervated, in which case the mechanism is perplexing (e.g., anginal pain referred to the jaw, gallbladder pain felt in the chest or shoulder). Various theories have been suggested to account for referred pain. Such theories as division of the same nerve into deep (visceral) and superficial branches, release of chemical mediators in the nervous system, and convergence of cutaneous and visceral nerves into common synaptic pools at the spinal cord all might explain the dermatomal referral of pain but fail to explain pain at remote sites.

HEADACHE AND OTHER HEAD PAIN

Headache is one of man's most common afflictions. The frequency of disabling headache is

TABLE 116–2. SOURCES OF HEAD AND FACE PAIN

SENSITIVE	INSENSITIVE
Intracranial	
Dural venous sinuses	Brain
Dura at base of brain	Dura (except at base)
Pial arteries (proximal)	Pia-arachnoid
Trigeminal, glossopharyngeal, vagus, and first three cranial nerves	Distal arteries
Periosteum of skull	Skull
Extracranial	
Skin, muscles, blood vessels, nerves, eye, ear, paranasal sinuses (ostia)	

TABLE 116–3. CLASSIFICATION OF HEAD AND FACE PAIN

No structural disease—pathophysiology poorly understood
  Migraine and other vascular headaches
  Tension type headaches
  Cluster headaches
  Trauma and post-traumatic headache
  Miscellaneous unexplained headache
Intracranial structural disorder
Extracranial structural disorder
Toxic, metabolic, and systemic illnesses
Cranial neuralgias

TABLE 116–4. DIFFERENTIAL DIAGNOSIS OF MIGRAINE AND TENSION HEADACHE

	MIGRAINE	TENSION
Intensity	Moderate to severe	Mild to moderate
Duration	4–48 hours	Minutes to weeks
Location	Unilateral (parietotemporal)	Bilateral (variable)
Precipitating factors	Food, alcohol, menstruation, bright lights, exercise	Fatigue, anxiety
Age	Children, adolescents, and young adults	Any
Sex	Females more than males	Either
Associated symptoms	Nausea, vomiting, photophobia, phonophobia, malaise	Tight, tender muscles
Treatment	Dark room, sleep, ergot; prophylactic drugs available	Analgesics and/or antidepressants
Diurnal pattern	Morning, often awakens one from sleep	Anytime, usually afternoon or evening, rarely awakens one from sleep

explained in part by the rich nerve supply to the head (including efferent nerve fibers from trigeminal, glossopharyngeal, vagus, and upper three cervical nerves) and in part by the psychological implications of head pain, causing anxiety about even modest headache, whereas a pain of equal severity elsewhere in the body might be ignored. Head pain can result from distortion, stretching, inflammation, or destruction of pain-sensitive nerve endings as a result of either intra- or extracranial disease in the distribution of any of the aforementioned nerves (Table 116–2). Most head pain, however, arises from extracerebral structures and carries a benign prognosis. Table 116–3 classifies the common causes.

Because headache is so common and so rarely due to structural disease, excessive application of expensive and highly technical laboratory procedures to its diagnosis and management substantially increases unnecessary medical costs. Nevertheless, in some instances a timely brain image by CT or MR scan or a lumbar puncture can give life-saving information about an otherwise undiagnosable problem. The following principles may help to manage the individual patient:

1. A complete history, with special attention to the location and character of the pain, associated symptoms (e.g., nausea, paresthesias), precipitating, exacerbating, and relieving factors, and previous history of headache, can usually establish the diagnosis. The physical and laboratory examinations are rarely helpful unless the history suggests structural disease. The vast majority of patients complaining of headache suffer from either vascular headache of the migraine type or tension type headaches. Their characteristics are defined in Table 116–4. Even when the unilateral prodromes and headache of long-standing, classic migraine consistently affect the same side, the incidence of associated intracranial lesions remains so low that brain imaging is unnecessary and angiography unjustified.

2. Headaches that are of recent origin or progression deserve investigation by brain imaging. This principle especially applies to headaches that have a consistently focal distribution, follow trauma, or begin after the age of 30 years.

3. The EEG and radioisotope brain scan are almost never useful in the diagnosis of headache. Skull x-rays are useful in diagnosing headache only (a) when searching for abnormalities involving the base of the brain such as sellar or suprasellar lesions or (b) immediately following head trauma. CT or MR scans have superior discriminating capacities and, when available, eliminate the need for radiographs.

4. Diagnostic lumbar puncture should be performed with any acute headache that (a) is accompanied by fever or (b) is explosive or the most severe headache ever suffered (a history typical of acute subarachnoid hemorrhage). Lumbar puncture should, if possible, be deferred until after CT scanning with other forms of acute headache, especially if stiff neck but no fever is present. (This combination may indicate partial herniation of cerebellar tonsils into the for-

amen magnum secondary to an intracranial mass lesion.)

Migraine and Other Vascular Headaches
(Table 116–5)

The term *vascular headache* applies to a group of clinical syndromes of unknown etiology in which the final step in pathogenesis of the pain appears to be dilatation or irritation of one or more branches of the carotid artery (especially the external carotid and its branches), leading to stimulation of nerve endings supplying that artery. The pain threshold of these nerve endings is lowered by release of neurotransmitters or other substances from nerve endings in the vessel wall. A typical vascular headache is unilateral, throbbing in quality, and recurs over months or years. Individual headaches are frequently precipitated by identifiable environmental or psychological factors. During a vascular headache, the involved arteries may be tender to touch, and compression of the carotid artery may temporarily relieve the pain, only to have it return with increased severity when compression is released. Common migraine may affect as many as 25 per cent of the population. Other vascular headache syndromes are less common, but each has distinctive clinical findings. Most acute vascular headaches last only several hours and are best treated by rest in a quiet, dark room accompanied by a mild analgesic agent such as aspirin, if the patient is not too nauseated to take it. Occasionally more potent analgesics such as codeine or Demerol may be required, but such drugs should generally be avoided, in part because they add to the nausea frequently accompanying vascular headaches and in part because of their potential for abuse. Patients with prolonged or severe migraines usually respond to vasoconstrictive agents such as ergotamine given orally, rectally, or subcutaneously. If the headaches recur frequently (twice a week or more), prophylactic agents such as beta-adrenergic blockers (e.g., propranolol), methysergide, calcium channel blockers, or sometimes tricyclic antidepressants (e.g., amitriptyline) may provide effective prophylaxis.

Migraine is characterized by recurrent headaches, often severe, frequently beginning unilaterally, and usually associated with malaise, nausea and/or vomiting, and photophobia. The disorder often begins in childhood, affects women more often than men, and runs in families. Identifiable factors that often precipitate individual headaches are holidays and weekends, menstrual periods, foods (especially chocolate, nuts, and aged cheese), alcohol (especially red wine), and environmental stimuli (such as bright sunlight, too much sleep, and undue emotional stress or resentment). Medical conditions and their treatment may also precipitate attacks. Vasodilators such as nitroglycerin and antihypertensives, serotonin releasers such as reserpine, as well as estrogens and oral contraceptives have all been reported to cause migraine attacks in susceptible individuals. Important historical points that help distinguish migraine from the equally common tension headaches (see below) include their unilaterality, their association with nausea or vomiting, the tendency of migraine to awaken one from sleep, a positive family history, and a favorable response to ergot preparations.

In *classic migraine* (about 15 to 20 per cent of migrane patients), well-defined symptoms of brief (up to 30 minutes) neurological dysfunction precede or, less often, accompany headache. The neurological symptoms are usually visual, most often consisting of bright flashing lights (scintillation or fortification scotomas) beginning in the center of a homonymous visual half-field and radiating over 10 to 30 minutes outward toward the periphery. Other neurological disturbances include unilateral paresthesias of the hand and perioral area, aphasia, hemiparesis, and hemisensory defects. Neurological symptoms usually disappear before the headache begins. If the symptoms are unilateral, the headache almost always affects the other side. When there is no neurological prodrome, the same disorder is called *common migraine*. If the neurological dysfunction continues into or outlasts the duration of the headache, the disorder is called *complicated migraine*. In rare instances, a neurological disorder may be permanent, the vasoconstriction having resulted in cerebral infarction. Specific types of complicated migraine include familial hemiplegic migraine, ophthalmoplegic migrane, and basilar artery migraine; the last occurs predominantly in children and adolescents and is characterized by vertigo, ataxia, and diplopia, sometimes with hemiparesis or hemisensory changes and rarely stupor, confusion, or even coma. *Migraine equivalents* are of two kinds. Young children sometime suffer from episodic nausea and vomiting or episodic vertigo. The headache may be absent. Adults, including the elderly, may suffer recurrent attacks of neurological dysfunction which mimic migraine prodromes but do not culminate in headache. Migraine equivalents are often confused with transient ischemic attacks or focal seizures and differ from both in their slower evolution, among other variables.

Cluster headaches are short-lived attacks of extremely severe, unilateral head pain that occur in clusters, often occurring several times daily and lasting several weeks, only to disappear for months or years

TABLE 116–5. CLASSIFICATION OF VASCULAR HEADACHES

Migraine headache
  Classic migraine
  Common migraine
  Complicated migraine
  Migraine equivalents
Cluster headache
  Episodic cluster
  "Chronic" cluster
  Chronic paroxysmal hemicrania
Miscellaneous vascular headaches
  Carotidynia
  Hypertension
  Orgasmic, exertional, and cough headache
  Occlusive vascular disease

before recurring. Their pathogenesis is unknown, although they are believed to be vascular headache related to migraine. The diagnosis is established by the characteristic history. The disorder affects men much more than women and usually starts between the third and sixth decades. Clusters characteristically occur in the spring and fall and last three to eight weeks. Each attack, which lasts 30 minutes to 2 hours, is characterized by the rapid onset of a knifelike pain in the nostril or behind the eye which spreads to involve the forehead. During the attack, the ipsilateral nostril waters and the eye may tear. About 20 per cent of cases develop a homolateral Horner's syndrome. The headache disappears as abruptly as it came, usually leaving no residua. Unlike migraine, patients with cluster headaches neither feel systemically ill nor suffer nausea, vomiting, or exhaustion when the headache ceases. During a cluster epoch, but not otherwise, alcohol invariably induces an attack. The individual cluster headache is so brief that there is insufficient time for pharmacological agents to be absorbed. Inhalation of pure oxygen often aborts the headache. Since the headaches frequently recur at known times, the ingestion of ergotamine tartrate prophylactically an hour or two before the expected headache may abort the headache. The serotonin inhibitor methysergide also is often successful in preventing cluster headaches.

Several uncommon types of headaches probably have vascular origin. Headache associated with a tender carotid artery (carotidynia) may occur spontaneously or follow carotid endarterectomy. Headaches associated with physical exertion, cough, or orgasm probably also have an extracranial vascular basis and are more likely to occur in people who suffer from migraine. Occlusive vascular diseases, particularly cerebral emboli, are sometimes accompanied by headache.

True hypertensive headaches are rare except in patients with severe, episodic hypertension, such as occurs with pheochromocytoma or reflex sympathetic hyperactivity such as is induced from an isolated distal spinal cord in paraplegics.

Tension Headache (Table 116–6)

So-called tension headaches are characterized by a steady, nonpulsatile, unilateral or bilateral aching pain, usually beginning in the occipital region but often involving frontal or temporal regions as well. Their pathogenesis is unknown, but they are frequently accompanied by tender posterior cervical,

temporalis, and masseter muscles. Tension headaches often recur daily, usually in early afternoon or evening, with a dull occipital or frontal pain that, vicelike, may grip the entire head in a constricting band. Unique among headaches, the pain may be constantly present for days, weeks, or months. Patients rarely complain of nausea, vomiting, or malaise, but modest dizziness, blurring of vision, and sometimes tinnitus are frequent symptoms. Tension headaches are more frequent in women, in individuals who are tense and anxious, and in those whose work or posture requires sustained contraction of posterior cervical, frontal, or temporal muscles. There is much overlap between the symptoms of common migraine and tension headaches, and many patients suffer from both. Similar headaches are often associated with depression or other severe psychological abnormalities.

Tension headache variants include the so-called temporomandibular joint syndrome with unilateral or bilateral head pain, usually in the temporal region and in the jaw, often radiating into the ear. Tenderness affects the masseter and temporalis muscles and may be exacerbated by chewing. Accompanying symptoms often include limitation of full movement at the temporomandibular joint when opening the jaw, bruxism, and malocclusion. The disorder occasionally responds to dental manipulation, particularly use of a mouth guard that prevents bruxism. For most patients analgesics and antianxiety manipulation effectively treat the muscle contraction head pain. *Post-traumatic headaches* are dull, generalized, aching head pains that follow head injury. The disorder can blend into *depressive headache*, a chronic generalized headache, usually vaguely described, sometimes associated with giddiness and unsteadiness, that occurs as a frequent and sometimes predominant manifestation of depression. The headache may have muscle contraction and tension as its pathogenesis or may be a *somatic delusion* in a severely depressed patient. The treatment of choice is an antidepressant drug.

Atypical facial pain or atypical facial neuralgia is a term used to describe a syndrome characterized by steady aching face pain, usually unilateral, localized to the lower part of the orbit, maxillary area, and sometimes the jaw. The pain begins without a known precipitating episode and may last for hours or indefinitely. It may spread to involve the head or neck, and the muscles of the jaw and neck often become tender. Sometimes autonomic symptoms including sweating, flushing, rhinorrhea, and pallor are present. The disorder almost exclusively affects tense, anxious, and often chronically depressed women, often in early middle age. The importance of diagnosis lies in minimizing expensive laboratory tests and avoiding addicting drugs or mutilating surgical or dental procedures.

TABLE 116–6. CLASSIFICATION OF TENSION HEADACHES

Common tension headache
Depressive equivalent
Conversion reaction
Post-traumatic headache
Temporomandibular joint dysfunction
Atypical facial pain

Headache from Intracranial Disorders

Most of the intracranial disorders that cause headache (Table 116–7) are discussed under their respective headings.

TABLE 116–7. HEADACHE FROM INTRACRANIAL DISORDERS

Increased intracranial pressure
    Benign intracranial hypertension
    High-pressure hydrocephalus
Increased venous pressure
    Septic or aseptic intracranial thrombophlebitis
    Extracranial venous occlusion
Decreased intracranial pressure
    Cerebrospinal fluid leakage
    Post–lumbar puncture headache
Infection
    Meningitis
    Encephalitis
    Subdural abscess
    Empyema
Vascular disorders
    Subarachnoid hemorrhage
    Intracranial hematoma
Tumors
    Brain
    Pituitary

Acute and subacute meningitis causes gradually developing headache resulting from inflammation of pain-sensitive structures surrounding the brain. The headache is usually generalized, throbbing, and very severe. It may be rapid or gradual in onset, and by the time it is fully developed is associated with nuchal rigidity. The diagnosis is established by lumbar puncture. In *subarachnoid hemorrhage* (p. 778), the initial sudden headache is caused by an abrupt alteration of intracranial pressure. This immediate pain is succeeded by a chronic persistent headache, often accompanied by gradually increasing nuchal rigidity that results from a chemical meningitis caused by the blood.

Intracranial hypotension, usually from loss of spinal fluid from lumbar puncture or a dural tear, decreases the buoyancy of the brain so that the organ descends when the upright position is assumed, exerting traction on structures at its apex and compression on structures at its base. (In rare instances, the small bridging veins that enter the sagittal sinus may rupture and cause subdural hematomas.) *Intracranial hypertension* causes headaches when vascular and neural structures over the apex or at the base of the brain are compressed by tumor or edematous brain. The most common cause of headache related to intracranial hypertension is brain tumor. The characteristics of brain tumor headache are discussed on page 798. Another cause of increased intracranial pressure headache is pseudotumor cerebri (benign intracranial hypertension).

Headache caused by *pituitary tumors* is the result of compression and distortion of pain-sensitive structures at the base of the skull, particularly the diaphragma sellae. Pain is generally referred to the frontal or temporal regions bilaterally and may on occasion be referred to the vertex or occipital regions. Acute headache occurring with known pituitary lesions (pituitary apoplexy) usually results from infarction or hemorrhage into the tumor. Sudden expansion of the tumor may compromise the overlying optic chiasm, leading to visual loss, or invade the laterally lying cavernous sinus, producing ocular palsies. Pituitary apoplexy should be treated surgically by emergency drainage of the hemorrhagic or infarcted material.

Extracranial Structural Headache (Table 116–8)

Nasal and Sinus Headache. Sinus headache, like headache caused by "eye strain," is uncommon. True sinus headache results from acute inflammation of the paranasal sinuses, which produces pain localized over the involved sinus and is associated with the stigmata of acute infection, including fever, swelling, and tenderness over the sinus and engorgement of the turbinates, ostia, nasofrontal ducts, and superior nasal spaces. Most patients diagnosed by a physician or self-diagnosed as having sinus headaches are in fact suffering from either vascular or muscle contraction headache. Sinus radiographs and a physical examination are diagnostic.

Dental Pain. Noxious stimuli in a tooth usually evoke local toothache, but severe dental pain can be extremely difficult to localize because pain may spread to other teeth or distant tissues, which exhibit surface hyperalgesia, tenderness, and vasomotor reactions, such as tender eyeballs, reddening of the conjunctivae, and tenderness of the auricular and temporal tissues. Secondary muscle contraction produces other sites of tenderness and pain behind the ears, behind the lower border of the mastoid process, and in the muscles of the occiput, neck, and shoulders. Patiently tapping each tooth for tenderness, using a blunt object or rod, often gives a localizing clue.

Aural Pain. Pain in the vicinity of the ear can be caused by disease of the teeth, tonsils, larynx and nasopharynx, temporomandibular joint, or cervical spine and its soft tissues. Pain in the ear can be associated with vascular headaches, atypical facial pain, and herpes zoster of the fifth and seventh cranial nerves as well as, rarely, the glossopharyngeal nerve. True glossopharyngeal neuralgia causes severe pain radiating from the tonsil into the ear. Primary ear disease is relatively infrequent—but important—as a source of headache, because it almost always indicates inflammation or destructive disease.

Eye Pain and Headache. Errors of refraction (hypermetropia, astigmatism, anomalies of accommodation), ocular muscle imbalance (strabismus), glaucoma, and iritis are universally described as causing

TABLE 116–8. HEADACHE FROM EXTRACRANIAL STRUCTURAL LESIONS

Paranasal sinusitis and tumors
Dental infections
Otitis
Ocular lesions
Cervical osteoarthritis
Cranial arteritis

headache. For most, the headache is mild in degree and usually starts around and over the eyes and subsequently radiates to the occiput and back of the head. The pain of glaucoma or iritis begins in the eye, can become severe, and then later extends to include a periorbital distribution.

Cervical Osteoarthritis. Any of the pain-sensitive structures of the upper neck (see p. 713) can cause pain that radiates toward or is referred to the cranium. The pain is usually precipitated or exacerbated by active or passive movement of the neck and is relieved by resting the neck with a cervical collar or bedrest. At times the pain is chronic and difficult to differentiate from tension headache. Lidocaine block of the C2-C3 zygapophyseal joint may help establish the diagnosis by identifying the source of pain.

Cranial Neuralgias

The term *cranial neuralgias* refers to several distinctive, extremely severe, paroxysmal head pains that appear to result from sudden episodic, intrinsic, and excessive discharges from the involved nerve. The best known is trigeminal neuralgia. Similar but much rarer disorders than trigeminal or glossopharyngeal neuralgia have been reported to involve the greater occipital nerve and the nervus intermedius portion of the facial nerve. The clinical features and treatment of these rare disorders are similar to those of trigeminal neuralgia.

Trigeminal Neuralgia. Trigeminal neuralgia is characterized by sudden, lightning-like paroxysms of pain in the distribution of one or more divisions of the trigeminal nerve. Most trigeminal neuralgia is probably caused by compression of the trigeminal nerve by tortuous arteries of the posterior fossa. Occasionally the syndrome can result from a gasserian ganglion tumor, multiple sclerosis, or a brain stem infarct.

The history is diagnostic. The pain occurs as brief, lightning-like stabs, frequently precipitated by touching a trigger zone around the lips or the buccal cavity. At times, talking, eating, or brushing the teeth serves as a trigger. The pains rarely last longer than seconds, and each burst is followed by a refractory period of several seconds to a minute in which no further pain can be precipitated. The pains, however, often occur in clusters so that affected patients may report that each pain lasts for hours. The pain is limited to the distribution of the trigeminal nerve, usually involving the second or third division or both. Spontaneous remissions are common. Exacerbations tend to occur in the spring and fall. Between paroxysms of pain, the patient is asymptomatic. The pain rarely occurs at night. Ordinarily, the neurological examination is entirely normal. Sensory changes in the distribution of the trigeminal nerve should prompt a careful search for structural disease such as tumor.

Carbamazepine is the initial treatment of choice for the treatment of trigeminal neuralgia; phenytoin and baclofen are also sometimes effective. The drugs are not analgesics and are effective only for specific kinds of pain such as trigeminal neuralgia, glossopharyngeal neuralgia, and the lightning pains of tabes dorsalis. If medical treatment fails, surgery, either radiofrequency lesions of the gasserian ganglion (to block sensory conduction) or posterior fossa craniotomy (to relieve the trigeminal nerve of compression by vascular structures), is indicated.

Glossopharyngeal Neuralgia. Glossopharyngeal neuralgia is characterized by pain similar to that of trigeminal neuralgia but in the distribution of the glossopharyngeal and vagus nerves. The trigger zone usually lies in the tonsil or posterior pharynx, and the pain spreads toward the angle of the jaw and the ear. Occasionally patients suffer cardiac slowing or brief arrest (syncope) during attacks of pain as a result of the intense afferent discharge over the glossopharyngeal nerve. Carbamazepine is often effective, but, if drugs fail, glossopharyngeal nerve roots are sectioned in the posterior fossa. Symptomatic glossopharyngeal neuralgia is occasionally the presenting complaint in a patient with a tonsillar tumor, and careful examination of the pharynx and tonsillar fossa for mass lesions must be carried out.

Miscellaneous, less frequent causes of headache are listed in Table 116–9.

NECK AND BACK PAIN

Neck and/or back pain is one of man's most common afflictions. About 80 per cent of individuals suffer significant low back pain at least once during their life. The annual incidence is 5 per cent. Next to alcoholism, back pain is the leading cause of time lost from work. Most neck and back pain, although incapacitating, is transient and neither life-threatening nor associated with obvious pathological abnormalities. In most instances, the symptoms are more severe than abnormalities found on physical examination or imaging studies. Because the pathophysiology of most such pain is poorly understood, the physician often encounters patients in whom he can neither make a certain diagnosis nor prescribe rational therapy. Fortunately, most patients suffering from back pain recover within a few weeks regardless of the treatment. Only 4 per cent of patients suffering from back pain are disabled longer than six months.

Pain in the neck or back may arise from one or more of several pain-sensitive structures (Table 116–10), including the periosteum of the vertebral body (explain-

TABLE 116–9. MISCELLANEOUS CAUSES OF HEADACHE

Headache associated with substances or their withdrawal
  Ergotamine abuse and withdrawal
  Analgesic abuse
  Alcohol abuse and withdrawal (hangover)
  Caffeine withdrawal
  Nitrates/nitrites (hot dog headache)
  Monosodium glutamate (Chinese restaurant syndrome)
  Carbon monoxide
Headache associated with systemic infection or fever
Headache associated with metabolic abnormality
  Hypoxia and ischemia
  Dialysis

ing why compression fractures of the spine are at least initially painful), posterior longitudinal ligament (one source of pain from herniated disc), the nerve roots exiting the intervertebral foramina (the source of dermatomal pain from nerve root compression by herniated discs), the facet joints (a common cause of acute back pain after unaccustomed bending), the sacroiliac joints, and the paravertebral muscles. Table 116–11 lists some common causes of neck or back pain. Most acute neck or back pain is probably caused by muscle strain and spasm due to unaccustomed exercise or stretching, is transient, and is not life-threatening (see also myofascial pain, below). Patients suffering from such pain usually recover within a few weeks no matter what the treatment, but a few suffer chronic disability. Most chronic neck or back pain is either myofascial in origin or associated with vertebral arthritis and/or intervertebral disc disease, the former causing pain by compression of small nerve twigs supplying the facet joints and the periosteum of the vertebral bodies, the latter causing pain by compression of the nerve root. More rarely, tumors and inflammatory or degenerative arthritic lesions of the spine may be responsible.

In patients with acute neck or back pain, particularly when the precipitating cause (such as unaccustomed exercise) cannot be identified, heat and rest suffice without further diagnostic work-up. In patients with persistent or recurrent pain, meticulous diagnostic evaluation and vigorous therapy often prevent or reverse serious or potentially lethal neurological damage.

The diagnostic evaluation begins with a history. Most benign back or neck pain is of acute or subacute onset and frequently follows by minutes to hours some unaccustomed physical activity, particularly lifting or bending. Other patients awaken feeling stiff and sore the morning after unusual exercise. Sometimes low back pain begins acutely, frequently on arising in the morning, without any obvious precipitating event. Most neck pain begins as a stiff neck, often on awakening in the morning, without a previous history of unusual activity. Many patients' neck or back pains occur episodically over many years. Most benign neck or back pain is dull or aching in quality, exacerbated by movement, and relieved by rest. The majority of patients are comfortable when recumbent and immobile or at least are able to find one position that relieves the pain. Pain that is present when the patient is immobile and that cannot be relieved by postural manipulation should lead the physician to search for a serious disorder. Likewise, pain that radiates in a clear dermatomal distribution is probably a result of nerve root compression, especially if there are paresthesias or loss of sensation. Radiating pain in a nondermatomal distribution often accompanies neck and back muscle spasms; it usually does not portend serious neurogenic disease.

A careful physical and neurological examination may reveal an obvious cause for the pain. Systemic disease such as cancer, urinary tract infection, pelvic disease, or abdominal aneurysm may be a cause of

TABLE 116–10. PAIN SENSITIVE STRUCTURES IN AND AROUND THE SPINE

SENSITIVE	INSENSITIVE
Ligaments	Ligaments
Anterior and posterior longitudinal ligaments	Intraspinous and ligamentum flavum
Facets	Vertebral body
Articular cartilage	Intervertebral disc
Capsule	
Nerve roots	
Paraspinal muscles	

TABLE 116–11. COMMON CAUSES OF NECK AND/OR BACK PAIN

Trauma
  Muscle strain or spasm
  Subluxed facet joints
  Compression fractures (osteoporosis)
Psychophysiological
  Muscle tension and spasm
  Fibromyalgia
Degenerative disorders
  Herniated disc
  Spondylosis
    Spinal stenosis
  Osteoarthritis
Neoplasm
  Extradural (usually malignant)
  Intradural extramedullary (usually benign)
  Intramedullary (either benign or malignant)
Inflammation
  Arthritis
  Osteomyelitis of vertebral body
  Disc infection

back pain because a lesion impinges on the vertebral body or paravertebral structures. Evidence for neurological disease such as weakness, sensory loss, or reflex abnormalities suggests spinal cord or nerve root dysfunction. Such evidence of neurological disability requires a careful laboratory examination, including plain radiographs, CT scan of vertebral and paravertebral structures, and, if clinically indicated, myelography. Specific findings resulting from intervertebral disc disease are found on p. 750 and those from spinal tumor and congenital anomalies on p. 742.

In the absence of a clear abnormality on physical examination, conservative treatment of back pain with immobility, heat, analgesics, and sometimes physical therapy will ameliorate symptoms in a short period of time without the necessity of substantial laboratory evaluation. Even in the absence of neurological signs, however, if pain persists after conservative treatment, radiographic and laboratory evaluation become mandatory.

MYOFASCIAL PAIN

A major part of head, back, and neck pain arises from skeletal muscle, particularly from the paravertebral muscles. Unaccustomed exercise causes soreness and tenderness in the involved muscles but is rarely a source of patient complaint. Prolonged tonic contraction of skeletal muscles, however, has a pathogenesis that originates in psychological tension, resentment, and anxiety and may produce pain whose cause is not immediately apparent to the patient. Examples are tension headache arising from chronic contraction of muscles at the base of the skull, anterior chest pain from contraction of the pectoralis majors, posterior thoracic or lumbar pain from paraspinous muscle contraction, and abdominal pain from rectus muscle contraction. The pain is initially localized over the area of muscle contraction but may spread widely in a distribution characteristic for the muscles involved. The affected muscles are usually tender to palpation, and one often finds a particularly tender area somewhere in the muscle, called a trigger zone, which, when palpated, reproduces the distribution of the spontaneous pain. One common variant of myofascial pain is the fibrositis/fibromyalgia syndrome, a disorder of middle-aged women characterized by generalized musculoskeletal pain, morning stiffness, disturbed sleep and fatigue (nonrestorative sleep), and at times vague complaints of swelling paresthesias. Headache and "irritable bowel" symptoms are common, and most patients are concurrently anxious and/or depressed. Tender points can be found on examination in most or all of the 14 sites illustrated in Figure

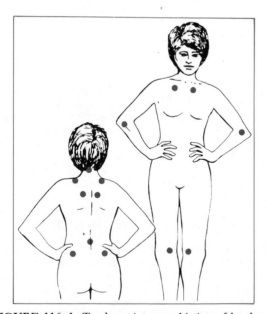

FIGURE 116–1. Tender point map: 14 sites of local tenderness. The unilateral sites are at the intertransverse and/or interspinous ligaments of C4 to C6 and the interspinous ligament at L4 to L5, the bilateral sites at the upper borders of the trapezius, the supraspinatus origins at the medial border of the scapula, the upper outer quadrants of the buttocks, the second costochondral junctions, the lateral epicondyles, and the medial fat pads of the knees. (From Wolfe F: The clinical syndrome of fibrositis. *In* The fibrositis-fibromyalgia syndrome. Am J Med 81 (Suppl 3A): 1986.)

116–1. It is likely that other myofascial and referred pain syndromes are fragments of the fibromyalgia syndrome.

The pathophysiology of myofascial pain is poorly understood. Some observers have reported microscopic changes at trigger points (so-called fibrous nodules), suggesting that a tonic contraction may lead to structural changes in the muscle. Others have suggested that release of noxious substances such as lactic acid, potassium, or kinins from chronically contracting muscles might be responsible for the pain and tenderness associated with this syndrome. The treatment of myofascial pain is often difficult and frustrating. In some patients mild analgesic drugs (aspirin), heat, and massage yield temporary or long-term relief. In other patients, massage or even injection of trigger points with local anesthetics gives relief. Biofeedback with the patient trying consciously to relax contracted muscles recorded by surface EMG has been reported to be useful. Antidepressants are modestly effective and produce at least a short-term remission in about 20 per cent of patients. For most patients, a combination of the above physical methods with investigation and treatment of the underlying psychological disorder is necessary if long-term relief is to be achieved.

REFLEX SYMPATHETIC DYSTROPHY

Reflex sympathetic dystrophy is a painful disorder that usually follows a major or minor injury to an extremity and is characterized by a constellation of symptoms including sustained neuropathic pain, hyperesthesia and hyperalgesia, and autonomic changes in skin, subcutaneous tissue, and joints. When the inciting injury involves a peripheral nerve, particularly the sciatic or median nerve, the syndrome is called *causalgia* (hot pain). Other synonyms include posttraumatic painful osteoporosis, Sudeck's atrophy, and shoulder-hand syndrome, the particular diagnostic term depending on the outstanding symptom. Severe pain, usually of a burning quality, is the first symptom after the injury. The pain is continuous, worsened by emotional stress, and sometimes associated with such severe hyperpathia that moving or touching the limb is intolerable. At first the pain is localized to the site of injury or the distribution of the nerve injured, but with time it often spreads to involve the entire extremity. Along with the pain there develop vasomotor changes, first vasodilation (warm and dry skin) and later vasoconstriction (edema, cyanosis, and cool skin). Other autonomic abnormalities include either hyper- or hypohidrosis, atrophy of the skin and subcutaneous tissues, and osteoporosis. The entire symptom complex is rarely present in any one patient, and one sign or symptom usually predominates. Untreated, the disorder leads eventually to muscle atrophy, fixation of joints, and a useless extremity. The mechanism of the pain and sympathetic changes is poorly understood.

Treatment is sometimes effective, particularly if begun early. Repeated local anesthetic infiltration of the painful site with lidocaine sometimes leads to relief. If local measures fail, most patients are relieved by sympathetic ganglion block, which, if repeated, may give permanent relief. A short course of corticosteroids has been reported to be effective. Analgesic drugs usually offer little relief.

REFERENCES

Rose FC: The Management of Headache. New York, Raven Press, 1988.

Vinken PJ, Bruyn GW, Klawans HL (eds): Handbook of Clinical Neurology. Vol 48: Headache. Amsterdam, Elsevier Science, 1985.

Wall PD, Melzack R (eds): Textbook of Pain. Edinburgh, Churchill Livingstone, 1984.

B.   THE SPECIAL SENSORY SYSTEM

EXAMINATION OF THE PATIENT

Special (i.e., nonsomatic) sensation is subserved by several of the cranial nerves and their central extensions. In most instances, even the most subtle abnormality of special sensory function is immediately apparent to the patient. Such disorders, which include visual loss, hearing loss, dizziness, and abnormalities of smell or taste perception, are a frequent cause for physician consultation. It follows then that, with a few exceptions, unless the patient reports symptoms, meticulous physical evaluation of this system is likely to be unrewarding. However, a brief screening examination, even in asymptomatic patients, may yield some important findings of which the patient is unaware.

Odor perception (olfactory nerve) is best tested by having the patient, with eyes closed, obstruct the naris on one side and sniff with the other. The patient is alternately presented with nothing and an odoriferous object (e.g., coffee, toothpaste, soap, perfume) and asked both to identify if an odor is present and its nature. Many normal persons can detect but not identify odors. Unilateral anosmia in the absence of nasal obstruction may be unrecognized by the patient and should lead to further neurological work-up. Most bilateral anosmia is due to nasal disease. If malingering (as in litigation) is suspected, try a pungent substance such as ammonia, since this stimulates trigeminal nerve endings and the patient should perceive it even with total olfactory loss.

Taste abnormalities are usually complained of by the patient. Most patients can recognize even unilateral loss of taste (such as associated with facial nerve lesions). Bedside testing of taste by applying sweet, sour, salty, or bitter objects to the tongue is rarely helpful. Some patients who complain of taste loss can perceive the primary tastes on the tongue. Such patients usually have olfactory loss and are misinterpreting the symptom.

Visual acuity should be tested in each eye with the patient wearing his glasses and, if necessary, by the addition of a pinhole held against the lens. Corrected vision in either eye of less than 20/40 suggests a cataract or a retinal or neurological disorder, and further work-up is indicated. Most patients are immediately aware of unilateral central visual loss but some patients may fail to notice such amaurosis, particularly in the nondominant eye, until they inadvertently close the other one. Color sensation in each eye should be tested. Acquired diminution of color vision strongly suggests a lesion of the optic nerve; even when visual acuity is normal the patient may note that colors appear "washed out" in the involved eye. *Visual fields* in all four visual quadrants should be tested, comparing the patient's field with the examiner's. Many patients, particularly with cerebral lesions, may be unaware of the visual field defect although the astute patient may report that he bumps into things or has had an automobile accident on the "blind side." The field should be tested first with unilaterally and then bilaterally presented objects. In particular, bitemporal defects should be sought, as they may be unrecognized by the patient and be the only sign of a pituitary tumor. Normal visual fields with unilateral testing but an abnormal field (in particular a left field defect), when tested bilaterally (extinction), suggest a central defect. Suspicious findings on bedside confrontation or a positive history warrant formal perimetry, which should be performed by a specialist.

The *pupils* should be inspected in both dim and bright light (significant anisocoria may be present in only one). Pupillary inequalities of 1 mm or less are rarely significant (15 per cent of normal individuals have some anisocoria). At the same time as pupillary size is evaluated, the size of the palpebral fissure should also be noted. Ptosis with a small pupil suggests a Horner syndrome; ptosis with a large pupil, a partial third nerve palsy. Pupillary reactions should be tested using a bright light in a relatively dim room. The reaction should be brisk and symmetrical. The bright light is moved quickly from one eye to the other. If there is dilatation of one pupil as the light is moved to it from the other side, one should suspect an abnormality of the optic nerve in that eye. The accommodative pupillary response can be tested by asking the patient first to look into the distance and then at the examiner's finger held a foot from his nose. The pupils should constrict symmetrically and rapidly.

Eye movements are examined first by asking a patient to voluntarily move his eyes laterally up and down and then to track a flashlight in the same directions. Failure of voluntary movement with normal following movements suggests a supranuclear brain disorder (e.g., a progressive supranuclear palsy). Failure of conjugate movement, either voluntarily or on tracking, also suggests a supranuclear disorder. Disconjugate movements suggest a brain stem or peripheral disorder. One should inquire about double vision and look for nystagmus both on forward and on eccentric gaze. Diplopia identified at extremes of gaze but not complained of by the patient is probably not pathological. Unsustained nystagmus on extremes of gaze is usually physiological. Sustained nystagmus unassociated with vertigo is probably due to a central lesion.

Patients with ocular paralyses complain either of blurred vision ("like a ghost on a television set") or frank diplopia. The former may supersede the latter with progressive weakening of the ocular muscle such as is caused by damage of one of the ocular nerves. Horizontal diplopia implies either lateral rectus (abducens nerve) or medial rectus (oculomotor nerve) dysfunction. Vertical or oblique diplopia must involve other muscles. The patient should be closely questioned about the onset of the diplopia (progressive worsening after onset suggests compressive lesions; sudden onset, vascular lesions). Inquire about diurnal pattern (most diplopia worsens with fatigue but diplopia absent in the morning and present later in the day suggests myasthenia gravis) and about relationship to other neurological symptoms. In a patient complaining of diplopia, one should try to determine by examination the position in which the diplopia is most marked. This defines the ocular muscle(s) involved. Deviations of ocular muscles too subtle to be seen by the examiner may be perceived as diplopia to the patient. Red glass testing should be left to the expert, since in the hands of a nonspecialist it is often more misleading than helpful. Intermittent diplopia suggests myasthenia gravis, and one should attempt to fatigue the muscles by sustained action to produce the abnormality. All patients complaining of diplopia in whom an immediate cause is not apparent should have a Tensilon test (see p. 760). Frank abnormalities of ocular movements on examination without diplopia suggest a slowly developing, long-standing lesion such as ocular myopathy with compensation on the part of the patient suppressing the experience of diplopia. Monocular diplopia is usually caused by disease of lens or retina and only rarely by psychogenic or cerebral disease.

Hearing should be tested by having the patient listen to a softly ticking watch or by rubbing one's fingers a few inches from the ear. The examiner can use his own hearing as a standard. If hearing is diminished, the Weber test (see p. 721) should be carried out. Lateralization to the poorly hearing side suggests conductive loss. Lateralization to the normally hearing side suggests a sensorineural abnormality. More thorough evaluation of hearing requires audiometry.

Dizziness. This exceedingly common symptom is only sometimes due to abnormality of the vestibular

TABLE 116–12. DIFFERENTIAL DIAGNOSIS OF DIZZINESS

Vertigo
  Physiological
  Pathological
Lightheadedness or syncope (see Table 9–9)
Ataxia
  Cerebellar dysfunction
  Proprioceptive loss
Diplopia or other visual abnormalities
Anxiety
Hyperventilation
Dissociative episodes
Partial complex seizures

system (vertigo) (Table 116–12). The physician's first task in a dizzy patient is to distinguish vertigo from other symptoms and then, if the patient is suffering from vertigo, to assign a cause (Table 116–12). Since in most patients dizziness is an episodic and not a continuous symptom, a patient usually has neither symptoms nor signs when examined by the physician. Thus, the physician must try to evoke the symptom or sign in order to determine its cause: The heart and blood pressure examination deserve special attention, since orthostatic hypotension or cardiac arrhythmias may lead to syncope. Cerebellar or peripheral nerve dysfunction may cause ataxia. The visual and ocular motor system should be examined for diplopia or other visual distortions. Provocative tests may be used to simulate the patient's dizziness.

Hyperventilation lowers the P_{CO_2} and decreases cerebral blood flow, causing a "lightheaded" sensation. Ask the patient to hyperventilate maximally for 3 minutes. If the procedure exactly mimics the patient's symptoms, it suggests that anxiety and hyperventilation may be playing an important role. In addition, during the course of hyperventilation the patient may suffer dry mouth, chest tightness, and paresthesias which he may then recognize are part of his spontaneous attacks, thus helping in the diagnosis. Tandem walking (heel to toe) with eyes open or closed intensifies ataxia and simulates the sensation of dysequilibrium. The Bárány rotation maneuver (rotating the patient about a vertical axis 10 times over 20 seconds), caloric tests (see below), and positional tests (see below) simulate the symptoms of vestibular vertigo.

Examine the patient carefully for nystagmus. The patient should fix upon a light successively requiring horizontal and vertical gaze in both the erect and supine positions. Nystagmus and vertigo can sometimes be precipitated by rapid movements of the head (*Nylen-Bárány test*). The examiner tilts the seated patient so that the head is hanging 45 degrees below horizontal, with first one ear and then the other dependent. He observes for nystagmus and vertigo. In some patients rapid head turning (once from center to side or vice versa or from supine to erect) suffices to bring out positional nystagmus and vertigo. A latency of 15 seconds or so characteristically separates the abrupt head movement from the appearance of the nystagmus.

SMELL AND TASTE

Smell. Most acquired disturbances of smell result from transient or sustained diseases of the nasal mucous membranes that obstruct access to or dry out or deaden the receptor areas. Such disorders seldom are complete and commonly respond to local treatment. More severe and often permanent anosmia results from, respectively, basal skull fractures avulsing the olfactory nerves, frontal fossa brain tumors affecting the central pathways, and, much less often, herpes zoster, vitamin B$_{12}$ deficiency, diabetes, and multiple sclerosis. Specific alterations of olfactory function can also be found by quantitative testing of patients with Alzheimer's disease, Parkinson's disease, Huntington's chorea, and Korsakoff's psychosis. Sudden idiopathic anosmia usually associated with loss of taste has been reported, probably a result of a local neurotropic viral infection. No satisfactory treatment has been found for such neurogenic anosmias. Affected patients must be warned explicitly to avoid gas heating and to install smoke alarms to compensate for the life-threatening hazards of the defect. *Dysosmia* is a distortion of olfactory perception (normal odors perceived as a foul smell) that may occur without prior anosmia or during the recovery phase from anosmia. The cause most often lies in paranasal infections or, sometimes, in psychiatric illness. Hallucinations of smell, usually of a foul quality, occur with epileptogenic lesions affecting the region of the amygdala and are termed uncinate fits.

Taste. Much of what is perceived as taste derives indirectly from olfaction, which should be checked in any patient complaining of taste loss. Disorders that directly cause taste abnormalities include Bell's palsy, an acute, unilateral loss of facial nerve function that usually reduces taste perception on the involved side. Trigeminal dysfunction with somatosensory loss on the tongue sometimes affects taste. Epileptic discharges occasionally cause gustatory hallucinations. Psychologically depressed or paranoid patients often complain of a foul taste, but taste perception is usually normal. Aging, hepatitis, cancer, and several drugs reduce or distort taste. Unilateral taste loss should prompt a search for facial nerve disease; bilateral taste loss demands investigation of local tongue disease, followed by a systematic review of medications, and, if still necessary, an inquiry into systemic illness. Treatment depends on cause; zinc therapy is not helpful.

DISORDERS OF VISION AND OCULAR MOVEMENT

VISION

Introduction and Definitions

A knowledge of the anatomy of visual pathways is of great importance in clinical diagnosis, because lesions damaging or interrupting the visual sensory system can usually be discretely localized by history and visual field examination (Fig. 116–2). Partial or complete visual loss in one eye, sparing the other, implies damage to the retina or optic nerve anterior to the chiasm, whereas a visual field abnormality affecting both eyes originates at the chiasm or posterior; the more congruent the visual field, the more posterior. *Scotomas* are areas of relative or complete visual loss. *Central scotomas* severely decrease vision because the macular fibers are damaged, whereas scotomas away from the macula may hardly be noticed by the patient. Visual field abnormalities impairing half or nearly half of the field are termed hemianoptic. A *homonymous*

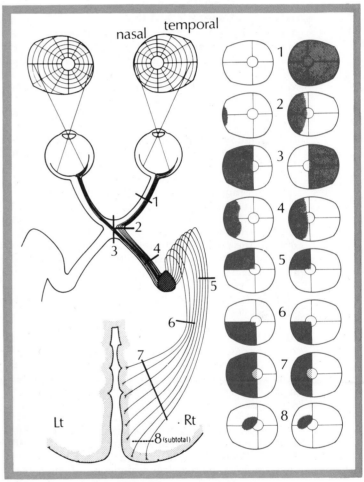

FIGURE 116–2. Visual fields that accompany damage to the visual pathways. 1. Optic nerve: Unilateral amaurosis. 2. Lateral optic chiasm: Grossly incongruous, incomplete (contralateral) homonymous hemianopia. 3. Central optic chiasm: Bitemporal hemianopia. 4. Optic tract: Incongruous, incomplete homonymous hemianopia. 5. Temporal (Meyer's) loop of optic radiation: Congruous partial or complete (contralateral) homonymous superior quadrantanopia. 6. Parietal (superior) projection of the optic radiation: Congruous partial or complete homonymous inferior quadrantanopia. 7. Complete parieto-occipital interruption of optic radiation. Complete congruous homonymous hemianopia with psychophysical shift of foveal point often sparing central vision, giving "macular sparing." 8. Incomplete damage to visual cortex: Congruous homonymous scotomas, usually encroaching at least acutely on central vision. (From Plum F: Neuro-ophthalmology. *In* Wyngaarden JB, Smith LH Jr (eds): Cecil Textbook of Medicine. 18th ed. Philadelphia, WB Saunders Co, 1988, p 2111.)

hemianopia implies a postchiasmal lesion, a *bitemporal hemianopia* a chiasmal lesion, and an *altitudinal hemianopia*, whether unilateral or bilateral, implies vascular damage to retinal structures. Smaller defects involving only a quarter of the visual field are called *quadrantanopia*. Homonymous *superior quadrantanopia* implies temporal lobe damage, whereas homonymous *inferior quadrantanopia* implies parietal lobe damage. *Scintillating scotomas* refer to hallucinations of flashing lights. Such abnormalities imply an abnormal discharge of the visual system anywhere along its course. The disorder is common in migraine and also in seizures originating from the occipital lobe.

Diseases Causing Visual Impairment

Corneal, lenticular, or vitreous diseases large enough to produce visual symptoms can usually be detected by funduscopic inspection. *Glaucoma* with high intraocular pressure causes either slow or rapid visual loss associated with ring or annular scotomas and a deeply cupped optic disc. Visual loss may be preceded by halos seen around illuminated lights and pain in the affected eye. Diagnosis can be made only by tonometry. *Retinal detachment* gives rise to unilateral distortion of visual images that may be mistaken for monocular scintillating scotomas. Detachment can be usually identified by irregularities seen in the retina on funduscopic examination.

Unilateral Visual Loss. Serious visual loss from optic nerve lesions affects either one eye or both eyes asymmetrically, leading to nonhomonymous visual defects; the pupillary light reflex is diminished to the same degree as is vision. Most acute or subacute optic nerve disease is due to demyelinating disease (optic neuritis), vascular disorders (retinal or optic nerve ischemia from arterial embolism or occlusion), or neoplastic lesions. The history is important: If the visual loss is abrupt in onset, whether transient or permanent, the cause is usually vascular. A slower onset over hours or days suggests demyelination; progressive visual loss over weeks or months implies a compressive lesion (e.g., tumor). If the disorder is at the nerve head, it produces papillitis, but if more posteriorly the same disease process can cause a central scotoma or even blindness with no visible change in the optic nerve. *Demyelinating optic neuritis* is usually unilateral. It may be a symptom of multiple sclerosis, but many patients with optic neuritis recover and do not develop other neurological dysfunction. Demyelinating lesions of the optic nerve appear to have a particular predilection for the myelinated fibers that supply the macula, thus leading to central scotomas. Visual acuity is severely impaired, but the peripheral vision may remain intact. *Ischemic optic neuropathy* may be a symptom of *cranial arteritis* or more often occurs in late middle-aged, usually hypertensive individuals as a result of arterial embolism. Blinded patients with giant cell arteritis are usually elderly and suffer from headache, malaise, fever, and an elevated sedimentation rate. Emergency treatment with corticosteroids may prevent blindness in the other eye. In patients with ischemic optic neuropathy, the second eye also tends to become involved, but there is no treatment

to prevent it. *Tumors* can usually be identified by either funduscopic examination, brain imaging, or both. Acute and *transient monocular blindness* is usually a result of embolization of the central retinal artery or one of its branches. The emboli may originate from an atherosclerotic plaque in the carotid or ophthalmic artery or from thrombotic material in the left heart or on cardiac valves such as may complicate rheumatic heart disease and mitral valve prolapse.

Bilateral Visual Loss. Bilateral retinal or optic nerve disease occurs with heredodegenerative conditions, vascular diseases such as diabetes, idiopathic (senile) macular degeneration, or diseases such as retinitis pigmentosa. These conditions can be diagnosed by funduscopic or sometimes slit lamp examination. Acute *transient bilateral blindness* (bilateral visual obscuration) is usually a symptom of increased intracranial pressure; it is almost always associated with severe papilledema and can occur with either brain tumors or pseudotumor cerebri (p. 804).

Acute or subacute bilateral optic neuritis may reflect a demyelinating process, but most examples are due to toxic-nutritional problems or inherited optic atrophy rather than multiple sclerosis. Most chiasmal lesions in the adult result from tumors compressing that structure; the most common are pituitary adenomas, but also include craniopharyngiomas, meningiomas, and large aneurysms of the carotid artery. In small children, optic gliomas are a major cause of chiasmal visual loss. Lesions of the optic tract producing incongruous homonymous field defects are usually caused by infarcts or less commonly tumors. Disorders posterior to the optic tract produce congruent field defects that usually involve macular fibers. When the lesion is occipital, sparing the occipital pole (which often has a bilateral supply from both the middle and the posterior cerebral artery), macular fibers may be spared. The phenomenon cannot be detected at bedside but can be detected by careful visual field testing. Most postchiasmal visual loss is caused by vascular disease or tumor.

Bilateral damage to the visual radiation or occipital cortex produces *cortical blindness*. Such blindness is characterized by a normal funduscopic examination, normal pupillary light reflexes, and often unawareness on the part of the patient that he is, in fact, blind. Most transient cortical blindness is a symptom of basilar artery insufficiency, hypertensive encephalopathy, or more rarely of migraine. The disorder may also occur in the postictal state after a generalized seizure. The reason for the vulnerability of the cerebral cortex to these diffuse cerebral disorders is not clear. Cortical blindness, because of the preservation of pupillary reflexes, may at first be confused with a conversion reaction (hysteria). If there is any question, however, visual evoked responses will establish the diagnosis.

Any complaint of visual loss, particularly unilateral and transient, is an emergency. Lesions that involve one eye can often soon involve the second, and transient or incomplete lesions can become permanent or complete. Many disorders of the visual system are caused by vascular disease, inflammation, or tumors and are thus potentially treatable. Accordingly, a rapid

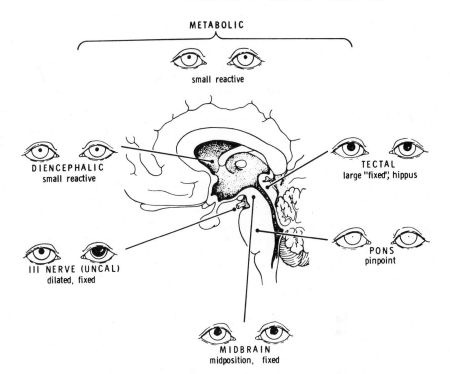

FIGURE 116–3. Pupillary responses in comatose patients. The schematic shows abnormalities resulting from damage to various areas of the central pupillary pathways. In patients with metabolic encephalopathy, pupils are small and reactive, as are pupils resulting from diencephalic damage such as occurs with early herniation. Lesions of the upper brain stem usually produce unilaterally or bilaterally large or mid-position fixed pupils, whereas pontine lesions result in pinpoint pupils. (From Plum F, Posner JB: Diagnosis of Stupor and Coma. 3rd ed. Philadelphia, FA Davis Co, 1980.)

and meticulous examination is necessary first to localize the site of the lesion by funduscopic and visual field examination, and then to identify its pathogenesis (that is done usually by a CT scan or angiography). These steps may lead to appropriate treatment that preserves vision. Examples of sight-saving procedures include reduction of pressure in acute glaucoma, the early use of corticosteroids for the treatment of cranial arteritis, anticoagulation for crescendo carotid or basilar insufficiency, and prompt surgical decompression for the treatment of tumors.

PUPILS

The size of the pupil is determined by the balance between discharges of the sympathetic and parasympathetic (oculomotor nerve) fibers (Fig. 116–3). The pupillary light reaction is determined on the afferent side by visual sensory fibers originating in the retina and traveling through the optic nerve, chiasm, and tract to the midbrain and on the efferent side by parasympathetic fibers that arise in the oculomotor nucleus of the midbrain (Table 116–13).

When *sympathetic fibers* are damaged, the pupil narrows (the light reaction is still normal) and the palpebral fissure becomes smaller as the upper lid descends and the lower lid elevates (Horner's syndrome). The eye, however, does not close as it does with oculomotor nerve lesions. Sweat fibers may be involved as well, leading to anhidrosis on the entire half of the body if the damage is central, on the ipsilateral face and neck if the damage is between the spinal cord and the superior cervical ganglion, or on the medial side of the forehead only if the damage is above the superior cervical ganglion.

Horner's syndrome may be caused by vascular damage to the hypothalamus or brain stem but then is associated with other neurological signs that point to the disorder. An isolated Horner's syndrome may be the first sign of a lung cancer of the superior sulcus or may occur with tumors or other diseases involving the carotid artery. In some instances the cause of the disorder is not found. Horner's syndrome is valuable as a localizing diagnostic sign but in and of itself does not require treatment in that it impairs neither vision nor ocular motor function.

Parasympathetic disorders occur unilaterally with

TABLE 116–13. COMMON CAUSES OF PUPILLARY ABNORMALITIES

SIZE		REACTION TO LIGHT
SMALL PUPILS	LARGE PUPILS	
Argyll Robertson pupil	Holmes-Adie pupil	Nonreactive
Pontine hemorrhage	Post-traumatic iridoplegia	
Opiates	Mydriatic drops	
Pilocarpine drops	Glutethimide overdose	
	Cerebral death	
	Atropine or scopolamine poisoning	
	Amphetamine or cocaine poisoning	
Old age	Childhood	Reactive
Horner's syndrome	Anxiety	
	Physiological anisocoria	

Modified from Patten J: Neurological Differential Diagnosis. New York, Springer-Verlag, 1983.

any lesion of the oculomotor nerve, particularly those that compress the nerve, such as tumors or aneurysms. Cerebral herniation leads to pupillary dilatation if it affects the third nerve or to bilaterally midpositioned and fixed pupils if it affects the midbrain.

The pupils are not always equal in size. Essential anisocoria (lifelong difference in the sizes of the pupils with a normal light reaction) occurs in about 15 per cent of normal people. Tonic (Adie's) pupil is a somewhat larger than normal pupil that constricts little or not at all to light and shrinks slowly on accommodation. It constricts more than normal when dilute pilocarpine is instilled, suggesting that the pupil is parasympathetically denervated (denervation hypersensitivity). The disorder may be unilateral or bilateral and when symptomatic is characterized by a long delay in focusing when the patient attempts to move from far to near vision. There may be pain or a dazzling sensation when affected patients exit from a dark to a light room. In some persons the disorder is associated with absent deep tendon reflexes (Adie's syndrome), but neither the pupillary nor the reflex disorder causes serious disability.

Argyll Robertson pupils are small (1 to 2 mm), unequal, irregular, and fixed to light. They constrict briskly on accommodation. Their principal cause is neurosyphilis, although partial Argyll Robertson pupils occur with diabetes and certain of the autonomic neuropathies. Unexplained unilaterally or bilaterally dilated pupils with visual blurring can result from accidental or intentional instillation of mydriatics such as scopolamine or atropine. Such an abnormality is characterized by failure of the pupil to constrict promptly with 1 per cent pilocarpine.

Damage to visual fibers (the afferent arc of the pupillary light reflex) leads to the "paradoxical pupillary response," in which the direct reaction to light is impaired (because the afferent information is not carried to the oculomotor nerve), but the consensual reaction is normal (since the efferent information reaches both oculomotor nerves). The response is best seen when a bright light is rapidly moved from a normal to a visually impaired eye; the consensually constricted pupil in the impaired eye then dilates.

OCULAR MOVEMENT

Definitions

Abnormal disjunctive eye movements can result from disturbances at several levels of the neuraxis. These include abnormalities in the action of individual muscles (ocular myopathies), the myoneural junction (myasthenia gravis), the oculomotor nerve, the three paired nuclei in the brain stem, or the internuclear medial longitudinal fasciculus that yokes the eyes in parallel movement. The term *strabismus* describes an involuntary deviation of the eyes from normal physiological position. Nonparalytic strabismus is due to an intrinsic imbalance of the ocular muscle tone and is usually congenital. Paralytic strabismus results from defects in ocular muscle innervation and thus implies a neuromuscular disorder. A congenital strabismus

may be compensated during life only to become manifest with aging, fatigue, or systemic disease. With strabismus, the patient often suppresses vision in one eye in order to prevent diplopia. If this occurs in early infancy, the suppressed eye will develop permanent reduction of vision (amblyopia ex anopsia). This does not occur if strabismus develops later in life.

Defects in ocular movement resulting from faulty action of the eye muscles or their peripheral innervation (such as the third, fourth, and sixth cranial nerves) are called ocular paralyses. Abnormalities of conjugate gaze are called gaze paralyses and result from disease of central structures.

Ocular Paralyses

The *abducens* (sixth cranial) nerve subserves the lateral rectus muscle. Selective involvement of the abducens nerve anywhere along its pathway, in or outside the brain stem, leads to isolated weakness of abduction of the affected eye. If the nucleus itself is involved, there is also a gaze paresis to the ipsilateral side as a result of damage to supranuclear structures in the same area. The *trochlear* (fourth cranial) nerve subserves the superior oblique muscle, which intorts the eye and moves it down when it is medially deviated. All other muscles, including the pupilloconstrictor and the levator of the upper lid, are controlled by the *oculomotor* (third cranial) nerve. Abnormalities of the cranial nerves in the brain stem are almost always associated with other neurological signs and are usually caused by vascular disturbances, tumors, or demyelinating disease. The peripheral nerves may be involved individually or together by lesions anywhere from their site of exit in the brain stem to their site of entry to the muscle. The nerves are most widely separated in the posterior fossa and run closest to each other in the cavernous sinus and superior orbital fissure. Accordingly, compressive lesions in the cavernous sinus usually cause multiple unilateral ocular palsies, whereas those in the posterior fossa may cause single (sometimes bilateral) nerve dysfunction. Intrinsic lesions of the third nerve (e.g., diabetic vasculopathy) often spare the pupil, whereas compressive lesions (tumors and aneurysms) involve the pupil early. Table 116–14 lists the major causes of acute ophthalmoplegia.

Conjugate Paralysis

Conjugate movement of the eyes is regulated by supranuclear pathways that descend from the forebrain to reach the medial longitudinal fasciculus in the brain stem. Unilateral hemispheral disease resulting from hemorrhage, infarct, or tumor acutely paralyzes conjugate gaze to the contralateral side and often causes deviation of the eyes to the ipsilateral side. Sometimes, particularly in deep-lying hemispheral hemorrhages involving the thalamus, the eyes deviate in the opposite direction. The eye deviation can usually be overcome by vestibular stimulation (p. 724) and is generally transient. Lesions of brain stem pathways cause more permanent conjugate paralysis to the ipsilateral side, with slight eye deviation to the contralateral side. This abnormality usually cannot be overcome by vestibular stimulation.

Lesions of the medial longitudinal fasciculus (MLF), which connects the third and sixth nerves in the brain stem, lead to *internuclear ophthalmoplegia*, in which the eyes at rest may either be parallel or show a mild skew deviation but move disjunctively on lateral gaze. (Skew deviation results from any of a number of lesions involving the brain stem and has little localizing value.) A characteristic of internuclear ophthalmoplegia is that during lateral gaze toward the side of the MLF lesion, the ipsilateral eye abducts and shows nystagmus (see below), whereas the contralateral adducting eye partially or completely fails to move nasally because of the failure of ascending impulses to reach the opposite third nerve nucleus. Internuclear ophthalmoplegia may be caused by an infarct from small vessel disease (e.g., systemic lupus erythematosus) or by demyelinating disease. Bilateral internuclear ophthalmoplegia is almost always a result of multiple sclerosis.

HEARING AND ITS IMPAIRMENTS

Symptoms of Auditory Dysfunction

Only two symptoms result from disease of the auditory system: The first is hearing impairment, sometimes associated with pitch distortion (diplacusis) as well as a decrease in the intensity of sound, and the second is tinnitus, a sound heard in the ear or head not arising from the external environment. Hearing loss is termed conductive (external and middle ear), sensorineural (cochlea and auditory nerve), or central (brain stem and cerebral hemispheres). The approach

TABLE 116–14. MAJOR CAUSES OF ACUTE (<48 HOURS) OPHTHALMOPLEGIA

CONDITION	DIAGNOSTIC FEATURES
Bilateral	
Botulism	Contaminated food, high altitude cooking, pupils involved
Myasthenia gravis	Fluctuating degree of paralysis; responds to edrophonium chloride IV
Wernicke's encephalopathy	Nutritional deficiency; responds to thiamine IV
Acute cranial polyneuropathy	Antecedent respiratory infection; elevated CSF protein
Brain stem stroke	Other brain stem signs
Unilateral	
Carotid-posterior communicating aneurysm	Third cranial nerve, pupil involved
Diabetic-idiopathic	Third or sixth cranial nerve, pupil spared
Myasthenia gravis	As above
Brain stem stroke	As above

to the patient complaining of hearing loss is illustrated in Figure 116–4.

Conductive hearing loss is characterized by equal loss of hearing at all frequencies and by well-preserved speech discrimination once the threshold for hearing is exceeded. The ear often feels full, as if "blocked." Bone conduction exceeds air conduction and, if unilateral, the Weber test (tuning fork in the center of the head) is referred to the deaf ear. With *sensorineural hearing loss*, one typically hears better for low- than for high-frequency tones, and it may be difficult to hear speech that is mixed with background noise; small increases in the intensity of sound may cause discom-

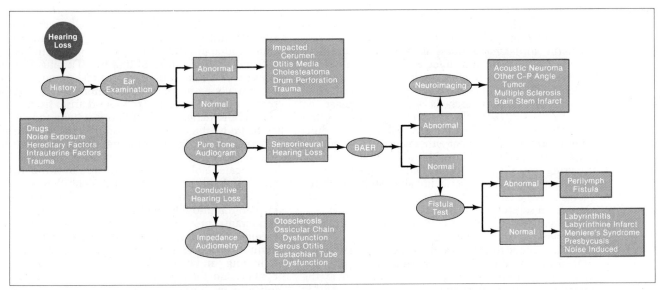

FIGURE 116–4. Evaluation of deafness (unilateral and bilateral). (From Baloh RW: The special senses. *In* Wyngaarden JB, Smith LH Jr (eds): Cecil Textbook of Medicine. 18th ed. Philadelphia, WB Saunders Co, 1988, p 2118.)

fort (recruitment). Air conduction exceeds bone conduction and the Weber test refers to the hearing ear. With hearing loss resulting from cochlear disease (usually due to selective destruction of hair cells), diplacusis and recruitment are common. *Central hearing loss* is uncommon and usually characterized by loss of speech more than of pure tone perception. Substantial central hearing loss requires bilateral lesions of such areas as inferior colliculus, medial geniculate bodies, or temporal lobe. When the primary receiving areas (Heschl's gyrus) are destroyed, hearing is diminished or absent even for pure tone. If association areas in the superior temporal gyrus are damaged, a patient may hear the sounds but be unable to comprehend their meaning.

Causes of Hearing Loss

Conductive hearing loss arises from abnormalities of the external or middle ear and can raise hearing threshold no more than 60 dB, since bone conduction is intact. Otoscopic examination may reveal obstruction in the external auditory meatus (the most common cause of conductive hearing loss) which impairs sound wave transmission to the tympanum. This benign condition is most often caused by *impacted cerumen*, but it occasionally results from canal infection or similar causes. A *fluid-filled middle ear*, a result of middle ear infection (otitis media), reduces movement of the ossicles against the oval window. If the otoscopic examination is negative, *otosclerosis*, a process in which the annular ligament that attaches the stapes to the oval window overgrows and calcifies, is a likely diagnosis. Chronic tinnitus sometimes marks the early stages of this process, which reduces ossicular transmission via the window to the cochlear basement membrane.

Sensorineural hearing loss from genetically determined deafness may be present at birth or develop in adulthood. The diagnosis of *hereditary deafness* rests on the finding of a positive family history.

Acute unilateral deafness usually has a cochlear basis. Bacterial or viral infections of the labyrinth, head trauma with fracture or hemorrhage into the cochlea, or vascular occlusion of a terminal branch of the anterior inferior cerebellar artery can damage the cochlea and its hair cells. An acute, idiopathic, often reversible, unilateral hearing loss strikes young adults and is presumed to reflect either a viral infection or a vascular disorder of the cochlea. Sudden unilateral hearing loss, often associated with vertigo and tinnitus, can result from a perilymphatic fistula. Such fistulae may be congenital, follow stapes surgery, or result from severe or mild trauma to the inner ear.

Drugs fairly often cause sudden bilateral hearing impairment. Salicylates, furosemide, and ethacrynic acid can cause intense tinnitus and transient deafness when taken in high doses. Aminoglycoside antibiotics can destroy cochlear hair cells in direct relation to the height of their serum concentrations, thereby causing permanent hearing loss. Some anticancer chemotherapeutic agents, particularly cisplatin, cause severe ototoxicity by a similar mechanism. Subacute, relapsing cochlear deafness occurs with *Meniere's syndrome*, a condition associated with fluctuating hearing loss and tinnitus, recurrent episodes of abrupt and often severe vertigo, and a sensation of fullness or pressure in the ear. Recurrent endolymphatic hypertension (hydrops) is believed to cause the episodes. Pathologically, the endolymphatic sac is dilated and contains atrophic hair cells. The resulting deafness is subtle and reversible in the early stages but subsequently becomes permanent. What hearing remains is characterized by *diplacusis* (a different pitch heard in the affected ear) and loudness recruitment (quiet sounds are not heard but loud sounds are heard as loud as or louder than in the good ear). The disorder is usually unilateral. When bilateral (< 20 per cent of cases), it begins in one ear before the other.

Gradually progressive hearing loss with age (*presbycusis*) reflects deterioration in the cochlear receptor system with degeneration of the hair cells, especially at the base. As a result, higher tones are lost early, a change similar to that which follows the recurrent trauma of noise-induced hearing loss from exposure to loud military or industrial noises or loud blaring modern music. Unilateral hearing loss that begins and progresses insidiously is characteristic of a benign neoplasm of the cerebellopontine angle (e.g., acoustic neuroma); a high-resolution CT or MR scan usually establishes that diagnosis.

Treatment of Hearing Loss. The best treatment is prevention. Early detection of noise- or drug-induced hearing loss and removal of the offending agent often preserves hearing. Otosclerosis can often be corrected by surgery; closure of a perilymph fistula may improve hearing. Hearing aids are helpful in patients with conductive hearing loss, and sometimes newer hearing aids help patients with cochlear or other sensorineural abnormalities.

Tinnitus

Tinnitus is the term applied generally to extraneous noises heard in one or both ears. Figure 116–5 illustrates the approach to the patient with tinnitus and lists most of the causes of tinnitus. Tinnitus is either *objective*, i.e., the patient hears a real sound, one that can usually be heard by the examiner with a stethoscope, or *subjective*, i.e., the sound arises from an abnormal discharge of the auditory system and cannot be heard by the observer. Most objective tinnitus has a benign cause, but the finding may also be an early sign of increased intracranial pressure. Such tinnitus, which can be obliterated by pressure over the jugular vein, probably arises from turbulent flow of compressed venous structures at the base of the brain. The symptom is also relieved transiently by decreasing the intracranial pressure, e.g., by lumbar puncture.

Subjective tinnitus can arise from anywhere in the auditory system. A faint, moderately high-pitched metallic ring can be observed by almost everyone if they concentrate their attention on auditory events in a quiet room. Sustained, louder tinnitus accompanied by audiometric evidence of deafness occurs in association with either conductive or sensorineural disease. The phenomenon can be a manifestation of sal-

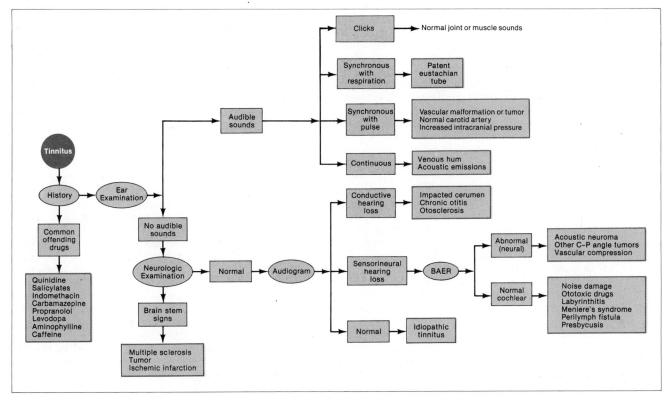

FIGURE 116–5. Evaluation of tinnitus. (Modified from Baloh RW: The special senses. *In* Wyngaarden JW, Smith LH Jr (eds): Cecil Textbook of Medicine. 18th ed. Philadelphia, WB Saunders Co, 1988, p 2120.)

icylate, quinine, or quinidine toxicity. Tinnitus observed with otosclerosis tends to have a roaring or hissing quality, while that associated with Meniere's syndrome often produces sounds that vary widely in intensity with time and quality, sometimes including roarings or clangings. Tinnitus with other cochlear or auditory nerve lesions tends to be higher-pitched and ringing in quality. Clanging or tonally fluctuating tinnitus or formed auditory hallucinations can be manifestations of temporal lobe seizures.

Treatment. If the underlying disorder causing objective tinnitus can be corrected, tinnitus may disappear. Most tinnitus is chronic, of no pathological importance, and can be overcome by the physician's reassurance and the patient's withdrawing attention from the symptom. Otherwise, masking noises placed into the ear sometimes make the patient more comfortable and better able to function.

DIZZINESS AND VERTIGO

Symptoms of Vestibular Dysfunction

The vestibular system, consisting of the bilateral semicircular canals and otolithic apparatus of the inner ear as well as their central connections, is a finely tuned discharging system. Any imbalance in input-output between the paired vestibular end organs or their primary receiving areas in the vestibular nuclei that is not caused by a true movement of the head or body produces a mismatch between vestibular stimulation and that going to other sense organs (especially the eyes and proprioceptive organs). This mismatch leads to an illusory sensation of movement in space, called vertigo. Vertigo is the only direct symptom of a vestibular abnormality, but because the vestibular system influences other neural systems, vertigo may be accompanied by autonomic symptoms (nausea, vomiting, diaphoresis), motor symptoms (ataxia, past pointing, falling), or ocular symptoms (oscillopsia—a visual sensation that the environment is moving). The clinical sign of a vestibular abnormality is *nystagmus*, a rhythmic to-and-fro movement of the eyes. Patients suffering from vertigo and nystagmus have an abnormality, either physiological or pathological, of the labyrinthine-vestibular system. As indicated on page 716, many patients are unable to distinguish vertigo from lightheadedness or other dizziness, and the physician must first determine whether the patient is truly vertiginous (see Table 116–12).

Nystagmus reflects an imbalance in the complex neural network that involves the visual pathways, the labyrinthine proprioceptive influences from neck muscles, the vestibular and cerebellar nuclei, the reticular formation of the pontine brain stem, and the oculomotor nuclei. It can be of two types: *Jerk nystagmus* consists of a slow phase away from the visual object followed by a quick saccade back toward the target. The quick eye movement describes the direction of jerk nystagmus. Benign jerk nystagmus, at the extremes of lateral gaze, is a common finding without pathological significance. It is more common with fatigue or poor lighting. Sustained gaze-evoked nystagmus with combined horizontal and torsional components inhibited by fixation suggests a peripheral lesion, whereas vertical nystagmus, particularly that which is not inhibited by fixation, suggests a central lesion. With rebound nystagmus there is nystagmus on lateral gaze that either disappears or reverses direction as the gaze position is held and then rebounds in the opposite direction when eyes are returned to the primary position. It is believed to be the only kind of nystagmus that specifically implicates cerebellar disease. *Pendular nystagmus* describes nystagmus usually slow and coarse and equal in rate in both directions. It is usually congenital in origin or develops after birth as a result of severe visual impairment but can occasionally be a symptom of cerebellum or brain stem disease.

Purely horizontal fine nystagmus at the extremes of gaze is a common finding without pathological significance. It is more common with fatigue or poor lighting. When bidirectional gaze-evoked nystagmus is prominent or involves vertical as well as horizontal movements to an equal degree, excessive sedative or anticonvulsant drug ingestion is most often the cause.

Several unusual forms of nystagmus have neurological localizing qualities: *Dissociated nystagmus*, i.e., unequal in the two eyes, implies a brain stem lesion. *Periodic alternating nystagmus* consists of a horizontal jerk nystagmus that changes its direction periodically. It has been associated with a variety of posterior fossa abnormalities, especially those involving the region of the craniocervical junction. *Downbeat nystagmus* produces downward jerks with the eyes in the primary gaze position; it often reflects a craniocervical abnormality such as the Arnold-Chiari malformation but can occur with parenchymal lesions such as multiple sclerosis. Some subjects have the capacity to induce *voluntary nystagmus*, which is extremely rapid, occurs in short bursts of 10 to 15 seconds or so, is present on the extremes of gaze, and may be unequal in the two eyes.

Other abnormalities of conjugate eye movements include *ocular bobbing*, consisting of fast conjugate downward eye jerks followed by a slow return to the primary gaze position. The phenomenon accompanies severe displacement or destruction of the pons or, much less often, metabolic CNS depression. *Ocular myoclonus* consists of continuous, rhythmic, pendular oscillations, most often vertical, with a rate of two to five beats per second. Often it accompanies palatal myoclonus and has a similar pathogenesis. Square wave jerks (defined by electronystagmography) and *ocular flutter* consist of brief, intermittent, horizontal oscillations arising from the primary gaze position. The abnormalities blend into *opsoclonus*, a pattern of rapid, chaotic, conjugate, repetitive saccadic eye movements ("dancing eyes"). Both of these disorders reflect cerebellar or brain stem dysfunction and also can emerge as a remote effect of systemic neoplasm, especially neuroblastoma in children. *Ocular dysmetria* consists of saccadic overshoots or undershoots of conjugate eye movement during rapid saccadic shifts of visual fixation. The phenomenon reflects cerebellar dysfunction.

Laboratory Tests of Vestibular Function

Bedside *caloric tests* (Fig. 116–6) induce vertigo. With the patient lying supine and the head elevated approximately 30 degrees, water either 7 degrees above or below body temperature is douched against the tympanic membrane. In the normal situation, cold water produces nystagmus away from the side of stimulation (because of inhibition of the horizontal semicircular canal) and warm water nystagmus to the side of stimulation (because of stimulation of the semicircular canal). An astute patient suffering from labyrinthine vertigo can often tell which stimulation reproduces the symptoms, thus assisting in the localization of the lesion. Absence of the caloric response on one side suggests ipsilateral labyrinthine failure. Because most peripheral nystagmus is partially inhibited by the visual fixation of the open eyes, accurate quantitative evaluation requires electrical recording of the eye movement with the eyes closed. *Electronystagmography* can be performed in the resting position, with the head rotated into various positions to provoke nystagmus, and before, during, and after caloric stimulation. Electronystagmography is often helpful in identifying the pathology of the vestibular system and localizing it when identified.

Causes of Vertigo

Vertigo can be either physiological or pathological. *Physiological vertigo* occurs when there is a mismatch among the vestibular, visual, and somatosensory systems induced by an external stimulus. Common examples of physiological vertigo include motion sickness, height vertigo (the sensation that occurs when one looks down from a great height), and visual vertigo (the sensation sometimes felt when one views a motion picture of a roller coaster or other violent movement). In almost all instances, the diagnosis is clear from the history. One exception may be head extension vertigo, a sensation of vertigo or postural imbalance induced with the head maximally extended while standing; the sensation abruptly stops when the head is flexed to a neutral position. The symptoms may mistakenly be attributed to vertebral artery insufficiency. Head extension vertigo does not occur when the head is extended in the lying position and appears rarely when sitting. If physiological vertigo becomes a clinical problem, it is best treated by supplying sensory cues that help to match the various sensory systems. Thus, motion sickness, which is often exacerbated by sitting in a closed space or reading, giving the visual system the miscue that the environment is stationary, may be relieved by looking out at the environment and watching it move.

CONDITION: OCULAR REFLEXES IN UNCONSCIOUS PATIENTS

FIGURE 116–6. The upper section illustrates the oculocephalic (*above*) and oculovestibular (*below*) reflexes in an unconscious patient whose brain stem ocular pathways are intact. Lateral conjugate eye movements (*upper left*) to head turning are full and opposite in direction to the movement of the face. A stronger stimulus to lateral deviation is achieved by douching cold water against the tympanic membrane(s). There is tonic conjugate deviation of both eyes toward the stimulus. Because the patient is unconscious, there is no nystagmus. Extension of the neck in a patient with a similar condition produces conjugate deviation of the eyes in the downward direction, and flexion of the neck produces deviation of the eyes upward. Bilateral cold water against the tympanic membrane likewise produces conjugate downward deviation of the eyes, whereas warm (38–42 °C) water causes conjugate upward deviation of the eyes. The middle drawing shows the effects of bilateral medial longitudinal fasciculus lesions on oculocephalic and oculovestibular reflexes. The left portion of the drawing illustrates that oculocephalic and oculovestibular stimulation deviates the ipsilateral eye laterally and brings the contralateral eye only to the midline, since connections between the abducens and oculomotor nuclei are interrupted. Vertical eye movements often remain intact. The lower portion of the drawing illustrates the effects of a low brain stem or severe metabolic lesion. Neither oculovestibular nor oculocephalic movements cause deviation of the eyes. (From Plum F and Posner JB, Diagnosis of Stupor and Coma, 3rd ed. Philadelphia, FA Davis, 1982.)

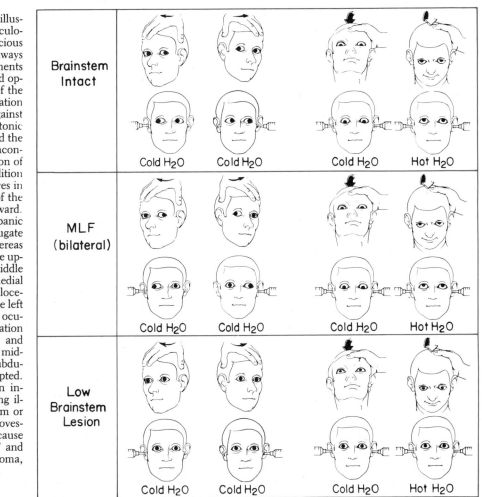

Brainstem Intact — Cold H₂O — Cold H₂O — Cold H₂O — Hot H₂O

MLF (bilateral) — Cold H₂O — Cold H₂O — Cold H₂O — Hot H₂O

Low Brainstem Lesion — Cold H₂O — Cold H₂O — Cold H₂O — Hot H₂O

Height vertigo caused by a mismatch between sensation of normal body sway and lack of its visual detection can often be relieved by the patient either sitting or visually fixing a nearby stationary object.

Pathological vertigo usually arises from an abnormality of the vestibular system but less commonly can be produced by visual or somatic sensory disorders. Vestibular vertigo can be caused by disease of either the peripheral or central vestibular apparatus (Table 116–15). In general, peripheral vertigo is more intense, more likely to be associated with hearing loss and tinnitus, and often leads to nausea and vomiting. Nystagmus associated with peripheral vertigo is frequently inhibited by visual fixation. Central vertigo is generally less severe, more sustained, and often associated with other signs of central nervous system disease. The nystagmus of central vertigo is not inhibited by visual fixation and frequently is disproportionately prominent to the degree of vertigo. Figure 116–7 illustrates the diagnostic approach to the vertiginous patient.

Benign positional vertigo is an extremely common disorder of middle and old age which accounts for the symptoms of at least 25 per cent of such patients with vertigo. Typically, the patient first experiences severe whirling vertigo when turning over, first lying down in bed at night, or arising in the morning. Less commonly, the patient may experience similar symptoms when he turns suddenly while standing or walking. Usually the symptoms are greatest when the patient lies on his side with the affected ear undermost. The vertigo is delayed for several seconds following the motion, sudden in onset, very severe, and may be accompanied by nausea or vomiting. The patient usually reports that the vertigo ceases when he moves out of the position that causes it, but in fact if he remains in that position, it rarely lasts more than a minute. The pathophysiology of the disorder is not established. Some investigators have postulated that debris from otoliths may enter the posterior canal to artificially stimulate it in the dependent position. The diagnosis is made by the characteristic history and the reproduction of the attack by the Nylen-Bárány maneuvers

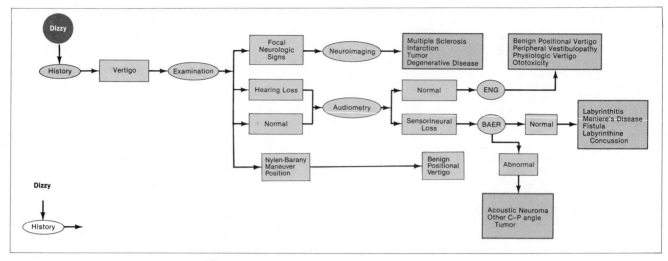

FIGURE 116–7. Evaluation of vertigo. (From Baloh RW: The special senses. *In* Wyngaarden JW, Smith LH Jr (eds): Cecil Textbook of Medicine. 18th ed. Philadelphia, WB Saunders Co, 1988, p 2122.)

(p. 716). The illness usually lasts several weeks and then resolves, but may recur. If the patient has the classic history and physical findings, no further evaluation is necessary. If the history or findings are atypical, the condition must be distinguished from other causes of vertigo and nystagmus, such as tumor or infarct of the posterior fossa. Typical benign positional vertigo is very rarely associated with such conditions. The treatment for most patients is simple reassurance. Since the vertigo can be fatigued, many patients find that repetitively reproducing the sudden head movement each day gives them prolonged relief.

    Peripheral Vestibulopathy. This disorder, also called acute labyrinthitis or vestibular neuronitis, may occur as a single bout or may recur repeatedly over months or years. The vertigo is acute, severe, and often associated with nausea and vomiting. Attacks sometimes follow a respiratory infection. The vertigo may be so severe that the patient is unable to sit or stand without vomiting and ataxia. He prefers to lie absolutely still in bed with the involved ear uppermost. Nystagmus is invariably present, usually horizontal or rotatory, and directed away from the involved labyrinth. The severe symptoms usually improve substantially within 48 to 72 hours, allowing the patient to be up and about. However, many patients report that for weeks or months following the episode sudden movements of the head produce mild vertigo or nausea. Although the disorder is called *acute labyrinthitis,* suggesting a viral infection of the labyrinth, EMG evoked potential studies suggest that in many patients there are accompanying eighth nerve or brain stem abnormalities, leading some to refer to the disorder as *vestibular neuronitis.* Labyrinthine fistulae have been reported to produce episodic vertigo. Fistula testing by a skilled otolaryngologist should establish that diagnosis. There has been a recent suggestion that some vertigo results from compression of the vestibular nerve by blood vessels of the posterior fossa in a manner analogous to trigeminal neuralgia (p. 712). *Other peripheral causes of vertigo* include Meniere's syndrome (p. 722) and the taking of vestibulotoxic drugs, most of which are also ototoxic (p. 722). Vertigo may be an additional symptom in patients suffering from *sudden hearing loss.* The pathogenesis of the disorder is unknown but may be vascular in some, viral infections in others. Bacterial infection of the labyrinth or occasionally otitis media causes vertigo. Degenerative and genetic abnormalities of the labyrinthine system can cause vertigo. *Cervical vertigo* is the term given to the feelings of dysequilibrium associated with head movement described by some patients with cervical osteoarthritis or spondylosis. The disorder probably is caused by unbalanced input from cervical muscles to the vestibular apparatus. Acute neck strain may be occasionally associated with vertigo. Local anesthetics injected into one side of the neck can produce vertigo and ataxia by a similar lack of balanced input. There is no nystagmus in these disorders.

TABLE 116–15. CAUSES OF VESTIBULAR VERTIGO

PERIPHERAL CAUSES	CENTRAL CAUSES
Peripheral vestibulopathy*	Brain stem ischemia
Labyrinthitis and/or vestibular neuronitis	Cerebellopontine angle tumors
Acute and recurrent peripheral vestibulopathy	Demyelinating disease
	Cranial neuropathy
"Benign" positional vertigo*	Seizure disorders (rare)
Meniere's syndrome*	Heredofamilial disorders
Vestibulotoxic drugs	Spinocerebellar degeneration
Focal labryrinthine–third cranial nerve disease	Friedreich's ataxia
Trauma	Olivopontocerebellar atrophy, etc.
Cancer	Other central causes
Infection	Brain stem tumors
Otosclerosis	Cerebellar degenerations
Perilymph fistula	Paraneoplastic syndromes

* Common causes of acute severe vertigo.

CENTRAL VERTIGO

Central causes of vertigo, less common than peripheral causes, are characterized by less severe vertigo than that resulting from peripheral lesions, no hearing loss or tinnitus, and concomitant neurological signs of brain stem or cerebellar dysfunction.

Cerebrovascular Disease. If ischemia, infarction, or hemorrhage affects the brain stem or cerebellum, vertigo accompanied by nausea and vomiting is a relatively common symptom. Occipital headache as well as nystagmus and other neurological signs suggesting brain stem or cerebellar dysfunction usually accompany vertigo. Rarely, vertigo (nonpositional) is the sole symptom of *transient ischemic attacks* of the brain stem, but most patients suffering such attacks will, if carefully questioned, report headache, diplopia, facial or body numbness, and ataxia as well.

Cerebellopontine Angle Tumors. Most tumors growing in the cerebellopontine angle (e.g., acoustic neuroma, meningioma) grow slowly, allowing the vestibular system to accommodate, and thus they usually produce vague sensations of dysequilibrium rather than acute vertigo. Frequently such neoplasms produce complaints of tinnitus, hearing loss, and a sensation that the person is being pulled or pushed when he walks. Occasionally episodic vertigo or positional vertigo will herald the presence of a cerebellopontine angle tumor. Virtually all affected patients will have retrocochlear hearing loss and decreased or absent caloric responses on the involved side. Careful CT or MR scans through the temporal bone and posterior fossa usually reveal the tumor.

Demyelinating Disease. Acute vertigo may be the first symptom of *multiple sclerosis*, although only a small percentage of young patients with acute vertigo eventually develop multiple sclerosis. Vertigo may also be a symptom of *parainfectious encephalomyelitis* or, rarely, *parainfectious cranial polyneuritis* of the Guillain-Barré type. In this instance, the accompanying neurological signs establish the diagnosis.

Cranial Neuropathy. A variety of acute or subacute illnesses affecting the eighth cranial nerve can produce vertigo as an early or sole symptom, the most common being *herpes zoster*. The *Ramsay Hunt syndrome (geniculate ganglion herpes)* is characterized by vertigo and hearing loss, variably associated with facial paralysis and sometimes pain in the ear. The typical lesions of herpes zoster, which may follow the appearance of neurological signs, are found in the external auditory canal and sometimes over the palate. Whether herpes zoster is ever responsible for vertigo in the absence of the full-blown syndrome is not certain. *Granulomatous meningitis* or *leptomeningeal metastases* and cerebral or systemic *vasculitis* may involve the eighth nerve, producing vertigo as an early symptom. In these disorders, cerebrospinal fluid analysis usually suggests the diagnosis.

Seizure Disorders. Patients suffering from temporal lobe epilepsy occasionally suffer vertigo as the aura. Vertigo in the absence of other neurological signs or symptoms, however, is never caused by epilepsy or other diseases of the cerebral hemispheres.

Other Central Causes. Many structural lesions of the brain stem or cerebellum, particularly if rapid in onset, may cause vertigo. In a few instances, vertigo may initiate the symptoms of *paraneoplastic brain stem or cerebellar degeneration*. As with *brain stem tumors, cerebellar degenerative diseases* and other structural disease of the brain stem and posterior fossa, there are usually other neurological symptoms, almost always including signs of brain stem or cerebellar dysfunction in addition to the vertigo and nystagmus.

Treatment

The best treatment of symptomatic vertigo is to cure the underlying disease. In many instances, however, that is not possible and one must resort to symptomatic treatment only. In acute vertigo, such as occurs with labyrinthitis, most patients insist on being at bedrest. Vestibulosedative drugs such as meclizine or diazepam may be helpful. Prochlorperazine suppositories can be used to circumvent vomiting. Vestibulosuppressive drugs such as meclizine also sometimes help more chronic vertiginous disorders. Scopolamine, 0.4 to 0.8 mg, together with methylphenidate, 5 mg orally, may give relief of vertigo, particularly motion sickness. Recently, transdermal scopolamine paste-on units placed behind the ear have been reported to be effective in preventing motion sickness for up to 72 hours. These, like all scopolamine products, may produce anticholinergic side effects. If head or neck movement precipitates vertigo, a cervical collar sometimes relieves the symptoms.

REFERENCES

Baloh WR: Dizziness, Hearing Loss, and Tinnitus: The Essentials of Neurotology. Philadelphia, FA Davis Co, 1984.
Zee DS, Leigh RJ: Disorders of Ocular Movement. Philadelphia, FA Davis Co, 1983.

C. DISORDERS OF SOMATIC SENSATION

EVALUATION OF SYMPTOMS AND SIGNS

Disorders of somatic sensation can arise from dysfunction that involves sensory pathways anywhere along their course from receptors in skin, subcutaneous tissue, muscle, or viscera to the somatosensory areas of the parietal lobe of the cerebral cortex. Between these extremes, sensory fibers traverse peripheral nerves to reach their cell bodies in the dorsal root ganglia and then enter the spinal cord. Pathways subserving the sensations of pain and temperature synapse in the posterior horn, cross, and ascend contralaterally to reach the thalamus. Those subserving proprioception and light touch ascend ipsilaterally in the spinal cord to synapse in the brain stem and then cross to reach the contralateral thalamus. Because sensory fibers are so intimately associated with fibers subserving other neurological functions in almost their entire anatomical pathway, isolated disorders of somatic sensation are uncommon. Furthermore, although somatic sensory symptoms are a source of many patient complaints, testing sensation often yields uncertain results, leading physicians to depend on more objective motor or reflex abnormalities to establish anatomical localization and etiology of the disorder. Thus, most abnormalities of somatic sensation are discussed along with their accompanying motor abnormalities (e.g., peripheral nerve disorders) or under the various causative diseases (e.g., neoplasms or vascular disease of the brain or spinal cord). Only a few purely sensory disorders are discussed here. Abnormalities of sensory pathways causing pain are discussed in Section A of this chapter.

EVALUATION OF THE PATIENT

Somatosensory disorders may diminish, increase, or distort sensation depending on the pattern and intensity of the damage to sensory pathways: Diminution of function is readily recognized by the patient as an inability to perceive normally touch (hypesthesia or anesthesia), pain (hypalgesia or analgesia), or temperature. Hyperfunction of a disordered sensory system is perceived as tingling sensations (paresthesias) that are present spontaneously or when the disturbed area is stimulated either by increased sensitivity to touch or a noxious stimulation such as sometimes occurs following a sunburn (hyperesthesia or hyperpathia). Dysesthesias are unpleasant or painful sensations produced by stimuli that are ordinarily painless (allodynia).

Mild sensory abnormalities, readily perceived by the patient, often cannot be confirmed on examination. In this situation the patient should be asked to describe the abnormality as precisely as possible and to map its distribution. Many patients will gently rub the affected part, using both temporal and spatial summation to produce an after-discharge (paresthesia) and map the distribution. Such careful mapping allows the physician to determine whether the sensory abnormality is in the distribution of a single nerve (e.g., meralgia paresthetica), many nerves (sensory peripheral neuropathy), a nerve root, or a portion of the central nervous system. The physician should attempt to document sensory complaints by careful sensory testing. The point of a safety pin suffices to test pain sensation (many patients with intact touch sensation can distinguish the sharp from a dull end of a pin even though the pin does not feel "sharp," i.e., painful). Sensory testing for all modalities should be carried from the area of impaired sensation to a normal area, asking the patient to carefully note the boundary. The threshold for each sensation is best compared with the examiner's threshold, recognizing that threshold for vibration and touch sensation may diminish somewhat with age. Touch can be tested with light cotton, vibration with a 128-Hz tuning fork, and position sense by moving the joints through a small range of motion and asking the patient the direction in which the joint moves. All patients should be tested to see if they can identify objects in the hands (stereognosis) and if they can distinguish two points 2 to 3 mm apart in the fingertips. Sensory examinations are difficult to perform and particularly fail in patients who are fatigued. Thus, one may have to do the examination at several sittings, recognizing that the boundaries of a sensory abnormality may change from time to time even with a fixed defect.

Deep tendon reflexes disappear early in patients with large fiber sensory abnormalities, because dysfunction of the large fiber afferent arc impairs simultaneous firing of the monosynaptic stretch reflex. The clinical implication is that patients with normal deep tendon reflexes (in particular the ankle reflexes) are not suffering a substantial large fiber sensory neuropathy.

SPECIFIC DISORDERS OF SENSATION

Isolated disorders of somatic sensation occur in two settings. The first is when a focal structural disorder strikes a portion of the nervous system that is restricted to subserving sensation. Examples are entrapment neuropathies of pure sensory nerves (e.g., lateral cutaneous nerve of the thigh), compression of the sensory portion of a nerve root in a herniated disc, a small syrinx damaging only spinal thalamic fibers crossing in the anterior commissure of the spinal cord, and small infarcts or tumors restricted to the sensory thalamus, or, less often, the somatosensory cortex. All of these disorders except sensory mononeuropathies are described under appropriate headings in later chapters. The second instance is when a genetic, metabolic, or degenerative disorder affects sensory fibers as a system, sparing intermixed motor fibers. The best example of widespread diseases of the sensory system are the acute and subacute sensory neuropathies in which either axonal damage affects sensory nerves or a direct attack damages dorsal root ganglion cells (see Fig. 117–6). A second example is a very rare disorder called *congenital universal indifference to pain*, which is characterized by normal sensation except for a lifelong absence of appreciation of pain anywhere in the body. The pathophysiological basis of this condition is not known.

Mononeuropathies or monoradiculopathies are usually caused by entrapment of nerves passing through small spaces (e.g., intervertebral foramen, thoracic outlet, carpal tunnel) and may cause only somatic sensory manifestations. The most common pure sensory disorder is *meralgia paresthetica*, an entrapment neuropathy resulting from compression of the lateral cutaneous nerve of the thigh which passes under the inguinal ligament. Obese persons wearing tight belts and those with pendulous abdomens are especially prone to develop numbness or burning sensations over the lateral thigh. Sometimes prolonged standing or walking provokes the symptoms. Weight reduction may help, but in many cases the condition subsides spontaneously. Because there are no motor fibers in the lateral cutaneous nerve of the thigh, weakness never develops. A similar syndrome can affect the dorsal aspect of the thumb when a tight watchband compresses a cutaneous branch of the radial nerve. Carpal tunnel and thoracic outlet syndromes may be purely sensory in the beginning; they cause serious disability only if motor fibers are involved as well.

Compression of sensory nerve roots or sensory pathways in the spinal cord, such as occurs with herniated discs or cervical or lumbar spondylosis, is discussed on page 750. Herpes zoster may cause sensory loss (and pain) in the distribution of the affected nerve root.

Polyneuropathies (p. 756) may begin with sensory loss or, less often, remain purely sensory. *Acute inflammatory sensory neuropathy*, or neuronopathy, is probably the sensory counterpart of the motor polyradiculopathy of the Guillain-Barré syndrome. The disorder, which is substantially rarer than the Guillain-Barré syndrome, may follow a banal infection by several weeks and is characterized by rapid onset of sensory loss and pain. Any region of the body may be affected, usually symmetrically. Such patients often are severely incapacitated by dysesthesias and proprioceptive loss to hands and legs which prevent walking or fine movements. Tendon reflexes usually disappear. Examination of the cerebrospinal fluid may yield an increased protein level. Nerve conduction velocities are often normal, whereas sensory reaction potentials cannot be elicited. Unlike with the Guillain-Barré syndrome, the prognosis for recovery is poor, patients usually being left with substantial disability resulting from the sensory loss.

A clinical picture similar to that of the above inflammatory sensory neuropathy is sometimes encountered as a "remote effect" of cancer on the nervous system. This disorder is also subacute in onset, generally is nonremitting, and may be associated with other signs of central nervous system dysfunction (encephalomyelitis). It is usually associated with a localized and often occult small cell carcinoma of the lung. Patients rarely recover even if the underlying cancer is successfully treated. The pathology is that of dorsal root ganglion cell destruction, accompanied by local inflammatory infiltrates.

Hereditary sensory neuropathies are rare inherited disorders of sensory fibers. Type I is a dominantly inherited radicular neuropathy that affects pain and temperature sensation more than touch and proprioception. It may lead to perforating ulcers of the feet. The disorder is slowly progressive, and the diagnosis is made by the family history. Types II and III are recessive disorders that begin in childhood. Type III (dysautonomic or Riley-Day) is also associated with autonomic dysfunction. Familial amyloid disease similarly causes maximal damage to pain and autonomic fibers.

Many of the metabolic and toxic neuropathies (p. 757) begin as or remain predominantly sensory disorders. This is true of diabetic and uremic neuropathies as well as those caused by cisplatin, pyridoxine, isoniazid, and thalidomide (Table 116–16).

TABLE 116–16. PREDOMINANTLY OR EXCLUSIVELY SENSORY POLYNEUROPATHY

Metabolic	Toxins
Diabetes	Arsenic
Uremia	Acrylamide
Paraproteinemia	Thallium
Amyloidosis	Trichlorethylene (face)
Drugs	**Miscellaneous**
Pyridoxine	Parainfectious
Cisplatin	Paraneoplastic
Thalidomide	Rheumatoid arthritis
Isoniazid	

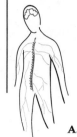

A. INTRODUCTION AND EVALUATION OF THE PATIENT

Muscles move the world, directed by the brain and its efferent motor pathways. Dysfunction anywhere along the line, including muscle, myoneural junction, efferent motor nerve plexus or nerve roots, cranio-spinal motor neuron pool, descending corticospinal systems, basal ganglia, or cerebellum, can interfere with the normal strength, coordination, and automatic postural controls that are required to complete the voluntary motor act. Furthermore, disordered somatic perception, in particular proprioception, often disables the motor system as much as true paralysis.

At the supraspinal level, the corticospinal system includes the premotor and primary motor cortex of the cerebrum as well as the red and vestibular nuclei of the brain stem and the reticular formation of the brain stem and spinal cord. Collectively, these cortical and subcortical areas transmit *parallel* motor signals that descend to converge upon the segmental craniospinal interneurons and lower motor neurons (Fig. 117–1). In varying degrees, depending upon the individual case and the anatomical distribution of the lesion, their dysfunction results in the syndromes of the *upper*

motor neuron as described in a subsequent paragraph.

In contrast to the parallel descending upper motor neuron systems, both the basal ganglia and the cerebellum normally exert their major controls on voluntary movement *in series* with the cerebral cortex (Fig. 117–1); i.e., they project their signals to the latter structure before it sends its final commands caudally to the segmental neuron pools. During the initiation of voluntary movement, signals from the frontal and parietal lobes flash to the basal ganglia and cerebellum and back again to the cortex a few milliseconds before the motor cortex transmits its final message spinalwards. The process guarantees normal postural supports and the coordination of movement. Furthermore, the arrangement means that both basal ganglia and cerebellar hemispheric (neocerebellar) diseases express their symptoms through the descending upper motor neuron systems rather than by directly influencing the spinal motor neuron pool. This feature helps to explain why signs of basal ganglia and cerebellar abnormality tend to disappear during sleep or if a corticospinal hemiplegia develops.

HISTORY

The examination of the motor system begins with the taking of a history. Most persons promptly recognize a recently developing or rapidly progressing muscle motor loss but tend to ignore insidiously developing, painless weakness until it produces substantial functional disability (e.g., inability to climb stairs). Families or physicians may sometimes detect such gradually evolving limitations that do not cause functional disability (e.g., limping or dragging a leg) before the patient does. Most patients with motor system disorders complain of "weakness," although an occasional patient uses the term "numbness" to indicate that objects drop from the weak hand. Some patients use the term "weakness" to mean fatigability, asthenia, or even incoordination. Patients should be pressed to be specific about the terms they use and, if they are truly weak, to describe which motor acts are limited. In the legs, proximal muscle weakness is usually characterized by difficulty getting out of low chairs or off the toilet seat or climbing stairs, whereas distal motor weakness is characterized by tripping because of failure to dorsiflex the foot while walking on irregular ground or climbing stairs or curbs. Proximal motor weakness in the upper extremity is characterized by difficulty using a hair dryer or lifting heavy objects above the head and distal weakness by inability to turn ignition keys or door knobs or to press a stiff aerosol can. Facial weakness is appreciated by the appearance of the face in the mirror, a tendency to drool from the paralyzed lips, or mild dysarthria caused by failure of the lips to move normally during speech.

An observant patient can help the physician distinguish upper from lower motor weakness (Table 117–1) by recognizing that in upper motor neuron weakness skilled movements are disabled out of proportion to crude strength (e.g., a patient with lower motor neuron weakness can type if his fingers move; a patient with upper motor neuron weakness, even if strength is adequate, cannot achieve the rhythm necessary for typing). Patients with lower motor neuron or muscle disorders do not complain of stiffness (the exception is myotonic dystrophy). Patients with upper motor neuron disorders (and some disorders of basal ganglia) recognize that their movements are limited by increased tone. They use the term "stiffness" to mean either spasticity or rigidity. Clonus and flexor spasms (do your legs jump in bed at night?) complicate only cortical spinal tract disease and not basal ganglia disorders. Muscle cramps occurring spontaneously at night or with attempted exercise suggest lower motor neuron disability.

The patient usually recognizes the presence of most adventitious movement (Table 117–2). Most of these abnormal movements are also present when the physician examines the patient and are easier to define by direct inspection than by the patient's report. The exceptions are fasciculations that the patient may note from time to time but that may not be present during the examination (fasciculations unaccompanied by weakness are always benign but may concern a patient

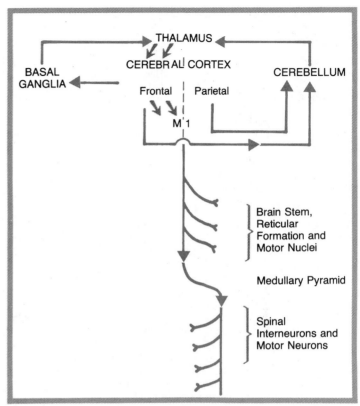

FIGURE 117–1. The principal supranuclear influences on motor control, greatly simplified. The cerebral cortex sends signals to both the basal ganglia and the cerebellum before initiating movement. The latter two structures, in turn, predominantly feed signals forward via the thalamus to the cortex, which guarantee the programming of postural activity that makes possible the subsequent skilled movement and automatic acts. The brain stem reticular formation and other major motor nuclei receive corticospinal and cerebellar projections and, in turn, send additional descending fibers that join the corticospinal pathway to make up the upper motor neuron system.

TABLE 117–1. CLINICAL SIGNS OF UPPER AND LOWER MOTOR NEURON LESIONS

	UPPER	LOWER
Paralysis	Mostly distal, distributed in major body part	Proximal or distal, distributed by nerve root or anterior horn cell anatomy
Atrophy	Minimal, late, disuse	Prominent, early, neurotropic
Fasciculations	Absent	Often present
Spasticity	Present	Absent
Deep tendon reflexes	Increased	Decreased or absent
Babinski reflex	Present	Absent

TABLE 117–2. MAJOR MOVEMENT DISORDERS

Tremor	Dystonia (Table 117–3)
Parkinson's	Athetosis (congenital)
Cerebellar	Dyskinesia
Familial—senile	Hemifacial spasm
Chorea	Levodopa-associated
Huntington's	Tardive
Sydenham's	
Lupus- or pregnancy-related	

who recognizes their relationship to motor neuron disease).

EXAMINATION

The examination of the motor system is a part of the general neurological examination and in the absence of specific complaints proceeds as indicated on page 670. If the history suggests disease of the motor system, individual muscles of the face, neck, trunk, and each extremity must be tested for *strength* and *fatigability*. Most patients with motor system diseases fatigue only modestly. Patients with myasthenia gravis may have normal strength with initial contraction but after several seconds of sustained contraction become weak. Patients with a Lambert-Eaton myasthenic syndrome, on the other hand, may gain strength over a few seconds and become essentially normal. Facial weakness is usually obvious to the physician during the interview. Lower motor neuron facial weakness is characterized by inability to raise the brow, close the eyes, or move the corner of the mouth. On the other hand, unilateral upper motor neuron facial weakness is characterized by drooping of the corner of the mouth and decreased definition of the nasolabial fold. Eye closure, although weak, appears normal on blinking, and elevation of the brow is usually possible as well. Neck muscles can be individually tested by having the patient rotate his chin against resistance (contralateral sternocleidomastoid) and flex the neck against resistance (bilateral sternocleidomastoids) or extend the head against resistance. Patients with myasthenia gravis often complain of difficulty holding the head upright, whereas with other myopathies neck flexion tends to be weaker than neck extension.

Tone is tested by passively flexing, extending, and rotating the resting extremities. *Spasticity* is marked by length and shortening reactions so that increased resistance at the beginning of the movement may suddenly cease (clasp-knife phenomenon). *Rigidity* associated with basal ganglia disease, on the other hand, demonstrates the same increase in tone throughout the full range of the movement. Paresis from lower motor neuron dysfunction is generally associated with a decrease in tone. A similar decrease in tone may mark cerebellar disease.

Deep tendon reflexes should be normally symmetrical. Hyperactive reflexes, including clonus, if symmetrical, can result from anxiety as well as from upper motor neuron disease. Hypoactive or absent deep tendon reflexes may also be physiological if symmetrical. Pathologically absent reflexes with relatively normal strength commonly is an early sign of peripheral nerve disease (either afferent or efferent) but is rare with disease of the neuromuscular junction or the muscle itself (the Lambert-Eaton syndrome, in which lower extremity reflexes are usually absent, is an exception). Conversely, substantial weakness with preservation of deep tendon reflexes suggests that the disorder is in the neuromuscular junction or muscle rather than the peripheral nerve. The masseter reflex (jaw jerk) is usually difficult to elicit but, if grossly hyperactive, suggests a disorder of the cortical spinal tracts above the foramen magnum, useful in distinguishing spinal cord from cerebral hemisphere disease. Superficial abdominal and cremasteric reflexes are rarely helpful diagnostically in and of themselves but their reduction or absence may add to other evidence of unilateral dysfunction of lower motor neuron or cortical spinal tract. The Babinski and related responses are nociceptive withdrawal reflexes that are elicited by delivering a noxious stimulus (usually a scrape or a scratch) to the lateral aspect of the sole or foot. A positive response (dorsiflexion of the great toe), sometimes accompanied by dorsiflexion of the foot and flexion of the knee and hip (the triple flexion response), is pathognomonic of cortical spinal tract dysfunction. Unfortunately, the response is often made equivocal by voluntary withdrawal, so that in the absence of other unequivocal evidence of cortical spinal tract disease the Babinski test is rarely diagnostic. In fact, in the absence of confirming evidence on the neurological examination, an equivocal Babinski test is more likely to be misleading than helpful.

The patient should be examined for *rapidly alternating movements* by having him rapidly pronate and supinate the outstretched arms, rapidly tap the examiner's hand, or repeatedly oppose the thumb and index finger. In the lower extremities rapidly alternating movements can be tested by having the patient tap the examiner's hand with his foot. Rapidly alternating movements are slow and sometimes awkward with cortical spinal tract disease and with diseases of the basal ganglia. Lower motor neuron, neuromuscular, or muscular dysfunction should not affect rapidly alternating movements unless the extremity is paralyzed. Extremely awkward rapidly alternating movements, in which the movement breaks up, suggests cerebellar disease. *Point-to-point* tests, including having the patient rapidly place his index finger on his nose and then touch the examiner's index finger held at arm's length from the nose, are slow and awkward with cortical spinal tract and basal ganglia disease but are performed accurately. In cerebellar disease or loss of proprioception the movements break up, usually with a side-to-side tremor-like movement as the patient attempts to correct errors in range and rate. If the disorder is proprioceptive it will worsen substantially with the eyes closed, whereas if the disorder is cerebellar the worsening is only moderate. The same phenomenon can be tested in the lower extremities by having the patient place his heel on his knee and run it down the shin or by having him attempt to stand with the feet either opposed to each other or one in front of the other (tandem stand).

Adventitious movements are usually apparent during the course of the interview. A patient with chorea, athetosis, or dystonia is in almost constant movement during the interview. More subtle chorea can be detected by watching the patient hold his arms outstretched or asking him to continuously squeeze the examiner's fingers with his hand. Repetitive break-up in the squeezing movements suggests chorea, as do jerky movements of the outstretched fingers. An alternating tremor with the patient sitting relaxed suggests Parkinson's disease, particularly if the tremor is inhibited by attempted motion. On the contrary, if the tremor is absent at rest and is exacerbated by motion, it more likely is due either to cerebellar disease or essential tremor. Fasciculations can often be elicited by a gentle tapping of the muscle with a reflex hammer. Asterixis and other movement disorders are described later.

PATHOPHYSIOLOGY OF MOTOR SYMPTOMS AND SIGNS

Asthenia consists of an inner sense of lassitude conveying feelings of undue weakness or motor fatigue before any activity is initiated. The symptom can arise acutely or subacutely during the course of a number of acquired illnesses, including viral infection, hepatitis, myocardial infarction, and endocrine disorders. Several neurological diseases, including multiple sclerosis, parkinsonism, and acute polyneuritis, produce symptoms of asthenia. Most chronic asthenia unassociated with objective evidence of somatic disease has a psychogenic basis.

Fatigue refers to an abnormal rate or degree of exhaustion following brief or sustained voluntary activity. The symptom tends to be more specific in its associations than asthenia and accompanies many of the systemic and neurological disorders listed above, as well as post-traumatic syndromes and chronic sedative drug abuse. Local fatigability most often reflects a regional disorder or deconditioning of the nerves or muscles; when accompanied by detectable, exercise-induced, local reductions in muscle strength, the symptom is characteristic of myasthenia gravis.

Weakness refers to an impaired capacity to carry out a voluntary motor act due to a loss of muscular power. The term *paresis* is synonymous. *Paralysis* designates a more complete loss of motor function. Most weakness or paralysis results from disease or dysfunction of the central or peripheral nervous system or the muscles. Muscle guarding and immobility that surround injured or inflamed areas of the trunk or extremities sometimes can produce pseudoparalysis when motion accentuates the pain. The quality of hysterical weakness is described below.

Patterns of Weakness

Upper motor neuron lesions arising at the cerebral level typically produce focal weakness predominating in the hand and arm, the lower face, or the foot and leg, in that order of frequency. A hemiparesis (face, arm, and leg) can originate from the cerebrum, as can face-hand-arm weakness. Face-leg weakness, sparing the arm, implies two anatomically distinct lesions, whereas arm-leg weakness sparing the face can originate anywhere along the corticospinal pathway between the internal capsule and the upper cervical cord. Upper motor neuron weakness typically affects skilled movement, with paresis being more marked distally than proximally in the limbs (Table 117–1). Various components of spasticity emerge, including increased muscular resistance to passive stretch with lengthening and shortening reactions, increased deep tendon reflexes, abnormal postural responses to stimulation, including decorticate, decerebrate, and spinal flexor responses, and the classic Babinski sign. Upper motor neuron lesions seldom severely paralyze the face and never completely so. As a result the brow and orbicularis oculi, like other midline muscle groups, are relatively spared. Atrophy of the limbs, if it occurs at all, is mild and due to disuse. The EMG usually shows no abnormality beyond loss of voluntary contraction.

Among *basal ganglia diseases,* asthenia is prominent in parkinsonism and chorea. Some patients in the early stages of parkinsonism complain of a hemiparetic weakness that can misleadingly suggest corticospinal tract dysfunction. Most persons with Parkinson's disease, however, suffer only mild to moderate weakness but report disproportionately prominent difficulty in initiating and continuing movements, "as if starting through molasses." Their limbs show rigidity rather than spasticity, their deep tendon reflexes are at most only moderately increased, and they lack Babinski signs or other evidence of pathological reflex spasticity.

Cerebellar diseases, especially those of the hemisphere and dentate nuclei, cause ipsilateral asthenia and weakness. Ataxia and incoordination, however, are more prominent. Muscle resistance to passive stretch is, if anything, reduced, but deep tendon reflexes may be moderately hyperactive, and impaired cerebellar regulation of the stretch reflex can cause pendularity. Pathological reflexes and muscle atrophy are lacking.

Disease of the lower motor neuron, including the anterior horn cells, the motor nerve root, or the motor nerve, causes a classic syndrome (Table 117–1). Weakness is regionally distributed according to areas of denervation, so that a major clue to anatomical diagnosis lies in distinguishing among the respective paralytic patterns produced by damage to spinal cord, ventral motor root, plexus, or peripheral nerve. Characteristic sensory defects will be added at many of these locations. With severe denervation-weakness, muscle atrophy begins within days. Motor resistance is subnormal, deep tendon reflexes diminish or disappear, and with proximally originating denervation, fasciculations may, in time, become visible through the skin. Electrical signs of denervation, including first fibrillation and later fasciculation, begin within three to four weeks of the time of injury.

Nerve-muscle junctional disease is of two kinds. The more frequent, myasthenia gravis (MG), consists of an autoimmune blockage of the acetylcholine receptor in the muscle. The other, the Lambert-Eaton myasthenic syndrome, involves immunological blockage of presynaptic calcium channels, reducing release of neurotransmitter from the nerve terminals. Weakness in MG affects most often the oculomotor, bulbar, and proximal limb muscles, which rapidly fatigue with quick successive action. Weakness in the Lambert-Eaton syndrome, by contrast, affects mainly the distal limbs, is maximal with first effort, and lessens with repeated tries. Atrophy occurs in neither disorder except when severe chronic MG induces muscle disuse. Muscle tone is normal, deep tendon reflexes are usually preserved or reduced, and sensation is unaffected. EMG changes are diagnostic.

Myopathies, diseases intrinsic to muscle, produce insidiously beginning weakness that symmetrically affects anatomical groups characteristic of the particular variant of degenerative (dystrophy), metabolic (e.g., thyrotoxic), or inflammatory (myositis) diseases. Weakness occasionally remains constant (congenital myopathy) but usually progresses either slowly (dystrophy), rapidly (metabolic or inflammatory myopathy), or episodically (periodic paralysis). Resistance to passive stretch is normal, but the muscles may be tender (myositis), show myotonia (congenital myotonia, myotonic dystrophy), be abnormally soft (thyrotoxicosis), look abnormally large (pseudohypertrophy), or feel unduly firm (connective tissue infiltration). Deep tendon reflexes are preserved until late except in hypokalemic myopathy. Serum enzymes often are abnormal in muscular dystrophy and EMGs in many instances are characteristic. Sensation remains intact.

Major Abnormal Movements

Table 117–2 lists the major conditions causing nonparoxysmal, focal, or generalized abnormal gross skeletal muscle movements. Several of the focal movements can be confused with epileptic attacks (Chapter 120). The reader also will recognize that categories overlap, especially those of dystonia, chorea, athetosis, and dyskinesia.

Myotonia comprises a prolonged (seconds) involuntary contraction of a group of adjacent muscle fibers following a self-limited, voluntary effort or an abrupt local percussion as with a reflex hammer. An abnormality of the postsynaptic muscle membrane producing self-repetitive depolarizations and muscle after discharges causes the sustained fiber shortening.

Cramps are a sudden, painful, abrupt shortening of muscles. Motor units during cramps fire at about 300 per second, much faster than the most vigorous voluntary contraction. The high rate of discharge probably causes the palpable muscle tautness and pain. The pain may be relieved by stretching the affected muscle or by massage. Central mechanisms may also be involved, since certain conditions are associated with a propensity to cramps: denervation (especially amyotrophic lateral sclerosis), pregnancy, and electrolyte disorders (especially water intoxication and hyponatremia). Cramps attributed to hypo-osmolarity are seen in some patients treated by maintenance hemodialysis. They respond to treatment with hypertonic solutions of glucose or sodium.

Cramps occur commonly in otherwise normal individuals, and some people with or without a family history of cramps are more susceptible than others for unknown reasons. Cramps that occur only at night can sometimes be prevented by quinine sulfate, 0.3 gm orally at bedtime. Others can occur frequently during the day, occasionally so often that the individual is effectively crippled. Phenytoin, 0.3 to 0.6 gm daily, may be helpful in these patients, but some are resistant to this as well as to other drugs that may be tried, including diazepam, carbamazepine, and diphenhydramine. Patients with benign fasciculations (lacking weakness, wasting, or other signs of motor neuron disease) seem especially prone to have frequent cramps.

Tetany is a special form of cramp, identified by its predilection for flexor muscles of the hand and fingers, its association with laryngospasm, and its relationship to hypocalcemia. Tetany can be painful. It differs from other cramps electromyographically because of a characteristic rhythmic grouping of discharging potentials. Hyperventilation-induced tetany is likely to be overlooked as a cause of cramps or laryngospasm.

Muscle fibrillation describes continuously recurrent, spontaneous contractions of single muscle fibers due usually to denervation but sometimes to dystrophic degeneration of single fiber membranes. In either event, the phenomenon reflects membrane and contractile hypersensitivity to circulating or locally diffusing acetylcholine (ACh). *Fasciculations* represent spontaneous, synchronous, recurrent depolarization-contraction of the fibers of a single motor unit or of a group of partially denervated motor units that have been reinnervated by sprouting from adjacent, still conducting motor axons. The pathogenesis reflects denervation hypersensitivity to ACh of the damaged motor axon. Fasciculation of larger motor units and grouped motor units is visible through the skin. Fibrillations and fasciculations produce characteristic EMG changes (p. 674).

Myokymia has been used to describe a variety of apparently different disorders characterized by cramps in association with continuous spontaneous twitching of muscle. The EMGs of some cases show prolonged trains of spontaneous potentials, whereas in others grouping of potentials is found. Some of these patients have difficulty in relaxing grip, a phenomenon called neuromyotonia, since, unlike myotonia, the muscular activity is abolished by neuromuscular blocking agents, indicating a neural rather than a muscular origin. Hyperhidrosis is prominent in some patients and is secondary to the increased muscular activity.

In patients with severe myokymia, continuous shortening of muscle leads to abnormal postures and abnormally increased resistance to passive movement. Such abnormalities are often due to central neurological disorders. There are other patients who suffer fluctuating rigidity of axial and limb muscles and continuous electromyographic activity despite authentic attempts to relax. This syndrome has been called the *stiff-man syndrome* (or Isaac's syndrome, quantal squander, armadillo disease, neuromyotonia, and continuous muscle fiber activity). Ordinary cramps may be superimposed upon the persistent stiffness. Phenytoin, carbamazepine, or diazepam in therapeutic doses may bring dramatic relief. The condition may have several causes; a defect in central gamma-amino butyric neurotransmission has been postulated.

Tremor exists in three major forms. *Essential tremor* or *benign familial tremor* is an accentuation of a physiological, 8- to 12-Hz rhythmic oscillation that can affect the distal arms, the head, or, less often, the vocal apparatus. Coarse in its pattern but absent at complete rest, the tremor begins with the maintenance of posture and is accentuated by voluntary movement, sometimes to an incapacitating degree. The abnormality depends on cerebellar mechanisms as well as basal ganglia dysfunction and can be blocked by lesions placed in the ventrolateral nucleus of the thalamus. Essential tremor varies widely in intensity and can appear at any age but becomes more common and prominent in elderly life (*senile tremor*). Accompanied by neither rigidity, akinesia, nor ataxia, its predisposition is transmitted as an autosomal dominant trait. Alcohol in small amounts and, less often, anxiolytic agents suppress the movement. The beta-blocker propranolol reduces the intensity of the tremor in about 25 per cent of affected persons. Primidone and baclofen are useful for some patients.

Resting or parkinsonian tremor, a 4- to 7-Hz oscillation, reflects the alternating contractions of agonist-antagonist muscles, most often of the distal extremities, especially the hand ("pill rolling"). Less frequently the lower facial muscles, the tongue, or the lower extremities are involved. The tremor worsens with anxiety or fatigue and tends to quiet down or briefly disappear with relaxation or periods of intense manual concentration. As with all abnormal movements of basal ganglia origin, parkinsonian tremor disappears during sleep. Its genesis is believed to reflect excess cholinergic activity in the striatum, leading to an abnormally high GABA output from the putamen to the pallidum. The tremor can be abolished by lesions of the thalamic ventrolateral nucleus and is improved by antiparkinsonian drugs, as discussed below.

Intention (cerebellar) tremor can take three patterns. One relates to damage of the vermis and anterior lobe and results in an oscillating, rhythmic ataxia of the trunk and lower limbs during attempts to walk (titubation). A second, associated with lesions of the afferent spinocerebellar input, produces a more irregular high-steppage shaking ataxia of the lower extremities, which can blend into titubation. The third, resulting from damage to the dentate outflow pathway of the superior peduncle, produces the classic manual intention tremor, consisting of an irregular, coarse 3- to 6-Hz distal oscillation that increases in amplitude and irregularity as the voluntarily moving hand approaches its object. In all instances, cerebellar tremor reflects a disruption in the balance between afferent impulses to the roof nuclei of the cerebellum and the immediately following inhibitory loop that normally feeds back on these roof nuclei from the Purkinje cells. Cerebellar intention tremor so far has resisted efforts at pharmacological control.

Asterixis is an irregular, flap-like tremor, distributed more distally than proximally, that involves the extremities, less often the tongue, with a frequency varying from less than 1 to as high as 3 Hz. It is most often observed to accompany the metabolic encephalopathies and usually is accompanied by an accentuated physiological tremor. Its mechanism reflects a brief loss of muscle contraction in muscles controlling extension of the involved member, followed by a rapid myoclonus-like recovery.

Chorea describes involuntary, nonrhythmic, irregularly distributed, coarse, quick twitching movements affecting the face, tongue, and proximal and distal extremities. Slower athetoid twistings sometimes intersperse themselves concurrently. Mild cases may resemble little more than anxiety-provoked fidgets, while the appearance of severe examples blends into generalized dystonia. Efforts at sustained muscular contraction accentuate the disorder, which possesses features of both basal ganglia and cerebellar dysfunction. Pharmacologically, the phenomenon most closely resembles the effects of central dopamine hyperactivity. *Ballism* consists of irregular, abrupt, repetitive, wide-amplitude flinging movements of the limbs initiated predominantly by proximal girdle muscles. Less prominent distal choreiform movements often accompany the condition, which involves body parts opposite to an infarcted or, rarely, otherwise damaged subthalamic nucleus. Usually unilateral in distribution (hemiballismus), the condition is ameliorated by haloperidol or reserpine. Ordinarily it subsides spontaneously within a few weeks after onset.

Dystonia can accompany several basal ganglia disorders and is the major sign of a primary movement disorder of late childhood, adolescence, or adult life, as discussed more extensively in a later section (see Table 117–3). The abnormality is characterized by bizarre twisting or turning motions, most but not all of which affect more distal body parts. The distinctive feature of the movements is that they involve the simultaneous tonic co-contraction of agonist and antagonist muscle groups. Brief dystonia usually lasts for a second or more, a rate somewhat faster than in *athetosis*, a slow, proximally distributed twisting observed most commonly in children who have suffered perinatal or infantile basal ganglia–thalamic damage. Most dystonic movements also tend to recur in longer spasms, sometimes lasting minutes to hours at a time. Dystonia can be generalized or restricted, inherited or acquired. It can arise as a distinct, idiopathic disorder or as an accompaniment to several basal ganglia diseases, including Huntington's chorea and Wilson's disease. The pathophysiology and pharmacological basis of dystonic movements are poorly understood. Several phenothiazine derivatives, however, can induce acute dystonia as an idiosyncratic response in susceptible hosts. Structural lesions involving the basal ganglia–thalamic motor pathways sometimes cause a contralateral hemidystonia. The anticholinergic, antihistamine drug diphenhydramine hydrochloride blocks drug-induced dystonia but not the naturally occurring form.

Motor tics are sudden, quick, irregular, stereotyped

movements of variable complexity that repetitively involve similar but not identical groups of muscles. They can come on at any age, most often in adolescence or young adulthood, and most frequently involve the face, eyes, or mouth, seldom the extremities. Some mild forms represent psychologically generated habit patterns. More severe examples, often combined with bizarre barkings or the shouting of scatological and other obscenities, comprise *Gilles de la Tourette's syndrome.*

Myoclonus describes sudden, abrupt contractions of single muscles or restricted groups of muscles, most frequently affecting the limbs, less often the trunk. The phenomenon has many causes and can arise from abnormally excitable gray matter at any level of the nervous system. Single generalized myoclonic jerks occur normally as startle responses or when drifting off to sleep. Myoclonic seizures generated from the cerebrum usually occur in distal muscles, while myoclonus generated in the lower brain stem or spinal gray matter usually has a proximal distribution that affects the pectoral girdle, trunk, or pelvic girdle. Myoclonic jerks accompany several forms of epilepsy (see page 789). They also occur in a multifocal pattern in association with several metabolic encephalopathies, especially those associated with uremia or penicillin intoxication, and they can follow severe cerebral anoxia or slow virus infection (Creutzfeldt-Jakob disease).

Palatal myoclonus relates more to a form of continuous tremor than to true myoclonus. The condition consists of rhythmic, regular, 2- to 3-Hz contractions of the soft palate and, less commonly, the adjacent pharynx. It arises in association with infarction or degeneration of the pathway that links together the dentate, red nucleus, and inferior olive. Unlike tremor of basal ganglia or cerebellar origin, palatal myoclonus persists during sleep. The serotonin precursor 5-hydroxytryptamine sometimes ameliorates the contractions, which have been attributed to denervation hypersensitivity of olivary neurons.

Hemifacial spasm can affect the motor distribution of either facial nerve, producing rapidly recurring, painless, nonstereotyped fragmentary twitching of any of the facial muscles. The condition persists into sleep and has been attributed to ephaptic cross-conduction of fibers within the nerve secondary to damage caused by its long-standing intracranial compression from an overlying branch of the basilar artery. Surgical decompression sometimes relieves the condition, which is disfiguring but neither painful nor dangerous.

B. MOVEMENT DISORDERS

The term *movement disorders* refers to a group of neurological conditions generated by abnormalities that arise in the brain and affect resting skeletal muscles in a nonparoxysmal manner so as to produce gross, functionally inappropriate activity in the face, limbs, or trunk. All appear only during the waking state and all are believed to represent dysfunction or damage related largely to or confined to the basal ganglia and its subcortical connections in the thalamus. Included anatomically are the symmetrically placed deep cerebral nuclei of the caudate nucleus and putamen (together known as the striatum), the globus pallidus or pallidum, the subthalamic nucleus, and the substantia nigra of the midbrain (Fig. 117–2). The functions of the basal ganglia are best deduced from their diseases. The ganglia especially influence the control of trunk and proximal appendicular movement by feeding information forward to the frontal cortex before that region sends its final signals to the craniospinal motor neurons via the corticospinal tract. Interruption of the corticospinal pathway ameliorates or interrupts signs of basal ganglia dysfunction. This observation has led to diseases of the basal ganglia being termed "extrapyramidal disorders." The basal ganglia also exert a major influence on the planning of movement and in establishing the postural "set" or "platform" upon which corticospinal influences erect learned motor activity.

The basal ganglia contain a distinct neurotransmitter anatomy. Corticostriatal and thalamostriatal afferents are both excitatory in their action, probably employing glutamate as a transmitter (Fig. 117–2). The well-known nigrostriatal input employs dopamine. Dopaminergic synapses probably exist on all neuronal types within the striatum, although the functionally

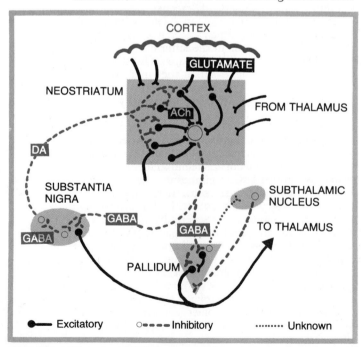

FIGURE 117–2. Simplified diagram of the principal connections and known transmitters of the basal ganglia. ACh = Acetylcholine; GABA = gamma-aminobutyric acid; DA = dopamine.

most important receptors appear to lie on the axon terminals of incoming corticostriate fibers. The striatum also contains many cholinergic interneurons believed functionally to oppose the dopaminergic input. This latter action may help to explain why anticholinergic drugs often improve the symptoms of parkinsonism. The major outputs of the basal ganglia to all of their known projection areas predominantly employ the inhibitory transmitter GABA. A number of neuropeptides have been identified in the nuclei, but their functional significance remains unknown.

PARKINSONISM

Parkinsonism is a syndrome consisting, in variable combinations, of slowness in the initiation and execution of movement (bradykinesia), increased muscle tonus (rigidity), tremor, and impaired postural reflexes. The movement disorder results primarily from a defect in the dopaminergic pathway that connects the substantia nigra to the striatum. In idiopathic or postencephalitic parkinsonism, the deficiency results from degeneration of the pigmented dopamine-secreting neurons in the substantia nigra, while most drug-induced parkinsonism reflects a blocking of dopamine receptors in striatal neurons. Several rare diseases that cause degeneration of striatal receptor neurons also produce clinical parkinsonism but fail to improve with the use of levodopa or its congeners. Similar therapeutic limitations apply to the parkinsonian manifestations that sometimes accompany advanced vascular diseases, neoplasms, and certain degenerative disorders such as progressive supranuclear palsy, the Shy-Drager form of generalized idiopathic autonomic insufficiency, and some of the progressive cerebellar degenerations. In most of these conditions treatment with dopamine agonists confers only small benefits.

Parkinson's Disease

This idiopathic disorder of adults has its highest incidence in males over 40 years. The cause is unknown. Epidemiological studies have traced some cohorts to long-preceding influenzal epidemics, while a few others have been poisoned by the illegally synthesized opiate MPTP. Most patients, however, relate no hint of a specific cause or a family predisposition. The early motor deficits can be traced to incipient degeneration of nigral dopamine-transmitting cells. Later, refractory motor, autonomic, and mental abnormalities develop in many cases, implying degeneration of striatal receptor mechanisms plus, sometimes, degeneration of the locus ceruleus and the basal nucleus of Meynert.

Symptoms and Signs. Most cases of idiopathic parkinsonism begin with either weakness, tremor, or both. Patients describe motor slowness, stiffness, or easy fatigability in a single limb or hemiparetic distribution. The typical 4- to 7-Hz resting tremor affects approximately 70 per cent but may not present at all in some patients, especially those affected by prominent rigidity.

Patients with parkinsonism often have a diagnostically typical appearance. The body stoops stiffly forward, bent at the knees, hips, and neck, with arms held close to the sides and flexed at the elbows. Steps are small or shuffling, turns are taken slowly, and patients with advaced cases tend to accelerate their steps (festination) or suffer retropulsion. The outstretched, often trembling hands are extended at the wrist and thumb and flexed at the metacarpophalangeal joints (pill rolling posture). The face becomes masklike, unblinking, and often greasy. Speech becomes slurred, monotonous, and sometimes barely understandable. Handwriting becomes cramped and small in size. Deep tendon reflexes can be of average, slightly increased, or decreased amplitude. Myerson's sign, the failure of the blink reflex to adapt to repeated gentle percussions of the brow, is present. Other abnormal motor reflexes are absent early, but Babinski signs sometimes emerge late, reflecting the development of corticospinal tract dysfunction. The limbs of most patients display a nonspastic, steadily increasing resistance to movement, often interrupted by an 8-Hz tremor, conferring the classic "cogwheel" rigidity. Behavioral disorders are common. Many if not most patients become depressed in the early stages, and as many as half develop dementia by seven or more years after onset.

Postencephalitic parkinsonism was particularly a problem in the 1930's and 1940's following the worldwide epidemic of lethargic encephalitis that occurred during the years 1918 to 1926. Persons involved with that illness, in addition to the above-mentioned classic signs and symptoms, also suffered a variety of acute behavioral disorders, as well as autonomic abnormalities, oculogyric crises, and various dystonias, choreiform movements, and tics. The illness tended to affect younger persons but progressed less rapidly than idiopathic parkinsonism. In the latter disease, an average duration of 5 to 10 years usually separates the first symptoms from an advanced stage of drug-resistant disability and, often, mental decline.

Drug-induced parkinsonism can follow the taking of several antipsychotic agents given chronically in high doses. Chief present offenders are the phenothiazines and butyrophenones, both of which pharmacologically block dopamine receptors in the striatum and may interfere with the dopamine output of nigral cells as well. Various toxic syndromes can occur with these agents, including a diffuse motor restlessness; acute dystonic reactions that dissipate with anticholinergic, antihistamine, or diazepam therapy; oculogyric crises, which reflect an oculomotor dystonia; and parkinsonism. The last-mentioned can be clinically typical in all respects except that it fails to subside with levodopa. The late complication of tardive dyskinesia is discussed below.

Treatment. The treatment of Parkinson's disease consists of general measures and specific drugs. These increasingly disabled and fearful patients need considerable emotional support and vigorous encouragement to continue their physical activity. Every dimension of personal life may require assistance in the later stages.

Drug therapy includes three mainstays that usually are given in some combination. *Amantadine HCl,* 100 mg two to three times daily, usually is tried first in all patients. The agent possesses low toxicity, modestly helps almost two thirds of patients, and sometimes can be used alone in early cases. If no benefit is noted by one week, the drug is discontinued. Most authorities consider *levodopa* the drug of second choice. The agent usually is given combined with a peripheral dopa decarboxylase inhibitor so as to minimize systemic toxicity and provide more drug for CNS absorption. When taken early in the disease, levodopa restores many patients to an asymptomatic state. No satisfactory evidence indicates that such an early usage accelerates the disease or shortens the duration of the drug's effectiveness. *Anticholinergic drugs* occasionally are used alone in an effort to control the symptoms of early Parkinson's disease. Most often, however, they serve in low doses as a useful adjunct to levodopa therapy. The anticholinergics often benefit tremor, whereas levodopa predominantly ameliorates rigidity and some of the postural abnormalities. Several dopamine agonist drugs, e.g., bromocriptine, have also been employed to treat parkinsonism in its various stages. They are more expensive than levodopa, and their superiority as treatment has not been clearly established.

Given over a long period of time or in high doses, both levodopa and the anticholinergic drugs can produce limiting side effects. Full benefits of levodopa seldom last more than five to seven years, and large doses or long usage eventually produces uncontrollable abnormal movements of the trunk and extremities, termed dyskinesias. Furthermore, with time, the dose acts more briefly and is followed by intermittent, unpredictable periods of immobility (the "off" effect). Anticholinergic drugs are prone to cause dry mouth, visual blurring, and, occasionally, urinary retention in almost any subject; nightmares or daytime delirium can be a distressing consequence in the elderly.

Many patients become depressed during the course of Parkinson's disease, some suicidally so. Tricyclic or other antidepressant medications may ameliorate these symptoms. Recently, efforts have been made to ameliorate parkinsonism by homotransplanting adrenal medullary tissue into the brain or implanting dopaminergic cells from tissue culture or fetal sources. Too little time has elapsed to judge the effect of these bold attempts.

Progressive Supranuclear Palsy

This is an uncommon disorder of middle-aged or older persons marked by insidiously developing and progressive degenerative changes in the basal ganglia, basal nuclei, and cerebellum. Clinical features include a Parkinson-like rigidity and a loss of postural reflexes combined with considerable rigidity of the body and a postural dystonia marked by extension of the head. Masked facies are absent and a progressive external ophthalmoplegia, consisting of paralysis first of voluntary conjugate vertical gaze and later of lateral gaze, is diagnostic. Full-range tonic abnormal oculocephalic reflex responses emerge concurrently and are easily elicited by bedside examination. A moderate dementia usually accompanies the motor changes. Dopamine agonist drugs occasionally bring symptomatic improvement.

Huntington's Disease

Huntington's disease, sometimes called Huntington's chorea, is an uncommon inherited disorder transmitted as an autosomal dominant trait with complete penetrance. Recent research has succeeded in bracketing the Huntington gene, on the short arm of chromosome 4, and it seems likely that specific genetic identification soon will be available. If so, it should be possible to identify those at risk for trials of therapy and to offer appropriate genetic counseling.

Huntington's disease affects striatal neurons, especially the small GABA-transmitting cells and scattered nerve cells in the frontal lobe cortex, claustrum, subthalamus, and cerebellar Purkinje and dentate systems. Gliosis is prominent. Neurochemically, GABA, acetylcholine, and angiotensin II decline in the striatum, with less severe reductions affecting substance P, cholecystokinin, and enkephalin. Somatostatin-containing neurons are selectively preserved.

The principal clinical changes include dyskinesia, altered behavior, and dementia. The age of onset averages 40 years, with most cases beginning between ages 30 and 50. Motor symptoms in the early stage often include dystonic posturing and rigidity, but these changes give way to prominent choreiform activity in most affected adults. Signs of corticospinal tract dysfunction or sensory changes are lacking. Eccentricity, inappropriateness, a loss of social amenities, excess irritability, and sexual hyperactivity can mark the early stages. Occasionally a schizophreniform illness precedes the motor abnormality by several years. Depression is common and suicide occurs frequently, since the progressing dementia often fails to blunt insight.

Diagnosis comes from recognizing the characteristic progressive generalized choreiform activity accompanied by behavioral or personality changes, especially in a person with a tell-tale family history. Spontaneous mutations are uncommon, but some affected persons inevitably lack knowledge of their true antecedents. CT or MR scans in fully developed cases show cerebral atrophy, especially of the caudate and putamen, to a degree that is almost specific to the disease. Symptomatic treatment is aimed at minimizing the distressing movements, reserpine or baclofen being the most useful agents. Psychological symptoms may require major antipsychotic drugs for their control. Until the specific gene is identified, genetic counseling remains based largely on statistical probabilities. The principal disorders to be considered in differential diagnosis are as follows: *Gilles de la Tourette's syndrome* (p. 736) occasionally is transmitted in an autosomal dominant pattern, but such patients show motor tics rather than chorea and lack the behavioral-mental changes. *Senile chorea* is a rare disorder beginning in persons older than 60 years. The abnormal movements usually are less prominent than in Huntington's, and there is no comparable degree of dementia. *Hemiballismus* is a disorder of older persons described on page 735. A benign adult chorea also can develop in association with lupus erythematosus or thyrotoxicosis. In both these instances, the chorea has an abrupt onset and gradually disappears within weeks or months.

Sydenham's Chorea

This now uncommon, self-limited disorder usually lasts two to six months and is related to rheumatic fever. It occurs most often in children under the age of 15 years but can sometimes affect pregnant women. In contrast to the flowing, more forceful movements in Huntington's disease, which commonly impair walking and standing to the point of causing falls, choreiform activity in Sydenham's chorea more often takes a fidgety, fragmented form, sometimes difficult to separate from habit tics. The children are clumsy and often dysarthric and walk unsteadily. An inability to sustain tonic movement, such as steadily protruding the tongue or sustaining an uninterrupted grasp of the examiner's fingers, is common to all the choreas.

Treatment is symptomatic. Recurrent attacks occur in as many as one third of affected children.

DYSTONIA

Dystonia can appear either as part of a primary basal ganglia disease or as a symptom secondary to a number of other conditions affecting those structures (Table 117–3). The chronic dystonias include a group of uncommon disorders of inherited or sporadic origin. The specific cause and pathophysiology are unknown for any of these conditions, and no neuropathological changes have been found consistently in the brain. An imbalance of neurotransmitter function in the basal ganglia has been postulated, but specific neurochemical candidates remain elusive, inasmuch as both dopamine excess and presumed dopamine receptor blockade can induce acute transient dystonic movement.

Severe generalized dystonia, sometimes called *dystonia musculorum deformans*, begins predominantly in young children and adolescents, most often beginning with an equinovarus posturing of the foot or a tonically flexed hand, then spreading to involve the neck, face, and trunk in nearly continuous, recurrent, intense, involuntary, asymmetrical contractions. The movements, which characteristically lead into prolonged spasms, eventually produce bizarre contortions with severe musculotendinous contractures. Ensuing bone deformities can produce scoliosis, chest deformities, and a foreshortening of natural height. Lesser degrees of the illness can arise during adulthood and tend to produce restricted impairments of the lower or upper extremities.

Spasmodic torticollis is the most common of the focal dystonias. It affects predominantly the muscles of the neck and shoulders, which bilaterally and simultaneously contract to produce recurrent unilateral head turning or head extension. Elevations of the shoulder and, often, platysmal contractions may accompany the movements of the head and neck. In mild cases the movement can be restrained by the sub-

TABLE 117–3. THE MAJOR DYSTONIAS

PRIMARY DYSTONIA

CONDITIONS	INHERITANCE	AGE OF ONSET
Generalized dystonia	Autosomal recessive	Childhood
	Autosomal dominant	Adolescence or adulthood
	Sporadic	
Focal dystonia Foot-leg or hand-arm	Inherited or sporadic	Mostly adulthood, occasionally late
Blepharospasm	Sporadic	Late adulthood
Facial mandibular (Meige's syndrome)	Sporadic	Late adulthood
Spasmodic dysphonia	Sporadic	Adulthood
Spasmodic torticollis	Mostly sporadic, occasionally autosomal recessive	Middle adulthood
Occupational dystonia Writer's cramp Musician's cramp	Sporadic	Early-middle adulthood

SECONDARY DYSTONIA

CHRONIC	ACUTE
Wilson's disease	Head trauma
Huntington's disease	Phenothiazines
Postencephalitic	Butyrophenones
Severe cerebral anoxia-ischemia	Levodopa
Manganese poisoning	

ject's placing gentle antagonistic pressure against the chin. More severe examples can spread to produce spastic dysphonia and hand-arm dystonia. Discussion of other forms of focal dystonia can be found in the references.

Treatment of the dystonias is unsatisfactory. High doses of the anticholinergic drug trihexyphenidyl somewhat relieve a few patients. The use of carbamazepine or diazepam occasionally has been reported favorably in others. Stereotaxic surgical attacks on the thalamus benefit some children with severe generalized dystonia but carry a high risk of complications and must be regarded as desperation measures. Recently, investigators have reported success with judiciously repeated fractional injection of botulinum toxin into the periocular muscles of patients with incapacitating blepharospasm.

DYSKINESIA

The dopamine-induced dyskinesia of chronic treated parkinsonism has been described above. *Tardive dyskinesia* consists of abnormal, semirhythmic involuntary movements affecting the mouth (lingual-oral-buccal), trunk, or extremities following the taking and, often, withdrawal of antidopaminergic antipsychotic drugs. Once it appears, the condition almost always remains permanently. A few cases are known to have succeeded upon no more than a few days of phenothiazine medication. More often, the complication follows prolonged drug use. Its appearance can be delayed until weeks, months, or even years after the drugs were taken. The facial movements most often consist of chewing, tongue darting, and grimacing. Other forms include repeated flexion and extension of the trunk, piano playing–like successive contraction of the fingers and toes, and repetitive steppings of the feet while standing erect. Supersensitivity of the dopamine receptors of the basal ganglia is believed to be the cause. Reserpine or, in the presence of continued psychosis, a higher dose of antidopaminergic antipsychotics sometimes bring partial relief. Tardive dyskinesia is a disfiguring, seriously disturbing, and frequent complication. The potential for producing it should discourage the use of phenothiazine drugs for any but serious medical-psychiatric problems. *Meigs' syndrome*, a dystonia involving the jaw and lower face, somewhat resembles tardive dyskinesia but produces slower, more twisting movements. There is no necessary history of antipsychotic medication. Baclofen or valproate has been reported to improve selective cases.

REFERENCES

Marsden CD, Fahn S (eds): Movement Disorders. London, Butterworths International Medical Reviews, 1987.
Vinken PJ, Bruyn GW, Klawans HL (eds): Handbook of Clinical Neurology. Vol 49: Extrapyramidal Disorders. Amsterdam, Elsevier Science, 1986.

C. THE MAJOR CEREBELLAR ATAXIAS

TABLE 117–4. PRINCIPAL DISEASES OF THE CEREBELLUM AND ITS CONNECTIONS

I. **Primarily spinocerebellar**
  A. Inherited spinocerebellar ataxias (childhood or adolescent onset, chronic course, few positive sensory symptoms)
    1. Molecular genetic defect uncertain: Friedreich's ataxia and its variants; Roussy-Lévy
    2. Genetic defect known: phytanic acid α-hydroxylase deficiency (Refsum); abetalipoproteinemia (Bassen-Kornzweig); arylsulfate and other deficiencies
  B. Acquired spinal sensory ataxia (acute, subacute, or insidious onset): polyneuropathy; sensory polyradiculopathy (tabes dorsalis); vitamin B_{12} deficiency; spinal cord damage (multiple sclerosis, neoplasm, etc.)

II. **Primarily cerebellar**
  A. Inherited degenerative (course progressive): restricted olivopontocerebellar atrophy (young to mid-adulthood); ataxia-telangiectasia (childhood onset)
  B. Developmental abnormalities (onset of signs varies, progressive): basilar impression; Arnold-Chiari malformation
  C. Nutritional-immunological (mostly adult onset, acute or subacute course)
    1. Acute, parainfectious cerebellar ataxia of children
    2. Alcoholic-nutritional cerebellar degeneration
    3. Paraneoplastic cerebellar–brain stem degeneration
  D. Structural cerebellar lesions (acute or subacute course): trauma, neoplasms, hemorrhage, anoxia-ischemia, etc.
  E. Intoxication (acute or subacute or chronic): alcohol; sedatives; anxiolytics; phenytoin; anticancer agents

III. **Cerebellar-plus disorders**
  A. Inherited-degenerative system degeneration (mid-adulthood onset, gradual progression)
    1. Olivopontocerebellar atrophy plus, variably, spasticity, parkinsonism, sensory changes, optic atrophy, retinitis pigmentosa, ophthalmoplegia, dementia
    2. Shy-Drager syndrome
    3. Generalized mitochondrial dysfunction with ataxia, ophthalmoplegia, myopathy
  B. Acquired disseminated disorders affecting cerebellar and other systems (disseminated cancer, abscess, etc.)

SIGNS AND MECHANISMS OF CEREBELLAR DYSFUNCTION

Disorders of the cerebellum or its principal connections produce characteristic symptoms and signs, including *asthenia* or easy fatigability; *ataxia* of gait; *dysmetria*, an inability to control the range of movement, producing under- or over-shoot; *dysdiadokokinesia*, the impairment of rapidly alternating movements; *decomposition of movement*, the inability to synergize motion around two or more joints; *postural* (*sustention*) or *intention tremor*; *dysarthria*; and, possibly, *nystagmus* with the fast component toward the side of the cerebellar lesion.

Ataxias linked to the cerebellum and its major afferent and efferent connections fall into three major groups (Table 117–4). These include (1) diseases affecting predominantly the afferent spinocerebellar and associated spinal pathways; (2) diseases or disorders involving the cerebellum proper and its immediate outflow tracts; and (3) diseases in which cerebellar involvement comprises only part of a widespread degeneration of central nervous system structures. Clinically the signs and symptoms of the three categories sometimes overlap, but distinction usually is possible. Mass lesions or demyelinating disorders affecting the cerebellar system usually can be identified by MR or CT imaging. The following paragraphs describe the principal degenerative disorders affecting the system.

Spinocerebellar disease produces a wide-based, lurching sensory ataxia due to involvement of ascending proprioceptors and spinocerebellar pathways. At their worst, patients stagger from side to side, stepping with high, irregularly placed feet that often pound the floor. Large afferent fibers carrying position and vibratory sense from the lower extremities degenerate, leading to rombergism and an accompanying loss of deep tendon reflexes. Involvement of descending corticospinal pathways results in pathological reflexes, while direct cerebellar involvement can impair oculomotor control as well as upper extremity coordination.

Within the cerebellum itself, damage or degeneration of the posterior midline *floccular nodular area* produces a narrow-based ataxia with a tendency to fall backwards plus nystagmus on lateral and, sometimes, downward gaze. Dysfunction of the more anterior midline *vermis and anterior lobe* is more common and accompanies especially deep midline cerebellar tumors and alcohol-nutritional or paraneoplastic degeneration. A broad-based, stiff-legged ataxia often is accompanied in severe cases by an oscillating, rhythmic sustention tremor of the trunk and lower extremities (titubation). Deep tendon reflexes tend to be accentuated, but nystagmus is uncommon unless the disease concurrently affects the vestibular nuclei.

Lateral hemispheric lesions characteristically produce subtle signs consisting of mild ipsilateral incoordination and perhaps hypotonia. If they directly involve the cerebellar roof nuclei or outflow pathways, they cause in the upper extremities the classic signs of cerebellar incoordination and tremor as described in the first paragraph of this section. Lesions that expand the cerebellum to compress the adjacent brain stem or infiltrate it add symptoms and signs of headache, nausea, vomiting, cranial nerve abnormalities, or long tract dysfunction to the above syndromes.

PRIMARY CEREBELLAR DEGENERATIONS

This category includes a heterogeneous group of largely genetically caused *system degenerations* in which neuroaxonal death variously affects afferent pathways to the cerebellum, the cerebellum itself, and, often, trans-synaptically connected central nervous system structures. Although one can identify more or less distinct syndromes of spinocerebellar and primary cerebellar degeneration, different diseases may overlap considerably in their neuropathology; and phenotypes can differ clinically in single kindreds. These considerations suggest molecular linkages among these disorders and several other degenerative central nervous system diseases. Related conditions include peroneal muscular atrophy, other degenerative neuropathies, hereditary spastic paraplegia, motor neuron disease, atypical forms of parkinsonism, and the Shy-Drager form of progressive autonomic insufficiency. Most of the CNS system degenerations are uncommon, and in only a few is the specific cause known. The following section describes the most frequent types; the references contain more extensive discussions as well as descriptions of the rarer entities.

Friedreich's Ataxia

Friedreich's ataxia, the prototypical spinocerebellar degeneration, affects children and young adults. The disease can be transmitted in autosomal dominant and autosomal recessive patterns, but sporadic cases are common. Neuronal loss involves the dorsal root ganglia and the spinal cells of origin of the spinocerebellar tracts, with degeneration beginning caudally and progressing rostrally. Axonal loss and demyelination affect the spinal nerves, the dorsal column, and the spinocerebellar tracts as well as the descending corticospinal tract. Some cases show cell loss in the cerebellum and occasionally in brain stem nuclei.

The molecular etiology of the spinocerebellar degenerations can vary from patient to patient despite considerable similarity in clinical presentations. Although the specific cause remains unknown in most instances, somewhat similar clinical disorders have been observed among small groups of patients showing abnormalities in several tissue enzymes as listed in section I.A.2 of Table 117–4.

Friedreich's ataxia typically begins insidiously, usually before age 10 years, and progresses steadily. Most patients become unable to walk unassisted during their third decade. Position and vibratory sense are lost initially in the lower extremities, and this plus the corticospinal defect leads to an increasing sensorimotor staggering ataxia. Concurrently, one finds atrophic, hypotonic lower limbs with areflexia and extensor plantar responses. By the time of their late teens or twenties, most patients develop dysarthria and many have nystagmus. Orthopedic changes include a characteristic pes cavus deformity (which can affect some family members as the sole mark of the abnormal trait) as well as a mild to moderate scoliosis and, sometimes, a high arched palate. Low intelligence affects some victims from the start, while a few appear to decline mentally as the disorder progresses. Associated, less common, abnormalities include optic atrophy, retinal degeneration, deafness, and anterior horn cell degeneration. Many victims develop cardiac enlargement and most show conduction defects on the ECG. Some develop heart failure; few survive beyond 40 years. Diagnosis usually is apparent from the patient's appearance and physical findings. Among laboratory tests, none is specific except in the specific deficiency syndromes, most of which clinically appear sufficiently distinctive to prompt appropriate biochemical study. Visual evoked potentials are abnormally slow in most cases of either spinocerebellar or primary cerebellar ataxia, while somatic evoked potentials tend to be particularly slowed in Friedreich's ataxia but not in olivopontocerebellar atrophy. The spinal fluid is normal.

Roussy-Lévy ataxia closely resembles Friedreich's except that the condition runs a much slower course, often with little progression into adulthood. Position and vibration sensations are spared, and extensor plantar responses fail to develop. Other family members may show evidence of the more common peroneal muscular atrophy or hereditary spastic paraplegia.

The Olivopontocerebellar Degenerations (OPCD)

This category includes a group of uncommon, progressive degenerative disorders of middle to late adult life producing cerebellar dysfunction with or without signs of degeneration in other motor-sensory systems, including spinal cord, cerebellar outflow pathways, basal ganglia, autonomic nervous system, optic nerves, and even cerebral cortex. The illnesses occur in both sporadic and hereditary patterns.

Pathologically, the most frequent denominator to the OPCD group includes degeneration of the inferior olive and the pontine cerebellar relay nuclei, with degeneration and demyelination of their respective climbing axons into the cerebellum. Trans-synaptic death occurs in the target cells of the cerebellar cortex. Less consistent abnormalities affect neurons and their axons in the more remote neurological structures mentioned above. Degeneration of the basal ganglia and central autonomic neurons usually is prominent in the Shy-Drager variant.

OPCD can affect either sex, most often between the ages of 40 and 60 years. Progression is relatively rapid, and most patients become totally dependent within six years of onset. Initial symptoms and signs include a relatively wide-based ataxia accompanied by incoordination of the upper extremities and dysarthria. Dysmetria usually remains worse in the lower than the upper extremities. The limbs become hypotonic, and deep tendon reflexes are preserved except when an associated spinal degeneration occurs. Most patients develop nystagmus. Among those with basal ganglia involvement, parkinsonian signs emerge during the moderately advanced stages of the illness. Babinski signs and other manifestations of corticospinal tract dysfunction occur late if at all. Some patients develop palatal myoclonus. A functional dementia accompanies the late stages of approximately one third of cases.

No specific test is diagnostic of OPCD. Brain stem auditory evoked potentials are abnormal in a majority. Differential diagnosis requires ruling out the conditions listed in sections II and III of Table 117–4. CT or MR imaging usually discloses cerebellar and pontine atrophy and rules out other structural lesions. Nutritional disease and possible drug intoxication can be identified by the history. Paraneoplastic syndromes are discussed on page 801.

The cause being unknown, only symptomatic treatment can be offered.

Ataxia-Telangiectasia

This disorder affects spinal cord, cerebellum, and basal ganglia functions. The illness begins in early childhood, inherited as an autosomal recessive trait. Progressive ataxia of gait, incoordinated upper extremities, facial and appendicular choreoathetosis, and opsoclonus are characteristic. Most children become wheelchair-bound and begin to show mental retardation by the second decade. Prominent telangiectases stud the conjunctivae, the ears, the nose, and the cheek areas. The disease includes thymic hypoplasia with a severe deficiency of IgA. Patients suffer a high incidence of endocrine abnormalities, respiratory infections, chromosomal aberrations, and neoplasms; most die before age 20 years.

REFERENCE

Andreas P: Cerebellar degenerations. *In* Appel SH (ed): Current Neurology, Vol 7. Chicago, Year Book Medical Publishers, 1987, pp 159–191.

D. DISORDERS OF THE SPINE AND SPINAL CORD AND NEUROCUTANEOUS SYNDROMES

The spinal cord may be affected by any of the numerous disorders that damage nervous system tissue. Some of these conditions represent only a portion of widespread involvement of the nervous system (e.g., spinocerebellar degenerations), whereas others are unique to the spinal cord (spinal neoplasms or arteriovenous malformations).

SPINAL CORD NEOPLASMS

Neoplastic growths that cause nerve root or spinal cord disorders can begin in the paravertebral, extradural, intradural, or intramedullary compartments. Most neoplasms that cause spinal cord compression are extradural and metastatic. Most extradural neoplasms originate in the vertebral body and compress spinal roots or cord without invading them. Most intradural neoplasms also cause symptoms by compressing spinal roots or cord without invading, but unlike extradural neoplasms, the majority are benign and slow growing. Intramedullary neoplasms cause symptoms by both invading and compressing spinal structures; the tumors may be either benign or malignant.

Paravertebral Tumors. Neoplastic lesions that begin in or metastasize to the paravertebral space often cause serious and perplexing neurological problems. The tumor may extend longitudinally within the paravertebral space, progressively compressing nerve roots as it grows. At times, the tumor may grow through an intervertebral foramen and compress not only the nerve root but also the spinal cord. Rarely, spinal cord symptoms may be caused by ischemia from compression of radicular arteries that supply the spinal cord. If the tumor lies lateral to the immediate paravertebral space, it may compress the brachial, lumbar, or sacral plexus, causing symptoms similar to root compression but with a different pattern of sensory and motor loss. The symptoms of extravertebral tumors begin insidiously with severe, unrelenting pain, often with a burning quality. The pain is localized just lateral to the spine and radiates, bandlike, in the distribution of the involved dermatome(s). If the lesion involves abdominal or thoracic roots, objective motor and sensory changes often are minimal, but autonomic changes may be prominent or the only neurological sign. *Hyperhidrosis* occurring in a band coinciding with the site of the pain strongly suggests the diagnosis. When the tumor involves cervical or lumbar roots, the pain may be soon followed by numbness in the fingertips or toes, with accompanying weakness and reflex diminution, depending on the roots involved. Autonomic changes, including anhidrosis or hyperhidrosis, can affect the arm or leg, while Horner's syndrome and/or diaphragmatic paralysis often accompany cervical or upper thoracic paravertebral tumors. The diagnosis of paravertebral tumors is best established by CT scan at the level suggested by the clinical findings. The CT scan also can determine whether the lesion has grown through the intervertebral foramen or has eroded vertebral bodies.

The differential diagnosis of paravertebral tumor includes a variety of other disorders that can cause paravertebral pain with or without compression of nerve roots. *Psychophysiological muscle tension* syndromes often cause paravertebral low back or neck pain. In some instances, there may be radiation of the pain, but usually in a nondermatomal distribution. On examination, there is often marked tenderness of muscle, which sometimes can be relieved by injecting the trigger point with saline solution or a local anesthetic. Temporary improvement of pain after such injections does not imply that structural disease is absent, since trigger points can equally well be a reaction to spinal or nerve root disease. In muscle tension syndrome, however, autonomic, sensory, or motor changes are not present. Disease of the kidneys and other viscera lying in the retroperitoneal space may cause pain similar to that of paravertebral tumors, but the pain usually does not radiate and is not associated with autonomic, motor, or sensory changes. Percussion of the involved viscera reproduces the pain that is described as a dull ache rather than a neurogenic burning pain. Entrapment neuropathies occasionally mimic the symptoms of paravertebral tumor. Chronic *post-thoracotomy pain* probably results from entrapment of nerve roots at the time of operation, perhaps with neuroma formation. The pain characteristically appears shortly after surgery and may be unremitting for many years. Motor, sensory, or autonomic changes are rare. Such pain sometimes can be relieved by paravertebral anesthetic blocks.

The management of paravertebral masses depends on the diagnosis. In patients known to have cancer, particularly lymphomas or carcinomas of the breast or lung, the tumor can be assumed to be metastatic and should be treated with radiation therapy and, if available, chemotherapy. If the patient has no known primary lesion, resection may be attempted, both to es-

tablish a diagnosis and to decompress the nerve roots. Once biopsy establishes diagnosis, further therapy such as radiation or chemotherapy can be chosen.

Extradural Tumors. Extradural neoplasms can compress spinal roots and cord in one of two ways. Either they arise in vertebrae surrounding the spinal cord and grow into the epidural space, or they arise in the paravertebral space and grow through the intervertebral foramen so as to compress the cord without involving either vertebral or paravertebral structures. Most extradural neoplasms are metastatic from carcinomas of the breast, lung, prostate, or kidney or from malignant melanoma. Some extradural neoplasms arise de novo in the vertebral bodies (e.g., chordoma, osteogenic sarcoma, myeloma, chondrosarcoma). A minority of extradural neoplasms are benign (e.g., chordoma, osteoma, osteoid osteoma, angioma). Pain, the first symptom, may precede other symptoms of spinal cord compression by weeks or months, depending on the rate of growth of the tumor. Rarely, extradural neoplasms may be painless, with the first symptoms being those of spinal cord dysfunction. The first spinal cord symptoms other than pain usually consist of corticospinal tract dysfunction with weakness, spasticity, and hyperreflexia, followed by paresthesias with loss of vibration and position sense. Unless the lesion compresses the conus medullaris or the cauda equina, bladder and bowel dysfunctions are late signs. As with other causes of spinal cord compression, extradural neoplasms cause symptoms first distally and later proximally. Thus, even thoracic and cervical neoplasms generally cause weakness and numbness in the legs before trunk and upper extremity muscles are involved. The diagnosis of extradural spinal cord compression must be suspected by the history of pain followed by signs and symptoms of spinal cord dysfunction and confirmed by radiographic study. In about 85 per cent of patients suffering from extradural spinal cord compression, plain radiographs reveal bone lesions at the site of compression. In the few remaining patients, radionuclide bone scan or CT or MR scan may demonstrate a bone lesion. The diagnosis of extradural spinal cord compression and its localization can be made by either MR scan or myelography. The differential diagnosis of extradural neoplasms includes inflammatory disease of bone and epidural abscess (e.g., vertebral tuberculosis, bacterial osteomyelitis), acute or subacute epidural hematomas, herniated intervertebral discs, spondylosis, and, very rarely, extreme extramedullary hematopoiesis (in patients with severe and chronic anemias) or epidural lipomatosis (in patients on chronic steroid therapy). Often a definitive diagnosis can be made only by biopsy of the lesion, either during the course of decompressive laminectomy or by percutaneous needle biopsy of the involved vertebral body.

The treatment of extradural neoplasms depends on the cause. Most neoplasms that cause extradural spinal cord compression are malignant and progress rapidly. Once spinal cord symptoms begin, paraplegia may develop in a matter of days. Complete paraplegia is usually irreversible, whereas patients with only moderate spinal cord dysfunction often recover. Thus, the early diagnosis and vigorous emergency treatment of extradural spinal cord compression is mandatory. The treatment includes corticosteroids (dexamethasone, 16 to 100 mg daily) to decrease spinal cord edema. In patients not known to be suffering from a primary cancer, metastatic disease is the most common cause of extradural spinal cord compression, but in these instances a definitive diagnosis must be made by biopsy. Such patients should begin corticosteroid therapy followed by surgery with removal of as much tumor as possible for both diagnostic and therapeutic purposes. When a primary cancer already has been diagnosed, treatment consists of radiation therapy and chemotherapeutic agents (if an effective agent is available). In patients in whom radiation therapy and chemotherapy are ineffective, resection of the vertebral body involved by tumor may delay the development of paraplegia. Benign extradural tumors require surgery and usually can be completely removed.

Intradural Extramedullary Tumors. Most intradural tumors are benign. Meningiomas and neurofibromas are the two most common types. Teratomas, arachnoid cysts, and lipomas are less common causes. Meningiomas occur especially in middle-aged and elderly women, predominantly in the thoracic spinal cord. Another common site is the foramen magnum. Meningiomas grow slowly. Pain is the first symptom in most patients, but in about 25 per cent the growth is painless, the first symptoms being those indicating gradually developing spinal cord compression. Because meningiomas are often located on the posterior aspect of the cord, paresthesias and sensory changes beginning distally in the lower extremities are a frequent early symptom and are often mistaken for peripheral neuropathy. As the disease progresses, however, the development of corticospinal tract signs indicates the spinal origin of the symptoms. Even when spinal cord signs and symptoms are obvious, the occasional lack of pain may lead one to suspect a degenerative or demyelinating disease such as multiple sclerosis rather than a neoplasm. In patients with meningiomas, the lumbar puncture reveals an elevated CSF protein content well above that found in degenerative or demyelinating diseases. CT, MR, or myelography usually establishes the diagnosis of a tumor. The treatment of spinal cord compression from meningiomas is surgical removal. Because the tumor grows so slowly and the cord has an opportunity to adapt to compression, even patients with severe neurological disability often recover fully.

The second most common cause of intradural spinal cord compression is neurofibroma. Because these tumors usually arise from the dorsal root, radicular pain is often the first symptom, preceding signs of spinal cord compression by months or years. When spinal cord compression develops, it progresses slowly. Some patients with spinal neurofibromas suffer from neurofibromatosis (see p. 747). That diagnosis may be suspected either by a positive family history or by the cutaneous stigmata of the disorder. As neurofibromas grow through the intervertebral foramen, they enlarge

it, a finding appreciated by an appropriately positioned radiograph. The CSF protein is almost always elevated. The diagnosis is established by myelography. Surgical extirpation of the lesion usually leads to recovery.

Occasionally metastatic tumors involving the leptomeninges produce intradural extramedullary mass lesions. Pain is almost always a prominent early symptom, and spinal cord compression develops more rapidly than it does with the more benign intradural tumors. In addition, malignant cells are usually found on cerebrospinal fluid examination. The glucose concentration may be low and the protein concentration elevated. The treatment of intradural malignant neoplasms is by radiation and chemotherapy, since complete surgical extirpation is almost always impossible.

Intramedullary Tumors. The most common intramedullary spinal tumors are astrocytomas (usually benign) and ependymomas. Other tumors that occasionally cause intramedullary spinal lesions are hemangioblastomas, lipomas, and metastases (Fig. 117–3). Pain is an early symptom of most intramedullary tumors, and signs of spinal cord dysfunction progress

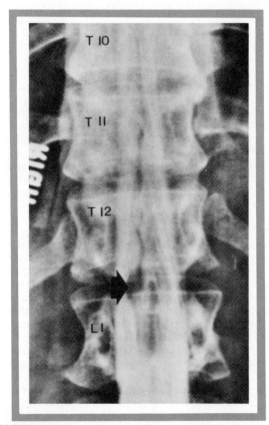

FIGURE 117–3. An intramedullary metastasis. A man with oat cell carcinoma of lung, in remission, complained of progressive weakness of the lower extremities and loss of bladder, bowel, and sexual function. A metrizamide myelogram revealed an area of enlargement at the conus medullaris (arrow), indicating a hematogenous metastasis to the spinal cord.

rapidly or slowly, depending on the growth characteristics of the tumor. Intramedullary tumors are often associated with syringomyelia, the syrinx sometimes lying at a distance from the primary tumor and producing its own symptoms of spinal dysfunction (p. 746). The so-called classic signs of intramedullary spinal cord lesions (dissociated sensory loss, sacral sparing, and early onset of bladder and bowel dysfunction) are not reliable enough clinically to distinguish intramedullary from extramedullary lesions; currently that diagnosis must be established by myelography or MR. In some patients with long-standing benign intramedullary lesions, plain radiographs of the spine may show widening of the spinal canal and erosion of the pedicles. If a syrinx is suspected, an MR is the test of choice. The differential diagnosis of intramedullary tumors includes intramedullary abscesses and syringomyelia without tumor. A definitive diagnosis is established by biopsy. Successful surgical removal of intramedullary tumors is possible, particularly with ependymomas and hemangioblastomas but sometimes with gliomas as well. A highly skilled and experienced surgeon, however, is necessary for tumors to be removed without producing increased neurological symptoms. If the tumor cannot be totally excised, postoperative radiation may delay recurrence.

Ependymomas have a predilection to involve the lower end of the spinal cord and the filum terminale. An unusual symptom sometimes produced by such tumors is *hydrocephalus*. Affected patients may present with headache, papilledema, and enlarged cerebral ventricles without signs of cauda equina dysfunction or with only minor signs such as mild sacral sensory loss or an absent ankle jerk. The pathogenesis of the hydrocephalus is believed to be the plugging of arachnoid granulations by protein exuded from the tumor into the spinal fluid. The diagnosis is suspected in a patient with papilledema and hydrocephalus accompanied by a high CSF protein; myelography establishes the diagnosis.

VASCULAR DISORDERS OF THE SPINAL CANAL

Extradural, intradural, and intramedullary vascular disorders all can cause spinal cord compression. The most common and serious extradural vascular disease is *spinal epidural hematoma*. Hemorrhage into the spinal epidural space may occur spontaneously or be associated with trauma, a bleeding diathesis, or a vascular malformation. The condition occurs particularly among patients being treated with anticoagulants. It may occasionally follow lumbar puncture, particularly in patients with bleeding abnormalities or those receiving anticoagulants. The hemorrhage usually arises from the epidural venous plexus and tends to collect over the dorsum of the spinal cord, covering several segments. The clinical picture is characterized by the sudden or rapid onset of severe localized back pain and spinal cord dysfunction, often leading to complete paraplegia in several hours. If the patient has a known

bleeding disorder, the clinical diagnosis is easily established. In patients without known bleeding or clotting disorders, the differential diagnosis includes acute epidural abscess and acute transverse myelopathy. Although occasional patients recover spontaneously from paraparesis related to epidural spinal cord compression, most require emergency surgical evacuation to save spinal cord function. The more rapidly the paralysis develops and the longer the delay in decompression, the less likely is recovery.

Spinal arteriovenous malformations may cause symptoms by hemorrhage (Fig. 117–4), compression, or ischemia. Spinal subarachnoid hemorrhage is characterized by the sudden onset of back pain, often with a radicular component, with or without the development of signs of spinal cord compression. A lumbar puncture reveals evidence of subarachnoid hemorrhage with red cells, xanthochromic spinal fluid, and usually an elevated protein concentration. In the absence of spinal cord signs, the differential diagnosis includes spontaneous intracranial subarachnoid hemorrhage. The diagnosis of spinal subarachnoid hemorrhage often can be suspected clinically because symptoms begin with back pain rather than with headache as in intracranial hemorrhage.

Vascular malformations within the substance of the spinal cord may give rise to intramedullary hemorrhage (hematomyelia) as well as subarachnoid hemorrhage. The sudden development of partial or complete transverse myelopathy is the most common onset. If there is bleeding into the subarachnoid space, pain in the neck and back and other signs of meningeal irritation occur.

Spinal arteriovenous malformations may also gradually compress the spinal cord or give rise to hemodynamic changes that result in spinal ischemia. In such cases, patients present with slowly progressive, sometimes episodically worsening symptoms of spinal

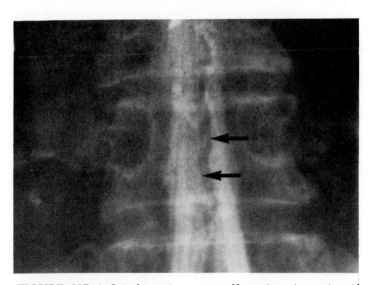

FIGURE 117–4. Spinal arteriovenous malformation. A metrizamide myelogram demonstrates a tangle of abnormal vessels (arrows) on the surface of the cord.

cord dysfunction. Transient exacerbation of symptoms may occur in association with menstrual periods or pregnancy.

Complete or partial recovery of function can follow episodes of spinal cord ischemia or even small hemorrhages. The unchanging localization of the attacks and the prominence of pain help differentiate symptoms caused by arteriovenous malformations from other recurrent neurological disorders such as multiple sclerosis. Rarely, a bruit may be heard by auscultation of the spine or back over the site of the malformation. Myelography often reveals vascular shadows suggesting the presence of arteriovenous malformation, but MR is a better screening test. Angiography with regional catheterization of radicular vessels is necessary as a preliminary step to surgical treatment. Advances in microsurgery have increased considerably the chances for satisfactory removal or obliteration of spinal vascular malformations. Embolization of the malformation or ligation of feeding arteries has been performed when the lesion cannot be removed surgically.

INHERITED AND DEVELOPMENTAL SPINAL STRUCTURAL DISORDERS

Congenital anomalies of the spine are common and are often encountered on radiographs of patients suffering from neck or low back pain. Some congenital anomalies such as spina bifida occulta are so common as to be considered variants of normal and are probably never responsible in and of themselves for low back pain. Other congenital anomalies that are usually asymptomatic but are potential causes of neck or back pain include *facet tropism* (misalignment of the facets on the two sides of the corresponding vertebral body; several authorities believe that this increases rotational stress on the facet joints and may cause back pain); *transitional vertebrae* (e.g., sacralization of a lumbar vertebra or lumbarization of a sacral vertebra) altering spinal mechanics, resulting in instability and stress, and sometimes producing back pain; and *spondylolisthesis* (forward slipping of one vertebral body onto another, caused by a defect between the articular facets). A third group of congenital anomalies of the spine consists of those that are likely to cause not only neck or back pain but also neurological disability. These include basilar impression, which is often associated with Arnold-Chiari malformation (see next section). Severe spinal scoliosis or kyphosis, congenital stenosis of the lumbar or cervical spinal canal, anterior and lateral spinal meningoceles, and diastematomyelia are other causes of back pain and neurological disability. *Diastematomyelia* is a bony abnormality that divides the spinal canal, leading to duplication of the spinal cord. It is usually associated with spina bifida. Sometimes the bony septum can be identified on plain x-rays. Patients who become symptomatic in adulthood almost always have some cutaneous abnormality, especially hypertrichosis over the sacral area. The dis-

order may be associated with other congenital abnormalities of the central nervous system as well.

Abnormalities of the Craniocervical Junction

Basilar impression consists of invagination of the odontoid process into the foramen magnum. Occasionally the condition arises from occipital bone softening due to Paget's disease, fibrous dysplasia, or cancer. Much more often basilar impression occurs as a congenital defect, often associated with anomalies of the foramen magnum, the Arnold-Chiari malformation, or syringomyelia. Symptoms of congenital basilar impression often first appear in the third or fourth decade of life and reflect the presence of either vertebral artery compression-ischemia or direct medullopontine compression-displacement. Occipital headache, vertigo, nystagmus, dysarthria, dysphagia, ataxia, abnormalities of central respiratory control, and long tract signs begin insidiously and progress gradually. Many patients develop a secondary obstructive hydrocephalus. Diagnosis is suggested by the clinical findings plus an abnormally short neck on inspection. MR reveals not only the protrusion of the odontoid process above the foramen magnum but also whether the Arnold-Chiari malformation is present (Fig. 117–5).

The *Arnold-Chiari malformation* type II consists of developmental displacement of the cerebellar tonsils through the foramen magnum, associated with elongation of the medulla and lower end of the fourth ventricle into the cervical canal. Symptoms can resemble

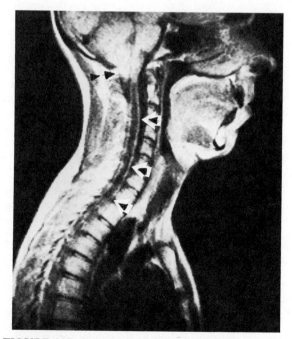

FIGURE 117–5. Midsagittal MR image of Chiari malformation (small black arrows) and syringomyelia (three white-black arrows) in a 33-year-old man. Note the cerebellar tonsils extending below the posterior rim of the foramen magnum (dark structure immediately above the black arrow). The syrinx extends from the medulla well into the thoracic cord.

those described for basilar impression, can be entirely due to obstructive hydrocephalus, or can reflect a progressive cerebellar ataxia. In any event, signs of spinal long tract dysfunction gradually become added to the above. MR imaging is diagnostic (Fig. 117–5). Treatment of either basilar impression or the Arnold-Chiari malformation causing progressive neurological deficits consists of surgical decompression or, when appropriate, ventricular shunting to relieve hydrocephalus.

Syringomyelia refers to a cavity within the central spinal cord, arising most often at the cervical level (Fig. 117–5). Syringomyelia can arise either as a congenital abnormality or in association with intra-medullary spinal neoplasms. In the congenital form, the lesions often extend into the medulla (syringobulbia) or can penetrate caudally into the thoracic and lumbosacral regions.

Pathologically, the syringomyelic cavity usually is associated anatomically with the central spinal canal; some communicate directly with the floor of the fourth ventricle. As life advances, the syrinx progressively replaces the centrally located gray matter of the posterior and anterior horns of the spinal cord and also interrupts the decussating spinothalamic pain-carrying fibers in the anterior commissure. Often, syringomyelia is associated with other congenital malformations, including the Arnold-Chiari malformation (Fig. 117–5), fusion of the cervical vertebrae, or malformations at the lumbosacral region, including spina bifida and associated meningomyelocele.

Clinical manifestations of congenital syringomyelia most often begin in the second or third decade, frequently affecting the hands or upper trunk with a typically dissociated impairment of pain and temperature sensation coupled with preservation of the senses of touch, vibration, and joint position. Progressive muscular atrophy usually develops in the involved segments, especially in the upper extremities, and commonly leads to kyphoscoliosis. The analgesia results in painless ulcers, burns, and traumatic arthropathy. As a rule, areflexia marks the upper extremities, while upper motor neuron signs eventually develop in the legs, accompanied in those members by reduced vibratory and position sensations. In most affected patients the disease process progresses slowly but relentlessly.

In patients with syringobulbia, dissociated impairment of pain and temperature develops over the face, along with nystagmus, pharyngeal and vocal cord paralysis, and lingual atrophy.

Clinical diagnosis is usually not difficult once considered. Leprosy, other rare and acquired peripheral neuropathies, and intramedullary destructive or neoplastic lesions of the spinal cord and brain stem are the only insidiously developing conditions that cause widespread dissociated loss of pain and temperature sensation. Leprosy can be dismissed if the subject has not been raised in an endemic area, and neither it nor other peripheral neuropathies produce signs of spinal cord dysfunction. The important consideration is whether or not an associated spinal neoplasm exists. MR imaging definitively outlines most syrinxes and neoplasms if present. Treatment generally is unsatis-factory unless a tumor is found and can be removed. Surgical drainage has been claimed to halt the disease process in some patients.

NEUROCUTANEOUS SYNDROMES

Neurofibromatosis, is a common disorder (1 in 3000 births) inherited as an autosomal dominant trait with a high spontaneous mutation rate (40 to 60 per cent of cases are clinically sporadic). There are two forms of the disorder. One (von Recklinghausen's neurofibromatosis) relates to a gene abnormality on chromosome 17. It is characterized by the occurrence of pigmented skin lesions (café au lait spots), multiple tumors of spinal or cranial nerves (neurofibromas composed of proliferating fibroblasts or neurilemmal sheath cells), skin tumors, and the frequent occurrence of intracranial meningiomas. There is an increased association with pheochromocytomas, cystic lung disease, renal vascular lesions causing hypertension, fibrous dysplasia of bone, and medullary thyroid carcinoma, as well as other tumors of endocrine glands. The tumors can overlap in the region of the brachial or sacral plexus to produce large plexiform neuromas that can evolve into malignant sarcomas. Intracranial astrocytomas and glioblastomas occur with a greater than normal frequency. Stenosis of the aqueduct with noncommunicating hydrocephalus is sometimes observed.

The presence of multiple cutaneous neurofibromas accompanied by nonraised café au lait spots represents the clinical hallmark. The pigmented skin lesions occur most commonly over the trunk and in the axilla. If greater than 1.5 cm in diameter and more than six in number, they indicate the presence of the disease. Nerve involvement can be solitary or multiple and diffuse. Multiple cranial nerves can be affected, resulting in facial weakness, numbness, deafness, and optic nerve atrophy. Local confluent tumors with associated fibrosis result in elephantiasis neuromatosa, as well as gross asymmetrical hypertrophy of body parts. Neurofibromas arising from nerve roots can invade the intervertebral foramina to compress the spinal cord or brain stem. A preliminary report suggests that ketotifen, a mast cell stabilizer, may slow tumor growth.

The second form, characterized by bilateral acoustic neuromas, is less common. Cutaneous manifestations may be absent, but meningiomas and spinal neurofibromas occur with increased frequency. The disorder is related to specific loss of alleles on chromosome 22.

Tuberous sclerosis is a neurocutaneous disorder inherited as an autosomal dominant trait. Its triad of findings, all present by late childhood, include facial nevi (adenoma sebaceum), epilepsy, and mental retardation. The importance of the disorder for adult medicine is that subtle cases occasionally produce problems in the differential diagnosis of early or late adolescent epilepsy, while funduscopic examination can disclose nodules or phakomas of the retina that look neoplastic but in fact are stable and similar in structure to the adenoma sebaceum. Some patients develop intracranial or optic gliomas. Rhabdomyomas of the heart as well as renal tumors and neoplasms of the endocrine organs can be observed.

Sturge-Weber disease produces a port wine–colored capillary hemangioma on the face accompanied by a similar vascular malformation of the underlying meninges and cerebral cortex. The cause is unknown. Diagnosis is made by observing the disfiguring stain involving the sensory dermatomal distribution of the first, second, or third portions of the trigeminal nerve. General or focal motor seizures may occur with or without associated mental retardation and require antiepileptic medication. The disfiguring stain deserves cosmetic repair if possible.

Hippel-Lindau disease is inherited in a simple autosomal dominant pattern and is characterized by hemangioblastomas of the cerebellar hemispheres with associated angiomas of the retina and cystic changes in the kidney and pancreas. Recent evidence maps the abnormal gene to chromosome 3 in the region associated with renal carcinoma. Hemangioblastomas can sometimes also be found in brain or spinal cord. An association with pheochromocytomas, polycythemia, and several forms of cancer has been noted.

REFERENCES

Callen JP, Meckler RJ: Neurocutaneous disorders. Neurol Clin, Vol 5, 1987.
Davidoff RA: Handbook of the Spinal Cord. Vols 4 and 5: Congenital Disorders, Trauma, Infections, Cancer. New York, Marcel Dekker, Inc, 1987.
Seizinger BR, Rouleau GA, Ozelius LJ, et al: Von Hippel-Lindau disease maps to region of chromosome 3 associated with renal cell carcinoma. Nature 332:268, 1988.

E. PERIPHERAL NERVE AND MOTOR NEURON DISORDERS

PERIPHERAL NERVES

General Considerations

Diseases of the peripheral nervous system may affect one (or more) of three structures: (1) the cell body (neuronopathy), (2) the axon (axonopathy), or (3) the Schwann cells and/or their metabolic product, the myelin sheath (demyelinating neuropathy). Any of these processes may be focal, leading to mononeuropathy (involvement of a single nerve) or multiple mononeuropathy (involvement of several different single nerves), or diffuse, causing polyneuropathy (a diffuse, predominantly symmetrical, and often distal involvement of the nerves of the extremities) (Table 117–5). The distal nature of most polyneuropathies reflects the fact that the longest nerves are the most metabolically active. Although each of the anatomical and pathological disorders listed in Table 117–5 can have distinctive clinical symptoms, there is considerable overlap. Furthermore, individual etiological agents, such as diabetes or cancer, may cause more than one type of neuropathy. Accordingly, in the pages that follow, the peripheral neuropathies are discussed first pathophysiologically and then etiologically. The same pathophysiological and etiological considerations apply to nerve roots that are the proximal extension of peripheral nerves and can be affected by focal (mono or multiple monoradiculopathy) or diffuse (polyradiculopathy) processes. One difference is that root lesions often extend to affect the spinal cord because of its proximity. This discussion covers focal nerve root lesions (and their accompanying spinal cord pathology, if any) before peripheral nerves.

In *demyelinating neuropathy* (Fig. 117–6) segments of myelin degenerate to a greater or lesser extent, usually due to immunological or infectious causes. Clinically, demyelinating neuropathy is characterized by functional failure of large myelinated fibers, leading to decreased light touch, position, and vibration sensation, as well as to weakness and reduction or absence of deep tendon reflexes. A relative sparing of lightly myelinated or unmyelinated fibers partially preserves temperature and pain sensation, although these modalities become involved if the disorder is severe. The onset of demyelinating neuropathy may be rapid, and with Schwann cell proliferation and remyelination, recovery may be equally rapid. Because the myelin sheath can be involved anywhere throughout its peripheral course, the disease, although usually symmetrical, sometimes affects both proximal and distal fibers to a similar degree. Cranial nerves are often involved, as well as peripheral nerves. The spinal fluid protein is elevated in diffuse demyelinating neurop-

TABLE 117–5. ANATOMICAL AND PATHOLOGICAL CLASSIFICATION OF PERIPHERAL NEUROPATHIES

LESION	CLINICAL EXAMPLES(S)
Focal	
Mononeuropathy or radiculopathy	Median nerve compression (carpal tunnel syndrome)
	Herniated disc
Multiple monoradiculopathies or radiculopathies	Periarteritis nodosa
	Lumbar spondylosis
Diffuse (Polyneuropathies)	
Axonopathies	
Distal	Diabetes, uremia
Central	Clioquinol poisoning
Myelinopathy	Guillain-Barré syndrome
Neuronopathies	
Sensory	Paraneoplastic sensory neuronopathy
Motor	Amyotrophic lateral sclerosis
Autonomic	Shy-Drager syndrome

Modified from Schaumburg HH, Spencer PS, Thomas PK: Disorders of Peripheral Nerve. Philadelphia, FA Davis Co, 1983.

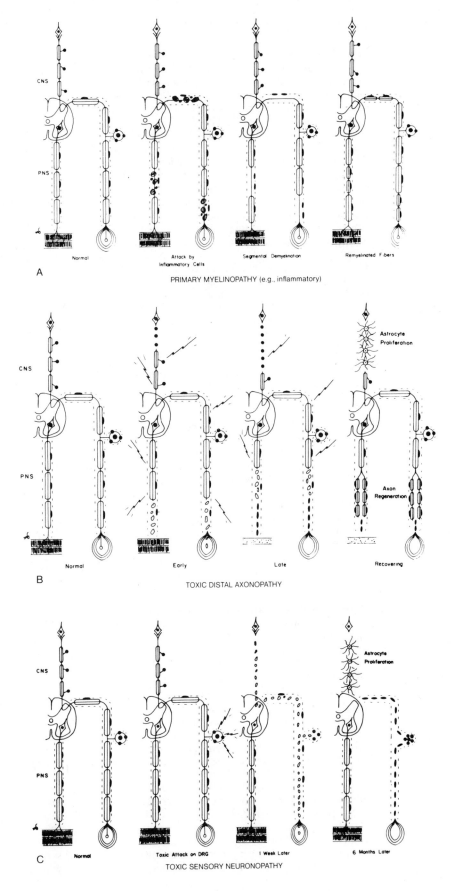

FIGURE 117–6. Pathological processes damaging the peripheral nervous system (PNS). *A*, A diagram of the cardinal pathological features of inflammatory PNS myelinopathy. Axons are spared, as in CNS demyelinating illness. Following the attack the remaining Schwann cells divide. The denuded segments of axons are remyelinated, leaving them with short internodes. *B*, The cardinal pathological features of a toxic distal axonopathy. The jagged lines (lightning bolts) indicate that the toxin is acting at multiple sites along motor and sensory axons in the PNS and CNS. Axon degeneration has moved proximally (dying-back) by the late stage. Recovery in the CNS is impeded by astroglial proliferation. *C*, The cardinal features of a rapidly evolving toxic sensory neuronopathy. The jagged lines (lightning bolts) indicate that the toxin is directed at neurons in the dorsal root ganglion (DRG). Degeneration of these cells is accompanied by a fragmentation and phagocytosis of their peripheral central processes. Schwann cells remain. There is no axonal regeneration. (From Schaumburg HH, Spencer PS, Thomas PK: Disorders of Peripheral Nerves. Philadelphia, FA Davis Co, 1983.)

athies because of damage to spinal roots. Electrical studies of demyelinated nerves reveal that conduction velocity is slowed, often to 20 or 25 per cent of normal values, and the amplitude of the action potential is small because it is dispersed over a longer duration.

Axonal neuropathy (Fig. 117–6) is characterized by degeneration of the distal ends of long axons, with secondary loss and degeneration of the myelin sheath. The disorder usually causes an equal loss of all sensory modalities, although in some instances small axons carrying pain and temperature suffer a loss disproportionate to larger axons. The first symptoms are usually sensory, with paresthesias or sensory loss of the tips of the fingers and toes. Only later, as the sensory loss spreads more proximally, does motor involvement occur in a typical "stocking and glove" distribution. Unlike with demyelinating neuropathy, recovery is usually slow because of the slow rate of regeneration of the damaged axons. Spinal roots usually are not involved and the CSF protein remains normal. Electrically, axonal neuropathies are characterized by normal or only slightly (10 to 15 per cent) slowed conduction velocity and by small sensory action potentials.

A recently described *central axonopathy* caused by several toxic substances may underlie some human degenerative diseases. This disorder is characterized by selective vulnerability of that portion of the sensory axon that lies between the dorsal root ganglion and the spinal cord, sparing the peripheral axon. There is a dying back of the axon in the posterior column, proceeding from distal to proximal, with secondary loss of the surrounding myelin sheath and gliosis of the posterior column. Central motor pathways may also be affected, with degeneration of distal portions of the corticospinal tract. The sensory loss usually begins subacutely with paresthesias and loss of large fiber function. Unlike with peripheral axonopathies, the deep tendon reflexes are usually hyperactive, and because of corticospinal tract damage, a spastic paraparesis may accompany the disorder.

Neuronopathies can also affect either sensory or motor nerves, or both. Neuronopathies cause either acute or gradual onset of sensory and/or motor loss with little or no recovery.

FOCAL RADICALOPATHY AND NEUROPATHY

The etiological agents that cause focal neuropathy usually differ from those causing polyneuropathy, although some diseases, such as diabetes and hypothyroidism, can cause either mononeuropathy or polyneuropathy. Most focal neuropathies result from vascular disease, compression, or trauma. Clinically, the mononeuropathies are characterized by sensory and/or motor loss (usually both) in the anatomical distribution of all or part of a nerve root, nerve plexus, or peripheral nerve (Fig. 117–7). One can determine the site of the injury clinically by observing the anatomical distribution of dysfunction (e.g., an injury to the radial nerve at the humerus causes weakness of the brachioradialis muscle and extensors of the wrist and fingers, but spares the triceps muscle because radial nerve fibers in the triceps depart from the nerve more proximally in the upper arm).

TRAUMA AND COMPRESSION

Most mononeuritides and monoradiculopathies are caused by trauma and result either from compression, transection, or stretching of nerve, or from chronic entrapment by various anatomical structures. Perhaps the most common disabling disorder is entrapment of a cervical or lumbar nerve root by a herniated intervertebral disc as the root passes through the intervertebral foramen. Mild injury to a nerve may leave the nerve structurally intact but cause a conduction block first by ischemia and subsequently by demyelination. Acute ischemic lesions recover rapidly when pressure is released; demyelinating lesions may recover more slowly. A more severe injury interrupts the axons but leaves the connective tissue sheaths intact. Such lesions are common in closed crush injuries. Depending on the degree of damage, recovery may be partial or complete, but it proceeds slowly. The most severe injury is transection of both axons and connective tissue sheaths, such as occurs with severe stretch injuries or penetrating wounds. Because of the interruption of the sheath, recovery does not occur unless the nerve is surgically repaired, and even then the prognosis is poor.

Acute Trauma

Any portion of the peripheral nervous system can be damaged by trauma. In wartime, penetrating wounds of peripheral nerves and nerve plexuses are major causes of disability. In peacetime, traumatic peripheral nerve lesions usually result from closed crush or traction injuries. The brachial plexus is a major site of stretch injuries, commonly resulting from motorcycle accidents or compression injury when the arm is hyperabducted, as under anesthesia. The former injuries are usually permanent, the latter transient. Other acute compression injuries that sometimes follow general anesthesia for surgery or are self-induced by alcohol or sedatives include radial nerve palsy from compression of the nerve in the radial groove of the humerus (Saturday night palsy), peroneal nerve palsy from compression between the surface and the head of the fibula (crossed-leg palsies), ulnar palsy (often from compression by an IV board in the ulnar groove at the elbow), and sciatic palsies from compression of the buttocks or ill-placed injections into that site.

Chronic Compression Radiculopathies and Myelopathies

Herniated Intervertebral Disc. With adequate trauma, the disc material herniates into the vertebral canal, generally lateral to the posterior longitudinal ligament, thereby compressing spinal roots as they enter the intervertebral foramen. Occasionally, the disc herniates more centrally, compressing either the spinal cord in the cervical or thoracic area or the cauda equina in the lumbar area. The specific signs and symptoms of herniated discs depend in part on whether the predominant compression is spinal cord

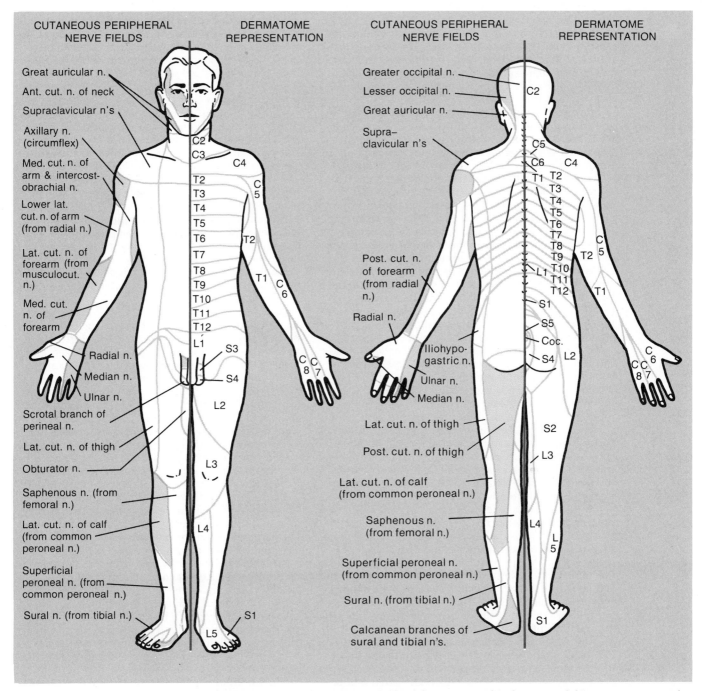

FIGURE 117–7. The cutaneous fields of the major peripheral nerves and dermatomes seen on the anterior (A) and posterior (B) surfaces of the body. (Redrawn from Haymaker W, Woodhall B: Peripheral Nerve Injuries. Philadelphia, WB Saunders Co, 1953.)

or nerve root, and in part on the level at which the neural structures are compressed. The most common sites of herniation are in the lumbar area, between L4 and L5 or L5 and S1, with the ensuing compression being upon the L5 and S1 roots. (Because of the anatomy, a laterally herniated disc between L4 and L5 compresses the L5 root, and a disc between L5 and

S1, the S1 root.) L3-L4 herniations are less common. In the cervical area, the common herniations occur between C5 and C6 (C6 root) and, most often, between C6 and C7 (C7 root). Less frequently, herniations appear between C3 and C4, C4 and C5, and C7 and T1. Thoracic disc herniations are rare, but when they occur they usually compress the spinal cord as well as the emerging root because of the narrowness of the thoracic vertebral canal. Although clinical localization in the diagnosis of disc disease is usually quite accurate, an extruded disc fragment at times may be large enough to affect several roots, or may migrate from the disc space in which it herniated, causing signs at a distance from the original herniation.

The most common symptom of herniated disc is pain. Local pain is felt as a dull aching in the neck or back, with an associated stiffness of those structures, frequently occurring episodically in response to minor trauma (or no discernible trauma at all) months or years prior to the development of radicular pain. The exact pathogenesis of the local back pain in disc disease is not known, but some believe that it results from compression of the sinuvertebral nerve, a recurrent branch of the nerve root that supplies the dura mater. Radicular pain may occasionally be the first sign of disc disease but is far more likely to follow repetitive bouts of local pain. Radicular pain is perceived as sharp and well-localized and may radiate from the back along the entire distribution of the involved root or affect only a portion of the root. Both local and radicular pain have the characteristics of being exacerbated by activity and relieved by rest.

With cervical disc herniation, most patients hold their necks stiffly and resist passive movement. Lateral bending, either to or away from the side of the herniated disc, frequently exacerbates both the local and the radicular pain. The patient may be more comfortable with his neck slightly flexed but is usually comfortable only when recumbent. Patients with lumbar disc disease are most comfortable lying, most uncomfortable sitting, and a little less uncomfortable standing. The back is held stiffly, reducing or erasing the normal lumbar lordotic curve, and pain is usually exacerbated by extension of the back. Slow forward bending sometimes relieves the pain. Muscle spasm is prominent with both cervical and lumbar disc disease. Raising the intraspinal pressure, as by coughing, sneezing, or straining, increases the pain sharply. Directly stretching the compressed root also aggravates the pain. In the upper extremities, extending the arm and laterally flexing the neck away from the extended arm often reproduces radicular pain. In the lower extremities, raising the extended leg with the patient in the recumbent position frequently reproduces the pain of an L5 or S1 radiculopathy and, if the pain is felt on the opposite side as well (crossed straight leg raising), the sign is very suggestive of herniated disc disease. Symptoms of L4 radiculopathy often can be reproduced by extending the hip or fully flexing the knee (stretching the femoral nerve) when the patient is lying in the prone position. Often tenderness is present along the entire distribution of the nerve(s) supplied by the compressed root, as well as in muscles supplied by the root. In patients with cervical disc disease, palpation or light percussion of the brachial plexus and the supraclavicular fossa or axilla often causes pain. In patients with lumbar disc disease, palpation over the femoral nerve (L4) in the groin or over the sciatic nerve (L5-S1) in the calf, thigh, or buttocks can cause severe pain. Occasionally tenderness in the calf (the posterior tibial nerve) can be so striking as to suggest that the patient is suffering from thrombophlebitis rather than disc herniation. Other neurological signs that commonly accompany disc disease include paresthesias and sensory loss in the distribution of the involved root and motor weakness in the myotome supplied by that root. The most important sign is a locally diminished or absent deep tendon reflex, giving objective evidence of neurological disease.

If an intervertebral disc herniates medially, rather than laterally, it may spare the root and involve the spinal cord or cauda equina directly. The lesion then mimics a spinal tumor (see p. 742) except that with disc disease there may be little or no pain. The diagnosis of herniated disc is deduced from the characteristic clinical symptoms and findings. Both CT and MRI are effective in identifying most disc disease (Fig. 117–7). Myelography may be performed before surgical extirpation to localize the site of disc herniation and to determine whether other disc lesions or tumors are present as well, but in most cases the CT or MR scan suffices.

No consensus exists about the preferred management of herniated discs. Most physicians believe that the first step is bed rest. Some investigators have reported that adrenocorticosteroids, either taken orally or injected into the epidural space, may hasten resolution of pain and other symptoms. A short course of oral steroids is safe, but there is no unequivocal evidence that it is efficacious. Steroids injected into the epidural or subarachnoid space, particularly those in depot form, may produce severe inflammatory reactions and are inadvisable. Surgery is indicated when (1) bed rest fails, and the patient is incapacitated by severe, intractable pain; (2) a centrally placed lumbar disc compresses the cauda equina, producing urinary dysfunction; or (3) there is motor weakness caused by compression of the spinal cord. Some believe that peripheral motor weakness caused by root compression is also an indication for immediate surgery. The best operation removes the involved disc, leaving intact as much bone as possible. Fusion of the lumbar spine is rarely necessary. Lumbar disc operations are done posteriorly via a laminotomy. Cervical disc operations may be done either posteriorly to decompress the cord or anteriorly to remove the disc without disturbing posterior bony elements. The surgical approach for myelopathy should probably be anterior if the disc is in the cervical area and lateral if the disc is in the thoracic area.

Disc dissolution by the injection of the enzyme chymopapain directly into the lumbar disc space is less widely used than formerly because of the complications of spinal damage and anaphylactic shock. A new technique in which disc material is suctioned out through a percutaneous catheter is currently under clinical trial.

Spondylosis. Spondylosis is a term applied to chronic degenerative disease of intervertebral discs associated with reactive changes in the adjacent vertebral bodies. Spondylotic changes in the neck and low back increase with increasing age and are almost invariably present in the elderly. Most spondylosis causes no symptoms, except when the reactive tissue compresses a nerve root or the spinal cord. When this occurs, the signs and symptoms resemble those of a herniated disc, but the onset is less abrupt and the treatment often more difficult. In both the cervical and lumbar areas, spondylosis is more likely to produce spinal cord or cauda equina symptoms if the sagittal diameter of the spinal canal is further impinged upon by osteophytes. The signs and symptoms of *cervical spondylosis* result from compression either of the spinal cord or its emerging roots and are thus similar to those of a herniated disc. Most patients suffer either radiculopathy or myelopathy (see p. 744) but not both. Pain is common in patients with spondylotic radiculopathy but usually less acute and severe than with herniated discs, and muscle spasm may be absent. However, the vertebral degenerative changes in the neck often lead to limitation of movement in all directions. The classic picture of cervical spondylotic *myelopathy* is one of little or no pain but slowly developing weakness, atrophy, and fasciculations in the upper extremities, particularly the small muscles of the hand, or an insidiously developing spastic paraparesis with decreased proprioception in the legs. At first the findings may suggest a diagnosis of amyotrophic lateral sclerosis (see p. 757). However, in cervical spondylosis there are sensory changes, particularly vibration loss in the lower extremities, and in amyotrophic lateral sclerosis there are fasciculations arising in areas different from motor roots compressed at the cervical level (e.g., the tongue). The differential diagnosis also includes other compressive lesions of root and spinal cord.

Plain radiographs of the cervical spine confirm the presence of cervical spondylosis, but many patients without symptoms have similar radiographic findings. When neurological signs suggest that cervical spondylosis is causing a myelopathy, magnetic resonance imaging is the examination of choice, often making more invasive myelography unnecessary (Fig. 117–8).

The natural history of cervical myelopathy and radiculopathy varies considerably among different individuals. Many patients experience long periods of pain relief and remission or stabilization of neurological symptoms. Such spontaneous improvement makes it difficult to evaluate the effect of a particular treatment. Many physicians prefer, once having established the diagnosis, to begin conservative treatment with a period of bed rest accompanied by cervical traction and stabilization of the neck with a soft collar. If these approaches are successful, they should be continued. However, if the patient develops progressive neurological signs, especially weakness and atrophy or spasticity, surgical therapy is indicated. Most neurosurgeons believe that if the spinal cord compression occurs at one or two segments, anterior removal of the disc material with spinal fusion is the preferred course. If more than a few segments are involved, laminectomy with foraminotomy is preferred.

In some patients with cervical spondylosis (or with congenital narrowing of the cervical spinal canal, or both), neurological symptoms are exacerbated by exercise, with pain, numbness, and weakness appearing

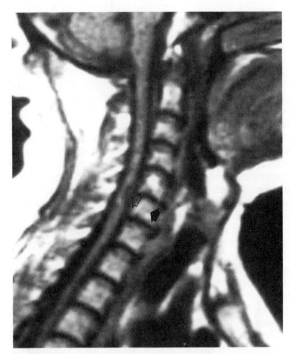

FIGURE 117–8. Cervical disc herniation causing myelopathy. MR image from a middle-aged patient with a one-year history of numbness in the right arm and progressive spastic weakness of both legs. There was no pain. Although magnetic resonance does not image bone, the bone marrow in the vertebral bodies is clearly visible (closed arrow). The herniated disc impinging on the cervical cord between C5 and C6 can be easily seen (open arrow).

when a particular extremity is exercised. The pathogenesis is thought to be compression of the spinal cord so severe that the blood supply to the area cannot increase during activity, leading to ischemia of the cord and root structures (pseudoclaudication).

The considerations described above under cervical spondylosis also apply to *lumbar spondylosis*. The symptoms of lumbar spondylosis are similar to those of herniated disc, often occurring at multiple levels. One outstanding difference is the frequent presence of pseudoclaudication from cauda equina compression in patients with spinal stenosis from either spondylosis or congenital narrowing. Typically, symptoms and signs are evoked or accentuated by walking and include pain, paresthesias, and weakness in the lower extremities. All of the symptoms may disappear when the patient ceases walking, even though he remains in the standing position. At times, however, the symptoms may be exacerbated by prolonged standing and relieved only by sitting or lying down. Pseudoclaudication of the cauda equina may be distinguished from intermittent vascular claudication in several ways. In vascular disease, the pulses in the lower extremities are usually absent or become absent as the patient begins to exercise. With vascular disease, the symptoms are usually reproducible and stereotypic; i.e., the patient can predict the exact distance he can walk at a given speed before symptoms develop. Symptoms of cauda equina pseudoclaudication are less stereotypic, so that on some days patients can walk much longer distances than on others. The reason for this variability is not known. In patients with pseudoclaudication, the neurological examination may be normal when the patient is at rest, but abnormal signs, particularly absence of deep tendon reflexes, may appear as the patient exercises. In patients with pseudoclaudication the lumbar canal is narrowed on either lateral x-ray, CT, or MR scan, and there is a substantial block to the passage of myelographic dye. With severe lumbar stenosis, conservative treatment usually fails and decompressive laminectomy is the treatment of choice.

Chronic Compression Neuropathies

In order to reach their peripheral targets, many nerves must pass through narrow channels where they can become chronically compressed in fibro-osseous tunnels, angulated and stretched over arthritic joints or bony structures, or recurrently compressed by repeated trauma. Table 117–6 lists the major compression neuropathies. The most common are discussed below.

Carpal Tunnel Syndrome. The median nerve is compressed at the wrist as it passes deep to the flexor retinaculum. The usual symptoms include numbness, tingling, and burning sensations in one or both hands and the fingers supplied by the median nerve, including the thumb, index, middle, and half of the ring finger. Some patients complain that all fingers become numb, but if tested this is usually found not to be the case. Pain and paresthesias are most prominent at night and often interrupt sleep. The pain is prominent at the wrist but may radiate to the forearm or at times to the shoulder. Both pain and paresthesias are relieved by shaking the hands. In some patients, symptoms may persist for years without objective signs of median nerve damage. In others, sensory loss may appear over the tips of the fingers and/or weakness can develop in the median nerve–innervated thumb muscles in association with atrophy of the lateral aspect of the thenar eminence.

The carpal tunnel syndrome occurs mostly in middle-aged and obese women. It may affect those who use the wrists and hands occupationally, as in gardening, house painting, meat wrapping, or typing. Other predisposing causes include pregnancy, myxedema, acromegaly, rheumatoid arthritis, and primary amyloidosis.

The diagnosis is based on clinical symptoms, the finding of Tinel's sign (paresthesias in the finger with a light tap over the nerve at the wrist), and the demonstration of a conduction block at the wrist by motor nerve velocity studies. The most effective treatment is section of the transverse carpal ligament, decompressing the nerve.

Ulnar Palsy. The ulnar nerve may be injured at the elbow, especially in persons with a shallow ulnar groove and those who rest on their elbows excessively. Injury may also occur years after a "malunited" supracondylar fracture of the humerus with bony overgrowth (*tardive ulnar palsy*). Contrary to the findings in the carpal tunnel syndrome, muscle weakness and atrophy characteristically predominate over sensory symptoms and signs. Patients notice atrophy of the first dorsal interosseous muscle and difficulty performing fine manipulations of the fingers. There may be numbness of the small finger, the contiguous half of the ring finger, and the ulnar border of the hand.

Cervical Rib and Thoracic Outlet Syndrome. The brachial plexus as it passes through the thoracic outlet can be compressed by a cervical rib or by normal bone, muscles, and fibrous tissue. The compression usually occurs when the arm is abducted and may involve the subclavian artery as well as the plexus. Symptoms include paresthesias of ulnar fingers and rarely weakness and wasting of the small hand muscles. The sensory abnormalities usually respond to avoiding the abducted position, but surgical removal of the first rib and fibrous band may occasionally be necessary if weakness persists.

Immune Focal Neuropathies

A few acute focal neuropathies are believed to have an immune cause. The most common is *acute brachial neuritis*, characterized by the acute onset of severe pain, usually in the distribution of the axillary nerve (over the lateral shoulder) but at times extending into the entire arm. It generally subsides after a few days to a week. Usually coincident with the subsidence of the pain, weakness of the proximal arm becomes apparent. The serratus anterior is the most commonly paralyzed muscle, but other muscles of the shoulder girdle, including the deltoid and muscles of the upper arm, may be paralyzed as well. Rarely, most of the arm and even the ipsilateral diaphragm are paralyzed. Sensory loss is usually restricted to the distribution of the axillary nerve. Weakness may last weeks to months and be accompanied by severe atrophy of the shoulder girdle. Total recovery occurs in most patients within several months to two or three years. The disorder has been reported to follow upper respiratory infection or an immunization, but often there is no antecedent illness. Considerably less common is a similar disorder affecting the *lumbosacral plexus*, causing pain and weakness of a lower extremity. As with acute brachial neuritis, although the pain may be severe and the weakness profound, recovery usually occurs. Differential diagnosis from acute disc herniation is made

---

TABLE 117–6. COMMON SITES OF NERVE ENTRAPMENT

Median nerve
  Carpal tunnel—wrist
  Pronator muscle—elbow
Ulnar nerve
  Elbow
  Wrist
Radial nerve—humeral groove
Brachial plexus—thoracic outlet
Sciatic nerve—buttock (sciatic notch)
Peroneal nerve—behind knee
Lateral femoral cutaneous nerve—inguinal ligament
Cervical and lumbar root—intervertebral canal

readily by identifying the distribution, which involves incomplete dysfunction of multiple nerve roots rather than a single root.

Infectious Focal Neuropathies

Cranial nerves and nerves of the cauda equina may be damaged by acute bacterial meningitis, subacute meningitis (e.g., tuberculosis), or less commonly chronic meningitis (e.g., fungal meningitis). Common infections of the peripheral nervous system include herpes zoster, leprosy, Lyme disease, and AIDS.

Vascular Neuropathies

Several diseases that affect small or medium-sized vessels may lead to ischemia or infarction of isolated peripheral nerves. The most common disorder is a mononeuropathy that complicates diabetes. Mononeuropathy or multiple mononeuropathies commonly arise as early complications or first symptoms of periarteritis nodosa. Less commonly, rheumatoid arthritis, systemic lupus erythematosus, hypersensitivity angiitis, Sjögren's syndrome, or Wegener's granulomatosis may cause a similar peripheral neuropathy. Vascular neuropathies are characterized by the acute onset of motor and sensory loss in the distribution of one or more single peripheral nerves. With the passage of time, other nerves become involved. Depending on the intensity of the vasculitis, the neurological deficit may resolve after weeks or months, only to affect another nerve at a distant place. Severe cases can involve so many nerves that the condition resembles a polyneuropathy rather than a mononeuritis multiplex. Usually a careful history will distinguish the focal onset of the latter.

MONO- AND MULTIPLE CRANIAL NERVE NEUROPATHIES

Several disorders cause acute or chronic dysfunction of one or more cranial nerves. *Acute cranial nerve mononeuropathies* include optic neuropathy, described on p. 718. Ocular motor mononeuropathies (i.e., sudden dysfunction of cranial nerves III, IV, or VI) usually have a vascular basis. An example is *diabetic ophthalmoplegia*, which generally occurs in mildly affected diabetics, sometimes before the diagnosis of diabetes is made. It is characterized by painful onset of single cranial nerve paralysis (most commonly the oculomotor, sparing the pupil). The pain resolves in a few days and the paralysis subsides over a few months. Similar disorders affecting nondiabetics are called acute ocular neuropathy, which likewise has a benign prognosis. The differential diagnosis includes compression lesions (i.e., tumor or aneurysm) and inflammatory lesions (meningitis). *Acute facial palsy* is usually of unknown cause and has a benign prognosis (Bell's palsy). The disorder may follow a banal infection or exposure to a draft and usually begins with mild pain behind the ear followed, within several hours, by paralysis of the muscles supplied by the facial nerve.

Unilateral loss of taste is commom (chorda tympani). Some patients complain of ipsilateral hyperacusis (from paralysis of the nerve to the stapedius), and a few patients develop a dry eye. More patients complain of excessive tearing because the muscle weakness leads the lower lid to turn out, allowing for overflow of normal tear production. Recovery usually begins within two months, and within nine months to a year 80 per cent of patients report virtually normal function. In a few patients there is no clinical recovery and some develop symptoms of aberrant regeneration, including synkinesis (e.g., eye closure when the patient attempts to smile, or grimacing when blinking) or crocodile tears (tearing during eating). The pathogenesis of the disorder is believed to be an infectious-inflammatory swelling of the facial nerve in the facial canal of the middle ear, leading to an acute compression neuropathy. Differential diagnosis includes herpes zoster as well as tumors and basal meningitis (e.g., Lyme disease, sarcoid). In herpes, the vesicles may be found only in the auditory canal behind the ear. Tumor or infection are especially likely in the case of bilateral acute-subacute facial nerve palsy. The most important aspect of management is to protect the cornea. Patients' with acute, severe facial paralysis cannot close the eye, and the cornea should be protected with a lens when out of doors and the eye should probably be patched at night. Although the evidence of efficacy is weak, many physicians who encounter a patient with Bell's palsy during the first 48 to 72 hours of paralysis treat the disorder with a short course of corticosteroids (60 mg of prednisone for one week, with gradual tapering over the next week) when not otherwise contraindicated. *Acoustic or vestibular nerve neuropathies* are believed to result from either vascular or inflammatory (viral) disorders and are discussed on page 926. Acute neuropathy of other cranial nerves occurs rarely. The etiology and pathogenesis are usually unexplained and recovery is common.

Multiple cranial nerve neuropathies are uncommon except as they complicate tumors at the base of the skull (e.g., nasopharyngeal carcinoma), leptomeningeal metastases, or meningitis (e.g., tuberculosis, sarcoid, Lyme disease). Idiopathic multiple cranial neuropathies typically begin with pain in the eye or face; paralysis develops acutely, often responds to treatment with corticosteroids, and may be recurrent. The most common well-defined syndrome is the Tolosa-Hunt syndrome, characterized by unilateral paralysis of muscles supplied by oculomotor, trochlear, and abducent nerve, sometimes accompanied by sensory loss in the first division of the trigeminal nerve. The disorder is thought to result from granulomatous inflammation of the superior orbital fissure or cavernous sinus. Similar syndromes can involve lower cranial nerves or a combination of oculomotor and lower cranial nerves. When the disorder is painless and symmetrical it may represent a restricted form or initial manifestation of the Guillain-Barré syndrome.

Chronic cranial mononeuropathies can affect the same nerves as their acute counterparts. In addition, a slowly developing sensory *trigeminal neuropathy* may occur unilaterally or bilaterally. The disorder can complicate the course of several collagen vascular diseases (e.g., Sjögren's syndrome, Chapter 103) or be idiopathic. *Trigeminal neuralgia* (see p. 712) and *hemifacial spasm* are disorders believed to result from compression of the cranial nerve by tortuous arteries in the posterior fossa.

POLYNEUROPATHY

Inflammatory/Immune Polyneuropathies

Several acute and chronic polyneuropathies are associated with inflammatory infiltrates in the peripheral nerves and roots. The mechanism of neurological dysfunction is usually demyelination, believed to be on an immune basis. Most of these disorders are rare, the exception being the Guillain-Barré syndrome (GBS, or acute postinfectious polyneuropathy). An acute disorder, GBS has a peak incidence in middle age but can affect all ages and races and both sexes. The disorder is characterized by a rapidly progressive, predominantly motor neuropathy that may paralyze all voluntary muscles, including those supplied by the cranial nerves and those controlling respiration. Sensory changes are usually milder than motor abnormalities and may include no more than tingling paresthesias in the hands and feet. Rarely, sensory loss may be profound and be more significant than motor weakness. Pain is common, as is some degree of autonomic dysfunction. Many patients suffer from hypertension or cardiac arrhythmias, the latter being the usual cause of death in the 5 per cent of patients who die. Bilateral facial paralysis is also common and helps distinguish the GBS from other polyneuropathies.

Characteristically, a previously healthy person who has suffered a mild respiratory infection in the past two or three weeks (other predisposing factors include surgical procedures and Hodgkin's disease) notes the painless onset of mild weakness in the lower extremities, often accompanied by tingling paresthesias in toes and fingers. Although the patient is aware of weakness, particularly when walking or climbing stairs, the examiner at this early stage may be unable to discern any abnormality save for diminished deep tendon reflexes. Over a matter of a few days in untreated cases, the weakness becomes more profound and often ascends from the lower extremities to the upper extremities and finally to the face (Landry's ascending paralysis). Deep tendon reflexes disappear, and the patient may complain of proprioceptive loss in arms and legs. It may become difficult for him to swallow and breathe. Examination now reveals symmetrical motor weakness of both proximal and distal muscles of all extremities. The spinal fluid protein concentration, which is normal during the first several days, rises often above 100 mg/dl, usually without an accompanying pleocytosis. In most instances the weakness progresses for several days to a couple of weeks and then stabilizes. After a period of stability, recovery begins and in 85 per cent of patients it is complete over several weeks to months. Some patients require respiratory support and careful monitoring of

cardiovascular function during the acute stages. Thus hospitalization is necessary until recovery is well under way. In a small minority of patients, neural function recovers only partially or not at all, and a few patients with persistently high spinal fluid proteins develop headaches and papilledema as a late complication of the illness. The pathogenesis of the latter is believed to be the plugging of arachnoid villi by the persistently elevated protein.

There is an unusual variant of GBS characterized by ataxia, oculomotor paralysis, and reflex absence. Other less common neuropathies that are probably GBS variants include a *chronic inflammatory neuropathy*, which may be progressive or relapsing and, unlike classic GBS, responds favorably to corticosteroid therapy, and acute neuropathies that predominantly involve either sensory or autonomic fibers.

There are two aspects to the treatment of the disorder. Plasmapheresis, particularly when applied early in the course of the illness, halts its progression and shortens its duration often in a dramatic manner. Supportive care, including respiratory support and careful monitoring of cardiovascular function, prevents the major complications that lead to death. Corticosteroids have no useful role in the treatment of the disorder, except when it relates to Hodgkin's disease.

Other immune polyneuropathies not related to the Guillain-Barré syndrome are those associated with multiple myeloma, particularly of the osteoblastic variety, and benign monoclonal gammopathies. The neuropathy in these instances slowly progresses and has a sensorimotor distribution with no distinct systemic signs other than the alterations of serum proteins. The pathogenesis is thought to be immune in that the gamma globulin produced in excess by the primary disorder deposits on the nerves to react with a myelin-associated glycoprotein and cause demyelination. In the case of multiple myeloma, treatment of the primary disease sometimes leads to amelioration of the neuropathy.

Metabolic Neuropathies

Several metabolic or nutritional diseases are associated with polyneuropathy (Table 117–7). Diabetic

TABLE 119–7. METABOLIC AND NUTRITIONAL DISEASES OF PERIPHERAL NERVES

Endocrine
  Diabetes (polyneuropathy)
  Hypothyroidism
  Acromegaly (usually entrapment neuropathies)
Nutritional
  Vitamin deficiency
    Thiamine (beriberi; Wernicke's disease)
    Pyridoxine (isoniazid toxicity)
    Vitamin B_{12} (pernicious anemia, gastrectomy)
  Multiple factors (alcohol)
  Malnutrition (Vitamins B_6 and E)
Renal (uremia)
Hepatic
  Porphyria
  Chronic liver failure

neuropathy (Table 117–8) can take several forms.

These subacute or chronic sensorimotor neuropathies have few individually characteristic signs, and the diagnosis is usually suggested by identifying the underlying systemic disease; e.g., most patients with the peripheral neuropathy of acute intermittent porphyria have mental changes and/or abdominal pain preceding the onset of the neuropathy. Likewise the characteristic slow reflexes of hypothyroidism are usually present in addition to the sensorimotor polyneuropathy. In any patient suffering from a chronic progressive sensorimotor polyneuropathy, a careful search for metabolic disorders is essential to establish the diagnosis.

Toxic Neuropathies

Table 117–9 lists some of the toxins known or believed to cause polyneuropathies. In general, polyneuropathies produced by toxins are sensorimotor in pattern, although a few, such as those caused by acrylamide and pyridoxine toxicity, produce predominantly sensory changes. In every instance of obscure polyneuropathy, a careful occupational history and search for intoxicants, either knowingly or unknowingly ingested, is warranted.

Hereditary Neuropathies

Hereditary neuropathies are slowly progressive inherited disorders in which the pathogenesis is not clearly defined. Hereditary disorders may produce sensorimotor neuropathies, relatively pure sensory neuronopathies, or autonomic neuropathies (Table 117–10). In addition to the obvious hereditary disorders of peripheral nerves and sensory and autonomic neurons, several motor neuropathies have a genetic basis and others are of unknown cause. These are considered in the next section on motor neuron diseases.

THE MOTOR NEURON DISEASES

The term motor neuron disease refers to a group of chronic neurological disorders affecting the anterior horn cells of the spinal cord and lower brain stem plus, in many instances, the large motor neurons of the cerebral cortex that give rise to the corticospinal tract. Sensory changes and cerebellar dysfunction are absent. Some apply the term amyotrophic lateral sclerosis to all of the motor neuron diseases of unknown cause beginning in adulthood. Others use the term motor neuron disease to apply to the general condition and subclassify the variations (Table 117–11). If both upper and lower motor neuron abnormalities are found, the disorder is called *amyotrophic lateral sclerosis* (ALS). *Progressive bulbar palsy* causes relatively rapidly advancing upper and lower motor neuron involvement of the muscles of the jaw, pharynx, and tongue. When there are no signs of upper motor neuron disease and only slowly progressive muscle wasting and weakness, the disorder is termed *progressive mus-*

TABLE 117–8. DIABETIC NEUROPATHIES

Polyneuropathy
  Rapidly reversible
  Distal, primarily sensory—small fibers predominant
  Distal, primary motor—large fibers predominant or mixed
  Autonomic
Focal neuropathy
  Cranial nerve lesions (especially oculomotor nerve)
  Focal peripheral nerve lesions
  Proximal lower extremity neuropathy (diabetic amyotrophy)

TABLE 117–9. SOME CAUSES OF TOXIC NEUROPATHIES

PHARMACEUTICAL AGENTS	OTHER AGENTS
Chloramphenicol	Acrylamide (truncal ataxia)
Dapsone*	Arsenic (sensory, brown skin, Mees' lines)
Dichloracetate	Carbon disulfide
Disulfiram	Cyanide
Ethionamide	Dichlorophenoxyacetic acid
Hydralazine	Biological toxin in diphtheritic neuropathy
Isoniazid†	Ethylene oxide
Lithium	n-Hexane
Metronidazole-misonidazole	Lead (wrist drop, abdominal colic)
Nitrofurantoin*	Methyl bromide
Platinum (cis-platinum)†	Organophosphates (cholinergic symptoms, delayed onset of neuropathy)
Pyridoxine†	
Sodium cyanate	Thallium (pain, alopecia, Mees' lines)
Vincristine	Trichloroethylene (facial numbness)

* Predominantly motor.
† Predominantly sensory.
  Modified from Schaumburg HH: Toxic neuropathy. *In* Wyngaarden JB, Smith LH Jr (eds): Cecil Textbook of Medicine. 18th ed. Philadelphia, WB Saunders Co, 1988, p 2265.

TABLE 117–10. MORE FREQUENT HEREDITARY NEUROPATHIES

Lipid Disorders
  Metachromatic leukodystrophy (sulfatide metabolism)
  Bassen-Kornzweig (beta-lipoprotein deficiencies)
  Refsum's disease (phytanic acid metabolism)
Unknown Cause (hereditary sensorimotor neuropathy)
  Charcot-Marie-Tooth peroneal muscular atrophy
  Dejerine-Sottas hypertrophic neuropathy

cular atrophy (PMA). The rarest form begins as bilateral upper motor neuron disease affecting the extremities (*progressive lateral sclerosis*), the bulbar muscles (*pseudobulbar palsy*), or both.

Motor neuron disease may first affect bulbar muscles, one or both of the extremities on one side of the body, the lower or upper extremities symmetrically, or all four limbs simultaneously. The disorder's incidence increases with advancing age and progresses over two to seven years until death. The bulbar form has the

TABLE 117–11. MOTOR NEURON DISEASES

Motor neuron disease (amyotrophic lateral sclerosis)
  includes:
Progressive muscular atrophy
Progressive bulbar palsy
Amyotrophic lateral sclerosis
  Sporadic forms
  Familial forms
  Western Pacific (Guam and Japan)
Spinal muscular atrophies
  Werdnig-Hoffmann disease
  Wohlfart-Kugelberg-Welander disease
  Facioscapulohumeral form
Motor neuron disease associated with other disease of the central
  nervous system
  Mental disorder
  Extrapyramidal disorders
  Spinal disease including the hereditary spinocerebellar ataxias
Miscellaneous diseases
  Viral poliomyelitides
  Metabolic, including hypoglycemia
  Toxicity—heavy metals, organophosphorus compounds
  Ischemic myelopathy, including radiation damage
  Trauma, including electrical injury
  Paraneoplastic

shortest course, PMA the longest (often more than 10 years), and ALS intermediate. The disease usually is sporadic, but familial groupings have occurred, indicating either a genetic predisposition or common exposure to an unknown causative agent. ALS was once the common cause of death among the indigenous population of the Mariana Islands. This disorder, which is now decreasing dramatically in incidence, has been related by some investigators to ingestion of a neurotoxin contained in the false sago plant, which was used in food and traditional medicine. Other endemic areas have been identified in Japan and New Guinea but in these areas the nature of possible etiologic agents is less clear. Familial cases tend to affect younger persons and to progress more rapidly than do sporadic ones. Despite extensive searches to establish ALS as an autoimmune (about 50 per cent of patients have an M protein in their serum) or slow virus disease, no firm leads exist, and the cause of the motor neuron degeneration remains unknown.

The typical patient with ALS develops progressive weakness distally more than proximally, especially affecting the small muscles of the hand. The disease may develop asymmetrically. There is prominent and early atrophy and fasciculations. Some patients may have muscle cramps, but sensory symptoms are rare. The deep tendon reflexes are usually preserved, at least in the upper extremities, in the early phase of the disease. Signs of upper motor neuron involvement may develop at any time but almost always appear by the time muscle involvement has lasted a year. These include spasticity, particularly in the lower extremities, with associated hyperreflexia, clonus, and extensor plantar responses on one or both sides. Characteristically, the superficial abdominal reflexes and the cremasteric reflexes as well as the bladder and bowel functions remain unaffected. Generalized fasciculations and mus-

cle atrophy in most instances involve the lower extremities later than the upper. ALS spares the extraocular muscles but in the late stages can interfere with supranuclear oculomotor control. Some patients show signs of emotional lability. Intellectual functions deteriorate in approximately 5 per cent. The cerebrospinal fluid is normal. EMG testing is helpful (see Table 113–10). The motor nerve conduction velocities remain normal even in the presence of severe atrophy, a finding that separates this disorder from the peripheral motor neuropathies, in which conduction velocities are reduced.

In its classic form, ALS, with painless weakness and atrophy of the hands, fasciculations in the entire upper extremities, and spasticity and reflex hyperactivity of the legs with extensor plantar responses, may be mistaken for a cervical spinal cord tumor or other myelopathy. However, in ALS the lack of sensory changes, the frequent presence of fasciculations in the tongue, and EMG findings of denervation in the lower extremities almost always establish the diagnosis. MRI easily rules out a cervical cord lesion. Likewise, in its typical form, PMA with its widespread weakness and atrophy affecting primarily distal muscles and both proximal and distal fasciculations is only rarely confused with peripheral neuropathy or muscle disease. The characteristic neurogenic EMG and the lack of creatine kinase elevation rule out muscle disease. Most peripheral nerve disorders cause sensory impairment and rarely cause fasciculations; they are also associated with slowing of electrical conduction velocity, a finding not found in PMA. Progressive bulbar palsy must be distinguished from myasthenia gravis and myopathies, in particular polymyositis. Upper motor neuron signs such as a hyperactive jaw jerk and emotional lability and spastic speech establish the presence of motor neuron disease. Marked atrophy and fasciculations of the tongue likewise establish that diagnosis. If these findings are absent, an edrophonium test (see p. 760) and EMG of bulbar muscles may be necessary to make the distinction. Early in its course, if motor neuron disease affects only a few contiguous muscles, it must be distinguished from nerve root, plexus disease or intramedullary neoplasms or syrinxes. Along with the absence of sensory changes, the finding of widespread electromyographic abnormalities, when clinical abnormalities are localized, usually establishes the diagnosis of motor neuron disease.

Werdnig-Hoffmann Disease

Werdnig-Hoffmann disease is a progressive impairment of the motor system occurring in infancy and early childhood, transmitted as an autosomal recessive trait. The lower motor neuron is exclusively involved, leading to paralysis of muscles innervated by motor cranial nuclei and anterior horn cells of the spinal cord. Infants and young children may present with this syndrome at birth or in the first few months of life with diffuse flaccidity, muscular atrophy, muscle fasciculations, and reduced to absent myotatic reflexes with associated respiratory and swallowing difficulties. There may be prominent lingual fasciculations and atrophy, and the cerebrospinal fluid is normal. Electromyography shows denervation with normal peripheral nerve conduction velocities.

Wohlfart-Kugelberg-Welander Disease

Wohlfart-Kugelberg-Welander disease begins during late childhood, adolescence, or early adulthood with symptoms that include progressive *proximal* muscle atrophy, weakness, and fasciculations. It progresses slowly and is usually compatible with a lifespan into the third or fourth decade. Typical examples have been described in families in which other children have Werdnig-Hoffmann disease. Thus, varying penetrance of a single genetic mutation inherited in an autosomal recessive manner may produce either an aggressive form of early childhood motor neuron disease (Werdnig-Hoffmann disease) or a more benign form of motor neuron disease in later childhood and early adulthood (Wohlfart-Kugelberg-Welander disease). The onset in the first and second decade of life of proximal weakness and atrophy with fasciculations but a very slow progression without evidence of upper motor neuron involvement separates this disorder clinically from amyotrophic lateral sclerosis. Both Wohlfart-Kugelberg-Welander disease and polymyositis may present with progressive proximal weakness and atrophy. If fasciculations are not prominent, electromyography (denervation with the insertional irritability of polymyositis) and muscle biopsy establish the diagnosis. These tests distinguish the neurogenic disease from acquired or inherited myopathies. The cause of the disorder is unknown, and specific therapy is not available.

Other Anterior Horn Cell Diseases

Monomyeleic (benign focal) amyotrophy is an uncommon disorder in which lower motor neurons supplying one extremity (usually an arm) are affected. The disease usually begins in the second or third decade and progresses over a period of two to four years and then stops. The patient is left with a variable degree of weakness in the involved extremity, but the disease does not generalize and is usually not disabling. *Poliomyelitis* is an acute, viral inflammatory disease affecting anterior horn cells which was a major cause of paralysis in the United States before the development of an effective polio vaccine. A similar but much less severe weakness can occasionally be caused by other neurotropic viruses. The *post-polio sydrome* is characterized by muscle weakness developing years after recovery from acute paralytic poliomyelitis. The disorder appears to be a "wear and tear" problem, resulting in increasing dysfunction of overburdened surviving motor neurons, causing a slow disintegration of the terminals of individual nerve axons. The disorder is not life-threatening. *Subacute motor neuronopathy*, a remote effect of Hodgkin's disease, is a rare cause of slowly progressive muscle weakness and wasting. The disorder is thought to be caused by a neurotropic virus.

REFERENCES

Asbury AK, Gilliatt RW (eds): Peripheral Nerve Disorders. A Practical Approach. London, Butterworths International Medical Reviews, 1984.

Dalakas M, Halle HM: The post-polio syndrome. *In* Plum F (ed): Advances in Contemporary Neurology. Philadelphia, FA Davis Co, 1988.

Vinken PJ, Bruyn GW, Klawans HL (eds): Handbook of Clinical Neurology. Vol 51: Neuropathies. Amsterdam, Elsevier Science, 1987.

F. DISORDERS OF MYONEURAL JUNCTION

Three kinds of abnormalities can cause myoneural junction dysfunction or disease. (1) Impaired postjunction receptor mechanisms produce the disease known as myasthenia gravis. (2) Deficiency of acetylcholine release characterizes the Lambert-Eaton myasthenic syndrome as well as the toxicity of botulism and the adverse effect of certain chemical poisons. (3) Depolarizing or nonpolarizing blockage of the action of acetylcholine at the muscle receptor mechanism can be caused by a variety of drugs and poisons, the most notorious being curare. Neuromuscular junction disorders are characterized by weakness and often by fatigability of muscle, so that repetitive use of the muscle often leads to increased weakness. In some, but not all, of the diseases, cranial and respiratory musculatures are peculiarly susceptible. Drugs may cause or exacerbate pre-existing neu-

TABLE 117–12. MAJOR DISORDERS OF NEUROMUSCULAR TRANSMISSION

Autoimmune
  Myasthenia gravis
  Lambert-Eaton myasthenic syndrome
Toxic
  Botulism
  Tick paralysis
  Drug-induced
  Pesticide poisoning
Congenital
  Familial infantile myasthenia*
  End-plate acetylcholinesterase deficiency†
  End-plate acetylcholine receptor deficiency*

---

* Autosomal recessive inheritance
† Autosomal or X-linked recessive inheritance

romuscular junction disorders. They are particularly likely to cause postoperative respiratory depression. The major disorders are listed in Table 117–12.

MYASTHENIA GRAVIS

Myasthenia gravis is an autoimmune disease caused by circulating antibodies that damage acetylcholine receptors lying within the postsynaptic muscle membrane. The disorder may occur in isolation or be associated with other autoimmune disorders, such as systemic lupus erythematosus and hyperthyroidism. The disorder is usually associated with an abnormality of the thymus gland, either hypertrophic germinal centers or a thymoma. It is accompanied by accumulation of lymphocytes in muscle and other organs, an increased frequency of nonspecific antibodies against nuclear antigens, and the presence of antithyroid antibodies. That a circulating substance plays a major role in production of the weakness is proved by two facts: (1) Transplacental passage of a substance occurs, so that infants born to myasthenic women suffer transient myasthenia-type bulbar weakness. Symptoms subside as the antibody supplied to the infant by the mother disappears, usually within a week to a month. (2) Plasmapheresis brings at least a transient relief of symptoms to patients with the disease.

Myasthenia gravis may begin at any time in life, including in the newborn, but there are two major peaks of onset, one in young adulthood, when the incidence is about three times more common in women than men, and another in older persons, with men and women about equally affected. There are occasional familial cases, but most are sporadic.

Clinically, the disease is characterized by weakness and fatigability. Weakness usually begins in the extraocular muscles, with ptosis and diplopia. The symptoms may be localized to the ocular muscles or be generalized, mild or severe (Table 117–13). Symptoms tend to become more prominent toward the end of the day, following fatiguing activity, or with continuous use of extraocular muscles, such as in driving or reading. Closing the eyes or relaxing the muscles for a few minutes makes the symptoms disappear. Other bulbar muscles may also be affected, with difficulty in swallowing, chewing, or speaking, becoming more noticeable after sustained activity of the involved muscles or when the patient is otherwise fatigued. If limb muscles are involved, weakness is more often proximal than distal. Respiratory weakness alone or in combination with swallowing paralysis is the most feared complication of myasthenia gravis. Because all symptoms of the disorder may be exacerbated by fatigue or infection, a patient who is otherwise not severely affected may develop sudden acute breathing failure during a respiratory infection.

The disorder is suggested by the history, and the diagnosis can usually be confirmed on physical examination, by observing weakness that develops in extraocular or other muscles as repetitive activity continues. The physician asks the patient to look fixedly at an object on the ceiling. After 30 or 40 seconds, the lids begin to droop and the eyes may diverge. Similarly, repetitive contraction of arm muscles may cause weakness of those muscles or may cause ptosis. In a symptomatic patient, an intravenous injection of *edrophonium chloride* (Tensilon), an anticholinesterase agent, leads to rapid amelioration of clinical symptoms and improved or normal muscle function for a few minutes, until the effects of the drug wear off. When positive, in a fully symptomatic patient, the results are so dramatic that they establish the diagnosis. False-positive tests can result from increased muscular effort by the patient during the test and can sometimes be identified by a similar positive response to a placebo. Occasionally, when the muscles are very weak, they may be refractory to edrophonium, giving rise to a false-negative test. Additional confirmatory evidence is provided by electromyographic response to nerve stimulation. With repetitive stimulation of the nerve, there is a rapid decline in the muscle action potential, the electrical counterpart of muscle fatigability. More recently, single fiber electromyography, which measures the interval between discharges of different fibers within the same motor unit, has been found to show excessive variation called jitter in patients with myasthenia gravis. Eighty to 90 per cent of patients with myasthenia gravis harbor auto-antibodies against the acetylcholine receptor. Such antibodies can be identified in at least half the patients with ocular myasthenia and in over 80 per cent of patients with generalized myasthenia. There are virtually no false-positive tests, although patients in remission from myasthenia may continue to have elevated levels of antibodies.

In a typical patient the diagnosis is not difficult to make once considered. However, the disorder must be distinguished from neurasthenia, a subjective feeling of weakness and fatigability caused by psychological disorders, as well as from other myopathies and neuropathies. Careful attention to the effects of pharmacological agents and studies of the electrical activity of muscle will almost always establish the diagnosis.

The treatment of myasthenia has three components: (1) One can increase the effectiveness of acetylcholine released at the myoneural junction by preventing its breakdown. The anticholinesterase drugs neostigmine and pyridostigmine rapidly ameliorate most myasthenic symptoms. Drugs are given in sufficient doses and with sufficient frequency to keep muscle function as close as possible to normal. An average dose of pyridostigmine is 60 to 120 mg every four to five hours.

TABLE 117–13. CLASSIFICATION OF MYASTHENIA GRAVIS

I.	Ocular myasthenia
IIA.	Mild generalized myasthenia with slow progression; no crisis; drug-responsive
IIB.	Moderate generalized myasthenia; severe skeletal and bulbar involvement, but no crisis; drug response less satisfactory
III.	Acute fulminating myasthenia; rapid progression of severe symptoms with respiratory crisis and poor drug response; high incidence of thymoma; high mortality
IV.	Late severe myasthenia; same as III, but takes two years to progress from Classes I or II; crisis; high mortality

Dosage is begun low and gradually adjusted upward to achieve maximal function. Unfortunately, excessive treatment itself can cause weakness because cholinesterase inhibitors may produce a depolarizing block at the neuromuscular junction. In addition, the augmented release of acetylcholine may cause distressing abdominal cramping. Because the autonomic acetylcholine receptors are muscarinic, they can be blocked by atropine-like agents (e.g., Pro-Banthine) without an effect on the nicotinic neuromuscular receptors. (2) The second approach is to remove the circulating antibody that produces the symptoms. Plasmapheresis has proved to be a safe and beneficial treatment for most patients with myasthenia. Patients who are severely weak may improve within minutes of completion of plasmapheresis and may be free of symptoms for days to weeks. In some patients who are refractory to other treatments, plasmapheresis given once a week to once every two weeks allows the patient to maintain relatively normal function. (3) The third approach is to suppress production of the antibody. That the thymus gland has had a causal role in myasthenia gravis has been known for a long time. Thymectomy is a well-established treatment that improves about 85 per cent of patients. All patients with generalized myasthenia should be considered for thymectomy, although that option may not be chosen in severely ill elderly patients. Another method of suppressing production of the antibody is to use immunosuppressive drugs, either steroids or azathioprine. Corticosteroids in high doses often produce an exacerbation of myasthenia symptoms (rarely even culminating in respiratory paralysis). The risk of exacerbation is minimized by starting the drug slowly and, in any event, after a few days or a week patients begin to improve. Many patients with myasthenia can be well-controlled on doses (20 to 50 mg) of prednisone every other day. Steroids, in addition to their effect in suppressing acetylcholine receptor antibody concentration, also have direct effects on neuromuscular transmission. Azathioprine is the other drug currently used to suppress antibody formation. Most investigators believe that in doses of 150 to 200 mg per day it can be helpful in the treatment of myasthenia.

Patients with myasthenia are prone to develop sudden worsening of symptoms, particularly associated with respiratory infections. These patients are best treated in intensive care units with respiratory support and without the use of anticholinesterase drugs. Plasmapheresis may be useful in hastening resolution of such *myasthenic crises*.

THE LAMBERT-EATON MYASTHENIC SYNDROME

The *Lambert-Eaton or myasthenic syndrome* is an uncommon autoimmune disorder of neuromuscular transmission that in many respects is the electrical opposite of myasthenia gravis. Repetitive stimulation of the nerve leads to a facilitation of the muscle action potential rather than a diminution. In about two thirds of instances, the myasthenic syndrome is a paraneoplastic phenomenon associated with oat cell carcinoma of the lung; in the remaining the disorder occurs without an underlying illness. Patients complain of proximal weakness of limb muscles, particularly in the lower extremities, and increased fatigability. They also complain of paresthesias in the thighs, a dry mouth and, in males, impotence. Cranial nerve muscles are almost never involved. Examination reveals proximal weakness that may increase as the patient attempts to sustain a contraction (the clinical counterpart of the electrical facilitation) and hypoactive or absent deep tendon reflexes, particularly at the knees and ankles. The diagnosis is confirmed by the electrical response. The presence of the Lambert-Eaton syndrome should prompt a careful search for oat cell carcinoma of the lung, since the neuromuscular symptoms occasionally precede other evidence of the cancer by months to years. The disorder results from impaired release of acetylcholine when autoantibodies react with voltage-dependent calcium channels to block these functions. As in myasthenia gravis, plasmapheresis often relieves the symptoms.

OTHER JUNCTIONAL DISORDERS

Botulism is caused by the exotoxin of *Clostridium botulinum* and occurs following the ingestion of contaminated, improperly canned food. The toxin interferes with adequate release of acetylcholine at the neuromuscular junction. Symptoms usually begin within a few days of ingestion with blurring of vision, diplopia, and difficulty in swallowing and chewing. Gastrointestinal symptoms may precede the neurological symptoms, and the weakness spreads rapidly to cause paralysis of cranial and respiratory muscles and lesser paralysis of arms and legs. Autonomic fibers, particularly the pupilloconstrictor fibers, are affected early in the disorder, and there is loss of visual accommodation. If electrical neuromuscular transmission studies are performed early, the findings may resemble the myasthenic syndrome. The disease may produce death from respiratory paralysis unless artificial respiration is started promptly. The history, its explosive onset and progression, and its normal spinal fluid protein distinguish botulism from the ophthalmoplegic form of the Guillain-Barré syndrome, which it can resemble closely. If the patient's physiological functions, particularly respiration, are supported, there is usually full recovery.

Tick paralysis is a disorder caused by a tick neurotoxin that blocks transmission at the neuromuscular junction. Most cases of tick paralysis occur in children, particularly girls, in whom the tick embeds in the skin near the hairline and goes unnoticed. After five or six days of embedding, paresthesias and progressive weakness develop, which may progress to flaccid paralysis of cranial and respiratory muscles and the extremities, resembling botulism or the Guillain-Barré syndrome. Spinal fluid protein is normal and the pa-

TABLE 117–14. DRUG-INDUCED NEUROMUSCULAR BLOCKADE

CLINICAL PRESENTA- TION	ANTIBIOTICS	CARDIOVAS- CULAR DRUGS	ANTIRHEU- MATIC DRUGS	PSYCHO- TROPIC DRUGS	ANTICONVUL- SANTS	HORMONAL AGENTS	OTHER DRUGS
Postoperative res- piratory depres- sion	Clindamycin Colistin Kanamycin Lincomycin Neomycin Streptomycin Tobramycin	Lidocaine Quinidine Trimethaphan	Chloroquine	Lithium Phenelzine Promazine			Aprotinin Cholinesterase in- hibitors Oxytocin
Aggravation or unmasking of myasthenia gravis	Colistin Kanamycin Streptomycin Tetracyclines	Procainamide Propranolol Quinidine	Chloroquine(?)	Chlorpromazine Lithium	Phenytoin	ACTH Corticosteroids Thyroid hor- mones	Acetylcholines- terase inhibitors Methoxyflurane
Drug-induced myasthenic syndrome	Colistin Gentamicin Kanamycin Neomycin Polymyxin B Streptomycin	Oxprenolol Practolol Trimethaphan	D-Penicillamine		Phenytoin Trimethadione	Oral contracep- tives(?)	Tetanus antitoxin

From Argov Z, Mastaglia FL: Medical intelligence: Drug therapy. N Engl J Med 301:8, 1979.

ralysis subsides promptly following removal of the embedded tick.

Aminoglycoside antibiotics, including neomycin, streptomycin, colistin, and kanamycin, can interfere with neuromuscular transmission (Table 117–14). The most common manifestation is postoperative apnea without other evidence of paralysis in patients who have received the antibiotics, particularly in those who have renal failure, leading to high antimicrobial drug levels. Some patients may have a flaccid quadriplegia that responds to administration of calcium and quinidine.

Pesticides containing long-acting anticholinester-

ases cause weakness from acetylcholine receptor de-sensitization and may also cause delirium. Atropine and pralidoxime reverse the symptoms.

Several rare congenital or hereditary disorders of function of the neuromuscular junction can cause weakness in infants and newborns (Table 117–14).

REFERENCE

Engle AG, Banker B (eds): Myology. New York, McGraw Hill Book Co, 1986.

G. DISORDERS OF SKELETAL MUSCLE

Muscle, the largest organ in the body, can be di-rectly affected by several diseases primary to the struc-ture itself or by the secondary effects of a number of systemic diseases. Furthermore, since weakness is so easily recognized by the patient, the muscular dys-function can lead to early consultation with the phy-sician even when the primary disease is elsewhere. Table 117–15 classifies the myopathies. This text places its emphasis on disorders that are common or that have characteristic clinical findings.

MUSCULAR DYSTROPHIES

Muscular dystrophies (Table 117–16) are inherited myopathies characterized by progressive weakness, usually beginning early in life. The genetics are well-established for most of the dystrophies, and the gene product has been identified in Duchenne dystrophy, making it the only dystrophy in which the biochemical defect is known.

Duchenne dystrophy is an X-linked recessive disor-der of boys (rarely girls) characterized by painless weakness that is maximal in the pelvic girdle and thighs, less prominent about the shoulders, and least prominent in the distal extremities. The abnormal gene positioned on band Xp21 fails to produce *dys-trophin*, a protein of skeletal muscle, although the mechanism by which absence of the protein causes muscle breakdown is unknown. The disorder reveals itself with abnormal and increasing clumsiness when the child begins to walk (beyond 18 months). Affected boys run awkwardly and rise from the floor by placing hands on knees and using the hands to walk up the thighs (Gowers' sign). With time the calf muscles ap-pear abnormally enlarged (pseudohypertrophy). Grad-ually the weakness becomes more severe, and adoles-cents are usually wheelchair-bound. Even with scrupulous care, death occurs in early adulthood, usu-ally from pneumonia. The diagnosis can be made early in life before symptoms appear by an elevated serum creatine kinase. The mutation rate is high, and in about two thirds of individuals, no other family member is affected. The disorder must be distinguished from two similar dystrophies: *Becker's dystrophy* reflects the presence of an abnormality in dystrophin rather than its absence. The disease also is X-linked but has its onset later in childhood or adolescence and has a slower or more variable tempo (some patients functioning well into adult life). *Emery-Dreyfuss dystrophy* also begins later and is more benign than Duchenne dystrophy; pseudohypertrophy is lacking and serum enzymes are normal or only slightly increased. This form is also characterized by cardiac arrhythmias that can lead to sudden death.

Limb-girdle dystrophy, an autosomal recessive disorder with a high mutation rate, affects muscles of the pelvic and shoulder girdle, usually begins late in childhood or adolescence, affects girls as often as boys, and progresses at extremely variable rates. Pseudohypertrophy is not common. Muscle biopsy and electromyography may be necessary to distinguish this disorder from a similar-appearing, also proximal neurogenic disorder—the Wohlfart-Kugelberg-Welander syndrome (page 759).

Facioscapulohumeral dystrophy is characterized by prominent weakness in the perioral muscles of the face and eventually weakness of eye closure. Latissimus dorsi degeneration leads to scapular winging, and the sternal head of the pectoral muscle is affected more than the clavicular. The shoulder and pelvic girdle muscles are affected as well. Weakness of the trunk muscles may cause severe scoliosis. The disorder is transmitted as an autosomal dominant trait with variable but usually extremely slow progression.

Ocular muscular dystrophy is a slowly progressive disorder characterized by ptosis and progressive external ocular paralysis. The pupils are spared, and both eyes are usually affected symmetrically, so that diplopia is not common. Other muscles of the head, neck, and limbs may be affected, but this varies from family to family. Because each oculomotor nerve fiber supplies only a few muscle fibers, it is exceedingly difficult to distinguish neuropathies from myopathies by either EMG or histological examination of the eye muscles. As a result, the clinical distinction between ocular myopathies and neuropathies rests on findings in other skeletal muscles. In some disorders producing ocular myopathy, the skeletal muscles of the neck or limbs contain abnormally large mitochondria in increased numbers, producing a characteristic "ragged red fiber" appearance on trichrome stains.

Distal myopathy, unlike most muscular dystrophies, affects distal leg and hand muscles first. It is rare and can be identified only by characteristic signs of myopathy on electromyography and muscle biopsy. *Scapuloperoneal dystrophy*, with its distal weakness in the legs, resembles neurogenic peroneal atrophy, but there is no sensory loss and proximal weakness often affects the shoulder girdle. The disorder is transmitted as an autosomal dominant trait with relatively slow progression.

TABLE 117–15. MYOPATHIES

Muscular dystrophy (see Table 117–16)
Myotonias (see Table 117–17)
Inflammatory myopathies
    Infections (e.g., toxoplasmosis, trichinosis, viral)
    Immune processes: polymyositis, sarcoidosis, polymyalgia rheumatica
        (see Ch. 104)
Endocrine myopathies
    Hyperthyroidism and hypothyroidism
    Hyperparathyroidism
    Hyperadrenalism
    Hyperpituitarism
Periodic paralysis (see Table 117–18)
Biochemical disorders
    Glycogen storage diseases
    Lipid storage and mitocondrial myopathies
Congenital muscle disorders
Drugs and toxins

TABLE 117–16. MUSCULAR DYSTROPHIES

X-linked recessive dystrophies
    Duchenne dystrophy
    Becker dystrophy
    Emery-Dreifuss dystrophy with joint contractures and atrial paralysis
Autosomal recessive dystrophies
    Autosomal recessive childhood (limb-girdle) muscular dystrophy
    Scapulohumeral (limb-girdle) muscular dystrophy
    Autosomal-recessive distal muscular dystrophies
    Congenital muscular dystrophies
Autosomal dominant dystrophies
    Facioscapulohumeral dystrophy
    Autosomal dominant scapuloperoneal dystrophy
    Dominantly inherited adult-onset limb-girdle dystrophy
    Oculopharyngeal dystrophy
    Autosomal dominant distal dystrophy

Modified from Engel AG: Muscular dystrophies. *In* Wyngaarden JB, Smith LH Jr (eds): Cecil Textbook of Medicine. 18th ed. Philadelphia, WB Saunders Co, p 2273.

Treatment

There is no treatment for any of the inherited muscular dystrophies. Physical therapy along with splints and braces may keep many patients walking who would otherwise be confined to a wheelchair. Carriers of Duchenne dystrophy can sometimes be identified by increased creatine kinase serum levels and deletions in the gene sequence for Duchenne dystrophy can be detected prenatally using 4cDNA probes. Accordingly, genetic counseling is valuable in preventing the disease.

OTHER INHERITED MYOPATHIES

Several rare congenital or inherited biochemical defects cause muscle weakness, which is usually lifelong. Among these are congenital myopathies, glycogen storage diseases, lipid storage diseases, and mitochondrial myopathies.

Congenital myopathies are a group of disorders characterized by mild weakness that generally persists unchanged throughout life. The cause is not known:

a few are familial and many are sporadic. The disorders are present at birth, and their chief importance lies in distinguishing them from the more severe progressive muscular dystrophies and neonatal anterior horn cell disorders. A number of glycogen storage diseases cause muscle symptoms. *McArdle's disease*, type 5 glycogen storage disease, results from an absence of muscle phosphorylase, so that patients are unable to break down glycogen during anaerobic exercise. They are usually asymptomatic until early adolescence or early adulthood when they develop painful muscle cramps (actually contractures) after exercise. Myoglobinuria and renal failure may ensue, and patients may eventually become weak. A similar deficit results from phosphofructokinase deficiency. The diagnosis of both is established by the failure of venous lactate to rise during ischemic exercise. Biochemical study of biopsied muscle will define the exact enzyme deficiency. *Lipid storage* and *mitochondrial myopathies* usually become symptomatic in childhood and can be responsible for neurological symptoms in addition to muscle weakness. The references provide sources that discuss these myopathies more extensively.

MYOTONIAS

Table 117–17 classifies muscle diseases associated with myotonia. Myotonia results from an abnormality of the muscle membrane leading to delayed relaxation. The diagnosis is easily made clinically by asking a patient to grip one's fingers and then quickly let go. There is also a characteristic electromyogram, displaying repetitive action potentials that may wax or wane over many seconds when the needle is inserted or after the patient attempts to relax from a voluntary contraction. The most common myotonic abnormality is *myotonic dystrophy*, occurring once in 7500 births, an autosomal dominant disorder characterized by progressive, primarily distal muscle weakness, myotonia, cranial muscle weakness, and endocrine abnormalities. The gene is on chromosome 19 with linkage to the gene encoding complement C3. The disorder may begin early in life or be delayed into adulthood. Affected persons have facial weakness with ptosis, difficulty puckering the lips, and dysarthria. In addition, wasting involves the temporalis and masseter muscles, which, when combined with the ptosis, gives the face a characteristic appearance. Selective weakness and wasting affect the sternocleidomastoid muscles, giving the neck a long and thin appearance (swan neck).

Extremity muscles are affected distally. The my-

TABLE 117–17. MYOTONIAS

Myotonic muscular dystrophy
Myotonia congenita
  Autosomal dominant
  Autosomal recessive
Paramyotonia congenita
Hyperkalemic periodic paralysis
Chondrodystrophic myotonia
Acquired myotonia

otonia occurs primarily in the hands and usually is the first symptom. It becomes less severe as weakness develops and may not be easy to identify clinically in the late stages. In addition to the muscle symptoms, almost all patients eventually develop cataracts, and males experience early frontal baldness and testicular atrophy. Conduction defects in the heart may lead to cardiac arrhythmias, and cardiac myopathy may cause congestive heart failure. The disease runs a long course and does not generally cause disability until well into adulthood. The clinical and electromyographic features are characteristic. There is no effective treatment. *Myotonia congenita* is rarer and occurs in both autosomal dominant and recessive forms. The disease begins early in life and is characterized by diffuse myotonia, which makes the patient stiff when he begins to exercise but loosens as activity continues. Affected persons move clumsily and have a stiff and wooden appearance. Cold generally makes their symptoms worse. The disorder is annoying more than disabling. Drugs such as phenytoin and quinine, which affect neuromuscular transmission, may relieve the symptoms. *Paramyotonia congenita* is a rare disorder of autosomal dominant inheritance that differs only slightly from myotonia congenita. Facial muscles and muscles of the forearm and hand are predominantly involved; the myotonia shows extreme sensitivity to cold, and indeed may be present only when the patient is exposed to cold. Similar myotonias sometimes occur in hyperkalemic paralysis, and paramyotonia may simply be a manifestation of the more common periodic paralysis. In addition to the congenital disorders, myotonia can be acquired after exposure to a number of toxins, including cholesterol antagonists and the herbicide 2-4D.

ENDOCRINE MYOPATHIES

Disorders of thyroid, parathyroid, adrenal, and pituitary can cause profound changes in muscle function. Mild proximal weakness accompanies most cases of florid *hyperthyroidism*, but sometimes myopathy may be the predominant symptom without obvious clinical evidence of either hypermetabolism or ocular changes of Graves' disease. Rarely, muscle twitches accompany the weakness, the so-called fasciculating myopathy of thyrotoxicosis. The shoulder girdle is sometimes weaker than hip muscles, and creatine kinase levels in the serum may be normal. Weakness always responds to the treatment of the hyperthyroidism. In young Asian males, hypokalemic periodic paralysis may complicate hyperthyroidism (p. 765). Hyperthyroidism also can precipitate exacerbations of myasthenia gravis.

In *hypothyroidism*, like thyrotoxicosis, weakness predominantly affects proximal muscles. Owing to increased muscle viscosity, the deep tendon reflexes relax slowly in a characteristic fashion, and affected patients can experience difficulty in relaxing muscles. The phenomenon lacks the characteristic EMG changes of myotonia. Percussion myoedema of the muscles (a mounding of the percussed muscle associated with the electrical silence of a focal contracture) is also characteristic of hypothyroid myopathy. Muscle enzyme levels in the serum can rise high enough to suggest polymyositis. Hypothyroid myopathy can occur in the absence of other stigmata of hypothyroidism, and the diagnosis must be suspected from the muscle findings and confirmed by appropriate laboratory tests. In children, the hypothyroid state may be associated with muscle hypertrophy. Exacerbations of myasthenia gravis are also occasionally associated with hypothyroidism.

Hypoparathyroidism with its resulting hypocalcemia can cause tetany, usually without associated myopathy. A few reports also suggest that hypoparathyroidism may be associated with anterior horn cell disease, with amyotrophic lateral sclerosis–like weakness affecting both bulbar and axial muscles. *Hyperparathyroidism* commonly produces weakness, and proximal muscle wasting, with the hips more involved than the shoulders, may be the presenting complaint. Myalgias often accompany the myopathies of hyperparathyroidism, potentially causing the endocrine disorder to be mistaken for polymyositis. Usually, however, other signs of hyperparathyroidism, including renal stones, encephalopathy, and peptic ulceration, accompany the weakness and represent a clue to its pathogenesis. A proximal myopathy is also part of the clinical picture of *hyperpituitarism*, but in this disorder acromegalic features overshadow the muscle weakness. *Hyperadrenocorticism*, whether spontaneous or induced by the ingestion of adrenocorticosteroids as part of therapy for another disorder, also causes proximal weakness and mild muscle wasting involving hips more than shoulders. Muscle enzymes usually remain normal. This so-called *steroid myopathy* complicates the course of almost every patient treated for more than a few weeks with pharmacological doses of corticosteroids and can even occur after a long period of doses that are considered close to replacement. Patients receiving every-other-day steroid therapy seem to have less myopathy. *Adrenal insufficiency* (Addison's disease) causes weakness only when the serum potassium rises to above 7 to 9 mEq/L.

DRUG, NUTRITIONAL, AND TOXIC MYOPATHIES

With the exception of corticosteroids, only a few drugs cause myopathy. These include vincristine, chloroquine, bretylium, emetine, ipecac, carbenoxolone, guanethidine, epsilon-aminocaproic acid, penicillamine, and clofibrate. Thiazide diuretics, the repeated use of laxatives, or the ingestion of other drugs that cause potassium loss may lead to chronic hypokalemia and a proximal myopathy that may be acute at onset, with elevated serum enzymes and even necrosis on muscle biopsy. For severe weakness to occur, the serum potassium concentration must fall below 2 mEq/L.

Nutritional deprivation of vitamin E or selenium ingestion causes a myopathy in animals, but these are not clinical problems in humans. However, chronic alcoholism can lead to severe proximal muscle weakness.

PERIODIC PARALYSES

Periodic paralyses are disorders characterized by recurrent attacks of flaccid weakness, often associated with an abnormally high or low serum potassium concentration, although rarely is the potassium level sufficiently abnormal to produce weakness in an otherwise normal individual (Table 117–18). Many of the cases are familial, usually inherited in a pattern consistent with an autosomal dominant trait. Periodic paralysis has two major forms: hypokalemic and hyperkalemic. The former is characterized by sudden attacks of flaccid weakness, usually beginning in late childhood or adolescence and frequently occurring at night after a large carbohydrate meal. The attacks may totally paralyze the extremities and trunk, sparing the respiratory, bulbar, and cranial muscles, and may last a day or more before spontaneously resolving. During the course of the attack, the serum potassium is usually low (e.g., 2.5 to 3 mEq/L), and the patient may respond to oral or intravenous potassium. Repeated attacks can lead to permanent weakness. Muscle biopsy shows vacuoles within muscle fibers. The hyperkalemic variety generally begins in early childhood with attacks that occur more frequently than the hypokalemic variety, are usually milder, and generally last only minutes to hours rather than days. Typically, the hyperkalemic attack begins while the patient is resting after vigorous exercise. Hyperkalemic attacks may begin with paresthesias in the extremities, but no sensory changes are found on examination. Lid lag and Chvostek's sign may be present along with prominent myalgias. During attacks, the serum potassium usually rises to between 5 and 7 mEq/L, and some patients develop myotonia, often limited to percussion myotonia of the tongue. Although the serum potassium levels and the clinical symptoms separate typical examples of the hypo- and hyperkalemic disorders, the conditions overlap, and many patients suffer periodic paralyses without alteration of the serum potassium.

TABLE 117–18. PERIODIC PARALYSIS

Primary
  Hypokalemic
  Hyperkalemic (including those with cardiac arrhythmias)
  Normokalemic
Secondary
  Hypokalemic
    Thyrotoxic
    Potassium-losing states
      Urinary potassium wastage
        Hyperaldosteronism
        Licorice intoxication
        Various renal diseases
        Thiazide diuretics
      Gastrointestinal potassium wastage
  Hyperkalemic
    Renal failure
    Adrenal failure
    Drug-induced: triamterene, spironolactone
    Self-induced: geophagia
    Iatrogenic: potassium supplements

The diagnosis of periodic paralysis is made by the typical history and confirmed by finding an abnormal serum potassium level during an acute attack. If an acute attack is not observed, one may be precipitated (in the hypokalemic form by glucose and insulin or in the hyperkalemic form by potassium), but this should be done only in a hospital setting where one is prepared to deal with complications. Thyroid function should be assessed in all patients suffering hypokalemic periodic paralysis; diuretic ingestion should be suspected if the serum potassium is below 2.5 mEq/L.

MYOGLOBINURIA

Myoglobinuria results when major injuries to muscles lead to *rhabdomyolysis* and release of myoglobin into the serum and urine, giving the urine a brown-rust color. Myoglobinuria either can occur as a hereditary disease or can complicate a variety of sporadic muscle injuries. Crush injury, such as occurs in accidents, is a common cause, as is pressure injury to muscles, resulting from a patient's lying immobile after poisoning from sedatives or carbon monoxide. Prolonged unconsciousness in the snow likewise can lead to myoglobinuria, as can arterial occlusion by tourniquet or embolism. Snake bites and binge alcohol ingestion also can cause myoglobinuria, as can malignant hyperthermia. Even normal people may develop some degree of myoglobinuria after vigorous exercise. Strenuous exercise among army recruits, during ritual hazing, or in marathon runners leads to myoglobinuria in a small percentage of individuals. In addition to the discoloration of the urine, the clinical syndrome is characterized by muscle aches and swelling as well as some weakness. Symptoms may persist for several days, even though the pigment in the urine rarely lasts more than four hours. The muscles most affected are those most vigorously exercised or crushed, but cranial musculature and respiratory muscles are almost never affected. The major potential problem is kidney injury due to myoglobin plugging the renal tubules. The disorder should be considered as a possible cause of acute renal failure of uncertain etiology. Myoglobin can be identified spectrophotometrically in the urine.

REFERENCES

Engle AG, Banker B: Myology. New York, McGraw Hill Book Co, 1986.
Layzer RB: Neuromuscular Manifestations of Systemic Disease. Philadelphia, FA Davis Co, 1985.

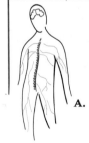

118

CEREBROVASCULAR DISEASE

Cerebrovascular diseases include disorders of the arterial or venous circulatory systems or their contents which produce or threaten to produce injury to the central nervous system. The general term *stroke* describes the functional neurological injury. The cause of stroke can be either *anoxic-ischemic*, the result of vasogenic failure to supply sufficient oxygen and substrate to the tissue, or *hemorrhagic*, the result of abnormal leakage of blood into or around central nervous system structures. *Arteriovenous malformations* of the brain or spinal cord can produce neurological abnormalities by bleeding, by producing ischemic damage, or by acting as space-occupying lesions.

Anatomy and Pathophysiology of the Cerebral Circulation

Anatomy. The cerebral arterial circulation derives from four major extracerebral (neck) arteries, the paired internal carotids, and the vertebrals. Acute, complete occlusion of these extracranial arteries can result at any age from atherosclerosis, embolization, inflammation, intrinsic arterial disease, or trauma. Age and the effectiveness of the anastomotic pattern of the large arteries at the base of the brain determine whether ischemic brain damage ensues.

The *circle of Willis* provides in most persons a potentially effective intracranial anastomotic pathway to compensate for sudden focal reductions in blood flow at the base of the brain. Sometimes, however, the circle loses its effectiveness because of congenital asymmetry of the vertebral arteries or narrowing or absence of its anterior or posterior communicating segments. Beyond the circle, the major intracranial arterial beds anastomose over the surface of the brain through tiny interconnecting pial arterioles, most of which are too small to compensate for major arterial occlusions. Penetrating arteries, descending from the pial surface into the deep white matter or subcortical nuclei, enjoy little anastomotic protection.

Physiology. Cerebral arteries contain less muscle, no elastic tissue, and less adventitia than do systemic arteries. The reduced musculature especially affects the junctions where major branches diverge from the large arteries at the base of the brain, creating vulnerable points from which most intracranial aneurysms arise. The absence of elastic tissue as an antigen may explain the invulnerability of the intracranial arteries to the common late-life immunological-inflammatory vascular disease cranial arteritis (Chapter 107).

The *blood-brain barrier* insulates the brain and its extracellular fluid, including the cerebrospinal fluid (CSF), from many of the chemical perturbations that can affect the systemic circulation, including circulating drugs, immunogenic antigens, and electrolyte changes. The anatomical barrier lies in the intracranial endothelium, where tight intercellular junctions weld the entire inner surface into a continuous membranous sheet. As a result, only nonpolar materials that either have a small molecular size, are lipid soluble, or are transported across the membrane by specific carrier systems or pumps penetrate the endothelium with any rapidity. Transient breaches of the barrier occur under a variety of circumstances and have little ill effect on brain function. Sustained, partial barrier alteration occurs in areas of cerebral neoplasms, inflammation, or necrosis and contributes to the formation of edema associated with such conditions. Severe damage to barrier transport mechanisms is a factor contributing to brain infarction during ischemia.

Autoregulation is the intrinsic functional capacity of the brain's resistance arterioles to adjust their degree of constriction according to the metabolic requirements of the tissue. The arterioles automatically and locally dilate or constrict in response to, respectively, increases or decreases in local brain functional activity, as well as to decreases and increases in systemic blood pressure. Although the two responses are independently regulated, they synergize in order to adjust to the brain's metabolic need. The normal limits of cerebral autoregulation to pressure extend between approximately 60 and 160 mm Hg of systemic mean pressure. Impaired autoregulation to pressure changes can contribute to brain injury in several circumstances, especially with disorders that cause an increased intracranial pressure (ICP). At such times widespread abnormal vasodilatation allows the ICP to rise, sometimes to alarming levels that can approach the arterial blood pressure. Impaired arterial autoregulation also can accompany severe hypertension (mean BP greater than 160 torr), in which case intense elevations of systemic blood pressure cause focal breakthroughs of the resistance vessels to produce vascular and brain tissue injury.

Epidemiology and Risk Factors

Stroke takes a worldwide toll, affecting especially persons age 55 years and older. Although the incidence has declined somewhat in recent years, only heart disease and cancer exceed stroke as a cause of death and disability in developed countries.

Stroke has several specific causes, listed in Table 118–1. In addition, a number of systemic conditions

TABLE 118–1. CAUSES OF ACUTE CEREBRAL ISCHEMIA

Mainly Focal
  Arterial disease, thrombotic or embolic
  Cardiac emboli
  Functional arterial spasm or constriction
    a. Migraine
    b. Subarachnoid hemorrhage
  Intracranial sinus or venous thrombosis

Mainly Global
  Absolute or functional (ventricular fibrillation) asystole >8 sec in duration
  Severe decline in cardiac output
    Shock; bradycardia <30–40 per minute; cardiac tamponade; severe heart failure
  Three- or four-vessel stenosis of cervical arteries plus TIA
  Profound anemia, HCT usually <20
  Profound hypoxemia: PaO_2 <35–40 mm Hg
  Carbon monoxide poisoning
  Prolonged status epilepticus
  Disseminated intravascular coagulation
  Fat embolization

TABLE 118–2. MAJOR RISK FACTORS IN STROKE

Hypertension	Congestive heart failure
Diabetes	Smoking
Hyperlipidemia	Alcohol abuse
Myocardial infarction	Obesity
Atrial fibrillation	

and social habits predispose to stroke (Table 118–2). Early medical or behavioral attention to several of these conditions can reduce an individual's stroke risk. *Hypertension* both adversely affects the heart and induces progressive narrowing of the cerebral arterioles; it creates the greatest risk factor. The increasingly widespread successful treatment of hypertension probably deserves the greatest credit for the decline in stroke incidence. Population studies show an especially strong association among dietary salt intake, hypertension, and cerebral hemorrhage. Both the length and degree of *smoking* correlate with an increased incidence of stroke as well as of myocardial infarction.

Alcoholic excess increases stroke risk, with several studies reporting an increase of severe strokes immediately following bouts of heavy intoxication. Modest alcohol ingestion on the order of one to two glasses of wine per day may actually reduce stroke risk. Combined progesterone/estrogen *oral contraceptives*, especially if combined with smoking, increase the risk of stroke among women of child-bearing age to about three times the normal rate.

TABLE 118–3. VASCULAR FACTORS CONTRIBUTING TO STROKE

Mural Abnormalities
A. Extracranial-intracranial atherosclerosis
  1. Thrombotic narrowing or occlusion of cervical vessels
  2. Ulcerated aortocervical plaques generating platelet-fibrin or cholesterol emboli
  3. Thrombotic occlusion of intracranial vessels
B. Inflammatory-immunological vascular occlusions
  1. Extracranial only—cranial arteritis
  2. Extracranial and intracranial
    a. Generalized polyarteritis
    b. Septic emboli (bacterial endocarditis)
  3. Intracranial only
    a. Accompanying bacterial or granulomatous arteritis
    b. Amphetamine—cocaine-like drugs
    c. Idiopathic
C. Invasion or compression of arterial or venous vascular walls by trauma, neoplasms, etc.

Embolic disorders
A. Artery to artery: platelet or cholesterol emboli from aortocervical atherosclerotic plaques
B. Cardiogenic
  1. Mural (post–myocardial infarction)
  2. Atrial
  3. Valvular
    a. Septic (endocarditis)
    b. Nonseptic (rheumatic, atherosclerotic, mitral prolapse, nonbacterial endocarditis)
  4. Neoplastic—arterial myxoma, etc.

TABLE 118–4. HEMATOLOGICAL ABNORMALITIES PREDISPOSING TO STROKE

Hematocrit > 55	Sickle cell disease
WBC > 500,000	Paraproteinemia
Thrombocytosis > 600,000	Lupus anticoagulant
Platelet hyperaggregability	Cardiolipin antibody

ISCHEMIC STROKE

Etiology and Mechanisms

Focal ischemic stroke is caused by either embolic or thrombotic occlusion of a major artery in the neck or head. *Global ischemic stroke* results in total failure of blood supply, e.g., following cardiac arrest or, rarely, from severe impairments of the oxygen supply alone to the brain.

Vascular Factors. These can be either primarily thrombotic or embolic, as listed in Table 118–3. In either case, the critical event is reduction of blood flow to the brain.

Hematogenous Factors. Table 118–4 lists the major causes. Except for anesthetic or industrial accidents that result in severe reductions in inhaled oxygen, or carbon monoxide poisoning which blocks oxyhemoglobin formation, uncomplicated hypoxemia and anemia are uncommon causes of ischemic stroke, inasmuch as arterial oxygen supplies must be reduced to about 40 per cent of normal before cerebral insufficiency develops; this level of anoxemia is likely to produce cardiac as well as cerebral difficulties. In the absence of severe hypotension or of anatomical abnormalities in the cervicocranial circulation, isolated hemoglobin levels greater than 7 to 8 gm/dl or Pao_2 values greater than 40 to 45 mm Hg seldom can be incriminated as primary causes of stroke. Indeed, because of blood flow adjustments, even lower hemoglobin values may cause no symptoms in chronically anemic persons. When combined with hypoxemia or electrolyte or biochemical abnormalities, however, anemia can contribute in a major way to a metabolic encephalopathy.

Among the coagulopathies causing stroke, physiological platelet aggregation deserves specific attention. Vascular changes producing partial or complete ischemia in brain stimulate an immediate increase in platelet aggregation in the abnormally irrigated areas. Similarly, ulcerated arteriosclerotic plaques attract fibrin-platelet aggregations to their surface as part of the healing process. The ensuing detritus provides a potential source for the extension of a thrombosis or the formation of artery-to-artery emboli.

Blood Flow and Tissue Factors. The brain and spinal cord possess the highest basal rate of metabolism of any large organ in the body, consuming approximately 20 per cent of the body's resting oxygen requirement. The brain contains practically no reserves of oxygen and only tiny stores of glucose, its normal substrate. As a result, any severe reduction of blood supply threatens the organ's vitality. The blood supply to the brain normally averages about 55 ml per 100 gm of tissue per minute. In the absence of anemia (Hb < 12 gm) or hypoxemia (Pao_2 < 65 mm Hg), cerebral autoregulation and increased tissue oxygen extraction can support normal or nearly normal cerebral functions in the face of blood flow reductions down to about 40 per cent of normal. Below this threshold physiological dysfunction appears, and only a small additional decline causes membrane failure and death of brain cells. Partial or complete vascular occlusion (focal ischemia) and profound hypotension (global ischemia) represent the most common causes of such catastrophes. Any significant degree of anemia, hypoxemia, or hypercoagulability accentuates the hazards of reduced blood flow.

Just how long severe anoxia or ischemia must last to cause irreversible brain damage is uncertain. Humans faint by about the eighth second of asystole, but both clinical and experimental evidence suggests that brain tissue sometimes can recover from severe partial ischemia lasting as long as an hour or more.

Heart disease is the single most important associated factor causing clinical stroke (Table 118–5). Most focal stroke results from emboli lodging in the intracranial arteries, with about 40 per cent coming from the heart. Cardiac arrhythmias account for most instances of syncope or global cerebral ischemia among older persons. Furthermore, since atherosclerosis commonly affects the cardiac and cerebral circulation concurrently, the statistical risk of future myocardial infarction in stroke patients is as great as or greater than the risk of a repeated cerebral event. Mitral valve prolapse, which can cause valvular or subvalvular thrombi, is found six times more frequently than normal among persons below age 45 with acute stroke. Similarly, a greatly increased incidence of focal stroke is associated with atrial fibrillation of whatever cause. Anterior wall myocardial infarction (MI) produces a high incidence of left ventricular thrombi; if not treated prophylactically with anticoagulants, as many as 40 per cent of such patients suffer stroke during convalescence from the MI. Bacterial endocarditis, prosthetic heart valves, nonbacterial (marantic) endocarditis, indwelling pacemakers, mitral or aortic calcific disease, and atrial myxomas all represent additional potential sources of cardiogenic emboli.

Neuropathology of Ischemic Brain Damage. *Cerebral infarction* is a pathological process that damages or destroys all tissue elements, including neurons, glial cells, and blood vessels. Within a matter of hours after onset, water leaks into the ischemic-necrotic tissue, increasing the mass by edema. Tissue lactacidosis added to the oxygen lack may be a factor in extending the damage. Infarction characteristically follows prolonged anoxia-ischemia such as occurs with vascular occlusion and can be focal or multifocal in nature depending on the pattern of affected vessels. Large infarcts involve the vascular territory of the major intracranial arteries. Small infarcts, 5 to 8 mm or so in diameter, sometimes called *lacunes*, result from occlusion of arteriolar branches. Lacunes may arise anywhere in the brain but especially result from occlusion of the deep end arteries that arise from the deeper circulatory beds of the middle cerebral and basilar arteries.

Hemorrhagic infarcts are marked by scattered areas of escaped red cells in the ischemic tissue, occurring most often at the periphery of an infarcted area. The mechanism is thought to represent reperfusion of an artery in which transient embolization damages the endothelium, allowing diapedetic bleeding to occur.

Selective neuronal necrosis is damage that is restricted to nerve cells, sparing glial and vascular elements. When caused by anoxia, the process especially affects selectively vulnerable neurons located in the hippocampus, the deeper level of the cerebral cortex (laminar necrosis), and the cerebellar Purkinje cells. Selective neuronal death characteristically follows brief periods of acute cardiac arrest, prolonged status epilepticus, and profound hypoglycemia. Severe hippocampal damage represents the most frequent cause of memory loss following cardiac arrest, while Purkinje cell damage is a major factor in causing the distressing condition of postanoxic myoclonus.

Postanoxic demyelination of the brain is an unusual condition wherein prolonged exposure to severe hypoxemia, usually associated with severe systemic hypotension, leads to diffuse damage to hemispheric white matter. The process largely spares the cerebral neurons. The demyelination produces signs and symptoms similar to those of a severe metabolic encephalopathy and often develops only after a delay of a few days to as much as three weeks following anoxic exposure. Although occasionally fatal, most patients recover at least partially. Many, however, suffer residual movement disorders from small, associated infarcts affecting the basal ganglia.

Clinical Definitions of Stroke

Ischemic strokes vary according to their size, anatomical location in the brain, and temporal pattern. *Transient ischemic attacks* (TIA's) are periods of focal, acute neurological insufficiency lasting from a few minutes to as much as an hour or so, followed by complete functional recovery. Most such short-lived, reversible events are caused by emboli composed of fibrin, platelets or, rarely, cholesterol crystals that arise in the heart or large cervical arteries to lodge in the retinal or small cerebral arteries and then rapidly dissolve. Less frequent sources include fragments of cardiac valvular vegetations or hematogenous abnormalities within the affected vessels. Severe narrowing of 85 per cent or more of a common or internal carotid artery in the neck possibly may account for some cases on a hemodynamic basis. The symptoms caused by a TIA depend on whether it involves the territorial distribution of the internal carotid–middle cerebral artery system or the vertebral-basilar system, as described below.

Completed stroke refers to a sustained ischemic event sufficient to produce neuronal necrosis or infarction in at least part of the territory of the affected artery. The ensuing neurological defect can last days, weeks, or permanently; even after maximal recovery,

TABLE 118–5. FINDINGS SUGGESTING CARDIAC ORIGIN FOR FOCAL STROKE

Persons <45 years of age with no evident systemic risk factors (mitral prolapse)
Known heart disease: Rheumatic aortic or mitral valve; atrial fibrillation; recent anterior wall infarction; murmur plus unexplained fever (SBE); chronic cardiomyopathy; mitral annular calcification
Multiple cerebral arteries involved
Emboli in other organs
Hemorrhagic infarct

at least minimal neurological difficulties often remain. The clinical severity of completed strokes depends upon the size of the affected arterial bed, the relative balance between lethal and critical flow reduction to the tissue, and the functional neuroanatomy of the lesion. Completed *minor strokes* involving only distal branches of the middle cerebral or basilar artery, for example, produce restricted neurological damage compared to *major strokes* that involve the main drainage areas of the middle cerebral or basilar arteries. A clinically important point is that minor strokes causing limited neurological impairment in a vascular territory sometimes warn of impending thrombosis of the larger parent artery. Accordingly, in the early hours following onset of neurological damage, minor completed strokes may be difficult or impossible to distinguish from reversible ischemic neurological deficits or even the beginning of a more serious stroke in evolution, as described below.

Between the extremes of TIA's and completed stroke lie two less common conditions. Briefly lasting, completed ischemic events, sometimes called *reversible ischemic neurological defects* (RIND's), produce neurological abnormalities similar to acute completed stroke, but the deficit disappears within 24 to 36 hours, leaving few or no detectable neurological residua. Although less severe in their initial clinical damage than most completed strokes, the favorable outcome of RIND's usually cannot be predicted until rapid recovery begins.

Stroke in evolution refers to a condition wherein ischemic neurological deficits begin in a focal or restricted distribution but over the ensuing hours spread gradually in a pattern reflecting involvement of more and more of the territory of a middle cerebral or basilar artery. Since the neurological deficit of about 15 per cent of patients with acute stroke increases measurably within 24 hours after admission to hospital, this represents an important time period for attempted therapy. Occasionally, stroke can evolve for longer periods, up to a week or so, but such a pattern more often reflects ischemia or bleeding related to a neoplasm or arteriovenous malformation. The pathogenesis of most evolving strokes probably consists of extension of thrombus from an initial clot along the affected artery. Some, especially in the vertebral basilar system, may reflect hemodynamic instability with insufficiency spreading into the penumbral margin of ischemic zones at the edge of the initially hypoperfused area. Evolving stroke must be differentiated from the less specific and temporary neurological worsening that results from cerebral edema complicating large, completed strokes (see below).

Major Stroke Syndromes

Ischemia of the Internal Carotid Artery (Anterior Circulation) System. Both thromboses and emboli can occlude the anterior cerebral circulatory system. Emboli are especially common because of the large size of the system and the fact that so many emboli from the heart find their first escape up the large common carotid arteries.

Transient Ischemic Attacks Affecting the Internal Carotid Artery (ICA) Distribution. About half the time, these events are associated with *stenosis-ulceration* or severe stenosis (> 75 per cent) in the ipsilateral common or internal carotid artery, usually at its bifurcation. Thrombi that arise from either the heart or the proximal aorta cause most of the rest. A few carotid TIA's may be caused by hematogenous abnormalities producing small, spontaneously arising endovascular clots.

Anterior circulation TIA's almost entirely affect either the retinal or middle cerebral artery (MCA) circulation, with the two involved concurrently about 10 per cent of the time. Isolated ophthalmic artery TIA's have the least serious prognosis, often appearing with no accompanying evidence of associated carotid or cardiovascular disease. Symptoms consist of a rapidly developing (10 seconds or so) unilateral graying-out of vision of one eye. Appropriately called *amaurosis fugax*, the episodes usually last for seconds, rarely for more than a few minutes. Retinal examination during the attack may disclose conspicuous narrowing of both arteries and veins, sometimes with blood flow being so slow that venous filling appears segmented. Occasionally one can observe fragments of white or yellow emboli slowly moving outward through the arteries as the attack clears, usually leaving no residua. Yellow, refractile, residual retinal arterial spots represent cholesterol crystals. Their presence implies cholesterol in an upstream arterial plaque and a greater potential risk for future irreversible embolic ischemia.

Symptoms of TIA's affecting the MCA distribution depend upon the functional neuroanatomy of the ischemic field. Peripheral cerebral branch occlusions characteristically cause transient, restricted hand-arm or face-hand-arm paresis with or without accompanying somesthetic sensory loss. Occlusions distal to the point where the lenticulostriate artery branches from the MCA in the dominant hemisphere can cause transient aphasia, while those lodging proximal to or within the lenticulostriate arteries produce transient motor hemiparesis with or without associated language defects. Neither altered consciousness nor confusion ordinarily accompanies ICA-MCA TIA's, most of which last less than 10 to 20 minutes. Seizures are rare.

ICA OCCLUSION. *Acute* occlusion of the previously fully patent vessel can occur at any age due to atherosclerosis, immunological-inflammatory disease, trauma, arterial dissection, massive embolism, or surgical ligation performed in an effort to halt traumatic bleeding or entrap an intracranial aneurysm. The resulting neurological effects depend upon the patient's age and the anastomotic anatomy of the circle of Willis. In persons under 50 years, acute closure often can be tolerated asymptomatically. Beyond that age occlusion increasingly causes small or large infarcts in MCA distribution, even when cerebral arteriography shows an apparently adequate collateral arterial supply. Most spontaneous ICA occlusions develop at the site of a previously severe stenosis, either at the carotid bifurcation or, less frequently, in the intracranial siphon.

The neurological effects of either severe stenosis or total ICA occlusion depend on the patient's age, the rate at which closure occurs, whether or not ulcerated plaques stud the surface of the endothelial lesion, and the degree of intracranial anastomotic compensation. Stenoses that narrow the ICA orifice by less than 85 per cent usually cause little or no reduction in blood flow across the lesion and few symptoms unless ulcers on the stenosing plaque shed TIA-causing emboli. Plaques containing calcification are especially dangerous. Complete occlusions vary widely in their resulting symptoms. Autopsy and arteriographic studies suggest that many ICA occlusions that evolve gradually cause neither symptoms nor structural brain damage. Neurological injury with the remainder ranges from small, deep focal infarctions to massive strokes that involve the entire distribution of the ipsilateral middle and, sometimes, anterior cerebral arteries.

TIA's or small completed strokes precede symptoms of major acute stroke due to ICA occlusion in as many as 20 per cent of cases, usually reflecting progressive stenosis or plaque formation. If a major hemispheric lesion does occur, neurological symptoms and signs affecting the MCA distribution characteristically develop rapidly, with their intensity depending on the size of the subsequent brain lesion. Ipsilateral or bitemporal headache may accompany the onset of occlusion. Whether or not language disorders, sensory impairments, confusional states, or altered levels of consciousness develop depends on the distribution and size of the infarct as well as on the associated cerebral tissue reactions. Focal motor or generalized seizures accompany the acute stage of about 5 per cent of large ICA-MCA distribution infarcts.

Diagnosis of a middle cerebral artery distribution stroke usually is made relatively easily on clinical grounds plus a confirming CT or MR image. Clinical diagnosis of internal carotid artery occlusion, by contrast, is not reliable and in most cases requires imaging studies by noninvasive methods (ultrasound or Doppler flow estimates) or arteriography.

External palpation of the neck is an unreliable sign in diagnosis of ICA occlusion, since internal and external carotid arteries cannot reliably be distinguished from one another. A total absence of cervical arterial pulsations in the region of the angle of the jaw or over the facial arteries suggests the uncommon event of common carotid or combined internal-external carotid artery occlusion. Bruits heard predominantly or entirely over the carotid bifurcation area below the angle of the jaw suggest an underlying stenosis of either the ICA or ECA or both. Generally, the harsher the bruit the more likely that it reflects severe stenosis, especially if accompanied by a palpable thrill. Note, however that only bruits which disappear as auscultation moves down the neck from the angle of the jaw toward the clavicle can be regarded confidently as emanating from the carotid bifurcation.

MIDDLE CEREBRAL ARTERY (MCA) OCCLUSION. Embolism represents the most frequent cause of MCA occlusion. Other mechanisms include extension of clot from an occluded internal carotid artery, intrinsic atherosclerosis, and endovascular thrombosis. The onset of symptoms and signs usually is rapid, taking seconds or minutes to evolve, and commonly silent, producing no more than a sense of paralysis or "deadness" in contralateral body parts. Affected patients, if asleep at onset, may notice no difficulty until they attempt to arise after awakening. Those who are awake may suddenly find without warning that they cannot speak or use an extremity in some common motor act. The immediate neurological deficit, as with carotid occlusion or ICA-MCA TIA's, depends upon where along the MCA the occlusion rests. Major MCA strokes in either hemisphere tend to produce contralateral hemiplegia. Those affecting the dominant hemisphere tend to cause aphasia, while those lying in the nondominant right hemisphere tend to produce confusional states, spatial disorientation, and various degrees of sensory and emotional neglect. Severe inattentiveness, stupor, or coma with unilateral cerebral stroke is limited to patients in whom acute, large, dominant-hemisphere lesions produce global aphasia or those who develop severe secondary brain edema and diencephalic compression-herniation.

ANTERIOR CEREBRAL ARTERY (ACA) OCCLUSION. The anterior cerebral artery has two major parts: (a) the basal portion extends from the ICA to join the anterior communicating artery and (b) the interhemispheric portion supplies the ipsilateral medial frontal lobe as far posteriorly as the sensorimotor foot area. Occlusion of the interhemispheric branch produces an acute focal sensorimotor defect in the contralateral foot and distal leg. Bilateral ACA occlusion distal to the anterior communicating artery causes a moderate spastic paraparesis, urinary incontinence, and behavioral and mental changes consistent with dysfunction of the association cortex of the frontal lobes. Proximal ACA occlusion may cause no neurological deficits so long as a stout and patent anterior communicating artery carries blood from the opposite carotid supply. Lacking such collateral, ischemia may affect deep frontal lobe nuclei to cause (in the dominant hemisphere) Broca's or anterior conduction aphasia. TIA's rarely affect the ACA distribution; recurrent paresthesias or weakness involving a single foot-leg is more consistent with cerebral seizures or, occasionally, recurrent ischemia in the vertebral-basilar system.

Ischemia of the Vertebral-Basilar (Posterior Circulation) System. The basilar artery (BA) and two intracranial vertebral arteries (VA) are supplied rostrally by the posterior communicating arteries and caudally from the cervical vertebral arteries, which originate from the subclavians. Variation in the patency of these sources has several possible effects. With both ends of the double supply open, narrowing or even occlusion of a vertebral or even the basilar artery sometimes can occur without causing symptoms. Emboli are less frequent in the posterior than the anterior circulation, whereas primary atherosclerotic occlusion affects the BA and VA's more frequently than the carotid systems.

TABLE 118–6. MOST COMMON SYMPTOMS OF VERTEBRAL BASILAR TIA'S

PARAMEDIAN ARTERIES	CIRCUMFERENTIAL ARTERIES
Transient global amnesia	Nonpositional vertigo
Diplopia	Unilateral face or body paresthesias
Episodic, paroxysmal drowsiness	Episodic hemianopia or scintillations
Paraparesis or tetraparesis	Unilateral posterior headache
Ataxia	
Dysarthria	

Vertebral-basilar TIA's can produce complex and variable symptoms and signs, the nature of which depends upon the anatomical distribution of ischemia. Often the neurological changes vary from attack to attack in the same person (Table 118–6). This variability contrasts with carotid TIA's, in which recurrent episodes in the same patient tend to remain stereotyped.

Occlusion of VA or BA and their main branches can cause several different syndromes depending on the rostral-caudal brain level of the arterial stoppage, the point of occlusion along the length of the vessel, and whether or not the involvement includes the paramedian vessels, circumferential arteries, or both.

Posterior cerebral artery (PCA) occlusions most often are due to atherosclerosis located at the basilar takeoff. More distal occlusions also can result, sometimes from emboli but also from inflammatory arteritis or compression during transtentorial herniation. Neurological effects depend on the site of PCA closure. Distal obstructions result in homonymous or quadrantic hemianopias, while more proximal stoppage produces infarction of the sensory thalamus and sometimes the lateral midbrain as well.

BA occlusion at the apex has several possible outcomes depending upon whether the obstruction includes the posterior cerebral arteries, the arteries supplying the overlying diencephalon, the vessels feeding the midbrain, or some combination thereof. Loss or reduction of consciousness at the onset is common and is often associated with a variety of pupillary, gaze, and oculomotor paralyses. If the cerebral peduncles are affected, decorticate or decerebrate motor posturing and paralysis ensue. During convalescence one finds varying combinations of inattention, dementia, memory loss, visual field defects, gaze palsy, and sensory or motor impairments, which individually or together reflect the extent of the eventual damage to the occipital lobe, the diencephalon, and the midbrain. More caudally placed occlusions of the BA, if they selectively affect paramedian vessels, impair consciousness and produce dysconjugate eye movements, unequal pupils, and signs of bilateral upper motor neuron dysfunction. Bizarre irregularities in breathing patterns often emerge. Obstruction of individual superior, anterior, and posterior cerebellar arteries characteristically produces contralateral sensory impairment on the body combined with variable lower motor neuron and sensory changes involving ipsilateral cranial nerves V through XII. Ipsilateral cerebellar ataxia and some degree of contralateral upper motor neuron deficit affecting at least the lower extremity often are associated.

Complete basilar occlusion affecting both paramedian and circumferential vessels usually produces incomplete ischemic transection of the brain stem. Affected patients usually are in a coma and show pinpoint, irregular, or unequal pupils, bilateral conjugate gaze paralysis, or internuclear ophthalmoplegia and tetraplegia. Mercifully, few survive more than a few days.

Unilateral VA occlusion occurs asymptomatically in about 50 per cent of cases. When symptoms do occur, they produce the syndrome of the posterior inferior cerebellar artery. Signs of mild ipsilateral cerebellar dysfunction are accompanied by ipsilateral lower motor neuron paralysis of cranial nerves IX, X, and XII, coupled with pain and temperature loss contralaterally on the body and ipsilaterally on the face. An ipsilateral Horner's syndrome usually is present. Hiccup is common.

Acute cerebellar infarction can occur more or less independently of other neurological difficulties when occlusion strikes any of the three main cerebellar arteries, principally the inferior branch. A grave complication ensues if the cerebellum swells sufficiently from ischemic edema to distort the brain stem and obstruct the normal CSF outflow. Initial symptoms in this instance include ipsilateral occipital headache and signs of mild cerebellar dysfunction followed by increasing occipital head pain, often vomiting, and the development of ipsilateral cranial nerve defects, including oculomotor changes. Progression, if it occurs, usually develops within 12 to 36 hours and is marked by more severe bilateral headache and drowsiness or stupor, as well as the appearance of bilateral upper motor neuron signs in the extremities. CT scans show an enlarged, hypodense cerebellar hemisphere with obstruction of the fourth ventricle together with dilatation of the third and lateral ventricles. Urgent treatment, consisting of lateral ventricular drainage or occipital decompression, can prevent further damage or death.

Spinal Stroke. Ischemic infarction due to atherosclerotic arterial occlusion rarely affects the spinal cord. More common is spinal infarction associated with prolonged hypotension (shock) or compression by intraspinal mass lesions. Arterial lesions, when they occur, almost always involve the anterior spinal artery, atherosclerotic obstruction striking most often at the level of the cervical radicular artery or one or two segments below. Inflammatory and immune arteritides are, if anything, more frequent than atherosclerotic obstructions, especially in younger persons, and tend to occur at the T4 level. In both instances, neurological damage develops acutely or rapidly, usually reaching a maximum within 24 hours of onset, and produces a transverse myelopathy of the anterior half of the cord. Lower motor neuron abnormalities sometimes can be detected at the level of the lesion combined with bilateral impairment of pain and temperature sensations beginning one or two dermatomes below.

Injury to corticospinal pathways results in upper motor neuron dysfunction caudal to the level of occlusion. Dysfunction of bowel, bladder, and male sexual activities usually accompanies these abnormalities.

Cerebral Venous Thrombosis. Obstruction to the cerebral venous sinuses or their main tributaries has several potential causes (Table 118–7). Most spontaneous examples appear either during the postpartum period, as an idiopathic phenomenon related to little understood "physiological" hypercoagulability, or as a complication of disease-related coagulopathy, especially that associated with cancer or infection. The clinical findings are discussed on page 808.

Hypertensive Encephalopathy (HE). HE represents a serious complication of severe hypertension, now made uncommon by the widespread use of effective antihypertensive drugs. The abnormal cerebral state accompanies an acute rise in blood pressure in excess of previous levels, precipitated most often by acute or chronic renal disease, eclampsia, or the abrupt withdrawal of previously taken antihypertensive drugs. Foods high in tyramine content can precipitate HE in patients taking monoamine oxidase inhibiting drugs for psychiatric illness. Recurrent crises sometimes reflect the presence of an underlying pheochromocytoma and can occur rarely for unexplained reasons in individuals with otherwise only moderate chronic hypertension.

The pathogenesis of HE relates to the effect of the high systemic intravascular pressure on the brain's arterioles. The elevated tension exceeds the upper limits of normal cerebral autoregulation, so that a combination of multifocal arteriolar vasodilatation and vasoconstriction occurs, producing diffusely distributed small zones of microhemorrhages and ischemia.

Florid multifocal and usually transient clinical changes characterize HE and include headache, nausea, vomiting, and sometimes, cortical blindness. Focal or generalized seizures, confusional states, stupor, or coma can mark the course of severe attacks. Focal, often evanescent monoplegia or hemiplegia may be present. The retinal arterioles usually show abnormal hypertensive changes and sometimes are barely visible owing to spasm. Hemorrhages and papilledema can occur but nowadays are no longer the rule. The BUN is less than 100 mg/dl and often normal. CSF values are usually elevated for pressure (above 180 mm CSF), protein (above 60 mg/dl), and cells (both RBC and WBC). CT is not diagnostic except to rule out an intracranial mass lesion or hemorrhage as the cause of illness.

Differential diagnosis of HE includes acute uremia (BUN > 100 mg/dl), encephalitis (fever, no severe hypertension, usually slower course), cerebral venous sinus thrombosis, and acute lead encephalopathy. Less common causes of acute multifocal encephalopathy must be considered, including disseminated intravascular coagulation and acute bacterial endocarditis.

HE requires urgent treatment using intravenously regulated sodium nitroprusside to lower blood pressure promptly to levels within the upper range of autoregulation (mean 130 ± 10 mm Hg). Later, within

TABLE 118–7. MAJOR CAUSES OF CEREBRAL VENOUS AND SINUS THROMBOSIS IN APPROXIMATELY DECLINING ORDER OF FREQUENCY

Late pregnancy and postpartum state
Contraceptive medication
Coagulant factors associated with malignancy, disseminated intravascular coagulation, thrombotic purpura
Idiopathic
Severe dehydration or intrinsic hyperviscosity
Septic extension from face, sinus, mastoid

12 hours or so, systemic pressures can be brought further down more gradually so as to allow arterioles to adapt to the reduced pressure and thereby reduce the risk of inducing focal cerebral hypoperfusion. Convulsions can be controlled acutely using diazepam, 10 to 20 mg intravenously. Long-term control of the underlying hypertension must be pursued vigorously.

Diagnosis and Differential Diagnosis in Ischemic Stroke

The major diagnostic questions are several: Has an ischemic event occurred? If so, is it transient, progressive, or completed? If completed, is it minor or major? Finally, what is its cause and what immediately and subsequently must be done?

Clinical understanding plus judiciously chosen confirmatory laboratory tests give accurate diagnosis in nearly all instances. Age, mode of onset, the presence or absence of known risk factors or previous vascular events, and whether or not the neurological deficit fits a known vascular distribution provide the chief clues. The first minutes or hours of observation show whether a stroke is a TIA, is progressing, or, for the moment, has completed its ravages. The general history and physical examination often disclose the presence or absence of stroke-causing systemic diseases (see Table 118–1), especially those of the heart or great vessels. These steps, combined with routine laboratory studies (urinalysis, CBC and smear, standard chemical and electrolyte screening, ECG, chest radiograph) provide accurate diagnosis in perhaps 90 per cent of instances. A CT or MR head scan should be obtained for any first completed or progressive stroke, since about 4 per cent of such patients turn out to have other disorders such as a neoplasm or hematoma. Imaging is also indicated to verify possible strokes with unusual anatomical patterns. CT or, if unavailable, lumbar puncture should be done before initiating anticoagulant therapy, since some cerebral hemorrhages have a stroke-like onset. One should recall, however, that even large cerebral infarcts may not produce abnormalities on the CT scan until as late as 24 to 48 hours after onset. Some strokes never disfigure the scan.

Ischemic stroke affects persons less than age 50 rarely, and those less than 70 uncommonly, except in association with specific risk factors or identifiable toxic or systemic causes. Patients lacking such apparent antecedents deserve especially careful appraisal.

Differentiation among TIA's, progressive stroke, minor completed stroke, and severe completed stroke is implicit in their presentations. TIA's must be differentiated from seizures, usually not a difficult matter, since TIA's rarely cause positive motor signs, are less long-lasting, and produce no postictal effects. Nevertheless, with stereotyped recurrent hemispheric attacks a CT scan is desirable to rule out a structural cause. Glaucoma or other local diseases of the eye, cranial arteritis, and migraine represent alternate potential causes of unilateral visual loss. Basilar migraine, an illness most common in young persons and carrying a strong family predisposition, can produce symptoms suggesting VB TIA's; age, family history, and a longer duration all are distinctive. Benign positional vertigo differs from basilar TIA's by its strict link to positional stimuli and its lack of associated symptoms of brain stem dysfunction. Similar considerations rule out the nonspecific dizzy feelings experienced by many elderly persons. Cardiac arrhythmias rarely cause symptoms resembling TIA's, just as TIA's rarely cause syncope (page 682). Subdural hematomas or large, unruptured intracranial aneurysms sometimes produce attacks that are indistinguishable from carotid TIA's and that may have a similar embolic pathogenesis. Such episodes rarely occur, however, in the absence of other symptoms of the primary disorder. Minor or major progressive or completed stroke must be distinguished from deep cerebral hemorrhage. Usually, the latter produces more headache, a faster evolution, a higher incidence of seizures, and prominent autonomic changes. Brain tumors can resemble stroke in occasional instances when they internally bleed and suddenly enlarge. Afebrile brain abscesses or granulomas can provide a similar problem. CT or MR imaging differentiates in all three instances. Postictal paralysis can give the appearance of stroke, but the history is distinctive. When the seizure is unobserved, age and rapid recovery usually serve to differentiate. Cervical-cerebral angiography has little usefulness in evaluating acute stroke. Its place in managing aftercare is described below.

Etiological diagnosis in stroke is important for guiding both acute and chronic management. All patients deserve careful evaluation of the cardiovascular system, with one basing the extent of the investigation upon preliminary findings and known risk factors. Echocardiography and cardiac wall motion studies can identify potential sources of emboli in patients with mitral prolapse, valvular stenosis, or anterior wall infarctions and detect the rare unsuspected atrial myxoma. EEG's and other clinical neurophysiological studies seldom provide useful information. Noninvasive investigations, such as ultrasonic or Doppler flow studies, applied to the carotid systems become more useful in planning convalescent than acute management. Generally speaking, the more restricted and reversible the initial neurological injury, the more assiduously one searches for specific causes for which treatment might reduce the risk of future brain damage.

Management of Acute Stroke

Once ischemia has damaged the brain, no currently available treatment favorably influences the outcome of the injury. Management consists of providing good general medical and nursing care, reducing hypertension or hyperviscosity if present, and taking steps to prevent acute or future worsening of the neurological deficit. Acutely, one attempts to halt progressing stroke, to prevent recurring cerebral emboli, and to stabilize with the least possible deficit patients with fluctuating neurological changes. In 24 hours or so after onset, the problem of ischemic brain edema may require therapeutic attention.

The Use and Choice of Anticoagulants. The use of these drugs in acute stroke is a somewhat controversial subject. The treatment can cause dangerous bleeding of about 1 to 2 per cent per year in experienced hands. Anticoagulation is contraindicated in the presence of uremia, any bleeding diathesis, and a diastolic blood pressure greater than 100 mm Hg. In other circumstances, the choice and use of anticoagulants are guided by theoretical considerations plus a limited number of incompletely controlled studies and the experience of the therapist. We describe here the approach employed at the New York Hospital.

Heparin therapy, unless specifically contraindicated, is initiated at the time of admission to hospital in patients describing repetitive, closely spaced TIA's, in those with progression of specific weakness during the hours before hospitalization, in those observed to have increasing neurological deficits (not due to early transtentorial herniation) during the first 12 to 18 hours following admission, and in patients demonstrating fluctuating signs and symptoms of vertebral, basilar, or carotid ischemia. A CT scan is obtained first to rule out hemorrhage. If lumbar puncture has been performed, heparin is thereafter delayed for at least two hours to reduce the risk of spinal epidural bleeding. Heparin is also given to patients with minor or restricted completed strokes of less than 8 to 12 hours' duration as well as to patients suffering a first stroke accompanied by conditions such as atrial fibrillation that threaten to cause recurrent embolism.

Heparin therapy is stopped usually within three to five days in patients who turn out to have no neurological progression or instability, in those who complete a severe stroke with massive cerebral, brain stem, or cerebellar infarction, and in patients with partial defects that clear quickly (RIND). Heparin is replaced gradually by coumadin derivatives in patients whose evolving stroke halts when they receive the drug as well as in those with a high risk of future embolization. Anticoagulation is stopped in most patients, except those with atrial fibrillation (AF), after two to three months and is continued out of hospital only when adequate supervision can be guaranteed. Chronic anticoagulation is reserved for patients with chronic AF, valvular prostheses, and a limited number of other specific thrombogenic disorders.

Platelet Antiaggregant Therapy. Several large trials have suggested that aspirin given to persons previously susceptible to TIA's or coronary artery disease reduces the risk of recurrent cerebral TIA's as well of both cerebral and cardiac thromboembolism. Two other agents, dipyridamole and sulfinpyrazone, also possess theoretically beneficial effects against platelet aggregation. Aspirin exerts long-lasting effects on the arachidonate cascade so as to inhibit platelet aggregation and is given in single daily doses ranging from 80 mg to as much as 1.5 gm. Empirical confirmation of the ideal dose awaits clinical trial. Dipyridamole and sulfinpyrazone possess shorter durations of action than salicylates and are given in divided doses, three to four times daily. Their benefit is unproved.

When not specifically contraindicated, platelet antiaggregants are currently used by most authorities to treat all patients experiencing infrequent carotid or vertebral basilar TIA's, for chronic treatment of patients who have had a completed stroke, and for patients considered at high risk for stroke.

Ischemic Cerebral Edema. Some degree of edema surrounds all cerebral infarcts. The necrosis of cells and vascular endothelium releases osmols into the extracellular space while the associated death of astrocytes removes their normal osmotic pumping action. The combined factors draw water into the extracellular space, sometimes in dangerous proportions. Ischemic edema generally becomes detectable within 12 to 24 hours following infarction and continues to increase for as long as 48 hours thereafter.

Cerebral edema produces hypodense areas by CT scanning surrounding a more or less distinct region of recent infarction. Such changes usually cannot be detected until at least 48 hours after the ictus and by themselves neither produce symptoms nor require treatment. Large, edematous hemispheric infarcts, however, can lead to transtentorial herniation, while similar enlargement in the cerebellum may compress the brain stem or obstruct CSF outflow pathways. Either can be fatal.

Systemic metabolic derangements and pulmonary or urinary infections appear to intensify the degree and ill effects of post-stroke edema. Treatment consists of correcting or treating these complications and, if herniation threatens, giving intravenously a dehydrating agent such as mannitol in an effort to shrink the brain. Passive hyperventilation briefly reduces the intracranial volume by inducing one to two hours of arterial vasoconstriction. Diuretic drugs produce minimal benefit except as they treat systemic fluid overload. The induction of anesthetic coma has no therapeutic value. Corticosteroid drugs are contraindicated in the treatment of stroke; they do not benefit necrotic edema and may accentuate neurological damage.

Convalescent Management. Most patients whose neurological disability improves incompletely within two to three weeks will benefit from an organized rehabilitation program. Little improvement can be expected beyond 8 to 12 weeks, making prolonged rehabilitation measures unjustified. The additional value of speech therapy is uncertain.

Preventive Measures. Even after a first stroke, epidemiological studies indicate that treatment of hypertension and cessation of smoking reduce the risk of recurrence. Weight loss for the obese and at least some exercise for everyone may be beneficial. Otherwise, careful medical supervision plus daily platelet an-

tiaggregants form the mainstay of most medical treatment.

Arteriography and Vascular Surgery in Stroke Prevention

Arteriography carries a risk of 1 to 2 per cent of serious complications in the stroke age group but may be indicated (1) when diagnosis is in doubt, (2) to seek the source of an arteriovenous malformation or an unexplained lobar cerebral hemorrhage, and (3) to search for potentially surgically treatable stenoses or ulcerations in the carotid arterial system.

Operative repair of internal carotid artery stenosis in the neck has become widely and probably excessively practiced in recent years as a putative preventive measure against strokes. Uncertainty surrounds both the indications for such procedures and their results, the only existing controlled study on the subject showing no benefit from surgery. The Stroke Research Center at The New York Hospital–Cornell Medical Center takes the following approach to this controversial therapy.

Treatment of Recurrent Anterior Circulation TIA's and Partial or Minor Strokes. A substantial fraction of patients with these disorders have lesions of the carotid arteries. If the ipsilateral internal carotid artery in the neck contains an ulcerated plaque or is stenosed more than 80 per cent, carotid endarterectomy is recommended so long as no contraindications exist as discussed below. The presence of surface calcium in the ulcer strengthens the recommendation. Patients with exclusively basilar TIA's or partial strokes involving the posterior circulation are not subjected to arteriography or considered for surgery, since no evidence suggests that benefits would follow.

Carotid Bruits and Neurologically Asymptomatic Internal Carotid Lesions. Several studies indicate that careful physical examination discloses a carotid bruit unassociated with cerebrovascular symptoms in about 5 per cent of the population over age 50 years. Only about half of such patients show appreciable internal carotid artery narrowing by arteriography. Present evidence indicates that in asymptomatic patients whose arteriograms show neither ulcerated plaques nor a greater than 80 per cent stenosis of the internal carotid artery the morbidity-mortality risk of arteriography plus surgery is probably higher than the risk of naturally occurring stroke. Accordingly, the ideal approach to patients with asymptomatic cervical bruits is to obtain noninvasive Doppler or sonographic flow studies of the carotid arteries. If these studies disclose severe ulcerations or tight narrowing, arteriography can then be carried out to determine whether or not a lesion exists that is appropriate for surgical treatment.

Contraindications for Carotid Surgery. These consist of circumstances in which either surgical treatment has no shown measurable benefit or potential complications exceed possible benefits. They include complete internal carotid artery occlusions; acutely evolving strokes; totally asymptomatic carotid narrowing in patients destined for coronary bypass or other major surgery; the presence of an already massive cerebral infarct involving the ICA-MCA vascular field; plaques or narrowing in the intracranial portion of the carotid artery, and unstable general medical conditions such as recent myocardial infarction, congestive heart failure, uncontrolled hypertension, or severe systemic metabolic problems. Such factors double or triple the surgical risk.

Some surgeons have attempted other vascular operations such as bypassing a superficial temporal artery to a distal branch of the middle cerebral artery in efforts to prevent future stroke. Controlled studies indicate that such operations have no therapeutic value.

Prognosis in Stroke

About one fourth of patients with acute completed stroke die during hospitalization. Advanced age, severe brain stem dysfunction, coma, and severe associated heart disease all worsen the outlook. Among survivors, about 40 per cent of all patients with acute stroke make a good functional recovery. The degree and rate depend on the initial severity, the amount of improvement within the first two weeks, age, and how much language or cognitive difficulty persists. Few patients with pronounced Wernicke aphasia or functional dementia regain full independence. Motor flaccidity or dense hemisensory defects persisting past the first weeks similarly reduce the chances for future independence.

Prognosis for patients with TIA's depends on the presence or absence of associated risk factors, especially cardiac. A variety of studies indicate a combined risk of about 12 per cent per year for either stroke, myocardial infarction, or death (from either) following the onset of these minor cerebrovascular events. The annual risk of such consequences climbs to about 20 per cent among patients with major strokes.

CEREBRAL HEMORRHAGE

Spontaneous (nontraumatic) cerebral hemorrhage may occur primarily into the substance of the brain (intracerebral or parenchymal) or over its surface (subarachnoid). Most examples arise from one of three causes: (1) progressive damage and finally rupture into the parenchyma of a brain-penetrating artery due to hypertension, atherosclerosis, or intrinsic arterial degeneration, (2) "spontaneous" rupture of a penetrating artery associated with either an intrinsically caused or therapeutic excess of anticoagulation; (3) rupture of a congenital or acquired arterial anomaly into the subarachnoid space (berry and mycotic aneurysm) or the parenchyma (arteriovenous malformation). Other uncommon mechanisms include hemorrhage into brain tumors, bleeding from degenerative amyloid (congophilic) angiopathy in the elderly, and bleeding from inflammatory vasculopathies such as periarteritis nodosa or that associated with amphetamine usage. Hemorrhagic infarction secondary to arterial or venous obstruction has been discussed in a previous section. Cerebral hemorrhage totals about 15 per cent of all clinically detectable strokes but assumes greater medical importance because of the serious consequences that often result.

Hypertensive-Atherosclerotic (H-A) Cerebral Hemorrhage. Roughly 90 per cent of spontaneous parenchymal cerebral hemorrhages fall into this category. Long-standing hypertension antedates the bleed in about two thirds of cases, with the incidence of bleeding generally paralleling the intensity and duration of that disorder. With or without hypertension, rupture reflects an area of weakening leading to bleeding from penetrating arterioles of approximately 100 to 150 µm in diameter. Spontaneous bleeding can affect almost any part of the brain, although the most common sites for hypertensive-atherosclerotic hemorrhages are into the deep cerebral regions of the internal capsule, basal ganglia, and thalamus, as well as into the central pons and the deep nuclear regions of the cerebellum (Figs. 118–1 and 118–2). Among patients over age 70, congophilic amyloid angiopathy becomes an increasing cause of cerebral hemorrhage, affecting most often the more peripheral or polar regions of the hemisphere. Such bleeds often produce few symptoms or cause mild symptoms that resemble ischemic stroke.

In contrast to ischemic stroke, which commonly occurs during sleep, most H-A cerebral hemorrhage begins during wakefulness, often associated with exertion. Sudden severe headache, "the worst in my life," announces the onset, followed within minutes to hours by neurological signs whose nature and severity reflect the site and extent of the bleeding. Characteristically, systemic examination discloses hypertension, sometimes to a temporarily severe degree, and, commonly, cardiac enlargement as well as hypertensive or atherosclerotic changes in the retinal arteries.

Basal Ganglia–Internal Capsular Hemorrhage. The onset headache commonly arises ipsilateral to the bleed and is followed shortly by a progressive contralateral hemiparesis, often accompanied by the eyes deviating toward the side of the lesion owing to damage to the adjacent frontal eye fields. Convulsions are common and can take either a generalized grand mal pattern or be focal and involve the body contralateral to the bleeding. In the latter case, the eyes often deviate away from the lesion during the seizure. Rupture into the lateral ventricle is frequent and precipitates autonomic symptoms of shivering, nausea, and vomiting. Large hemorrhages greater than 2.5 to 3 cm in diameter frequently cause coma within a few hours, and many such cases go on to transtentorial herniation followed by severe disability or death. Smaller hematomas cause proportionately less neurological damage, and ultimate improvement may be considerable.

Thalamic Hemorrhage. While serious, these often are smaller and less devastating than the ones discussed previously. Contralateral sensory loss, hemianopia, and hemiparesis or hemiplegia are characteristic. Compression of the tectum-midbrain commonly induces drowsiness, which proceeds to coma only in rapidly fatal cases. Gaze palsies are common and include defects in upward gaze. Eyes cast down and laterally at rest provide an almost pathognomonic sign

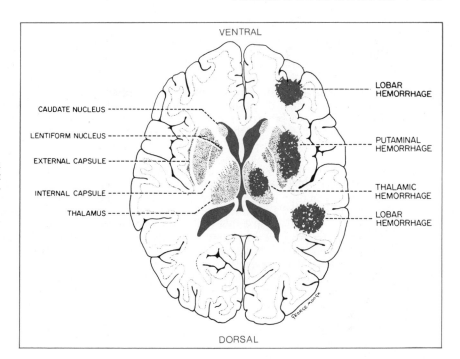

FIGURE 118–1. Horizontal section through the cerebral hemispheres illustrating frequent sites of thalamic, putaminal, and lobar hemorrhages.

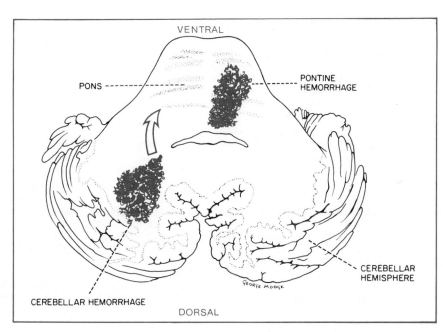

FIGURE 118–2. Horizontal section through pons and adjacent cerebellum showing common hemorrhage sites. The arrow shows a frequent line along which cerebellar hemorrhage can dissect into the pons.

of bleeding in this area. Midbrain compression may transiently cause pupillary inequality or fixation.

Pontine Hemorrhage. The onset usually is cataclysmic, with sudden headache followed within seconds to minutes by coma accompanied by stertorous or irregular breathing, pinpoint pupils, bilateral conjugate gaze paralysis or ocular bobbing, tetraparesis and, often, decerebrate or decorticate rigidity. Most patients die, and those who survive usually are left quadriplegic and totally dependent.

Cerebellar Hemorrhage. Unilateral occipital headache often announces the onset followed by ipsilateral incoordination-ataxia of the extremities, slurred speech, and sometimes nausea and vomiting. Disequilibrium, ipsilateral facial weakness, and diplopia with ipsilateral conjugate gaze paralysis often follow within a matter of hours and may reflect either dissection of the hematoma into the lateral pons or only compression of that structure. The development of a reduced level of consciousness or of signs of upper motor neuron dysfunction affecting the extremities suggests the development of brain stem compression, due to direct enlargement of the hematoma or secondary to acute obstruction of the fourth ventricle, producing hydrocephalus.

Diagnosis

Only acute ischemic stroke represents a frequent source of potential diagnostic uncertainty, although hemorrhage into brain tumors occasionally may be indistinguishable. Headache, severe hypertension, acute prostration, nausea and vomiting, convulsions, autonomic signs, and loss of consciousness are all more characteristic of deep cerebral hemorrhage than of ischemia. If blood reaches the subarachnoid space or if downward or upward herniation threatens, the neck will stiffen. CT scan is diagnostic, leaving only the cause of bleeding in doubt. Patients who are not hypertensive, who are young, or who have less than devastating neurological deficits deserve arteriography to seek a potentially treatable vascular anomaly. Lumbar puncture can precipitate fatal intracranial herniation and should be avoided unless no CT scan is available and acute bacterial meningitis seems a strong possibility.

Treatment

Treatment consists of lowering the blood pressure deliberately as described under hypertensive encephalopathy and applying supportive measures. Where clinical signs and CT examination suggest that a cerebellar hemorrhage is compressing the brain stem or causing acute hydrocephalus, lateral ventricular decompression may be life-saving. Occasionally, posterior fossa decompression may become necessary. Efforts to drain acute cerebral hemorrhages surgically usually remove viable brain in the process and worsen rather than improve the eventual outcome.

Few patients in coma from cerebral hemorrhage survive, and those with extensive brain stem damage usually remain neurologically devastated. Considerable neurological recovery, however, often follows even moderately large hemorrhages in the peripheral parts of the cerebral or cerebellar hemispheres, since the blood dissects between much of the tissue rather than totally destroying it.

INTRACRANIAL ANEURYSMS

Intracranial aneurysms occur in three characteristic forms: fusiform, mycotic, and congenital "berry" aneurysms.

Fusiform aneurysms represent ectatic dilatations of the basilar or intracranial portion of the carotid artery. They develop a sausage-like or irregular bulbous shape, sometimes reaching a size of 5 to 10 cm in diameter. Usually they produce no symptoms, but sometimes their large size compresses adjacent tissues or cranial nerves to cause local neurological dysfunction. Large basilar artery aneurysms characteristically cause multiple bilateral asymmetrical cranial nerve dysfunction extending anywhere from the third to the tenth nerve, while those of the carotid artery can cause ipsilateral visual loss or contralateral hemiparesis reflecting their parapituitary position. Such ectatic aneurysms seldom rupture, and they are rarely amenable to successful surgical therapy.

Mycotic aneurysms arise in the course of bacterial endocarditis when septic emboli lodge in a peripherally located cerebral vessel, producing endothelial ischemia at the embolic site. Infecting bacteria subsequently invade the arterial wall, and the resulting weakening invites aneurysmal blowout. Mycotic aneurysms often are multiple and characteristically are located peripherally on the cerebral arterial tree. Some resolve with antibiotic treatment, but those that remain after systemic infection is brought under control should be surgically treated.

Congenital berry aneurysms arise at bifurcation points along the circle of Willis at the base of the brain. In the anterior circulation they form especially at the junctions between the anterior cerebral and anterior communicating arteries; and between the middle cerebral and either the posterior communicating or carotid arteries (Fig. 118–3). Less frequently, similar aneurysms balloon out at one of the several major tributary points along the basilar-vertebral axis. Berry aneurysms vary considerably in size from a few millimeters to 1, 2, or more centimeters in diameter. Those larger than 1.5 to 2 cm in diameter are commonly termed "giant" and carry a particular risk of rupture.

The pathogenesis of berry aneurysms is thought to reflect a congenital defect that affects elastic tissue and muscle at arterial branch points along the base of the brain. The weak point allows aneurysmal formation and eventual rupture secondary to accumulated wear and tear. Similar aneurysms also occur in association with certain brain tumors. Congenital aneurysms are more common in persons with long-standing hypertension, especially those suffering from coarctation of the aorta and polycystic kidney disease. Some persons have multiple intracranial aneurysms. A low but definite family incidence suggests a hereditary factor.

Most intracranial aneurysms are detected only when they rupture, an event that can occur at any age but which is most common between the ages of 40 and 65. Most rupture takes place during the waking hours, many examples occurring in association with vigorous physical activity.

Clinical Manifestations of Aneurysmal Rupture and Subarachnoid Hemorrhage (SAH)

These can be divided into five phases: onset, the first week of acute symptoms, the risk of secondary ischemic infarction, the development of communicating hydrocephalus, and the indications for and outcome of surgery.

The usual first symptom is sudden excruciating headache, sometimes followed by brief syncope or a seizure. The latter symptoms result either from a neurogenically induced cardiac arrhythmia or from the brief concussion that accompanies the sudden rise in intracranial pressure. Subsequent effects depend on the locus and extent of the bleeding. Small warning leaks sometimes occur, causing a uniquely severe

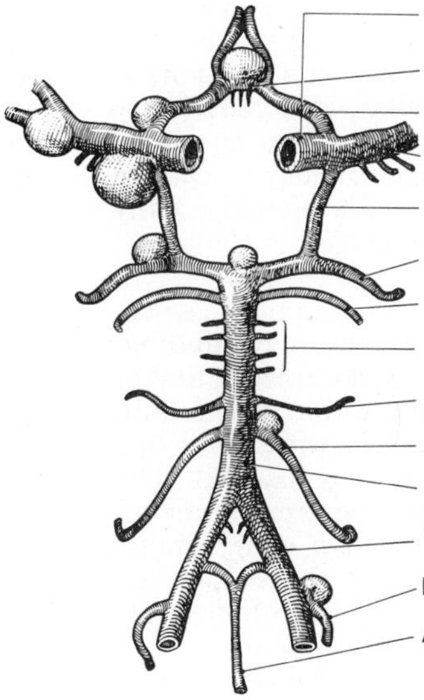

FIGURE 118–3. The more common sites of berry aneurysm. The diagrammatic size of the aneurysm at the various sites is directly proportional to its frequency at that locus.

INTERNAL CAROTID ARTERY
ANTERIOR COMMUNICATING ARTERY
ANTERIOR CEREBRAL ARTERY
MIDDLE CEREBRAL ARTERY
POSTERIOR COMMUNICATING ARTERY
POSTERIOR CEREBRAL ARTERY
SUPERIOR CEREBELLAR ARTERY
PARAMEDIAN ARTERIES
CIRCUMFERENTIAL ARTERY
ANTERIOR INFERIOR CEREBELLAR ARTERY
BASILAR ARTERY
VERTEBRAL ARTERY
POSTERIOR INFERIOR CEREBELLAR ARTERY
ANTERIOR SPINAL ARTERY

headache that then subsides over the following few days. Larger bleeds confined to the subarachnoid space produce more severe and sustained head pain, followed in 12 to 24 hours by signs of meningeal inflammation as red blood cells lyse and release irritating bile pigments into the CSF. Severe bleeds can immediately produce coma, sometimes caused by a high intracranial pressure, but more often because bleeding dissects into the brain or ruptures into the ventricular system. Persistent coma implies transtentorial herniation and a bad prognosis.

Stiff neck at onset implies a large hemorrhage, perhaps with descent of the cerebellar tonsils. Subhyaloid retinal hemorrhages can appear within minutes of the onset of the subarachnoid bleeding. If either focal neurological signs or a reduced state of consciousness develops immediately, it implies that blood has dissected into the brain, worsening the prognosis. After the first day, the development of new focal motor or neurological abnormalities reflects either an episode of rebleeding or a secondary cerebral infarction caused by arterial vasospasm induced by the subarachnoid blood.

After the first few hours of bleeding a variety of systemic and secondary changes complicate the picture. The autonomic storm that accompanies the initial headache releases systemic catecholamines, which produce diffuse myocardial micronecrosis and infarction-like ECG abnormalities. Acutely, systemic hyperglycemia, leukocytosis, and fever have a similar pathogenesis. Subsequently, fever, leukocytosis, and delirium can last a week or more owing to the continuing hemorrhagic chemical meningitis. Most severely

ill patients with acute SAH secrete inappropriately high levels of antidiuretic hormone, predisposing to hyponatremia. Late symptoms of lethargy, continued delirium, stupor, or diffuse, mild upper motor neuron abnormalities may reflect the development of communicating hydrocephalus.

Diagnosis

The first principle is to respect thoroughly the development of sudden severe headache in a previously well adult. Discrimination about an abrupt, new headache may be difficult in persons of known hypochondriacal disposition, but when in serious doubt, even if neurological findings are absent, it is wise to obtain lumbar puncture, taking care to identify intrinsic bleeding by centrifuging bloody fluid and looking for a discolored supernatant.

For more obviously acutely ill patients with typical symptoms, CT scan is the laboratory procedure of first choice and will detect an SAH large enough to threaten transtentorial herniation; if none is visualized, lumbar puncture can then be done to identify other potentially serious causes of sudden acute headache. CT scans also show the presence of large clots in the subarachnoid space or brain (they increase the risk of arterial spasm) and provide a baseline for future comparison in the event of subsequent unexplained worsenings. Contrast CT scans or MR images obtained with contemporary instruments often outline aneurysms of greater that 5 mm in diameter as well as arteriovenous abnormalities that may have caused the hemorrhage.

Arteriography is indispensable for identifying the

presence and location of aneurysms and, where more than one is found, for estimating which has bled. In hospitals staffed by neurosurgeons skilled in aneurysm work, radiographs should be obtained on suitable surgical candidates as soon as possible after admission. In poor-risk patients or when it is anticipated that surgery will be done elsewhere, no value is gained by adding the hazards of arteriography to the already precarious state. The latter patients should be transferred as early as possible to a tertiary care center.

Prognosis and Management

Prognosis is poor in acute SAH owing to ruptured aneurysm. Careful population studies indicate that of all such patients, two thirds die within one month (many without reaching a hospital), with about one fourth of the survivors being severely disabled. The first two weeks after onset carry the greatest risk of rebleeding, amounting to about 30 per cent. Among patients whose aneurysms cannot be treated successfully, rebleeding with a two thirds risk of mortality continues at a rate of about 3 per cent per year.

The above considerations imply that as soon as acute SAH is recognized patients should be placed in the hands of an experienced neurological-neurosurgical team for definitive management. Initially, patients are placed at bed rest, kept quiet with mild benzodiazepine sedatives, and given analgesics short of opiates for pain. Stool softeners or enemas are important for preventing straining. Gentle movement in bed and turning should be emphasized to prevent the complications of immobility. Blood pressure should be controlled at nearly normal levels, but blood volume should be maintained by adequate fluids using 3 per cent saline solutions if necessary to correct hyponatremia.

Most experienced centers do four-vessel cerebral angiography within 24 hours of onset. Definitive treatment consists of surgical isolation and clipping of the leaking aneurysm. Such procedures are technically difficult and carry a high perioperative risk of inducing even more brain damage. Currently, surgical opinion differs as to whether operation is better done immediately, risking more frequent complications, or after 10 to 14 days when the risk of spasm and associated infarction declines but the greatest risk of rebleeding already has passed. Surgery should be deferred or avoided in patients who are neurologically unstable, in those with major neurological deficits, and in those who are stuporous or comatose. Similarly, most authorities avoid immediate surgery for patients whose arteriograms show arterial vasospasm. Continued obtundation not explained by focal damage and associated with CT evidence of progressive hydrocephalus sometimes can be relieved by ventricular shunting. It is not established whether or not operating on intracranial aneurysms more than 30 days following the bleed confers any advantage over the natural history of the disease.

ARTERIOVENOUS MALFORMATIONS (AVM's)

In addition to congenital aneurysms, four types of vascular malformations can affect the brain. These include: (1) Capillary telangiectases, seldom a cause of clinical abnormalities. (2) Venous angiomas. One form comprises the Sturge-Weber syndrome (p. 748); larger ones may rupture or, when in the spinal cord, can produce tissue compression. (3) Small vessel *cavernous angiomas*, which sometimes provide an occult source of intracerebral hemorrhage. (4) AVM's consisting of snakelike vascular tangles in which arteries connect directly with veins. AVM's can affect any part of the brain or spinal cord. They can range in diameter from a few millimeters to structures that occupy most of a cerebral lobe. Most form at the junction points of two or more major intracranial arteries, such as in the deep frontoparietal area where anterior, middle, and posterior artery circulations converge. Most AVM's gradually increase in size and characteristically produce their symptoms in persons over age 30 years.

AVM's can cause three kinds of neurological disability. As many as half leak intermittently, producing various-sized parenchymal or subarachnoid hemorrhages. These usually are smaller and less dangerous than those resulting from either hypertensive hemorrhage or ruptured berry aneurysm. Of the remaining, some cause focal epileptic seizures, while others, in the process of their slow enlargement, generate progressive neurological deficits. A small percentage of AVM's are associated with unilateral headaches resembling classic migraines; among all migraine, however, this is a rare cause.

Surgical treatment of AVM's is technically difficult because many of the lesions reside in neurologically indispensable areas of brain. Moderate-sized AVM's discovered incidentally by CT scan or arteriography and causing no symptoms are best left alone. Although symptomatic lesions lying in the poles of the frontal or occipital lobes often can be amputated safely, larger AVM's usually have many arterial sources and may be difficult or impossible to remove without producing severe postoperative deficits. The risk of neurological damage or fatal bleeding in intracranial AVM's is relatively low, and cases should be judged individually by experienced neurological centers. Appropriate nonsurgical treatment is necessary to treat seizures and other neurological deficits.

REFERENCES

Barnett HJM, Moler JP, Stein BM, Yatsu FM (eds): Stroke. Pathophysiology, Diagnosis and Management. New York, Churchill Livingstone, 1986.

Millikan CH, McDowell FH, Easton JD: Stroke. Philadelphia, Lea & Febiger, 1987.

119

TRAUMA TO THE HEAD AND SPINE

Severe craniofacial and spinal injuries create a huge public health problem in the United States. The annual incidence exceeds 100,000 cases, almost half of whom die. Many of the survivors suffer chronic intellectual or motor-sensory limitations. Furthermore, most of the victims are in the younger, most productive decades of their lives. Since emergency and early general medical care influence both mortality and morbidity, an understanding of these disorders becomes important to almost every physician.

HEAD INJURY

Pathophysiology of the Injury

Severe head trauma threatens life and future well-being in direct proportion to the degree that it injures the brain. Open, *focal brain injuries* caused by crush or penetrating objects affect specific regions, usually of the cerebrum. In addition, high-velocity penetrating missiles can emit shock waves that injure more remote areas of the hemispheres and brain stem. Most focal injuries however, produce relatively restricted problems requiring largely acute surgical treatment. *Closed head injury* is a more frequent form of trauma affecting the brain diffusely with consequences that depend upon the intensity of impact, the direction of the resulting movement of the cranium, and whether or not complications arise. Certain factors beyond the immediate cerebral trauma also affect outcome. Heavy alcohol or illicit drug intoxication predisposes to carelessness and sedation. The effect increases the incidence of accidental head trauma and worsens its subsequent severity and complications. Furthermore, the presence or absence of serious systemic effects of trauma strongly influences acute and postacute management and outcome.

Acceleration-deceleration forces received at the time of impact cause most of the brain damage that comes from the closed head injury. When, for example, the forward-accelerating head strikes the immobile dashboard in a speeding automobile accident, inertia carries the gelatinous brain forward to injure structures both under the point of injury and at their polar opposite, 180 degrees away (contra coup) (Fig. 119–1). In such circumstances, the presence or absence of a fracture is relatively irrelevant. What counts against the patient is the degree to which implosive-explosive forces have produced capillary and neuronal damage in the brain and how much shearing of white matter has resulted from severe rotational movements at the time of the trauma.

Severity and Complications of Diffuse Head Injury

As a rule, one judges the severity of brain trauma usually by whether or not consciousness has been lost and by the presence or absence of associated neurological abnormalities, especially those that relate to neuro-ophthalmological function, motor activities, and breathing patterns. Later on, severity can be judged in retrospect by the duration of coma and how long anterograde or retrograde amnesia lasts. These latter indices, however, have little immediate application in the acute situation.

Cranial injuries in which persons report feeling only dazed or syncopal and have normal neurological findings and no localized headache usually need neither hospitalization nor laboratory testing so long as the patient can be depended upon to maintain close medical contact to report potential complications. If doubt exists, one is wise to obtain a CT or MR scan to rule out incipient extradural or parenchymal hematoma. When such are available, skull radiographs can be omitted.

Concussion describes brief loss of consciousness with no immediate or delayed neurological residua detectable by radiographic or clinical study. The boxer's

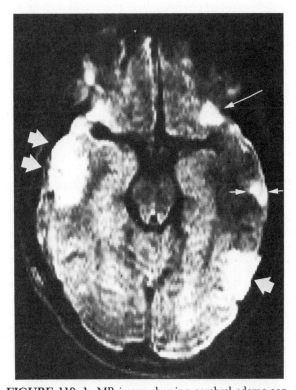

FIGURE 119–1. MR image showing cerebral edema-contusion at point of impact (two large arrows) and 180 degrees opposite (one large arrow) in a 22-year-old woman. An extradural hematoma had been removed at the impact site six days earlier. Small arrows indicate additional contusions. The patient recovered completely.

knockout, which derives from an abrupt sagittally delivered force, epitomizes the abnormality. One observes immediate, evanescent autonomic paralysis: consciousness disappears, the pupils dilate and fix, breathing stops, the heart slows, and muscles become flaccid. In concussed experimental animals petechial hemorrhages and scattered neuronal loss appear in the lower brain stem. Clinical recovery begins within seconds to minutes and completes itself within hours except that psychosensory symptoms such as giddiness, anxiety, and apprehension, may remain for days or longer. Brain imaging studies show no abnormality and no treatment is indicated other than reassurance.

Intermediate diffuse brain injuries extend the level of unconsciousness to as much as an hour or so and are followed by a proportionately slower recovery of orientation and behavior. Permanent residua can follow. Associated drunkeness can make appraisal difficult, but in the earliest stages safe evaluation requires that one attribute any neurological changes directly to the trauma. Patients with moderate brain injuries often remain lethargic for a day to a week or more and many go through an agitated stage. Temporarily, they may be partially disoriented, and many transiently show mild or moderate focal neurological abnormalities such as extensor plantar responses or unilateral weakness. Clinical signs of brain stem damage are lacking, but the CSF may be bloody, reflecting the presence of cerebral contusions or lacerations. CT or, especially, MR scans show scattered petechiae or contusions (Fig. 119–1), often with small contra coup hematomas. Even with severe closed injury, however, imaging studies can be normal. Patients affected with intermediate level injuries require hospitalization to guard against complications and to control possible agitated behavior. More active treatment seldom is necessary unless complications arise as discussed below. Most patients younger than about age 40 years recover completely within days to weeks. Loss of consciousness for as little as 24 to 36 hours in persons older than that age is a serious matter, however, and often is followed by permanent psychological and intellectual limitations.

Severe diffuse injury is judged by the patient's response rather than the nature of the trauma. Serious neurological damage usually is apparent from the start, although exceptions exist. For example, following seemingly mild to moderate head trauma, an occasional child or adolescent can develop within minutes to an hour or so massive and sometimes fatal brain edema. More commonly, in all age groups severe brain edema or ischemic infarction can be delayed for several hours or more after injury, and even hemorrages can make a late appearance. Such patients who "talk and die" comprise as many as 20 per cent of the fatalities in some series of head trauma.

Excepting the above, most patients who suffer from severe brain trauma become deeply unconscious from the onset; many almost immediately develop decerebrate or decorticate posturing responses to noxious stimuli. Signs of systemic bodily trauma are common, and at least partial respiratory obstruction due to aspiration of vomitus or oral secretions is almost the rule.

Evidence of brain stem damage indicated by bilateral pupillary fixation or impaired oculovestibular responses signifies especially severe injury and a poor prognosis, with fewer than 15 per cent making a satisfactory recovery. Almost half of all patients with such severe trauma show intracranial hemorrhages by CT scan; it is debatable whether or not early operative removal improves ultimate functional outcome in such instances.

Management of Acute Head Trauma and Its Complications

Emergency Management. Whether at the accident scene or hospital emergency room, proper immediate steps may save both lives and brains. Patients who are awake and do not appear to be seriously injured must be kept quiet and watched until it is certain that no occult damage silently creates delayed deterioration. At the accident, the more seriously injured should be placed flat and supine, taking care to avoid flexing or twisting a potentially fractured spine or neck. Pulmonary ventilation should be evaluated and guaranteed immediately, and systemic hemorrhage should be stopped. The victim must be transported promptly and, if not in shock, to the most effective rather than merely the nearest emergency facility. Opiates are contraindicated. One must evaluate emergency personnel respectfully: some trained paramedics are more skilled in managing acute trauma than are untrained or partially trained physicians. In the emergency room, unresponsive persons should be intubated and given 30 to 100 per cent oxygen with or without assisted ventilation depending on circumstances (see Table 114–12). A large-gauge intravenous needle should be placed to draw necessary blood and to treat the potential development of hemorrhage or shock. Dehydration is not an advantage, but one must guard against inducing hyponatremia or excess hyperglycemia by inappropriate fluid therapy. Seizures, if present, should be treated urgently with diazepam and a full phenytoin dose given intravenously (see Table 120–8). This is the time to complete the emergency neurological and systemic examinations and to obtain, if possible, brain images and any radiographs. Decisions as to the priority of treating systemic vs. intracranial lesions and whether or not to evacuate intracranial masses are best left to experts in trauma care.

Hospital Management. Patients with severe head trauma should be treated in an intensive care setting possessing appropriate facilities for monitoring vital functions. The level of consciousness, neuro-ophthamological status, and motor responses should be monitored at 30- to 60-minute intervals in potentially unstable cases so that complications can be met quickly. Arterial blood gases and electrolytes need close attention. Most brain-injured patients either aspirate gastric contents or suffer neurogenic pulmonary edema, so antimicrobial agents are prescribed after obtaining appropriate cultures. Corticosteroid drugs are contraindicated: they counteract immunity and may worsen traumatic tissue damage. Unless specific complications need attention, the medical care of head injuries focuses on maintaining good physiological balance and allowing the brain and systemic tissues spontaneously to recover their full potentials.

Certain general problems recurrently arise in caring for patients with intermediate or severe head injury. Ventilatory difficulties require constant attention to the upper airway, any associated thoracic trauma, pulmonary edema-pneumonitis, and infection. Renal or bladder trauma often accompanies head injuries, and urinary retention or incontinence is almost universal. Patients with altered consciousness should be placed on indwelling catheterization during the early stages, with the urine cultured at 48-hour intervals. The fluid intake should be balanced against output, and if renal failure is absent, urinary volume should reach at least 1500 ml a day to minimize infection and calculi. Serum electrolytes should be monitored concurrently. Effective bowel emptying may require enemas.

Pain is common as patients recover consciousness, and if severe may require codeine to supplement milder analgesics. Opiates should not be given to spontaneously breathing patients because of the risks of inducing hypoventilation and associated increases in intracranial pressure. Mild agitation is best controlled with diazepam, severe boisterousness with haloperidol. In alcoholics or those addicted to sedative drugs, delirium tremens or withdrawal seizures should be anticipated and counteracted with benzodiazepines at the first sign of motor tremulousness.

Management of Complications. *Cerebral edema* accompanies almost all severe head injuries, causing an increase in brain mass that interferes with the cerebral circulation and threatens to cause central or lateral transtentorial herniation (see Table 114–3). *Traumatic hematomas* can arise acutely in either the subdural, extradural, or parenchymal regions, creating additional space-occupying lesions and producing further blood-induced irritation to the tissue. Such hemorrhages most often signify their presence with signs of increasing neurological disability that begin at a time when improvement might otherwise be expected. Some centers routinely measure the intracranial pressure in an effort to detect and guide the treatment of these complications. With or without such steps, CT or MR imaging can be invaluable in detecting either intracranial shifts or hypodensities that indicate the development of edema and the presence and size of hematomas. Arteriography offers a poor substitute for such images. In the presence of known or suspected edema, giving a 20 per cent solution of mannitol intravenously, plus applying passive hyperventilation to reduce cerebral blood volume, can serve as an emergency measure to lower intracranial pressure in preparation for surgery. Few patients who require such acute surgical treatment make a fully satisfactory social-vocational recovery.

Where imaging is not available, skull radiographs must be done. Fractures by themselves indicate only that severe head trauma but not necessarily a brain injury has occurred. Fractures do, however, have several potential complications that may demand attention. Bony breaks across the middle meningeal artery

groove in the temporal bone can lacerate the artery, leading to delayed middle temporal fossa *extradural hematomas*. Typically, such clots enlarge progressively to produce signs of neurological worsening beginning from 12 hours to three days following the initial injury. Unilateral headache followed by restlessness, agitation, or greater obtundation is characteristic, Unless surgically treated, such hematomas can lead to transtentorial herniation and death. *Basal skull fractures* can open channels from the subarachnoid space into the paranasal sinuses or the middle ear. CSF rhinorrhea or secondary meningitis are risks; some authorities treat such CSF leaks with prophylactic antibiotics until the rhinorrhea stops spontaneously or is surgically repaired. *Depressed skull fractures* displace pieces of skull to a level below the surrounding bone surface. Such lesions confer an increased risk of post-traumatic epilepsy and are best treated by surgical elevation.

Acute bacterial *infections* can follow open skull or spine injuries, infecting the subdural space or deeper tissues to cause meningitis or brain abscess. Diagnosis is suspected from the nature of the injury and is discussed, along with treatment, in Chapter 122.

Cranial nerve paralyses are common following cranial-facial trauma, especially when it affects the ocular structures and the facial nerve. Incurable anosmia is common. The management of more serious injuries often requires surgical facial reconstruction.

Carotid-cavernous fistulas result when basal skull fractures lacerate the artery within the cavernous sinus. The condition also may occur spontaneously or in association with intracavernous aneurysms or connective tissue diseases. Orbital chemosis, a painful semi-immobilized eye, and pulsating exophthalmos develop ipsilaterally to the fistula and occasionally contralaterally as well. Vision can decline in either eye associated with secondary glaucoma and stretching of the optic nerve. Treatment, often difficult, consists of surgical ligation or efforts to patch the leak.

Post–Head Injury Problems

Postconcussion syndrome is a common disorder that characteristically follows mild to moderate, often subconcussional head injuries as well as other forms of potentially severe, psychologically threatening trauma. Headache, giddy sensations, irritability, difficulty in concentration, and vague apprehension comprise the major symptoms. Physical and laboratory signs of biologically significant neurological or systemic dysfunction usually are lacking, and the condition gradually passes with time, medication having no specific effect. No cause is known, although the nature of the symptoms suggests reversible brain stem dysfunction. Contrary to common opinion, compensation or psychological issues appear not to influence the incidence of the disorder, although they may prolong the period of disability.

Incomplete intellectual and motor recovery affects many patients with severe head injury, including nearly all adults over age 30 who remain in coma for more than one week. Comprehensive rehabilitation efforts in specialized centers offer the best hope for social and vocational restoration.

Post-traumatic epilepsy, mainly associated with generalized tonic-clonic attacks, ranges in incidence from a maximum of 50 per cent after penetrating brain injuries down to about 5 per cent following unconsciousness-producing closed head injury. Most authorities treat both groups of patients prophylactically with full phenytoin therapy for periods up to two years following severe injury. If no seizures occur, treatment is gradually discontinued. If patients do have seizures, antiepileptic medication is strengthened or treatment is lengthened according to the frequency and intensity of the attacks.

Delayed post-traumatic encephalopathy, an unusual syndrome affecting principally children or young adults, begins 15 minutes to two hours or more following usually minor head injuries. The young person becomes obtunded or stuporous, often with nausea or vomiting. Despite these potentially alarming early symptoms, most patients recover uneventfully, but focal neurological deficits including cortical blindness sometimes can last for several hours or, very rarely, permanently. The cause is not known although the visual loss may be secondary to posterior cerebral artery compression during transient edema-induced transtentorial herniation. Similarly unexplained are rare instances of parenchymal cerebral hemorrhage that can arise from hours to a matter of a week or more following relatively mild, initially uncomplicated cerebral trauma.

Chronic subdural hematoma is a late complication that can arise weeks to months after head injuries that are usually mild and sometimes so trivial as to have been forgotten. Older age, alcoholism, and the anticoagulated state are important predisposing factors. Many patients give no history of relevant risk factors or even injury. A sustained, new headache and mental dullness are the most common symptoms, often blending into hypersomnia and confusion with or without hemiparesis. The symptoms often fluctuate, presumably because of small rebleedings or the development of abnormal intracranial pressure waves (transient pressure elevations associated with impaired cerebral arterial autoregulation). Diagnosis is best made by brain imaging, which in symptomatic cases shows brain shift or, with bilateral hematomas, smaller than normal ventricles and few sulci at the vertex. One must interpret CT films cautiously, since at certain stages within a matter of a few weeks after injury, the hematoma itself becomes isodense with the surrounding brain and may not be outlined (Fig. 119–2). MR scanning circumvents this problem. Small or moderate hematomas can be treated by observation with or without the concurrent giving of steroid drugs to relieve brain swelling. Larger clots, particularly those causing abnormal neurological signs or symptoms, are best treated surgically.

Dementia pugilistica, the "punch drunk" syndrome, affects former boxers. Most reported instances have been in men older than age 55 years, although psychological tests show a high incidence of intellectual deterioration even under age 40. The old fighters develop progressive motor slowness, clumsiness, dysarthria, ataxia, memory loss, and incontinence. Development of the syndrome relates directly to the number of former fights, with the subsequent incidence being about 20 per cent among those who box for six to nine years or more. Brain images show cerebral atrophy and ventricular dilatation. Postmortem findings include neurofibrillary tangles in the brain along with neuronal loss, especially in the cerebellum and temporal lobes. Some subjects improve after ventricular shunt procedures.

SPINAL CORD INJURY

Severe spinal cord injury is relatively uncommon but often devastating and prolonged in its consequences, since most cases affect persons younger than 30 years of age. The intraspinal contents can be concussed, contused, lacerated, macerated, or sheared, depending upon the nature of the initiating injury. Road traffic accidents, domestic falls, and diving accidents are frequent causes. The spinal levels most susceptible to trauma lie at the upper and lower ends of the cervical canal and at the thoracolumbar junction, regions of maximal mobility. Any level, however, can be affected by injuries that strike the spinal column directly or penetrate into the spinal canal.

The principal mechanisms of spinal injury are dislocation with or without fracture at the atlas-axis junction, fracture-dislocations with or without bony fragmentation at other spinal levels, and penetrating missile or stab wounds that either concuss the cord and its roots or injure it directly. Less frequent causes are severe hyperflexion or hyperextension injuries that damage the cervical cord in persons who suffer from an abnormally narrow spinal canal (stenosis) caused by congenital or age-related factors.

Patterns of Spinal Cord Injury and Their Resulting Disabilities

Complete vs. partial cord injury can usually be discerned almost immediately following injury. With complete injury, neurological findings reflect functional cord transection. With the occasional exception of priapism, flaccid motor paralysis develops below the level of damage accompanied by pananesthesia in the same distribution. Spinal shock generally lasts for at least days and sometimes weeks or more; extensor plantar responses ordinarily do not appear for several days. Bladder and bowel functions are lost, and prognosis for neurologic recovery is poor, irrespective of treatment.

Partial spinal injury is more common with cervical than thoracic cord trauma and can take several forms. Any discernible voluntary movement or sensory perception that is found distal to the injury at the time of accident means that the injured cord or roots possess a capacity for recovery that only time will define.

Concussion most often follows high-velocity missile wounds that pass close to the spinal canal but fail to damage the cord structurally. Distal neurological loss never is complete, and recovery occurs within hours

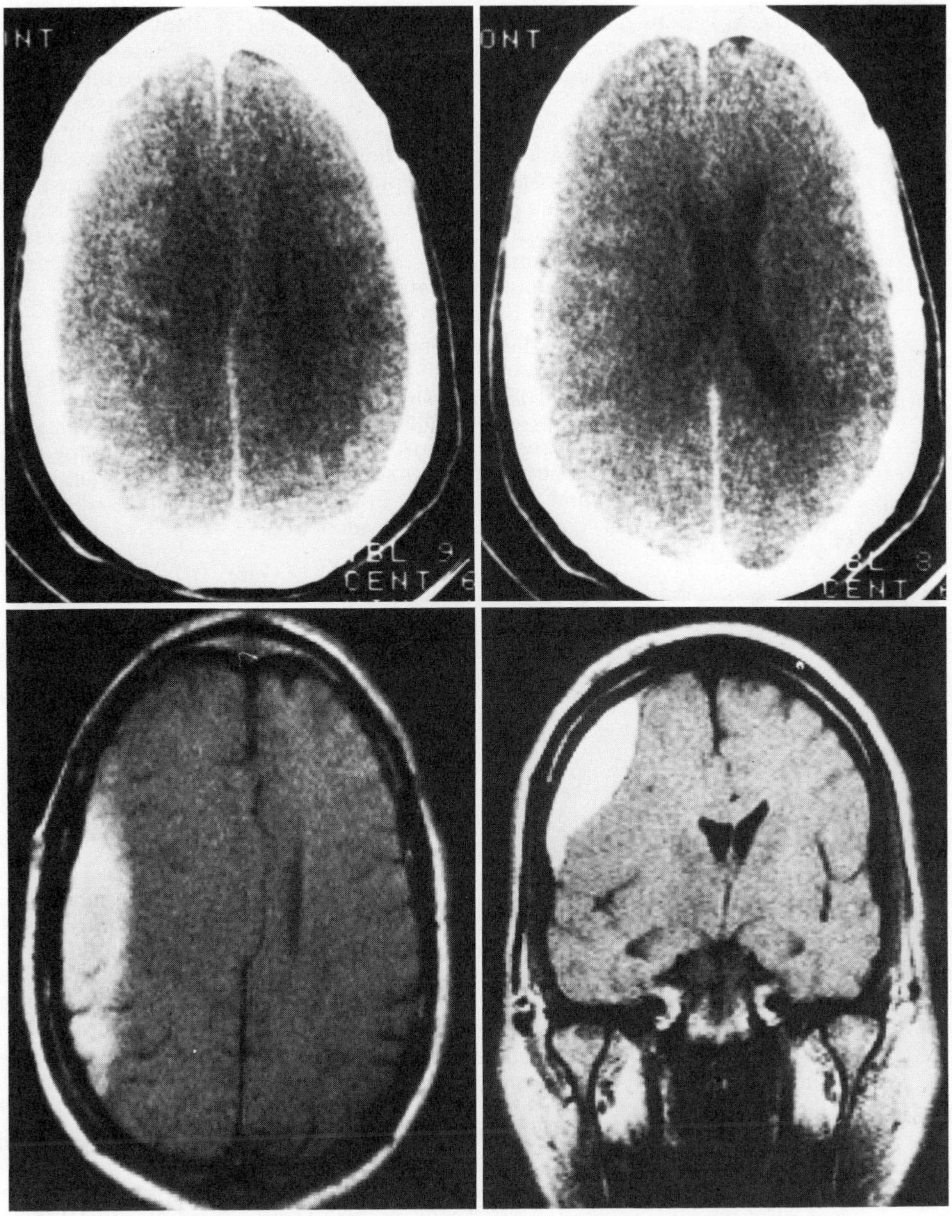

FIGURE 119–2. An isodense subdural hematoma invisible on CT scan (*A* and *B*) is readily disclosed by a concurrently obtained MR image (*C* and *D*). The patient, a 61-year-old man with a history of partial complex seizures and a single generalized convulsion one year earlier, had suffered from headache, loss of mental acuity, fatigue, and dysequilibrium for four months. He was unable to tandem walk, but examination otherwise was unremarkable. He recovered completely following drainage of the hematoma.

to days, occasionally leaving episodic residual paresthesias in the lower extremities secondary to dorsal column scarring (Lhermitte's sign).

Central cord damage due to trauma affects primarily the lower cervical segments, usually with patchy hemorrhage centered along or adjacent to the spinal central canal (hematomyelia). Severe external blows or local fractures without serious canal displacement are the most common causes. The upper extremities become more paralyzed and insensate than the lower; sensory changes at and immediately below the cervical level affect pain and temperature more than touch; bladder and male sexual paralysis are common.

Cervical hyperextension injury typically produces mild or inconsequential paraparesis affecting legs more than arms, coupled with painful paresthesias in the arms and hyposensitivity to position and vibratory testing below the lesion. *Hyperflexion injury*, on the other hand, may simulate the effects of anterior spinal artery occlusion, producing tetraparesis or tetraplegia accompanied by bilateral pain and temperature impairment below the lesion, often associated with acute urinary retention. Both hyperextension (posterior cord) and hyperflexion (anterior cord) injuries can vary widely in severity and many patients enjoy considerable functional recovery. Mixed or unilateral injuries produce variants of the *Brown-Séquard syndrome* of hemicord damage.

Intraspinal damage at or distal to the first lumbar level injures the *conus medullaris* or *cauda equina*, resulting in various mixtures of flaccid paralysis, distal mixed sensory loss, and autonomic-sexual paralysis affecting the pelvic girdle and lower extremities.

Treatment

Management at the scene of the accident consists of preventing flexion or twisting of the spinal column and placing the patient on a hard, flat surface for examination and transportation. Patients with cervical injury commonly require immediate ventilatory assistance, if necessary by mouth-to-mouth breathing. Transport to an experienced center should be arranged immediately, with special attention in patients with cervical injuries being given to immobilizing the neck and counteracting hypoventilation and/or hypotension. In the absence of neurological damage, patients with cervical fractures or fracture-dislocations should be placed in head traction and managed conservatively pending expert consultation. For patients with partial cervical cord injury and evidence of compression by radiograph or imaging studies, immediate surgical decompression sometimes is beneficial. For most severe cord injuries, however, including all examples of functional transection, open surgical treatment confers little benefit and only adds another trauma. Acute and postacute management for quadriplegics or paraplegics requires elaborate attention to pulmonary, cutaneous, autonomic, musculoskeletal, and psychosocial problems, employing techniques that are best carried out in specialized rehabilitation units.

REFERENCES

Becker DP, Miller JD: Grade diagnosis and treatment of head injury in adults. *In* Youmans JR (ed): Neurological Surgery. 3rd ed. Philadelphia, WB Saunders Co, 1988.
Cooper P (ed): Head Injury 2nd ed. Baltimore, Williams and Wilkins, 1987.

120

EPILEPSY

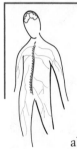

Definitions

An *epileptic seizure* is an episode of uncontrollable, abnormal motor, sensory, or psychological behavior caused by hyperactive, hypersynchronous, abnormal brain electrochemical activity. *Epilepsy* is a chronic disorder characterized by recurrent seizures in which the attacks themselves become the target for specific therapy. Many seizures occur sporadically in conditions that are not part of the disease of epilepsy. These can result from a variety of causes such as electro-convulsive therapy, profound syncope, the ingestion or withdrawal of certain drugs or toxins, or any of several kinds of infections of the brain.

Seizure disorders fall into two general etiological groups: (1) *Primary or idiopathic epilepsy* whose cause remains largely or entirely unknown. Most primary epilepsy reflects genetic predisposition. (2) *Secondary or symptomatic epilepsy*, in which a known structural or metabolic disease of the brain generates the seizures.

Incidence and General Etiology

Seizures can begin at any time of life. Neonatal seizures represent a special problem linked to brain injuries or developmental insufficiency. In children under age two, perinatal injury, metabolic disorders, and congenital malformations represent the most frequent causes. Genetic factors act most strongly in older children and adolescents. After the age of 20 years, intracranial space-occupying lesions, drug or alcohol withdrawal, and scarring from strokes or trauma become important mechanisms. Encephalitis or meningitis can initiate chronic epilepsy at any age.

Population studies in several developed countries worldwide indicate that from 2 to 4 per cent of all persons suffer from recurrent seizures at some time during their lives. Third-world areas show incidence rates almost twice as high.

Pathophysiology

Focal seizures are restricted to abnormal unilateral movements or sensations as well as to stereotyped behavioral patterns that express the pathological excitation of specific parts of the cerebral hemispheres. Most often, they originate in association with anatomically restricted lesions of gray matter such as scars, tumors, arteriovenous malformations, or focal areas of inflammation. (An exception to this rule of structural abnormality sometimes occurs in children with a benign and self-limited form of focal motor seizure called rolandic epilepsy.) Generalized seizures, by contrast, express themselves with bilateral motor abnormalities accompanied in most instances by at least a brief loss of consciousness. They reflect either a diffuse hyperexcitable propensity of brain cells or the presence of a deep, cryptic epileptogenic abnormality involving centrally located subcortical activating mechanisms. Focal and generalized seizures can overlap, since focally originating ictal discharges can become generalized when they anatomically project back into the diencephalic reticulum. In this instance, the remote focus quickly transmits its hyperactive hypersynchrony to a central electrophysiological pacemaker, which in turn excites both sides of the forebrain to produce a generalized attack. Certain anatomical areas of the cerebrum are especially epileptogenic, including the frontal lobes, the medial temporal lobes (limbic system), the diencephalic reticular formation, and, to a lesser degree, the occipital lobes.

Genetic factors influence susceptibility to both generalized and focal epilepsy. Intrinsic generalized epilepsies, such as petit mal absences and febrile convulsions, are usually transmitted as an autosomal dominant trait with variable penetration. The blood relatives of patients with chronic focal seizures originating in the temporal lobe also show an above-normal incidence of seizure disorders of all kinds.

The specific brain mechanisms that cause seizure discharges to start, spread, or stop are poorly understood. Abnormalities that have been suggested include (1) intrinsic neuronal membrane changes that could induce an abnormality in ionic conductance; (2) abnormal neurotransmitter synthesis leading to deficiencies of inhibitory or excesses in excitatory neurotransmitters; and (3) deficiencies in genetically regulated intracellular enzymes that normally affect the capacity of the neurons or glial cells to pump ions and repolarize. None has been proven to underlie all cases.

Clinical Seizure Patterns (Table 120–1)

Individual epileptic attacks commonly evolve in their patterns. Episodes can last from a few seconds to several minutes in duration, with the pattern of the symptoms often reflecting the physiological anatomy of the seizure focus. Seizures and their effects can be divided into several stages: the *aura* is the first self-experienced symptom. It usually reflects the anatomical focus where the seizure begins. The *attack* itself follows and subsequently gives way to the *postictal period*, during which headache, drowsiness, or focal neurological abnormalities can remain, often for minutes and sometimes for hours or even days.

Partial seizures consist of attacks of focal neurological dysfunction. The attacks are described as *simple* if only one restricted form of behavior is expressed (equivalent to the aura) and self-aware consciousness remains throughout. They are called *complex* if the pattern of neurological symptoms and signs changes during the attack (e.g., a hallucination of smell gives way to visceral automatisms or complex motor acts) or if consciousness is lost as the attack evolves. With any seizure the initiating signs and symptoms offer the best localizing evidence for the area of the brain that contains the epileptogenic lesion.

Partial motor seizures arise from epileptogenic foci in the primary motor or the premotor, supplementary motor, or prefrontal areas of either frontal lobe. Lat-

TABLE 120–1. CLASSIFICATION OF EPILEPTIC SEIZURE PATTERNS

I. **Partial seizures** originate from a focal lesion in brain, usually structural, and may occur either with a single symptom (simple) or symptoms that change in type as well as degree (complex).
   A. Motor (includes monomyoclonic)
   B. Sensory
   C. Psychological
   D. Partial complex. Seizures with changing patterns, usually of limbic-temporal lobe origin.

II. **Generalized seizures** (All but some myoclonic attacks cause at least momentary loss of consciousness)
   A. *Nonconvulsive*
      Absence (petit mal)
      Atypical absence
      Atonic
      Myoclonic
   B. *Convulsive*
      Tonic-clonic (grand mal)
      Tonic only
      Clonic only

III. **Atypical or unclassified seizures.** Consciousness usually remains intact.
   A. Paroxysmal tonic spasms
   B. Spinal myoclonus

eral prefrontal, supplementary motor, and premotor foci all cause adversive seizures, with only moderate differences distinguishing the respective movement patterns. The frontal lobe possesses many anatomical transcortical and thalamic interconnections. As a result, frontal seizure discharges can either spread to produce progressively larger amounts of contralateral motor activity or fire directly into the diencephalon to precipitate generalized convulsions. With lesions lying far anterior in the frontal lobes, consciousness may be lost concurrently with or even slightly before any focal movements begin. Most patients with focal seizures arising from supplementary or premotor areas, however, retain awareness for at least the beginning of the attack. Motor components in partial motor seizures can begin and remain as simple aversion of the head and eyes away from the side of the focus, can include extension or raising of the contralateral arm and turning of the trunk, and occasionally include crude vocalizations or, in the dominant hemisphere, speech arrest. Head turning alone is not a reliable lateralizing sign.

Primary motor (rolandic) seizures produce the classic *jacksonian* epileptic attack, named for the English neurologist who first deduced the significance of the pattern. Rhythmic, clonic twitching begins in the contralateral thumb or corner of the mouth and slowly spreads to produce adjacent movements, most often from thumb to hand to arm to face, but sometimes jumping in the reverse direction. Spread to a generalized convulsion is common. Many jacksonian seizures are followed by transient or sustained postictal (Todd's) paralysis of the limb affected by the seizure.

Partial sensory seizures produce the classic epileptic aura: a sensory presentiment or fragment that represents the ictal beginning and advertises its origin. Most common are epigastric rising sensations that emanate from discharges affecting the insular cortex, followed in frequency by somatosensory tingling or numbness (postcentral gyrus), simple visual phenomena (mostly occipital), vertigo (superior temporal gyrus), or vague cephalic or generalized body sensations (no localizing value). Lesions in and around the temporal uncus cause foul smelling, olfactory hallucinations that often blend into other temporal lobe symptoms.

Partial complex seizures of temporal lobe—limbic cortex origin represent the most frequent form of chronic epilepsy, amounting to about 40 per cent of total cases. About half begin before age 25 years, and most are associated with discernible structural lesions in the temporal limbic area. Frequent causes are developmental anormalies, residua of early life brain infection or severe febrile convulsions, head trauma, neoplasms, and in later life stroke or focal atrophy. Most partial complex seizures begin in foci that lie along the medial portion of the temporal lobe or the adjacent inferior frontal limbic area and spread posteriorly along the temporal lobe limbic cortex. They often project transcallosally to the opposite medial temporal area. Secondary generalization can spread into deep diencephalic structures to produce generalized convulsions but they are less common than complex automatisms. In either event, consciousness and memory are severely dulled or lost during the evolution of the attack.

TABLE 120–2. FREQUENT EARLY SYMPTOMS OF LIMBIC-TEMPORAL LOBE SEIZURES

SYMPTOM	LOCUS OF ORIGIN
Foul odor, "uncinate fit"	Temporal uncus-amygdaloid area
Micropsia or macropsia	Middle-inferior temporal gyrus
Déjà vu (intense familiarity)	Parahippocampal-hippocampal area
Jamais vu (environmental unfamiliarity)	
Fragments of voices, phrases, songs	Auditory association cortex
Lip smacking, abdominal pain, borborygmi, epigastric rising, cardiac arrhythmia	Insular, temporal-polar limbic cortex
Dreamy feelings, fear, pleasure, anger	Parahippocampal and septal areas

TABLE 120–3. COMMON ICTAL MANIFESTATIONS OF LIMBIC PARTIAL COMPLEX SEIZURES

Autonomic:	Flushing, pallor, tachypnea, nausea, eructation-borborygmi, sweating, cardiac arrhythmia
Cognitive:	Intense déjà vu (familiarity), jamais vu (spatial amnesia), forced thinking, dreamlike states, depersonalization
Affective:	Laughing, fear, rage, depression, elation
Sensory:	Olfactory hallucinations; macropsia, micropsia, familiar voice fragments, visualized objects or scenes, emotional experiences (dreamy states)
Motor:	Staring with lip smacking, chewing, semipurposeful rubbing; confused, bizarre behavior; walking or, occasionally, running; postictal confusion or drowsiness

The aura of partial complex seizures (Table 120–2) commonly reflects their anatomical origin and sometimes comprises the entire episode. More often, it spreads into stereotyped automatic movements that can take several forms, alone or in combination (Table 120–3). Partial complex seizures usually last 1 to 2 minutes, seldom as long as 5, and are followed by the patient's slow reorientation, with headache and drowsiness. The interictal EEG of affected patients shows temporal lobe spikes or slow foci in about 80 per cent, provided that records during sleep are obtained. The frequency of abnormalities increases during or after an attack, but even then deep limbic discharges may go undetected by skull surface electrodes.

Many patients suffering from partial complex seizures display abnormal interictal behavior, including ruminative obsessiveness, religiosity, circumstantiality, hypersensitivity, and self-absorption, as well as hypergraphia.

Differential diagnosis of partial complex seizures includes mainly petit mal absences and psychiatric fugue states. Absence attacks are abrupt in onset and offset, last only a few seconds, usually are unaccompanied by subjective self-awareness, do not produce auras or automatisms, and are associated with a diagnostic EEG abnormality. Psychiatric fugues can be more difficult to distinguish, especially when patients with psychomotor attacks have normal EEG's. Psychiatric states, however, include a past history of sustained psychiatric or behavioral aberration, they last longer than seizures, they lack the characteristic evolution from aura to attack to a drowsy and confused postictal state, and they often have a self-rewarding relationship to life situations that is lacking in true epilepsy. Partial complex seizures rarely offer a satisfactory explanation for unprovoked violence or planned crime.

GENERALIZED EPILEPSIES

SECONDARY GENERALIZATION

Many partial seizures, especially those that begin in the frontal lobe, but also some that begin in the temporal lobe or other areas, can evolve rapidly into generalized convulsions before the epileptic discharge burns itself out. Occasionally, as noted above with deep frontal lesions, the generalized seizure explodes before any focal behavioral sign has time to appear. In such instances meticulous EEG study, brain imaging, or identifying restricted postictal weakness may be needed to discover the focus and the lesion causing it.

PRIMARY GENERALIZED EPILEPSIES

These can take several forms depending upon the patient's age at onset and the extent and nature of any associated structural or metabolic disease of the brain. Since the clinical features are what most attract the physician's attention and serve as the principal focus for treatment, this chapter divides the generalized epilepsies according to whether or not they produce major convulsions.

Nonconvulsive Generalized Epilepsy

Absence Seizures (Petit Mal). Absence seizures begin in childhood, usually between the ages of 2 and 12 years, and in most instances cease by age 20. They represent the classic example of primary epilepsy: no structural or known metabolic disease exists in the brains of these youngsters. Genetic studies show an approximately 40 per cent incidence of EEG abnormalities among first-degree relatives. Intelligence is not impaired, and other neurological abnormalities are absent.

Simple absence attacks are brief, lasting no more than one to two seconds, and are characterized by a blank stare, often accompanied by mild 3- to 4-Hz blinking of the eyelids. Unprepared observers commonly note no abnormality, and the child remains unaware of the event. In severely affected children, dozens to 100 or more such episodes can occur in a single day. More protracted, *complex absence attacks* can last for 15 to 30 seconds, rarely as long as a minute. Such spells are readily detected: the child's head droops, the lids and sometimes the arms jerk rythmically but mildly, and there may be brief motor automatisms and even enuresis.

Both the clinical pattern and the EEG in classic absence epilepsy run true to form. The EEG contains repeated bursts and runs of symmetrical 3.5-Hz activity. In addition, both the electrical abnormality and the seizures often can be brought on by having the child overbreathe for 60 to 180 seconds. Atypical seizures that differ from the above or an EEG that is asymmetrical or contains faster or slower frequencies makes one consider an alternate diagnosis of one of the less benign generalized childhood epilepsies.

About half the children with petit mal seizures develop generalized tonic-clonic, grand mal convulsions before the age of 20. Status epilepticus with petit mal seizures is described in a later section.

Myoclonus, a brief, unexpected, and uncontrollable jerk of the entire body or a focal portion of the trunk or one of the extremities, is a common, normal phenomenon that often occurs during pre-sleep drowsiness. Diffuse or multifocal myoclonus, however, is abnormal and occurs in several degenerative toxic and infectious neurological disorders as well as in several of the severe childhood epilepsies (see below). A more benign form of restricted myoclonus, discussed below, affects the upper extremities and is closely related to generalized primary epilepsy. Partial myoclonus, with distally or proximally located repetitive focal twitchings, can be associated with several disorders of the cerebrum or spinal cord (see Partial Focal Motor Status Epilepticus in a later section).

Bilateral benign epileptic myoclonus is an uncommon condition consisting of bilateral repetitive mild myoclonic jerks affecting girls more than boys and often beginning at the menarche. The symmetrical jerks especially involve the shoulders and arms. Often, the EEG contains bifrontal 3.5- to 4-Hz sharp and slow activity similar to that found in absence seizures. The disorder pathogenetically and genetically lies close to petit mal and carries a similar risk of future tonic-

clonic seizures. It responds to similar medication, especially sodium valproate, but may be so mild as to require no treatment. A more serious form of symmetrical or multifocal massive myoclonus epilepsy affects children with inherited degenerative diseases (Unverricht-Lundborg disease; ceroid lipofuscinosis). Multifocal myoclonus also frequently accompanies progressive encephalitis in either children (subacute sclerosing panencephalitis) or adults (Creutzfeldt-Jakob disease). A variety of other degenerative disorders of the brain can produce multifocal or intention myoclonus, including postanoxic encephalopathy, the Ramsay Hunt form of cerebellar degeneration, and several dementias, including Alzheimer's disease, Hungtington's chorea, and occasionally Wilson's disease.

Atonic-akinetic seizures often accompany severe myoclonic epilepsy in young children between the ages of one and six years. Head dropping attacks, falls, staring spells, prolonged episodes of minor motor seizures, generalized tonic-clonic convulsions, and mental retardation can occur. Treatment is difficult and often incompletely successful.

Infantile spasms consist of brief, frequently repeated massive flexor spasms of the head and extremities. About half the cases are associated with a cerebral degenerative or metabolic disorder, with the remainder being of unknown cause. About 9 out of 10 affected children become mentally retarded, some severely so.

Generalized Convulsive Epilepsy

Generalized convulsive epilepsy can take two forms, tonic-clonic and tonic.

Tonic-clonic (grand mal) seizures can begin at any age. Most produce loss of consciousness at onset, although a fraction of patients report a brief rising epigastric sensation as the attack begins. Any focal manifestations in the evolution of the attack or in the postictal period suggest a localized structural cause rather than a generalized basis for the seizure. Prodromal warnings (not auras) sometimes precede the attacks by several hours and can include a change in mood, a sense of apprehension, insomnia, or loss of appetite. Sometimes episodes of repetitive myoclonus anticipate a convulsion. As the convulsion begins, many patients cry out unconsciously. They stiffen tonically in extension, usually with muscles contracted so tightly that breathing is arrested. Deep cyanosis occurs before relaxation and a first post-tonic breath ensues. Such vigorously tonic phases seldom last as much as a minute but may be repeated several times over. Gradually, hyperextension gives way to a minute or so of rapid successive clonic jerks of neck, trunk, and extremities. Finally, flaccid relaxation ensues, accompanied by stertorous breathing, pallor, and heavy salivation. Hypertension, tachycardia, and heavy perspiration accompany the motor changes. The pupils may be briefly fixed and moderately dilated during the tonic convulsions. Absent oculocephalic reflexes, hyperactive deep tendon reflexes, and extensor plantar responses can outlast the seizure for several minutes but these changes usually disappear along with the reappearance of arousal two to three minutes after the relaxation phase begins. Many patients bite their tongues or lose sphincter control during attacks. In addition, the tonic contractions may exert sufficient force to compress dorsal or upper lumbar vertebrae. Other serious injuries are relatively uncommon, but susceptible patients must be warned about tub bathing, since drowning is a hazard, as is suffocation against the bedclothes if a convulsion interrupts sleep. Fatigue, muscle weakness and soreness, generalized headache, and drowsiness follow grand mal attacks. Sometimes confusion can last for several hours. Most patients sleep postictally and awaken several hours later with only muscle soreness to remind them that a convulsion has occurred. Severe residua can follow multiple successive convulsions or status epilepticus, as discussed below.

During the convulsive movement of generalized seizures EEG recordings disclose rapidly repeating spike discharges followed by sharp-slow activity as clonic contractions supervene. Postictally the record becomes abnormally slow, sometimes for several hours. The interictal EEG can be normal in about 20 per cent but usually contains spike-slow complexes, bursts of abnormally slow activity, or mixtures of spike and slow activity in bursts or short, 10- to 20-second runs appearing symmetrically over the scalp.

Unusual Seizures and Other Conditions Responding to Antiepileptic Medication

Reflex epilepsy can affect predisposed persons in response to a variety of sensory stimuli. Photogenic seizures can be triggered by stroboscopic lights, driving past a stand of trees that filters the sun, or even waving the hand in front of eyes fixed upon bright illumination. The ensuing generalized seizure can take the form of myoclonus, an absence attack, or a tonic-clonic convulsion. Closely related are seizures elicited by looking at certain geometric patterns or, rarely, by reading. Polarized glasses may reduce the stimulus intensity of photosensitive attacks; valproic acid is the most effective anticonvulsant. Other rarer forms of responses to sensory stimuli consist of unduly violent, repetitive startle responses to noise as well as partial complex seizures triggered by particular musical themes.

Familial paroxysmal choreoathetosis is a rare disorder, inherited as an autosomal dominant or recessive trait and characterized by paroxysms of choreiform, dystonic, and athetoid body torsions occurring during full consciousness. Stress or sudden movement can precipitate the episodes. Phenytoin or carbamazepine relieves most cases.

Recurrent torsion spasms consist of episodic dystonic spasms affecting the face, trunk, and extremities in patients with multiple sclerosis. Sometimes attacks include ataxia and dysarthria rather than dystonia. Body movement or startling stimuli can precipitate the attacks, which do not interfere with consciousness. The EEG remains normal, but phenytoin or carbamazepine treatment prevents the episodes, which presum-

ably are caused by plaques involving the lower brain stem reticular formation.

Anticonvulsants also can favorably affect other conditions, including myokymia (page 734) and *lightning pains*—episodic, severe, flashlike pains affecting the extremities, associated most often with neurosyphilis or diabetic neuropathy. Trigeminal neuralgia, a condition in which lightning pains affect one or more divisions of the fifth cranial nerve, is described on page 712.

DIAGNOSIS

Given evidence that a seizure, automatism, or other brief episode of altered brain function has occurred, the major questions are whether it is epileptic and, if so, of what type and cause. Since the physician rarely can observe the attack itself, most of the evidence derives from the history and supplementary, mostly inferential evidence.

The patient's description of his experience plus, if available, a witness's accurate observation of an attack usually provides the most diagnostically rewarding information. The setting of the attack immediately suggests acute causes such as drug withdrawal, CNS infection, trauma, or stroke, while a history of past similar seizures implies a more chronically sustained, intrinsically epileptic, disorder. Any partial (focal) feature observed either as an aura or during or following the seizure suggests a structural brain lesion and demands appropriate investigation and, possibly, specific treatment. The pattern of an attack as well as the patient's age immediately limits the possible types and causes of the reported episode (Table 120–4).

The physical and neurological examinations are useful chiefly for identifying evidence of either systemic illness or acute or chronic structural neurological disease. Having susceptible patients hyperventilate during the examination often induces diagnostically typical absence attacks and sometimes precipitates partial complex seizures. Laboratory studies should include lumbar puncture in children with seizures of acute onset as well as in any adolescent or adult suspected of developing meningitis or encephalitis. Single seizures seldom affect the CSF fluid content, but major motor status epilepticus can raise the protein concentration and generate up to 100 white cells per cu mm. Anyone in whom either the history, findings, or EEG suggests a focal abnormality, as well as all persons whose seizures begin after childhood, deserves an MR or CT scan with contrast enhancement. The older the patient, the higher the yield from such images.

The electroencephalogram is particularly helpful in diagnosis. The normal EEG contains fairly rhythmic, bilaterally symmetrical potentials that range in frequency from 1 to 50 Hz, with amplitudes ranging from about 20 to 200 mV. The typical EEG frequencies recorded in healthy adults are 8.5 to 13 Hz, called alpha; 13 to 30 Hz, called beta; 4 to 7 Hz, called theta; and 0.5 to 4 Hz, called delta. Wakeful persons at rest typically show a dominant alpha rhythm, which accelerates into less rhythmic, faster frequencies during concentrated attention and after ingesting certain drugs. Frequencies of 8 Hz and slower occur normally during drowsiness or sleep; such slowing during wakefulness commonly reflects an abnormality of brain function. Regionally localized bursts of slowing, sharp waves, or spikelike waves characteristically reflect focal disturbances in brain function, while paroxysmal and symmetrical slow, sharp, or sharp-slow activity is typical of primary epilepsy. One must recall, however, that as many as 20 per cent of patients with clinically typical epilepsy can have normal records, whereas 2 to 5 per cent of persons who never have a seizure can evidence epileptic-like sharp waves or sharp-slow activity in the EEG. Most laboratories routinely employ hyperventilation and stroboscopic stimulation as EEG-activating measures. Special electrode placements, sleep studies, and telemetry are diagnostic tools utilized by specialists.

Chief to be considered in the differential diagnosis of epilepsy are syncope at all ages, pseudoseizures and other factitious attacks among adolescents and younger adults, and cerebral transient ischemic attacks in older patients.

Syncope (p. 682) provides the biggest problem, since one seldom can observe the attack and retrospective histories incline toward ambiguity. Furthermore, the disorder often recurs and, if severe, sometimes is punctuated at the maximum of hypotension by a brief, tonic seizure. As Table 120–5 indicates, however, syncope always occurs when sitting or standing except when associated with episodic cardiac arrest. Furthermore, attacks of syncope last a shorter time than seizures, produce characteristic changes in the patient's appearance and motor behavior, cause no postictal confusion or headache, and often are linked to emotional or visceral stimulation. Persons with syncope characteristically lack EEG abnormalities, and neither anticonvulsants nor other medications reliably induce improvement.

Factitious seizures or pseudoseizures provide a diagnostic challenge, since they sometimes occur in persons who suffer from organic epilepsy as well. Hysterical seizures most often take place in emotionally stressful settings or to achieve secondary gain. Certain features suggest pseudoseizures: rapidly rolling the head or body from side to side, an alternating thrashing of the extremities or pelvic thrusting. Few hysterics soil or injure themselves during attacks, while many epileptics do. Nevertheless, hysterics or malingerers can be good actors and produce attacks that fool even experienced observers. A dependable but expensive way to differentiate organic from hysterical major motor seizures is to obtain a serum prolactin level immediately postictally: true convulsions but not hysterical attacks abnormally elevate the value. In most instances, observing the pattern of the attack coupled with obtaining a normal postictal EEG and employing diagnostic common sense yields the answer.

Episodic fugue states or attacks of behavioral dyscontrol sometimes become confused with partial complex seizures (p. 694). Most such behavioral-psycho-

TABLE 120–4. MAJOR CLINICAL FEATURES OF POSTINFANTILE EPILEPSY

AGE	MAJOR CAUSE	TYPES OF SEIZURES
Children < 15 years	Idiopathic epilepsy	Generalized (grand mal) Febrile convulsions Petit mal absence Adolescent polymyoclonia Partial complex attacks (uncommon)
	Genetic and developmental defects: birth trauma; inherited biochemical disorders; acute CNS infection-inflammation; post-traumatic or post-infectious	Generalized grand mal Partial motor, sensory, or psychological attacks, simple or complex Disseminated or multifocal myoclonus
	Brain tumors (uncommon)	Partial or generalized
Adults 15–25 + years	Idiopathic epilepsy	Generalized (grand mal) convulsions Polymyoclonia Partial complex seizures
	Acute CNS infection-inflammation; traumatic–post-traumatic; drug intoxication or withdrawal; brain tumor or arteriovenous malformation	Generalized or partial seizures
Adults > 25 years	Brain tumor; CNS infection-inflammation; traumatic–post-traumatic; withdrawal; acute or post-stroke	Generalized or partial seizures

genic episodes bear little resemblance to the stereotyped automatisms of temporal lobe epilepsy. As with major convulsion-like attacks, a strongly abnormal EEG inclines one toward a diagnosis of epilepsy. In difficult cases, telemetric monitoring of behavior concurrently with EEG recording can assist diagnosis.

Cerebral TIA's (p. 769) only rarely produce symptoms resembling epilepsy, since their principal effects consist of ischemic hypofunction rather than epileptic hyperfunction. Occasionally, however, aphasic speech arrest can occur with TIA's, and a few patients develop contralateral or generalized trembling of the extremities which may resemble epileptic phenomena.

TABLE 120–5. MAJOR DISTINCTIONS OF SYNCOPE FROM SEIZURES

SIGN	SYNCOPE	SEIZURES
Prodromes	Usually nausea, "swimming" sensation, faintness, sometimes none	Aura or epigastric rise. Often none
Onset	Sitting or erect	Any position
Self-awareness	Always present	Sometimes absent (petit mal absences)
Motor activity	Usually none, occasionally brief clonic. Rare convulsions with cardiac arrests	Focal, tonic, clonic, sustained
Duration	Seconds	0.5 to 2 minutes
Cardiovascular	Pulse slow, weak	Pulse fast, strong
Appearance	Deathly pale, sweating	Flushed, salivating
Postictal	Oriented, sweaty, nauseated, sometimes vomiting, diarrhea	Confused, headache, drowsy
EEG	Normal	Abnormal

The recent development of symptoms, the vascular distribution of the changes, the lack of an epileptogenic lesion by clinical evaluation or brain imaging, and the presence of other signs of systemic or cerebral vascular disease almost always lead to the correct diagnosis.

Several other kinds of episodic events may briefly suggest seizures but can be dismissed by obtaining a careful history or description of the attack. These include breath-holding attacks in young children; migraine, which in children sometimes causes ataxia, vomiting, visual hallucinations or delirium, and stupor; narcolepsy-cataplexy; hyperventilation spells; and drop attacks in older adults. Nonepileptic causes of recurrent seizures include hypocalcemia, which can occur spontaneously in children and following parathyroidectomy in adults, hypoglycemia at any age, and recurrent alcohol or depressant drug withdrawal in adults.

MANAGEMENT

The initial management of recurrent seizures consists of efforts to halt the attacks completely. With symptomatic epilepsy this is followed by efforts to eradicate the cause, whereas in idiopathic seizure disorders antiepileptic therapy must be supplemented by efforts to help the patient adjust to a disease that brings fear to most and shame to many.

Control of Seizures

The ultimate goal is to achieve complete seizure control with minimal or absent antiepileptic drug toxicity. At present, about 60 per cent of patients with chronic epilepsy can have their seizures completely suppressed by medication, and another 15 to 20 per cent can be improved substantially. Many of the uncontrollable patients suffer from a serious underlying disease of the brain, whereas others for psychological reasons fail to comply with therapeutic instructions. Certain principles guide optimal prescribing of antiepileptic drugs and enhance the likelihood of their success.

1. Many persons have a single seizure with no recurrence. Accordingly, one starts long-term treatment on patients after a single, first attack only when a defined cause can be found that is likely to generate recurrences. Special social or vocational circumstances may override this rule. The principle of avoiding chronic treatment for only a single event also applies to uncomplicated febrile convulsions (see below).

2. Diagnose accurately the probable type of epilepsy and give the single preferred medication in full recommended therapeutic dose.

3. If a single drug does not control the seizures, even at toxic levels, try another. Similarly, if the first anticonvulsant causes serious side effects, withdraw it but rapidly initiate the next most effective agent. If efforts at single drug therapy fail, most patients are best referred to a specialized center for consultation, since combined therapy is often difficult to regulate without producing toxicity. In any event, adjust medications gradually so as to accomplish the maximum of seizure control with a minimum of side effects.

4. Never stop anticonvulsant medications for generalized seizures abruptly. Status epilepticus may result.

Choice of Anticonvulsants. Table 120–6 lists in order of preference the effective anticonvulsants for the various types of chronic epilepsy. Table 120–7 summarizes some of the major toxicities of these agents. As with any potent medication, physicians should read package inserts before prescribing. Notwithstanding these precautions, one must never forget

TABLE 120–6. CHOICE OF DRUGS IN EPILEPSY

Generalized Tonic-Clonic Seizures
  Phenytoin
  Phenobarbital
  Carbamazepine
  Primidone
Absence Seizures
  Ethosuximide
  Valproate
  Trimethadione
  Clonazepam
Partial Epilepsies
  Carbamazepine
  Phenytoin
  Primidone
  Clonazepam
  Valproate (adjunctive)
Myoclonic Epilepsies
  Infantile spasms
    ACTH or corticosteroids
      clonazepam
      valproate
  Others:
    valproate
    clonazepam

that recurrent seizures constitute a physically dangerous, emotionally devasting, and intelligence-threatening risk. By comparison, the incidence of potential complications of antiepileptic therapy is almost trivial.

Use of Drug Levels in Management. The determination of blood levels can be a valuable adjunct to treatment. "Therapeutic" blood levels reflect empirically established values at which most patients acquire seizure control without toxic side effects. Many patients become well-controlled (or occasionally toxic) below the therapeutic level, while others show no ill effects despite blood values above this point. In all instances the clinical response, not the blood level, defines the goal of the treatment.

Drug level determinations are especially useful within two to three weeks after beginning therapy so as to determine the patient's compliance, to judge his metabolic response to the medication, and to compare the pharmacological and clinical effects. They also can be helpful when drug dosage is changed, since some individuals quickly saturate their detoxification mechanisms when one increases an antiepileptic drug or drop their levels rapidly to subtherapeutic ranges when the dose is reduced. Blood levels should be rechecked when patients are placed on an additional anticonvulsant or receive another drug that may influence hepatic enzyme systems.

An occasional blood level determination obtained during the course of chronic, effective therapy helps to reinforce to the patient the need for continued compliance. Most patients with controlled seizure disorders need blood levels checked no more than annually.

STATUS EPILEPTICUS

The rapid succession of seizures so that one begins before the postictal symptoms of the previous attack have passed is termed *status epilepticus.* Attacks that follow in close succession but with brief periods of reawakening between are designated *serial seizures.* Each condition can occur with either partial or generalized epilepsy. Status epilepticus is of a special concern because in several of its forms the successive or continuous epileptic activity can damage the brain permanently. Without actually knowing that several seizures have occurred in rapid succession, however, the diagnosis cannot be made. Accordingly, if an accurate witness is unavailable, one must be sure that epileptic attacks are still continuing before initiating the treatment outlined in Table 120–8.

Partial motor status, an uncommon condition sometimes known as *partial continuous epilepsy,* occurs in several forms and can last for hours, days, or even as long as a year or more. The seizure frequency can range from as little as one every three seconds to as many as several per second. The motor attacks can consist of as little as a highly focal, myoclonic, repetitively localized twitch to jerks that involve most of the limb or even half the body, not always affecting precisely the same muscles. In general, cerebral lesions cause distally distributed partial motor seizures, whereas brain stem or spinal lesions tend to cause

TABLE 120–7. TOXICITY OF COMMON ANTIEPILEPTIC DRUGS

Phenytoin
  Dose excess: Tremor, vertigo, nystagmus, ataxia, drowsiness
  Hypersensitivity: Gingival hyperplasia, hirsutism, coarse features, exanthema
Phenobarbital
  Dose excess: Drowsiness, mental slowing, dysarthria, ataxia, nystagmus.
  Idiosyncratic: Exanthema
Primidone
  Same as Phenobarbital.
Carbamazepine
  Dose-related: Mental slowing, nausea, drowsiness, ataxia, nystagmus
  Idiosyncratic: Exanthema, inappropriate ADH secretion, leukopenia, aplastic anemia (rare), hepatic toxicity (rare)
Valproate
  Dose-related: Increased appetite, hair loss, tremor, ataxia, drowsiness
  Idiosyncratic: Toxic hyperammonemia, hepatic toxicity
Ethosuximide
  Dose-related: Dyspepsia, hiccup, headache, insomnia
  Idiosyncratic: Psychotic behavior, aplastic anemia (rare)
Clonazepam
  Dose-related (in up to 50 per cent): Sedation, muscular hypotonia, ataxia, oral and tracheobronchial hypersecretion

proximal myoclonic activity. Large hemorrhagic or ischemic strokes cause about half the cases, whereas neoplasms, encephalitic processes, or trauma produce the rest. In some instances, particularly with chronic partial continuous seizures, the cause never becomes clear despite extensive searching. Whatever the cause the seizures often resist treatment. Phenytoin, carbamazepine, diazepam, and clonazepam all have been tried but often with only limited success.

Partial complex status produces a sustained state of confusion or delirium in which stereotyped motor and autonomic automatisms are associated with dull, slow, blunted behavior, often combined with semimuteness or total disorientation. Some attacks produce a

TABLE 120–8. TREATMENT OF ADULT STATUS EPILEPTICUS OR SERIAL SEIZURES

I. Convulsive tonic-clonic or complex partial status
  1. Assure the airway, give O_2, check blood pressure and pulse. Establish a venous line and draw blood for glucose, calcium, hyper- or hypo-osmolar indicants. If indicated, measure pH, PaO_2, $PaCO_2$.
  2. Start infusion and give 50 ml of 50% glucose.
  3. Infuse diazepam intravenously 5 mg/min until seizures stop or to total 20 mg. Also start phenytoin 50 mg/min to total 18 mg/kg.
  4. If convulsions persist, give *either* (1) phenobarbital 100 mg/min or as loading dose to 20 mg/kg, *or* (2) 100 mg diazepam in 500 ml dextrose 5% run in at 40 ml/hr. Monitor ventilation closely.
  5. If convulsions persist, start anesthesia with halothane and neuromuscular blockade. If latter not immediately available, give lidocaine 50–100 mg intravenously.
II. Serial tonic-clonic or partial motor status
  Steps 3 and 4 above but not to induce coma.
III. Petit mal status
  Diazepam as in step 3 followed by oral ethosuximide, valproic acid, or both

schizophreniform or stuporous state, whereas others are marked by bizarre, detached activity. Patients may resist assistance in their fugue-like state, which can last for hours and sometimes days. The EEG usually shows continuous slow and spike activity predominanting over one or both temporal areas, commonly in an asymmetrical distribution. Occasionally, surface recordings can be normal, but abnormal activity can be detected on nasopharyngeal leads or from electrodes placed deep in limbic system structures of the brain. Treatment should be initiated promptly, as the effects of prolonged seizures can permanently impair memory and intellect.

Absence status (petit mal status) occurs in two forms. The more common is an extension of complex absence seizures discussed earlier in which semiconfused automatic behavior occurs accompanied by closely fused or continuous runs of 3- to 4-Hz spike and wave activity on the EEG. The condition occurs in patients with known petit mal and usually is confined to adolescents or occasionally young adults. Most episodes last less than 30 minutes. Somewhat similar in behavior are attacks of prolonged (days to months) automatisms associated with confusion and sometimes gradual interictal mental deterioration. These are more likely to occur in older persons, aften with no history of epilepsy. Most such later life attacks can be halted with diazepam given intravenously. Some, however, strongly resist antiepileptic therapy and are accompanied by progressive intellectual deterioration.

Major generalized motor status epilepticus with tonic-clonic convulsions creates a medical emergency, since continuation of the convulsions beyond an hour or so commonly produces residual brain damage. The most frequent cause is abrupt withdrawal of anticonvulsant medications from a known epileptic. Other precipitants include withdrawal of alcohol or drugs in a habitual user, cerebral infection, trauma, hemorrhage, or neoplasms. Treatment of the convulsions and the protection of the brain are of immediate concern and should take the form outlined in Tables 120–8 and 114–7. Specific diagnostic steps to identify and treat the seizures must be undertaken as soon as possible after seizures have been controlled.

Special Management Problems

Febrile Convulsions. Convulsions caused by fever occur mainly in neurologically otherwise healthy children between the ages of six months and five years who recurrently develop single generalized seizures when affected by an acute, fever-producing illness. Factors that increase the chance of having a future chronic epileptic disorder include age less than one year at onset, convulsions lasting longer than 15 minutes or coming in clusters, any pre- or postictal sign of neurological abnormality, or a family history of epilepsy. Ten per cent of children with two or more of these risks go on to have chronic epilepsy, while recurrent nonfebrile seizures affect less than 2 per cent of the remainder. Present practice is to do everything

possible to limit the course of the single convulsion but to place only children who have high risk factors on medication, usually phenobarbital.

Menstruation, Genetic Counseling, and Pregnancy. A number of women with epilepsy suffer an increase in seizures during the days immediately preceding and following the onset of menses. Acetazolamide, 250 to 500 mg daily, taken prophylactically or a modest increase in medication during the susceptible days often counteracts the problem.

Persons with seizure disorders inevitably ask about the hereditary risks to the fetus. Best available evidence suggests that during their lifetime 4 to 10 per cent of the offspring of patients with generalized primary epilepsy suffer one or more seizures. This compares to an incidence of approximately 1.5 per cent of the general population. Rates in the partial epilepsies are less clearly different from the norm.

Chronic anticonvulsant medication often requires adjustment during pregnancy, since blood volume increases and drug pharmacokinetics change. Blood level monitoring during the latter half of pregnancy can be useful in managing the difficult-to-control woman. During pregnancy, it is advisable to give vitamins and supplements, including folic acid and calcium. Vitamin K, 5 mg twice weekly, should be given orally during the final six weeks, with a parenteral supplement administered to the mother and infant at the time of delivery. Breast feeding is not contraindicated in women taking antiepileptics.

Teratogenic Effects. The overall incidence of important birth defects in children of mothers or fathers taking antiepileptic medication is two to three times higher than in the general population. The exact role of medication in these figures is uncertain. Seizures offer a greater risk to the mother and fetus than does the generally low rate of birth defects associated with antiepileptic drugs. Two agents, however, trimethadione and valproate, have been incriminated with especially high teratogenicity in experimental studies, and their use in pregnancy should be avoided if at all possible. Phenytoin carries a demonstrated risk, but the exact rate is unknown. Data on phenobarbital and carbamazepine are too few to allow firm recommendations.

Surgical Therapy. In addition to attempting to remove specific mass or destructive brain lesions that include seizures among their symptoms, several surgical treatments have been developed in efforts to halt or ameliorate medically intractable, chronic seizure disorders. Procedures include, for particular indications, local resection of seizure foci, anterior temporal lobe resections, section of the corpus callosum, and, rarely, in as many as two thirds or more of cases, provided that meticulous preoperative evaluation and selection are carried out. The procedures are largely confined to large medical centers sponsoring specialized programs for the cause and treatment of seizure disorders.

Psychosocial Management. The presence of incompletely controlled epilepsy and the frequent association between seizures and other neurologic limitations often create large emotional problems for the patient. In addition, some patients with partial complex seizures may possess aberrant personality traits that intensify their social isolation. Outbreaks of frustration are common, and depression and suicide are more frequent among patients with epilepsy than in the general population. A reduced libido and hyposexuality have been noted in males with partial complex seizures. These limitations notwithstanding, in the absence of associated brain damage most persons with epilepsy score in the normal range on standard intelligence tests. One can cite examples of persons with epilepsy who have performed in an outstanding manner in every level of professional, governmental, artistic, and business life.

Patients with seizure disorders are helped most by bringing the attacks under control, but reassurance, empathy, and optimistic social guidance by the physician aid immeasurably. Once seizures are under control, affected persons should be encouraged to live a normal life using mainly common sense as their guide. Sports carrying a high risk of injury are best avoided unless seizures have been completely controlled for well over a year; high diving, deep water or underwater swimming, high alpine climbing, boxing, and head-contact football are ill-advised. Most states grant automobile driver's licenses to patients with epilepsy provided that no seizures have occurred for at least a year. Educational and vocational opportunities depend upon whether or not seizures are controlled and upon the person's innate capabilities. Life and health insurance policies are available under special circumstances. The Epilepsy Foundation of America can assist patients with these and other social considerations.

Discontinuation of Medication. One considers stopping antiepileptic medication either (1) because seizures continue and patients believe the drugs are ineffective or (2) because seizures have been completely controlled for a long time. The first condition is uncommon and must be approached cautiously because of the dangers of precipitating status epilepticus. The latter decision can be considered between patient and doctor when absence seizures have been fully suppressed for two or three years and other types of seizures for three to five years. Patient's value systems, economic and social factors, and knowledge of risks all should contribute to the decision. Between 20 and 50 per cent of those who do discontinue treatment will undergo recurrent seizures, which may be more difficult to control than the original attacks. Particularly likely to relapse are persons whose initial seizures lasted longer than six months, were difficult to control, or were associated with any evidence of a focal defect or other neurologic abnormality. A moderate or severely abnormal EEG is an additional sign suggesting recurrence if treatment stops. In general, we advise most adult epileptics not to stop anticonvulsant medication no matter how long they have been well-controlled. For most, the cost of relapse is just too high.

REFERENCES

Delgado-Escueta AV, Treiman DM, and Walsh GO: The treatable epilepsies. N Engl J Med 308:1508, 1983.

Pedley TA, Meldrum BS (eds): Recent Advances in Epilepsy. Edinburgh, Churchill Livingstone, vol 2, 1985; vol 3, 1986.

121

INTRACRANIAL NEOPLASMS, CNS COMPLICATIONS OF CANCER, AND STATES OF ALTERED INTRACRANIAL PRESSURE

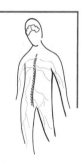

A. INTRACRANIAL NEOPLASMS
CLASSIFICATION
NEUROECTODERMAL TUMORS
MESODERMAL TUMORS
METASTATIC TUMORS
SYMPTOMS AND SIGNS
GENERALIZED
FOCAL

FALSE LOCALIZING SIGNS AND SYMPTOMS
DIAGNOSTIC TESTS
TREATMENT

B. SPINAL NEOPLASMS

C. PARANEOPLASTIC SYNDROMES
REMOTE EFFECTS

D. INJURY FROM THERAPEUTIC RADIATION

E. NON-NEOPLASTIC ALTERATIONS OF INTRACRANIAL PRESSURE

INTRACRANIAL HYPERTENSION
Pseudotumor Cerebri
Hydrocephalus
INTRACRANIAL HYPOTENSION

INTRACRANIAL NEOPLASMS

INTRODUCTION AND DEFINITIONS

Intracranial tumors can arise from any structure within the intracranial cavity. Most begin in the brain, but the pituitary, the pineal region, cranial nerves, and leptomeninges are also sites of neoplastic degeneration. Furthermore, any of these structures may be the site of metastatic spread from tumors that arise outside the nervous system. Intracranial tumors are not rare; they are the second most common cancer in children, and in adults malignant brain tumors are more common than Hodgkin's disease. Recent studies indicate

TABLE 121–1. CLASSIFICATION OF BRAIN TUMORS

I. Tumors of Neuroepithelial Tissue
  A. Astrocytic Tumors (25%)*
    1. Astrocytoma
    2. Anaplastic (malignant) astrocytoma
  B. Oligodendroglial Tumors (2%)
    1. Oligodendroglioma
    2. Anaplastic (malignant) oligodendroglioma
  C. Ependymal and Choroid Plexus Tumors (4%)
    1. Ependymoma
    2. Anaplastic (malignant) ependymoma
    3. Choroid plexus papilloma
    4. Anaplastic (malignant) choroid plexus papilloma
  D. Pineal Cell Tumors
    1. Pineocytoma
    2. Pineoblastoma
  E. Neuronal Tumors
    1. Gangliocytoma
    2. Ganglioglioma
  F. Poorly Differentiated and Embryonal Tumors
    1. Glioblastoma (30%)
    2. Medulloblastoma (4%)
    3. Primitive neuroectodermal tumors
II. Tumors of Nerve Sheath Cells (5%)
  A. Neurilemmoma (schwannoma, neurinoma)
  B. Anaplastic (malignant) Neurilemmoma
  C. Neurofibroma
  D. Anaplastic (malignant) Neurofibroma
III. Tumors of Meningeal Tissues (20%)
  A. Meningioma
  B. Meningeal Sarcoma
IV. Germ Cell Tumors
  A. Germinoma
  B. Embryonal Carcinoma
  C. Choriocarcinoma
  D. Teratoma
V. Tumors of the Anterior Pituitary (5%)
  A. Pituitary Adenoma
  B. Pituitary Adenocarcinoma

Modified from World Health Organization: International Histologic Classification of Tumors, No. 21, Geneva, Switzerland, 1979. Used with permission.

* Approximate percentages encountered in neurosurgical practice. All others total about 5%.

an incidence of 14.1 primary intracranial and spinal tumors per 100,000 population per year in the United States, or about 35,000 new patients. Evidence suggests that the incidence is increasing as the population ages. Of the various brain tumors approximately 12,000 are malignant. The incidence of symptomatic metastatic intracranial tumor is equal to or greater than that of primary neoplasms.

Intracranial tumors can be classified both by site of origin and by histological type (Table 121–1). Most arise from neuroectodermal elements (the precursor of both neurons and glia) of the brain. The commonly encountered brain tumor of adults is glial in origin, a benign or malignant astrocytoma (glioblastoma multiforme). The terms *benign* and *malignant* applied to brain tumors reflect histological criteria that in turn reflect local growth rate rather than propensity to metastasize. Even highly malignant primary brain tumors rarely metastasize, although they may spread locally from the parenchyma to seed the leptomeninges and spinal cord. Many "benign" brain tumors recur despite treatment and eventually lead to the demise of the patient. Others may undergo "malignant degeneration" that alters their biological potentiality.

CLASSIFICATION

Neuroectodermal Tumors. The most common neuroectodermal tumor is the *astrocytoma*. Astrocytomas can arise anywhere in the brain or spinal cord and infiltrate surrounding normal structures. Tumor cells can often be found several centimeters from the main bulk of the tumor. Furthermore, in some instances, astrocytomas may have a multicentric origin or, more rarely, infiltrate the entire neuraxis (gliomatosis cerebri). Some, particularly cerebellar astrocytomas of childhood, may become quiescent for decades after only partial resection. About half of astrocytomas are relatively benign. The others consist of rapidly growing tumors that include the anaplastic astrocytoma and, most malignant of all, the glioblastoma multiforme. In adults, benign astrocytomas have a prognosis of four to seven years, anaplastic astrocytomas one and a half to two and a half years, and glioblastoma usually a year or less. *Oligodendrogliomas* may be either benign or malignant. In general, oligodendrogliomas usually grow more slowly than astrocytomas and tend to calcify. Glial tumors are often mixed, so that elements of oligodendroglioma may be found within a tumor that is primarily astrocytic in origin, and areas of benign astrocytoma may be found within a malignant glioblastoma. Because of the heterogeneity of such tumors, small biopsies may give misleading diagnostic and prognostic information. *Ependymomas* also can be either benign or malignant. Common sites of ependymomal growth include the fourth ventricle in children and the spinal cord in children and adults. Malignant ependymomas of the fourth ventricle tend to spread to involve the leptomeninges. *Medulloblastomas* arise from a primitive neuroectodermal cell, usually in the cerebellum, and likewise may seed throughout the CSF. They are predominantly tumors of childhood and are highly malignant, but 50 per cent of children treated by surgery and radiation therapy now survive more than five years. In children, astrocytomas represent half of all cerebellar tumors, medulloblastomas and ependymomas making up the rest.

Mesodermal Tumors. The most common mesodermal tumor is *meningioma*. Meningiomas are usually benign and arise in certain favored sites: along the dorsal surface of the brain, the base of the skull, the falx cerebri, the sphenoid ridge, or within the lateral ventricles. Although these tumors are benign, they often reach a large size before they are discovered and may be difficult to remove. Furthermore, they may recur even after apparently complete surgical extirpation. The most common cranial nerve tumor is the *acoustic schwannoma* (neurilemmoma, neuroma). Early discovery of such tumors has been possible in recent years because of the development of refined auditory tests and computed tomographic (CT) scans, thereby enabling these tumors to be removed frequently via a translabyrinthine approach. *Pituitary adenomas* may begin as intrasellar masses and extend into extrasellar locations, causing visual loss. *Microadenomas*, asymptomatic except for their hormone secretion, can now be identified by high-resolution CT or MR scan of the pituitary. *Craniopharyngiomas* are developmental tumors derived from Rathke's pouch and may be intrasellar or suprasellar in location; they are frequently calcified and often cystic. *Pineal region tumors* occur primarily in children. They rarely truly originate from the pineal gland itself but instead are germinomas, often curable by radiation therapy. The benign *colloid cyst* usually grows in the anterior third ventricle. Vascular tumors include *arteriovenous malformations*, which are not truly neoplastic, and the *hemangioblastomas*, which are. The latter tumors, when located in the brain stem or cerebellum, may be part of the von Hippel-Lindau syndrome that includes hemangioblastomas elsewhere in the body. Congenital tumors include the craniopharyngiomas, *chordomas* (which arise at the base of the brain or the lumbosacral area from the primitive notochord), *dermoids*, and *teratomas*. Granulomas and parasitic cysts come from tuberculomas, cryptococcosis (toruloma), sarcoidosis, and cysticercosis.

Metastatic Tumors. These can spread to any part of the intracranial cavity and tend to exhibit growth characteristics similar to their parent neoplasm. There is some clinical and a great deal of experimental evidence, however, to suggest that the same tumor may grow somewhat more slowly in the brain than in the primary organ of origin. Metastatic tumors, unlike primary tumors, tend to be well-circumscribed rather than infiltrative and are easier to remove in toto than are primary neoplasms.

SYMPTOMS AND SIGNS

Because they arise within the closed box of the skull, intracranial tumors tend to cause symptoms and signs while still relatively small. Symptoms may be caused because (1) the tumor invades, irritates, or replaces normal tissue (Fig. 121–1). This probably accounts for only a minority of symptoms in brain tumors and is particularly characteristic of low-grade infiltrating gliomas. (2) The tumor growth compresses normal tissues. As intracranial tumors grow, they compress surrounding tissues and cause shift of normal brain structures. Blood vessels are compressed as well, leading to ischemia of the surrounding tissue. (3) New vessels formed in the growing brain tumor do not possess a blood-brain barrier (that anatomical-physiological structure that excludes proteins, ionized substances, and many water-soluble chemotherapeutic agents from the normal central nervous system). The blood-brain barrier also breaks down in compressed tissue surrounding a brain tumor. As a result, edema forms both within and around the tumor, which adds to the

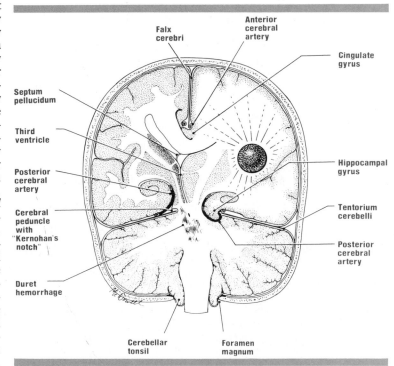

FIGURE 121–1. Schematic representation of the pathophysiology of clinical symptoms caused by a brain tumor. A mass lesion (black sphere) and surrounding edema (dashed lines) enlarge the hemisphere, obliterating normal sulci and shifting normal structures caudally and across the midline. The tumor and surrounding edema destroy and displace normal tissue in the hemisphere, producing contralateral neurological signs (e.g., weakness and sensory loss). Obliteration of subarachnoid spaces by the mass lesion raises intracranial pressure, producing generalized signs (e.g., headache and papilledema). Shifts of normal brain cause symptoms at a distance and may lead to cerebral herniation (see Chapter 114). (From Cairncross JG, Posner JB. *In* Yarbro JW, Bornstein RS (eds): Oncologic Emergencies. New York, Grune and Stratton, 1981.)

mass in the brain. Furthermore, because the brain has no lymphatics, removal of edema is slow. That edema produces many of the symptoms of intracranial tumors is attested to by the dramatic response that most brain tumor symptoms show to corticosteroids. These drugs, which decrease brain edema by restoring the integrity of the blood-brain barrier, substantially ameliorate symptoms for most patients with brain tumors without having a biologically significant effect on the growth of the tumor. (4) Large or small strategically located tumors (third ventricular and fourth ventricular tumors, leptomeningeal tumors) obstruct spinal fluid pathways, leading to hydrocephalus. The resulting inability of normally formed spinal fluid to escape from the ventricular system or the subarachnoid space further adds unwanted mass and raises intracranial pressure.

The mass of a brain tumor plus the attendant edema and hydrocephalus all may lead to herniation of normal cerebral structures under the falx cerebri, through the tentorium or foramen magnum (p. 679).

The symptoms and signs caused by brain tumors depend on the location of the tumor and its histopathology (rapidity of growth). Sudden changes in tumor size resulting from hemorrhage, necrosis, or sudden obstruction of spinal fluid pathways can cause additional symptoms. Symptoms and signs may be divided into three major categories: (1) *generalized*, largely due to increased intracranial pressure, (2) *focal*, a result of ischemia and/or compression of normal brain at the site of the tumor, and (3) *false localizing*, a result of shifts of cerebral structures, causing neurological abnormalities at a distance from the tumor.

Generalized Symptoms and Signs

The most common symptom of increased intracranial pressure is *headache*. Headache results from compression or distortion of pain-sensitive dural and vascular structures surrounding the brain; the brain itself is insensitive to pain. The head pain may be felt at the site of the tumor but more commonly is diffuse. In its early stages, the typical brain tumor headache is mild, tends to occur early in the morning when the patient first awakens, and disappears as the patient assumes an upright posture and breathes more deeply, thus lowering intracranial pressure. As the tumor enlarges, headaches become more constant and severe and are often exacerbated by coughing, bending, or sudden movement of the head. Later, headaches may awaken the patient at night. Headaches are common symptoms, only occasionally caused by brain tumors, but their onset in a patient not previously prone to headache or a recent change in headache pattern should alert the physician to the possibility of increased intracranial pressure. *Papilledema* occurs in about one tenth of patients with an intracranial neoplasm, probably as a result of obstruction of CSF pathways. Papilledema is much more common in children and young adults than it is in the elderly. *Vomiting*, with or without preceding nausea, is a common symptom of intracranial hypertension in children but less so in adults. Vomiting usually occurs early in the morning before breakfast. It is often, but not always,

accompanied by headache. Vomiting is more common in posterior fossa tumors but can occur with any tumor that raises intracranial pressure. *Mental changes* are also common. Patients first become irritable and then later quiet and apathetic. They retire to bed early and arise later (unless the early morning is accompanied by headache) and nap during the day. They are forgetful, seem preoccupied, and often appear psychologically depressed. Psychiatric consultation is frequently procured before the diagnosis of brain tumor is suspected. In patients with mass lesions and intracranial pressure, *plateau waves* are a common phenomenon. Plateau waves are increases in intracranial pressure that last between 5 and 20 minutes. They are caused by failure of normal cerebral vascular autoregulation so that an abrupt increase in cerebral blood volume occurs, causing the intracranial pressure to rise. Such pressure waves can increase an already high intracranial pressure by as much as 60 to 100 mm Hg. The wave may be asymptomatic but more commonly is accompanied by neurological symptoms including headache, visual obscurations, altered consciousness, and sometimes weakness of the extremities. These episodic changes in neurological function usually last only a few minutes and may be precipitated by a sudden rise from a lying position, by alterations in intracranial pressure associated with coughing, sneezing, or straining, or even by tracheal suctioning.

Focal Symptoms and Signs

The location of a brain tumor determines not only whether the tumor is more likely to produce generalized or focal signs but also the type of focal signs it will produce. Tumors arising in relatively silent areas of the brain (such as the frontal pole) may grow to large size, raise intracranial pressure, and cause severe signs of generalized brain dysfunction before focal signs are evident. Similarly, tumors arising in the ventricular system, particularly at the outflow of the third and fourth ventricles, also produce generalized signs before focal signs become evident. On the other hand, tumors arising in primary rather than association cortex are more likely at their outset to produce focal symptoms and signs: Tumors of the visual system, whether optic nerve, optic chiasm, or occipital cortex, cause visual loss or visual field deficits before generalized signs develop. Tumors of the sensorimotor cortex cause weakness and sensory change. In addition, because certain areas of the frontal lobe, temporal lobe, and sensorimotor cortex have a relatively low threshold for epileptic discharge, seizures are often an early symptom. If the tumor is in the sensorimotor cortex, the seizures take a focal sensory or motor pattern. Tumors arising in more silent areas can cause unrecognized focal epileptogenic discharges, which generalize to produce a grand mal seizure. Seizures are the most common presenting symptom of meningiomas and of low-grade infiltrating astrocytomas.

Frontal lobe tumors often grow to a huge size before producing symptoms. Focal symptoms of frontal lobe tumors include personality change, either irritability and facetiousness or depression and apathy (or a combination of both), abnormalities of gait, and sometimes urinary urgency and incontinence. Frontal lobe gliomas are often bilateral, arising in the corpus callosum and infiltrating the white matter of both frontal lobes. Posterior frontal lobe tumors involving the motor cortex lead to monoparesis or hemiparesis, and if in the dominant hemisphere to Broca's aphasia.

Parietal lobe lesions cause cortical sensory abnormalities in the contralateral half of the body. If the tumor extends to involve the thalamus, all sensory modalities including pain are impaired contralaterally. Large parietal lesions often give rise to apraxia and, if in the nondominant hemisphere, to anosognosia (the failure to recognize the presence of a neurological deficit). Difficulty with visual-spatial orientation, including inability to dress oneself, is characteristic of nondominant parietal lobe lesions.

Temporal lobe tumors often produce seizures as their first symptom. Hallucinations of smell or hearing as well as déjà vu phenomena are typical focal symptoms of temporal lobe tumors, often followed by a psychomotor or generalized seizure. Superior quadrantanopsia is common in temporal lobe seizures. If the tumor is on the dominant side, patients develop Wernicke's aphasia.

Occipital lobe tumors cause contralateral visual field defects and often contralateral visual seizures. In their early stages, the latter may be mistaken for migraine attacks (see p. 709).

Brain stem tumors are marked by upper and lower neuron signs (e.g., in brain stem gliomas, a common problem in children, symptoms such as facial diplegia and ocular palsies appear with or without involvement of sensory and motor long tracts).

Cerebellar tumors are particularly common in children and produce early signs of increased intracranial pressure by compressing the fourth ventricle. Focal signs include ataxia of gait with midline tumors such as medulloblastoma or ataxia of ipsilateral extremities with laterally placed tumors such as cerebellar astrocytomas.

Cranial nerve tumors include trigeminal and acoustic schwannomas or meningiomas. Fifth nerve tumors are characterized by pain and sensory loss in the face, the pain sometimes resembling that of trigeminal neuralgia. Eighth nerve tumors are characterized by slowly progressive hearing loss with or without loss of balance. Both can be treated surgically.

A number of different tumors growing in the *pituitary fossa* and/or the *suprasellar cistern* lead to a combination of neurological and endocrinological abnormalities. The most common sellar tumor is the pituitary adenoma, a benign growth that often secretes excessive amounts of the hormone made by its parent cell. The tumors often remain very small, the only symptoms produced being those of hypersecretion of prolactin (amenorrhea-galactorrhea syndrome in women), growth hormone (acromegaly), or adrenocorticotropic hormone (Cushing's disease). Other adenomas, however, can grow to a large size, compressing and destroying the normal pituitary gland and leading to hypopituitarism and diabetes insipidus. As such tumors grow superiorly, they compress the diaphragma sella, a pain-sensitive structure, and cause headache. Immediately above the diaphragma sella is the optic chiasm, compression of which leads to bitemporal hemianopsia. If the tumor grows laterally, it encounters the oculomotor nerves in the cavernous sinus, producing ocular palsies. Some pituitary tumors outgrow their blood supply. In this instance, patients suffer sudden hemorrhage or a necrosis into the tumor, producing the syndrome of *pituitary apoplexy*. A previously asymptomatic patient presents to the physician with acute headache, visual changes (bitemporal hemianopsia or blindness), and sometimes oculomotor palsies. The patient is often febrile, with a stiff neck from spillage of blood and necrotic tissue into the subarachnoid space. A CT scan usually reveals a pituitary mass, often hemorrhagic. Emergency treatment with hormonal replacement and, often, decompression usually leads to a good outcome. Tumors arising in the *parasellar area* may cause visual loss simultaneous with or even before pituitary failure. The first sign of pituitary failure in these instances is usually diabetes insipidus; in children, failure of sexual development and obesity are common problems, probably resulting from compression of the hypothalamus. Craniopharyngiomas, optic gliomas, meningiomas, and sometimes large carotid aneurysms cause masses in this area, as do germinomas (ectopic pinealoma).

Most tumors arising in the *pineal area* are germinomas, teratomas, or other embryonal growths. These tumors are common in children, boys more than girls. They produce their symptoms by compression of the sylvian aqueduct, leading to hydrocephalus. Compression of fibers in the upper brain stem leads to loss of upward gaze and sometimes pupillary fixation, early signs of pineal region compression. Occasionally compression of the inferior colliculus causes deafness. A definitive diagnosis of pineal region tumor is important, since the germinomas are usually curable with radiation therapy, whereas most of the others are not. *Leptomeningeal* tumors usually result from spread of a primary brain or systemic tumor to the leptomeninges; primary lymphomas or melanomas of the leptomeninges are rare. Metastatic leptomeningeal invasion, however, is common from lymphomas, leukemias, or solid tumors such as carcinomas of the breast or lung and malignant melanoma. Primary tumors of the nervous system that commonly seed the meninges include medulloblastomas, malignant ependymomas of the fourth ventricle, and germinomas. Symptoms of leptomeningeal involvement may occur before the primary tumor has declared itself. The first symptoms are often those of increased intracranial pressure from hydrocephalus (see Fig. 114–2). Additional symptoms include seizures from invasion of the cortex, cranial nerve palsies from infiltration of nerves passing through the subarachnoid space, and spinal root dysfunction, often involving the lower extremities and the bladder as a result of infiltration of the cauda equina. The diagnosis is suspected by the presence of diffuse or multifocal signs of central nervous system dysfunction and usually can be established by the identification of malignant cells in the spinal fluid.

False Localizing Symptoms and Signs

Growing tumors mold the surrounding normal brain and displace adjacent and remote structures from their normal positions. When these structures are shifted, they may be compressed by nearby dura, by bone at the base of the skull, or by the bony foramina through which the cranial nerves pass. Compression of normal structures at a distance from the growing tumor leads to focal neurological signs that may incorrectly localize the tumor. These false localizing signs usually occur with slow-growing tumors arising in relatively silent areas. Examples of well-recognized false localizing signs include diplopia from abducens nerve palsy as a result of displacement compression of the sixth nerve at the base of the brain, hemianopsia caused by tentorial herniation that compresses the posterior cerebral artery and produces ischemia to the occipital lobe, and tinnitus, vertigo, or hearing loss from compression of the eighth nerves as they pass through the internal auditory canal. False localizing signs rarely produce a diagnostic problem nowadays because of the availability of new imaging techniques. False localizing signs can also occur with pseudotumor cerebri or intracranial hypotension, where their recognition is particularly important if one is to avoid unnecessarily exhaustive laboratory evaluation or inappropriate surgery.

DIAGNOSTIC TESTS

In any patient clinically suspected of harboring an intracranial neoplasm, magnetic resonance imaging (MR scan) is the test of choice (Fig. 121–2). It can identify tumors sometimes missed by CT scan (low-grade gliomas and small posterior fossa lesions) and often helps differentiate tumor from arteriovenous malformations better than does CT. Meningiomas are often difficult to distinguish from normal structures

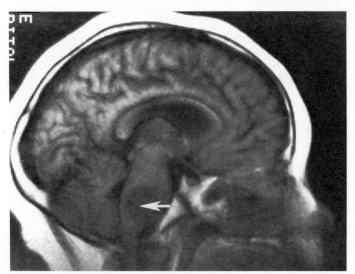

FIGURE 121–2. MR scan of an 18-year-old man with progressive cranial nerve symptoms suggesting a brain stem tumor. The CT scan was normal. Sagittal magnetic resonance image reveals a mass (arrow) in the pons.

by MR scan, but the newly available intravenous contrast material, gadolinium, largely solves that problem. Radionuclide brain scan, skull radiograph, and electroencephalography add nothing to the diagnosis. If a leptomeningeal tumor is suspected by the presence of unexplained hydrocephalus or a diffuse encephalopathy without focal abnormalities on a brain image, lumbar puncture should be performed to look for the characteristic changes of pleocytosis, malignant cells in the spinal fluid, elevated protein, and hypoglycorrhachia (low glucose content). At times, myelography identifies small tumors on the nerve roots.

Imaging techniques reveal the presence but not the exact nature of a lesion. Thus, neither CT nor MR can definitively distinguish between the histological types of tumors, nor can they reliably differentiate between neoplasms and other tumors such as abscesses or granulomas. Angiography is useful primarily to assist the surgeon in defining the proximity of the tumor to nearby arteries and veins. If a lesion is present and cannot clearly be identified on clinical grounds, biopsy is necessary before treatment is undertaken. When the lesion is accessible, surgical excision not only establishes the diagnosis but also provides the first step in the treatment of the patient. If the lesion is not accessible, CT- or MR-directed stereotactic needle biopsy often can establish the diagnosis definitively.

TREATMENT

The treatment of intracranial neoplasms varies, depending on the nature of the neoplasm, its location, and the general condition of the patient. Certain general principles apply: When there is a single lesion and it is surgically accessible, it should be removed to whatever degree possible. Although some patients undergoing surgery of intracranial neoplasms suffer increased neurological dysfunction, the majority improve after compression of brain structures is relieved. The advantages of surgery are that it cures some patients (pituitary adenoma, most meningiomas, cerebellar astrocytomas), that it ameliorates symptoms in the majority of patients, and that the debulking of a large malignant lesion allows time for other slower-acting therapeutic modalities to be effective. It also definitively establishes the diagnosis.

Most intracranial neoplasms cannot be cured surgically (Fig. 121–3). For them the second line of treatment is radiation therapy (RT). RT is delivered either to the local site of the tumor (some recurrent meningiomas) or by a combination of whole-brain and local radiation (most malignant gliomas) to the entire neuraxis (medulloblastomas, malignant ependymomas). RT improves both survival and the quality of life in most patients with highly malignant tumors. It probably also favorably affects the course of more benign tumors such as astrocytomas and recurrent meningiomas.

Chemotherapy, when added to RT, enhances both survival and quality of life of some patients with malignant astrocytomas, but its role in other intracranial neoplasms is not yet well-established.

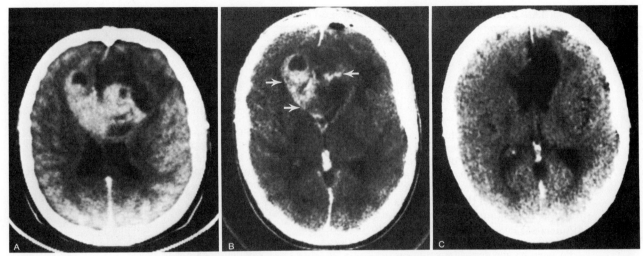

FIGURE 121–3. Results of treatment of glioblastoma multiforme. A 32-year-old man presented in the fall of 1982 with headaches, seizures, and papilledema. A large contrast-enhancing bifrontal mass was partially extirpated and then treated with radiation therapy and chemotherapy. A, The mass prior to therapy. B, The mass shortly postoperatively, indicating that there had been a major but incomplete resection. A residual tumor is indicated by the arrows. C, CT scan 2.5 years later. The site of surgical extirpation is indicated by the lucent area. There is no evidence of contrast enhancement, suggesting that the residual tumor has been eradicated. The patient became asymptomatic.

SPINAL NEOPLASMS

Spinal tumors originate from the same cell types as do intracranial tumors, and the same principles of diagnosis and treatment apply to them as to intracranial tumors. They are discussed in detail on pages 742–745.

PARANEOPLASTIC SYNDROMES

When patients with systemic cancer (i.e., cancer that arises outside the central nervous system) develop nervous system dysfunction, metastasis is usually the cause. However, cancer also exerts deleterious effects on the nervous system in the absence of direct metastatic involvement (paraneoplastic syndromes). Recognition of these nonmetastatic neurological complications can prevent inappropriate and perhaps harmful therapy directed at a nonexistent metastasis. Since at times the nervous system symptoms precede the discovery of the cancer, they can also lead the physician to the diagnosis of an otherwise occult neoplasm. An almost bewildering variety of neurological disorders have been ascribed to effects of systemic cancer (Table 121–2). Most patients with nervous system dysfunction not caused by metastases are eventually found to be suffering from systemic infections, from vascular or metabolic disorders that affect the nervous system secondarily, or from unwanted side effects of cancer therapy. This section discusses two types of nervous system damage related to cancer and not described elsewhere in this book: "remote effects" and radiation injury.

REMOTE EFFECTS

Remote effects of cancer on the nervous system is a term used to describe nervous system dysfunction of unknown cause occurring either exclusively or with greater frequency in patients with cancer.

Remote effects are not common, probably affecting less than 1 per cent of patients with cancer. Circulating antibodies against the target nervous system organ can be found in some patients suffering from remote effects. In a few instances, injection of the antibody or extracts of tumor into experimental animals has reproduced portions of the clinical syndrome, suggesting an autoimmune mechanism, with the antigen originating in the tumor. Not all patients harbor such antibodies, and other suggestions for etiology have included viral infections, toxins secreted by the tumor, and nutritional deprivation.

A few neurological syndromes are highly characteristic of remote effects. These include subacute cerebellar degeneration, subacute sensory neuronopathy, and the myasthenic syndrome. These are discussed in the paragraphs below.

Subacute cerebellar degeneration caused by cancer has a clinical picture sufficiently characteristic to suggest strongly that cancer is present even if the neurological symptoms predate the appearance of the tumor. There is usually subacute onset of bilateral and symmetrical cerebellar dysfunction, the patient being equally ataxic in arms and legs. Severe dysarthria is usually present, and vertigo and diplopia are common, but nystagmus may be absent. Many patients have neurological signs pointing to disease outside the cerebellum: extensor plantar responses are common; tendon reflexes may be either diminished or exaggerated; and dementia occurs in about half. The cerebrospinal fluid is usually normal, but there may be as many as 40 lymphocytes per cubic milliliter and an elevated protein and IgG concentration. The disease, which

TABLE 121–2. NONMETASTATIC EFFECTS OF CANCER ON THE NERVOUS SYSTEM

I. "Remote effects"
  A. Brain and cranial nerves
    1. Dementia
    2. Bulbar encephalitis
    3. Subacute cerebellar degeneration—opsoclonus*
    4. Optic neuritis—retinal degeneration
  B. Spinal cord
    1. Gray matter myelopathy
      a. Subacute motor neuropathy
      b. "Autonomic insufficiency"
    2. Subacute necrotic myelopathy
  C. Peripheral nerves and roots
    1. Subacute sensory neuronopathy (dorsal root ganglionitis)*
    2. Sensorimotor peripheral neuropathy
    3. Acute polyneuropathy, "Guillain-Barré" type
    4. Autonomic neuropathy
  D. Neuromuscular junction and muscle
    1. Polymyositis and dermatomyositis (dermatomyositis in older men*)
    2. Lambert-Eaton "myasthenic" syndrome
    3. Myasthenia gravis (thymoma)
    4. Neuromyotonia
II. Metabolic encephalopathy
  A. Destruction of vital organs
    1. Liver (hepatic coma)
    2. Lung (pulmonary encephalopathy)
    3. Kidney (uremia)
    4. Bone (hypercalcemia)
  B. Elaboration of hormonal substances by tumor
    1. "Parathormone" (hypercalcemia)
    2. "Corticotropin" (Cushing's syndrome)
    3. Antidiuretic hormone (water intoxication)
  C. Competition between tumor and brain for essential substrates
    1. Hypoglycemia (large retroperitoneal tumors)
    2. Tryptophan (carcinoid)
  D. Malnutrition
III. Infections (usually associated with lymphomas)
  A. Parasites
    1. Toxoplasma cerebral abscess
  B. Fungi
    1. Meningitis (cryptococcosis)
    2. Encephalitis (aspergillosis, mucormycosis)
  C. Bacteria
    1. Meningitis (*Listeria monocytogenes*)
  D. Viruses
    1. Herpes zoster (radiculitis, myelitis, encephalitis, granulomatous vasculitis)
    2. Progressive multifocal leukoencephalopathy
IV. Vascular disease
  A. Intracranial hemorrhage
    1. Subdural hematoma
    2. Subarachnoid hemorrhage
    3. Intracerebral hemorrhage
  B. Cerebral infarction
    1. Thrombotic (due to "hypercoagulability")
    2. Embolic nonbacterial thrombotic endocarditis
V. Side effects of therapy
  A. Chemotherapy
    1. Central nervous system
    2. Peripheral nervous system
  B. Radiation therapy
    See Table 121–3

* Neurological disorders that may precede diagnosis of cancer and strongly suggest its presence.

may be associated with any cancer, precedes the discovery of the neoplasm by a few weeks to three years in more than half the patients, and it tends to run a progressive course over weeks to months, rendering the patient severely disabled. Cerebellar atrophy may be seen on a CT scan, particularly if done late in the course of the illness. Characteristic pathological changes consist of diffuse or patchy loss of Purkinje cells in all areas of the cerebellum. There may be lymphocytic cuffs around blood vessels, particularly in the deep nuclei. This illness can be distinguished from cerebellar metastases by the symmetry of its signs and the absence of increased intracranial pressure, and from alcoholic-nutritional cerebellar degeneration because dysarthria and ataxia in the upper extremities are prominent in the carcinomatous cerebellar degenerations and are usually mild or absent in the alcoholic variety. The hereditary cerebellar degenerations rarely run so rapid a course. At times the disorder stabilizes or improves with successful treatment of the tumor. Antibodies to cerebellar Purkinje cells have been found in the serum of some patients.

Another, less common cerebellar syndrome is that of *opsoclonus* (spontaneous, conjugate, chaotic eye movements most severe when voluntary eye movements are attempted). Opsoclonus is frequently associated with cerebellar ataxia and myoclonus of the trunk and extremities. It is most common in children as a remote effect of neuroblastoma. In children, the neurological symptoms respond to adrenocorticosteroid therapy and to therapy of the tumor.

Subacute sensory neuronopathy is marked by loss of sensation with relative preservation of motor power. The illness sometimes precedes the appearance of the carcinoma and progresses over a few months, leaving the patient with a moderate or severe disability. The cerebrospinal fluid protein is usually elevated. Pathologically, there is destruction of posterior root ganglia with perivascular lymphocytic cuffing and wallerian degeneration of sensory nerves. Many of the patients have inflammatory and degenerative changes in brain and spinal cord as well. The entity is rare and there is no treatment. Some patients harbor an antibody that reacts with an antigen found in the nuclei of neurons throughout the central nervous system. Dorsal root ganglion cells also harbor the antigen.

The *myasthenic syndrome* (Lambert-Eaton syndrome) is associated with small cell lung cancer in about two thirds of patients; the other one third do not have cancer. It is discussed on p. 761.

INJURY FROM THERAPEUTIC RADIATION

When parts of the nervous system are included within an ionizing irradiation portal, adverse effects may result (Table 121–3). The likelihood of adverse effects is related to the total dose of radiation, the size of each fraction, the total duration over which the dose is received, and the volume of nervous system tissue irradiated. Other factors such as underlying nervous system disease (e.g., brain tumor, cerebral edema), previous surgery, concomitant use of chemotherapeutic agents, and individual susceptibility make it impossible to define precisely a safe dose for any given individual. However, certain guidelines allow the radiation therapist to calculate generally safe nervous system doses. Adverse effects may involve any portion of the central or peripheral nervous system and may occur acutely or be delayed weeks to years following irradiation.

Clinical Manifestations

Acute encephalopathy may follow large radiation doses to patients with increased intracranial pressure, particularly in the absence of corticosteroid prophylaxis. Immediately following treatment, susceptible patients develop headache, nausea and vomiting, somnolence, fever, and occasionally worsening of neurological signs, rarely culminating in cerebral herniation and death. Acute encephalopathy usually follows the first radiation fraction and becomes progressively less severe with each ensuing fraction. This disorder is believed to result from increased intracranial pressure and/or brain edema from radiation-induced alteration of the blood-brain barrier. It responds to corticosteroids. Acute worsening of neurological symptoms does not occur after spinal cord irradiation.

Early delayed encephalopathy or *myelopathy* appears 6 to 16 weeks after therapy and persists for days to weeks. In children, the encephalopathy commonly follows prophylactic irradiation of the brain for leukemia and is called the "radiation somnolence syndrome." The disorder is characterized by somnolence, often associated with headache, nausea, vomiting, and sometimes fever. The electroencephalogram may be slow, but there are no focal signs. In adults, the syndrome usually follows whole-brain irradiation for brain tumors and is characterized by lethargy and worsening of focal neurological signs. Both disorders usually respond to steroids but if untreated will resolve spontaneously. In adults, the syndrome may be distinguished from recurrent brain tumor by CT scan. In children, lumbar puncture rules out the potential diagnosis of meningeal leukemia. *Early delayed myelopathy* follows radiation therapy to the neck or upper thorax and is characterized by Lhermitte's sign (an electric shock–like sensation radiating into various parts of the body when the neck is flexed). The symptoms resolve spontaneously. Early delayed radiation syndromes are believed to result from demyelination, possibly due to radiation-induced damage to oligodendroglia.

Late delayed radiation injury appears months to years following radiation and may affect any part of the nervous system. In the brain, there are two clinical syndromes. The first follows whole-brain irradiation either to patients without brain tumors (prophylactic irradiation for oat cell carcinoma) or in some patients

TABLE 121–3. RADIATION INJURY TO THE NERVOUS SYSTEM

TIME AFTER RT	ORGAN AFFECTED	CLINICAL FINDINGS
Primary Injury		
Immediate (min to hrs)	Brain	Acute encephalopathy
Early delayed (6–16 wks)	Brain	Somnolence, focal signs
	Spinal cord	Lhermitte's sign
Late delayed (mos to yrs)	Brain	Dementia, focal signs
	Spinal cord	Transverse myelopathy
	Peripheral nerves	Paralysis, sensory loss
Secondary Injury (years)	Several	Brain, cranial, and/or peripheral nerve sheath tumors
	Arteries (atherosclerosis)	Cerebral infarction
	Endocrine organs	Metabolic encephalopathy

with primary and metastatic brain tumors. The disorder is characterized by dementia without focal signs. There is cerebral atrophy on CT scan and pathological changes are nonspecific; there is no treatment. The second disorder affects patients who receive either focal brain irradiation during therapy of extracranial neoplasms or whole-brain irradiation for intracranial neoplasms. Neurological signs suggest a mass and include headache, focal or generalized seizures, and hemiparesis. Brain CT scans reveal a hypodense mass, sometimes with contrast enhancement. Neuropathological features include coagulative necrosis of white matter, telangiectasia, fibrinoid necrosis and thrombus formation, and glial proliferation and bizarre multinucleated astrocytes. The clinical and CT or MR findings cannot be distinguished from brain tumor, and the diagnosis can be made only by biopsy. Corticosteroids sometimes ameliorate symptoms. The treatment, if the disorder is focal, is surgical removal. *Late delayed myelopathy* is characterized by progressive paralysis, sensory changes, and sometimes pain. A Brown-Sequard syndrome (weakness and loss of proprioception in the extremities of one side with loss of pain and temperature sensation on the other) is often present at onset. Patients occasionally respond transiently to steroids, and the disorder may stop progressing, but generally patients become paraplegic or quadriplegic. Pathological changes include necrosis of the spinal cord. *Late delayed neuropathy* may affect any cranial or peripheral nerve. Common disorders are blindness from optic neuropathy and paralysis of an upper extremity from brachial plexopathy after therapy for lung or breast cancer. The pathogenesis is probably fibrosis and ischemia of the plexus. There is no treatment.

Radiation-induced tumors, including meningiomas,

sarcomas or, less commonly, gliomas, may appear years to decades after cranial irradiation and may follow even low-dose radiation therapy. Malignant or atypical nerve sheath tumors may follow irradiation of the brachial, cervical, and lumbar plexuses. The central nervous system may also be damaged when radiation alters extraneural structures. Radiation therapy accelerates *atherosclerosis*, and cerebral infarction associated with carotid artery occlusion in the neck may occur many years after neck irradiation. Endocrine (pituitary, thyroid, parathyroid) dysfunction from radiation may be associated with neurological signs. Hypothyroidism or hyperparathyroidism from radiation may also cause an encephalopathy.

NON-NEOPLASTIC ALTERATIONS OF INTRACRANIAL PRESSURE

INTRODUCTION AND DEFINITIONS

Intracranial pressure is determined by rates of cerebrospinal fluid (CSF) formation and absorption and by cerebral venous pressure, the last a reflection of systemic venous pressure. Lumbar puncture pressure in the lateral decubitus position accurately reflects intracranial pressure in most instances. The normal CSF pressure is usually between 65 and 195 mm of CSF (5 to 15 mm Hg), although pressures as high as 250 mm of CSF have been reported in apparently normal individuals. Nevertheless, pressures above 170 are suspect, and pressures above 200 should be considered abnormal until proven otherwise. CSF pressure is not affected by obesity. Elevated CSF pressure measured at lumbar puncture does not necessarily reflect neurological disease; e.g., elevation of the head of the bed can raise the lumbar CSF pressure, although it lowers intracranial pressure. Elevation of systemic venous pressure, such as occurs acutely with coughing, straining, crying or chronically with congestive heart failure or venous obstruction of the superior vena cava or jugular veins, raises intracranial pressure. Hypercapnia (e.g., pulmonary disease, excessive sedation) increases the cerebral blood volume and thus CSF pressure. Conversely, if the patient is positioned with the head down, lumbar puncture pressure is lower, although intracranial pressure becomes higher. The loss of CSF around the needle hole between the time the needle enters the subarachnoid space and the manometer is placed also lowers intracranial pressure. When all of these artifactual causes of altered intracranial pressure are eliminated, the most common cause of intracranial *hypertension* is intracranial tumor and the most common cause of intracranial *hypotension* is a CSF leak following lumbar puncture or myelogram. This section discusses several other disorders that can alter intracranial pressure.

INTRACRANIAL HYPERTENSION

Pseudotumor cerebri, as the name suggests, is a disorder characterized by increased intracranial pressure in the absence of a tumor or obvious obstruction of CSF pathways. The cause is usually not established, although a number of central nervous system or systemic illnesses appear to play an etiological role. Pseudotumor can follow head trauma, middle ear disease, internal jugular vein ligation, oral contraceptive use, pregnancy, and polycythemia vera, all conditions that suggest possible cerebral venous occlusion. In a few such patients, MR scans or angiograms show sagittal or lateral sinus occlusion. The disorder has also been reported in patients on prolonged corticosteroid therapy, after steroid withdrawal, with Addison's disease or hypoparathyroidism, and with ingestion of drugs such as vitamin A, nalidixic acid, and tetracycline. Most cases, however, are idiopathic.

The disorder usually affects young (ages 20 to 30), usually obese females, is characterized by headache, papilledema, and at times visual obscurations (sudden momentary, usually bilateral visual loss), and has a benign prognosis.

Most patients with pseudotumor present to the physician with headache and papilledema. In a few, headaches are absent and the disorder is discovered because of either visual obscurations or papilledema found on routine ophthalmological examination. Sometimes there is no papilledema or only unilateral papilledema even though intracranial pressure is grossly elevated. Visual obscurations do not portend visual loss. However, whether or not patients have visual obscurations, 10 to 15 per cent of patients lose some vision during the course of the disease, varying from small scotomata to total blindness. Other clinical symptoms that are less common but that may concern the physician include vomiting, diplopia, vertigo, tinnitus, neck pain and stiffness, orbital pain, drowsiness, and dysesthetic sensation. These false localizing signs probably result from minor shifts of normal structures engendered by the intracranial hypertension. The disorder usually runs a benign course, with the headache and papilledema resolving in several weeks to several months, although in many patients intracranial pressure as measured at lumbar puncture remains elevated for months to years.

The diagnosis is suspected clinically and established by the presence of elevated intracranial pressure in a patient with a normal MR or CT scan. The CSF pressure is usually above 300 mm and its composition is otherwise normal, although in some patients there may be a relatively low protein (below 15 mg/dl). Venous occlusions can usually be detected by MR. A few errors in diagnosis occur in patients with an anomalous elevation of the optic discs (pseudopapilledema) or, very rarely, in patients with diffuse infiltrating gliomas of the brain (gliomatosis cerebri). The first can be ruled out by appropriate ophthalmologic tests, including fluorescein angiography, and the second usually by MRI and time.

Treatment is symptomatic. Repeated lumbar punctures sometimes relieve the headaches, and some physicians believe that corticosteroids are helpful. Only if there is evidence of progressive visual loss is therapeutic intervention mandatory. In that instance, the best treatment appears to be shunting the CSF from the lumbar sac into the peritoneum.

Hydrocephalus refers to an enlargement of the cerebral ventricular system by an increase in the amount of ventricular fluid. Obstructive hydrocephalus can result from either stenosis or occlusion of CSF pathways within the ventricular system (noncommunicating) or from stenosis or occlusion of subarachnoid pathways outside the ventricular system (communicating). Nonobstructive hydrocephalus results from passive enlargement of the ventricular system because of atrophy of brain substance (hydrocephalus ex vacuo). Obstructive hydrocephalus is often but not always associated with intracranial hypertension and, when acute, may be rapidly fatal. The more chronic the hydrocephalus, the more likely the intracranial hypertension is to be either mild or undetectable (normal pressure hydrocephalus) and the more likely the symptoms are to be indolent.

Acute hydrocephalus, such as occurs with sudden obstruction of the ventricular system (e.g., colloid cyst of the third ventricle, subarachnoid or cerebellar hemorrhage), is characterized by sudden severe headache, vomiting, lethargy, and sometimes coma. If the system is not decompressed, herniation and death can occur. Subacute (subarachnoid hemorrhage, meningitis, leptomeningeal neoplasia) or chronic hydrocephalus (congenital aqueductal stenosis, spinal cord tumors, idiopathic normal pressure hydrocephalus) is usually characterized by progressive lethargy, apathy, and dementia, often associated with an unsteady gait and urgency incontinence of urine. There may be bilateral corticospinal tract signs, particularly in the lower extremities, with hyperactive knee and ankle jerks and extensor plantar responses. If the pressure is grossly elevated, patients may develop headache and papilledema, but these are uncommon.

The presence of enlarged ventricles is detected easily by MR or CT scan. Unfortunately, it is not always easy to distinguish on the CT scan between obstructive hydrocephalus and hydrocephalus ex vacuo unless the cause (e.g., tumor) can be identified. A lumbar puncture revealing an elevated intracranial pressure assists in the diagnosis, but because some patients with obstructive hydrocephalus have a relatively normal intracranial pressure, that test likewise may not give a definitive diagnosis. In patients with classic symptoms of chronic hydrocephalus (i.e., dementia, gait unsteadiness, and incontinence), removal of CSF at lumbar puncture sometimes relieves symptoms, indicating both that CSF obstruction is producing the symptoms and that ventricular shunting will be therapeutic.

INTRACRANIAL HYPOTENSION

Intracranial hypotension usually follows lumbar puncture but occasionally results from spontaneous or traumatically induced tears of the dura, leading to leakage of subarachnoid fluid. The resulting low CSF pressure is characterized by headache beginning occipitally and radiating frontally when the patient assumes the erect posture. The headache is sometimes associated with nausea, vomiting, photophobia, and a stiff neck. Some patients develop diplopia from abducens nerve paralysis. Auditory symptoms such as tinnitus and vestibular symptoms such as dizziness also can occur. The symptoms probably result because the brain, unsupported by CSF, shifts downward when the erect posture is assumed. The diagnosis is easily made on clinical grounds if the patient has undergone a lumbar puncture or myelogram a few days previously, but can be established only by performing a lumbar puncture and noting the low CSF pressure if no such history is present. Symptoms usually resolve spontaneously but in a few instances may persist, in which case a search for the site of the leak should be made. Some investigators have recommended epidural injection of a few milliliters of the patient's blood to patch a dural leak following lumbar puncture, and in a few instances of spontaneous or traumatic dural tears, surgical repair of the leak has been necessary.

REFERENCES

Kornblith PL, Walker MD, Cassady JR (eds): Neurologic Oncology. Philadelphia, JB Lippincott Co, 1987.

Vick, NA, Bigner DD: Neuro-Oncology. Neurol Clin, Vol 3, No 4, Nov, 1985.

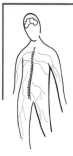

Despite its sequestration from the rest of the body by the blood-brain barrier, the central nervous system is subject to attack by many of the same infectious agents and antigen-antibody reactions that affect the remainder of the body. As with systemic infections, bacterial, fungal, and parasitic infections of the nervous system are particularly likely to occur when the body's resistive mechanisms have been breached. Viral infections of the nervous system are also common. Although more frequent in immunosuppressed hosts, many viruses (e.g., that causing herpes zoster) are neurotropic (i.e., have a predilection for invasion of the nervous system). Except for slow viruses, discussed in this section, virus diseases of the nervous system are described in Chapter 86. When managing inflammatory disease of the nervous system, one has the obligation not only to identify and treat the invading organism but also to search for host factors that may predispose to further infections. Chapter 81 discusses such factors.

BACTERIAL INFECTIONS OF THE BRAIN

Bacteria reach the nervous system from a prior site of infection in a systemic organ. The only exception occurs when a communication connects the central nervous system and the surface of the body, such as can follow central nervous system trauma, surgical procedures, or the development of spontaneous CSF fistulae. A careful search for the last is always warranted in a patient with repetitive central nervous system bacterial infections. The offending organism is often *Streptococcus pneumoniae*.

Bacterial infections of the central nervous system may be meningeal or parameningeal. The most common infection, acute bacterial meningitis, is discussed in detail in Chapter 86. Less common *parameningeal infections* include brain and spinal epidural abscesses and brain and spinal subdural abscesses (subdural empyema). This chapter discusses these, along with parenchymal brain and spinal abscesses and certain unusual neurological complications of bacterial infections resulting from bacterial endocarditis and secondary venous sinus thrombosis.

INTRACRANIAL ABSCESSES

Intracranial abscesses are pockets of pus localized to one of the intracranial compartments (i.e., the epidural space, the subdural space, or the brain itself).

Epidural abscesses

Epidural abscesses usually arise by direct extension from adjacent osteomyelitis, mastoiditis, or infection of the paranasal sinuses. In the early stages, signs and symptoms are usually those of infection of the extracranial site from which they arose. Thus, head pain and often local swelling and redness commonly overlie the site of the epidural abscess. Fever usually is present accompanied by leukocytosis with a preponderance of polymorphonuclear leukocytes. Focal neurological signs are uncommon, and increased intracranial pressure is not usually present. In the early stage the cerebrospinal fluid usually contains at most a few lymphocytes with a slightly elevated protein. If the initial disorder is untreated, the infection may breach the dura to produce a subdural empyema, bacterial meningitis, or brain abscess. If the epidural inflammation lies close to a large venous sinus, thrombophlebitis with sinus occlusion (page 808) often complicates the infection. The extent of an epidural abscess is usually easily defined by CT scan, a contrast-enhancing mass being identified in the epidural space compressing the underlying brain. In their early stages, such abscesses can be treated successfully with appropriate antibiotics (the organism having been identified by culture of purulent material from the ear or sinuses). In some instances, particularly when the abscess is large or when it fails to shrink rapidly with antibiotic therapy, surgical drainage is required.

Subdural Abscess

Most subdural abscesses (subdural empyemas) arise from infection of paranasal sinuses or the middle ear (otitis media). Organisms from the primary infection follow cranial venous channels, often producing thrombophlebitis as they go through the dura into the subdural space. Occasionally, traumatically induced subdural hematomas become secondarily infected to form subdural empyemas. The site of the empyema depends on the site of the primary infection. Those of the paranasal sinuses usually extend over the frontal lobe, while those from ear infections penetrate the skull posteriorly both above and below the tentorium. The inflammatory reaction excited by the organism may form a membrane that completely walls off the collection of pus.

Most patients with subdural empyema suffer the signs and symptoms of sinusitis or otitis prior to the onset of the empyema. As the intracranial abscess develops, the pain of the primary process usually worsens, with more severe headache spreading widely from its original site. Fever, if not already present, develops, the white count rises, and patients often become drowsy and may vomit. Secondary thrombophlebitis of the brain often develops and causes focal neurological signs of seizures or hemiparesis. Eventually the intracranial pressure rises, and a fulminant course may produce death within a few days if no treatment is undertaken. The diagnosis is suggested by a history of pre-existing infection combined with local physical abnormalities. CT scans define both the site of primary infection and the subdural collection of pus. If obtained, the cerebral spinal fluid is usually under increased pressure and may contain several hundred cells with an elevated protein but normal glucose concentration. Lumbar puncture, however, should not be performed in patients suspected of subdural empyema, since no organisms will be recovered and the rapidly increasing intracranial pressure threatens to produce cerebral herniation.

Subdural empyema almost always requires surgical drainage. Drainage combined with appropriate antibiotic therapy usually relieves the symptoms and cures the patient if the disease is detected in its earliest stages. Unfortunately, diagnosis is often delayed, resulting in a mortality of about 25 per cent. Most patients die as a result of venous sinus thrombosis with secondary cerebral infarction or meningitis.

Brain Abscess

Brain abscess is the most common intracranial abscess. Like those of the epidural and subdural space, parenchymal abscesses of the brain can arise by direct extension along venous channels from infections in the paranasal sinuses or the ear. Currently, however, most arise by hematogenous spread from infections elsewhere in the body. Metastatic abscess probably originates from a transient bacteremia with organisms lodging in capillary vessels of the brain. The process begins as a focal encephalitis, followed in days or weeks by encapsulation of pus to form a true abscess. Unlike epidural or subdural abscesses, in which one almost always can identify the primary site of the infection, in a substantial number of patients with brain abscesses the systemic infection may already have resolved without having produced symptoms. Some patients with brain abscess give a history of dental manipulation or mild urinary tract infection several weeks earlier; others have had lung infections. Congenital cyanotic heart disease and arteriovenous shunts in the lungs increase the risk of brain abscess because the lungs normally filter out circulating bacteria. Immunosuppressed patients often develop multiple rather than the single brain abscesses that most often affect patients with normal immunity.

The primary site of the infection determines the offending organism. Common agents include an aerobic or microaerophilic *Streptococcus* as well as enteric bacteria. In traumatic abscesses, staphylococci are common; *Clostridium* occasionally is present. Many of the infections are mixed. Rarer causes of abscesses include *Actinomyces* and *Nocardia*. Tuberculous abscesses are uncommon in the United States but frequent in less developed countries.

The site of a brain abscess depends partly on its source. Those that originate in the middle ear generally invade the temporal lobe or cerebellum, those in the paranasal sinus penetrate the frontal lobe, and those from penetrating injuries involve the wound site. Hematogenous abscesses can affect any part of the brain, although most are in the distribution of the middle cerebral artery.

Most abscesses produce symptoms similar to but more rapidly progressive than those of a brain tumor. It is uncommon for patients to suffer from fever, substantial tenderness of the skull, or an elevated white blood cell count. Instead, patients present with headache, signs of increased intracranial pressure, and focal signs that depend on the site of the lesion. Focal or generalized seizures are a common accompaniment.

The differential diagnosis includes brain tumor and less often cerebral infarct. Abscess should be suspected if a patient suffers one of the predisposing causes (e.g., immune suppression, cyanotic heart disease, arteriovenous shunting in the lungs) or if a systemic bacterial infection has occurred in the recent past. A history of a draining ear or evidence of otitis media, particularly when clinical symptoms and signs point to a lesion in the temporal lobe or cerebellum, strengthens the likelihood of brain abscess, as does a history of purulent sinusitis. If fever exists or the white blood cell count is elevated (neither usually is the case), the diagnosis favors abscess. Lumbar puncture should not be performed because of the risk of cerebral herniation. CT scans are helpful but not always diagnostic. Abscess on CT scan is characterized by a hypodense lesion surrounded by a contrast-enhancing ring. The abnor-

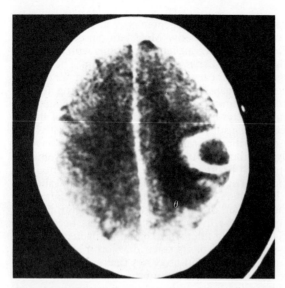

FIGURE 122–1. CT scan showing a brain abscess. A woman presented to physicians after a focal seizure followed by headache and weakness of the arm. Dental work had been performed several weeks before. CT scan revealed a contrast-enhanced, ringlike mass surrounded by edema. It is not possible on this scan to differentiate tumor from abscess. At surgery a well-encapsulated abscess was encountered.

mality can resemble rings that sometimes rim primary and metastatic brain tumors as well as recent cerebral infarcts. A thin, smooth-walled ring suggests an abscess, whereas a thick, irregular ring is more common with brain tumor (Fig. 122–1). However, it usually requires surgical exploration to make the diagnosis.

The treatment begins with antibiotics. For abscesses 3 cm or smaller, antibiotics alone usually suffice, the choice depending on the suspected causal organism. If the organism is not known, a combination of penicillin and metronidazole in high doses for a period of about six weeks is usually effective. CT scanning helps greatly in judging the effectiveness of antibiotic therapy and deciding when, if ever, surgical extirpation is necessary. Even after full recovery the contrast-enhancing ring may persist for many weeks and does not imply that the abscess is still active. Large abscesses, failure of the lesion to shrink or the patient to improve with antibiotic therapy, or the presence of a doubtful diagnosis mandate surgical removal or, for surgically inaccessible lesions, stereotactic needle biopsy and drainage. With early detection and vigorous antimicrobial treatment most patients do not need surgery and recover with few sequelae other than a tendency to seizures, which can be controlled by anticonvulsants. This approach has reduced the mortality from brain abscesses in some series to about 5 per cent.

VENOUS SINUS AND CORTICAL THROMBOPHLEBITIS

Bacterial infections of the central nervous system may cause thrombophlebitis with secondary occlusion of the large dural sinuses. Similarly, occlusion of large dural sinuses may occur in the absence of infection in patients with disorders of clotting (see Table 118–7). The most common sites of infective sinus occlusion are the lateral sinus (a complication of acute or chronic otitis media), cavernous sinus (a complication of orbital or nasal sinus infection), and the superior sagittal sinus, usually occluded by direct extension of the infected clot from the first two. Cortical veins may be involved either by direct contact with an infection in the epidural or subdural space or by extension of infective clot from the sinuses.

The symptoms of lateral sinus occlusion depend on the rapidity of the occlusion and the importance of that sinus in draining the brain's blood. Since the two lateral sinuses are often different sizes, slowly developing occlusion of the smaller one usually causes no symptoms at all. Occlusion of the dominant lateral sinus is often heralded by headache and papilledema. There are usually no focal signs unless the occlusion spreads to involve the jugular vein, in which case there may be pain, swelling, and a palpable cord in the neck. If the occlusion spreads to the inferior petrosal sinus, abducens and trigeminal nerve involvement (Gradenigo's syndrome) can be added and, if the jugular bulb is involved, dysarthria, dysphagia, and neck weakness (jugular foramen syndrome) ensue.

Cavernous sinus occlusion causes a more florid picture, often resulting from staphylococcal infection of the face or sinus. Symptoms begin with fever, headache, nausea, vomiting, and seizures. Proptosis affects the ipsilateral eye with chemosis and ophthalmoplegia, to which sensory loss in the distribution of the first division of the trigeminal nerve sometimes is added (all result from the third, fourth, fifth, and sixth nerves passing through the cavernous sinus). Papilledema is a late event.

Sagittal sinus occlusion is characterized by headache and, often, papilledema. If acute in onset and involving the posterior sinus, bilateral hemorrhagic infarction of the brain develops, sometimes producing bilateral hemiparesis more marked in the leg and proximal arm than in the hand and face.

The diagnosis of sinus occlusion or corticothrombophlebitis should be suspected in a patient with a head or neck infection who develops signs of increased intracranial pressure with or without focal neurological signs. The diagnosis of sinus occlusion can easily be made by MR scan, which distinguishes clot from flowing blood in vessels, or by a digital intravenous angiogram (Fig. 122–2); the tests do not distinguish between infective and noninfective thromboses.

Infective sinus thrombosis is usually successfully treated with appropriate antibiotics; sometimes despite treatment the clot propagates to cause severe cerebral infarction and even death. Although anticoagulant treatment for sinus thrombosis was at one time a controversial matter, recent evidence indicates that prompt diagnosis, followed by heparin-coumadin therapy, substantially reduces mortality and prevents or reverses neurological damage.

BACTERIAL ENDOCARDITIS

The disseminated emboli of subacute bacterial endocarditis affect the nervous system of a quarter to a third of patients with that disease (Table 122–1). The most common symptom is that of an embolic stroke characterized by the acute onset of focal motor weakness. Multiple small emboli may lead to a clinical picture resembling a toxic encephalopathy with confusion, hallucinations, and lethargy with or without fleeting focal signs. Infected emboli lodged in cerebral blood vessels may lead to aneurysm formation (mycotic aneurysm). These aneurysms typically form in the distal portion of arteries in contradistinction to congenital aneurysms, which locate themselves more proximally. The aneurysms may rupture to cause severe cerebral or subarachnoid hemorrhage. Resolution of the aneurysms after antibiotic therapy has been reported, but in many patients surgical clipping is necessary to prevent recurrent hemorrhage. As in other disorders causing sepsis, brain abscesses can result from either acute or subacute bacterial endocarditis.

SPINAL INFECTIONS

The spinal leptomeninges contiguous with those of the intracranial cavity are bathed by the same cerebrospinal fluid and share in all of the meningeal infections and inflammatory processes that affect the brain. Subdural and epidural collections of pus, however, can be localized to the spinal canal and present with clinical pictures that differ from their counterparts in the intracranial cavity. Spinal cord parenchymal abscesses are exceedingly rare. They usually reach the spinal cord, as they do the brain, by hematogenous spread.

Spinal Abscess

Most *spinal epidural abscesses* occur at either the cervical or lumbar level and extend from an infected focus in an adjacent vertebral body (osteomyelitis), *Staphylococcus aureus* being the most common organism. Other abscesses arise either by hematogenous spread to the epidural space or by direct extension from a paravertebral infected focus. Depending on the virulence of the organism, clinical signs may develop either rapidly or slowly. In either case, neck or back pain is the most prominent symptom. The pain is usually severe and, in its early stages, well-localized. One finds marked tenderness of the spine over the site of the infection. As the illness develops, pain may spread in a dermatomal distribution as nerve roots are irritated by the inflammatory process. Unless effective treatment is started, the patient develops progressive weakness and sensory loss below the site of the lesion (myelopathy), which may lead to paraplegia in hours to days. Most patients with acute epidural abscesses are febrile and toxic, with an elevated white count. In the more chronic processes these findings may be absent, but the erythrocyte sedimentation rate is usually elevated. X-rays of the vertebral body may not become abnormal for several weeks following the onset of symptoms even when the patient is suffering from osteomyelitis. Traditionally, the diagnosis has been made by myelography. Spinal fluid obtained at the time of myelography is characterized by pleocytosis

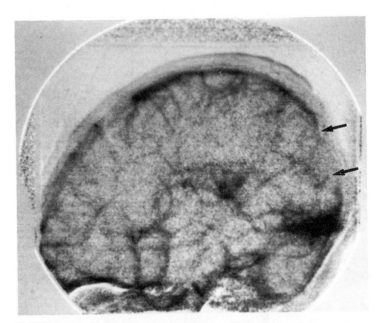

FIGURE 122–2. Digital venous angiogram (DIVA), lateral view patient facing left, in a patient with sagittal sinus occlusion. The procedure is generally more effective in demonstrating the cerebral venous system than is an arteriogram, because the cerebral hemispheres are filled with contrast material simultaneously. The patient had a bland occlusion of the posterior sagittal sinus (arrows). Inflammatory sinus occlusions have a similar appearance.

(up to several hundred white cells), elevated protein, and a normal glucose concentration; organisms are rarely cultured. In more chronic processes the pleocytosis may be absent. Recently, some workers have reported a high diagnostic accuracy using CT scans, which show an extradural lesion leading to either a complete or a partial block in most cases, plus percutaneous tapping of the abscess for bacteriological diagnosis.

Spinal subdural empyemas, usually caused by *Staphylococcus aureus,* are more likely to be associated with meningitis and spinal cord infarction than are epidural abscesses but otherwise are similar in clinical presentation. The diagnostic and therapeutic approaches are also similar.

Antibiotic therapy should be started as soon as the

TABLE 122–1. MAJOR NEUROLOGICAL COMPLICATIONS OF BACTERIAL ENDOCARDITIS*

Cerebral infarction
Multiple microemboli (diffuse encephalopathy)
Meningeal signs and symptoms
Seizures
Microscopic brain abscesses
Visual disturbances
Cranial or peripheral neuropathy
Mycotic aneurysm
Subarachnoid hemorrhage (without identifiable mycotic aneurysm)

* Signs of cerebral infarction or embolic encephalopathy affect as many as one third of cases, in many producing the first symptoms.

diagnosis is suspected. In the past, surgical drainage has been considered imperative in acute abscesses. Recently, a nonsurgical approach similar to that employed in brain abscess has been suggested, but too few results yet exist to judge the effectiveness of this approach. Chronic abscesses sometimes respond to antibiotics alone, but if signs of myelopathy appear, the patient should be surgically decompressed. The outcome is usually satisfactory in patients who are not completely paralyzed at the time treatment is undertaken.

Acute or subacute spinal abscesses must be differentiated from acute (subacute) transverse myelitis (see p. 816) and from spinal epidural or subdural hematomas (usually a disorder of patients with abnormal coagulation). Chronic spinal abscesses must be distinguished from tumor. In the acute disorder, fever, toxicity, and a history of prior infection support the diagnosis of abscess, and a carefully done myelogram or CT scan reveals the lesion to be extradural. Acute transverse myelopathy is associated either with a normal myelogram or with swelling of the spinal cord itself. In the more chronic form, differentiation between tumor and abscess may be more difficult. Both conditions can produce radiographic changes in the vertebral bodies, inflammation being more likely to affect two contiguous vertebral bodies across an intravertebral disc, whereas tumors are usually restricted to individual vertebral bodies. If the diagnosis is in doubt, biopsy of the vertebral body or decompression of the epidural space is necessary to make the differentiation.

OTHER BACTERIAL INFECTIONS

Two bacterial diseases of the nervous system, syphilis and tuberculosis, once common in the United States, are now rare, adding to the difficulty in making a definitive diagnosis when they are encountered. A discussion of the systemic manifestations of syphilis can be found in Chapter 95 and tuberculosis in Chapter 88.

Syphilis

The spirochete causing syphilis invades the central nervous system in most instances of systemic infection. The organism then may either be cleared by host defenses or persist to produce a more chronic infection expressed symptomatically only years later. The most common form of neurosyphilis is asymptomatic; patients harbor in the CSF a few white cells and have a positive serological test for syphilis. Symptomatic neurosyphilis can appear as acute or subacute meningitis (meningitic form) resembling that of other bacterial infections and usually occurring during the stage of secondary syphilis when there are cutaneous changes as well. The diagnosis is suspected by the history of syphilis as well as by the cutaneous changes, if present, and established by positive serological tests in the CSF. Patients respond promptly to antisyphilitic therapy.

Vascular syphilis begins two to ten years after the primary lesion. The disorder is characterized by both meningeal inflammation and a vasculitis of small arterial vessels, the latter leading to arterial occlusion. Clinically the disorder produces few signs of meningitis but results in monofocal or multifocal cerebral or spinal infarction. The disorder may be mistaken for an autoimmune vasculitis or even arteriosclerotic cerebral vascular disease. The early and prominent spinal cord signs should lead one to expect syphilis, while the findings in the CSF of pleocytosis, elevated gamma globulin, and a positive serological test for syphilis establish the diagnosis. Patients respond to antibiotic therapy, although recovery from focal abnormalities may be incomplete.

General paresis, once a common cause of admission to mental institutions, is now rare. The disorder results from syphilitic invasion of the parenchyma of the brain and begins clinically 10 to 20 years after the primary infection. Paresis is characterized by progressive dementia, sometimes with manic symptoms and megalomania and often with coarse tremors affecting facial muscles and tongue. The diagnostic clue is the presence of Argyll Robertson pupils (p. 720). The spinal fluid is always abnormal. The diagnosis is made by serological tests. Early treatment with antibiotics usually leads to improvement but not complete recovery.

Tabes dorsalis is a chronic infective process of the dorsal roots which appears 10 to 20 years after primary syphilitic infection. The disorder is characterized by lightning-like pains and a progressive sensory neuropathy affecting predominantly large fibers supplying the lower extremities. There is profound loss of vibration and position sense as well as areflexia. Autonomic fibers are also affected, causing postural hypotension, trophic ulcers of the feet, and traumatic arthropathy of joints. Argyll Robertson pupils are usually present. Spinal fluid serological tests are usually positive. The disorder responds only partially to treatment by antibiotics.

Rare complications of syphilis include *progressive optic atrophy, gumma* (a mass lesion in the brain), *congenital neurosyphilis*, and syphilitic infection of the *auditory* and *vestibular system*. Descriptions can be found in appropriate texts.

Tuberculosis

Central nervous system tuberculosis can occur in several forms, sometimes without evidence of active infection elsewhere in the body. The most common form is *tuberculous meningitis*. This disorder is characterized by the subacute onset of headache, stiff neck, and fever. After a few days, affected patients become confused and disoriented. They often develop abnormalities of cranial nerve function, particularly hearing loss due to the marked inflammation at the base of the brain. Most patients if untreated lapse into coma and die within three to four weeks of onset. An accompanying arteritis may produce focal signs, including hemiplegia, during the course of the disorder. Tuberculous meningitis must be distinguished from other causes of acute and subacute meningeal infection, a process that often is not easy even after examination of the spinal fluid. The pressure and cell count are elevated with up to a few hundred cells, a mixture of leukocytes and lymphocytes. The protein is elevated, usually above 100 mg/dl and often to very high levels, and the glucose is depressed. Smears for acid-fast bacilli are positive in only about 25 per cent of samples. Tuberculosis organisms grow on culture but only after several weeks. Recently, accurate CSF markers for the rapid diagnosis of the disease have been reported and are available through the Centers for Disease Control in the United States. Pending complete availability and accuracy of such measures, patients with subacutely developing meningitis suspected of having tuberculosis should be treated with antituberculous agents prior to definitive diagnosis. Large samples of CSF should be sent for culture, and a careful search should be made for tuberculosis elsewhere in the body. Seventy-five per cent of such patients have a positive tuberculin skin test, and in most a careful search yields evidence of systemic tuberculosis.

Tuberculomas of the brain produce symptoms and signs either of the mass lesion or of meningitis, the tuberculomas being found incidentally. One or multiple lesions are identified on CT scan, but the scan itself does not distinguish tuberculomas from brain tumor or other brain abscesses. In the absence of evidence of meningeal or systemic tuberculosis, biopsy is necessary for diagnosis. Patients with tuberculomas, as those with tuberculous meningitis, respond to antituberculous therapy, but brain lesions may remain visible in the CT scan long after the patient has improved clinically; the clinical course and not the scan predicts the outcome.

Less common manifestations of tuberculosis include *chronic arachnoiditis* characterized by a low-grade inflammatory response in the spinal fluid and progressive pain with signs of either cauda equina or spinal cord dysfunction. The diagnosis of arachnoiditis is suggested by a myelogram showing evidence of fibrosis and compartmentalization instead of the usually smooth subarachnoid lining. The disorder responds poorly to treatment. *Tuberculous myelopathy* probably results from direct invasion of the organism from the subarachnoid space. Patients present with a subacutely developing myelopathy characterized by sensory loss either in the legs or in all four extremities, depending on the site of the spinal cord invasion. Many patients have additional signs of meningitis, including fever, headache, and stiff neck. The spinal fluid usually contains cells and tuberculous organisms. Myelogram may show evidence of arachnoiditis and frequently demonstrates an enlarged spinal cord or complete block to the passage of contrast material in the thoracic or cervical region.

SLOW AND LATENT VIRUS INFECTIONS OF THE NERVOUS SYSTEM

Acute viral meningitis and encephalitis are discussed in Chapter 86. The term *slow virus infection* describes a group of transmissible disorders in which a long latent period separates the time between first inoculation and the subsequent development of dis-

TABLE 122–2. SLOW VIRUS INFECTIONS OF THE NERVOUS SYSTEM

DISORDER	VIRUS
AIDS (see Ch. 97)	Human immunodeficiency virus I (HIV)
Progressive multifocal leukoencephalopathy	JC virus
Subacute sclerosing panencephalitis	Measles virus
Progressive rubella panencephalitis	Rubella virus
Creutzfeldt-Jakob disease	? Prion
Kuru	? Prion

ease in the host (Table 122–2). *Latent infection* occurs with the herpes-varicella virus when, after an acute infection, the virus becomes quiescent (in sensory ganglia), only to become reactivated years later as herpes zoster.

Slow virus infections are of two kinds. One is caused by transmissible agents not fully characterized that resist usual sterilization procedures and thus far have escaped morphological identification. The agent is unlike any known virus and has been called by some a prion. The other results from conventional viral forms and is related to an abnormal host immune response. The illnesses caused by the first agents include kuru and Creutzfeldt-Jakob disease (CJD). The slow infections caused by otherwise typical viruses include subacute sclerosing panencephalitis, progressive rubella panencephalitis, and progressive multifocal encephalopathy. A chronic progressing or relapsing viral infection also has been proposed but never proved as a cause of several rare neurological disorders, including chronic focal epilepsy, Mollaret's relapsing meningitis, Behçet's syndrome, and the Vogt-Koyanagi-Harada syndrome, all of which have some dimension of inflammation in their natural history. A slow virus cause also has been sought, so far unsuccessfully, in several other neurological disorders, including multiple sclerosis, Parkinson's disease, and motor neuron disease.

Kuru, a disease of the primitive Fore tribe of New Guinea, provided the prototype for the existence of the nonimmunogenic infectious particle of subviral form. The illness causes a progressive ataxia, ophthalmoplegia, and dementia leading to death in 3 to 20 months. It appears to have been transmitted from person to person by tribal cannibalism. Passage of a similar disorder by inoculation of patient brain material into, at first, chimpanzees and subsequently several other mammalian species led to the discovery of the unique infectious agent. Since the Fore tribe has abolished ritual cannibalism, kuru has almost disappeared.

Creutzfeldt-Jakob disease develops mainly after age 40 in a worldwide distribution. The illness is characterized by progressive myoclonus, signs of upper motor neuron dysfunction, ataxia, and intellectual decline, all evolving rapidly, over a period of weeks to a few months. Neither fever, blood nor spinal fluid abnormalities occur, but the EEG early on undergoes diffuse slowing and later shows repeated short bursts of sharp waves. Although CJD is relatively rare and sporadic in its distribution, a slight familial predisposition is observed. The disorder can be transmitted to a variety of animal species. Medical personnel appear to carry little or no risk of contamination by affected patients, but person-to-person transmission has taken place via transplanted contaminated corneas or the successive use of intracerebral electrodes from affected persons and, apparently, via other neurosurgical instruments as well. There is no effective treatment.

The neurological problems associated with human acquired immunodeficiency syndrome (AIDS) are discussed in Chapter 97. *Human immunodeficiency virus* infection which causes AIDS (see Chapter 97) is associated with a variety of neurological abnormalities (Table 122–3). The most common nervous system complication results from direct invasion of the brain by the virus, causing an encephalopathy referred to as the AIDS dementia complex. This disorder usually begins insidiously and progresses over months or even a few years. Occasionally the disorder may be acute or subacute in onset. AIDS dementia complex is characterized by poor concentration and memory, slowing of thought processes, and behavioral abnormalities, usually social withdrawal and apathy. A few patients become agitated, confused, or paranoid or develop hallucinations. Motor signs are common but usually mild, including impaired rapidly alternating movements, impaired ocular motility, and mild gait ataxia. As the disease progresses, the patients become more and more demented and may develop a myelopathy characterized by spastic weakness of the lower extremities and incontinence. The patients eventually become completely withdrawn and bedridden before dying from systemic illness.

The AIDS dementia must be distinguished from opportunistic infections or neoplasms that also affect the brain (Table 122–3). CT and MR scans in the AIDS dementia complex usually yield evidence of cerebral atrophy. On MR scan, identified patchy white matter abnormalities are seen in a significant number of patients. There may be mild mononuclear pleocytosis of the spinal fluid with an elevated protein. The virus has been cultured from the spinal fluid.

There is no established treatment, but early evidence suggests that AZT may retard progression of the disorder. Anxiolytic agents may reduce anxiety associated with early dementia. More potent neuroleptic agents (butyrophenones or phenothiazines) may be required to control behavior later in the illness.

FUNGAL AND PARASITIC CNS INFECTIONS

Fungal and parasitic infections of the central nervous system are less common than viral and bacterial infections and often affect immunosuppressed patients. Table 122–3 lists the more common of these infections. Like bacterial infections, fungal and parasitic infections may cause either meningitis or parenchymal abscesses. The meningitides, when they occur, present with clinical symptoms that, while similar, are usually less severe and abrupt than those of acute bacterial meningitis. The common causes of meningitis are fungal and include especially cryptococcosis, coccidioidomycosis, and histoplasmosis. *Cryptococcal meningitis* is a sporadic infection that affects both immunosuppressed patients (50 per cent) and nonimmunosuppressed patients. The disorder is characterized by headache and sometimes fever and stiff neck. The clinical symptoms may evolve for periods as long as weeks or months; diagnosis can be made only by identifying the organism or its antigen in the cerebrospinal fluid. Histoplasma and coccidioidomycosis menigitis occur in endemic areas and often affect nonimmunosuppressed individuals. The diagnosis is suggested by a history of residence in the appropriate geographical area and confirmed by spinal fluid evaluation. Antifungal treatment, particularly in the nonimmunosuppressed patient, is usually effective.

Parasitic infections of the nervous system usually produce focal abscesses rather than diffuse meningitis. The most common to affect the nonimmunosuppressed host is cysticercosis, a disorder caused by the *Taenia solium* tape worm contracted by eating inadequately cooked pork. The disorder is common in the underdeveloped world and parts of the United States having a large Hispanic population. The brain may be invaded in as many as 60 per cent of infected persons. Invasion of the brain leads to formation of either single or multiple cysts, which often lie in the parenchyma but sometimes reside in the ventricles or subarachnoid space. Seizures and increased intracranial pressure are the most common clinical symptoms. CT scanning identifies small intracranial calcifications and hypodense cysts. Serum indirect hemagglutination tests are usually positive and confirm the diagnosis. Where cysts obstruct the ventricular system to cause symptoms, shunting procedures may be necessary. Recent evidence suggests that the anthelmintic praziquantel is effective therapy.

Toxoplasmosis of the brain, when it occurs in the adult, is a manifestation of immunosuppression. Patients with abnormal cellular immunity may develop single or multiple abscesses (Fig. 122–3), which appear usually as ring-enhancing lesions on CT scan. The le-

TABLE 122–3. SOME FUNGAL AND PARASITIC CAUSES OF CNS INFECTIONS

FUNGAL INFECTION	HELMINTHS PARASITIC INFECTION	PROTOZOAN INFECTION
Cryptococcosis	Trichinosis	Toxoplasmosis
Coccidioidomyocosis	Cysticercosis	Amebiasis
Aspergillosis	Echinococcosis	Malaria
Mucormycosis	Schistosomiasis	Chagas' disease
Actinomycosis	Angiostrongyliasis	Trypanosomiasis
Histoplasmosis	Ascariasis	(African)
Blastomycosis		
Candidiasis		

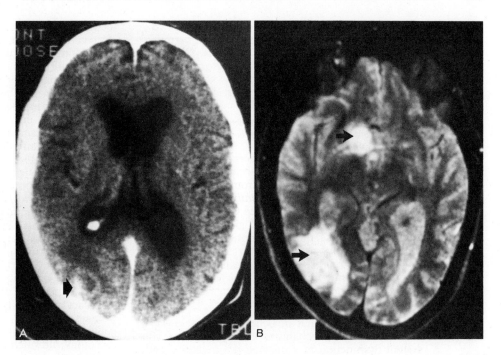

FIGURE 122–3. Toxoplasma abscesses in a patient with acquired immune deficiency syndrome (AIDS). *A*, CT scan shows one contrast-enhanced mass (arrow). *B*, Magnetic resonance image reveals multiple masses (arrows) not seen on CT scan, leading physicians to suspect abscesses rather than tumor.

sions cannot be distinguished from brain tumors or other infections, so that stereotactic directed needle biopsy often is required to make the diagnosis. Toxoplasma abscesses can be effectively treated with a combination of pyrimethamine and sulfadiazine.

CHRONIC MENINGITIS

Most cases of meningitis due to common viral and bacterial agents either resolve spontaneously or respond promptly to treatment. The diagnosis is usually rapidly established by appropriate CSF studies. Some patients, however, suffer from a subacute or chronic meningitis in which the diagnosis is not easily made. In addition to infectious agents, the clinical picture of subacute or chronic meningitis can be caused by neoplasms, sarcoidosis, or a variety of other illnesses of unknown cause. Table 122–4 lists the differential diagnosis of chronic meningitis. A definitive diagnosis can be established only by identifying definitive systemic manifestations of the underlying disease or by repeatedly examining the spinal fluid for evidence of malignant cells, organisms, abnormal antibodies, or antigens. If a diagnosis cannot be made by lumbar puncture it often is useful to perform a cisternal puncture, since many inflammatory and granulomatous infections of the meninges are most prominent at the base of the brain. Careful search for illness outside the central nervous system may disclose the hilar adenopathy of sarcoidosis or the genital ulcers of herpes simplex or the Behçet syndrome. In a few instances, one never ferrets out a diagnosis, and some patients suffer continuous or recurrent symptoms and signs of meningeal inflammation for months or years.

DEMYELINATING AND OTHER CNS INFLAMMATORY DISORDERS OF PROBABLE IMMUNE CAUSE

Demyelinating Disorders

Disorders with a relative predilection for damaging central nervous system (CNS) myelin are listed in Table 122–5. Those that have an immune basis are discussed here. Others, if they affect primarily adults, are described elsewhere in the text under appropriate headings.

TABLE 122–4. CAUSES OF SUBACUTE AND CHRONIC MENINGITIS

I. Bacterial Infections
 Partially treated acute bacterial meningitis
 Parameningeal infections
 Syphilis and tuberculous meningitis
II. Viral Meningitis and Meningoencephalitis
III. Fungal and Parasitic Meningitis
IV. Neoplasm
 Primary and metastatic leptomeningeal tumor
 Epidermoid cyst with rupture
V. Vascular Lesions
 Subdural hematoma
 Subarachnoid hemorrhage (late)
 Granulomatous arteritis
VI. Unknown
 Systemic lupus erythematosus
 Behçet's syndrome
 Mollaret's meningitis
 Sarcoidosis
 Vogt-Koyanagi-Harada syndrome
 Benign lymphocytic meningitis

TABLE 122–5. DEMYELINATING DISORDERS

A. Unknown Cause
1. Multiple sclerosis
2. Devic's disease
3. Optic neuritis
4. Acute transverse myelopathy
B. Parainfectious Disorders
1. Acute disseminated encephalomyelitis
2. Acute hemorrhagic leukoencephalopathy
C. Viral Infections
1. Progressive multifocal leukoencephalopathy
2. Subacute sclerosing panencephalitis
D. Nutritional Disorders
1. Combined systems disease (vitamin B_{12} deficiency)
2. Demyelination of the corpus callosum (Marchiafava-Bignami)
3. Central pontine myelinolysis
E. Anoxic-Ischemic Sequelae
1. Delayed postanoxic cerebral demyelination
2. Progressive subcortical ischemic encephalopathy

Several disorders that are believed to operate via abnormal immune mechanisms cause central nervous system dysfunction by damaging the myelin sheaths covering axons. The conditions appear to have their primary effect on the oligodendroglial cells, which are responsible for the production and maintenance of the myelin sheaths. The acute lesions of these demyelinating disorders usually contain inflammatory infiltrates, particularly lymphocytes, at the site of subsequent demyelination. There is usually production of IgG within the central nervous system characterized by an elevated cerebrospinal fluid–to–serum IgG ratio. In their severe forms, the disorders also can damage other structures in demyelinated areas, including axons and astrocytic cells.

Multiple Sclerosis (MS). This is by far the most common of the presumed immune demyelinating disorders of the CNS. It usually causes its first symptoms between the ages of about 20 and 40 years and classically is characterized by remissions and exacerbations of neurological dysfunction affecting several different sites in the central nervous system over many years (lesions disseminated in space and time). Typically, at onset an otherwise healthy person suffers an acute or subacute attack of unilateral loss of vision, true vertigo, ataxia, paresthesias, incontinence, diplopia, dysarthria, or paralysis (Table 122–6). The symptoms result from a focus of inflammatory demyelination (which later scars to form a "plaque") in the white matter of the brain (usually periventricular), brain stem, or spinal cord, which acts to slow or block conduction of nerve impulses. The symptoms usually are painless, remain for several days to weeks, and then partially or completely resolve. After a period of relative freedom, new symptoms appear. Although individual frequencies vary widely, the average rate of exacerbations is about one every other year. In some patients the clinical course consists of progressive neurological dysfunction; this usually takes the form of a slowly progressive myelopathy characterized by spasticity and ataxia, predominantly of the lower extremities. In other instances one or two attacks may characterize the disease of an entire lifetime, with significant disability never developing. On average, about 60 per cent of patients remain fully functional 10 years after the first attack, and 25 to 30 per cent remain functional 30 years after the onset. Statistically, the disorder does not greatly decrease life expectancy, although some patients become severely disabled and die from recurrent infections and the complications of being bedridden.

ETIOLOGY. The etiology of multiple sclerosis is unknown, although clues point to infectious (viral), immunological, and genetic factors. The disease is far more common in the northern and southern temperate latitudes than in the more equatorial regions. Young children who move from a tropical to a temperate area increase their likelihood of contracting multiple sclerosis. The findings suggest an infective agent acquired early in life (a slow or retrovirus, or exposure to a childhood infection). An immune disorder is suggested not only by the inflammatory infiltrates sometimes seen in the perivascular areas of the demyelinated plaques but also by the fact that a decrease in suppressor lymphocytes in the serum usually precedes acute attacks. A relapsing encephalomyelitis resembling multiple sclerosis has been produced by injection of antigen into experimental animals. Genetic predisposition is suggested by the fact that haplotype DW2 is found in about 65 per cent of MS patients, compared with 15 per cent of control subjects, and there is a high coincidence in monozygotic twins. In addition, the disorder is uncommon in Orientals and African blacks including those who are born in the United States.

DIAGNOSIS. The diagnosis depends upon identifying, in persons of appropriate age, clinical evidence of central nervous system lesions that affect different areas of CNS white matter separated in time by at least two months. Whenever doubt exists, laboratory evidence of CNS immune dysfunction or of imaged white matter lesions should be sought. Otherwise healthy persons who suffer relapsing and remitting neurological dysfunction over a long period of time (e.g., diplopia in year one, sensory loss in an arm in year three, urgency incontinence in year five, etc.) almost certainly have multiple sclerosis. Furthermore, evidence

TABLE 122–6. SYMPTOMS AND SIGNS OF MULTIPLE SCLEROSIS LISTED IN DECLINING ORDER OF FREQUENCY

SYMPTOMS	SIGNS
Fatigue	Spasticity or hyperreflexia
Muscle weakness	Babinski sign
Ocular disturbance, especially internuclear ophthalmoplegia	Absent abdominal reflexes
	Dysmetria or intention tremor
Urinary disturbance	Nystagmus
Gait ataxia	Impairment of sensation (Lhermitte's sign)
Paresthesias	Labile or changed mood
Dysarthria or scanning speech	
Mental disturbance	
Vertigo	

of more than one widely spaced lesion in the nervous system (e.g., optic neuritis plus internuclear ophthalmoplegia) strongly suggests disseminated sclerosis in a younger person who lacks evidence of other disease. In patients with unifocal lesions, laboratory tests such as abnormal visual or auditory evoked responses may detect a subclinical lesion residing elsewhere in the nervous system.

Certain symptoms strongly suggest the diagnosis of multiple sclerosis. These include bilateral internuclear ophthalmoplegia (see p. 721), Lhermitte's sign (electric shock–like sensation radiating to the extremities initiated by neck flexion), and a marked exacerbation of neurological symptoms associated with acute febrile illness. Although all neurological dysfunction becomes worse with fever, raising the body temperature characteristically both exacerbates the present signs of multiple sclerosis and uncovers new signs not detected during normothermia.

The laboratory examination is helpful but not definitive. Most patients have an elevated gamma globulin in their spinal fluid, and separate, discrete (oligoclonal) bands are found in the gamma region on agarose or polyacrylamide gel electrophoresis in about 90 per cent of patients. Multiple oligoclonal bands (more than two) strongly support a diagnosis of multiple sclerosis in an appropriate clinical case, although inflammatory diseases of the nervous system can also produce oligoclonal bands. Spinal, auditory, or visual evoked responses can give evidence of additional subclinical lesions in doubtful cases. Most helpful from a laboratory standpoint is MR imaging, which usually reveals characteristic white matter lesions scattered through brain and/or spinal cord (Fig. 122–4). CT scanning provides less sensitive detection.

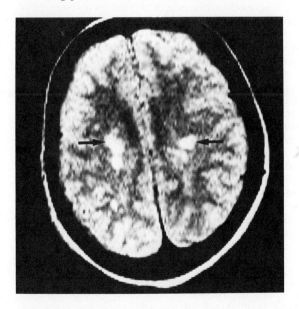

FIGURE 122–4. A magnetic resonance image from a patient with multiple sclerosis. Multiple lesions of the white matter (arrows) with a predilection for periventricular areas strongly support the diagnosis of multiple sclerosis in a patient with an appropriate history and physical findings.

Early diagnosis can be difficult in some cases, particularly in the absence of the typical remitting and exacerbating history, and when neither spinal fluid nor MR findings are characteristic. Often, early symptoms are primarily sensory and sometimes in bizarre and "nonanatomical" distribution, leading the physician to worry about a conversion reaction. Occasionally signs in MS may be severe and apparently unifocal, at first suggesting a brain or spinal cord tumor or vascular disease. Particular difficulty arises with brain stem disorders. A small, single brain stem lesion can give rise to a potentially misleading collection of cranial nerve, sensory, cerebellar, and motor signs that at first suggest demyelination. To prove a disseminated disorder in a patient with prominent brain stem signs requires evidence of dysfunction of structures not represented in the brain stem (e.g., optic neuritis, visual field deficit, or aphasia). Visually evoked responses often help because the optic nerve is a common site of multiple sclerosis, causing abnormalities of conduction in the optic nerve, often without clinical symptoms. A difficult differential diagnosis is between multiple sclerosis with remitting and exacerbating symptoms and small arteriovenous anomalies of the medulla or pons, which can produce remitting and exacerbating symptoms by recurrent small hemorrhages.

TREATMENT. One can treat the symptoms of multiple sclerosis, but so far not the disease. Many physicians believe that acute bouts of neurological dysfunction resolve more quickly when treated with short-term administration of corticosteroids. No evidence indicates that such treatment brings long-term benefit. Some therapeutic trials suggest the potential efficacy of immunosuppressive agents in chronic progressive multiple sclerosis, but firm evidence is lacking. Patients minimally affected by the disorder require no specific treatment. The illness understandably frightens patients, however, and sympathetic reassurance and follow-up supervision provide considerable support. Patients severely disabled by late symptoms, which generally include spasticity and bladder and bowel dysfunction (Table 122–6), often are best treated in multidisciplinary clinics or centers where physical therapy, psychological support, family counseling, and supportive medical therapy are all available.

Acute Disseminated Encephalomyelitis. This monophasic demyelinating inflammatory disorder can appear after viral infections or as a complication of vaccination. The disorder usually produces multifocal brain and spinal cord symptoms but may be restricted to one area, particularly optic nerve (acute optic neuropathy) or spinal cord (acute transverse myelopathy). When the disorder is related to an antecedent viral infection, it usually occurs 6 to 10 days after the appearance of the other systemic symptoms. When it follows vaccination, it usually begins 10 days to three weeks after the injections. At times a similar syndrome can appear in the absence of any identifiable exposure. The pathogenesis is believed to reside in an antigen-antibody response, the antigen being either the injected vaccination protein or the infecting virus. Clinically the disorder is usually characterized by the acute development of headache and fever and multifocal neurological signs. The most severely affected patients develop delirium, stupor, or coma. Seizures are relatively common. The spinal fluid is characterized by pleocytosis of 20 to 200 lymphocytes and usually an elevated gamma globulin. Protein concentration may be a little elevated, but glucose concentration is usually normal. Myelin basic protein can be identified in the spinal fluid in some of the patients. The electroencephalogram is usually diffusely abnormal, with widespread slowing, but does not have the characteristic focal slow and sharp wave activity of herpes simplex encephalitis.

Acute disseminated encephalomyelitis produces clinical and spinal fluid manifestations similar to those of acute viral encephalitis and cannot, in fact, be distinguished from that disorder by clinical findings. Since neither acute encephalomyelitis nor acute viral encephalitis, save for herpes simplex, can be treated definitively, such a differentiation is not crucial. Despite its presumed immune mechanism, neither corticosteroids nor other immunosuppressive agents have proved efficacious in treatment.

Acute hemorrhagic leukoencephalitis is a fatal, rare variant of acute encephalomyelitis. The illness usually occurs after an upper respiratory infection and is characterized by sudden headache, seizures, and rapid progression to coma. Patients often die within a few days. CSF often shows more polymorphonuclear leukocytes than lymphocytes. The brain at autopsy is swollen, with bilateral and asymmetrical hemorrhages scattered throughout the white matter. There is no known treatment.

Acute Transverse Myelopathy (Myelitis). Acute transverse myelopathy is a clinical syndrome characterized by the rapid onset of ascending or transverse spinal cord dysfunction, usually involving primarily the midthoracic or high thoracic cord. The disorder usually begins with abrupt, severe back pain and sometimes fever and malaise. In a matter of 12 to 24 hours, the patient complains of weakness and paresthesias in the lower extremities, sometimes associated with radicular pain at the level of the uppermost involved cord segments. Occasionally the disease is painless. In its severest form, complete paralysis and loss of sensation and autonomic function develop below the highest level of the lesion. In less severe forms there may be patchy loss of sensation with bilateral corticospinal tract signs predominating or a Brown-Sequard syndrome. In a few patients, the spinal cord signs ascend for hours to a week or two and reach a stable level, usually in the upper thoracic cord. In about half the patients there is a preceding history of banal infection, usually upper respiratory, or of a vaccination, the myelopathy presumably being a delayed immune response. Rarely, the illness is associated with an occult neoplasm. Late recurrences occasionally occur.

The spinal fluid usually contains 50 to 100 white cells and a slightly elevated protein concentration. The diagnostic problem is to distinguish acute transverse myelopathy from parameningeal infection with secondary involvement of the cord. The history and findings in transverse myelopathy may mimic those of epidural or subdural infections, in which diagnosis can be established by myelography. In patients with acute transverse myelopathy, however, the spinal cord may be sufficiently swollen to produce a complete block to myelographic dye, so that care must be taken to distinguish the swollen cord from an epidural or subdural block. Magnetic resonance imaging eventually will replace myelography as the diagnostic test of choice. There is no effective treatment for the disorder. About one third of patients make a spontaneous recovery.

Other Demyelinating Disease. Devic's disease (neuromyelitis optica) is a clinical syndrome characterized by transverse myelopathy and optic neuropathy, usually bilateral. The two symptoms usually occur within days or weeks of each other. The disease is generally thought to be a variant of multiple sclerosis, but in many instances, particularly when the myelopathy is severe, there may be necrosis of the cord far more intense than the demyelinating plaques seen in most examples of multiple sclerosis.

Acute optic neuritis can either occur as a symptom of multiple sclerosis or arise in isolation independently. This disorder is described on p. 718.

Reye's Syndrome. Reye's syndrome is a parainfectious encephalopathy, primarily affecting children, which follows viral infection, usually influenza type A or B or varicella. The syndrome is characterized by failure of liver and brain function and is thought to result from a mitochondrial disturbance of those organs, leading to metabolic derangements including serum hyperammonemia, lactic acidosis, and elevation of free fatty acids. Recent evidence suggests that in children with primary viral illness such as influenza and varicella, ingestion of aspirin may play a role in the pathogenesis. Reye's syndrome usually begins as the initial viral illness clears. The onset is with headache, intractable vomiting, and lethargy or stupor. Patients may rapidly become comatose. The diagnosis is confirmed by evidence of hepatic dysfunction without hyperbilirubinemia, the presence of an elevated arterial ammonia level, and, in children, hypoglycemia (in the few cases reported in adults hypoglycemia has been uncommon). The CSF is normal save for increased pressure. Liver biopsy reveals a noninflammatory panlobular hepatocellular accumulation of lipid droplets and both histochemical and ultrastructural evidence of inflammation. At postmortem examination the brain shows marked swelling accompanied by ultrastructural changes in mitochondria similar to those found in liver. Mortality is high in comatose patients. Careful control of increased intracranial pressure using hyperosmolar agents and correction of hypoglycemia and electrolyte abnormalities may allow for recovery. Adults with the syndrome appear to have a lesser mortality than children.

REFERENCES

Booss J, Thornton GF: Infectious diseases of the central nervous system. Neurol Clin, Vol 4, No 1, Feb. 1986.

McDonald WI, Silberberg DH: Multiple Sclerosis. London, Butterworths International Medical Reviews, 1987.

Vinken PJ, Bruyn GW, Klawans HL (eds): Handbook of Clinical Neurology. Vol 3: Demyelinating Diseases. Amsterdam, Elsevier Science, 1985.

INDEX

Note: Page numbers in *italics* refer to illustrations; page numbers followed by the letter t refer to tables.

The colophon on the front cover and spine is an abstraction which symbolizes the universal aspects of medicine. The circle represents the world. The stylized triangle in the upper area is the classic image of positive and negative forces—the Law of Life. The vertical line with the upper right staff suggests the staff of Æsculapius and Hermes, and the horizontal bar connects all three symbols into the total summation of medicine as Art and Science.